Developmental-Behavioral Pediatrics:
Evidence and Practice

Developmental-Behavioral Pediatrics: Evidence and Practice

MARK L. WOLRAICH, MD
CMRI/Shaun Walters Professor of Developmental and Behavioral Pediatrics
Section Chief of Developmental and Behavioral Pediatrics
University of Oklahoma Health Sciences Center
Oklahoma City, Oklahoma

DENNIS D. DROTAR, PhD
Professor
Department of Pediatrics
Case Western Reserve University School of Medicine
Chief, Division of Behavioral Pediatrics and Psychology
Department of Pediatrics
Rainbow Babies and Children's Hospital
Cleveland, Ohio

PAUL H. DWORKIN, MD
Professor and Chairman
Department of Pediatrics
University of Connecticut School of Medicine
Farmington, Connecticut
Physician-in-Chief
Connecticut Children's Medical Center
Hartford, Connecticut

ELLEN C. PERRIN, MA, MD
Professor
Department of Pediatrics
Tufts University School of Medicine
Director
Division of Developmental-Behavioral Pediatrics
The Floating Hospital for Children
Tufts–New England Medical Center
Boston, Massachusetts

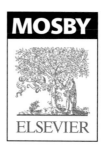

MOSBY

ELSEVIER

MOSBY
ELSEVIER

1600 John F. Kennedy Blvd.
Suite 1800
Philadelphia, PA 19103-2899

DEVELOPMENTAL-BEHAVIORAL PEDIATRICS: EVIDENCE AND PRACTICE

ISBN: 978-0-323-04025-9

Library of Congress Cataloging-in-Publication Data
Developmental-behavioral pediatrics : evidence and practice / [edited by] Mark Lee Wolraich . . . [et al]—1st ed.
    p. ; cm.
Includes bibliographical references and index.
ISBN 978-0-323-04025-9
    1. Pediatrics. 2. Pediatrics—Psychological aspects. I. Wolraich, Mark.
[DNLM: 1. Child Behavior Disorders. 2. Child Behavior. 3. Child Development. WS 350.6 D48865 2007]
RJ47.D484 2007
618.92'89—dc22
                                                                    2007018064

Acquisitions Editor: Judith Fletcher
Developmental Editor: Martha Limbach
Publishing Services Manager: Frank Polizzano
Senior Project Manager: Peter Faber
Design Direction: Gene Harris

Printed in Canada

Last digit is the print number: 9 8 7 6 5 4 3 2 1

Contributors

HOOVER ADGER, JR., MD
Professor of Pediatrics
Johns Hopkins University School of Medicine
Baltimore, Maryland
The Effect of Substance Use Disorders on Children and
    Adolescents

GEORGINA M. ALDRIDGE
Graduate student
Neuroscience program
University of Illinois at Urbana–Champaign
Urbana, Illinois
The Origins of Behavior and Cognition in the Developing
    Brain

GLEN P. AYLWARD, PhD, ABPP
Professor
Pediatrics and Psychiatry
Director, Division of Developmental and Behavioral
    Pediatrics
Southern Illinois University School of Medicine
Springfield, Illinois
Screening and Assessment Tools: Measurement and
    Psychometric Considerations; Screening and Assessment
    Tools: Assessment of Development and Behavior

MARCIA A. BARNES, PhD
Professor and University Research Chair
Psychology
University of Guelph
Guelph, Ontario
Adjunct Scientist
The Hospital for Sick Children
Toronto
Professor (Adjunct)
Department of Pediatrics
University of Toronto Faculty of Medicine
Toronto, Ontario, Canada
Learning Disabilities

ROWLAND P. BARRETT, PhD
Associate Professor of Psychiatry
Brown Medical School
Providence
Director
Center for Autism and Developmental Disabilities
Emma Pendleton Bradley Hospital
East Providence, Rhode Island
Atypical Behavior: Self-Injury and Pica

TAMMY D. BARRY, PhD
Assistant Professor
Department of Psychology
University of Southern Mississippi
Hattiesburg, Mississippi
Externalizing Conditions

HAROLYN M. E. BELCHER, MD, MHS
Associate Professor of Pediatrics
Johns Hopkins University School of Medicine
Research Scientist
Kennedy Krieger Institute
Baltimore, Maryland
The Effect of Substance Use Disorders on Children and
    Adolescents

JAMES E. BLACK, MD, PhD
Assistant Professor
Department of Psychiatry
School of Medicine, Southern Illinois University
Springfield, Illinois
The Origins of Behavior and Cognition in the Developing
    Brain

STEPHANIE BLENNER, MD
Fellow
Developmental and Behavioral Pediatrics
Boston University School of Medicine/Boston
    Medical Center
Boston, Massachusetts
Feeding and Eating Conditions: Food Insecurity and Failure to
    Thrive

BARBARA L. BONNER, PhD
CMRI/Jean Gumerson Professor
Director
Department of Pediatrics Center on Child Abuse
    and Neglect
University of Oklahoma Health Sciences Center
Oklahoma City, Oklahoma
Child Maltreatment: Developmental Consequences

CAROLINE L. BOXMEYER, PhD
Research Psychologist
Department of Psychology
The University of Alabama
Tuscaloosa, Alabama
Externalizing Conditions

JEFFREY P. BROSCO, MD, PhD
Associate Professor of Clinical Pediatrics and History
University of Miami
Director
Clinical Services
Mailman Center for Child Development
Chair
Pediatric Bioethics Committee
Jackson Memorial Hospital
Miami, Florida
Ethical Issues in Developmental-Behavioral Pediatrics: A
     Historical Approach

EUGENIA CHAN, MD, MPH
Instructor in Pediatrics
Harvard Medical School
Assistant in Medicine
Developmental Medicine Center
Children's Hospital Boston
Boston, Massachusetts
Treatment and Management: Complementary and Alternative
     Medicine in Developmental-Behavioral Pediatrics

BENARD P. DREYER, MD
Professor and Vice Chairman
Department of Pediatrics
Director
Developmental-Behavioral Pediatrics
New York University School of Medicine
New York, New York
Research Foundations, Methods, and Issues in
     Developmental-Behavioral Pediatrics

DENNIS D. DROTAR, PhD
Professor
Department of Pediatrics
Case Western Reserve University School of Medicine
Chief
Division of Behavioral Pediatrics and Psychology
Department of Pediatrics
Rainbow Babies and Children's Hospital
Cleveland, Ohio
Diagnostic Classification Systems

PAUL H. DWORKIN, MD
Professor and Chairman
Department of Pediatrics
University of Connecticut School of Medicine
Farmington, Connecticut
Physician-in-Chief
Connecticut Children's Medical Center
Hartford, Connecticut
Screening and Assessment Tools: Surveillance and Screening
     for Development and Behavior

ROBIN S. EVERHART, MA
Department of Psychology
Center for Health and Behavior
Syracuse University
Syracuse, New York
Family Context in Developmental-Behaviorial Pediatrics

HEIDI M. FELDMAN, MD, PhD
Ballinger-Swindells Endowed Professor of
     Developmental and Behavioral Pediatrics
Department of Pediatrics
Stanford University School of Medicine
Stanford
Medical Director
Mary L. Johnson Development and Behavior Unit
Lucile Packard Children's Hospital at Stanford
Palo Alto, California
Screening and Assessment Tools: Assessment of Speech and
     Language; Language and Speech Disorders

BARBARA H. FIESE, PhD
Professor and Chair
Department of Psychology
Syracuse University
Adjunct Professor
Department of Pediatrics, Psychiatry, and Behavioral
     Sciences
State University of New York Upstate Medical
     University
Senior Scientist
Center for Health and Behavior
Syracuse University
Syracuse, New York
Family Context in Developmental-Behaviorial Pediatrics

DEBORAH A. FRANK, MD
Professor of Pediatrics
Division of Developmental and Behavioral Pediatrics
Boston University School of Medicine
Director
Growth Clinic for Children
Boston Medical Center
Boston, Massachusetts
Feeding and Eating Conditions: Food Insecurity and Failure to
     Thrive

MARY A. FRISTAD, PhD, ABPP
Professor
Departments of Psychiatry and Psychology
Director, Research and Psychological Services
Division of Child and Adolescent Psychiatry
The Ohio State University
Columbus, Ohio
Internalizing Conditions: Mood Disorders

LYNN S. FUCHS, PhD
Nicholas Hobbs Professor of Special Education and
    Human Development
Vanderbilt University
Nashville, Tennessee
Learning Disabilities

SARAH R. FUCHS, BS
Mailman Center for Child Development
Miami, Florida
Ethical Issues in Developmental-Behavioral Pediatrics: A
    Historical Approach

SHEILA GAHAGAN, MD
Professor of Pediatrics and Communicable Diseases
University of Michigan Medical School
Assistant Research Scientist
Center for Human Growth and Development
University of Michigan
Ann Arbor, Michigan
Feeding and Eating Conditions: Infant Feeding Processes and
    Disorders

SANDRA L. GARDNER, RN, MS, CNS, PND
Director and Neonatal/Perinatal/Pediatric
    Consultant
Professional Outreach Consultants
Aurora, Colorado
Developmental-Behavioral Aspects of Chronic Conditions:
    The Effects of Adverse Natal Factors and Prematurity

FRANCES P. GLASCOE, PhD
Adjunct Professor of Pediatrics
Department of Pediatrics
Vanderbilt University School of Medicine
Nashville, Tennessee
Screening and Assessment Tools: Surveillance and Screening
    for Development and Behavior

EDWARD GOLDSON, MD
Professor
Department of Pediatrics
University of Colorado Denver and Health Sciences
    Center
Staff Physician
Child Development Unit
The Children's Hospital
Denver, Colorado
Developmental-Behavioral Aspects of Chronic Conditions:
    The Effects of Adverse Natal Factors and Prematurity;
    Child Maltreatment: Developmental Consequences

KENNETH W. GOODMAN, PhD
Associate Professor of Medicine and Philosophy
University of Miami
Director, Bioethics Program
University of Miami
Miami, Florida
Ethical Issues in Developmental-Behavioral Pediatrics: A
    Historical Approach

WILLIAM T. GREENOUGH, PhD
Swanlund Professor of Psychology and Psychiatry
Swanlund Professor of Cell and Developmental
    Biology
Center for Advanced Study Professor
University of Illinois at Urbana-Champaign
Urbana, Illinois
The Origins of Behavior and Cognition in the Developing
    Brain

SAURABH GUPTA, MD
Child Psychiatrist
Rockford Center
Newark, Delaware
Treatment and Management: Psychopharmacological
    Management of Disorders of Development and Behavior

KRISTIN M. HAWLEY, PhD
Assistant Professor
Department of Psychological Sciences
University of Missouri–Columbia
Columbia, Missouri
Treatment and Management: Evidence-Based Psychological
    Interventions for Emotional and Behavioral Disorders

GRAYSON N. HOLMBECK, PhD
Professor and Director of Clinical Training
Department of Psychology
Loyola University Chicago
Chicago, Illinois
Theoretical Foundations of Developmental-Behavioral
    Pediatrics

KHIELA J. HOLMES, MS
Graduate Student
Department of Psychology
The University of Alabama
Tuscaloosa, Alabama
Externalizing Conditions

JEFFREY I. HUNT, MD
Associate Professor (Clinical)
Department of Psychiatry and Human Behavior,
    and Associate Training Director
Child and Adolescent Psychiatry Fellowship and
    Triple Board Programs
Brown Medical School
Providence
Director
Adolescent Program
Emma Pendleton Bradley Hospital
East Providence, Rhode Island
Treatment and Management: Psychopharmacological
    Management of Disorders of Development and Behavior

BARBARA JANDASEK, MA
Graduate Student
Department of Psychology
Loyola University Chicago
Chicago, Illinois
Theoretical Foundations of Developmental-Behavioral
    Pediatrics

NORAH JANOSY, MD
Resident
Department of Anesthesiology and Peri-Operative
    Medicine
Oregon Health and Science University
Portland, Oregon
Pain and Somatoform Disorders

LYNN M. JEFFRIES, PT, PhD, PCS
Clinical Assistant Professor
Department of Rehabilitation Sciences
University of Oklahoma Health Sciences Center
Oklahoma City, Oklahoma
Screening and Assessment Tools: Assessment of Motor Skills

VALERIE L. JENNINGS
Graduate student
Beckman Institute
University of Illinois at Urbana–Champaign
Urbana, Illinois
The Origins of Behavior and Cognition in the Developing
    Brain

AMANDA JENSEN-DOSS, PhD
Assistant Professor
Departments of Educational Psychology and
    Psychology
Texas A&M University
College Station, Texas
Treatment and Management: Evidence-Based Psychological
    Interventions for Emotional and Behavioral Disorders

CHRIS PLAUCHÉ JOHNSON, MEd, MD
Clinical Professor
Department of Pediatrics
University of Texas School of Medicine at San
    Antonio
Neurodevelopmental Pediatrician
Village of Hope Medical Center for Children with
    Disabilities
University of Texas Health Sciences Center
San Antonio, Texas
Cognitive and Adaptive Disabilities; Autism Spectrum
    Disorders

MARIA A. JONES, PT, PhD
Clinical Assistant Professor
Department of Rehabilitation Sciences
Oklahoma University Health Sciences Center
Oklahoma City, Oklahoma
Screening and Assessment Tools: Assessment of Motor Skills

DESMOND P. KELLY, MD
GHS Professor of Clinical Pediatrics
University of South Carolina School of Medicine
Columbia
Medical Director
Division of Developmental-Behavioral Pediatrics
Donald A. Gardner Family Center for Developing
    Minds
Children's Hospital
Greenville Hospital System
Greenville, South Carolina
Developmental-Behavioral Aspects of Chronic Conditions:
    Sensory Deficits

KERI BROWN KIRSCHMAN, PhD
Assistant Professor
Department of Psychology
University of Dayton
Dayton, Ohio
Internalizing Conditions: Anxiety Disorders

NICOLE M. KLAUS, PhD
Postdoctoral Fellow
Clinical Child Psychology
Department of Child and Adolescent Psychiatry
University of Michigan
Ann Arbor, Michigan
Internalizing Conditions: Mood Disorders

HEATHER KRELL, MD, MPH
Private Practice
Los Angeles, California
Pain and Somatoform Disorders

KATHLEEN L. LEMANEK, PhD
Associate Clinical Professor of Pediatrics
Ohio State University College of Medicine
Pediatric Psychologist
Department of Psychology
Columbus Children's Hospital
Columbus, Ohio
Internalizing Conditions: Anxiety Disorders

JOHN E. LOCHMAN, PhD
Professor and Doddridge Saxon Chairholder in
   Clinical Psychology
Department of Psychology
Director
Center for Prevention of Youth Behavior Problems
The University of Alabama
Tuscaloosa, Alabama
Externalizing Conditions

THOMAS M. LOCK, MD
Associate Professor of Pediatrics
University of Oklahoma School of Medicine
Oklahoma City
Director of Clinical Services
Oklahoma University
Child Study Center
Oklahoma City, Oklahoma
Attention-Deficit/Hyperactivity Disorder

JULIE C. LUMENG, MD
Assistant Professor of Pediatrics
Department of Pediatrics
Assistant Research Scientist
Center for Human Growth and Development
University of Michigan
Ann Arbor, Michigan
Feeding and Eating Conditions: Introduction; Feeding and
   Eating Conditions: Obesity and Restrictive Eating
   Disorders

IRENE R. McEWEN, PT, PhD, FAPTA
Ann Taylor Chair in Pediatrics and Developmental
   Disabilities in Physical Therapy
Professor
Department of Rehabilitation Sciences
Oklahoma University Health Sciences Center
Oklahoma City, Oklahoma
Screening and Assessment Tools: Assessment of Motor Skills

LAURA McGUINN, MD
Assistant Professor of Pediatrics
Section of Developmental and Behavioral Pediatrics
Oklahoma University Health Sciences Center
Oklahoma City, Oklahoma
Treatment and Management: Family-Centered Care and the
   Medical Home

CHERYL MESSICK, PhD
Director of Clinical Education
Communication Science and Disorders Department
University of Pittsburgh
School of Health and Rehabilitation Sciences
Speech/Language Pathologist
Children's Hospital of Pittsburgh
Pittsburgh, Pennsylvania
Screening and Assessment Tools: Assessment of Speech and
   Language; Language and Speech Disorders

PAUL STEVEN MILLER, JD
Henry M. Jackson Professor of Law
Director
University of Washington Disability Studies Program
University of Washington School of Law
Seattle, Washington
Ethical Issues in Developmental-Behavioral Pediatrics: A
   Historical Approach

SCOTT M. MYERS, MD
Assistant Professor of Pediatrics
Jefferson Medical College of Thomas Jefferson
   University
Philadelphia
Associate
Neurodevelopmental Pediatrics
Geisinger Medical Center
Danville, Pennsylvania
Autism Spectrum Disorders

ROBERT E. NICKEL, MD
Professor of Pediatrics
Child Development and Rehabilitation Center
Oregon Health and Science University
Portland, Oregon
Motor Disabilities and Multiple Handicapping Conditions

SONYA OPPENHEIMER, MD
Professor of Pediatrics
University of Cincinnati School of Medicine
Staff Physician
Division of Developmental and Behavioral Pediatrics
Cincinnati Children's Hospital Medical Center
Cincinnati, Ohio
Treatment and Management: The Interdisciplinary Team
   Approach

JUDITH A. OWENS, MD, MPH
Associate Professor
Department of Pediatrics
Warren Alpert School of Medicine at Brown
   University
Director, Pediatric Sleep Disorders Clinic
Hasbro Children's Hospital
Providence, Rhode Island
Sleep and Sleep Disorders in Children

TONYA M. PALERMO, PhD
Assistant Professor
Department of Anesthesiology and Peri-Operative
    Medicine
Oregon Health and Science University
Portland, Oregon
Pain and Somatoform Disorders

ROSE ANN M. PARRISH, BSN, MSN
Assistant Professor
Department of Pediatrics
University of Cincinnati
Assistant Professor of Pediatrics
Division of Developmental and Behavioral Pediatrics
Cincinnati Children's Hospital Medical Center
Cincinnati, Ohio
Treatment and Management: The Interdisciplinary Team
    Approach

MARIA J. PATTERSON, MD, PhD
Professor
Department of Microbiology/Molecular Genetics
    and Pediatrics
College of Human Medicine
Michigan State University
East Lansing
Attending Physician
E. W. Sparrow Health System and Ingham Regional
    Medical Center
Lansing, Michigan
Developmental-Behavioral Aspects of Chronic Conditions:
    Developmental and Behavioral Outcomes of Infectious
    Diseases

ELLEN C. PERRIN, MA, MD
Professor
Department of Pediatrics
Tufts University School of Medicine
Director
Division of Developmental-Behavioral Pediatrics
The Floating Hospital for Children
Tufts-New England Medical Center
Boston, Massachusetts
Sexuality: Variations in Sexual Orientation and Sexual
    Expression

MARIO C. PETERSEN, MD, MSc
Associate Professor of Pediatrics
Child Development and Rehabilitation Center
Oregon Health and Science University
Portland, Oregon
Motor Disabilities and Multiple Handicapping Conditions

NICOLE R. POWELL, PhD, MPH
Research Psychologist
Department of Psychology
The University of Alabama
Tuscaloosa, Alabama
Externalizing Conditions

LEONARD A. RAPPAPORT, MD, MS
Mary Demming Scott Associate Professor
Department of Pediatrics
Harvard Medical School
Chief
Division of Developmental Medicine
Children's Hospital Boston
Boston, Massachusetts
Elimination Conditions

MARSHA D. RAPPLEY, MD
Dean
College of Human Medicine
Pediatrics and Human Development Professor
Michigan State University
East Lansing, Michigan
Developmental-Behavioral Aspects of Chronic Conditions:
    Developmental and Behavioral Outcomes of Infectious
    Diseases

JULIUS B. RICHMOND, MD
Professor of Health Policy
Emeritus
Department of Social Medicine
Harvard Medical School
Advisor
Child Health Policy
Emeritus
Children's Hospital Boston
Boston, Massachusetts
The History of Child Developmental-Behavioral Health Policy
    in the United States

JAMES J. RIVIELLO, JR., MD
Professor of Neurology
Harvard Medical School
Director
Epilepsy Program
Division of Epilepsy and Clinical Neurophysiology
Department of Neurology
Children's Hospital Boston
Boston, Massachusetts
Developmental-Behavioral Aspects of Chronic Conditions:
    Central Nervous System Disorders

OLLE JANE Z. SAHLER, MD
Professor of Pediatrics,
Psychiatry, Medical Humanities, and Oncology
Department of Pediatrics
University of Rochester School of Medicine and
    Dentistry
Rochester, New York
Adaptation to General Health Problems and Their Treatment

DEAN P. SARCO, MD
Instructor in Neurology
Harvard Medical School
Division of Epilepsy and Clinical Neurophysiology
Department of Neurology
Children's Hospital Boston
Boston, Massachusetts
Developmental-Behavioral Aspects of Chronic Conditions:
    Central Nervous System Disorders

DAVID J. SCHONFELD, MD
Thelma and Jack Rubinstein Professor of Pediatrics
University of Cincinnati College of Medicine
Director
Division of Developmental and Behavioral Pediatrics
Cincinnati Children's Hospital Medical Center
Cincinnati, Ohio
Research Foundations, Methods, and Issues in
    Developmental-Behavioral Pediatrics

ALISON SCHONWALD, MD
Instructor in Pediatrics
Harvard Medical School
Assistant in Medicine
Children's Hospital Boston
Boston, Massachusetts
Elimination Conditions

JANE F. SILOVSKY, PhD
Associate Professor
Department of Pediatrics
Center on Child Abuse and Neglect
University of Oklahoma Health Sciences Center/
    Children's Hospital of Oklahoma
Oklahoma City, Oklahoma
Sexuality: Sexual Development and Sexual Behavior Problems

MARY SPAGNOLA, MA
Department of Psychology
Center for Health and Behavior
Syracuse University
Syracuse, New York
Family Context in Developmental-Behavioral Pediatrics

CAITLIN SPARKS, BS
Graduate Student
Department of Psychology
Loyola University Chicago
Chicago, Illinois
Theoretical Foundations of Developmental-Behavioral
    Pediatrics

TERRY STANCIN, PhD
Professor of Pediatrics, Psychiatry, and Psychology
Case Western Reserve University
Cleveland
Head
Pediatric Psychology
Department of Pediatrics
MetroHealth Medical Center
Cleveland, Ohio
Screening and Assessment Tools: Measurement and
    Psychometric Considerations; Screening and Assessment
    Tools: Assessment of Development and Behavior

MARTIN T. STEIN, MD
Director of Developmental and Behavioral Pediatrics
University of California San Diego School of
    Medicine
La Jolla
Staff Physician
Rady Children's Hospital
San Diego, California
Strategies to Enhance Developmental and Behavioral Services
    in Primary Care

MARSHALL L. SUMMAR, MD
Associate Professor
Center for Human Genetics Research and
    Department of Pediatrics
Vanderbilt University School of Medicine
Nashville, Tennessee
Developmental-Behavioral Aspects of Chronic Conditions:
    Metabolic Disorders

LISA M. SWISHER, BA, MS, PhD
Clinical Assistant Professor
Department of Pediatrics
Clinical Assistant Professor
Department of Psychiatry and Behavioral Sciences
University of Oklahoma Health Sciences Center
Oklahoma City, Oklahoma
Sexuality: Sexual Development and Sexual Behavior Problems

DOUGLAS L. VANDERBILT, MD
Assistant Professor
Department of Pediatrics
Boston University School of Medicine
Medical Director
NICU Follow-up Program
Division of Developmental and Behavioral Pediatrics
Boston Medical Center
Boston, Massachusetts
Developmental-Behavioral Aspects of Chronic Conditions:
    Central Nervous System Disorders

WILLIAM O. WALKER, JR., MD
Associate Professor of Pediatrics and Director
Developmental Behavioral Pediatrics Fellowship
  Program
University of Washington School of Medicine
Director
Neurodevelopmental/Birth Defects Clinics
Children's Hospital and Regional Medical Center
Seattle, Washington
Cognitive and Adaptive Disabilities

PAUL P. WANG, MD
Director
Clinical Research and Development
Pfizer Global Research and Development
Groton, Connecticut
Developmental-Behavioral Aspects of Chronic Conditions:
  Genetics in Developmental-Behavioral Pediatrics

MARYANN B. WILBUR, BS
Department of Pediatrics
Boston University School of Medicine/Boston
  Medical Center
Boston, Massachusetts
Feeding and Eating Conditions: Food Insecurity and Failure to
  Thrive

PAUL H. WISE, MD, MPH
Richard E. Behrman Professor of Child Health and
  Society
Department of Pediatrics
Centers for Health Policy/Primary Care and
  Outcomes Research
Stanford University
Stanford
Professor
Department of Pediatrics
Lucile Packard Children's Hospital
Palo Alto, California
The History of Child Developmental-Behavioral Health Policy
  in the United States

MARK L. WOLRAICH, MD
CMRI/Shaun Walters Professor of Developmental
  and Behavioral Pediatrics
Section Chief of Developmental and Behavioral
  Pediatrics
Director
OU Child Study Center
Department of Pediatrics
University of Oklahoma Health Sciences Center
Oklahoma City, Oklahoma
Diagnostic Classification Systems; Attention-Deficit/
  Hyperactivity Disorder

KIM A. WORLEY, MD
Oklahoma City, Oklahoma
Attention-Deficit/Hyperactivity Disorder

LOUIS E. WORLEY, BSEd
Director
Sooner SUCCESS
University of Oklahoma
Department of Pediatrics
Section of Developmental and Behavioral Pediatrics
Child Study Center
University of Oklahoma Health Sciences Center
Oklahoma City, Oklahoma
Treatment and Management: Family-Centered Care and the
  Medical Home

LONNIE K. ZELTZER, MD
Professor of Pediatrics,
Anesthesiology, Psychiatry and Biobehavioral
  Sciences
David Geffen School of Medicine at UCLA
Director, Pediatric Pain Program
Mattel Children's Hospital at UCLA
Los Angeles, California
Pain and Somatoform Disorders

KENNETH J. ZUCKER, PhD
Professor
Department of Psychiatry and Psychology
University of Toronto Faculty of Medicine
Head, Gender Identity Service
Child, Youth, and Family Program
Centre for Addiction and Mental Health
Toronto, Ontario, Canada
Sexuality: Gender Identity

JILL M. ZUCKERMAN, MA
Graduate Student
Department of Psychology
Loyola University Chicago
Chicago, Illinois
Theoretical Foundations of Developmental-Behavioral
  Pediatrics

LAUREN ZURENDA, BS
Graduate Student
Department of Psychology
Loyola University Chicago
Chicago, Illinois
Theoretical Foundations of Developmental-Behavioral
  Pediatrics

Introduction

The field of developmental-behavioral pediatrics is a newly recognized subspecialty of pediatrics, formalized by the American Board of Pediatrics (ABP) in 1999. As a field of study and clinical service, its roots go back to the two separate strands within its name—development and behavior. Early work started in the 1940s and 50s. The number of prominent contributors to the field is too large to enumerate here, and any listing probably would not do justice to all prominent participants.

The impetus for a major focus on developmental conditions began in 1962, when President Kennedy established the President's Panel on Mental Retardation. From that panel grew the concept of the University-Affiliated Facility (UAF). The Maternal and Child Health Mental Retardation Amendments and the Mental Retardation Facilities and Community Mental Health Construction Act (88-164) were passed in 1963, and construction began in 1966-1967. The Kennedy Foundation and the Mental Retardation Branch of the Public Health Service provided planning grants, and approximately 30 universities received grants to assist in the development of strong interdisciplinary programs and to construct 19 separate facilities. The programs focused on providing interdisciplinary services for children with mental retardation, as well as relevant training and research. Programs evolved to be dually funded by the Maternal and Child Health Bureau (MCHB) and the Administration on Developmental Disabilities (ADD). In accordance with these developments, the designation *University-Affiliated Facility* was changed to *University-Affiliated Program* (UAP) and, most recently, to *University Center of Excellence in Developmental Disabilities* (UCEDD). The program funding sources also diverged: The MCHB maintained a focus on children and the health aspects, now called Leadership Education in Neurodevelopmental Disabilities (LEND) programs, whereas the ADD funding focused on the broader life span and less on the health aspects. Currently, 35 LEND programs provide a resource for fellowship training in developmental-behavioral pediatrics, as well as in other disciplines (e.g., neurodevelopmental disabilities, nursing, occupational therapy, physical therapy).

The major initiative related to behavioral pediatrics was implemented with funding from the W.T. Grant Foundation to the University of Maryland, starting in 1976. The W.T. Grant Foundation subsequently funded 11 programs across the country in 1978. The requirements of these programs were commitments from department chairs for faculty support, space, and clinical care facilities. These programs initiated the creation of the Society of Behavioral Pediatrics in 1982, renamed the Society for Developmental and Behavioral Pediatrics (SDBP) in 1994. The MCHB later funded 12 behavioral pediatric fellowship training programs beginning in 1986. After the American Board of Pediatrics brokered the development of the certifiable subspecialty of developmental-behavioral pediatrics, the MCHB training program was expanded to encompass developmental-behavioral pediatrics fellowship training programs.

A third important component of the development of the field has been the evolution of pediatric psychology. The Society of Pediatric Psychology (SPP) was founded in 1967 and began publishing the *Journal of Pediatric Psychology* in 1975. The publication of the *Handbook of Pediatric Psychology* in 1988[1] defined the SPP's field. The third edition of the *Handbook* reflects the continued growth of that discipline within psychology, as does the incorporation of the SPP into the American Psychological Association as Division 54. Many common members of the SDBP and the SPP have played an important role in helping to shape and define both fields.

Both behavioral and developmental pediatrics contributed impetus to extend the amount of training in these areas within pediatric residency programs. Members of both disciplines were integral members of the Task Force on Pediatric Education of 1978,[2] which encouraged increased education in both developmental and behavioral pediatrics. Part of the charge of the 11 centers funded by the W.T. Grant Foundation was to help provide curriculum direction and training in behavioral pediatrics for pediatric residents and to develop fellowship training programs. For the developmental aspects, a grant from the Federal Bureau for Handicapped Children sponsored a National Invitational Conference in 1978 to describe model programs. The result of that conference was the development of a project to create and publish a Curriculum in Developmental Pediatrics for residency training programs.[3]

Subsequently, the SDBP published a residency curriculum as a supplement in the SDBP journal.[4] The continued need for more and improved training of primary care pediatricians in developmental-behavioral pediatrics was emphasized again in the second Task Force Report (Future of Pediatric Education II).[5] The importance of training in developmental–behavioral pediatrics also has been emphasized by the American Academy of Pediatrics (AAP), which presents many continuing medical education (CME) courses every year in this discipline. The AAP convened a Task Force on Mental Health in 2004 and has supported several major initiatives relating to attention-deficit/hyperactivity disorder (ADHD), autism, developmental screening, and medical homes.

The AAP has had a consistent interest in behavioral and developmental issues. Five years after its formation in 1930, the AAP set up a Committee on Mental Hygiene and in 1949 formed a Section on Mental Health, changed to the Section on Child Development in 1960 and to the Section on Developmental and Behavioral Pediatrics in 1988. Other AAP committees and similar groups pertinent to the field have included the Committee on Psychosocial Aspects of Child and Family Health; the Committee (now Council) on Children with Disabilities; the Committee on Early Childhood, Adoption and Dependent Care; the Committee on Adolescence; the Task Force on Coding for Mental Health Disorders; the Task Force on Mental Health; and the ADHD Guidelines and Advisory Committees.

An initiative to develop the *Journal of Developmental and Behavioral Pediatrics* was started in the 1950s and came to fruition in 1980, separate from the SDBP. This publication was adopted and sponsored by the SDBP in 1985 and continues as a successful and high-quality journal.

In 1991 the SDBP's Executive Council voted to pursue formal recognition of the subspecialty of developmental-behavioral pediatrics from the ABP. Movement toward that goal was delayed in 1992, owing to a restraint on the creation of any more subspecialties. Through persistent efforts on the part of a number of SDBP members, who clearly identified the need for and clarified the definition of this new field, and with support from a majority of pediatric department chairpersons, developmental-behavioral pediatrics was approved by the American Board of Medical Specialties (ABMS) and the ABP as the 13th formal subspecialty of pediatrics in 1999. Subsequently, the Accreditation Council of Graduate Medical Education (ACGME) developed criteria for training in this new subspecialty. The first cohort of successful applicants were certified in 2002. As of 2006, 520 certified developmental-behavioral pediatricians and 45 fellowship training programs were accredited by the ACGME.

As part of the process of creating an examination for purposes of certifying physicians, a comprehensive content listing was developed by the ABP's Subboard of Developmental-Behavioral Pediatrics to describe the expected content of the new subspecialty. This textbook reflects the scope of the field as defined by that process.

Our goal in writing this book was that the content be clinically extensive and based on the most current evidence available. The four co-editors, all past presidents of the SDBP, considered that we were in a good position to develop such a text.

Several basic assumptions underlie our approach to the content of the book. The first is that the previous distinctions made between *development* and *behavior* are artificial and no longer useful. *Development* is characterized by various manifestations of the maturation of the central nervous system and the biological and environmental influences on it. *Behavior* is characterized by the normal relationships and functions of children and the environmental and psychosocial factors that enhance or disturb them. The two are so entwined that neither theoretical frameworks nor clinical interventions are possible without full understanding of both the developmental and behavioral aspects. Evidence of *development* in a child is seen through that child's behavior; children's *behavior* can be understood only in the context of their developmental level. Furthermore, we believe that clinical interventions, research, and training require a biopsychosocial perspective in order to effectively study, understand, and intervene with families and children. We have selected the topics for the chapters to provide a comprehensive picture of this perspective. We also asked all of the contributing authors to reflect this perspective in writing their chapters.

The book provides the theoretical, policy, and research underpinnings of the field including cultural, biological, and classification issues, because any scientific body of knowledge must be supported on a sound theoretical and research base. We have provided information on both developmental and behavioral assessment procedures, tools and evidence for their reliability and validity. The treatment and management sections begin with management principles such as family-centered and interdisciplinary care and then provide current evidence-based information on the range of conditions that constitute developmental–behavioral pediatrics. Rounding out the content of the book are chapters related to special ethical issues in developmental–behavioral pediatrics and the contributions of the field to innovations in primary care pediatrics.

We hope that you find the book informative, helpful, and authoritative and that it is a worthy representation of the recently formalized subspecialty of developmental–behavioral pediatrics.

REFERENCES

1. Routh DK: *Handbook of Pediatric Psychology.* Guilford Press, New York, 1988.
2. Task Force on Pediatric Education: *The Future of Pediatric Education.* American Academy of Pediatrics, Evanston, IL, 1978.
3. *Curriculum in Developmental Pediatrics.* Handicapped Children's Early Education Program Department of Education, Washington, DC, 1982.
4. Coury DL, Berger SP, Stancin T, et al: Curricular guidelines for residency training in developmental–behavioral pediatrics. *J Dev Behav Pediatr* 20:S1-S38, 1999.
5. Collaborative Project of the Pediatric Community: The Future of Pediatric Education II: Organizing pediatric education to meet the needs of infants, children, adolescents and young adults in the 21st century. *Pediatrics* 105:161-212, 2000.
6. Perrin EC, Bennett FC, Wolraich ML: Subspecialty certification in developmental–behaviorial pediatrics: Past and present challenges. *J Dev Behav Pediatr* 2:130-132, 2000.

Contents

The History of Child Developmental-Behavioral Health Policy in the United States

PAUL H. WISE ▪ JULIUS B. RICHMOND

Policies regarding child development are inherently responsive to a broad spectrum of societal influences. Historical reviews of these policies have tended to focus on only one aspect of child development policies, usually defined by a particular discipline or select set of professional interests. We instead consider this history broadly with an explicit objective of linking advances in developmental science to current popular sensibilities regarding children and our collective capacity to improve their health and well-being.

There are many ways to define public policy. For this discussion, we adopt a rather simple construction, one that underscores policy's inherently pragmatic nature: the transformation of societal intent into societal action. For a scientific audience, it would be affirming to suggest that this process of transformation begins with scientific insights and then proceeds logically to an evaluated pilot program and on into broad policy. The reality of policy development, of course, follows a far broader logic than that of scientific inquiry. Rather, policy requires collective action, which on some level requires consensus, and consensus is not discovered but created. In this discussion, we examine the context in which remarkable progress in the science of child development has influenced the interpretation of this science, as well as public perceptions of society's responsibilities and capacities to use this science in the best interest of children.

Different analytical perspectives have been used to assess the history of developmental-behavioral pediatrics. Some assessments have been disciplinary, focused on the professionalization of the field.[1-3] Others have been concerned with progress in the science of child development and have chronicled the nature and cadence of scientific discovery and its conceptualization.[4] Still other authors have examined historical currents in the perception of childhood itself, recognizing at least indirectly the central importance of development in shaping these broad social perceptions.[5,6]

In this discussion, we attempt to address all these analytical perspectives. This broad approach is mandated by the focus on policy, an arena of social endeavor that is shaped by not one but all these historical trends. In accordance with this comprehensive mandate, we employ a comprehensive policy model that provides an integration of the many factors that shape policy. This model suggests that public policies are determined by three broad domains of influence:

1. Knowledge base. Policy requires some empirical basis for taking action. Knowledge is necessary to help identify the nature of problems to be addressed, their prevalence and scope of effect, and, of significance, effective means of ameliorative response.
2. Social strategy. Policy requires strategies for implementing ameliorative responses in large populations. This entails the development of funding mechanisms, systems of provision and accountability, and ultimately a means of ensuring sustainable political support.
3. Political will. At some level, all policies must have sufficient political support to ensure their implementation and maintenance. This often requires not only a public awareness of the issue but also the political framing of issues in ways that lead to the development of sufficient consensus to enable enactment and the appropriation of resources.

Because this model treats policy as intensely interactive, it helps identify thematic continuities that transcend the science, the structure of public and private programs, and the dominant political perceptions and sensibilities. These themes evolve and, if coherent enough, come to characterize the policies of the historical period in which they occur. In this manner, we examine the evolution of child development policy with a special focus on the knowledge base, social strategy, and political will that have shaped its course and cadence.

DEVELOPMENT AS STATE INTEREST

The modern concern for child development has its roots in the public reaction to the rapid industrialization that characterized the United States in the 19th century. Waves of immigration and the mass relocation of families from rural areas into large urban centers overwhelmed existing housing, sanitation, and virtually all municipal services, which resulted in tragically high rates of illness and death among children. Public apprehension for the well-being of children was broadly framed by these general living conditions, but of special concern was the widespread employment of children in a variety of industrial and street occupations, many of them extremely hazardous in nature. Although the peril urban life posed to children took many forms, the exploitation of children working in factories, mills, and on the street was seen as a particularly egregious threat and ultimately served as a distilled image for the development of requisite political will to ultimately address what in fact was a variety of societal threats to children's well-being at the turn of the 20th century.

Critics of child labor could draw on only a fledgling knowledge base to support their positions. Heavily influenced by Darwin's theories of evolution, G. Stanley Hall advocated childhood as a series of progressive stages, each requiring freedom from deleterious societal pressures and an emphasis on play and guided exploration.[7] John Dewey, although conceptualizing on a different basis, also emphasized the need to create environments that would optimize children's psychological and social development.[8] However, far more important in shaping public perceptions of vulnerable children was less science than, quite literally, fiction. Following a romantic thread woven earlier by Jean Jacques Rousseau and William Wordsworth, 19th century authors such as Charles Dickens in England, Victor Hugo in France, and Mark Twain in the United States cast, in deeply emotional terms, the transcendent innocence of children mistreated by a harsh and unfeeling adult world.[9] This body of literature, coupled with the work of reformist photographers, particularly Jacob Riis, Lewis W. Hine, and Wallace Kirkland at Hull House, created powerful public images of children as "innocent victims" and moved the affective center of the prevailing political will to a new position, one far more sympathetic to

children and, of significance, to public action on their behalf.

There remained, however, a need to provide social strategies that could transform this political will into effective programs and policies. Ultimately, this was supplied by the emergence at the end of the 19th century of a strong women's movement in shaping local programs to assist poor children and their families through education, social assistance, and health interventions. Under the leadership of remarkable women such as Jane Addams and her associates at Hull House in Chicago,[10] community-based social work, which Skocpol[11] termed *maternalistic* social reform strategies, provided an alternative to "paternalistic" reform efforts, such as improved wages, worker's compensation, and safety legislation, which at the time met heavy resistance at both the state and federal levels.

The influence of Addams and her Hull House associates quickly extended beyond local social work. Their studies and advocacy led to a successful campaign to pass the Illinois Juvenile Court Act in 1899. Realizing that judges knew little about the developmental capacities and backgrounds of the children appearing in their court, these advocates helped to establish the Illinois Juvenile Psychopathic Institute in 1909, which pioneered clinical studies of children and their families. They recruited Dr. William Healy to direct the research, and in the process, the discipline of child psychiatry was established, perhaps the only instance in which a medical specialty grew out of community action.

The convergence of these political, scientific, and programmatic forces led to the first White House conference on children, convened by President Theodore Roosevelt in 1909, and ultimately the establishment of the Children's Bureau in 1912. The Bureau was directed to "investigate and report . . . upon all matters pertaining to the welfare of children and child life among all classes of our people and shall especially investigate the questions of infant mortality, the birth rate, orphanages, juvenile courts, desertion, dangerous occupations, accidents and diseases of children, employment, legislation affecting children."[12] Under its first director, Julia Lathrop (an alumna of Hull House), the Bureau embarked on a series of research and support activities to help state and local groups address the general health and well-being of children and mothers.[13,14] However, from the beginning, the Bureau emphasized assisting children "who were abnormal or subnormal or suffering from physical or mental ills" both because of the urgent needs these children demonstrated and in the contention that such assistance ". . . also serves to aid in laying the foundations for the best service to all children of the Commonwealth" (Bradbury,[15] pp 17, 15, 39). The pediatrician Ethel Dunham was recruited to develop studies for the better prevention and management of prematurity, which paved the way for the development of neonatology as a medical specialty.

Although the Children's Bureau's influence was manifold, perhaps its most enduring function was to represent and ultimately to embody a recognition of the federal government's responsibility to promote the health and welfare of the nation's children. Until establishment of the Bureau, federal efforts on behalf of children were relatively isolated and idiosyncratic, based mostly on a long-standing reliance on familial provision and local charity. With each new report and local initiative, the Children's Bureau emphasized and eventually solidified the proposition that there was indeed a state interest in the well-being of children, and that that interest was best served by action at the federal level.

The nature of this initial federal action was to establish a grants-in-aid program to assist agencies at the state level to expand services for young children and their mothers. Passed in 1920, the Sheppard-Towner Act created the means by which the expertise developed at the Children's Bureau could be transmitted throughout the country. This extended the Bureau's actions far beyond what its meager budget could ever have allowed in isolation. Among the many improvements that occurred at this time were the establishment or growth of state child hygiene agencies, which incorporated for the first time the latest views on child health and development into its programs; the proliferation of maternal and child health centers, which provided direct health and development services to local communities; and a remarkable increase in the scale and expertise of visiting nurse services throughout the country. Unfortunately, the success of the Sheppard-Towner Act became its undoing, as opposition from conservative politicians and the organized medical establishment blocked its renewal in 1929. Although this was a major setback, the Act, and through it the Children's Bureau, had already begun the transformation of the well-being of children into a public good, and therefore even the termination of the Act could not reinstate federal indifference to the needs of children. Indeed, the Sheppard-Towner Act's goals foretold the coming of a new era of public provision, and its structure ultimately provided the basic architecture for federal initiatives for child development to this day.

DEVELOPMENT AS CASUALTY

The period between 1930 and 1950 was defined by two predominant events: the Great Depression and World War II. Although these events were associated with a variety of complex political changes, among the most far-reaching was the popular embrace of the government's role in advancing social welfare in general and the well-being of children in particular.

The social strategies developed during the years of the Sheppard-Towner Act continued to provide a blueprint for translating this public support into actual programs and services. The recommendations of the 1930 White House Conference on Child Health and Protection gave considerable support for a comprehensive approach to the public provision of maternal and child health services, particularly, for what was then termed "crippled children." The Conference specifically recommended that "Grants-in-aid constitute the most effective basis for national and state cooperation in promoting child welfare and in securing the establishment of that national minimum of care and protection which is the hope of every citizen."[8] This argument was embraced fully with the passage of the Social Security Act of 1935, as it included as Title V ("Promoting Informed Parental Choice and Innovative Programs") of the Act federal grants to the states for maternal and child health services, including services specifically for "crippled children."

This period also witnessed a rapid growth in the knowledge base regarding child development. With financial support from private philanthropy, particularly the Laura Spelman Rockefeller Fund and the Commonwealth Fund, a number of child guidance centers and research institutes were created, including the Child Research Council in Denver; The Fels Research Institute at Yellow Springs, Ohio; the Yale Child Study Center in New Haven; and the Berkeley Institute of Child Welfare Research. These programs produced more scientific observations of normal child development, as well as explorations of the determinants of mental retardation and behavioral problems in children. Work done at developing programs in child psychiatry, such as the Judge Baker Foundation in Boston, added to these insights.

Perhaps the most influential early scientific observer and analyst of child development was Arnold Gesell (1880-1961), a psychologist and pediatrician. Working in the early part of the 20th century, Gesell conducted a variety of studies on children with normal development and those with specific physiological challenges, such as children with Down syndrome and those experiencing harmful perinatal events. Although his techniques of observation and analysis were to shape the methods of a broad range of developmental scientists for years to come, Gesell's theoretical bearings were set by a clear embrace of biological determination and were largely descriptive. Not only did he view the effect of experience as relatively trivial but he also looked with skepticism on the potential of interventions to alter developmental pathways.[16,17]

This emphasis on biological determinants included both inherited etiologies of developmental disabilities and nonhereditary biological mechanisms, particularly adverse fetal and perinatal events. This focus attracted a growing body of empirical observations linking early adverse events to later neurodevelopmental outcomes. Much later, this "continuum of reproductive casualty" was a framework that served not only as a conceptual tool for scientific analysis but also as a means for representing the determinants of adverse developmental disorders to the broader public.[18-20] Other events tended to strengthen the public acceptance of biologically determined disabilities, including the impression of casualty transmitted by the large-scale return of disabled soldiers after World War II and later, the tragedy of birth defects caused by the ingestion of thalidomide during pregnancy in the late 1950s.

A strong alternative perspective was being advanced at approximately the same time by those who endorsed the primacy of environmental influences. Generally framed as behaviorism, this perspective was boldly articulated by one of its prominent, early spokesmen, John B. Watson (1878-1958):

> Give me a dozen healthy infants, well-formed, and my own specified world to bring them up in and I'll guarantee to take any one at random and train him to become any type of specialist I might select—doctor, lawyer, artist, merchant-chief, and yes, even beggar-man and thief, regardless of his talents, penchants, tendencies, abilities, vocations, and race of his ancestors.[21]

This alternative to biological determinism became even more fashionable as behaviorism became more technically grounded by the experiments of B. F. Skinner (1904-1990). Psychoanalytical thought was attracting much attention at this time as well. Although Freud's concepts were grounded in biology, social interaction was seen as forming the basis for the emergence of emotions and behavior. Erik Erikson (1902-1994) built on this psychoanalytical base to emphasize periods of transition or crisis, heavily shaped by social contexts and culture.[22]

Alongside this core tension between biological and environmental determination, the history of child development policies has also been heavily informed by a second arena of research: the extent to which and the mechanisms by which child development is influenced by early life experiences.[23] The research community's response to these questions was first based in examining the effect of profound early deprivation on later developmental outcomes, primarily among institutionalized infants. These studies suggested that profound isolation and the lack of a nurturing environment could interfere with normal development and result in a variety of adverse conditions, including growth retardation and social maladjustment.[24] Spitz,[24] Bowlby,[25] and others in the 1950s provided observations of early social deprivation in a variety of settings, which ultimately led to a theoretical framework underscoring the importance of early attachment processes between parent and child in shaping developmental outcomes later in life.[26,27]

The tension between the biological and environmental models of developmental influence grew as more scientific evidence was generated in support of each of these two perspectives. The child development laboratories and guidance centers continued to increase the knowledge base regarding brain development and adverse biological insults and, at the same time, confirmed the sensitivity of the child to caregiving practices and social pressures. A new formulation was needed, one that could make sense of the disparate findings, powerful enough to engage the complexity of child development, and yet disciplined enough to offer a basis for popular understanding and ultimately for constructive action.

DEVELOPMENT AS JUSTICE

In the 1960s, the directions of political will and the knowledge base began to converge in ways that dramatically altered the nature and scale of child development programs in the United States. Politically, the civil rights movement was elevating public awareness of the profound racial inequalities that had so long characterized American society.[28] The publication of Michael Harrington's *The Other America* in 1963 extended this awareness to broader economic stratification affecting all racial and ethnic groups.[29] These powerful challenges to the status quo were interpreted in a variety of ways and led to a variety of disparate political arguments and movements. What resonated most profoundly in the mainstream of American politics was the notion that existing policies did not facilitate, much less guarantee, equal *opportunity* for the requirements of a fulfilled life. Indeed, the rhetoric of opportunity permeated the public justification of major ameliorative legislation such as the Civil Rights Act of 1964 and an array of initiatives that were included in President Johnson's "war on poverty." Indeed, the legislation enabling the war on poverty was the Economic *Opportunity* Act of 1964 (our italics).

This political embrace of opportunity as the central theme of policy reform in the early 1960s also began to find support in the scientific community's reframing of early child development. The antagonism between biological and environmental explanations for adverse developmental outcomes began to lessen as more integrative models became more widely accepted. Empirical and theoretical support grew for the important role of both biological determinants and early life experiences in shaping later developmental outcomes. In addition, a series of studies suggested that many of these outcomes were difficult to predict with certainty and that many were potentially amenable to later remedial interventions.[30,31]

Jean Piaget (1896-1980), whose work became well known in the United States in the 1950s and 1960s, challenged the sharp distinctions between biologically determined and behaviorist visions of child development by stressing the dynamic character of cognitive capacities in children. According to his theories, children were not blank slates waiting to be written on but active participants, builders of understanding, constantly creating and testing their own theories of the world.[32] This more integrative perspective revealed a more complex and interactive model of child development, one that could incorporate new insights into biological maturation without reducing the potential for environmental influence. Also at this time, there was growing evidence that the developmental consequences of many early deprivations were modifiable by purposeful intervention.[33,34] These findings converged with research that suggested far more pliability in the determination of intelligence than had been widely presumed.[35,36]

Together, these observations gave scientific weight to the political argument that early deprivation resulted in more than hardship; it altered life opportunities. This in turn transformed observations of young children's development and behavior into questions of justice and thereby elevated the realm of child development into the highest reaches of political discourse.

This coupling of early child experiences with broad political debate marked a major shift in the political context of developmental-behavioral policy in the United States. Although this linkage of development science to direct political advocacy generated new policy activity, it had in fact, deep roots in earlier thinking on the relationship between childhood and human freedom. John Locke (1632-1704), drawing on a long thread of philosophical speculation, had popularized the perspective that children were a tabula rasa (translated from the Latin approximately as a "blank slate"), on which experience writes the narrative of an individual's personality, skills, and ideas (Locke,[37] p 26). Jean Jacques Rousseau (1712-1778) argued that children are born into a natural state of relative peace and selflessness and that the many evils of society were the result of dehumanizing social and political structures (Rousseau,[38] pp 61-62).

However, unlike the debates of the 1960s, these arguments regarding children were not directly concerned with the unfairness of early life deprivation per se; rather, they were the requisite stepping stones to far broader challenges to the then widely accepted view that human competence and merit were the products of innate forces.

At the middle of the 20th century, child development moved from merely offering evidence that societal inequality interacted with child outcomes to directly targeting this relationship for ameliorative intervention. Justice mandated equal opportunity, a "level playing field," and this had generated a variety of attempts to guarantee such opportunities for adults in voting, employment, and legal protections. Meanwhile, the new science of child development was suggesting that reaching the age of majority was an artificial starting point for guaranteeing equal opportunity. This had the effect of extending into childhood justice arguments that traditionally had been confined to the adult world. Justice mandated equal opportunity and for the first time, this guarantee was cast as inherently developmental.

The influence of this emerging reframing of child development was apparent in the progression of social strategies that were employed. President John F. Kennedy appointed a Panel on Mental Retardation to consider how best to use the growing knowledge base in shaping new public programs. Its recommendations led to the enactment in 1963 of Public Law 88-156, the Maternal and Child Health and Mental Retardation Planning Act, in which the Title V funding mechanism was used to support at the state level a variety of special projects related to mental retardation. In many ways, the Panel's work and the resulting legislation were transitional. The law was a gesture to the reproductive casualty perspective by focusing on prenatal and newborn prevention interventions, including Maternity and Infant Care Projects and neonatal screening for phenylketonuria and other metabolic disorders. It was also a recognition that poor developmental outcomes occurred disproportionately in "families who are deprived of the basic necessities of life, opportunity and motivation" and enhanced community-based services for affected children and their families.[39] The Panel in its findings was even more explicit as it pronounced that "Society [has a] special responsibility to persons with extraordinary needs . . . . to permit and actually foster the development of their maximum capacity."[40] It also articulated explicitly the role of social and material deprivation in shaping poor developmental outcomes and recommended the establishment of educational programs for young children in economically disadvantaged communities throughout the country. In order to implement these developing programs, Public

Law 88-156 and, in particular, Public Law 90-538, the Handicapped Children's Early Education Assistance Act, enacted in 1968, set in motion research and training initiatives designed to produce personnel with expertise in education, developmental science, and the special needs of children with disabling conditions, a field now generally known as early childhood special education. These efforts were augmented by subsequent legislation and served to professionalize the providers of early child developmental services. That these programs were influencing pediatric research, education, and practice was evident in the growing pediatric literature on child development.[41] These, in turn, helped improve the quality of these expanding programs and the efforts of the workers charged with implementing them.

The linkage of child development to opportunity and justice concerns culminated with the development of the Head Start program in 1965. Begun as a summer preschool project as part of the war on poverty, Head Start quickly became a national movement with an explicit commitment to parent and community involvement. A basic requirement was that the program be governed by local community boards. It was conceived as a comprehensive program designed to provide early educational experiences for young children in disadvantaged communities, but it also included nutritional guidance, social services, health, and mental health components.[42] Its goals, its administrative home in the Office of Economic Opportunity, and even its name were shaped by the public concern for equal opportunity, even as its operation was grounded in the daily substrate of child development.

As early childhood demonstration and outreach programs multiplied through the 1970s, the framing of development as justice continued to evolve. Far greater emphasis began to be placed on the civil rights of disabled persons (including children) and, consequently, on political advocacy for greater inclusion in employment and public life, with legal remedies when such inclusion did not occur.[43] In response to a variety of constituencies, but particularly to the exceptional advocacy from parents of children with developmental disorders, the passage in 1975 of Public Law 94-142, the Education of All Handicapped Children Act and now named the Individuals with Disabilities Education Act, established the right of all children, regardless of disability and developmental needs, to a free and appropriate public education. It required individual assessments of special needs and that an Individual Education Plan (IEP) be developed for each eligible child. These were to be constructed to provide each child with a comprehensive educational plan to be implemented in the least restrictive environment possible. Significantly, the law stipulated

that the IEP assessments be conducted in a nondiscriminatory manner and that procedural and legal recourse was available if parents were dissatisfied with the IEP process.

What followed was a series of state and federal laws challenging long-standing discrimination against disabled persons, including Public Law 93-112, the Vocational Rehabilitation Act, passed in 1973, and its amendment, Public Law 93-516, enacted a year later, which together outlawed discrimination against disabled persons in employment, institutions of higher learning, and access to public facilities. These and other similar pieces of legislation laid a foundation for enhanced services, as well as a basis for subsequent case law protecting the rights of disabled persons in virtually all aspects of daily life.[44]

During this period, developmental disorders were attracting new attention from the medical profession. Many of the traditional threats to child health, particularly acute infectious disease, had been dramatically reduced, and, as a result, developmental disorders became more prominent in pediatric practice.[45] Although known as the "new morbidity," these developmental and behavioral disorders were not in fact new but newly discovered by a profession long focused on acute disease. This shift in focus set in motion an important new dynamic by which pediatrics became more intimately involved with the identification and response to developmental disorders and strengthened its training and organization to deal with these issues.[46]

This new attention from the medical profession coincided with the rapid expansion of the Medicaid program, the primary publicly funded health insurance program for poor children in the United States. Not only did Medicaid mandate a variety of screenings and services as part of the Early and Periodic Screening, Diagnostic and Treatment program, but as an entitlement program, its funding levels quickly dwarfed other public programs concerned with child health and development. This had the effect of shifting the center of gravity for developmental services from local programs supported by Title V funds to medical practices, particularly as more effective medications and behavioral treatment strategies were developed to treat developmental and behavioral disorders. Although the stronger medical presence was long overdue, it also put new strains on the systems that had been developed to coordinate services for children with developmental disorders.

This challenge was addressed in part with the passage of the Education for All Handicapped Children Act Amendments of 1986. This legislation required "a statewide, comprehensive, coordinated, multidisciplinary, interagency program of early intervention services for all handicapped infants and their families" (see a cogent discussion of this Act by Shonkoff and Meisels[23]). The focus was on providing developmental services in the broadest context with the expressed goal of enhancing the coordination of the full range of services to better assist young children with special needs and their families. The importance of these early intervention services cannot be overstated, inasmuch as they continue to represent among the most generally available and focused interventions for children with a wide array of developmental conditions.

Although it did not provide formal funding streams, the Americans with Disabilities Act of 1990 provided the most comprehensive federal civil rights law ever enacted to protect individuals with mental or physical disabilities from discrimination. The law prohibits discrimination in employment (Title I); in state and local government services (Title II); in public accommodations, including preschools, daycare facilities, and Head Start programs administered by private agencies (Title III); in public transportation (Title IIIB); and in telecommunications (Title IV).[47]

The social strategies to implement child development policies under a rubric of equal opportunity and justice have continued to rely on federal-state partnerships and legal challenges to discrimination. The rapid growth of these programs has generated repeated calls for greater coordination among them and even the elimination of the categorical funding streams associated with these varied pieces of legislation. Although greater efficiency and improvements in the quality of delivered services remain important goals and may require new approaches to funding and organization, there can be no doubt that the convergence of the more integrative scientific base, the political framing as opportunity and justice, and the programmatic strategies through federal legislation and legal action produced the most dramatic expansion in public commitment to the needs of young children in U.S. history.

DEVELOPMENT AS IDENTITY

Although it is difficult to predict how science will affect the field of child development in the near future, there is little doubt that rapid advances in the technology of investigation will generate rapid advances in specific arenas of understanding. Progress in genetics, neuroimaging, and the observational and statistical assessments of environmental influence are already shedding light on developmental processes that have long evaded productive scrutiny.

Among the most important areas of scientific progress has been in the genetics of development and behavior, including the mapping of the human genome. The field of quantitative genetics has made great strides in quantifying the relative and combined contributions of genetic and nongenetic influences on a variety of developmental and psychological disorders in large or special populations (twins and adopted children, for example). Because of the tortured history of statistically partitioning intelligence or behavioral attributes into genetic and nongenetic determinants, these quantitative genetics studies must be viewed critically, particularly in their interpretation by and representation to the broader public.[48] Of critical importance are the findings that underscore the profound interactions among genetic and environmental influences in generating observed phenotypes and developmental outcomes. These gene-environment interactions have emerged as potentially crucial mechanisms of mediating, if not determining outright, the ultimate phenotypic expression of genetic predisposition.[49] In addition, explorations of epigenetic phenomena have demonstrated that environmental influences early in life can alter the lifelong expression of a genetic profile.[50] These studies underscore the urgent need to expand and update more traditional transactional[51] or ecological models[52] of child development that have served as a useful theoretical base for integrating new insights from a variety of disciplines.

Developments in neuroscience are also likely to have important implications for child development policy. Advances in neuroimaging have permitted detailed examinations of both the structure and function of children's brains as they grow and develop. Specific patterns of abnormal brain functioning have begun to be associated with a variety of developmental or psychological disorders.[53] Of equal usefulness have been new insights into the ways genetic and environmental phenomena shape the molecular and cellular events through which brains develop.

There has also been a growing awareness of the role that culture plays in shaping child development and the appreciation of differences in children's capacities. Child-rearing beliefs, patterns of caregiving, feeding practices, and approaches to discipline, among many other elements, can all potentially affect developmental processes.[54] These observations have not only highlighted the need for greater study of these factors[55] but also have served as an important reminder that child development remains deeply woven into the fabric of family and community life.

Among the most far-reaching effects of this new science is the collapse of the strict boundaries between normal and abnormal that has long characterized the public impression of developmental outcomes. Improved tools of measurement have recast many arenas of behavioral and developmental outcomes as continuums of strengths, weaknesses, or just differences. Detailing the complexity of causation inherent in any broad developmental capacity (such as school performance) or behavior (such as antisocial behavior) has tended to disaggregate these outcomes into a network of component capacities and behaviors, each of which can be tested and assessed. This, virtually by definition, has expanded the potential to identify components that are below or above some expected distribution in the larger population.

There may also be trends in the science and practice patterns of developmental clinicians and psychiatrists that have helped blur the boundaries of normalcy in child development. The emergence of the *Diagnostic and Statistical Manual of Mental Disorders* as a basis for categorizing diagnoses and, significantly, for billing for services in many jurisdictions, has tended to reify developmental concerns as specific diagnoses. The trends in the knowledge base provide an important context for documenting a rising prevalence of developmental disorders in children.[56] It is difficult to identify what portion of this increase resulted from increased public awareness, an improved ability to identify problems and specific disorders, changes in the demands on children, or actual increases in the underlying prevalence of these disorders. Regardless of its causes, the high prevalence itself has altered public perceptions of child development by bringing the issue into more homes, making it a more integral component of family and community life. This rise in the prevalence of developmental disorders has occurred at the same time that many of the traditional threats to the health of children continue to be dramatically reduced. This has created an epidemiological scenario in which most children will never experience any major medical illness necessitating hospitalization, much less result in death. Indeed, these trends have generated a kind of "dichotomization" in patterns of child health and disease in which most children are unlikely to experience a serious health problem and the remaining portion of children accounting for a growing portion of services and expenditures.[45] Accordingly, pediatricians interact mostly with children increasingly unlikely ever to experience a serious acute illness.[57] This pattern has focused heightened attention on detailed developmental issues of concern to parents and is likely to have the effect of blurring traditional definitions of normalcy, of redefining "well" children to emphasize that they are not necessarily free from a variety of developmental and social problems and disorders.

The rapid growth in the medical involvement in the management of developmental disorders has made child development services vulnerable to pressures occurring in the larger health care system. The intense focus on cost reduction has created strong incentives for implementing strategies that reduce the use of health services through changes in financing and practice. Among the most important has been the direction of children with a variety of disabilities into managed care, particularly if they are enrolled in Medicaid or other public insurance programs. There remains a striking paucity of empirical insight into whether this trend has benefited or harmed this vulnerable population of children. Theoretically, managed care could enhance the coordination of services for these children. However, when cost containment is emphasized, the restrictions on referral for specialty care, medications, and coverage for medical equipment such as wheelchairs and eyeglasses raise deep concerns that this strategy could erect new barriers to appropriate care for these children and their families.

In association with this growing capacity to describe developmental attributes, there has been a dramatic shift in the kinds of capacities required in the workforce and, therefore, in schools. The growing need for communication and information-based skills has placed new demands on the developmental capacities of children and youth in ways that are likely to unmask even subtle problems in learning or cognitive performance. Therefore, as the capacity to test for developmental problems has grown, so too has the apparent need for this testing.

The rapid expansion in the science of child development, the growing accessibility of developmental testing, and the increased prevalence of developmental disorders have occurred at the same time that health issues have become among the most prominent domains of popular culture. News programs, magazines, and the Internet offer new discoveries regarding health as a central staple for their audiences. The science of health, including the science of development, has been elevated into the public consciousness in unprecedented ways. Medical research that would just a few years ago have remained the province of a highly specialized audience is now widely accessible through virtually all forms of public media.

The rapid dissemination of research findings into the general culture has meant that the identification of new developmental syndromes, genetic predispositions, or environmental risks for behaviors or development problems is now far more likely to generate public concerns than ever before—perhaps even prematurely, before their complexity has been adequately explored.

SUMMARY

Any review of the history of child development policies in the United States must conclude that the 20th century was one of enormous progress.

Remarkable strides in understanding the biology of child development have been accompanied by empirical insights into the role of the social environment in shaping developmental outcomes. Although these advances in the knowledge base of child development have fueled long-standing tensions between biological and social explanations for developmental outcomes, they have also been associated with new, integrated conceptual reframings of biological and environmental interactions. These in turn, have helped to ground the new professional discipline of developmental-behavioral pediatrics in scientific evidence and methodological rigor.

The translation of this knowledge base into policy requires both practical social strategies for implementation and the political will to act. The historical development of social strategies designed to optimize child development has been characterized by rapid progress. The emergence of federal-state partnerships for a variety of specialized programs for children with developmental disorders has been linked to strong legal provisions to help ensure the inclusion of such children in the mainstream of educational and other aspects of community life.

The actual implementation of child health policies, however, is always dependent on political will. Advocates for enhanced child development policies have always lamented that children cannot directly influence the political process in the United States. This is often voiced as "Children don't vote." Perhaps the real question is "Why should they have to?" Children's political voices have always been defined by the development of proxy constituencies. Repeatedly, these political proxies have been motivated parents and professionals, particularly those affected by the tragic inadequacy of programs and policies available for children. Broader political proxies are almost always required and depend on larger currents of political perceptions and sensibilities, which in turn emerge from a variety of economic, demographic, and cultural forces.

Together, the evolution of the knowledge base, social strategies, and political will continue to shape both the nature and scope of children's health policies in the United States. In spite of many obstacles, services for children with developmental disorders generally improved greatly over the course of the 20th century. However, old challenges remain and new ones have developed. Programs for children have generally fared poorly amid intense competition for public funding. In part, this reflects the current pressures on social spending in general. However, perhaps more troubling is the lack of a compelling public argument for an enhanced commitment to children's development and behavioral health. As highlighted in *From Neurons to Neighborhoods*,[55] a remarkably cogent review of advances in child development science, the rapidly emerging biological insights into the determinants of developmental and behavioral outcomes have yet to generate a clear message that is accessible to wide public understanding. It will be the task of the now broad array of professional disciplines concerned with child development to create the policy-based strategies and services that are not only increasingly effective but also ultimately reach all children in need.

DEVELOPMENTAL AND BEHAVIORAL PEDIATRICS TIMELINE

1838: First U.S. kindergarten established in Columbus, Ohio

1880: American Medical Association establishes Section on Diseases of Children

1888: American Pediatric Society founded

1889: Hull House founded

1909: First White House Conference on Children
First American Medical Association conference on infant mortality
American Association for the Study and Prevention of Infant Mortality founded

1912: Foundation of the U.S. Children's Bureau

1915: Perkin's Law passed: federal government funds programs that provide services to crippled children

1916: Keating-Owen Child Labor Act passed

1917: Healy established Child Guidance Clinics in Boston

1919: The American Association for the Study and Prevention of Infant Mortality becomes the American Child Hygiene Association and later (in 1923 under President Herbert Hoover) becomes the American Child Health Association

1921: Sheppard-Towner Maternity and Infancy Act passed

1924: American Orthopsychiatric Association established

1925: Society for Research in Child Development founded

1929: Sheppard-Towner Act repealed Children's Fund established in Michigan by Senator James Couzzens

1930: American Academy of Pediatrics founded the White House Conference on Child Health and Protection, which led to creation of the Children's Charter

1931: Department of Special Education established within U.S. Office of Education

1933: Roosevelt's Child Health Recovery Program implemented

1935: Social Security Act passed
  Title IV: Aid to Dependent Children
  Title V: Maternal and Child Welfare—The Crippled Children's Services Program
1938: Fair Labor Standards Act passed
  Milton J. E. Senn establishes Human Developmental residency program at New York Hospital
1943: Emergency Medical and Infant Care Program established
1946: National School Lunch Program established
1948: Senn develops child development training and research program at Yale Child Study Center
1954: Brown v. Board of Education
1961: Surgeon General establishes Center for Research in Child Health
1962: National Institute for Child Health and Human Development founded
1963: Community Mental Health and Mental Retardation Act
  Association for Children with Learning Disabilities holds first conference in Chicago
  Leadership in Neurodevelopmental Disabilities Training Program initiated (Maternal and Child Health Bureau)
1964: Economic Opportunity Act
  Civil Rights Act
1965: Medicaid program established
  Head Start established
  Maternal and Infant Care Programs established
  Community Health Centers established
  Division of Handicapped Children and Youth established within U.S. Office of Education
1966: International Smallpox Eradication Program established
1967: Bureau for Education of the Handicapped replaces Division of Handicapped Children and Youth in Office of Education
1969: Children with Specific Learning Disabilities Act passed (Public Law 91-230)
1971: Mondale-Brademas Child Development Bill (vetoed by President Richard S. Nixon)
1974: Sudden Infant Death Syndrome Act passed
1975: The Education for All Handicapped Children Act passed
  Child Support Enforcement Act passed
  National Joint Committee on Learning Disabilities formed
  Federal government establishes the Center for Research for Mothers and Children
1979: Healthy People, The Surgeon General's Report on Health Promotion and Disease Prevention of 1979, published

1980: Federal funds allotted to states to provide adoption assistance and foster care
1981: The Maternal and Child Health Services Block Grant established
1983: Public Law 98-199, federal commitment to educate handicapped pupils, passed
  International Health Efforts for Children Act passed
1984: Emergency Medical Services for Children program established
  1986 Behavioral Pediatrics Training Programs initiated (Maternal and Child Health Bureau)
1987: Omnibus Budget Reconciliation Act (Public Law 100-203)
1988: Federal support for child care
  Child Abuse Prevention, Adoption, and Family Services Act
  Hawkins-Stafford Elementary and Secondary School Improvements Amendments
1990: National Institutes of Health begins national program of Child Health Research Centers
1991: Healthy Start program established
1992: Back to Sleep campaign started
1993: Vaccines for Children program established
  National Institutes of Health Revitalization Act
1994: Medical Home Initiative implemented by the Maternal and Child Health Bureau
  Improving America's Schools Act
  Healthy Meals for Healthy Americans Act
1997: State Children's Health Insurance Program established
  Child Health Improvement Act
  Milk Matters campaign
  National Institute of Child Health and Human Development (NICHD) establishes the Network on the Neurobiology and Genetics of Autism
  Adoption and Safe Families Act
2000: Children's Health Act
  Developmental Disabilities Assistance and Bill of Rights Act
2001: Muscular Dystrophy Community Assistance, Research and Education Amendments
2002: United Nations Convention on the Rights of the Child
  U.S. Department of Education holds "Learning Disability Summit"
  No Child Left Behind Act
  The Best Pharmaceuticals for Children Act
2003: Pediatric Research Equity Act
2004: Individuals with Disabilities Education Act

REFERENCES

1. Richmond JB, Janis JM: Ripeness is all: The coming of age of behavioral pediatrics. *In* Levine M, Carey W, Crocker A, Gross T, eds: Develpmental-Behavioral Pediatrics. Philadelphia: WB Saunders, 1983, pp 15-23.

2. Haggerty RJ, Friedman SB: History of Developmental-Behavioral Pediatrics. Dev Behav Pediatr 24:S1-S18, 2003.

3. Smuts AB: Science in the Service of Children: 1893-1935. New Haven, CT: Yale University Press, 2006.

4. Pinker S: The Blank Slate. New York: Viking Press, 2002.

5. Mintz S: Huck's Raft: A History of American Childhood. Cambridge, MA: Belknap Press, 2004.

6. Aries P: Centuries of Childhood. New York: Vintage Press, 1962.

7. Hall GS: Aspects of Child Life and Education. Boston: Ginn & Company, 1907.

8. Dewey J: My pedagogic creed [originally published 1897]. *In* Hickman LA, Alexander TM eds: The Essential Dewey, vol 1. Bloomington: Indiana University Press, 1998.

9. Pifer E: Demon or Doll: Images of the Child in Contemporary Writing and Culture. Charlottesville: University of Virginia Press, 2000.

10. Richmond JB: The Hull House era. Vintage years for children. Am J Orthopsychiatry 65:10-20, 1995.

11. Skocpol T: Protecting Soldiers and Mothers: The Political Origins of Social Policy in United States. Cambridge, MA: Belknap, 1995.

12. "A bill to establish a children's bureau in the Department of Commerce and Labor:" U.S. Statutes, 62nd Congress, 1911, second session, Pt 1, 73:79-80, 1912.

13. Lesser AJ: The origin and development of maternal and child health programs in the United States. Am J Public Health 75:590-598, 1985.

14. Parker J, Carpenter D: Julia Lathrop and the Children's Bureau: The emergence of an institution. Soc Serv Rev 55:60-77, 1981.

15. Bradbury D: Five Decades of Action for Children. Washington, DC: U.S. Department of Health, Education and Welfare, Children's Bureau, 1962.

16. Gesell A: The Mental Growth of the Preschool Child. New York: Macmillan, 1925.

17. Gesell A: Infancy and Human Growth. New York: Macmillan, 1929.

18. Lilienfeld AM, Parkhurst E: A study of the association of factors of pregnancy and parturition with the development of cerebral palsy: A preliminary report. Am J Hygiene 53:262-282, 1951.

19. Lilienfeld AM, Pasamanick B: Association of maternal and fetal factors with the development of epilepsy, I: Abnormalities in the prenatal and paranatal periods. JAMA 155:719-724, 1954.

20. Knobloch H, Rider R, Harper P, et al: Neuropsychiatric sequelae of prematurity: A longitudinal study. JAMA 161:581-585, 1956.

21. Watson JB: Behaviorism [originally published 1924]. New Brunswick, NJ: Transaction, 1998.

22. Erikson EH: Childhood and Society. New York: WW Norton, 1950.

23. Shonkoff JP, Meisels SJ: Early childhood intervention: The evolution of a concept. *In* Meisels SJ, Shonkoff JP, eds: Handbook of Early Childhood Intervention. Cambridge, UK: Cambridge University Press, 1998.

24. Spitz RA: Hospitalism: An inquiry into the genesis of psychiatric conditions in early childhood. *In* Eisler RS, ed: Psychoanalytic Study of the Child. New Haven: Yale University Press, 1945.

25. Bowlby J: Maternal Care and Mental Health. Geneva: World Health Organization, 1951.

26. Bowlby J: Attachment and Loss, vol 1. New York: Basic Books, 1969.

27. Ainsworth MDS: Object relations dependency and attachment: A theoretical review of the mother-infant relationship. Child Dev 40:969-1025, 1969.

28. Branch T: Pillar of Fire: America in the King Years 1963-65. New York: Simon & Schuster, 1999.

29. Harrington M: The Other America. New York: Simon & Schuster, 1963.

30. Graham FK, Ernhart CB, Thurston DL, et al: Development three years after perinatal anoxia and other potentially damaging newborn experiences. Psychol Monogr 76:522, 1962.

31. Fishler K, Graliker BV, Koch R: The predictability of intelligence with Gesell developmental scales in mentally retarded infants and young children. Am J Ment Defic 69:515-525, 1964.

32. Piaget J: The Origin of Intelligence in Children. New York: International University Press, 1952.

33. Kirk SA: Early education of the mentally retarded. Urbana, IL: University of Illinois Press, 1958.

34. Skeels HM: Adult status of children with contrasting early life experiences. Monogr Soc Res Child Dev 31: 1-65, 1966.

35. Hunt JM: Intelligence and Experience. New York: Ronald Press, 1961.

36. Bloom BS: Stability and Change in Human Characteristics. New York: Wiley, 1964.

37. Locke J: An Essay Concerning Human Understanding, Book II [originally published 1690]. New York: EP Dutton, 1947.

38. Rousseau J-J: Discourse upon the Origin and Foundation of Inequality among Mankind [originally published 1755]. New York: Oxford University Press, 1994, pp 61-2.

39. Kennedy JF: Special message to the Congress on Mental Illness and Mental Retardation [originally presented February 5, 1963]. *In* Bremner RH, ed: Children and Youth in America: A Documentary History. Cambridge, MA: Harvard University Press, 1974, pp 1544-1550.

40. U.S. President's Panel on Mental Retardation: A proposed program for national action to combat mental retardation [originally published 1962]. *In* Bremner RH, ed: Children and Youth in America: A Documentary History. Cambridge, MA: Harvard University Press, 1974, pp 1536-1544.

41. Richmond JB, Janis JM: Ripeness is all: The coming of age of behavioral pediatrics. *In* Levine M, Carey W,

Crocker A, et al, eds: Developmental-Behavioral Pediatrics. Philadelphia: WB Saunders, 1983, pp 15-23.

42. Zigler E, Valentine J, eds: Project Head Start: A Legacy of the War on Poverty. New York: Free Press, 1979.

43. Gliedman J, Roth W: The Unexpected Minority: Handicapped Children in America. New York: Harcourt Brace Jovanovich, 1980.

44. Martin EW, Martine R, Terman DL: The legislative and litigation history of special education. Future Child 6:25-39, 1996.

45. Wise PH: The transformation of child health in the United States. Health Aff 23:9-25, 2004.

46. Haggerty RJ, Friedman SB: History of developmental-behavioral pediatrics. Dev Behav Pediatr 24:S1-S18, 2003.

47. Americans with Disabilities Act of 1990, Public Law 101-336, S.933.

48. Rutter M: Nature, nurture, and development: From evangelism through science toward policy and practice. Child Dev 73:1-21, 2002.

49. Moffit TE, Caspi A, Rutter M: Strategy for investigating interactions between measured genes and measured environments. Arch Gen Psychiatry 62:473-481, 2005.

50. Cushing BS, Kramer KM: Mechanisms underlying epigenetic effects of early social experience: The role of neuropeptides and steroids. Neurosci Biobehav Rev 29:1089-1105, 2005.

51. Sameroff AJ, Chandler MJ: Reproductive risk and the continuum of caretaking casualty. *In* Horowitz FD, Hetherington M, Scarr-Salapatek S, et al, eds: Review of Child Development Research, vol 4. Chicago: University of Chicago Press, 1975, pp 187-244.

52. Bronfenbrenner U: The Ecology of Human Development. Cambridge, MA: Harvard University Press, 1979.

53. Nelson CA, Bloom FE: Child development and neuroscience. Child Dev 68:970-987, 1997.

54. Garcia Coll C, Magnuson K: Cultural differences as sources of developmental vulnerabilities and resources. *In* Shonkoff JP, Meisels SJ, eds: Handbook of Early Childhood Intervention. Washington, DC: National Academies Press, 2000, pp 94-114.

55. Shonkoff JP, Phillips DA: From Neurons to Neighborhoods. Washington, DC: National Academies Press, 2000.

56. National Center for Health Statistics: National Health Interview Survey, Various years, 1962, 1972, 1982 and 2001.

57. Schor EL: Rethinking well-child care. Pediatrics 114:210-216, 2004.

Theoretical Foundations of Developmental-Behavioral Pediatrics

GRAYSON N. HOLMBECK ■ BARBARA JANDASEK ■ CAITLIN SPARKS ■
JILL ZUKERMAN ■ LAUREN ZURENDA*

What is the role of "theory" in the field of developmental-behavioral pediatrics? To answer this question, it is useful to imagine how clinical work and research endeavors would be affected if there were no theoretical or conceptual models to explain observed phenomena in practice or in research. Without conceptual models, *practitioners* would have no basis for suggesting specific interventions or understanding why some interventions are successful and why others fail. More to the point, practitioners would not be able to explain to families why certain recommendations are indicated or why the suggested interventions are likely to be helpful. In discussing nonadherence to treatments for chronic illness, Riekert and Drotar[1] argued that conceptual models serve several purposes for the practitioner. Specifically, these models (1) guide the practitioner in the information gathering process, (2) guide communications between patients and practitioners, (3) aid the practitioner in determining the goals and targets of interventions, and (4) help the practitioner anticipate potential barriers to treatment success.

In the absence of theory, pediatricians may be inclined to develop new interventions for each specific physical condition and may assume that mechanisms that underlie certain difficulties are unique for each illness group. For example, without a general guiding theory, medical adherence issues for asthma may be treated entirely differently from medical adherence issues for type 1 diabetes. Alternatively, available developmentally oriented, family-based theories of medical adherence would indicate that similar processes underlie medical adherence across populations and that an intervention that works well for one illness may also work well for a different population. For example, on the basis of theory, a developmental-behavioral pediatrician may suggest that families make developmentally gauged changes in how responsibilities for adherence to aspects of the medical regimen are shared between parent and child, particularly as the child begins to transition into early adolescence.[2]

With theoretical frameworks, *researchers* would be more able to generate testable hypotheses or determine which variables are critical and should be examined in the context of their research programs. Indeed, a conceptual model facilitates the development of a program of research (as opposed to a set of unrelated studies), and it drives all aspects of the research endeavor, including participant selection, the design of the study, specification of independent and dependent variables, specification of relationships between variables, data-analytic strategies, and potential recommendations for clinical practice.[1,3]

The goal of this chapter is to demonstrate the importance of theory development and the role of conceptual models in the field of developmental-behavioral pediatrics. Throughout, we take the "developmental" aspect of developmental-behavioral pediatrics very seriously. Indeed, an exciting but also challenging aspect of studying and providing clinical services to children is that they are developmental "moving targets." Moreover, the course of developmental change varies across individuals, so that two children who are the same age may differ dramatically with regard to neurological, physical, cognitive, emotional, and social functioning.[4] For example, two

*All authors after the first are listed in alphabetical order by last name; the contributions of these authors were similar. Completion of this manuscript was supported by research grants from the National Institute of Child Health and Human Development (R01-HD048629) and the March of Dimes Birth Defects Foundation (12-FY04-47). All correspondence should be sent to: Grayson N. Holmbeck, Loyola University at Chicago, Department of Psychology, 6525 N. Sheridan Road, Chicago, IL 60626 (gholmbe@luc.edu).

12-year-old boys may differ dramatically with regard to pubertal status, one boy being prepubertal and the other experiencing the latter stages of pubertal development; such interindividual differences have significant effects on their physical and social functioning. Similarly, consider two 9-year-old girls, one of whom is functioning at a lower level of cognitive ability. The child with more cognitive impairment may misinterpret social cues from her peers and fail to express her emotions verbally, which results in aggression with peers. The other 9-year-old child may respond to challenging social situations by questioning her peer and verbally expressing her feelings in a socially appropriate manner. It is also the case that the same behaviors that are developmentally normative at a younger age are often developmentally atypical at a later age.[5] For example, temper tantrums may be an expected outcome when a young child lacks the language abilities to express his or her frustration. In older children, and after language skills develop, tantrums are expected to be less likely. Frequent tantrums in an older child would be considered atypical.

In attempting to understand better such developmental variation and change, theories have been advanced to explain both the general rules of development, as well as individual variation.[6] In general, developmental-behavioral pediatricians may have the opportunity to educate primary care pediatricians, who would benefit greatly from attention to and extensive knowledge of the theory and research focused on these developmental issues. In their work, developmental-behavioral pediatricians have opportunities to observe the same children frequently and repeatedly over the course of individual development. Thus, if pediatricians are equipped with the proper knowledge, they are in a unique position to identify early risk factors that portend later, more serious difficulties. Moreover, they can intervene early while the difficulties are still manageable. They also have opportunities to follow up with these same children to determine whether a particular early intervention had a sustained and positive impact.

Since the appearance of a similar volume on developmental-behavioral pediatrics in the late 1990s,[7] the field of developmental-behavioral pediatrics has witnessed extensive progress in theory development across several areas (e.g., biological bases of behavior, behavioral genetics and gene-environment interactions, developmental psychopathology). Concurrent with these developments, both the quantity and quality of research focused on such issues have increased as well. The purpose of this chapter is to review current theories relevant to the field of developmental-behavioral pediatrics. We begin with a discussion of "What makes a good theory?" in which we discuss features of theories that have had a major influence on the field. Second, we provide an historical perspective on theories in the field of developmental-behavioral pediatrics, followed by a discussion of more contemporary theoretical and empirical work. Finally, we conclude with a discussion of directions for future theory development.

WHAT MAKES A GOOD THEORY?

Influential theories in the field of developmental-behavioral pediatrics tend to share many features: (1) a clarity of focus; (2) a developmental emphasis; (3) the ability to address limitations of previous research; (4) specifications of predictors (i.e., independent variables) and outcomes (i.e., dependent variables), with a clear rationale for each; (5) a clear articulation of links between predictors and outcomes (that sometimes involves specification of mediational and moderational effects) with accompanying testable hypotheses; and (6) clear implications for interventions. We review these features in turn in this section.

Before a discussion of components of useful theories, it is important to define our use of the term *theory* and to note similarities between our use of this term and other related terms, such as *framework* and *model*. A strict (but also ideal) definition of theory is as follows:[8-10] "[A theory is] a set of interconnected statements-definitions, axioms, postulates, hypothetical constructs, intervening variables, laws, hypotheses ... usually expressed in verbal or mathematical terms .... [The theory] should be internally consistent ... testable and parsimonious ... [and] not contradicted by scientific observations" (Miller, 1983, pp 3-4).[11] In general, most scientific theories fall short of this ideal definition. For this book, we have chosen a "soft" definition of *theory*. In our view, a theory is a model or framework that guides clinical work or research endeavors. It could be considered a metaphor for how two or more variables are related or how a causal process is likely to unfold over time (e.g., a camera is a metaphor for how the human eye functions; such a metaphor could serve as a guide for future investigations of the eye). Despite their limitations, "soft" theories provide more guidance than if there were no theories. In the absence of theory, physicians would be forced to rely on past experience and common sense. However, as noted by Lilienfeld, the more widely held the belief is and the more that a belief is based on common sense (e.g., parents have more influence on children than children have on parents), the more crucial it is that such beliefs be carefully scrutinized and subjected to empirical evaluation.[12]

Clarity of Focus

Useful conceptual models are often focused on a phenomenon that is important to professionals working in the field and are very specific in their focus, rather than overly general. For example, suppose an investigator wanted to develop a model of communication between practitioner and patient. It would be tempting to include all possible variables in this model. With regard to the patient, the investigator could include variables such as past medical experiences, type of condition, temperament, communication style variables, personality variables, historical and family system variables, and variables that focus on beliefs and expectations. With regard to the practitioner, the investigator could include a similar number of variables. Although all of these variables may be relevant to the phenomenon of interest, inclusion of all relevant variables would make for a very unwieldy conceptual model. From the perspective of a practitioner, there would be too many variables to integrate, making it difficult to consider any one of them during an actual interaction with a patient. From a research perspective, the model would likely be highly exploratory and require "everything but the kitchen sink" data-analytic strategies. Findings based on such strategies would not necessarily be validated across research programs. Thus, a more focused model would be needed. Such a model would explain a smaller aspect of the phenomenon of interest, but it would probably have more clinical and research usefulness. Continuing with the example just given, the investigator might develop a model that proposes a typology of practitioner and patient communication styles that delineates the best fitting matches between different practitioner and patient communication styles.[1]

Developmental Emphasis

A developmental emphasis is crucial for the work of the developmental-behavioral pediatrician and should, therefore, be an integral part of any theoretical or conceptual model. At the most general level, a model is developmentally oriented if (1) it includes developmentally relevant constructs (which could be biological, cognitive, emotional, or social), (2) the constructs are tied to the age group under consideration, and (3) it emphasizes *changes* in the proposed constructs.[11] Such a model also takes into account the critical developmental tasks and milestones relevant to a particular child's or adolescent's presenting problems (e.g., level of self-control, ability to regulate emotions, the development of autonomy, a child's ability to share responsibilities for medical treatments with parents).

The Model Addresses Limitations of Previous Models and Research

A useful theory-driven model seeks to move the field forward by addressing gaps in prior theorizing.[3] The process by which conceptual models are derived is often a cumulative process by which older conceptual models are integrated with new empirical findings to generate new conceptual models. For example, Thompson and Gustafson reviewed prior models of psychological adaptation to chronic illness.[3] Older models[13] specified important constructs of interest (e.g., stress, coping style, response to illness), but later models[14,15] were more focused on identifying particular components of these constructs that were relevant (for an example involving palliative vs. adaptive coping and specific cognitive processes concerning illness appraisal and expectations, see Thompson and colleagues[15]). Later, these more focused models were refined in response to research findings and critiques[16] (see Wallander et al for revised versions of these models[17]).

Specification of Independent Variables and Dependent Variables

A conceptual model should not only be based on a clear articulation of the relevant constructs but should also include a clear rationale for each of these constructs. Within the context of research, it is not enough to say "construct X is being examined in this study because it has never been studied in the context of this chronic physical condition." Indeed, "lack of study" is not an adequate rationale for the inclusion of a variable in a program of research. For example, the researcher might include a specific patient personality variable (e.g., neuroticism) in a study of adherence, stating that this personality variable has not received any attention in this literature. Instead, it is more useful if the researcher provides a theory-driven rationale for why this variable is likely to be linked with adherence and how investigators might take this variable into account when conducting an adherence intervention.

Conceptual models rarely account completely for a medical phenomenon; thus, there is usually variance in the outcome that the predictors do not adequately explain. For example, in attempting to understand causes of spina bifida (a congenital birth defect that produces profound effects on neurological, orthopedic, urinary, cognitive/academic, and social functioning), investigators have recently determined that low levels of maternal folic acid before conception are causally related to the occurrence of spina bifida. Unfortunately, this single variable does not account for all cases of spina bifida. Thus, comprehensive models of causation for this condition often include other variables as well, including genetic and behavioral factors.

Articulation of Links between Independent Variables and Dependent Variables

Perhaps the most important aspect of a conceptual model is the articulation of links between the predictors and outcomes. Models vary considerably in their levels of sophistication; at the simplest level, main (or direct) effects of predictor on outcome (e.g., parenting behaviors → child adjustment) are proposed. As the number of predictors increases, scholars often seek to test multiple pathways between predictors and outcomes. Researchers who study pediatric populations have begun to posit more complex theoretical models to explain phenomena of interest. These models include longitudinal developmental pathways, mediational and moderational effects, genetic × environment interaction effects, risk and protective processes, and intervening cognitive variables (e.g., cognitive appraisal[3]). This enhancement of the theoretical base has necessitated an increase in terminological and data-analytic sophistication. Research focused on mediational and moderational models (and particularly the definitions of risk and protective factors) has emerged as a crucial method for testing competing theories about developmental pathways and other concepts central to developmental-behavioral pediatrics (see Rose et al for a more in-depth discussion[18]).

MEDIATOR

A *mediator* is an explanatory link in the relationship between two other variables (Fig. 2-1). Often a mediator variable is conceptualized as the mechanism through which one variable (i.e., the predictor) influences another variable (i.e., the criterion).[17,19,20] Suppose, hypothetically, that a researcher finds that parental intrusive behavior is negatively associated with child adherence to a medical regimen. Given these findings, a researcher could explore whether a third variable (e.g., child independence) might account for or explain the relationship between these variables. Continuing with the example, suppose that child independence mediates the relationship between intrusiveness and adherence (more intrusive parenting → less child independence → less medical adherence). In this case, parental intrusiveness would have a negative effect on level of child independence, which in turn would contribute to poor medical adherence.[21]

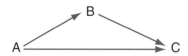

FIGURE 2-1 Mediated relationship among variables. A, Predictor; B, mediator; C, criterion/outcome. (From Rose BM, Holmbeck GN, Coakley RM, et al: Mediator and moderator effects in developmental and behavioral pediatric research. J Dev Behav Pediatr 25:1-10, 2004. Copyright 2004 by Lippincott Williams & Wilkins. Reprinted with permission.)

MODERATOR

A *moderator,* unlike a mediator, is a variable that influences the strength or the direction of a relationship between a predictor variable and a criterion variable (Fig. 2-2). Suppose a researcher is interested in examining whether familial stress (e.g., in the context of a child's chronic illness) is associated with the child's psychological adjustment and, more specifically, whether this effect becomes more or less robust in the presence of other contextual variables. For example, the strength or the direction of the relationship between stress and adjustment may depend on the level of uncertainty that characterizes the child's condition; that is, a significant association between stress and adjustment may emerge *only* when there is considerable uncertainty regarding the child's illness status. By testing "level of uncertainty" as a moderator of the relationship between stress and outcome, the researcher can specify certain conditions under which family stress is predictive of the child's adjustment.

Developmental-behavioral pediatric researchers often posit mediational and moderational processes when conducting studies of risk and protective factors. In general, research on risk and protective factors is focused on understanding the adjustment of children who are exposed to varying levels of adversity. There is evidence that both contextual factors (e.g., socioeconomic status, family level functioning, peer relationships) and developmental variables (e.g., cognitive skills, autonomy development) can significantly influence outcomes for individuals living under adverse conditions and thus serve a moderational role.[21-24] Risk and protective processes have been explored in the study of "resilience," a term used with increasing frequency in developmental and pediatric research

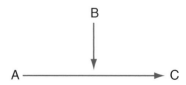

FIGURE 2-2 Moderated relationship among variables. A, Predictor; B, moderator; C, criterion/outcome. (From Rose BM, Holmbeck GN, Coakley RM, et al: Mediator and moderator effects in developmental and behavioral pediatric research. J Dev Behav Pediatr 25:1-10, 2004. Copyright 2004 by Lippincott Williams & Wilkins. Reprinted with permission.)

(see later section on resilience). *Resilience* refers to the process by which children successfully navigate stressful situations or adversity and attain developmentally relevant competencies.[25] More generally, appropriate application of these terms (i.e., *resilience, risk factors, protective factors*) is necessary for promoting terminological consistency.

PROTECTIVE VERSUS RESOURCE FACTORS

A protective factor either ameliorates negative outcomes or promotes adaptive functioning. To isolate a true "protective factor," however, there must be a particular stressor that influences the sample under investigation. The protective factor serves its protective role *only* in the context of adversity; a protective factor does not operate in low-adversity conditions.

Protective factors are contrasted with resource factors. Specifically, a factor that has a positive effect on the sample regardless of the presence or absence of a stressor is a *resource factor*[24] (sometimes referred to as a *promotive factor*[26]). For example, if a positive father-child relationship reduces behavior problems only in children of depressed mothers but has no effect on children of nondepressed mothers, then the father-child relationship would be conceptualized as a *protective factor* (Fig. 2-3).[18] However, if the positive father-child relationship reduces behavior problems in all children, regardless of the mother's level of depression, then it would be conceptualized as a *resource factor* (see Fig. 2-3).[18,24] A model may also identify a positive father-child relationship as both a protective and resource factor if it reduces behavior problems in children who have depressed mothers *more* than in children who have nondepressed mothers but if it also produces a significant reduction in behavior problems for all children, regardless of level of maternal depression. It is also important to note that a protective factor represents a moderational effect (see the statistically significant interaction effect in Fig. 2-3, *left*), whereas a resource factor represents an additive effect (i.e., two main effects; see Fig. 2-3, *right*).[18]

RISK VERSUS VULNERABILITY FACTORS

Risk and vulnerability factors operate in much the same way as resource and protective factors but in the opposite direction (Fig. 2-4).[18] A *vulnerability factor* is a moderator that increases the chances for maladaptive outcomes in the presence of adversity.[24] Like a protective factor, a vulnerability factor operates only in the context of adversity. In contrast, a variable that negatively influences outcome regardless of the presence or absence of adversity is a *risk factor.*[24] For example, witnessing violence in the home environment is conceptualized as a vulnerability factor if it increases behavior problems only in children who are also exposed to a stressor, such as viewing extreme violence on television (see Fig. 2-4, *left*).[18] A vulnerability factor is a moderator and is demonstrated statistically with a significant interaction effect. Witnessing violence in the home can be conceptualized as a risk factor if it results in an increase in child behavior problems for all children, regardless of the amount of television violence witnessed. As with resource factors, a risk factor represents an additive effect (i.e., two main effects; see Fig. 2-4, *right*).[18] A model may also identify a factor as being both a risk and vulnerability factor if it increases the chance of a maladaptive outcome in samples with and without

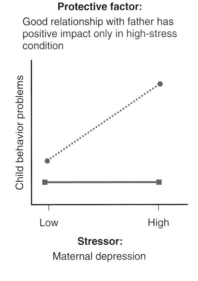

FIGURE 2-3 Protective factors (***left***) **and resource factors** (***right***). (From Rose BM, Holmbeck GN, Coakley RM, et al: Mediator and moderator effects in developmental and behavioral pediatric research. J Dev Behav Pediatr 25:1-10, 2004. Copyright 2004 by Lippincott Williams & Wilkins. Reprinted with permission.)

Protective factor:
Good relationship with father has positive impact only in high-stress condition

Resource factor:
Good relationship with father has positive impact in both low- and high-stress conditions

Child behavior problems

Stressor: Maternal depression

Stressor: Maternal depression

●•••••••••● Poor relationship with father   ■━━━━━━■ Good relationship with father

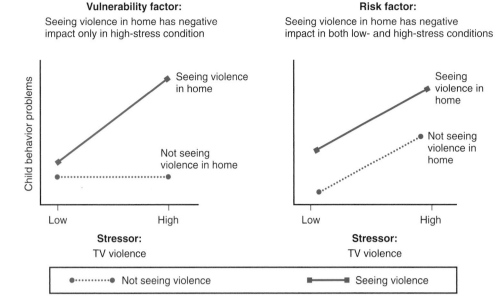

FIGURE 2-4 Vulnerability factors (*left*) and risk factors (*right*). (From Rose BM, Holmbeck GN, Coakley RM, et al: Mediator and moderator effects in developmental and behavioral pediatric research. J Dev Behav Pediatr 25: 1-10, 2004. Copyright 2004 by Lippincott Williams & Wilkins. Reprinted with permission.)

exposure to a stressor but also if it increases the chances for maladaptive functioning significantly more in the sample with the stressor.

In sum, if a factor significantly promotes or impairs the chances of attaining adaptive outcomes in the presence of a stressor, then it operates through protective or vulnerability mechanisms, respectively. In these cases, the factor serves a moderational role. However, if a factor significantly promotes or impairs the chance of attaining adaptive outcomes without differentiating between the presence or absence of a stressor, then it is conceptualized as operating through resource or risk mechanisms, respectively. Many examples of these types of effects have appeared in the literature. For example, in their study of maltreatment and adolescent behavior problems, McGee and associates found that the association between severity of physical abuse and internalizing symptoms was moderated by gender.[27] Specifically, the association was positive and significant for girls but not for boys. In other words, being male could be considered a protective factor against the development of internalizing symptoms when a person is exposed to high levels of physical abuse. Similarly, Gorman-Smith and Tolan found that associations between exposure to violence and anxiety/depression symptoms in young adolescents were moderated by level of family cohesion.[28] The effect was significant (and positive) only at low levels of cohesion. At high levels of cohesion, the effect was nonsignificant, which suggests that family cohesion buffers (or protects against) the negative effects of exposure to violence on adolescent mental health.

Some investigators have sought to examine risk factors as mediational causal chains over time. For

example, Tolan and colleagues examined a causal chain as a predictor of violent behaviors in adolescence, which included the following variables (in temporal order): community structure characteristics, neighborliness, parenting practices, gang membership, and peer violence.[29] Woodward and Fergusson examined predictors of increased rates of teen pregnancy and found a causal chain that began with early conduct problems; such problems were associated with subsequent risk-taking behaviors in adolescence, which placed girls at risk for teen pregnancy.[30]

In summary, we have attempted to demonstrate how the use of mediational and moderational models can lead to a deeper and more comprehensive knowledge about the relationship between predictors and outcomes by providing information about the conditions under which two variables are associated (moderation) and also about intervening processes that help to explain their association (mediation). At the most complex level, researchers can test competing theories about relationships among variables of interest. By directly comparing the utility of two or more alternative models, a researcher can determine which theoretical model best captures or explains an observed relationship among variables.

Clear Implications for Interventions

Perhaps, of most importance, a theory should have clear implications for interventions. Although many variables have potential intervention implications, some are clearly more relevant to practice than are others. For example, suppose a researcher is examining predictors of medical adherence during adolescence in children with type 1 diabetes. The researcher could examine parent and child adherence-relevant problem-solving ability as a predictor of subsequent levels of adherence, or the researcher could examine adolescent personality variables (e.g., neuroticism) as predictors of adherence. Clearly, it would be easier to imagine developing an intervention that targets problem-solving ability than one that targets a personality variable. Moreover, the researcher would speculate that problem-solving ability is also more likely to be responsive to an intervention than is a personality variable. Interestingly, some variables may not appear to be intervention-relevant at first glance but may become so on further examination. For example, demographic variables (e.g., gender, social class) would obviously not be targets of an intervention, but they may be important markers for risk. For example, the researcher may find that individuals from the lower end of the socioeconomic distribution are at increased risk for medical adherence difficulties; thus, this subpopulation could be targeted as an at-risk group and receive a more intense intervention.

Not only do predictor-outcome studies have implications for intervention work but also intervention studies themselves can be very instructive. Specifically, a research design that includes random assignment to intervention condition provides a particularly powerful design for drawing conclusions about causal mediational relationships.[31,32] These types of models have three important strengths. First, significant mediational models of intervention effects provide information about mechanisms through which treatments have their effects.[33-35] Simply put, with such models, researchers are able to ask how and why an intervention works.[33] Second, as noted by Collins and associates, if a manipulated variable (i.e., the randomly assigned intervention) is associated with change in the mediator, which is in turn associated with change in the outcome, there is significant support for the hypothesis that the mediator is a *causal* mechanism.[36] Researchers are more justified in invoking causal language when examining mediational models in which the predictor is manipulated (i.e., random assignment to intervention vs. no intervention) than in mediational models in which no variables are directly manipulated. With random assignment, many alternative interpretations for a researcher's findings can be ruled out, and thus it is more certain that changes in the outcomes (e.g., symptoms of attention-deficit/hyperactivity disorder [ADHD]) result from the intervention instead of from some other factor.

Third, when a researcher isolates a significant mediational process, the researcher has learned that the mediator may play a role in the maintenance of the outcome (e.g., problem behavior). In this way,

knowledge about mediational processes in the context of randomized clinical trials informs investigators about etiological theories of disorders.[33,37] As an example of this strategy, Forgatch and DeGarmo examined the effectiveness of a parenting-training program for a large sample of divorcing mothers with sons.[38] They also examined several parenting practices as mediators of the intervention → child outcome association. In comparison with mothers in the control sample, mothers in the intervention sample showed improvements in parenting practices. Improvements in parenting practices were linked with improvements in child adjustment. Thus, this study provides important evidence that certain types of maladaptive parenting behavior *maintain* certain maladaptive child outcomes.

Such intervention/mediation models not only allow researchers to test potential mediators within an experimental design but also allow researchers to examine the differential utility of several mediational variables. In other words, a researcher can determine which mediator best accounts for the effectiveness of a given treatment. For example, if researchers examined the effectiveness of parenting training for decreasing child behavior problems (as in the preceding example), they might target three areas of parenting with this intervention: parental consistency, positive parenting, and harsh/punitive parenting. By testing mediational models within the context of an intervention study, they could determine which of these three parenting targets accounts for the significant intervention effect. It may be, for example, that the intervention's effect on parental consistency is the mechanism through which the treatment has an effect on child outcome. This component of the treatment could then be emphasized and enhanced in future versions of the intervention (Fig. 2-5).[18]

Finally, how do investigators determine what variables are most intervention relevant? A useful place to start would be to consult with practicing developmental-behavioral pediatricians to gather information on their perceptions of major issues related to potential interventions. For example, practitioners are uniquely able to identify child- and family-related barriers that prevent satisfactory adherence to medical regimens. In addition, focus groups composed of patients and family members can help identify areas worthy of research that may not be apparent to the pediatrician. For example, certain struggles or conflicts surrounding adherence may occur in the family's home and may not be observable by or reported to the pediatrician. Such barriers could then be the targets of both basic and applied research that could be maximally informative to developmental-behavioral pediatricians.

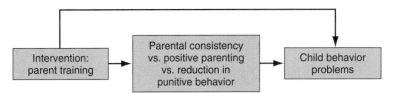

FIGURE 2-5 Mediators in intervention research. Parenting behaviors as mediators of the relationship between parent training (intervention) and child behavior (outcome). (From Rose BM, Holmbeck GN, Coakley RM, et al: Mediator and moderator effects in developmental and behavioral pediatric research. J Dev Behav Pediatr 25:1-10, 2004. Copyright 2004 by Lippincott Williams & Wilkins. Reprinted with permission.)

This overview of features shared by the most influential theories provides the basis for a focused review of theories relevant to the field of developmental-behavioral pediatrics.

THEORETICAL MODELS IN DEVELOPMENTAL-BEHAVIORAL PEDIATRICS

It would, of course, be impossible to provide an overview of all relevant theories in the field of developmental-behavioral pediatrics. Thus, we have chosen theories from five areas that are of primary concern to developmental-behavioral pediatricians: (1) theories that take into account biological, genetic, and neurological bases for behavior; (2) transactional models of development; (3) theoretical principles from the field of developmental psychopathology (a relatively new discipline through which investigators seek to understand how problem behaviors develop and are maintained across the lifespan); (4) theories of adjustment to chronic illness; and (5) models relevant to medical adherence. Some important models are not covered because they are highlighted in other chapters in this volume (e.g., for a review of family systems theory and models of cultural influence, see Chapter 5).

A Brief Historical Perspective on Child Development

Modern theories of developmental-behavioral pediatrics have their roots in early theories of child development. The purpose of this section is to trace the history of some of the important constructs that are now taken for granted in more recent theorizing. In an earlier review for a volume on developmental-behavioral pediatrics, Kessen provided a comprehensive overview of past theories and research on human behavioral development (beginning with work conducted as early as 1850).[6] Moreover, in the four-volume fifth edition of the *Handbook of Child Psychology,*

an entire volume (more than 1200 pages) is devoted to "theoretical models of human development." Thus, a complete overview of this area is well beyond the scope of this chapter.

The study of human development is a field devoted to identifying and explaining changes in behavior, abilities, and attributes that individuals experience throughout their lives. Because infants and young children change so dramatically over a relatively short time, they received intense empirical scrutiny in past research. However, in more recent years, research has been focused on developmental issues of relevance over the entire lifespan.[39] Although the field of developmental psychology has undergone many changes since its advent in the late 1800s, several themes have been revisited throughout the past century.[40] These include (1) the nature/nurture issue (i.e., what is the relative importance of biological and environmental factors in human development?), (2) the active/passive issue (i.e., are children active contributors to their own development, or are they passive objects, acted on by the environment?), and (3) the continuous/discontinuous issue (i.e., are developmental changes better seen as discontinuous or continuous?).[6,41] These themes emerge throughout the following discussion of some of the most influential early theorists.

Charles Darwin's *A Biological Sketch of an Infant* was the most influential of the "baby biographies" and is often cited as the impetus for the child study movement.[42] His theory of evolution could be considered the underlying theoretical force behind the entire discipline of developmental psychology, and its influence continues to inspire present-day thought in the field. For example, Boyce and Ellis's theory of biological stress reactivity (as discussed in a later section) is one example of a modern idea that is largely inspired by evolutionary theory.[43] However, before Boyce and Ellis's notion of biological stress reactivity, Darwinian theory influenced many other notable contributors, including one who would come to be known as the founder of American developmental psychology: G. Stanley Hall (1844-1924). Hall believed that human development follows a course similar to that of the evolution of the species.[44,45] He acknowledged the scientific shortcomings of the baby biographies (which were based on potentially biased observations of small numbers of children) and attempted to collect more objective data on larger samples. In 1891, he began a program of questionnaire studies at Clark University in what is often considered the first large-scale scientific investigation of developing youth. Although research has since cast doubt on his "storm and stress model" as described in *Adolescence,* Hall was instrumental in bringing recognition to this period as a distinct and defining time of growth and transition.[44]

Hall is also recognized for his role as a mentor and administrator. In 1909, he invited Sigmund Freud (1856-1939) to Clark University, thereby generating international recognition for psychoanalytic theory. Originally trained as a neurologist, Freud observed that many of the physical symptoms seen in his patients appeared to be emotional in origin.[46] Through a methodology much different from that employed by Hall, Freud used *free association, dream interpretation,* and *hypnosis* to analyze the histories of his emotionally disturbed adult patients. On the basis of his analyses, Freud proposed that development occurs through the resolution of conflict between what a person *wants* to do versus what the person *should* do. He suggested that everyone has basic biological impulses that must be indulged but that society dictates the restraint of these impulses. This notion formed the basis of Freud's theory of psychosexual development. Although many of Freud's ideas have not been supported by empirical evidence, no one would refute that his contributions changed clinicians' thinking within the field. For instance, he was the first to popularize the notion that childhood experiences affect adult lives, as well as the first to introduce the idea of a subconscious motivation. In addition, Freud advanced the field by addressing the emotional side of human experience, which previous theorists had neglected.[46]

Freud was also the first prominent theorist to endorse an interactionist perspective, which acknowledged both biological and environmental factors that influence human development (although he emphasized the impact of environmental factors, such as parenting). Insofar as most theorists today consider both genetic and environmental factors that contribute to a person's development (e.g., diathesis-stress model of psychopathology), Freud's influence continues. In contrast to Freud's interactionist viewpoint, the *maturational theory* of Arnold Gesell (1880-1961) represents a prominent biological theory of child development.[47] In Gesell's view, development is a naturally unfolding progression that occurs according to some internal biological timetable, and learning and teaching cannot override this timetable.[48] He maintained that children are "self-regulating" and

develop only as they are ready to do so. Gesell is noteworthy for the detailed studies of children's physical and behavioral changes that were carried out under his supervision throughout his tenure at the Yale Clinic of Child Development. The results of Gesell's observational studies revealed a high degree of uniformity in children's development. Although developmental milestones may not have occurred at the same age for all children, the pattern of development was largely uniform (e.g., children walk before they run and run before they skip). Gesell used his data to establish statistical norms to describe the usual order in which children display various early behaviors, as well as the age range within which each behavior normally appears. Interestingly, physicians still use updated versions of these norms as general guidelines for normative development. Gesell also made important contributions to methodology in the field of psychology. He was the first to capture children's observations on film, thereby preserving their behavior for later frame-by-frame study, and he also developed the first one-way viewing screens.

Although Gesell was influential in terms of his contributions to methodology and his establishment of developmental norms, his purely biological theory was deemed an oversimplification of the complex process of human development insofar as it neglected to account for the importance of children's experiences. However, his emphasis on similarities across children's development and his focus on patterns of behavior set the stage for Jean Piaget (1896-1980), who is often credited for having the greatest influence on present-day developmental psychology.[49] Unlike the theorists previously discussed, many of Piaget's general theoretical hypotheses are still widely accepted by developmental psychologists. One reason his theories are appealing is that they complement other theories well. For instance, more recent thinkers in developmental psychology combine aspects of Piagetian theory with information processing and contextualist perspectives to more thoroughly understand the process of cognitive development.

Piaget became interested in child cognitive development through the administration of intelligence tests. He was interested less in the answers that children provided to test questions than in the reasoning behind the answers they gave. He soon realized that the way children think is qualitatively different from how adults think. Piaget became immersed in the study of the nature of knowledge in young children, as well as how it changes as they grow older.[50-52] He termed this area of study *genetic epistemology.* Unlike Gesell's method, in which the researcher stood apart from his objects of study, Piaget developed a research technique known as the *clinical method.* This involved presenting children with various tasks and verbal problems that would tap into children's reasoning.

Although he would begin with a set of standardized questions, he would then probe children's responses with follow-up questions to reveal the reasoning behind their responses. According to Piaget's cognitive-developmental theory, children universally progress through a series of stages: the *sensorimotor stage* (birth to age 2 years), the *preoperational stage* (ages 2 to 7 years), the *concrete operational* stage (ages 7 to 11 years), and the *formal operational* stage (ages 11 years and beyond). Piaget's theory is extremely complex, and a discussion of the processes by which children progress from stage to stage is beyond the scope of this chapter.[50]

Perhaps his most important contribution to the field of developmental psychology is the emphasis that Piaget placed on the active role that children play in their own development. This contribution is particularly relevant to the more recent work in the area of behavioral genetics (see later section on behavioral genetics). Specifically, researchers who study gene-environment interactions consider the effect that children have in molding their own environments. In addition, researchers who study attachment styles have focused on the role that children play in eliciting various responses from their caregivers. In this way, children are seen not as passive objects to be acted on by their environments but as active participants who sculpt their environments.

Although Piaget's ideas about children are still widely accepted today, his theory has not gone without criticism. One major criticism of his theory concerns its lack of emphasis on cross-cultural factors that may play a role in development. Although Piaget acknowledged that culture may influence the *rate* of cognitive growth, he did not address ways in which culture can affect *how* children grow and develop. He is also criticized for overlooking the role of social interactions in cognitive development. This latter idea is the hallmark of Lev Vygotsky's (1896-1934) sociocultural perspective.[53,54] According to Vygotsky, cognitive development occurs when children take part in dialogs with skilled tutors (e.g., parents and teachers).[55] It is through the process of social interaction that children incorporate and internalize feedback from these skilled tutors. As social speech is translated into private speech and then inner speech, the culture's method of thinking is incorporated into the child's thought processes. Vygotsky is also noteworthy for his consideration of the way cognitive development varies across cultures. Unlike Piaget, who maintained that cognitive development is largely universal across cultures, Vygotsky argued that variability in cognitive development that reflects the child's cultural experiences should be expected. As such, Vygotsky played a role in the movement toward cross-cultural and contextually oriented studies in developmental psychology. His influence can also be seen in the more recent literature on child and adolescent development, in which various contexts (e.g., family, peers, school, work) are considered with regard to their unique influences on development.

Current Theories in Developmental-Behavioral Pediatrics

In this section, we provide a selective review of contemporary theories and models relevant to developmental-behavioral pediatrics across five areas: (1) biological, genetic, and neurological bases for behavior; (2) transactional models of development; (3) developmental psychopathology; (4) adjustment to chronic illness; and (5) medical adherence.

MODELS THAT FOCUS ON BIOLOGICAL, GENETIC, AND NEUROLOGICAL BASES FOR BEHAVIOR

Several models of child functioning that focus on biological, genetic, and neurological bases for behavior have been proposed. It is believed that biologically based vulnerabilities can account, at least in part, for the emergence of certain psychosocial difficulties (e.g., depression, anxiety). In this section, models in the areas of biological stress reactivity and behavioral genetics (including a discussion of shared and nonshared environmental effects) are emphasized. Neurodevelopmental factors relevant to developmental-behavioral pediatricians are discussed thoroughly in Chapter 4.

BIOLOGICAL STRESS REACTIVITY

Stress reactivity is an individual differences variable that refers to an individual's physical neuroendocrine response to stressful events and adversity.[43] Researchers measure such reactivity with a host of physiological assessment techniques, including measures of heart rate, blood pressure, salivary cortisol, and respiratory sinus arrhythmia. Early research and theorizing on stress reactivity suggested that heightened or prolonged reactivity in response to stressors is maladaptive and places the individual at risk for adjustment difficulties (including affective disorder, anxiety disorders, and externalizing symptoms) and medical illness (e.g., heart disease). On the other hand, such reactivity may be adaptive in the short term by preparing the individual to confront external threats. Moreover, when significant stressors occur early in an individual's life, such individuals appear to be at risk for heightened levels of stress reactivity.

In 2005, Boyce and Ellis proposed a complex and intriguing theory of biological stress reactivity.[43] On the basis of a comprehensive review of research findings (including anomalous findings) in this literature, they concluded that the relationship between reactivity and outcome is not so straightforward. Rather, they proposed, according to an evolutionary-developmental theory, that high reactivity can result from exposure to highly stressful environments *or* from exposure to highly supportive/protective environments. As in previous theorizing, they maintained that early exposure to highly stressful environments can cause heightened reactivity (such individuals are more prepared for future occurrences of highly stressful events). But they also proposed that environments with very low stress can also produce children with heightened reactivity because such reactivity levels enable such children to experience more completely the beneficial characteristics of a protective environment. They argued further that this curvilinear relationship between early stress and reactivity is a process that has evolved through natural selection and one that affords advantages to both of these highly reactive groups. They concluded, "Highly reactive children sustain disproportionate rates of morbidity when raised in adverse environments but *unusually low* (emphasis added) rates when raised in low-stress, highly supportive settings." Interestingly, in a empirical investigation that was a companion to their theoretical paper, Ellis and associates found support for many of their propositions.[56] Empirical support for this viewpoint has also emerged in studies of primates.[57]

Another intriguing theory of stress reactivity was proposed by Grossman and colleagues, who discussed longitudinal changes in stress reactivity in depressed individuals.[58] They argued that the interplay between stressful environmental events and genetic expression can produce "potentiated stress reactivity" over time.[58] They suggested that early stressful events may alter genetic expression, whereby depressive episodes are triggered by increasingly less intense environmental and psychological stressors over time. The term *kindling* is used to explain this process in which life experiences produce subtle changes in brain functioning, genetic expression, and stress reactivity. They also invoke Waddington's compelling concept of "canalization."[59] The argument here is that development progresses in a "canal" of normative development that increases in "depth" with age. Psychopathology (e.g., depression) is likely to result if the individual is pushed up the sides of the canal beyond a genetically determined threshold (i.e., the threshold is higher in the canal for some individuals than for other individuals). In typically developing individuals, and because of the increasing depth of the canal, early stressors are more likely to move the individual beyond the pathology threshold than are stressors that occur later in life. With regard to depres-

sion, a severe stressor early in childhood can produce a depressive episode. After recovery from this episode, the individual can experience a second episode (moving above the threshold in the canal) as a result of another, less intense stressor. Genetics may influence the severity of the stressor that is necessary for the initial episode and the pace at which the kindling process takes hold.[58] The following case example illustrates how such a process may unfold:

> When his parents divorced, 8-year-old Jonathan and his mother moved in with his grandmother. Around this time, he began exhibiting symptoms of depression. Jonathan's teachers reported that he appeared withdrawn, played by himself during free play, and had difficulty concentrating in the classroom. At home, Jonathan appeared more irritable than usual and would throw frequent temper tantrums. In addition, he had difficulty sleeping and appeared to lose interest in eating. After a couple of months, Jonathan's behavior began to improve. However, these symptoms resurfaced a year later, when Jonathan and his mother moved into their own apartment, which necessitated a change in schools.

BEHAVIORAL GENETICS

Two important areas of behavioral genetics are discussed in this section. First, a number of investigators have examined ways in which there are gene × environment interactions, whereby the effect of certain environmental conditions may be exacerbated (or buffered) depending on the level of genetic vulnerability. Second, the field of behavioral genetics has attempted to shed light on how behavioral variation observed among children and adolescents can be ascribed to either genetic or environmental processes or to both. Researchers in this area have contributed to the field by investigating how both "nature" and "nurture" are the precursors of normal as well as abnormal behavior.[60,61] We begin with a discussion of gene × environment interactions and later discuss how investigators have attempted to partition variance into genetic and environmental effects.

Whether an individual is more a product of his or her genetic makeup versus his or her environment has been long debated. However, research in the fields of medicine and psychology has indicated that these influences are rarely distinct from one another and that their effects are probabilistic rather than determinative.[62] For example, modifications in lifestyle can decrease the risk of heart disease in an individual who is genetically prone to this illness.

Investigators who study joint effects of genes and environment on psychopathology distinguish between gene-environment interactions and gene-environment correlations.[63] Gene-environment *interactions* represent the diathesis-stress model of psychopathology. According to this model, certain environmental stressors contribute to the emergence of psychopathology in individuals who have a genetic vulnerability (i.e., diathesis). In this way, associations between stress and outcome are moderated by genetic vulnerability. In a set of intriguing studies, Caspi and colleagues identified polymorphisms in specific genes that moderate the effects of negative life experiences on the emergence of both antisocial behavior and depression.[64,65]

Unlike gene-environment interactions, gene-environment *correlations* refer to significant associations between genetic vulnerabilities and environmental risk, whereby individuals with higher levels of genetic vulnerability are more likely to be exposed to higher levels of environmental risk.[63] Hypothesized mechanisms for gene-environment correlations include (1) a passive process, whereby environmental risk is beyond the individual's control; (2) an evocative process, whereby an individual with a certain genetic vulnerability elicits certain toxic characteristics from the environment; and (3) an active process, whereby an individual with a certain genetic vulnerability actively alters or promotes a specific type of environment. To illustrate these hypothesized mechanisms, consider the example of a child with a genetic vulnerability to ADHD:

> *George, a 6-year-old, is one of five siblings. His mother works at night and often sleeps during the day, leaving his 16-year-old sibling in charge. George's chaotic family environment and lack of routine make it difficult for him to learn important self-regulation skills (i.e., a passive process). In addition, George's mother often feels frustrated by his inability to follow directions, noisiness, and high degree of activity, and has difficulty managing his behavior. She finds herself frequently ignoring or reprimanding him, which ultimately results in either attention-getting or oppositional behavior on his part (i.e., an evocative process). In school, George enjoys playing with children who are very active, like him. Because his peers share his difficulties, his negative behaviors are reinforced (i.e., an active process).*

Studies of depression, anxiety, and antisocial behavior have supported the role of both gene-environment interactions and gene-environment correlations.[62,64-67]

The degree to which there is interplay between genetic and environmental factors may also be dependent on developmental timing and contextual influences. For example, studies of the roles of genes and environment on depressive symptoms have suggested that environmental factors are associated with depressive symptoms in childhood. However, during adolescence and adulthood, genes appear to play a more salient role.[68] In addition, in terms of gene-environment correlations, passive processes, such as family influences, may be more prominent during early childhood. Evocative and active gene-environment correlations may play a greater role later in development.[69] Finally, the strength of genetic influence may be dependent on environmental context. For example, genetic factors appear to play a weaker role in the intellectual development of children raised in impoverished environments than in those raised in more affluent environments.[70]

Grossman and colleagues noted that the manifestation of many pathological conditions that may, at first glance, appear to be produced entirely by genetic factors or environmental factors may, in fact, be produced by a combination of genetic and environmental factors.[58] Fetal alcohol syndrome is an example of a disorder that is caused environmentally (by fetal exposure to alcohol). Clinical outcomes associated with fetal alcohol syndrome result from disruption of several neurodevelopmental processes. On the other hand, the developmental processes that are affected depend on several factors. For example, large single-episode quantities of alcohol are more detrimental to fetal brain development than are several exposures to low levels of alcohol. Moreover, effects are greater in the later stages of pregnancy. Thus, although fetal alcohol syndrome is clearly caused by environmental factors, it is also true that environmental factors are interacting with "genetically determined developmental time courses" to produce varying detrimental effects on brain development.[58] Unlike fetal alcohol syndrome, fragile X syndrome is an example of how a genetically caused disorder can be influenced by environmental factors, inasmuch as individuals with fragile X syndrome vary widely in their presentation. Environmental factors, such as the quality of the home environment, can interact with genetic effects to lead to significant variability in outcomes for individuals afflicted with fragile X syndrome.[58]

With regard to the partitioning of individual variation (e.g., variation in childhood problem behaviors) into environmental and genetic effects, classic behavioral genetics research methods include family, twin, and adoption study designs. Adoption and twin studies, in which the family members of varying genetic relatedness are compared, are needed to disaggregate genetic and environmental sources of variance. For example, if heredity affects a behavioral trait, then it follows that monozygotic twins will be more similar to each other with regard to that trait than will dizygotic twins. A stepfamily design is also used in which monozygotic twins and dizygotic twins are compared, along with full siblings, half-siblings, and unrelated siblings living in the same household.[60,61,71]

Most of the work in behavior genetics has employed an additive statistical model. One basic assumption of the additive model is that genetic and environmental influences are independent factors that sum to account for the total amount of individual variation. This model partitions the variance of the characteristic being studied among three components: genetic factors, shared environmental influences, and non-shared environmental influences. A heritability estimate, which ascribes an effect size to genetic influence, is calculated. The variance left over is then ascribed to environmental influences.[36,60,61,71]

Environmental influences are then further subdivided into shared and nonshared types. The term *shared environment* refers to environmental factors that produce similarities in developmental outcomes among siblings in the same family. If siblings are more similar than would be expected from their shared genetics alone, then this implies an effect of the environment that is shared by both siblings, such as being exposed to marital conflict or poverty or being parented in a similar manner. Shared environmental influence is estimated indirectly from correlations among twins by subtracting the heritability estimate from the monozygotic twin correlation. Nonshared environment, which refers to environmental factors that produce behavioral differences among siblings in the same family, can then be estimated. Nonshared environmental influence is calculated by subtracting the monozygotic twin correlation from 1.0.[60,61,71] In the stepfamily design described previously, shared environmental influence is implicated when correlations among siblings are large across all types of sibling pairs, including those that are not related. On the other hand, nonshared environmental influence is implicated when sibling correlations are low across all pairs of siblings of varying genetic relatedness, including monozygotic twins.[72]

Results of multiple studies with genetically sensitive designs suggest that many aspects of child and adolescent psychopathology show evidence of genetic influence.[60,61,71] Autism and Tourette syndrome in particular have been demonstrated to be mostly genetically determined.[61,71] Genetic factors have also been found to strongly influence externalizing behaviors, including aggression.[73] Although the results are less clear, genetic influence has been associated with the development of internalizing problems as well.[74] However, genetic influence does not account for all of the variance in psychopathological disorders.[60,61,71] For example, the environmental conditions under which children and adolescents are socialized play an important role. Interestingly, however, it is the environmental factors that are not shared—those that create differences among siblings

and not shared environmental factors—that seem to contribute to a large portion of the variation. Environmental factors that have been postulated to be nonshared include differential treatment by parents, peer influences, and school environment.[60,61,71]

Nonshared environmental factors have been implicated in hyperactivity, anorexia nervosa, aggression, and internalizing symptoms.[71] In addition, the combination of nonshared and genetic influences may influence the adolescent's choice of peer group.[75] Juvenile delinquency appears to be one exception to the rule in that shared environmental factors have been shown to be more influential than nonshared environmental or genetic factors.[71]

Behavior genetics research has gone beyond the partitioning of variance into genetic and environmental components. For example, researchers have examined how differential parenting practices may produce differing developmental outcomes among siblings. One study revealed that more than 50% of the variance in antisocial behavior and 37% of the variance in depressive symptoms were associated with conflictive and negative parenting behavior that was directed specifically at the child.[76] However, research has also suggested that longitudinal associations between both parenting behavior and child adjustment may be explained partly by genetic factors,[77] which suggests that genetically influenced characteristics of the child may elicit specific types of parenting behavior. In this way, nonshared experiences of siblings may in fact reflect genetic differences, such as differences in temperament.[78] One adoption study demonstrated that those who were at genetic risk for the development of antisocial behavior, by virtue of having a biological parent with a disorder, were more likely than children without this risk to be exposed to coercive parenting by their adoptive parents.[79]

Another important question examined in behavioral genetics research is whether genetic influences are more prominent at the extreme range of a psychopathological condition. By examining the full range of symptoms rather than specific diagnoses, behavior genetics research may highlight the continuity or discontinuity between normal and abnormal development.[61] One study showed that although variation in subclinical depressive symptoms is influenced mostly by genetics, adolescent depressive disorder appears to be influenced mostly by shared environmental factors.[74] Behavior genetic research has also demonstrated that genetic influences may partly explain comorbidity among disorders.[60] One study demonstrated that half of the correlation between externalizing and internalizing behaviors can be explained by common genetic liability.[72]

Researchers have pointed to the many limitations of behavior genetics research that need to be considered when these findings are evaluated.[34,36,80,81] In particular, the additive statistical model, the assumption that lies at the heart of behavior genetics methodology, has been criticized as neglecting to consider the potentially important contribution of gene-environment interactions (see earlier discussion). As noted previously, genetic and environmental influences may also be correlated.[34,36,80-82] Stable heritability estimates are also difficult to calculate. These estimates are highly influenced by the range of genetic and environmental variations within the sample and also tend to be influenced by reporter. For example, parent reports of child characteristics tend to show lower heritability estimates than when the same characteristics are reported on by children or teachers or when observational measures are used.[81] If heritability estimates are unstable, then estimates of environmental influences, derived from heritability estimates, are also unstable.[81] Critics have suggested that environmental influences cannot be estimated without being measured directly. However, the methods used in studies of environmental factors, such as differential parenting, may also be difficult to interpret. For example, genetic similarity may be confounded with family structure in that full siblings are likely to have more congruent parenting experiences than are half-siblings or step-siblings.[80,81] Also, shared events, such as those found in similar family environments, may contribute to nonshared variance in that different siblings may be affected differently by the same experiences.[60]

TRANSACTIONAL MODELS OF DEVELOPMENT

Transactional models have been crucial in highlighting how children can have an effect on their environment (e.g., their parents). For example, parents may not be aware that their children can have significant effects on their parenting and that children are not merely passive recipients of their parenting behaviors and values. As one example, it is known that a child's temperament (i.e., adaptability, reactivity, emotionality, activity level, sociability) has a significant effect over time on the nature and quality of a parent's behaviors toward the child.[83]

Traditionally, child development was conceptualized in a linear manner, whereby risk and protective factors were believed to have a unidirectional influence on a child's developmental trajectory. From this perspective, the effects of individual and environmental factors on development were considered to be distinct from one another. In contrast, according to modern theories of child development, development is a dynamic process; these theories incorporate Piaget's notion of the child as an active participant in his or her development. Hence, transactional models of development emphasize the importance of bidirectional, interactional processes that unfold over time. Through this interplay, the child and the child's context function to alter one another and are therefore inseparable in terms of their collective effect on development.

Studies of temperament and attachment provided early support for a transactional model of development.[84,85] Theories that postulated that negative temperament was simply a result of poor parenting behaviors were replaced by the idea that specific child characteristics elicited maladaptive parenting, which later resulted in child behavioral difficulties.[86] Similarly, increasing emphasis has been given to the child's role in the development of attachment style, as illustrated in the following case example:

> Brenda has had a very difficult time parenting her 11-month-old daughter, Jocelyn. Since she was born, Jocelyn has been very fussy, irritable, and difficult to soothe. As a result, Brenda has felt exhausted, frustrated by her inability to comfort her baby, and has questioned her parenting skills. This has compromised her ability to be responsive and nurturing in her interactions with Jocelyn. Brenda complains that Jocelyn wants only to be with her and becomes overly upset if her mother leaves her, even for a short period of time.

Consistent with Bronfenbrenner's biopsychosocial model,[87] various levels of context can interact with one another and either directly or indirectly affect child development. For example, in the context of poor maternal social support, irritable infants may elicit unresponsive mothering, leading to insecure attachment.[88] However, when provided with adequate social support, mothers may be able to respond to their children in a more positive manner, thereby promoting secure attachment.

In addition, the relative importance of various contexts on development is dependent on developmental timing. Whereas the family context is primary during infancy and early childhood, interactions with teachers and peers take on increasing importance in late childhood and adolescence.[89,90] Research on conduct problems has supported this notion. In early childhood, children who exhibit difficult temperament and noncompliant behavior often elicit punitive and inadequate parenting practices, which may actually serve to reinforce noncompliant behaviors.[91,92] Over time, parents and child may engage in interactions in which parenting becomes increasingly harsh and child behavior more noncompliant and aggressive. This transactional pattern appears to be especially salient in the context of poverty, as inherent parental stress and lack of access to resources may compromise parenting ability.[89] In the school environment, the child's aggressive behavior may lead to negative teacher-child interactions, contributing to poor academic achievement and negative peer interactions, resulting in peer rejection and poor self-esteem.[89] Indeed, phenomena such as peer rejection have been found to both predict and be predicted by conduct problems.[89] Additional research has supported the role of transactional processes in disrupting parent-child interactions and peer functioning in other types of psychopathology, such as depression and ADHD.[66,93]

Transactional processes contribute to the understanding of continuity, or maintenance, of psychopathology and personality characteristics, over time, through these cyclical interaction processes between the individual and the environment.[94] Hence, lack of healthy adaptation over time is probably a reflection of continued dysfunctional interaction between an individual and his or her environment.[95,96] Some studies of depression have differentiated between dependent and independent negative life events, occurrences that are within versus beyond an individual's control, respectively. This research has demonstrated that whereas the onset of depression may result from the occurrence of independent negative life events, depressive symptoms may be maintained by dependent negative life events.[66]

The exacerbation and emergence of new psychosocial difficulties also can be understood through transactional processes. For example, aggressive individuals may be prone to peer rejection as a result of their aggressive behaviors. This "self-generated" peer rejection may create negative life events linked to depression.[66] In addition, these individuals may hold cognitive biases that lead them to expect and misperceive others' actions as rejecting, thereby further contributing to the negative cycle of aggression and depression.[66]

Transactional models of development are also suggestive of targets for interventions. Indeed, efforts to change perceptions, expectations, and child-environment interactions, through parent training, have proved successful in terms of promoting healthy attachment and reducing conduct problems in infants and children, respectively.[97-99]

DEVELOPMENTAL PSYCHOPATHOLOGY

Developmental psychopathology could be considered a *metatheory*, or a macroparadigm that integrates knowledge from many fields, including lifespan developmental psychology, clinical child psychology, family systems, neuroscience, and behavioral genetics, to name just a few.[100,101] As such, this section is the longest and most detailed of the "current theory" sections. Developmental-behavioral pediatricians can benefit greatly from knowledge of this field because of its emphasis on tracing the evolution of problems in development. In this way, informed pediatricians can play a key role in identifying children who are manifesting the beginnings of maladaptive developmental trajectories and who are probabilistically at risk for eventually developing more severe levels of pathological behavior. In view of the young ages of their patients, they also have the first opportunity to recommend or provide interventions designed to reduce risk.

Research based on a developmental psychopathology perspective has advanced the understanding of the developmental precursors and correlates of childhood psychopathology. By adopting a developmental perspective on psychopathology, physicians can begin to ask different kinds of questions. For example, the following questions might be posed: (1) Do prenatal and early childhood precursors differ for childhood-onset versus adolescent-onset versions of the same disorder? (2) How does the symptom presentation of a particular childhood-onset disorder change as the child negotiates certain developmental tasks? (3) What resilience processes make it less likely that certain symptoms will emerge in the future? (4) What types of developmental pathways lead to which types of psychopathologies, and are multiple antecedent developmental pathways possible for the same psychopathology? (5) What behaviors are typical for the age period (e.g., experimentation with drugs), and which are indicative of more serious psychopathology?

In the first section, we discuss the major assumptions and tenets of the developmental psychopathology perspective. After this, sections on issues relevant to a developmental psychopathology perspective are provided: developmental trajectories (including multifinality and equifinality), the onset and maintenance of psychopathology, age-at-onset research, resilience, comorbidity, person-environment fit research, and research on culture and contextualism.

Assumptions and Tenets of the Developmental Psychopathology Perspective

The goal of developmental psychopathology is to understand the unfolding of psychopathology over the lifespan and how the processes that lead to psychopathology interact with normative developmental milestones and contextual factors.[101,102] Some of the assumptions and tenets of this field are as follows:[101,102]

1. A given type of psychopathology is best understood through a complete examination of experiences

and trajectories leading up to the problem behavior, as well as trajectories that occur after the problem behavior.

2. It is assumed that *multifinality* (i.e., two children with the same symptoms or experiences at one point in time may have different outcomes later in development) and *equifinality* (i.e., two children with the same outcome may have developed this outcome along different pathways) are more the rule rather than the exception. A related assumption is that a single factor is usually not necessary or sufficient to produce a given psychopathology.[103]

3. Knowledge is enhanced when the understanding of normative child and adolescent development is used to further the understanding of child and adolescent psychopathology. Similarly, knowledge of normal development can be enhanced by the study of atypical development.[104]

4. It is of interest to understand the full range of child and adolescent functioning (including clinical, subclinical, and normative forms of behavioral functioning) across multiple domains.

5. It is of interest to understand why some children who are at risk for a disorder, or who have been exposed to adversity, do not show symptoms (i.e., resilient youth).

6. Relations between antecedent events/adaptations and subsequent psychopathology are assumed to be probabilistic.[103] One corollary of this assumption is that early historical adaptations (e.g., anxious attachment) may not themselves be psychopathological or even a sufficient condition for subsequent psychopathology.[105,106] Rather, such earlier adaptations and pathways are probabilistically associated with the quality of later functioning (i.e., continuity), but discontinuity is also possible (a process that Cicchetti and Rogosch refer to as *probabilistic epigenesis*[101]). With regard to early attachment difficulties, for example, such early experiences may have an effect on the child's neurophysiology and ability to regulate emotions, which may, in turn, be predictive of later social and individual pathology,[106] but such outcomes clearly do not occur in all cases.

7. Development occurs through continuous and multiple reorganizations across all domains of child and adolescent functioning (e.g., physical, social, cognitive, neurological, emotional).

8. It is assumed that children play an important role in determining their own development and outcomes of development (e.g., by the environments in which they choose to engage and by changing these environments over time) through transactional processes between individual and environment (see earlier discussion).

9. The large number of transitions during childhood and adolescence provide many opportunities for a redirection of prior maladaptive trajectories,[107] as well as more possibilities for movement onto maladaptive pathways.

10. Factors associated with the onset of a disorder may be distinct from those associated with the maintenance of a disorder.[102,108]

Given this overview of assumptions and tenets, we now provide more specific reviews of some of the major constructs from this field.

Developmental Trajectories during Childhood and Adolescence: Multifinality and Equifinality

As implied previously, proponents of the developmental psychopathology perspective attempt to understand how pathology unfolds over time, rather than examining symptoms at a single time point. As a consequence, developmental psychopathologists have found the notion of "developmental trajectories" very useful.[101] For example, researchers could examine alcohol use and isolate different developmental trajectories of such use over time (e.g., some youth may show rapid increases in alcohol use over time, some may show gradual increases, and others may show increases followed by decreases[109]).

It is also assumed that some developmental trajectories are indicative of a developmental failure that probabilistically increases the chances that a psychopathological disorder will develop at a later point in time.[101] Thus, there is an interest in isolating early-onset trajectories that portend later problems. As an example, Dodge and Pettit pointed out that children who have early difficult temperaments (i.e., an early trajectory) who are also rejected by their peers for 2 or more years by grade 2 have a 60% chance of developing a serious conduct problem during adolescence.[89] Again, this confluence of trajectory (i.e., difficult temperament) and risk factor (i.e., chronic peer rejection) does not automatically produce a conduct-disordered adolescent; rather, it merely increases the odds that the child will develop such a disorder.

In view of the vast individual differences in trajectories in any given domain of functioning, developmental psychopathologists have also been interested in the concepts of multifinality and equifinality.[110] Multifinality occurs when there are multiple outcomes in those who have been exposed to the same antecedent risk factor (e.g., maternal depression). After equivalent exposure to a parent who is depressed, not all children so exposed will develop along identical pathways. In a study of multifinality, Marsh and colleagues examined outcomes of adolescents with insecure preoccupied attachment orientations (i.e., they all had the same starting point).[111] Those adolescents with mothers who displayed low levels of autonomy in observed interactions were more likely to display internalizing symptoms. Conversely, those with mothers who displayed very high levels of autonomy were more likely to exhibit risky behaviors. Thus, multiple outcomes (i.e., multifinality) occur in those who all have the same initial risk factor (i.e., insecure preoccupied attachment orientation).

Equifinality occurs when individuals with the same level of psychopathology achieved such pathological outcomes through different pathways. Evidence for equifinality has emerged in research. For example, Harrington and associates found that suicidal behavior can be reached through different paths, one involving depression and another involving conduct disorder.[112] Similarly, in girls, it appears that several of the same outcomes (e.g., anxiety disorders, substance use, school dropout, pregnancy) emerge in those with depression *or* conduct disorder.[113] Finally, Gjerde and Block suggested that depressed adult women and men progress along very different developmental pathways before developing depression.[114] It is worth noting, from an intervention perspective, that the presence of equifinality suggests that different versions of a given treatment for a given problem may be needed, depending on the pathway by which an individual progressed toward a psychopathological outcome.

When investigators recognize the notion that multiple types of trajectories are possible, even when the starting point is the same (i.e., multifinality), they may be interested in devising a typology of such trajectories. It may be, for example, that some children exhibit increasing levels of aggression with development (an "increasing" trajectory), some children consistently display low levels of aggression (a "low and flat" trajectory), and other children initially exhibit high levels of aggression but then desist from such behaviors with increasing age (a "high and desist" trajectory). Such possibilities could be discussed with parents as a rationale for early intervention.

Interestingly, the existence of such diverse types of trajectories has been supported by past research. For example, Lacourse and colleagues were able to isolate different trajectories of delinquent group membership in boys and their association with subsequent violent behaviors[115] (see Zucker et al[116] for a similar example involving a typology of alcoholics or Broidy et al[117] for an example involving outcomes of typologies of childhood aggression). Such approaches have been termed *person-oriented* approaches (as opposed to *variable-oriented*), insofar as people are clustered into groups on the basis of the similarity of their characteristics or patterns of trajectories over time.[118] Trajectory groups are differentiated on the basis of their patterning or profile of scores on antecedent or outcome variables

of interest (e.g., maladaptive parenting, school failure). Moreover, such trajectories can assume quadratic forms (i.e., U-shaped or inverted ∩-shaped functions).[119]

From a clinical perspective, a typological approach is beneficial because professionals who are familiar with typologies can then use this information to guide their evaluations and subsequent recommendations. For example, a history of insecure attachment would prompt a more thorough assessment to elicit information, including early childhood medical history, family environment, parenting behaviors and beliefs, child temperament and behavior problems, and emergent social relationships.

The Onset versus Maintenance of Psychopathology

It appears that factors that lead to the *onset* or initiation of a developmental trajectory are often different from those that *maintain* an individual on a developmental trajectory.[108] This distinction has considerable clinical relevance. For example, a professional may be able to prevent the onset of sleep problems in young children by instructing parents on how to institute various behavioral plans early in development. Once a maladaptive sleep pattern emerges, other types of interventions may be needed.

With regard to maintenance of problem behaviors, an individual who has begun on a particular pathway may continue on the pathway or may be steered from the pathway.[105] Factors that steer an individual from a maladaptive trajectory may be chance events, developmental successes, or protective processes that serve an adaptive function.[102] In an analogous manner, other factors may steer individuals from adaptive trajectories onto maladaptive trajectories. It is an assumption of developmental psychopathology that maintenance on a pathway is more likely than steering away, particularly when an individual has moved through several developmental transitions on the same pathway.[108]

What do we know about factors that lead to the onset of maladaptive paths versus those that serve to maintain individuals on such pathways? Steinberg and Avenevoli argued that researchers have tended to confuse factors that lead to the onset of psychopathology versus those that lead to its maintenance and that this confusion has hampered progress in the field of developmental psychopathology.[108] With regard to "onset," Steinberg and Avenevoli argued (from a "diathesis-stress" perspective) that biological predispositions (e.g., temperament, level of autonomic arousal) can exacerbate or decrease the degree to which individuals are vulnerable to the effect of subsequent environmental stressors.[108] Thus, two individuals exposed to the same stressor may begin on different pathways (e.g., anxiety vs. depression vs. aggression vs. no pathology), depending on the specific nature of each individual's biological predispositions. Put another way, stressors appear to have *nonspecific effects* on the onset of pathology as a result of the moderating effect of particular biological vulnerabilities.[108] These authors argued that future research on the elicitation of psychopathology needs to begin to isolate particular combinations of biological vulnerabilities and environmental threats that precede engagement with maladaptive developmental pathways. Indeed, such evidence is beginning to emerge; Brennan and associates found that early-onset and persistent aggression are predicted by interactions of biological and social risks (see later discussion of early- vs. late-onset psychopathology).[120] Similarly, as noted earlier, Caspi and colleagues found support for a gene × environmental stress interaction effect in predicting depressive symptoms.[65]

With regard to "maintenance," Steinberg and Avenevoli argued that environmental stressors have *specific effects* on the course of psychopathology.[108] Thus, it is possible that two individuals may begin on the same pathway (as a result of having the same biological predispositions and same level of exposure to early stressors) but may have very different long-term outcomes if their environments differ. For example, two young children who have started on an early aggression pathway may diverge from each other over time because one of them is exposed to incompetent parenting, lack of structure, and deviant peers and the other is not (also see Dodge and Pettit[89]). Those who begin on an "early aggression" trajectory are probabilistically more likely to associate with deviant peers and "choose" maladaptive environments, but this is clearly not always the case for every affected child. Steinberg and Avenevoli also provided evidence that those who continue on certain paths and select certain environments are also more likely to strengthen the synaptic weights or connections of the original biological predisposition (e.g., the nature of the child's arousal regulation capacities), which makes it even less likely that the individual will desist from this behavior or be steered from the maladaptive developmental trajectory.[108] Put another way, psychopathology is likely to be maintained in individuals in whom the symptoms or the antecedents of the symptoms are repeated.[108] In the preceding example, "lack of structure" in the family environment may not be a factor in the onset of conduct problems, but it may help maintain these problems because it permits more exposure to deviant peers and permits the pathological process to become more ingrained and entrenched.[108]

Researchers in several areas have begun to distinguish between onset and maintenance in their research designs (e.g., in the area of substance use, see Brook et al[121]; in the area of antisocial behavior, see Patterson et al[122]). For example, Dodge and Pettit[89] provided a model of chronic conduct problems that is consistent with the notions advanced by Steinberg and Avenevoli.[108] Dodge and Pettit argued that the bulk of research on conduct problems in childhood and adolescence suggests that children with certain neural or psychophysiological predispositions are more likely than others to begin a trajectory leading to conduct problems in adolescence. Such children are more likely to be parented harshly or neglected, because of their early difficult temperament. Outside the family, such children are more likely to be aggressive and to engage in conflict with peers during early childhood. According to Dodge and Pettit, such children enter elementary school in an at-risk state (although this transition is also an opportunity for steering away from this trajectory).[89] Most often, such children experience peer rejection and have difficult relations with teachers. This combination of harsh parenting and peer rejection serves to stabilize the negative trajectory, which makes it less likely that steering away will occur. Although adolescence is another transitional opportunity, such children are at risk for affiliation with deviant peers. In fact, Dodge and Pettit provided evidence that such children react psychophysiologically in ways that make it uncomfortable for them to interact with typical peers.[89] At this point, other cognitive strategies also play a role (e.g., the greater likelihood of hostile attributions). Movement toward a diagnosis of conduct disorder is overdetermined in such adolescents; the probability of such an outcome increases rapidly with age because of a confluence of multiple contributing factors.

In describing a developmental psychopathology model of depression, Hammen argued that cognitive vulnerabilities (e.g., negative view of self and negative self-schema) may be developed over time as a consequence of problematic relations and attachments with parents. Such cognitions make affected individuals more vulnerable to subsequent stressors, depression being the eventual outcome.[123] Interestingly, Hammen provided evidence that depression-prone individuals are also more likely to generate new stressors or exacerbate existing ones, thus fueling the cycle[123] (see Petersen et al for a similar perspective on adolescent depression[124]).

From a clinical perspective, understanding factors that contribute to the onset and/or maintenance of psychopathology informs preventive interventions, as well as the need to involve families in the implementation of these interventions. Research has demonstrated that, beginning in infancy, children with difficult temperaments are at risk for negative or harsh parenting. Early identification of difficult temperament then becomes a critical time point for clinician intervention. At this stage, pediatricians have the opportunity to intervene and provide support to parents in order to prevent the onset of conduct problems. Suppose that this early opportunity is missed. The transition into elementary school can then become stressful for the child and lead to difficulties with peer interactions. However, the clinician can act to prevent the maintenance of psychopathological behavior by engaging the family in the process of intervention. The earlier a clinician can identify risk for pathological behavior, the sooner the opportunity for prevention or intervention occurs, which in turn, provides the child with the most opportunities to master developmental transitions successfully.

Although we have argued thus far that factors associated with the onset of psychopathological behavior may differ from those associated with its maintenance, this is not always the case. For example, Patterson and associates found that early-onset antisocial behavior (during preadolescence) is linked with early arrests (before age 14) which are, in turn, linked with chronic offending in later adolescence (at age 18).[122] Of most relevance to this discussion is that they also found that the factors that were associated with the onset of the trajectory (i.e., problematic parental discipline and monitoring, marital transitions, social disadvantage, deviant peer involvement) were the same factors that were associated with the maintenance of this "chronic offending" trajectory.

Age-at-Onset Research

A related line of research focuses on the age of the child or adolescent when symptoms of psychopathology begin. Interestingly, it appears that both the antecedents and long-term outcomes for children and adolescents with early onset of symptoms differ significantly from those for persons who have late-onset symptoms. This is important because it suggests that studies of adolescents that do not take age at onset into account in sampling procedures will probably combine across multiple subgroups of adolescents in whom severity and chronicity vary significantly.[101]

Perhaps the most widely cited example of such age-at-onset differences is Moffitt's distinction between "life course–persistent" and "adolescence-limited" delinquents.[125] The former exhibit earlier conduct problems than do the latter, and they are more likely to have neuropsychological problems, difficult early temperament, inadequate parenting and family dysfunction, hyperactivity, and psychopathic personality traits[126] (although there is some debate about whether the neuropsychological difficulties predate the conduct problems[127]).

The outcomes for the life course–persistent delinquents tend to be worse than for their adolescence-limited counterparts, with higher rates of adult criminality and violence, substance dependence, and adult work-related problems.[101,128] The conduct problems of adolescence-limited delinquents are more likely to abate over time than is the case for the life course–persistent delinquents (although the former are not without problems, inasmuch as they are also at risk for mental health problems and high levels of life stress).[127,128] Clearly, these are very different pathways with different antecedents and outcomes. On the other hand, if these two groups were studied together at only one point in time (e.g., middle to late adolescence), their behaviors may appear similar.[126] Finally, Moffitt and colleagues suggested that there is a third group of boys who are aggressive as children but exhibit low levels of conduct problems in adolescence (in earlier work, these boys were referred to as "recoveries").[128] These individuals are also at risk for problems in adulthood, but the risk is lower than in the other two groups just described. Moreover, their problems are more likely to be of the internalizing type (e.g., depression, anxiety). An analogous distinction has been made in the literature on adolescent alcohol use. Zucker and associates described three types of adolescent and young adult "alcoholisms," each with different ages at onset, antecedents, and long-term consequences[129] (see Schulenberg et al for a similar approach to adolescent alcohol use[130]).

Interestingly, it appears that Moffitt's distinction between the two types of delinquency in adolescents (i.e., childhood onset vs. adolescence limited) may apply only to boys.[125] Silverthorn and Frick proposed that the childhood-onset form may be the only one that applies to girls, but with one important difference.[131] Delinquent adolescent girls appear to have the same antecedents as boys with life course–persistent delinquency, but their conduct problems emerge later than in boys. Thus, it appears that adolescent girls are more likely to fit a "delayed-onset" life course–persistent subtype.

With regard to internalizing symptoms, there is some suggestion that the antecedents of childhood symptoms of depression differ from those of adolescent symptoms of depression.[132] Whereas variables indexing the overall family context are associated with symptoms in childhood, factors such as maternal depression (in girls) and lack of supportiveness in the early rearing environment (in boys) were more strongly associated with symptoms during adolescence. On the other hand, it is difficult to determine whether such differences in findings are related more to the question of onset versus maintenance (see previous discussion) or early versus late onset. In the literature on depression, distinctions have also been made between adolescent-onset and adult-onset depression. Those with the former are more likely than those with the latter to have perinatal problems, psychopathology in their family background, caregiver instability, and other mental health problems.[133]

Resilience

As noted previously, some children may exhibit adaptive behavior outcomes despite exposure to adversity. Knowledge of factors that promote resilience in affected children can bolster preventive efforts by developmental-behavioral pediatricians.

Developmental psychopathologists are interested in understanding the full range of normative and atypical functioning. In fact, researchers have examined a subset of individuals in the normative range: namely, those who function adaptively despite exposure to significant levels of risk and/or adversity (e.g., trauma, social disadvantage, marital transitions, difficult temperament, high genetic loading for psychopathology). Rather than engaging with a maladaptive developmental trajectory (as would be expected, in view of their history), these "resilient" children manage to defy their at-risk status. From a prevention and intervention perspective, children who exhibit resilience are of interest because they can provide much needed information to researchers and interventionists regarding factors that protect at-risk individuals from developing later problems. The issue of resilience is also relevant to the study of multifinality; in children with a particular risk factor (e.g., a substance-abusing parent), outcomes are likely to vary (e.g., substance use vs. normal functioning); one of these outcomes is resilience.[134] Moreover, a child may display resilience with regard to one outcome (e.g., academic achievement) but not necessarily with regard to another (e.g., peer relations). Indeed, researchers have found that some inner-city adolescents who have experienced high levels of uncontrollable stress may be resilient in some areas (e.g., school performance, behavioral conduct) but not in others (e.g., they may exhibit high levels of internalizing symptoms).[135]

How does resilience develop? Researchers and theorists agree that resilience is best viewed as a dynamic process that unfolds over time on the basis of transactions between the individual and the environment rather than as a single variable operating at a single time within a child.[102,105] Interestingly, past research suggests that individual and environmental factors that characterize resilient children are similar to those that provide developmental advantages to any child. Superior intellectual functioning, easy temperament, and close relations with caring adults are characteristics that can protect a child exposed to adversity,[136] but they provide advantages for other children as well. Also, research by Stouthamer-Loeber

and colleagues suggests that protective and risk effects often occur within the same variables, in such a way that scores on one end of a continuum (e.g., superior intellectual functioning) may be protective, whereas scores on the other end of the continuum (e.g., low intellectual functioning) produce higher risk status.[137] Also, a variable may be protective by increasing adaptation or by decreasing maladaptation (see more detailed previous discussion of risk, protective, vulnerability, and resource factors).[137]

Adaptive coping patterns are related to both physical and psychological well-being. Seeking social support has been identified as a beneficial contributor to stress tolerance and has been shown to function as both a mediator and a moderator of stress-illness relations.[136,138] Also, the use of problem-focused coping strategies in childhood has been tied to increased resilience to stress later in life.[139] The ability to minimize the threat of potential stressors by rationally reappraising oneself or the situation also contributes to stress tolerance.[140] In some cases, avoidance, blaming others, and wishful thinking have been shown to be maladaptive coping strategies.[141,142] Avoidant coping, specifically, has been linked to distress, depression, mood disturbance, poorer quality of life, and increased pain perception in medical patients.[143-145]

Key interventions that can build resilience and are especially appropriate as interventions with the chronically ill include creating a flexible narrative about the course of the illness and its effect and meaning for all family members; improving communication within the family to increase understanding and support; and helping the child and family develop a sense of health efficacy.[146] Health efficacy (the belief that a person can have a positive influence on his or her own health) can be enhanced when there is an accurate understanding of the illness and its medical and psychosocial consequences. In addition, a proactive stance, such as advocating for appropriate health services, can help families experience a sense of control.[146]

Comorbidity

Comorbidity involves the presence of two or more disorders within a single individual; the term *comorbidity* is typically used when disorders co-occur at rates higher than expected from each disorder's base rate (e.g., ADHD and conduct disorder).[102,147] Although some instances of comorbidity may be the result of definitional ambiguities or methodological artifacts,[102] comorbidity does seem to occur with regularity in childhood and adolescence. One well-known clustering scheme suggests that there are two broadband categories of psychopathology:[148] *internalizing* problems (i.e., disorders that represent problems within the self, such as depression, anxiety, somatic complaints, and social withdrawal) and *externalizing* problems (i.e., disorders that represent conflicts with the external environment, such as delinquency, aggression, and other self-control difficulties). Alternatively, Jessor and colleagues proposed that a "problem behavior syndrome" characterizes some children and adolescents, whereby there tend to be high intercorrelations among several types of problem behavior (e.g., drug use, sexual intercourse, drinking, and aggression).[149,150] According to problem behavior theory, such behaviors develop as a function of the same etiological factors and, therefore, tend to co-occur in the same individuals (such findings have been replicated in several laboratories; for examples, see Bingham and Crockett[151] and Farrell et al[152]; but see Loeber et al[153] for an alternative perspective).

Some studies have shown evidence for comorbidity that combines across the internalizing and externalizing dimensions. For example, Capaldi studied four groups of boys: those with depressed mood only, those with conduct problems only, those with both problems, and those with neither.[154] Findings suggested that the poorest adjustment occurred for those with the comorbid problems. Like many who study comorbidity, Capaldi was also interested in whether there was a temporal relationship between the two disorders (in which one disorder precedes the other or in which a common risk factor causes both comorbid disorders).[154] Specifically, she found that once a conduct disorder is in place, multiple failures across multiple contexts (i.e., family, peer) place such young adolescents at risk for subsequent depressive symptoms. Similarly, Aseltine and associates examined four groups of participants with presence versus absence of depression and substance use. They found distinctive risk factors for depression, substance use, and their comorbidity.[155]

The presence of comorbid disruptive disorders (oppositional defiant disorder or conduct disorder) in children with ADHD has been well established.[156,157] It has become apparent that internalizing disorders such as depression and anxiety also commonly co-occur with ADHD.[156,158,159] In a study of 6- to 12-year-old children with ADHD, a significant comorbidity was found to exist between ADHD-combined type and oppositional defiant disorder/conduct disorder.[160] On the other hand, children with ADHD with predominantly inattention symptoms are not as likely to have a comorbid diagnosis of oppositional defiant disorder or conduct disorder.[160-162]

Clinically, knowledge of such instances of comorbidity is important for several reasons. First, one of the disorders may complicate the treatment of the other disorder. For example, if a child has significant learning problems and a conduct disorder, the presence of a conduct disorder must be taken into account when the learning disability is treated. Second, it may be that the development of one of the disorders preceded development of the other disorder. In other words, the symptoms of one disorder promotes (or exacerbates) the development of the other. Continuing with the example just presented, it may be that the conduct disorder symptoms have developed as a response to (or as a way of coping with) the learning difficulties. If it can be ascertained that one disorder "drives" the other disorder, treatment of the first disorder may also lead to a decrease in the symptoms of the second disorder. (Alternatively, a single causal factor may be responsible for the development of both disorders.) Finally, and in view of the frequencies with which many disorders are comorbid with other disorders, physicians should routinely assess for comorbidity when a child or adolescent presents with significant psychopathology.

Person-Environment Fit Research

Person-environment fit theory focuses on the interaction between characteristics of the individual and the environment, whereby the individual not only influences his or her environment, but the environment also affects the individual (see earlier discussion of transactional models). The adequacy of this fit between a person and the environment can affect the person's motivation, behavior, and overall mental and physical health[163]; that is, if the fit is optimal, the individual's functioning may be facilitated; if it is unsuitable, the individual may experience maladaptation. For example, a developmental-behavioral pediatrician may learn that a particular school environment is not providing much needed academic programming for an academically at-risk child. The clinician can intervene, the goal being to maximize the fit between the child's needs and the schools programming. The importance of person-environment fit with parents can provide a useful rationale when a particular intervention is recommended.

The person-environment fit paradigm has been successfully integrated within a developmental framework. Within this developmental perspective, person-environment fit theory, or, more specifically, stage-environment fit theory, postulates that the combination of an individual's developmental stage and the surrounding environment produces adaptive change within the individual.[164] Proponents of this perspective maintain that synchronizing the trajectory of development to the characteristics and changes in the surrounding environment will encourage positive growth and maturity.[163] According to stage-environment fit theory, adaptation is more likely if changes within the individual are matched with supportive change within the child's three main environments: home, peer, and school.

One environmental change that marks early adolescence is the transition from elementary school to junior high, or middle, school. Several negative changes within the individual have been associated with this transition, such as decreases in motivation, self-concept, and self-confidence, as well as increased academic failure.[163] This phenomenon may be a result of several differences between elementary schools and junior high schools that make the latter less developmentally appropriate for students in this age range. In fact, the Michigan Study of Adolescent Life Transitions revealed that, in comparison with elementary schools, junior high schools were characterized by a greater emphasis on discipline and control, fewer opportunities for the students to participate in decision making, less personal and less positive teacher-student relationships, and lower cognitive requirements for assigned tasks.[163] Thus, a stage-environment mismatch within the school environment may be associated with some of the negative changes that often occur within the adolescent at this time.

Patterns of change in the adolescent's home environment are also supportive of the stage-environment hypothesis. During early adolescence, the process of establishing greater independence from parents results in greater conflict and modification of roles between the child and parents.[165] Collins postulated that maladaptive conflicts may occur when there is a poor fit between the child's desire for autonomy and opportunities for such independence.[166] Consideration of pubertal development has provided further support for this theory. In general, early-maturing girls report that they are less satisfied with levels of autonomy and decision making provided at home and in school than are their less physically mature peers.[163] For children who must adhere to complex medical regimens, the degree of fit between home environment and their readiness to assume some responsibility for self-care can be crucial for adaptive outcomes. Specifically, the degree to which parents can facilitate a sharing of responsibility when a child is developmentally ready can have an effect on subsequent health and important medical outcomes.

Another notable aspect of stage-environment fit is how congruence, or lack thereof, in one environment may affect functioning in another environment. Current research suggests that compatibility of stage-environment match in one setting is associated with functioning in other settings. For example, a positive home environment characterized by involvement in decision making was directly associated with higher intrinsic school motivation in one study.[167] This "spill-over effect" is appealing from a clinical perspective insofar as positive outcomes that result from an intervention (e.g., increased congruence in the home environment) may yield positive effects in other domains (e.g., academic performance), thus making the intervention more efficient.

Stage-environment fit theory has other clinical implications as well. Specifically, the clinician may be interested in maintaining a good fit between a specific child and the specific interventions that are implemented. For instance, interventions could be designed and implemented with the developmental stage of the target child in mind. Alternatively, interventions could be tailored to suit the unique strengths and weaknesses of the individual child. In short, interventions that are developmentally appropriate, syndrome specific, and modified to fit the specific needs of a particular child are most likely to be effective.

Culture and Contextualism

A major question in the literature is this: How do culture and context affect a child's development trajectory and the development of symptoms? Indeed, research on culture and contextual factors has revealed that there may be individual pathways to psychopathology that vary depending on type of neighborhood, ethnicity, or sociocultural circumstances.[168,169] Also, norms for appropriate behavior, as well as the types of processes that are protective, may vary across culture.[101] Even help-seeking behaviors appear to vary across cultures (e.g., initial problem identification, choice of treatment provider).[170] For example, in many cultures, discussing ailments is negatively viewed as a sign of weakness, particularly if those ailments are not entirely physical in nature. Members of those cultural groups are encouraged to manage their *pain* internally and often sacrifice the opportunity to receive beneficial support as a result of their silence. In this case, clinicians may miss an important opportunity to gather helpful information about a child's emotional or behavioral concerns because of the parents' or the child's cultural beliefs. In addition, cultural beliefs play a role in the timing of help-seeking behaviors, which perhaps explains a family's choice to delay treatment. Culture can also limit the types of treatment that clinicians are allowed to provide. Moreover, the effectiveness of interventions promoted by developmental-behavioral pediatricians may depend on the pediatrician's sensitivity to cultural context and how the intervention is presented to the family. In short, culture appears to play a complex role in all stages of the treatment process.

As a result of demographic changes, minority populations in the United States have steadily increased, which underscores the need to study acculturation and other cultural issues.[168] Although culture has been defined as the continual passing of socially transmitted patterns from one generation to another that govern the thoughts, values, and behaviors of individuals in all societies,[171] the continually changing role of culture in the lives of children makes it a difficult topic to investigate.[168] On the other hand, taking culture into consideration in developmental psychopathology research can help validate and extend current theories of normal development in a number of ways:[168] (1) Cultural research can reveal which developmental progressions or associations between predictors and outcomes are culture-specific and which are universal,[172] (2) such research can isolate pathways to adaptive and maladaptive outcomes that vary across cultural groups, and (3) research may suggest factors crucial for mental growth that are culture specific versus culturally invariant (e.g., parental warmth appears to be crucial across cultures,[172] but "kinship" may be particularly crucial for African-American children[173]). Garcia Coll and Magnuson called for a paradigm shift in research whereby culture and context would be placed at the core rather than the periphery of understanding and investigating developmental processes.[174]

A number of issues have yet to be addressed in investigating the role of contextualism in developmental psychopathology. First, more systematic and carefully crafted assessments of cultural context must be used. Future research must "unpack culture" to gain a better understanding of its role in developmental psychopathology.[175] Intervention is another area affected by the study of culture and context. Little work has been directed toward understanding and applying culturally sensitive modes of intervention, despite research showing that interventions that incorporate knowledge of cultural issues may be more effective.[176,177]

A Framework for Understanding Adolescent Development: An Application of Principles of Developmental Psychopathology

In this section, many of the guiding principles from the field of developmental psychopathology are integrated into a discussion of a single developmental period. The adolescent developmental period was chosen because of the dramatic developmental changes that characterize this period; because of the confluence of biological, social, and psychological factors in a single developmental stage; and because several of the theoretical principles discussed thus far regarding the field of developmental psychopathology can be illustrated when adolescent development is discussed. Moreover, several of the constructs in the framework to be discussed are relevant to interventions that may be implemented by developmental-behavioral pediatricians.

Adolescence is a transitional developmental period between childhood and adulthood that is characterized by more biological, psychological, and social role changes than is any other stage of life except infancy.[178,179] Indeed, change is the defining feature of adolescence. In view of the many changes that characterize adolescent development, it is not surprising that there are also significant changes in the types and frequency of psychological disorders and problem behaviors that are manifested during adolescence, in comparison with childhood. Moreover, distinctions between normal and abnormal are sometimes less clear during this developmental period than they are in earlier developmental periods.[101]

As noted, the influence of theories from the field of *developmental psychopathology* is evident in research on adolescent problem behaviors. Developmentally oriented research has documented the importance of the following for the psychosocial functioning of the child and adolescent:[107,126] the timing (early vs. late) of developmental events, the accumulation of multiple events that occur simultaneously and the effect of such accumulation on subsequent trajectories of psychopathology, and the fit between the developmental needs of an adolescent and the adolescent's environmental context. Contextual perspectives on adolescent psychopathology also have their roots in developmental theory.[87]

It is our contention that adolescent behavior and psychopathology are best understood within the context of the major tasks of this developmental period. We believe that an appreciation for the rapid developmental changes of adolescence and the contexts of such development will aid developmental-behavioral pediatricians in considering developmental issues in their clinical and research endeavors. The sample framework presented here summarizes major constructs that have been studied by researchers in this field and is based on earlier models presented by the American Psychological Association,[180] Hill,[181] Holmbeck and colleagues,[21,182,183] Steinberg,[184] and Grotevant.[185] The model is biopsychosocial in nature, insofar as it emphasizes the biological, psychological, and social changes of the adolescent developmental period (Fig, 2-6).[186]

At the most general level, the framework presented in Figure 2-6 indicates that the primary developmental changes of adolescence have an effect on the developmental outcomes of adolescence *through* the interpersonal contexts in which adolescents develop. In other words, the developmental changes of adolescence (puberty, cognitive, social) have an effect on the behaviors of significant others (family, peers, teachers), which, in turn, influence ways in which adolescents resolve the major issues of adolescence, such as autonomy, sexuality, and identity. Moreover,

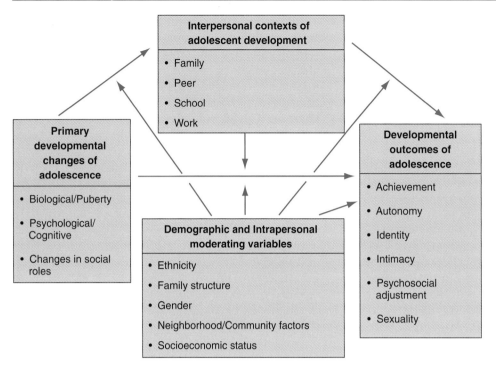

FIGURE 2-6 **A framework for understanding adolescent development and adjustment.** (From Holmbeck GN, Shapera WFA: Research methods with adolescents. *In* Kendall PC, Butcher JN, Holmbeck GN, eds: Handbook of Research Methods in Clinical Psychology, 2nd ed. New York: Wiley, 1999, pp 634-661. Copyright 1999 by John Wiley & Sons, Inc. Reprinted with permission.)

it is apparent that multifinality would be more the rule than the exception, in view of the multitude of factors noted in the framework that could influence developmental trajectories. Many of the contextual factors noted in the framework could buffer the adolescent from the effects of early risk factors, thus facilitating resilience.

For example, suppose that a young preadolescent girl begins to mature physically much earlier than her age mates. Such early maturity will probably affect her peer relationships, insofar as early-maturing girls are more likely to date and initiate sexual behaviors at an earlier age than are girls who mature on time.[187] Such effects on male peers may influence the girl's own self-perceptions in the areas of identity and sexuality. In this way, the behavior of peers in response to the girl's early maturity could be said to *mediate* associations between pubertal change and outcomes such as identity and the trajectories of sexual behaviors (and therefore account, at least in part, for these significant associations).

Such causal and mediational influences may also vary depending on the demographic and intrapersonal contexts in which they occur (see Fig. 2-6, "Demographic and Intrapersonal Moderating Variables"[186]). Specifically, associations between the primary developmental changes and the developmental outcomes may be *moderated* by demographic variables such as ethnicity, gender, and socioeconomic status. For example, if associations between pubertal change and certain sexual outcomes held only for girls, investigators could infer that gender moderates

such associations. In addition to serving a mediational role as described previously, the interpersonal contexts (i.e., family, peer, school, and work contexts) can also serve a moderating role in the association between the primary changes and the developmental outcomes. For example, early maturity may lead to poor adjustment outcomes only when parents react to early pubertal development in certain ways (e.g., with increased restriction and supervision); in this example, familial reactions to puberty moderate associations between pubertal development and adjustment.

In summary, we have attempted to demonstrate how a developmentally oriented theory (see Fig. 2-6[186]) can integrate across an array of potential linkages among many developmental changes for a given developmental period (in this case, adolescence). With such a theory, investigators can begin to explain the onset and maintenance of both adaptive and maladaptive behavior over time and formulate hypotheses regarding appropriate points for intervention. Such a model can also guide the developmental-behavioral pediatrician in the information-gathering process as the practitioner attempts to understand, in an organized way, the complex array of influences affecting a given child or adolescent.

In view of this overview of developmental psychopathology and the implications that this field has for the field of developmental-behavioral pediatrics, we now focus on two areas related to children who present with significant physical conditions: theories of adjustment to chronic illness and theories of medical adherence.

THEORIES OF ADJUSTMENT TO CHRONIC ILLNESS

Theories in this section help clinicians understand why different children with the same condition exhibit different levels of psychosocial adjustment to their condition. Some may be highly resilient in the presence of adversity, whereas others may exhibit clinically significant levels of depression or poor medical adherence.

In their comprehensive text on adaptation to childhood chronic illness, Thompson and Gustafson[3] trace the history of theorizing in the area of adjustment to chronic illness, beginning with Pless and Pinkerton's integrated model.[13] According to this early theory, adjustment to chronic illness is affected by numerous factors, including intrinsic attributes, coping, self-concept, the family and social environment, an individual's and others' responses to the illness, and disability characteristics. Thompson and Gustafson proposed that relations between predictors and adjustment were bidirectional (see previous section on transactional models of development) and cumulative over time. They also noted that an individual's functioning before diagnosis can have an effect on responses to his or her illness.

A similar early influential theory was Moos and Tsu's life crisis model.[188] They extended Pless and Pinkerton's work by detailing some of the cognitive events that underlie successful coping with chronic illness. Specifically, they detailed the explanatory importance of cognitive appraisal, or the individual's understanding and thoughts about his or her own illness. They also described several "adaptive tasks" that follow from appraisals, such as the manner in which a person manages his or her symptoms. Finally, they also identified a variety of coping strategies that individuals may use when adapting to a physical illness, a conceptualization that could be considered a precursor to later conceptualizations of coping (see Thompson and Gustafson for a thorough review[3]).

More recent conceptual work has expanded and integrated such early conceptual frameworks to account for variations in adjustment to chronic illness. Wallander and Varni's disability-stress-coping model is a risk-and-resilience framework that identifies a number of "resistance" factors (e.g., intrapersonal factors, stress processing variables, social-ecological factors) that buffer (or exacerbate) the effect of psychosocial stress (both illness-related and non–illness-related stressors) on child adjustment.[189] Similarly, Thompson and Gustafson's transactional stress and coping model identifies adaptational processes residing within the mother and child that buffer the effects of illness on adjustment outcomes.[3] Although both these theories have been very influential in providing

a basis for many programs of research, these models are not without conceptual difficulties (see Holmbeck for a review[16]). These models tend to be more "temporal" than causal (which makes them difficult to test). Moreover, there is some confusion over descriptions of moderational and mediational effects, and the focus of Thompson and Gustafson's model is on mothers, with the exclusion of fathers. With regard to the last point, and as noted by family systems theorists[190] and ecological theorists,[87] clinicians should take all contexts of the child's life into account when attempting to understand variations in psychosocial adjustment. Following is an example of a case in which the family, peer, and school contexts are all affected by a chronic condition:

Francine, a 16-year-old, was struggling in school and had a history of domestic and peer conflict. After suffering from nosebleeds, she was diagnosed with lupus. She did not feel that she could communicate with her family or friends about her anxieties related to her diagnosis, and her brother teased her when she began gaining weight from her medication. As a consequence of frequent hospitalizations, her school attendance was poor, which resulted in plummeting academic performance, and she withdrew from school. In addition, her arguments with her parents worsened when she avoided taking her medication and stopped going to school. When hospitalized, Francine verbalized anger toward hospital staff about how her illness prevented her from having a normal life.

THEORIES OF MEDICAL ADHERENCE

Theories of medical adherence have been proposed to explain individual differences in medical adherence behaviors, as well as why medical adherence difficulties are more likely to occur during certain stages of development (e.g., adolescence).

Models of medical adherence have been reviewed by several theorists.[1-3,191] One of the most influential theories is the Health Belief Model,[192] which focuses on individual perceptions of barriers to satisfactory medical adherence (e.g., cost, time considerations, the degree to which the medical regimen disrupts daily activities) and factors predictive of higher levels of adherence (e.g., realistic perceptions of susceptibility to complications, adequate understanding of the seriousness of the condition, appreciation of the benefits associated with adherence to a medical plan). Analysis of barriers and benefits can often yield a greater understanding of patient adherence across settings, as illustrated in the following case example:

Mark, a 10-year-old boy, with a diagnosis of type 1 diabetes, was exhibiting poor glycemic control, although his mother reported good adherence at home. Mark often forgot to check his blood glucose level at school, and when emembered, he felt too embarrassed to do it. Also, at ....ch, he did not want to stand out among his peers and therefore ate foods he knew he should not, believing that this behavior would not be harmful if he was "good most of the time." At home, Mark's mother helped him to manage his diabetes by reminding him to check his blood glucose level. In addition, she prepared food for the whole family that was acceptable for Mark to eat.

Although the validity of an individual's self-reports of barriers and benefits has been questioned, some support has been found for the Health Belief Model of medical adherence.[2] As yet, however, few interventions exist that have attempted to manipulate these types of "barrier" cognitions.[1] A related theory, based on Bandura's self-efficacy theory,[193] suggests that the degree to which individuals believe themselves capable of managing their medical regimen is likely to be predictive of higher levels of adherence.[2]

Another influential theory (although one that has not received much attention in studies of children with chronic physical conditions) is the transtheoretical model.[194] According to this perspective, an individual acquires adherence behaviors over five stages of change:[191] (1) precontemplation (i.e., not thinking about changing his or her behavior), (2) contemplation (i.e., thinking about changing his or her behavior at some point in the future), (3) preparation (i.e., considering a change in behavior in the near future), (4) action (i.e., changing his or her behavior), and (5) maintenance (i.e., maintaining the changes made to his or her health behaviors). One potential promise of this stage-oriented approach is that different interventions could be developed for different individuals at varying stages of change. On the other hand, this theory awaits empirical validation with samples of children (see Rapoff for a thorough critique[2]).

Behavioral theory has played a major role in facilitating a more complete understanding of adherence, especially in children. The term *operant conditioning* describes the effect that a consequence can have in terms of either strengthening (positively reinforcing) or weakening (negatively reinforcing) a behavior.[195] A close analysis of conditions that may support or undermine a person's adherence to a medical regimen can yield greater understanding and thereby help the professional make informed decisions and recommendations with the goal of improving adherence. Interventions, including behavioral components such as distraction, praise, and incentives, have been found to increase children's cooperation during painful medical procedures.[196]

Rapoff concluded his review of models of adherence by noting that theories tend to emphasize one of two processes: cognitive processes (e.g., individual perceptions of barriers, self-efficacy) or environmen-

tal contingencies (e.g., parental reinforcement for successful completion of adherence tasks).[2] Despite the differing theoretical perspectives, Rapoff argued that the interventions that have been developed on the basis of these various theories have more similarities than their underlying conceptual frameworks would suggest. Specifically, most interventions that focus on medical adherence include the following components: (1) verbal discussions with patients and family members concerning the importance of adherence, (2) a "role model" that demonstrates appropriate levels of adherence, (3) goal setting and goal monitoring, (4) teaching of adherence skills, and (5) strategies to help individuals put into place positive consequences for satisfactory adherence behaviors.

CONCLUSIONS AND FUTURE DIRECTIONS

In this chapter, we have sought to provide a convincing case regarding the relevance of theory to research and practice in the field of developmental-behavioral pediatrics. We have attempted to delineate the components of well-developed theories in the field and provide examples of both historical and contemporary models that can guide practitioners and researchers. By taking the "development" aspect of developmental-behavioral pediatrics seriously, we have attempted to discuss the importance of understanding normative development. Clearly, developmental-behavioral pediatricians are in a unique position to identify difficulties early in a child's life that may place the child at risk for more serious difficulties later in life. With extensive knowledge of developmentally oriented theories, they are able to identify such early risk factors and are also able to provide families with theory-based and developmentally appropriate explanations regarding potentially effective interventions.

What are some limitations of current theorizing? Our brief review of the history of developmental theory reveals that clinicians have come to appreciate the complexities involved in developmental-behavioral pediatrics and the many factors that may contribute to a given outcome. However, it is important to consider whether such increases in complexity have occurred at the expense of clarity of focus. Although a more focused model would not include all possible contributing factors, it may have more clinical and research utility. Future theorists should attempt to strike a balance between being comprehensive and developing theories that are clinically useful for developmental-behavioral pediatricians.

A second limitation of current theory concerns a lack of emphasis on the mechanisms that operate between the variables. For example, although clinicians know a lot about *what* risk and protective factors may contribute to various outcomes, they know little as to *how* these processes operate. More specifically, although they know that children with chronic illnesses are at a heightened risk for behavioral and psychosocial difficulties, they have not yet identified a causal mechanism.[197] Future research should aim to uncover processes by which these factors operate.

A third limitation of current theories is that they often lack a developmental component. Future theories should include constructs that are developmentally appropriate for a specified age group. Furthermore, the full range of developmental domains (e.g., biological, cognitive, emotional, social) that are relevant to a particular age group should be considered. This is particularly important with pediatric patient populations, because children within these populations may follow a developmental trajectory that is different from that of their healthy age mates.

With regard to theory development, what future directions would be fruitful? The field would benefit greatly from theories that provide seamless linkages between a clearly articulated research-driven, developmentally oriented theory *and* interventions that follow directly from the constructs and pathways specified in the theory.[1] In addition, increased focus on mechanisms of treatment and the delineation of which populations do and do not benefit from specific interventions are needed. Too often, theories lack clarity or include constructs that have little relevance to the interventionist. Simply put, theories should be conceived with the interventionist in mind.

As the ability to understand biological processes (e.g., genetics) is continually enhanced by improving technology, new theories describing the influence of these processes on psychosocial functioning must keep pace. Traditional theory in this field, which has focused on biological vulnerabilities, should be expanded to address the potentially protective role of genes and biological mechanisms.

Although the importance of Bronfenbrenner's biopsychosocial model[87] and the role of transactional influences have been recognized, the application of these theories has been limited. These theoretical models are especially salient in view of improved rates of survival in pediatric conditions that were previously considered fatal (e.g., spina bifida, cancer, human immunodeficiency virus [HIV] infection) and increased incidence rates of other chronic conditions (e.g., obesity). Therefore, more attention to transactional processes between pediatric conditions and various contexts surrounding the child throughout the lifespan is necessary. For instance, theories focusing on mechanisms of intervention should be expanded to include their influence on surrounding systems and their indirect effects on the child's adjustment.[198] In addition, more theory is needed to address (1) how cultural beliefs and practices used in various contexts interact over time, (2) the influence of the health care system on family and individual functioning, (3) transactional interactions between peers and children and their effects on psychosocial adjustment, and (4) effects of financial forces on the various contexts affecting the child's development.[199]

Another implication of the developmental focus of this chapter is the importance of considering the developmentally appropriate fit between the theory, the needs of children and adolescents, and the proposed interventions. Moreover, research in the field of developmental and behavioral pediatrics has begun to move beyond an interest in static diagnostic and clinical issues to an interest in understanding how pathological mental and physical processes unfold over time. It is our hope that this developmental perspective is useful to clinicians who wish to conduct research or develop prevention or intervention programs for children and adolescents who are navigating the challenges of these important developmental periods.

REFERENCES

1. Riekert KA, Drotar D: Adherence to medical treatment in pediatric chronic illness: Critical issues and answered questions. *In* Drotar D, ed: Promoting Adherence to Medical Treatment in Chronic Childhood Illness. Mahwah, NJ: Erlbaum, 2000, pp 3-32.
2. Rapoff MA: Adherence to Pediatric Medical Regimens. New York: Kluwer, 1999.
3. Thompson RJ, Gustafson KE: Adaptation to Chronic Childhood Illness. Washington, DC: American Psychological Association, 1996.
4. Eyberg S, Schuhmann E, Rey J: Psychosocial treatment research with children and adolescents: Developmental issues. J Abnorm Child Psychol 26:71-81, 1998.
5. Kazdin AE: Psychotherapy for children and adolescents: Current progress and future research directions. Am Psychol 48:644-657, 1993.
6. Kessen W: The development of behavior. *In* Levine MD, Carey WB, Crocker AC, eds: Developmental-Behavioral Pediatrics. Philadelphia: WB Saunders, 1999, pp 1-13.
7. Levine MD, Carey WB, Crocker AC: Developmental-Behavioral Pediatrics. Philadelphia: WB Saunders Company, 1999.
8. Meehl PE: Theoretical risks and tabular asterisks: Sir Karl, Sir Ronald, and the slow progress of soft psychology. J Consult Clin Psychol 46:806-834, 1978.
9. Platt JR: Strong inference. Science 146:347-353, 1964.

10. Popper KR: The Logic of Scientific Discovery. New York: Harper, 1965.

11. Miller PH: Theories of Developmental Psychology. San Francisco: Freeman, 1983.

12. Lilienfeld SO: When worlds collide: Social science, politics, and the Rind et al (1998) child sexual abuse meta-analysis. Am Psychol 57:176-188, 2002.

13. Pless IB, Pinkerton P: Chronic Childhood Disorders: Promoting Patterns of Adjustment. Chicago: Year Book Medical, 1975.

14. Wallander JL, Varni, JW, Babani L, et al: Family resources as resistance factors for psychological maladjustment in chronically ill and handicapped children. J Pediatr Psychol 14:157-173, 1989.

15. Thompson RJ, Gustafson KE, George LK, et al: Change over a 12-month period in the psychosocial adjustment of children and adolescents with cystic fibrosis. J Pediatr Psychol 19:189-203, 1994.

16. Holmbeck GN: Toward terminological, conceptual, and statistical clarity in the study of mediators and moderators: Examples from the child-clinical and pediatric psychology literatures. J Consult Clin Psychol 65:599-610, 1997.

17. Wallander JL, Thompson RJ, Alriksson-Schmidt A: Psychosocial adjustment of children with chronic physical conditions. In Roberts MC, ed: Handbook of Pediatric Psychology. New York: Guilford, 2003, pp 141-158.

18. Rose BM, Holmbeck GN, Coakley RM, Franks EA: Mediator and moderator effects in developmental and behavioral pediatric research. J Dev Behav Pediatr 25:1-10, 2004.

19. Baron RM, Kenny DA: The moderator-mediator variable distinction in social psychological research: Conceptual, strategic, and statistical considerations. J Pers Soc Psychol 51:1173-1182, 1986.

20. Holmbeck GN: Post-hoc probing of significant moderational and mediational effects in studies of pediatric populations. J Pediatr Psychol 27:87-96, 2002.

21. Holmbeck GN, Johnson SZ, Wills KE, et al: Observed and perceived parental overprotection in relation to psychosocial adjustment in preadolescents with a physical disability: The mediational role of behavioral autonomy. J Consult Clin Psychol 70:96-110, 2002.

22. Holmes CS, Yu Z, Frentz J: Chronic and discrete stress as predictors of children's adjustment. J Consult Clin Psychol 67:411-419, 1999.

23. Masten AS, Hubbard JJ, Gest SD, et al: Competence in the context of adversity: Pathways to resilience and maladaptation from childhood to late adolescence. Dev Psychopathol 11:143-169, 1999.

24. Rutter M: Psychosocial resilience and protective mechanisms. In Rolf J, Masten AS, Cicchetti D, et al, eds: Risk and Protective Factors in the Development of Psychopathology. New York: Cambridge University Press, 1990, pp 181-214.

25. Masten AS: Ordinary magic: Resilience processes in development. Am Psychol 56:227-238, 2001.

26. Stouthamer-Loeber M, Loeber R, Wei E, et al: Risk and promotive effects in the explanation of persistent serious delinquency in boys. J Consult Clin Psychol 70:111-123, 2002.

27. McGee RA, Wolfe DA, Wilson SK: Multiple maltreatment experiences and adolescent behavior problems: Adolescents' perspectives. Dev Psychopathol 9:131-149, 1997.

28. Gorman-Smith D, Tolan P: The role of exposure to community violence and developmental problems among inner-city youth. Dev Psychopathol 10:101-116, 1998.

29. Tolan PH, Gorman-Smith D, Henry DB: The developmental ecology of urban males' youth violence. Dev Psychol 39:274-291, 2003.

30. Woodward LJ, Fergusson DM: Early conduct problems and later risk of teenage pregnancy in girls. Dev Psychopathol 11:127-141, 1999.

31. Clingempeel WG, Henggeler SW: Randomized clinical trials, developmental theory, and antisocial youths: Guidelines for research. Dev Psychopathol 14:695-711, 2002.

32. Howe GW, Reiss D, Yuh J: Can prevention trials test theories of etiology? Dev Psychopathol 14:673-694, 2002.

33. Kraemer HC, Wilson T, Fairburn CG, et al: Mediators and moderators of treatment effects in randomized clinical trials. Arch Gen Psychiatry 59:877-883, 2002.

34. Rutter M, Pickles A, Murray R, et al: Testing hypotheses on specific environmental causal effects on behavior. Psychol Bull 127:291-324, 2001.

35. Weersing VR, Weisz JR: Mechanisms of action in youth psychotherapy. J Child Psychol Psychiatry 43:3-29, 2002.

36. Collins WA, Maccoby EE, Steinberg L, et al: Contemporary research on parenting: The case for nature and nurture. Am Psychol 55:218-232, 2000.

37. Kraemer HC, Stice E, Kazdin A, et al: How do risk factors work together? Mediators, moderators, and independent, overlapping, and proxy risk factors. Am J Psychiatry 158:848-856, 2001.

38. Forgatch MS, DeGarmo DS: Parenting through change: An effective prevention program for single mothers. J Consult Clin Psychol 67:711-724, 1999.

39. Dixon RA, Lerner RM: History and systems in developmental psychology. In Bornstein MH, Lamb ME, eds: Developmental Psychology: An Advanced Textbook. Mahwah, NJ: Erlbaum, 1999, pp 3-46.

40. Parke RD, Ornstein PA, Rieser JJ, et al: The past as prologue: An overview of a century of developmental psychology. In Parke RD, Ornstein PA, Rieser JJ, et al, eds: A Century of Developmental Psychology. Washington, DC: American Psychological Association, 1994, pp 1-72.

41. Shaffer DR: Developmental Psychology: Childhood and Adolescence. Belmont, CA: Thomson Learning, 2002.

42. Darwin C: A biological sketch of an infant. Mind 2:285-294, 1877.

43. Boyce WT, Ellis BJ: Biological sensitivity to context: I. An evolutionary-developmental theory of the origins

of stress reactivity. Dev Psychopathol 17:271-301, 2005.

44. Hall GS: Adolescence: Its Psychology and Its Relations to Psychology, Anthropology, Sex, Crime, Religion, and Education, vol 2. New York: Appleton-Century-Crofts, 1904.

45. White SH: G. Stanley Hall: From philosophy to developmental psychology. *In* Parke RD, Ornstein PA, Rieser JJ, et al, eds: A Century of Developmental Psychology. Washington, DC: American Psychological Association, 1994, pp 103-126.

46. Freud S: The Basic Writings of Sigmund Freud. New York: The Modern Library, 1938.

47. Thelen E, Adolph KE: Arnold L. Gesell: The paradox of nature and nurture. *In* Parke RD, Ornstein PA, Rieser JJ, et al, eds: A Century of Developmental Psychology. Washington, DC: American Psychological Association, 1994, pp 357-388.

48. Gesell A: Infancy and Human Growth. New York: Macmillan, 1929.

49. Beilin H: Piaget's enduring contribution to developmental psychology. *In* Parke RD, Ornstein PA, Rieser JJ, et al, eds: A Century of Developmental Psychology. Washington, DC: American Psychological Association, 1994, pp 257-290.

50. Piaget J: Genetic Epistemology. New York: Columbia University Press, 1970.

51. Piaget J: Intellectual evolution from adolescence to adulthood. Hum Dev 15:1-12, 1972.

52. Piaget J: Piaget's theory. *In* Kessen W, ed: Handbook of Child Psychology, Volume 1: History, Theory, and Methods (Mussen PH, series ed). New York: Wiley, 1983, pp 103-128.

53. Daniels H: Introduction: Psychology in a social world. *In* Daniels H, ed: An Introduction to Vygotsky. New York: Routledge, 1996, pp 1-27.

54. Wertsch JV, Tulviste P: L.S. Vygotsky and contemporary developmental psychology. *In* Daniels H, ed: An Introduction to Vygotsky. New York: Routledge, 1996, pp 53-74.

55. Vygotsky L: Mind in Society: The Development of Higher Psychological Processes. Cambridge, MA: Harvard University Press, 1978.

56. Ellis BJ, Essex MJ, Boyce WT: Biological sensitivity to context: II. Empirical exploration of an evolutionary-developmental theory. Dev Psychopathol 17:303-328, 2005.

57. Suomi SJ: Early determinants of behavior: Evidence from primate studies. Br Med Bull 53:170-184, 1997.

58. Grossman AW, Churchill JD, McKinney BC, et al: Experience effects on brain development: Possible contributions to psychopathology. J Child Psychol Psychiatry 44:33-63, 2003.

59. Waddington CH: The Strategy of the Genes. London: Allen & Unwin, 1957.

60. O'Connor TG, Plomin R: Developmental behavior genetics. *In* Sameroff AJ, Lewis M, eds: Handbook of Developmental Psychopathology. New York: Plenum Press, 2000, pp 217-235.

61. Rende R, Plomin R. Nature, nurture, and the development of psychopathology. *In* Cicchetti D, Cohen DJ, eds: Developmental Psychopathology, Volume 1: Theory and Methods. New York: Wiley, 1995, pp 291-314.

62. Rutter M, Sroufe LA: Developmental psychopathology: Concepts and challenges. Dev Psychopathol 12:265-296, 2000.

63. Plomin R, Rutter M: Child development, molecular genetics, and what to do with genes once they are found. Child Dev 69:1223-1242, 1998.

64. Caspi A, McClay J, Moffitt TE, et al: Role of genotype in the cycle of violence in maltreated children. Science 297:851-855, 2002.

65. Caspi A, Sugden K, Moffitt TE, et al: Influence of life stress on depression: Moderation by a polymorphism in the 5-HTT gene. Science 301:386-390, 2003.

66. Hankin BL, Abramson LY: Development of gender differences in depression: An elaborated cognitive vulnerability-transactional stress theory. Psychol Bull 127:773-796, 2001.

67. Silberg J, Rutter M, Neale M, Eaves L: Genetic moderation of environmental risk for depression and anxiety in adolescent girls. Br J Psychiatry 179:116-121, 2001.

68. Thapar A, McGuffin P: The genetic etiology of childhood depressive symptoms: A developmental perspective. Dev Psychopathol 8:751-760, 1996.

69. Scarr S, McCartney K: How people make their own environments: A theory of genotype to environment effects. Child Dev 54:1-19, 1983.

70. Rowe DC, Jacobson KC, Van Den Oord JCG: Genetic and environmental influences on vocabulary IQ: Parental education level as moderator. Child Dev 70:1151-1162, 1999.

71. Pike A, Plomin R: Importance of nonshared environmental factors for childhood and adolescent psychopathology. J Am Acad Child Adolesc Psychiatry 35:560-570, 1996.

72. O'Connor TG, McGuire S, Reiss D, et al: Co-occurrence of depressive symptoms and antisocial behavior in adolescence: A common genetic liability. J Abnorm Psychol 107:27-37, 1998.

73. Deater-Deckard K, Plomin R: An adoption study of etiology of teacher and parent reports of externalizing behavior problems in middle childhood. Child Dev 70:144-154, 1999.

74. Rende R, Plomin R, Reiss D, et al: Genetic and environmental influences on depressive symptomatology in adolescence: Individual differences and extreme scores. J Child Psychol Psychiatry 34:1387-1398, 1993.

75. Iervolino AC, Pike A, Manke B, et al: Genetic and environmental influences in adolescent peer socialization: Evidence from two genetically sensitive designs. Child Dev 73:162-174, 2002.

76. Reiss D, Hetherington EM, Plomin R, et al: Genetic questions for environmental studies: Differential parenting of siblings and its association with depression and antisocial behavior in adolescence. Arch Gen Psychiatry 52:925-936, 1995.

77. Neiderhiser JM, Reiss D, Hetherington EM, et al: Relationships between parenting and adolescent

adjustment over time: Genetic and environmental contributions. Dev Psychol 35:680-692, 1999.

78. Plomin R, Reiss D, Hetherington EM, et al: Nature and nurture: Genetic contributions to measures of the family environment. Dev Psychol 30:32-43, 1994.

79. O'Connor TG, Deater-Deckard K, Fulker D, et al: Genotype-environment correlations in late childhood and early adolescence: Antisocial behavioural problems and coercive parenting. Dev Psychol 34:970-981, 1998.

80. Jackson FJ: Human behavioral genetics, Scarr's theory, and her views on interventions: A critical review and commentary on their implications for African-American children. Child Dev 64:1318-1332, 1993.

81. Maccoby E: Parenting and its effects on children: On reading and misreading behavior genetics. Annu Rev Psychol 51:1-27, 2000.

82. Steinberg L, Morris AS: Adolescent development. Annu Rev Psychol 52:83-110, 2001.

83. Saudino KJ: Behavioral genetics and child temperament. J Dev Behav Pediatr 26:214-223, 2005.

84. Thomas A, Chess B, Birch HG, et al: Behavioral Individuality in Early Childhood. New York: New York University Press, 1963.

85. Bell RQ: A reinterpretation of the direction of effects in studies of socialization. Psychol Rev 75:81-95, 1968.

86. Thomas A, Chess B, Birch HG: Temperament and behavior disorders in children. Oxford, UK: New York University Press, 1968.

87. Bronfenbrenner U: The ecology of human development: Experiments by nature and design. Cambridge, MA: Harvard University Press, 1979.

88. Crockenberg SB: Infant irritability, mother responsiveness, and social support influences on the security of infant-mother attachment. Child Dev 52:857-865, 1981.

89. Dodge KA, Pettit GS: A biopsychosocial model of the development of chronic conduct problems in adolescence. Dev Psychol 39:349-371, 2003.

90. Sameroff AJ, Peck SC, Eccles JS: Changing ecological determinants of conduct problems from early adolescence to early adulthood. Dev Psychopathol 16:873-896, 2004.

91. Anderson KE, Lytton H, Romney DM: Mothers' interactions with normal and conduct-disordered boys: Who affects whom? Dev Psychol 22:604-609, 1986.

92. Patterson GR: Performance models for antisocial boys. Am Psychol 41:432-444, 1986.

93. Johnston C, Mash EJ: Families of children with attention-deficit/hyperactivity disorder: Review and recommendations for future research. Clin Child Fam Psychol Rev 4:183-207, 2001.

94. Wachtel PL: Cyclical processes in personality and psychopathology. J Abnorm Psychol 103:51-54, 1994.

95. Sameroff A: Developmental systems and family functioning. *In* Parke RD, Kellam SG, eds: Exploring Family Relationships with Other Social Contexts. Hillsdale, NJ: Erlbaum, 1994, pp 199-214.

96. Sameroff AJ: Developmental systems and psychopathology. Dev Psychopathol 12:297-312, 2000.

97. Kazdin AE: Problem-solving skills training and parent management training for conduct disorder. *In* Kazdin AE, Weisz JR, eds: Evidence-Based Psychotherapies for Children and Adolescents. New York: Guilford, 2003, pp 241-262.

98. Kazdin AE, Weisz JR: Identifying and developing empirically supported child and adolescent treatments. J Consult Clin Psychol 66:19-36, 1998.

99. Van Den Boom DC: Neonatal irritability and the development of attachment. *In* Kohnstamm GA, Bates JE, Rothbart MK, eds: Temperament in Childhood. Chichester, UK: Wiley, 1989, pp 299-318.

100. Cicchetti D, Rogosch FA: Conceptual and methodological issues in developmental psychopathology research. *In* Kendall PC, Butcher JN, Holmbeck GN, eds: Handbook of Research Methods in Clinical Psychology, 2nd ed. New York: Wiley, 1999, pp 433-465.

101. Cicchetti D, Rogosch FA: A developmental psychopathology perspective on adolescence. J Consult Clin Psychol 70:6-20, 2002.

102. Mash EJ, Dozois DJA: Child psychopathology: A developmental-systems perspective. *In* Mash EJ, Barkley RA, eds: Child Psychopathology, 2nd ed. New York: Guilford, 2003, pp 3-71.

103. Kazdin AE, Kraemer HC, Kessler RC, et al: Contributions of risk-factor research to developmental psychopathology. Clin Psychol Rev 17:375-406, 1997.

104. Sroufe LA: Considering normal and abnormal together: The essence of developmental psychopathology. Dev Psychopathol 2:335-347, 1990.

105. Sroufe LA: Pychopathology as an outcome of development. Dev Psychopathol 9:251-268, 1997.

106. Sroufe LA, Carlson EA, Levy AK, et al: Implications of attachment theory for developmental psychopathology. Dev Psychopathol 11:1-13, 1999.

107. Graber JA, Brooks-Gunn J: Transitions and turning points: Navigating the passage from childhood through adolescence. Dev Psychol 32:768-776, 1996.

108. Steinberg L, Avenevoli S: The role of context in the development of psychopathology: A conceptual framework and some speculative propositions. Child Dev 71:66-74, 2000.

109. Schulenberg J, Wadsworth KN, O'Malley PM, et al: Adolescent risk factors for binge drinking during the transition to young adulthood: Variable- and pattern-centered approaches to change. Dev Psychol 32:659-674, 1996.

110. Cicchetti D, Rogosch FA: Equifinality and multifinality in developmental psychopathology. Dev Psychopathol 8:597-600, 1996.

111. Marsh P, McFarland FC, Allen JP, et al: Attachment, autonomy, and multifinality in adolescent internalizing and risky behavioral symptoms. Dev Psychopathol 15:451-467, 2003.

112. Harrington R, Rutter M, Fombonne E: Developmental pathways in depression: Multiple meanings, antecedents, and endpoints. Dev Psychopathol 8:601-616, 1996.

113. Bardone AM, Moffitt TE, Caspi A, et al: Adult mental health and social outcomes of adolescent girls with

depression and conduct disorder. Dev Psychopathol 8:811-829, 1996.

114. Gjerde PF, Block J: A developmental perspective on depressive symptoms in adolescence: Gender differences in autocentric-allocentric modes of impulse regulation. In Cicchetti D, Toth SL, eds: Adolescence: Opportunities and Challenges, vol 7. Rochester, NY: University of Rochester Press, 1996, pp 167-196.

115. Lacourse E, Nagin D, Tremblay RE, et al: Developmental trajectories of boys' delinquent group membership and facilitation of violent behaviors during adolescence. Dev Psychopathol 15:183-197, 2003.

116. Zucker RA, Ellis DA, Fitzgerald HE, et al: Other evidence for at least two alcoholisms II: Life course variation in antisociality and heterogeneity of alcoholic outcome. Dev Psychopathol 8:831-848, 1996.

117. Broidy LM, Nagin DS, Tremblay RE, et al: Developmental trajectories of childhood disruptive behaviors and adolescent delinquency: A six-site, cross-national study. Dev Psychol 39:222-245, 2003.

118. Bergman LR, Magnusson D: A person-oriented approach in research on developmental psychopathology. Dev Psychopathol 9:291-319, 1997.

119. Garber J, Keiley MK, Martin NC: Developmental trajectories of adolescents' depressive symptoms: Predictors of change. J Consult Clin Psychol 70:79-95, 2002.

120. Brennan PA, Hall J, Bor W, et al: Integrating biological and social processes in relation to early-onset persistent aggression in boys and girls. Dev Psychol 39:309-323, 2003.

121. Brook JS, Kessler RC, Cohen P: The onset of marijuana use from preadolescence and early adolescence to young adulthood. Dev Psychopathol 11:901-914, 1999.

122. Patterson GR, Forgatch MS, Yoerger KL, et al: Variables that initiate and maintain an early-onset trajectory for juvenile offending. Dev Psychopathol 10:531-547, 1998.

123. Hammen C: Cognitive, life stress, and interpersonal approaches to a developmental psychopathology model of depression. Dev Psychopathol 4:189-206, 1992.

124. Petersen AC, Compas BE, Brooks-Gunn J, et al: Depression in adolescence. Am Psychol 48:155-168, 1993.

125. Moffitt TE: Adolescence-limited and life-course–persistent antisocial behavior: A developmental taxonomy. Psychol Rev 100:674-701, 1993.

126. Moffitt TE, Caspi A, Dickson N, et al: Childhood-onset versus adolescent-onset antisocial conduct problems in males: Natural history from ages 3 to 18 years. Dev Psychopathol 8:399-424, 1996.

127. Aguilar B, Sroufe LA, Egeland B, et al: Distinguishing the early-onset/persistent and adolescence-onset antisocial behavior types: From birth to 16 years. Dev Psychopathol 12:109-132, 2000.

128. Moffitt TE, Caspi A, Harrington H, et al: Males on the life-course–persistent and adolescence-limited antisocial pathways: Follow-up at age 26 years. Dev Psychopathol 14:179-207, 2002.

129. Zucker RA, Fitzgerald HE, Moses HD: Emergence of alcohol problems and the several alcoholisms: A developmental perspective on etiologic theory and life course trajectory. In Cicchetti D, Cohen D, eds: Developmental Psychopathology, Volume 2: Risk, Disorder, and Adaptation. New York: Wiley, 1995, pp 677-711.

130. Schulenberg J, Maggs JL, Hurrelmann K: Negotiating developmental transitions during adolescence and young adulthood: Health risks and opportunities. In Schulenberg J, Maggs JL, Hurrelmann K, eds: Health Risks and Developmental Transitions during Adolescence. Cambridge, UK: Cambridge University Press, 1997, pp 1-19.

131. Silverthorn P, Frick PJ: Developmental pathways to antisocial behavior: The delayed-onset pathway in girls. Dev Psychopathol 11:101-126, 1999.

132. Duggal S, Carlson EA, Sroufe LA, Egeland B: Depressive symptomatology in childhood and adolescence. Dev Psychopathol 13:143-164, 2001.

133. Jaffee SR, Moffitt TE, Caspi A, et al: Differences in early childhood risk factors for juvenile-onset and adult-onset depression. Arch Gen Psychiatry 59:215-222, 2002.

134. Cicchetti D, Rogosch FA: Psychopathology as risk for adolescent substance use disorders: A developmental psychopathology perspective. J Clin Child Psychol 28:355-365, 1999.

135. Luthar SS, Doernberger CH, Zigler E: Resilience is not a unidimensional construct: Insights from a prospective study of inner-city adolescents. Dev Psychopathol 5:703-717, 1993.

136. Masten AS, Coatsworth JD: The development of competence in favorable and unfavorable environments: Lessons from research on successful children. Am Psychol 53:205-220, 1998.

137. Stouthamer-Loeber M, Loeber R, Farrington DP, et al: The double edge of protective and risk factors for delinquency: Interrelations and developmental patterns. Dev Psychopathol 5:683-701, 1993.

138. Taylor SE, Klein LC, Lewis BP, et al: Biobehavioral responses to stress in females: Tend-and-befriend, not fight-or-flight. Psychol Rev 107:411-429, 2000.

139. Cederblad M, Dahlin L, Hagnell O, et al: Salutogenic childhood factors reported by middle-aged individuals. Eur Arch Psychiatry Clin Neurosci 244:1-11, 1994.

140. Isaacowitz DM, Seligman ME: Cognitive styles and well-being in adulthood and old age. In Bornstein MH, Davidson L, eds: Well-Being: Positive Development Across the Life Course: Crosscurrents in Contemporary Psychology. Mahwah, NJ: Erlbaum, 2003, pp 449-475.

141. Vitaliano PP, DeWolfe DJ, Maiuro RD, et al: Appraised changeability of a stressor as a modifier of the relationship between coping and depression: A test of the hypothesis of fit. J Pers Soc Psychol 59:582-592, 1990.

142. Vitaliano PP, Maiuro RD, Russo J, et al: Coping profiles associated with psychiatric, physical health, work, and family problems. Health Psychol 9:348-376, 1990.

143. Carver CS, Pozo C, Harris SD, et al: How coping mediates the effect of optimism on distress: A study of women with early stage breast cancer. J Pers Soc Psychol 65:375-390, 1993.

144. Culver JL, Arena PL, Antoni MH, et al: Coping and distress among women and under treatment for early stage breast cancer: Comparing African Americans, Hispanics, and non-Hispanic whites. Psychooncology 11:495-504, 2002.

145. Penedo FJ, Gonzalez JS, Davis C, et al: Coping and psychological distress among symptomatic HIV+ men who have sex with men. Ann Behav Med 25:203-213, 2003.

146. Shapiro ER: Chronic illness as a family process: A social-developmental approach to promoting resilience. J Clin Psychol 58:1375-1384, 2002.

147. Hinshaw SP, Lahey BB, Hart EL: Issues of taxonomy and comorbidity in the development of conduct disorder. Dev Psychopathol 5:31-49, 1993.

148. Achenbach TM: Assessment and Taxonomy of Child and Adolescent Psychopathology, Volume 3: Developmental Clinical Psychology and Psychiatry. Beverly Hills, CA: Sage Publications, 1985.

149. Jessor R, Donovan JE, Costa FM: Beyond Adolescence: Problem Behavior and Young Adult Development. New York: Cambridge University Press, 1991.

150. Jessor R, Jessor SL: Problem Behavior and Psychosocial Development: A Longitudinal Study of Youth. New York: Academic Press, 1977.

151. Bingham CR, Crockett LJ: Longitudinal adjustment patterns of boys and girls experiencing early, middle, and late sexual intercourse. Dev Psychol 32:647-658, 1996.

152. Farrell AD, Danish SJ, Howard CW: Relationship between drug use and other problem behaviors in urban adolescents. J Consult Clin Psychol 60:705-712, 1992.

153. Loeber R, Farrington DP, Stouthamer-Loeber M, et al: Antisocial Behavior and Mental Health Problems: Explanatory Factors in Childhood and Adolescence. Mahwah, NJ: Erlbaum, 1998.

154. Capaldi DM: Co-occurrence of conduct problems and depressive symptoms in early adolescent boys: I. Familial factors and general adjustment at grade 6. Dev Psychopathol 3:277-300, 1991.

155. Aseltine RH, Gore S, Colten ME: The co-occurrence of depression and substance abuse in late adolescence. Dev Psychopathol 10:549-570, 1998.

156. Bird H, Gould M, Staghezza-Jaramillo B: The comorbidity of ADHD in a community sample of children aged 6 through 16 years. J Child Fam Stud 3:365-378, 1990.

157. Hinshaw SP: On the distinction between attentional problems/hyperactivity and conduct problems/aggression in child psychopathology. Psychol Bull 101:443-463, 1987.

158. Biederman J, Newcorn J, Sprich S: Comorbidity of attention deficit hyperactivity disorder with conduct, depressive, anxiety, and other disorders. Am J Psychiatry 148:564-577, 1991.

159. A 14-month randomized clinical trial of treatment strategies for attention deficit hyperactivity disorder. The MTA Cooperative Group. Multimodal treatment study of children with ADHD. Arch Gen Psychiatry 56:1073-1086, 1999.

160. Eiraldi RB, Power TJ, Nezu CM: Patterns of comorbidity associated with subtypes of attention-deficit/hyperactivity disorder among 6- to 12-year-old children. J Am Acad Child Adolesc Psychiatry 36:503-514, 1997.

161. Barkley RA: Attention-Deficit Hyperactivity Disorder: A Handbook for Diagnosis and Treatment. New York: Guilford, 1990.

162. Cantwell DP, Baker L: Attention deficit disorder with and without hyperactivity: A review and comparison of matched groups. J Am Acad Child Adolesc Psychiatry 31:432-438, 1992.

163. Eccles JS, Midgley C, Wigfield A, et al: Development during adolescence: The impact of stage-environment fit in young adolescents' experiences in schools and in families. Am Psychol 48:90-101, 1993.

164. Eccles JS, Midgley C: Stage-environment fit: Developmentally appropriate classrooms for young adolescents. In Ames C, Ames R, eds: Research on Motivation in Education: Goals and Cognitions, vol 3. San Diego, CA: Academic Press, 1989, pp 139-186.

165. Fuligni AJ, Eccles JS: Perceived parent-child relationships and early adolescents' orientation toward peers. Dev Psychol 29:622-632, 1993.

166. Collins WA: Parent-child relationships in the transition to adolescence: Continuity and change in interaction, affect, and cognition. In Montemayor R, Adams G, Gullotta T, eds: Advances in Adolescent Development: From Childhood to Adolescence: A Transitional Period? Vol 2. Beverly Hills, CA: Sage Publications, 1990, pp 85-106.

167. Eccles JS, Buchanan CM, Flanagan C, et al: Control versus autonomy during early adolescence. J Soc Issues 47:53-68, 1991.

168. Garcia Coll CT, Akerman A, Cicchetti D: Cultural influences on developmental processes and outcomes: Implications for the study of development and psychopathology. Dev Psychopathol 12:333-356, 2000.

169. Rutter M: Antisocial behavior: developmental psychopathology perspectives. In Stoff DM, Breiling J, eds: Handbook of Antisocial Behavior. New York: Wiley, 1997, pp 115-124.

170. Cauce AM, Domenech-Rodriguez M, Paradise M, et al: Cultural and contextual influences in mental health help-seeking: A focus on ethnic minority youth. J Consult Clin Psychol 70:44-45, 2002.

171. Hallowell AI: Culture and mental disorder. J Abnorm Soc Psychol 29:1-9, 1934.

172. Greenberger E, Chen C: Perceived family relationships and depressed mood in early and late adolescence: A comparison of European and Asian Americans. Dev Psychol 32:707-716, 1996.

173. Taylor RD: Adolescents' perceptions of kinship support and family management practices: Association with adolescent adjustment in African American families. Dev Psychol 32:687-695, 1996.

174. Garcia Coll CT, Magnuson K: Cultural influences on child development: Are we ready for a paradigm shift? *In* Nelson C, Masten A, eds: Minnesota Symposium on Child Psychology, vol 29. Mahwah, NJ: Erlbaum, 1999, pp 1-24.

175. Cooper CR, Jackson JF, Azmitia M, et al: Multiple selves, multiple worlds: Three useful strategies for research with ethnic minority youth on identity, relationships, and opportunity structures. *In* McLoyd VC, Steinberg L, eds: Studying Minority Adolescents: Conceptual, Methodological, and Theoretical Issues. Hillsdale, NJ: Erlbaum, 1998, pp 111-125.

176. Sameroff A, Fiese B: Transactional regulation and early interaction. *In* Meisels S, Shonkoff J, eds: Handbook of Early Intervention. New York: Cambridge University Press, 1990, pp 119-149.

177. Toth SL, Cicchetti D: Developmental psychopathology and child psychotherapy. *In* Russ S, Ollendick T, eds: Handbook of Psychotherapies with Children and Families. New York: Plenum Press, 1999, pp 15-44.

178. Feldman SS, Elliott GR, eds: At the Threshold: The Developing Adolescent. Cambridge, MA: Harvard University Press, 1990.

179. Holmbeck GN, Colder C, Shapera W, et al: Working with adolescents: Guides from developmental psychology. *In* Kendall PC, ed: Child & Adolescent Therapy: Cognitive-Behavioral Procedures, 2nd ed. New York: Guilford, 2000, pp 334-385.

180. American Psychological Association: Developing Adolescents: A Reference for Professionals. Washington, DC: American Psychological Association, 2002.

181. Hill JP: Understanding Early Adolescence: A Framework. Carrboro, NC: Center for Early Adolescence, 1980.

182. Holmbeck GN: A model of family relational transformations during the transition to adolescence: Parent-adolescent conflict and adaptation. *In* Graber JA, Brooks-Gunn J, Petersen AC, eds: Transitions through Adolescence: Interpersonal Domains and Context. Mahwah, NJ: Erlbaum, 1996, pp 167-199.

183. Holmbeck GN, Updegrove AL: Clinical-developmental interface: Implications of developmental research for adolescent psychotherapy. Psychotherapy 32:16-33, 1995.

184. Steinberg L: Adolescence, 6th ed. Boston, MA: McGraw-Hill, 2002.

185. Grotevant HD: Adolescent development in family contexts. *In* Damon W, ed: Handbook of Child Psychology, vol 3: Social, Emotional and Personality Development (Eisenberg, N., Series ed.), New York: Wiley, 1997, pp 1097-1149.

186. Holmbeck GN, Shapera WFA: Research methods with adolescents. *In* Kendall PC, Butcher JN, Holmbeck GN, eds: Handbook of Research Methods in Clinical Psychology, 2nd ed. New York: Wiley, 1999, pp 634-661.

187. Magnusson D, Stattin H, Allen VL: A longitudinal study of some adjustment processes from mid-adolescence to adulthood. J Youth Adolesc 14:267-283, 1985.

188. Moos RH, Tsu UD: The crisis of physical illness: An overview. *In* Moos RH, ed: Coping with Physical Illness. New York: Plenum Press, 1977, pp 3-21.

189. Wallander JL, Varni JW: Effects of pediatric chronic physical disorders on child and family adjustment. J Child Psychol Psychiatry 39:29-46, 1997.

190. Fiese BH, Sameroff AJ: Family context in pediatric psychology: A transactional perspective. *In* Roberts MC, Wallander JL, eds: Family Issues in Pediatric Psychology. Hillsdale, NJ: Erlbaum, 1992, pp 239-260.

191. La Greca AM, Bearman KJ: Adherence to pediatric treatment regimens. *In* Roberts MC, ed: Handbook of Pediatric Psychology. New York: Guilford, 2003, pp 119-140.

192. Becker MH, Maiman LA, Kirscht JP, et al: Patient perceptions and compliance: Recent studies of the health belief model. *In* Haynes RB, Taylor DW, Sackett DL, eds: Compliance in Health Care. Baltimore, MD: The Johns Hopkins University Press, 1979, pp 78-109.

193. Bandura A: Self-Efficacy: The Exercise of Control. New York: Freeman, 1997.

194. Prochaska JL, DiClemente CC: The Transtheoretical Approach: Crossing Traditional Boundaries of Change. Homewood, IL: Dorsey, 1984.

195. Skinner BF: Science and Human Behavior. New York: Macmillan, 1953.

196. Powers SW: Empirically supported treatments in pediatric psychology: Procedure-related pain. J Pediatr Psychol 24:131-145, 1999.

197. Fiese BH, Wilder J, Bickham NL: Family context in developmental psychopathology. *In* Sameroff AJ, Lewis M, Miller SM, eds: Handbook of Developmental Psychopathology, 2nd ed. Dordrecht, The Netherlands: Kluwer, 2000, pp 115-134.

198. Sameroff AJ, MacKenzie MJ: Research strategies for capturing transactional models of development: The limits of the possible. Dev Psychopathol 15:613-640, 2003.

199. Brown RT: Society of pediatric psychology presidential address: Toward a social ecology of pediatric psychology. J Pediatr Psychol 27:191-201, 2002.

Research Foundations, Methods, and Issues in Developmental-Behavioral Pediatrics

DAVID J. SCHONFELD ▨ BENARD P. DREYER

THE UNIQUE NATURE OF DEVELOPMENTAL-BEHAVIORAL PEDIATRIC RESEARCH

The scope of research in the field of developmental-behavioral pediatrics (DBP) is as diverse and rich as the clinical field itself. A wide range of research methods and analytical techniques accounts for both its depth and its complexity. The same characteristics of research in the field that render the potential for its findings to be of such practical significance and relevance often pose critical challenges to ensuring its scientific validity.

The research and the associated research teams are often multidisciplinary, permitting an application of various methodological approaches. The field of DBP permits integration of complementary theoretical perspectives and methods, such as the blending or juxtaposition of quantitative methods characteristic of medical science with qualitative approaches more typical of social science research. Research training in the field is therefore more eclectic and broader than in subspecialties that rely almost exclusively on basic science techniques. The field does not have one well-circumscribed set of research methods that can be mastered in a relatively short time. For quality research in DBP, multidisciplinary teams must consist of individuals who can each contribute their own perspective and skills, and each team member must be adequately informed of the basic principles inherent in the research approaches of the other disciplines.

DBP research often aims to study the full spectrum of child development and behavior: from normal variations to concerns or problems to clinical disorders. One of the driving forces for establishing the American Psychiatric Association's *Diagnostic and Statistical Manual of Mental Disorders* was to standardize the diagnostic criteria for disorders to foster consistency in research in mental illness.[1] Research that incorporates the continuum of developmental and behavioral difficulties must establish reliable and valid outcome measures for subthreshold or problem conditions or criteria for identifying where on the bell-shape curve of behavior or development is the appropriate cutoff for defining a concern or a problem. Although achieving reliability in delineating the diagnostic criteria for a mental illness may be challenging, it is often even more elusive for a behavioral problem or personality trait. One common approach is to inquire whether the characteristic of interest (e.g., attention) is believed to occur significantly more often in one person than in typical peers of the same age or developmental level and to require an association with some perceived impairment (e.g., attention-deficit/hyperactivity disorder [ADHD]). This approach often introduces a reliance on subjective, self-reported measures of perceived impairment or relative deviation from perceived norms that can compromise validity and produce a reporting bias.

Research in DBP often addresses more abstract issues, such as community support or adjustment to illness. Because much of the research addresses such common topics, the researcher may assume that the methodology is therefore "simple." But, in fact, operationalizing these variables and developing and validating relevant measures are difficult. Much of the research in DBP involves measuring constructs for which validated measures do not already exist and for which objective, concrete biological outcome measures are not feasible.

Because DBP often assumes an ecological perspective, researchers are more apt to look critically at sociocultural influences on child development and behavior. Such factors are difficult to measure, even harder to report accurately, and far more difficult to interpret or explain. The use of race and ethnicity as explanatory variables illustrate the complexity of this issue.[2] Researchers who understand the complexity of social and cultural influences appreciate the futility of controlling for all relevant influences within an ecological model.

Despite these challenges, the complexity of research design issues in DBP fosters its richness. The multiple perspectives and theories and the diversity of available methodological approaches enable the construction of rich, multidimensional theoretical models. Researchers must necessarily explore not only outcome measures but also mediators and moderators (see Chapter 2). The complexity is increased by the factor of time and the challenges inherent in measuring one construct in the context of a child's developmental trajectory. For example, in studies of the influences of early childhood experiences on later language outcomes, investigators need to consider not only the multiple environmental, familial, cultural, and community factors that may influence language development but also the reality that developmental processes are not static in the individual child. Parsing out how much of change in language development is attributable to the normative process of child development ot to inherent deficits in the child, social, environmental, family or community factors, or the unanticipated effect of uncontrolled historical events (such as changes in preschool policy or educational interventions) can be daunting.

CROSS-CUTTING METHODOLOGICAL AND THEORETICAL ISSUES

The nature of DBP research introduces a range of cross-cutting methodological and theoretical concerns that must be addressed to ensure the validity of the findings. This section highlights select examples that illustrate the complexity of the issues that are involved.

Incorporating Child Development within Child Development Research

Central to any research in the area of child development is an appreciation that children's capabilities and behavior change over time as a result of developmental processes, independent of other factors or interventions. Measures of skills or capabilities therefore need to be adjusted and compared with norms for different ages/stages, introducing analytical concerns for cross-sectional studies involving children of different ages or developmental stages. Measurements of the effect of interventions provided over time may also

be compromised by analytical concerns inherent in measuring the same domain at different developmental stages, which may necessitate the use of different age/stage-appropriate instruments or, at the very least, correction for age/stage. In addition, measurement of children's abilities may be confounded by the child's developmental capacity to understand instructions and communicate comprehension. For example, young children have been described as having difficulty appreciating the perspective of someone else. It is possible that such difficulty may result, at least in part, from limitations in their ability to comprehend the task requested, their language ability to communicate their understanding, or the researcher's ability to communicate the task required. Research on young children's understanding of the concepts of human immunodeficiency virus (HIV) and acquired immunodeficiency syndrome (AIDS) initially suggested that young children's understanding of core concepts of illness was significantly limited developmentally, which seriously constrained their capacity to benefit from educational interventions; however, subsequent research demonstrated that a developmentally based educational intervention could result in dramatic gains in young children's conceptual understanding in this area.[3] In other words, what appeared at first to be a limitation in children's ability to learn was subsequently found to represent limitations in adults' understanding of how to teach effectively and/or in researchers' ability to measure validly children's underlying comprehension.

Inclusion of Children with Disabilities in Research Protocols

A child with a motor disability may engage in less play activities with peers during a play observation directly because of impairments in motor function. Alternatively, the child's motor disability may have resulted in fewer opportunities for social interaction in the past, which in turn resulted in less well-developed peer interactions that are subsequently manifested by decreased peer engagement in peer play activities during the observation period. It therefore becomes important to select measures of function (in this example, a measure of peer interaction) that are not confounded by the child's underlying disability. More subtle influences could be anticipated for the effect of sociocultural or personality factors, which would be difficult to identify and confirm.

The Biopsychosocial Model

The biopsychosocial model emphasizes the complementary influences of genetic predisposition, environmental factors, and experience on development and behavior. DBP research encompasses basic science and social science research methods, allowing the demonstration of causal mechanisms by which environmental and experiential factors alter basic biological processes. For example, to study the influence of early stressful experience on later hyperactivity of neurons that release corticotropin-releasing factor as a cause of adult anxiety or depressive disorders, both stressful experiences and neuronal function must be measured, and the potential confounders of both must be understood.

State versus Trait Measures

In accordance with the biopsychosocial model, many behavioral constructs represent both intrinsic traits of an individual and transient states influenced by recent circumstances and environmental factors. This poses measurement challenges. For example, changes in repeat measures of anxiety may reflect concerns with test-retest reliability or variations in state anxiety over time.

Instrument Development

Many of the outcomes of interest to the field of DBP lack well-validated and standardized measures. Researchers in DBP are therefore often faced with the additional challenge of developing and standardizing new measures and demonstrating their validity. Competing theoretical constructs pose a challenge for achieving construct validity; the absence of well-accepted "gold standards" and objective biological or physical endpoints (e.g., for a measure of coping with the death of a parent) is a major challenge for demonstrating criterion-related concurrent or predictive validity. Researchers must often select measures that were standardized for populations that differ from the current study population in critical ways (e.g., language, culture, social class) and require restandardization. This is highly relevant to testing of certain variables and domains that are central to DBP research, such as children's intelligence and language. Because the ecological perspective underlies much of DBP research, many instruments measure domains that are intrinsically sensitive to sociocultural influences.

Survey Development

Many of the variables of interest in DBP research relate to perceptions, feelings, or other constructs that rely on self-report. Surveys are often used to assess outcome measures. Researchers need to be able to construct effective and valid questionnaires. Method-

ological issues relate to sentence or instrument construction, such as question structure (e.g., open-ended vs. close-ended questions), formatting, or wording (e.g., clarity, neutrality, nonleading, reading level, culturally appropriate). Other issues include the construction of scales and summary scores and validation of the instrument, as well as variation introduced by the means of administration of the survey (e.g., self-administered, administered by interviewer, computer, or Web-based administration). Comparable issues of construction and administration are evident for structured and semistructured interviews. Knowing what to ask is the first step; knowing how to ask (and score the responses) is particularly challenging and relevant for DBP research.

Reliance on Parent Report

Young age and cognitive delays, when present, may preclude children's ability to provide independent reports of experiences, perceptions, or feelings. Self-report by children may also be constrained by their reluctance to disclose sensitive information. In these settings, parental report may be an acceptable proxy. Reliance on parental report often leads to an underestimate of children's exposure (such as that observed with parental report regarding young children's exposure to violence) and feelings and internalizing symptoms (e.g., depression, anxiety, fears, pain). The construction of more developmentally appropriate instruments for self-reports of young children (such as utilizing pictures or storytelling) allows even younger children to provide self-reports. In addition, parental reports of children's symptoms are influenced by the parents' own perceptions or state (e.g., parents who are themselves depressed may either attribute similar feelings to their children or be less sensitive to or aware of their children's difficulties). These limitations highlight the value of triangulation of data: the use of multiple instruments to provide reports from different reporters (e.g., child, parent, and teacher) and to compare results across these different perspectives. The validity of individual reports is thereby strengthened through the congruence of data from multiple sources.

Qualitative Methods

Qualitative research methods are most appropriate in situations in which little is known about a phenomenon or when attempts are being made to generate new theories or revise preexisting theories. Qualitative research is inductive rather than deductive and is used to describe phenomena in detail, without answering questions of causality or demonstrating clear relationships among variables. Researchers in

DBP should be familiar with common ethnographic methods, such as participant observation (useful for studying interactions and behavior), ethnographic interviewing (useful for studying personal experiences and perspectives), and focus groups (involving moderated discussion to glean information about a specific area of interest relatively rapidly). In comparison with quantitative research, qualitative methods entail different sampling procedures (e.g., purposive rather than random or consecutive sampling; "snow-balling," which involves identifying cases with connections to other cases), different sample size requirements (e.g., the researcher may sample and analyze in an iterative manner until data saturation occurs, so that no new themes or hypotheses are generated on subsequent analysis), different data management and analytic techniques (e.g., reduction of data to key themes and ideas, which are then coded and organized into domains that yield tentative impressions and hypotheses, which serve as the basis of the next set of data collection, continuing until data saturation occurs and final concepts are generated), and different conventions for writing up and presenting data and analyses. The strength of the findings is maximized through triangulation of data, investigator (e.g., use of researchers from different disciplines and perspectives or several researchers to independently code the same data), theory (i.e., use of multiple perspectives), or method (e.g., use of focus groups and individual interviews to obtain complementary data).

Intervention Fidelity and Treatment Dose

Interventions are often delivered in naturalistic and group settings by individuals who are not part of the research team, such as teachers, parents, and home visitors. Although this allows for the testing of interventions that are much more likely to generalize to the general population, distortions in the delivery of the intervention may occur. Research requires measures of the intervention fidelity (i.e., the degree to which the intervention is delivered in the manner intended by the researcher) and treatment dose (the extent to which the subject participates in or receives the full intervention). A study of a school-based intervention delivered by regular classroom teachers needs not only a strong method for teacher training and monitoring but also explicit measures of how the teachers delivered the intervention and the degree to which students attended and/or received the full intervention. Such monitoring may include a mix of quantitative measures (e.g., curriculum checklists, student attendance records, self-reports of teacher

satisfaction with the intervention) and qualitative assessments (e.g., ethnographic observations of classrooms while lessons are being taught, focus groups of teachers, or individual interviews). Other measures (i.e., triangulation) may be used to confirm teacher reports of intervention fidelity or treatment dose, such as asking students to complete a questionnaire about simple concepts or facts from the intervention, to test whether children were exposed to the relevant lessons.

Efficacy verses Effectiveness

Clinical trials involve optimal control in the selection of subjects, and the intervention and the dependent measures are applied so that the most rigorous application and observation of the results can be obtained. The intent is to determine the efficacy of the interventions. However, the evidence may be limited to a narrowly defined group of children, such as those with ADHD without comorbid conditions, or to an application of the intervention that is not practical to use in a real-world setting, such as one requiring too much time or training than is practical for most practicing clinicians. Determining effectiveness involves assessing the effects of an intervention in actual settings. Balancing the need for what is practical and what is rigorous is a creative challenge. Of importance is trying to maintain the elements of randomization, comparative groups, and independent measures. Effectiveness is one of the elements studied in what is now categorized as health services research.

Clustering and Nested Analyses

Interventions delivered in group settings may introduce variability caused by clustering: children are members of classes, which are parts of schools, which are parts of school districts, and so forth. In this manner, the variability in children's individual responses on outcome measures may be explained in part by variability in some of the group-level variables (e.g., the variability in teacher, school climate, school district practice). Nested analyses are then necessary to attempt to estimate the percentage of the variance attributed to the clustering, which requires larger sample sizes and the collection of group-level measures.

Placebo Effects

The use of a placebo in psychosocial interventions is less clear than in medication trials. Some studies utilize alternative interventions (e.g., the control group for a study of hypnosis to decrease pain in children with a chronic condition might receive education about an unrelated component of their condition). The limited empirical evidence on how "counseling" or "therapy" works contributes to difficulties in controlling for all components that may be involved in a therapeutic or placebo effect. Furthermore, if individuals report less pain or subjective discomfort after the use of an interpersonal placebo intervention, such as the psychoeducational component of the example just described, should the placebo then be considered as a possibly effective, alternative form of treatment (e.g., perhaps informal group support occurred as a result of the psychoeducational sessions that decreased parental anxiety, that in turn decreased the child's anxiety and perceptions of discomfort or pain)?

Advocacy

Intrinsic to the field of DBP is an explicit value placed on advocacy. Researchers have to be ever mindful of the potential for bias to influence study design or interpretation of results. Ethical concerns may also become evident if interventions valued by members of the professional or lay community (e.g., home visitation, early intervention, supportive psychotherapy, drug prevention curricula, infant daycare) are not supported by the findings of a research project or when "interventions" thought to be damaging to children (e.g., gang enrollment, parental divorce, employment during childhood) yield unexpected positive findings (e.g., increased self-esteem, decreased anxiety, increased problem-solving skills) or neutral results. The inclination to withhold publication or reporting of such "negative" studies may be quite strong, because of the desire to protect the interests of children and families. Researchers must engage in some introspection with regard to their biases, develop methods that limit the likely effects of such biases, and maintain the integrity to report findings, even if the findings run counter to the researchers' presumptions.

ETHICAL ISSUES

The nature of research in the field of DBP introduces some ethical issues that, although not necessarily unique, may occur with greater frequency or complexity than in other fields. This section illustrates the range of issues that may be encountered.

Socially Sensitive Topics

Research in DBP often involves exploring socially sensitive topics, such as bias against individuals with disabilities, stigma related to mental illness, and sexuality among individuals with developmental disabilities. The extreme sensitivity necessary to engage prospective study subjects and their communities may undermine the research team's willingness to conduct the open and frank discussions necessary to ensure informed consent. Presenting the results of such studies in a public forum is often met with considerable controversy that makes it particularly difficult to present objective findings in an atmosphere of open disclosure.

Prevention of Disclosure of Confidential Information

Inquiry into highly confidential information, such as mental health status or criminal or antisocial beliefs and behaviors, may heighten concerns about the accidental disclosure of highly confidential, personal information. Because the focus of these studies is often to explore the reasons for such outcomes or behaviors, subjects and other informants are typically asked a wide range of highly personal questions, not only about their behaviors but also about the possible reasons for these behaviors. This further increases the amount of highly confidential information obtained for research purposes and results in the need for extreme care to prevent unintended disclosure.

Withholding Explicit Intent of Studies

Informed consent protocols may need to include some element of withholding the explicit purpose of the research study, in order to permit a relatively unbiased collection of data. For example, if researchers are studying reporting bias and aim to compare the validity of self-reports of smoking in the presence or absence of concurrent measurement of salivary nicotine metabolites, it would be very difficult to obtain valid results after informing subjects of the study's intent. Clarifying the distinction between deception and providing accurate but less than complete information to avoid overly biasing subjects (e.g., in this example, stating that the purpose of the study is simply to measure individuals' tobacco use) is often difficult but crucial.

The Ability to Provide Consent and Assent

Research in DBP often involves participation of research subjects who have cognitive/developmental limitations that affect their ability to provide consent or assent. Studies may also involve the collection of data from individuals who report on characteristics of the family, community, or other groups. In such situations, ethical concerns may be raised about the ability of the individual (especially when that individual is a minor) to provide potentially sensitive information about others.[4]

The Use of a Placebo

Despite limited evidence for the efficacy of specific psychological or behavioral interventions, ethical concerns may be raised about random assignment of subjects to a nonintervention control group when such interventions are the community norm. For example, despite limited data to support the efficacy of supportive counseling after a traumatic experience, communities are unlikely to accept "sham" or "placebo" mental health interventions to document the efficacy and control for potential biases. The use of a placebo in medication trials is more commonly accepted than the use of a placebo in psychological or behavioral intervention trials.

IMPLICATIONS FOR RESEARCH TRAINING IN DEVELOPMENTAL-BEHAVIORAL PEDIATRICS

The eclectic and complex nature of research in DBP requires that research training be broad. The mixing of qualitative and quantitative methods, the need for the development of valid and reliable measures for complex constructs, the importance of sociocultural influences, and the need for repeated measurements over time mandate rich and varied educational experience in research methods. Training should include a strong foundation in the basics of research design, as well as a focus on qualitative methods, instrument and survey development, and the use of large datasets. Skills in clinical epidemiology and evidence-based medicine are important for performing research related to diagnosis, screening, and prevention, as well as for understanding the validity and strength of findings. An understanding of statistical methods for data analysis, both bivariate and multivariate, is important for both the appropriate design of studies and the evaluation of study results. DBP researchers should also be educated in the principles of the responsible conduct of research, especially the special protection necessary for children and other vulnerable populations. Finally, training in all aspects of scientific communication, for presentations, publications, and teaching, must be provided.

In addition to the need for a broad-based training in research methods, the specific issues elucidated previously have important and specific implications for research training of developmental-behavioral pediatricians. These implications are discussed as follows.

Training in Quasi-experimental and Observational (Epidemiological) Research Designs

The majority of research in DBP does not involve double-blind, randomized, controlled trials (RCTs). Double-blind RCTs are conducted in studies of psychopharmacological therapy for such conditions as ADHD and autistic spectrum disorders, and single-blind RCTs are conducted for behavioral and educational interventions for the treatment or the prevention of developmental and behavioral disorders. Examples of the latter include the High/Scope Perry preschool study[5] and the Hawaii home visiting study.[6] However, many important nonpharmacological interventions in DBP are difficult to randomize. New educational interventions in the school setting, for example, are likely to be offered to whole classes or schools rather than to randomly selected students, with other classes in the same school or other schools in the same district acting as controls after being matched on a variety of characteristics. These "quasi-experimental" designs play an important role in DBP research.

Research training should, therefore, include education in quasi-experimental designs. A quasi-experimental design is similar to an experimental design except that it lacks the important step of randomization.[7] The most common type of quasi-experimental design involves the use of nonequivalent matching groups. One cohort of children receives an intervention, whereas another matched cohort acts as a control or receives an alternative intervention. Quasi-experimental designs such as this, although frequently the only possible design for some nonpharmacological interventions, suffer from the threat to their validity of selection bias. Education concerning the identification of selection bias and methods to reduce its effect (such as matching, sample stratification, and adjusting for potential confounders) is important for the developmental-behavioral researcher.[8]

Furthermore, researchers in DBP frequently seek to study the effects of harmful and protective factors on childhood outcomes in normative or at-risk populations or to elucidate underlying constructs associated with or causing various outcomes. The study of naturally occurring constructs or of potentially harmful factors leads to choosing observational designs rather than experimental designs.[8]

Observational designs in DBP research are usually single- or double-cohort studies. Single-cohort studies usually involve monitoring a group of children and looking for factors that are predictive of outcomes. For example, the researcher may want to monitor a group of children with intrauterine exposure to cocaine, or with very low birth weight, and determine whether breastfeeding or maternal expectations lead to improved developmental outcomes. Double-cohort studies usually involve a comparison group. For example, a study may compare the incidence of behavior problems in cocaine-exposed infants when they reach preschool with that in a matched group of children. Single-cohort studies may lead to spurious results because of confounding factors. Double-cohort studies, like quasi-experimental designs, may be threatened by selection bias. The DBP researcher should receive in-depth training in these observational study designs and in methods to adjust for confounding and to minimize selection bias.

In addition, the researcher should receive training to understand concerns about inferring causality from results of observational studies and to devise strategies to enhance causal inference (e.g., inclusion and exclusion criteria, matching, and stratification). The principles of strength of evidence for causality—temporality, effect size, dose-response relationships, biological plausibility, reversibility, specificity of results, and consistency of results across studies—should be clearly understood.

Training in Qualitative Methods

Qualitative research designs play an important role in developmental-behavioral research. For example, in one study, investigators sought to understand Latina mothers' cognition and attitudes concerning stimulant medication for ADHD and how these factors might determine adherence to medication regimens and resistance to starting drug therapy.[9] Qualitative methods are the best approach to this type of research question, with which investigators seek to understand the perspectives of persons or groups and to develop and revise research hypotheses. Therefore, a strong foundation in qualitative methods is important for DBP researchers. Training should include providing an understanding of the types of research questions that qualitative methods are best suited to answer, skills in the use of common ethnographic methods, facility with methods used for data coding and data reduction, and familiarity with methods used to ensure trustworthiness of qualitative research results.[10-13]

Training in the Development and Validation of Testing Instruments and Scales

Many of the outcomes and constructs of DBP lack well-standardized or validated measures. Furthermore, even well-validated and reliable measures developed for a general population may not be appropriate for use in a special population. Therefore, the development and validation of such measures are frequent subjects of a research study or are common components of a larger research project. For example, in one study, investigators sought to measure self-efficacy and expectations for self-management among adolescents with chronic disease (diabetes) and to determine the effects of these factors on disease management outcomes.[14] However, there existed no scale for measuring self-efficacy or measuring expectations for self-management of diabetes. Therefore, the researchers had to develop their own scales and test the reliability and validity of those scales before answering the underlying research question. In another study, researchers wanted to determine whether the Pediatric Symptom Checklist,[15] a commonly used screen for behavior problems in a general population, was valid for use in a chronically ill population.[16] In this case, the researchers sought to test the construct validity of a well-validated scale on a new population.

Therefore, research training should include skills in test development, including testing for reliability (with measures such as test-retest reliability and interrater reliability), internal consistency, and validity. The researcher should be familiar with the different types of validity, including content and sampling validity, construct validity, and criterion-related validity, and be able to use methods that assess them.[17]

Training in the Use of Large Secondary Datasets

Research publications increasingly reflect the efforts of researchers to mine large secondary datasets, including federally funded national databases, administrative databases, and electronic medical records, for information related to delivery of care and outcomes in DBP. This type of research has been especially fruitful in the study of ADHD. In one published study, the researchers used the National Ambulatory Medical Care Survey and the National Hospital Ambulatory Medical Care Survey to study regional and ethnic differences in the diagnosis of ADHD and receipt of psychotropic medications for that diagnosis.[18] In another, investigators used health maintenance organization (HMO) data to compare total health care costs for children with and without ADHD.[19] Researchers at the Mayo Clinic have used their computerized medical records database, which has information on 95% of the population in Olmstead County, Minnesota, from 1977 to the present. They have studied ADHD, autism, psychostimulant treatment, and learning disabilities, among other topics.[20-22] Finally, Rappley and colleagues used Medicaid database information to sound an alarm about apparent excessive prescription of psychotropic medication for preschool children.[23]

These studies demonstrate that large datasets contain potential answers to clinical, epidemiological, policy, and health finance questions important to DBP. Research training should provide the knowledge and skills to evaluate these large datasets and to use appropriate sampling and statistical methods in subsequent data analysis. Training should also focus on the types of information collected by cross-sectional and longitudinal national survey datasets, as well as the advantages and disadvantages of using national survey data to answer research questions. Familiarity with health plan administrative datasets, electronic medical records, and disease registries may also be useful for the researcher interested in epidemiological questions concerning disease rates and distribution, utilization of resources, and resulting costs.

Training in Multivariate Statistical Analyses

As a consequence of the frequent use of quasi-experimental and observational study designs in DBP research, training in statistical methods that adjust for confounding factors and that determine unique and independent contributions of hypothesized factors to patient outcomes is essential. Research training should focus on such commonly used statistical techniques as multiple linear regression,[24] analysis of covariance (ANCOVA), and logistic regression.[25] Although training goals may vary in the level of expertise from "educated consumer" of statistical services to independent producer of statistical analyses, the DBP researcher should be skilled in the interpretation of the results of these analyses, knowledgeable about the different types of statistical models, and able to recognize the pitfalls and limitations of these techniques.

Measurement of psychological or behavioral characteristics with scales frequently necessitates an analysis of data for the underlying factors or constructs embodied by the measured variables. Factor analysis is employed to reduce measured variables to a smaller number of underlying "latent" variables. Factor analysis is frequently used to explore and confirm the construct validity of a new scale or a previously validated scale for use in a new population. In addition, factor scores may be used to substitute for variables in other statistical analyses. Because research in DBP often involves the development of new measures for abstract outcomes, factor analysis is a useful statistical method for DBP researchers. For example, factor analysis was used to develop new scales in the previously noted study[14] in which investigators sought to compare self-efficacy and expectations for diabetic management to diabetes self-management outcomes. They then used the scores on these scales, including a separate score for each of two identified factors, in multiple regression analyses of the relationships between these constructs. In another previously cited study,[16] researchers used factor analysis to compare items on the Pediatric Symptom Checklist[15] in a chronically ill population with those in a general population.

Therefore, an understanding of the role of factor analysis in the development and validation of testing instruments and scales is important for the DBP researcher. Familiarity with methods of extraction of factors from the collected data, procedures for keeping and discarding factors, and other aspects of factor analysis are an important part of research training.[26-28]

Training in Neurobiological and Genetic Science

The frequently used multidisciplinary approach to DBP, as well as the importance of the biopsychosocial model, requires the DBP researcher to collaborate with other scientists who use research techniques by which they attempt to elucidate the neurobiological and genetic bases for development, behavior, and learning. The researcher needs to be familiar with and understand these basic sciences and scientific methods in order to interpret the scientific literature and to generate new research questions for investigation.

A growing body of research has focused on the use of neuroimaging techniques to elucidate brain function and anatomical location of activation during behavioral and psychological tasks. Functional magnetic resonance imaging (fMRI) has become an important tool in developmental-behavioral research. Unlike positron emission tomography (PET) and single photon emission computed tomography (SPECT), fMRI does not include the injection of radioactive materials. Therefore, children can undergo imaging repeatedly, which allows for study during different disease states or throughout developmental changes. It also allows the researcher to study healthy children at low risk for the disorder under investigation. For example, using fMRI, researchers have sought to localize the areas of brain activation with attention or reading tasks in children with ADHD or dyslexia and compare those activation patterns with patterns in normal children.[29,30] Other researchers have used brain proton magnetic resonance spectroscopy to identify children with brain creatine deficiency who have global developmental delay.[31] It is likely that functional neuroimaging techniques will play an important role in the future study of the neurobiological basis of developmental and behavioral problems or conditions. Future researchers should receive training in the science of these techniques to enable them to collaborate with neuroradiologists in answering questions that span the spectrum of the biopsychosocial model.

Similarly, training in the genetics of developmental and behavioral disorders is important for researchers. Understanding the role of genetics will empower the researcher to incorporate genetics into research hypotheses and methods. One area that should be considered for inclusion in research training is quantitative behavioral genetics.[32] In this field, investigators seek to determine the proportion of variance in behaviors resulting from heritability, shared environment (family, neighborhood, home environment), and unshared environment (e.g., peers, teachers, differential parental treatment, illnesses). For example, one article focused on the quantitative behavioral genetics of child temperament.[33]

Another important area for research is the association of behavioral phenotypes with molecular genetic findings and variations. Behavioral and psychoeducational profiles have been elucidated through research for velocardiofacial, Williams, Down, Prader-Willi, fragile X, and Turner syndromes, among others.[34] Studies have shown associations of these behavioral and psychological characteristics with specific molecular genetic patterns. The availability of molecular genetic techniques has also allowed scientists to study behavioral phenotypes of subjects with "milder" genetic deficits. For example, in one study, researchers found an association of fragile X premutation (carriers) with autistic spectrum diagnosis through the use of molecular genetic studies.[35] Other researchers have been studying polymorphisms in specific genes, such as the dopamine D_4 receptor gene (*D4DR*) and the serotonin transporter promoter gene (*5-HTTLPR*), and finding associations with ADHD and temperamental traits.[36,37] Collaboration between DBP researchers and geneticists and the use of molecular genetics technology are likely to yield important findings concerning the etiology of developmental-behavioral disorders and normative behavior patterns.

SUMMARY

The field of DBP encompasses the full spectrum of child development and behavior, drawing from multiple theoretical orientations and incorporating the expertise of a wide variety of complementary disciplines. The biopsychosocial perspective requires an integration of basic and social sciences; the ecological perspective requires careful attention to sociocultural influences. As a result, research within the field is often multidisciplinary, eclectic in theoretical foundation, robust in methodological and analytical approach, and complex to perform. DBP researchers require a thorough and very broad understanding of research design and methods. In addition, the nature of DBP research requires research training to focus intensively on areas such as quasi-experimental and observational designs, qualitative methods, development of testing instruments, study of large secondary datasets, multivariate statistical analyses, neuroimaging, and genetics. In this way, DBP research is as rich and diverse as the field itself and uniquely able to advance the understanding of child development and behavior in all its complexity.

REFERENCES

1. American Psychiatric Association: Diagnostic and Statistical Manual of Mental Disorders, 4th ed, text revision. Washington, DC: American Psychiatric Association, 2000.
2. Rivara F, Finberg L: Use of the terms *race* and *ethnicity*. Arch Pediatr Adolesc Med 155:119, 2001.
3. Schonfeld DJ, O'Hare LL, Perrin EC, et al: A randomized, controlled trial of a school-based, multi-faceted AIDS education program in the elementary grades: The impact on comprehension, knowledge and fears. Pediatrics 95:480-486, 1995.
4. Understanding and agreeing to children's participation in clinical research. *In* Field MJ, Behrman RE, eds: Ethical Conduct of Clinical Research Involving Children. Washington, DC: National Academies Press, 2004, pp 146-210.
5. Schweinhart LJ, Montie J, Xiang Z, et al: Lifetime Effects: The High/Scope Perry Preschool Study through Age 40. Ypsilanti, MI: High/Scope Perry Press, 2005.
6. Duggan A, Windham A, McFarlane E, et al: Hawaii's healthy start program of home visiting for at-risk families: Evaluation of family identification, family engagement, and service delivery. Pediatrics 105: 250-259, 2000.
7. DeAngelis C: An Introduction to Clinical Research. New York: Oxford University Press, 1990.
8. Hulley SB, Cummings SR, Browner WS, et al: Designing Clinical Research: An Epidemiologic Approach, 2nd ed. Philadelphia: Lippincott Williams & Wilkins, 2001.

9. Arcia E, Fernandez MC, Jaquez M: Latina mothers' stances on stimulant medication: Complexity, conflict, and compromise. J Dev Behav Pediatr 25:311-317, 2004.

10. Morse JM, Field PA: Qualitative Research Methods for Health Professionals, 2nd ed. Thousand Oaks, CA: Sage Publications, 1995.

11. Patton MQ: Qualitative Research and Evaluation Methods, 3rd ed. London: Sage Publications, 2002.

12. Giacomini MK, Cook DJ: Users' guides to the medical literature: XXIII. Qualitative research in health care A. Are the results of the study valid? Evidence-Based Medicine Working Group. JAMA 284:357-362, 2000.

13. Giacomini MK, Cook DJ: Users' guides to the medical literature: XXIII. Qualitative research in health care B. What are the results and how do they help me care for my patients? Evidence-Based Medicine Working Group. JAMA 284:478-482, 2000.

14. Iannotti RJ, Schneider S, Nansel TR, et al: Self-efficacy, outcome expectations, and diabetes self-management with type 1 diabetes. J Dev Behav Pediatr 27:98-105, 2006.

15. Gardner W, Murphy M, Childs G, et al: The PSC-17: A brief Pediatric Symptom Checklist with psychosocial problem subscales. A report from PROS and ASPN. Ambul Child Health. 5:225-236, 1999.

16. Stoppelbein L, Greening L, Jordan SS, et al: Factor analysis of the Pediatric Symptom Checklist with a chronically ill pediatric population. J Dev Behav Pediatr 26:349-355, 2005.

17. Suen HK: Principles of Test Theories. Hillsdale, NJ: Erlbaum, 1990.

18. Stevens J, Harman JS, Kelleher KJ: Ethnic and regional differences in primary care visits for attention-deficit hyperactivity disorder. J Dev Behav Pediatr 25:318-325, 2004.

19. Guevara J, Lozano P, Wickizer T, et al: Utilization and cost of health care services for children with attention-deficit/hyperactivity disorder. Pediatrics 108:71-78, 2001.

20. Barbaresi WJ, Katusic SK, Colligan RC, et al: Long-term stimulant medication treatment of attention-deficit/hyperactivity disorder: Results from a population-based study. J Dev Behav Pediatr 27:1-10, 2006.

21. Katusic SK, Colligan RC, Barbaresi WJ, et al: Incidence of reading disability in a population-based birth cohort, 1976-1982, Rochester, Minn. Mayo Clin Proc 76:1081-1092, 2001.

22. Barbaresi WJ, Katusic SK, Colligan RC, et al: The incidence of autism in Olmsted County, Minnesota,

23. 1976-1997: Results from a population-based study. Arch Pediatr Adolesc Med 159:37-44, 2005.

23. Rappley MD, Eneli IU, Mullan PB, et al: Patterns of psychotropic medication use in very young children with attention-deficit hyperactivity disorder. J Dev Behav Pediatr 23:23-30, 2002.

24. Cohen J: Applied Multiple Regression/Correlation Analysis for the Behavioral Sciences, 3rd ed. Mahwah, NJ: Erlbaum, 2003.

25. Hosmer DW, Lemeshow S: Applied Logistic Regression, 2nd ed. New York: Wiley, 2000.

26. Kim J-O, Mueller CW: Introduction to Factor Analysis: What It Is and How to Do It. Newbury Park, CA: Sage Publications, 1978.

27. Kim J-O, Mueller CW: Factor Analysis: Statistical Methods and Practical Issues. Newbury Park, CA: Sage Publications, 1978.

28. Loehlin JC: Latent Variable Models : An Introduction to Factor, Path, and Structural Equation Analysis, 4th ed. Mahwah, NJ: Erlbaum, 2004.

29. Shafritz KM, Marchione KE, Gore JC, et al: The effects of methylphenidate on neural systems of attention in attention deficit hyperactivity disorder. Am J Psychiatry 161:1990-1997, 2004.

30. Pugh KR, Mencl WE, Jenner AR, et al: Neurobiological studies of reading and reading disability. J Commun Disord 34:479-492, 2001.

31. Newmeyer A, Cecil KM, Schapiro M, et al: Incidence of brain creatine transporter deficiency in males with developmental delay referred for brain magnetic resonance imaging. J Dev Behav Pediatr 26:276-282, 2005.

32. Plomin R, DeFries JC, McClearn GE, et al: Behavioral Genetics, 4th ed. New York: Worth Publishing, 2001.

33. Saudino KJ: Behavioral genetics and child temperament. J Dev Behav Pediatr 26:214-223, 2005.

34. Wang PP, Woodin MF, Kreps-Falk R, et al: Research on behavioral phenotypes: Velocardiofacial syndrome (deletion 22q11.2). Dev Med Child Neurol 42:422-427, 2000.

35. Goodlin-Jones BL, Tassone F, Gane LW, et al: Autistic spectrum disorder and the fragile X premutation. J Dev Behav Pediatr 25:392-398, 2004.

36. Mill J, Curran S, Kent L, et al: Attention deficit hyperactivity disorder (ADHD) and the dopamine D_4 receptor gene: Evidence of association but no linkage in a UK sample. Mol Psychiatry 6:440-444, 2001.

37. Auberbach J, Geller V, Lexer S, et al: Dopamine D_4 receptor (D4DR) and serotonin transporter promoter (5-HTTLPR) polymorphisms in the determination of temperament in 2-month-old infants. Mol Psychiatry 4:369-373, 1999.

The Origins of Behavior and Cognition in the Developing Brain*

JAMES E. BLACK ▨ VALERIE L. JENNINGS ▨ GEORGINA M. ALDRIDGE ▨ WILLIAM T. GREENOUGH

Pediatricians specializing in developmental, learning, and behavioral problems have a strong interest in how the brain develops. As clinicians, pediatricians are also interested in the related topic of neural plasticity, especially how development can go pathologically "off track" and how treatment can help correct its course. We have argued[1,2] that brain development can be described as a complex scaffolding of three categories of neural processes: gene-driven, experience-expectant, and experience-dependent. *Gene-driven processes,* which are comparatively insensitive to experience, serve to guide the migration of neurons, to target many of their synaptic connections, and to determine their differentiated functions. *Experience-expectant processes* correspond approximately to "sensitive periods," developmentally timed periods of neural plasticity for which certain types of predictable experience are expected to be present for all juvenile members of a species. Not all brain development, however, is determined by gene-driven processes. Some species have a survival advantage if they can adapt to the environment or incorporate information from it. Indeed, many mammalian species have evolved specialized structures that can incorporate massive amounts of information. Because they have a long evolutionary history, the specialized systems vary across species and occur in multiple brain regions, so that there is no single "place" or "process" for learning and memory. Some types of neural plasticity have evolved to be incorporated into the developmental schedule of brain development, whereas others have evolved to serve the individual's needs by incorporating information unique to their environment. This type of neural plasticity is termed *experience-dependent,* and it corresponds approximately to ordinary learning and memory: that is, encoding information that has adaptive value to an individual but is unpredictable in its timing or nature.

We emphasize a contemporary model of brain development that is derived from the study of dynamic, nonlinear systems. The dynamic systems perspective suggests that individuals use the interaction of genetic constraints and environmental information to self-organize highly complex systems (especially brains). Each organism follows a potentially unique and partly self-determined developmental path of brain assembly to the extent that the organism has unique experiences. The genetically determined restrictions (e.g., the initial cortical architecture) serve as constraints to the system, allowing the interaction of environmental information with existing neural structures to substantially organize and refine neural connections. In this chapter, which extends and amplifies earlier work by Black and colleagues,[3] we review the evidence for these three processes, integrate them into a general model of brain development, provide evidence that the human brain is similarly plastic, and then apply this information to issues of children's development and behavior.

GENE-DRIVEN PROCESSES

Gene-driven processes provide much of the basic structure of the brain and are intrinsically resistant to experience. Waddington[4] described this tendency to resist deviations from predetermined pathways of development as canalization. Some of these genetically determined structures have evolved to constrain and organize experiential information, facilitating its storage in the brain in massive quantities. We now know much of the molecular biological processes of cell differentiation, neuron migration, and cell regulation and signaling. These processes are capable of building enormously complex neural structures

*Preparation of this chapter was supported by National Institute of Mental Health MH35321, National Institute on Aging AG10154, and National Institute on Alcohol Abuse and Alcoholism AA09838.

without substantial input from the external environment. Evidence for the importance of gene-driven processes can be found in the tens of thousands of genes uniquely expressed in rat brain development.[5,6] Indeed, in order to protect brain development, much of the basic organization of most nervous systems is largely impervious to experience. Neural activity that is intrinsically driven, such as that arising from the retina in utero, can play a role in these organization processes, by means of some of the mechanisms that seem also to be used later in the encoding of experience. For example, myelination of the optic nerve appears to be initially driven by spontaneous retinal activity and subsequently influenced by visually generated stimulation of the retina.[7-10] Astrocytic development is also influenced by activity[11] and is discussed in more detail later in this chapter. This theme of molecules and mechanisms, borrowed for other purposes in brain development or plasticity, can be found many times in this chapter.

TISSUE INDUCTION AND FORMING THE BASIC BRAIN PATTERN

Early central nervous system (CNS) development involves an ordered sequence of processes, beginning with formation of the neural plate and followed by an orderly program of further inductions.[12] As in many embryological processes, brain tissue induction typically involves an organizer and its developmental target. Neural induction is familiar to physicians from the embryological process of gastrulation, in which the neuroectoderm just organizes itself. The signaling factors include activation of receptor tyrosine kinases, insulin-like growth factors and fibroblast growth factors, controlled inhibition of other signaling pathways (e.g., Noggin and Chordin), and the wingless pathway.[13] A region of the neuroectoderm becomes differentiated by these signals, and its lateral edges become the neural crest and, later, the peripheral nervous system. Thus, these early signals point the tissue toward neural development or toward other ectodermal development. Many molecular mechanisms of neuronal development and organization have been preserved across species and time, in such a way that they remain remarkably similar in species as diverse as the fruit fly, amphibian, and mouse.[14] We contend that some of these same mechanisms are then exploited later in development for analogous functions in critical periods and in learning and memory.

Some of the most important and unique characteristics of human brain structure appear to have evolved from relatively simple adjustments of genes control-

ling neuron number, modifying the rate of brain development, and regulating brain plasticity.[15] Within the neural ectoderm, the spatial pattern determines much of future brain anatomy.[16] The signals further differentiate the neural tube along an anteroposterior dimension and a mediolateral axis. After this point, each compartment has its own program of differentiation. The anteroposterior segments differentiate into the rhombencephalon (hindbrain), mesencephalon (midbrain), and prosencephalon (forebrain). Each of these subdivisions then follows a genetically controlled program of cell division and migration to swell into rhombomeres in the hindbrain and prosomeres in the forebrain, each of which becomes an important neural structure in the mature brain. Of course, early brain morphogenesis and control are very similar for many vertebrates. In contrast, analysis of genetic drift shows that the abnormal spindle-like microcephaly-associated (ASPM) gene, which affects overall brain size, began changing only in the past 5 million to 6 million years of human evolution to allow larger brain size.[17] This recent adaptive evolution in a gene controlling brain growth is consistent with the role of key, distinctive features in human brain development: the timing of maturation and regulation of size, connectivity and plasticity.

The mediolateral regionalization produces distinct tissues that are longitudinally aligned along the long axis of the CNS. Medial inductions are regulated by substances produced by axial mesodermal organizers: the notochord and the prechordal plate. These organizers are midline structures that lie underneath and produce substances such as sonic hedgehog that induce the medial neural plate to form the floor plate and basal plate. Growth factor proteins such as transforming growth factor–β mediate inductions from the lateral edge of the neural plate that are produced by the nonneural ectoderm. Lateral inductions are likely to be essential for the development of the neural crest, alar plate, and roof plate. Further patterning is determined in a checkerboard organization of brain subdivisions specified by the coordinates of anteroposterior and mediolateral location. Within the checkerboard, specific cues trigger the formation of swellings and vesicles that later become the telencephalon, eyes, and posterior pituitary gland. Although the process of regionalization subdivides the neural plate into the major brain structures, the process of morphogenesis transforms the shape of the neural plate into first a tube and then a complex tube with flexures and evaginations. As the neural plate transforms into the neural tube (neurulation), it converts the lateral-medial dimension of the neural plate into the dorsal-ventral dimension of the neural tube.[14] The fusing of the neural tube is complete 26 days after conception in humans.[18] The neural tube now has four ventral-to-dorsal subdivisions—the floor, basal, alar, and roof plates—each of which extends along much of the anteroposterior axis of the CNS and contributes to the distinct functional elements of the nervous system. The basal plate is the origin of the motor neurons, the alar plate is the origin of the secondary sensory neurons, and the floor plate is devoid of neurons and has several functions that are required during development. Like the notochord, the floor plate produces sonic hedgehog and is believed to serve as a secondary organizer guiding certain sensory neurons. Most of the roof plate forms the nonneuronal dorsal midline, including the choroid plexus and the pineal gland (Fig. 4-1).

HISTOGENESIS, MIGRATION, AND CELL FATE

As the neural tube organizes into regions that will become major structures (e.g., cerebrum, striatum, thalamus, cerebellum), tissue-specific genetic programs of histogenesis are begun within each region.

Histogenesis can be subdivided into two general parts: neuron proliferation and differentiation.[19] In general, each of these processes takes place in distinct zones within the wall of the neural tube. Proliferation takes place in the ventricular zone, which lines the inner surface of the neural tube and is adjacent to the ventricular cavity, whereas differentiation takes place largely in the mantle, which surrounds the ventricular zone. The ventricular zone cells are undifferentiated and mitotically active. Each brain region has distinct proliferation programs that regulate the rate of cell division, the number of cell divisions, and the character of cell division. Cell division can be symmetrical or asymmetrical. Symmetrical division produces cells that are identical; both the daughter cells either continue to proliferate or go on to differentiate. Asymmetrical division produces one daughter cell that differentiates and one that continues to proliferate. The regulation of these processes is integral to controlling how many cells are produced and when they are made, and local differences in replication rate give rise to the gross morphological structures of the forebrain, including the massive cerebral cortex.[20]

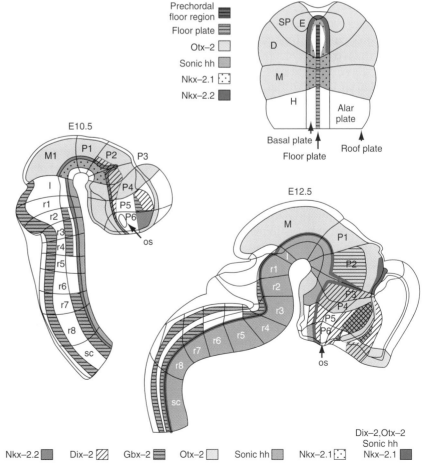

FIGURE 4-1 Six genes are expressed in different regions of the neural plate (E8.5), and neural tube (E10.5, E12.5) in the developing mouse brain. D, diencephalon; E, eyes; H, rhombencephalon-hindbrain; I, isthmus; M, mesencephalon-midbrain; os, optic stalk; p, prosomere; r, rhombomere; sc, spinal cord; SP, secondary prosencephalon. (From Lumsden A. Krumlauf R. Patterning the vertebrate neuraxis. Science 274:1109-1115, 1996.)

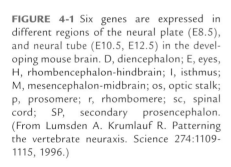

Like the ventricular zone, the subventricular zone is involved in the proliferation of brain cells, but it emerges somewhat later, between 8 to 10 weeks of gestation.[21,22] In the human, migration into the telencephalic region (destined to become the cerebral cortex, hippocampus, and associated structures) begins at approximately 8 weeks of gestation, when the progenitor cells engage in asymmetrical proliferation to create postmitotic neurons.[23] Proliferation ends at approximately 4.5 months of gestation, and the last cells begin their migration.[23] Two waves of neurons migrate, in such a way that postmitotic neurons from the ventricular zone are first to leave, and the neurons from the subventricular zone emerge next.[24] Cortical neurons migrate in an inside-out pattern, whereby neurons that developed earlier migrate to lower cortical layers, and the cells that developed later travel through and beyond previously migrated neurons for destinations in the outer cortex.[25] Therefore, neurons generated in the ventricular zone take up residence in the lower layers of the cortex, and neurons that are derived from the subventricular zone become located in the outer regions of the cortex.

Although neuroanatomy texts may display a dazzling array of brain cell types, all these cells belong to only two major cell classes: neurons and glia.[26] There are two major types of neurons: projection neurons, whose axons migrate to distant territories, and local circuit neurons (interneurons), whose processes ramify nearby. There are many distinct types of projection and local circuit neurons. There are two types of CNS-derived glia: astrocytes and oligodendrocytes. Astrocytes, which are believed to be derived from radial glia, probably regulate the local chemical milieu and have been shown in some cases to release neurotransmitters such as glutamate in ways that can affect neuronal activity. Oligodendrocytes produce the myelin sheaths that surround many axons; these sheaths function as insulators that increase the velocity of action potentials. As described later in the chapter, myelin appears to play key roles in regulating the plastic capacities of axons of neurons and the offset of sensitive periods for experiential organization of neuronal networks.[27] Thus, these CNS-derived glial cells are increasingly seen as partners of neurons in plasticity during development and neural repair. (Another major glial type, the microglia, is derived from mesoderm and performs a phagocytic and immune system role.) Early in development, the ventricular zone contains proliferative cells that have the potential to produce both neurons and glia. In general, neurogenesis precedes gliogenesis. Most regions of the CNS can produce both neurons and astrocytic glia. Different types of neurons are generated at distinct dorsal-ventral positions in the CNS. Motor neurons in the spinal cord, for example, are generated by ventral progenitors, whereas sensory neurons are generated by dorsal progenitors. Likewise, in the telencephalon, ventral progenitors produce the motor neurons of the basal ganglia, whereas dorsal progenitors produce sensory cortical neurons.

In addition to patterning the regions of the nervous system (e.g., cerebral cortex and basal ganglia), histogenesis also regulates where cells travel (migration) and their ultimate functional fate (differentiation). The mechanisms underlying cell fate decisions in the nervous system involve both intrinsic and extrinsic signals. These signals have integral roles in regulating whether these cells continue to divide, whether they undergo symmetrical or asymmetrical division, and what lineage they will follow. Notch signaling is an example of molecular genetic control of differentiation and is mediated by Notch receptors and their ligands.[28] Activation of Notch by its ligand biases a cell not to differentiate; thus, neurogenesis requires inhibition of Notch signaling.[29] Notch signaling can control the rate and timing of neuron production, or it can bias progenitors toward an astrocytic fate. Notch signaling activates a complex cascade of molecular switches that culminates in altered gene expression in the differentiating cell.[30] Many other types of transcription factors have important roles and serve as examples of gene-driven brain development, including the homeobox, helix-loop-helix, T-box, Winged-helix, and HMG-box families. Each of these families consists of subfamilies; for instance, key homeobox genes include Dlx, Emx, Kx, Otx, Pax, and POU, which control such processes as regional fate, cell type identity, neuronal maturation, and cell migration.[16]

Once neurons are generated, the next step in their differentiation is migration to the appropriate destination. Each brain region has a specific migration program. In some structures (e.g., cerebral cortex and superior colliculus), migrations are orchestrated to form layered or laminar structures. In most subcortical regions, migrations originate from nuclear structures that generally are not laminar. There are two general types of migration: radial and tangential. Radial migration is movement perpendicular to the wall of the ventricle toward the pial surface; tangential migration is movement parallel to the plane of the ventricle. Radial migration involves the interaction between elongated processes of radial glial cells and migrating immature neurons. Immature neurons are programmed to migrate to a specific location within the wall of the neural tube, where they disengage from the radial glial cell and continue to differentiate. One of the key molecules in regulating this process was identified through the analysis of the reeler mutant mouse, whose reeling behavior reflected the effects of its mutation on functional brain organization.[31] In the cerebral cortex of reeler mice, later born neurons fail to migrate past their earlier born counterparts, leading to partial inversion of the usual inside out lamination. The reeler gene encodes a large secreted molecule named Reelin that appears to promote dissociation of neuroblasts from radial glia. Mouse genetic studies have implicated two low-density lipoproteins (VLDLR and ApoER2) as the receptors for the Reelin molecule. Intriguingly, this pathway appears to be significantly disturbed in the neurodevelopmental disorder of schizophrenia.[32] Tangential migration of neurons has long been known to occur in the cerebellum and in the rostral migratory stream of the olfactory bulbs. Within the telencephalon, many of the γ-amino butyric acid (GABA)–based local circuit neurons are like cousins rather than like siblings, as they appear to have migrated tangentially from the basal ganglia primordial to the cerebral cortex and hippocampus.[19] Progress has also been made in identifying genes that control cytoskeletal processes that are essential for migration. Several of these genes were first identified as causing neuronal migration defects in humans, including *lissencephaly-1, doublecortin,* and *filamin.*[33] It is of clinical interest that a gene (DCDC2) associated with *doublecortin* has now been associated with heritable reading disabilities.[34]

NEURAL PATHWAYS AND SYNAPTIC CONNECTIONS

As the immature neurons and glia migrate from the proliferative ventricular zone to the mantle, they elaborate into more complex cellular structures. Neurons extend thin processes away from their cell body, including multiple dendrites and a single axon that can sometimes traverse long distances to find its targets. (For review, see Tessier-Lavigne and Goodman[35] and Grunwald and Klein.[36]) The growing tip of the axon is called the *growth cone.* This dynamic weblike structure contains filopodia that extend and retract in multiple directions, seeking potential targets. Certain molecules can attract or repel the growing axons through their specific receptor interactions, whereas other molecules provide paths for the growing axons. Other signals provide more specific information about local branching geometry and pathways. For example, glial cells serve as guideposts for axons. Through fasciculation, late-arriving axons adhere and are bundled together with earlier axons. Molecules on the surface of the axons, some of which are related to immunoglobulins, regulate the pattern of fasciculation and later defasciculation, when the bundle separates.

As axons grow and navigate, they express receptors for guidance molecules that are expressed by neighboring cells.[35,37] These processes operate as growth cones extending along specific pathways, the most well-studied of which involve crossing midline structures (commissures), such as the optic chiasm and corpus callosum. Activation of these receptors determines whether an axon grows toward or away from a target cell. At least four conserved families of guidance molecules have been identified: (1) The semaphorins, which constitute a large, 20-member family of soluble, membrane-bound molecules that elicit repulsive signals through two receptor families, neuropilins and plexins; (2) the Slit family of proteins, which consists of three members in mammals and acts through Robo receptors in commissural axons to prevent them from recrossing the midline; (3) the netrin family, whose members can be repulsive or attractive for a growth cone, depending on the receptor on the axon; and (4) the ephrin family, whose members are membrane bound and interact with two families of receptors, EphA and EphB.[38] In addition to regulating axonal path finding, these same guidance molecules (i.e., semaphorins, slits, netrins, and ephrins) are involved in controlling aspects of neuron migration. Upon reaching their target, some growth cones form specialized connections with dendrites to become synapses.[39] Presynaptic and postsynaptic signals induce the formation and stabilization of molecules on both sides to become specialized synaptic structures.[40] On the presynaptic side, for example, synaptic vesicles filled with neurotransmitter are grouped together; on the postsynaptic side, receptor molecules are grouped together into a dense domain that is sometimes located within a dendritic protrusion called a *synaptic spine.*[41]

The wiring of complex CNS systems requires a connection of multiple cell types that are located in different positions. The wiring diagram of the visual system is an example of this process that has received a massive amount of experimental attention. The retina contains primary sensory receptor neurons (rods and cones), interneurons (amacrine, bipolar, and horizontal cells), glia, and projection neurons called *retinal ganglion cells.* The retinal ganglion cells extend optic nerve axons that must make several choices as they proceed to their targets. As they pass the optic chiasm, axons from the temporal retina do not cross, whereas axons from the nasal retina do cross. Intrinsic signals that distinguish nasal and temporal cells (brain factor 1 and 2 transcription factors) help guide the growing axons. Upon exiting the chiasm, the optic axons grow caudally toward their two main targets: the thalamus and the superior colliculus. Branches perpendicular to the optic tracts enter the visual center of the thalamus and form synapses with the lateral geniculate nucleus (LGN). Other optic axons continue caudally to the midbrain into the superior colliculus, where they are sorted into a retinotopic map by the ephrin family receptors.

In the LGN, the optic axons form another retinotopic map. In higher mammals, the LGN is a laminar structure, with each layer connected to only one eye. During development, however, axons from both eyes have processes extending into many LGN layers. Neuronal activity related to visual experience is required for pruning back synapses and for axonal branches to segregate into layers specific for one eye or the other. The projection neurons in the LGN send axons anteriorly into the telencephalon, in which they traverse the striatum in the internal capsule and enter the cerebral cortex. The thalamocortical axons enter the cortex while neurogenesis is still actively occurring and grow into a layer called the *intermediate zone* that is interposed between the proliferative zones (ventricular zone and subventricular zone) and mantle zones (cortical plate). The thalamocortical fibers then innervate specific regions of neocortex. The neocortex is subdivided into functionally distinct areas, each with its own thalamic inputs. Primary visual cortex receives LGN axons. Cortical maps from other thalamic nuclei determine primary sensory cortex (e.g., auditory cortex), whereas other regions of cerebral cortex are described as associative, because their connections are primarily to other areas of cortex. In humans, some of these associative areas are both enormous and complex, including the dorsolateral prefrontal cortex, which is involved in executive function, and the ventromedial prefrontal cortex, which is involved in complex emotional/social reasoning. Both regions have late and lengthy developmental schedules, and maldevelopment of each is implicated in numerous psychiatric disorders (see Fuster[42]).

EXPERIENCE-EXPECTANT DEVELOPMENT

Although numerous examples of neural plasticity have been found in mammalian species, we have proposed that much of plasticity can be classified into two basic categories. Experience-expectant development involves a readiness of the brain to receive specific types of information from the environment. This readiness occurs during critical or sensitive stages in development during which there are central adaptations to information that is reliably present for all members of the species. This information includes major sensory experience, such as patterned visual information that drives the LGN axonal withdrawal

described previously, and information affecting social, emotional, and cognitive development. The overproduction of neural connections is one aspect of the brain's readiness to receive this expected information, of which a subset is selectively retained on the basis of experience.

A general process observed in many mammalian species is that a surplus of connections is produced, a large portion of which is subsequently eliminated. Evidence for overproduction and partial elimination of synapses during development has been found in many brain regions and species, including cats,[43] rodents,[44] monkeys,[45,46] and humans.[47] The overshoot in the number of synapses produced in cortical areas in many animals, including humans, has been estimated to be approximately double the number found in adults[48] (see Huttenlocher[49] for review). In humans, synaptic density and estimates of total synapse numbers in the visual cortex reach a peak at approximately 8 months of age, and synapse numbers decline thereafter.[48] Another important finding by Huttenlocher[50] is that the blooming and pruning of synapses in the frontal cortex is substantially delayed; its peak occurs during childhood. Although synapse density and absolute synapse number may differ, depending on other tissue elements, we assume for purposes of this discussion that they are equivalent. A measure that has been interpreted as reflecting synapse overproduction and loss is the volume of regions of the human cerebral cortex and other brain areas, measured by structural magnetic resonance imaging.[51] Heterosynchrony (i.e., staggered developmental timing with late development of prefrontal cortex) is unique in humans among the primates.[51] The clinical implications of late-developing prefrontal cortex are discussed in a later section.

The process of overproduction and selective elimination of synapses appears to be a mechanism whereby the brain is made ready to capture critical and highly reliable information from the environment. This possibility is supported by several lines of research (described in the following sections) indicating that the pruning into structured patterns of functional neural connections requires appropriate patterns of neural activity that are obtained through experience. These events occur during known critical or sensitive periods. Furthermore, the pruning appears to be driven by competitive interactions between neural connections, so that inactive neural connections are lost and connections that are most actively driven by experience are selectively maintained. "Most active" may refer to synchronous or correlated activation, such as presynaptic activity coincident with postsynaptic activity, as first proposed by Hebb,[52] or some mechanism other than the mere frequency of firing. In many cases, it appears that these plastic neural systems have evolved to take advantage of information that could be "expected" for all juvenile members (i.e., it has an adaptive value for the whole species, not just individuals). In many of the experiments described in this section, investigators used interventions that disturb some aspect of the "expected" experience, leading to substantial disruptions of further development. Many patients with developmental and behavioral disorders have had similarly disturbed experiences with subsequently disrupted development.

Visual Deprivation Experiments

Studies of the effects of early visual deprivation have provided some of the strongest examples of experience inducing neural structure during development. Together, they indicate a direct link between patterns of experience-expectant visual information and patterns of neural connectivity. Experimental visual deprivation falls into two main classes. Binocular visual deprivation can be complete, depriving animals of all visual stimuli, or partial, depriving animals of patterned visual stimuli but allowing diffuse, unpatterned stimulation. This deprivation may be achieved, for example, by suturing both eyelids shut (complete deprivation) or by raising animals in complete darkness (partial deprivation). Partial deprivation reduces or distorts visual experience in some manner but allows some effect of experience on neural activity. Complete deprivation in both eyes leads to a loss in complex visuomotor learning and in the precision of neuronal response properties, but it preserves balance in eye dominance and basic perceptual skills.[53] In contrast, selective deprivation in one eye during the critical period leads to a drastic reduction in its control over visual cortex neurons and behavior, whereas the nondeprived eye correspondingly gains in control. The degree of recovery from deprivation depends on the species and on the onset and duration of the deprivation period.

Binocular Deprivation

Studies of binocular deprivation have shown that appropriate visual stimulation during certain developmental stages is critical for the development of normal neural connectivity in the visual system. Dark rearing or bilateral lid closure in developing animals results in behavioral, physiological, and structural abnormalities in visual pathways.[54-56] The severity and reversibility of the visual impairments are dependent on the onset and duration of the deprivation, corresponding to defined sensitive periods of a given species.[57] Even short periods of early visual deprivation can result in impairments in visuomotor skills,

such as visually guided placement of the forepaw in cats.[58] The structural effects of dark rearing include smaller neuronal dendritic fields, reduced spine density, and reduced numbers of synapses per neuron within the visual cortex.[43,59-61] In kittens, for example, developmental binocular deprivation resulted in a 40% reduction in the number of adult visual cortex synapses.[43]

Selective Deprivation

Experiments in selective deprivation have indicated the importance of specific types of visual experience to normal brain development. For example, kittens reared in a strobe-illuminated environment have plentiful visual pattern experience but are selectively deprived of the normal experience of movement (i.e., movement in the visual field would appear jerky or disconnected). Specific impairments in motion perception have been found in such kittens.[62] These animals had visual cortical neurons that were insensitive to visual motion,[63] and they exhibited impairment on visuomotor behavioral tasks that involve motion.[64]

Other researchers limited visual experience to specific visual patterns, or contours. Hirsch and Spinelli[65] raised kittens in chambers with one eye exposed to only horizontal stripes and the other eye to only vertical stripes. Physiological recordings of visual cortical neurons from these kittens revealed that neurons were most responsive to stimuli oriented in the direction of the stripes they had experienced. These neurons also occupy twice as much of the visual cortex as neurons sensitive to stripes in nonexposed directions.[66] Behaviorally, stripe-reared animals performed best on tests involving stimuli in the orientation to which they were exposed during development.[67,68] Unlike dark rearing or bilateral lid closure, stripe rearing does not appear to result in an overall diminishment of neuronal size, but it does alter the orientation of the neuronal dendritic arbors.[69,70] Thus, neural function appears to be determined by the pattern, in addition to the overall number, of neural connections. A related, albeit debatable clinical finding in humans who have uncorrected astigmatism in a particular orientation in one eye is reduced acuity in that axis.[71]

Monocular Deprivation

A great deal of information about experience-expectant processes has been learned from one particular deprivation model. In species with stereoscopic vision, including cats and monkeys, binocular regions of the cortex receive information from each eye via projections from the LGN in adjacent stripes or columns within cortical layer IV, termed *ocular dominance columns*. With normal experience early in development, the cortical input associated with each eye initially projects in overlapping terminal fields within layer IV. During development in normal animals, these axonal terminal fields are selectively pruned, which results in sharply defined borders between ocular dominance columns in adult animals. The neurons of this layer send convergent input to other layers, made up in large part by binocularly driven neurons.[72]

Studies of monocular deprivation in stereoscopic animals have shown that the formation of the ocular dominance columns is dependent on competitive interactions between the visual input from each eye.[73] In monocularly deprived monkeys, the axons projecting from the deprived eye regress, whereas the axons from the experienced eye do not. This pruning back results in the thinning of the columns corresponding to the deprived eye, whereas the columns of the nondeprived eye are enlarged in relation to those of normal animals.[72,74] Thus, the axonal terminals from the dominant eye appear to be selectively maintained at the expense of the inactive input of the deprived eye, in which the excess synapses are eliminated. Physiologically, the number and responsiveness of cells activated by the deprived eye are severely decreased.[55] Functionally, monocular deprivation for an extended period during development results in near blindness to visual input in the deprived eye. In contrast, binocular deprivation results principally in a loss of visual acuity. Physiologically, it reduces but does not abolish the response of neurons to visual stimuli.[55] It also does not prevent the formation of ocular dominance columns, although the segregation of columns is well below normal.[72,75,76] Thus, in binocular deprivation, cortical input from the eyes may be partially maintained in the absence of competing information.

The physiological and anatomical effects of monocular deprivation occur fairly rapidly. Antonini and Stryker[74] found that the shrinkage of geniculocortical arbors corresponding to the deprived eye was profound in cats with only 6 to 7 days of monocular deprivation, similar to that found after 33 days of deprivation. Like binocular deprivation, the recovery from the deprivation is sensitive to the time of onset and duration of the deprivation. Monocular deprivation corresponding to the sensitive period of a given species results in enduring impairments and physiological nonresponsiveness,[55] whereas even very extensive deprivation in adult animals has little effect.[77] In humans, early monocular deprivation resulting from congenital cataracts can have severe effects on acuity, even after treatment, whereas adults who develop cataracts in one eye show little post-treatment impair-

ment.[78] The sensitive period for the effects of monocular deprivation can be affected by prior experience. For example, the maximum sensitivity to monocular deprivation in kittens is normally during the fourth and fifth weeks after birth.[79,80] Cynader and Mitchell[81] found that kittens dark-reared from birth to several months of age maintain a physiological sensitivity to monocular deprivation at ages that normal kittens are insensitive. Dark-reared animals do not, however, simply show normal visual development at this later age. With binocular deprivation early in life, the ocular dominance columns of layer IV do not segregate in a fully normal pattern and do not maintain a structural sensitivity to monocular deprivation effects.[75]

The implication of these studies is that the sensitive period for experience effects is self-limiting; that is, as supernumerary synapses are eliminated and/or as additional synapses cease to be generated, the capacity for responding, or the experience-sensitive phase, comes to an end. Alternative models might invoke changes in the synapses that survive, leaving them immutable to further pruning or to forces acting at a distance, such as the development of local GABA-based inhibitory systems[82,83] or the influence of modulatory axonal activity from other parts of the brain. There are a variety of such proposals, many with supporting data (e.g., α-amino-3-hydroxy-5-methyl-4-isoxazolepropionic acid [AMPA] and N-methyl-D-aspartate [NMDA] glutamate receptor distribution and subunit composition[84,85]), but one merits additional mention because it illustrates the interactions of neurons and glia and has been increasingly implicated in the regulation of synaptic plasticity in both development and adulthood (the latter in damaged or diseased nervous systems). It has long been known that mature axons in the brain and spinal cord show much less tendency to regrow connections after crush or transection than do seemingly equivalent axons outside of the central nervous system. Still-developing pathways in the CNS show greater flexibility. A search for the mechanism revealed an interacting series of signals typified by the molecule Nogo and its receptor. Nogo is produced by the oligodendrocytic myelin surrounding nerve cell pathways and inhibits axonal sprouting in vitro. A function blocking antibody to Nogo facilitates axonal growth after nerve injury to the adult rat spinal cord in vivo[86,87] and enhances recovery of behavioral function. Work by McGee and colleagues[27] has further implicated Nogo in the termination of visual sensitive periods; a mouse rendered genetically incapable of producing Nogo receptor exhibited sensitivity to monocular deprivation extending well beyond the normal age, which suggests that the Nogo mechanism limits postdevelopmental plasticity in multiple systems.

Investigators have proposed involvement of various signaling pathway mechanisms of synapse stabilization and maintenance similar to those described for genotype-driven development, such as α-calcium–calmodulin kinase type II (αCaMKII) for ocular dominance maturation.[88,89]

Deprivation in Other Sensory Systems

Research in other sensory systems has also demonstrated experience-expectant processes. Within layer IV of the somatosensory cortex in rodents, each whisker is represented by a distinctly clustered group of neurons arranged in what have been called *barrels.*[90] The cell bodies of these neurons form the barrel walls, and a cell-sparse region forms the barrel hollow. In adult animals, the input from each whisker (via the thalamus) terminates predominantly within the barrel hollows. Positioned to receive this input, most of the dendrites of the neurons lining the barrel wall are also oriented into the barrel hollow. This distinctive pattern of barrel walls surrounding a hollow forms postnatally, before which neurons in this region appear homogeneous. The simultaneous regression of dendrites inside the barrel walls and continued growth of dendrites in the barrel hollows mask the expected synapse overproduction and pruning back, inasmuch as the overall process is dendritic expansion.[44] Were it not for the location of information provided about the structure of the barrel, this dendritic pruning in the barrel walls would be entirely masked by the simultaneous dendritic extension in the hollows.

Many rodents use their highly developed whiskers, or *vibrissae,* to navigate in the dark (along with heightened olfactory perception). The whisker barrel region, with its overlapping blooming and pruning of synapses, might therefore be expected to be sensitive to experience. Indeed, Glazewski and Fox[91] were able to demonstrate experience-expectant plasticity in the barrel field cortex of young rats by reducing the complement of vibrissae on one side of the muzzle to a single whisker for a period of 7, 20, or 60 days. The vibrissa dominance distribution was shifted significantly toward the spared vibrissa, which gained control of more neurons in barrel cortex, whereas the deprived whiskers lost control. As the deprived whiskers grew back in, they progressively gained back some control of neurons from the spared whiskers. Whisker deprivation had the strongest effects in weanling animals and very little effect in adult rats. However, manipulations that are known to induce plasticity in sensory maps, such as the alternate trimming of individual whiskers, can cause changes in spine dynamics, even in adult animals.[92] Whisker deprivation alone has been shown to alter spine dynamics over time, dramatically decreasing elimina-

tion rates in young animals but having a more subtle effect on elimination rates in adult animals.[93]

Humans and some other species appear to have a critical period for attachment, during which the lack of expected nurturing behavior in a timely manner disrupts subsequent emotional development. Human and monkey studies have revealed substantial effects of disrupted attachment on behavior and endocrine function, but little is known about any underlying neural plasticity. The phenomenon known as *imprinting* (e.g., by which newly hatched chicks learn to recognize mothers) involves both the formation of new synapses and elimination of preexisting synapses.[94,95] Imprinting fits the definition of experience-expectant neural plasticity, but it is an example of social rather than perceptual development. Various primate species are differentially sensitive to maternal deprivation,[96] and humans appear to be relatively sensitive. For example, rhesus monkeys raised in isolation show enduring heightened responses to stress; abnormal motor behaviors, including stereotyped movements; sexual dysfunction; eating disorders; and various extreme forms of social and emotional dysfunction.[97-99] The effects of total social isolation are more severe than partial isolation, which permits visual and auditory interactions with other animals without direct physical contact. Dendritic arbors of neurons within the neocortex[100] and the cerebellum[101] have been found to be poorly developed in socially deprived monkeys in comparison with normal animals. Martin and associates[102] found that socially deprived rhesus monkeys show a marked reduction in the dopaminergic and peptidergic innervations within the caudate-putamen, substantia nigra, and globus pallidus. In addition to evidence of reduced neuronal growth and development, socially deprived monkeys show brain abnormalities more typical of neurological disorders. However, in many of the studies just mentioned, social deprivation was confounded with broader experiential deprivation; therefore, there is still relatively little knowledge about structural brain changes specifically related to social experience.

The fragile X mental retardation syndrome is another phenomenon that might involve a different type of disruption of the systems involved in attachment and social development that leads to pathology. This syndrome is caused by impaired or blocked expression of the fragile X mental retardation protein (FMRP), which results from a triplet repeat mutation in the regulatory region of the gene. In addition to cognitive impairment and learning disabilities, fragile X retardation is often accompanied by symptoms of attention-deficit/hyperactivity disorder (ADHD) and autism.[103] There is also abundant evidence for a link between the presence of the fragile X chromosome and psychiatric symptoms. Even individuals with a relatively small expansion of the cytosine-guanine-guanine repeat, who are "unaffected" cognitively, exhibit anxiety disorder (31%), bipolar disorder (23%), panic disorder (17%), and social phobia (11%).[104] Men with the fragile X syndrome exhibit elevated degrees of schizoid and schizotypal features.[105] "Mood lability" that does not reach criterion for bipolar diagnosis is also common in these patients.[106] Investigators frequently report social problems such as "gaze avoidance" and other disturbances.

The failure to develop normal social skills through experience is a plausible origin for these disturbances, and there is reason to suspect a failure of experience-expectant developmental mechanisms in the fragile X syndrome. There are indications that, at least in the cerebral cortex, the maturation and elimination of dendrites and synapses is developmentally delayed, both in humans with fragile X syndrome, according to studies of autopsy tissue and in the knockout mouse model for the syndrome, in which the fragile X gene has been rendered nonfunctional. Dendritic spines in visual, auditory, and somatosensory cortices of humans or mice exhibit an appearance suggestive of an immature structure: longer and thinner than typically developing spines.[107-111] In addition, the dendritic pruning typical in the previously described whisker barrel cortex fails to occur in the knockout mouse,[112] and a similar failure of typical dendritic pruning appears in the olfactory system.[113] Thus, a failure of an experience-expectant mechanism caused by an inherited genetic disorder may underlie some of the behavioral pathology described in the fragile X syndrome, a good example of an interaction, albeit a debilitating one, between genetic and experiential contributions to the development process.

FMRP is a messenger RNA (mRNA)–binding protein that appears to function by binding cargo mRNAs in the nucleus and accompanying them through cytoplasmic transport to where they are ultimately translated, often in response to local, synaptically associated signaling pathways.[114-117] To date, the mRNAs shown to associate with FMRPs represent a heterogeneous group of encoded proteins, although a number of them appear to be involved directly or indirectly in synaptic plasticity.[118-120] Investigators have speculated that FMRP may play a role in modulating protein synthesis and its effects on the synaptic plasticity process involved in developmental information storage,[117] but further work is needed to confirm these ideas. However, in view of the essential synaptic role of many of the proteins whose mRNA FMRP is hypothesized to regulate, it is possible that dysregulation of the distribution and accumulation of specific cargo mRNAs accounts for altered synaptic plasticity

in these patients. For example, Post-synaptic Density-95 (PSD-95) is a developmentally and environmentally regulated scaffolding protein thought to be intimately involved with plasticity at the synapse, being one of the most highly expressed synaptic proteins whose overexpression, in turn, has dramatic effects on synaptic structure and on spine maturation and dynamics.[121,122] In vivo studies in which expression of PSD-95 was tagged with photoactivatable green-fluorescent protein (paGFP) have demonstrated that the protein's presence in the spine is dynamic, especially in younger animals, and dependent on experience.[123] Although direct evidence is still lacking to tie modulation of PSD-95 to FMRP, the mRNA of PSD-95 contains a G-quartet motif thought to be a common feature of FMRP cargoes. In cultured neurons from FMRP knockout mice, metabotropic glutamate receptor (mGluR) activation–induced expression of PSD-95 appears to be deficient, and this lack of regulation could, in theory, explain many of the dendritic spine and plasticity abnormalities observed in the fragile X syndrome. However, the deficits observed in the fragile X syndrome are more likely to arise by the misregulation of a combination of mRNAs. This "cargo hypothesis" of the fragile X syndrome suggests that analysis of FMRP cargoes, in isolation and in combination, may lead not only to targets for treating fragile X symptoms but also to a potential understanding of overlap between fragile X symptoms and those of other genetically complex disorders such as autism.

EXPERIENCE-DEPENDENT DEVELOPMENT

Experience-dependent development involves the brain's adaptation to information that is unique to an individual. This type of adaptation does not occur within strictly defined critical periods, inasmuch as the timing or nature of such experience cannot be reliably anticipated. Therefore, this type of neural plasticity is likely to be active throughout life. Such systems, however, cannot be constantly "on" and recording information. They need to have some kind of regulatory process that helps filter important information from the extraneous material. Although this type of process does not have fixed "windows" of plasticity, there may be necessary sequential dependencies on prior development. For example, a child learns algebra before mastering calculus. Sometimes experience-dependent processes depend on prior experience-expectant ones, as in language development, in which a universal sensitive period is followed by more idiosyncratic expansion of grammar and vocabulary.

Manipulating Environmental Complexity

An additional, important mechanism for experience-dependent development is the formation of new neural connections, in contrast to the overproduction and pruning back of synapses often associated with experience-expectant processes. This idea was initially supported by experiments in which the overall complexity of an animal's environment was manipulated, as well as by experiments involving specific learning tasks. Modifying the complexity of an animal's environment can have profound effects on behavior and on brain structure, both in late development (e.g., after weaning in rats) and in adulthood. In experimental manipulations, animals are typically housed in one of three conditions: (1) individual cages, in which the animals are housed alone in standard laboratory cages; (2) social cages, in which animals are housed with another rat in the same type of cage; or (3) a complex or "enriched condition" environment, in which animals are housed in large groups in cages filled with changing arrangements of toys and other objects. Raising animals in an enriched environment provides ample opportunity for exploration and permits animals to experience complex social interactions, including play behavior, as well as experience with the manipulation and spatial components of complex, multidimensional arrangements of objects.

In accordance with a tradition established by the well-known Berkeley group (e.g., Bennett et al[124]), the experimental groups are often referred to as "enriched" and "impoverished." It is important to emphasize that these are more accurately described in terms of varying degrees of deprivation, in relation to the typical environment of feral rats. Barring considerations of stress or nutrition, we argue that rats in enriched environments experience something close to "normal" brain development and that their brains would more closely resemble those of rats raised in the wild. Although a great deal of useful information can be obtained from laboratory animals, it is important to understand that standard animals are generally overfed, understimulated, and physically out of shape.

Animals raised in complex environments have superior performance on many different types of learning tasks (reviewed by Greenough and Black[2]). Various studies have suggested that animals living in enriched environments may use more and different types of cues to solve tasks and may possess enhanced information-processing rates and capacities.[125-128] Their superiority in complex mazes may rely, in part, on a greater familiarity with complicated spatial arrangements obtained through their rearing environment. These abilities are generalized across a wide range of other learning tests, however, which suggests that the enriched environment's abilities do not simply reflect specific types of information gathered from the rearing environment. Rather, the brain adaptation to complex environment rearing involves changing how information is processed; that is, the rat in enriched environments appears to have learned to learn better. In the initial publication of this result, Hebb[52] noted that the enriched rats learned more quickly than do their laboratory cage–reared counterparts and improved more rapidly as they were subjected to consecutive tests.

Examination of brain structure in animals in complex environments reveals a growth of neurons and synaptic connections in comparison with siblings raised in standard cages. This has been most prominently studied in the visual cortex, which shows an overall increase in thickness, volume, and weight[124]; an increase in dendritic branching complexity and spine density[129,130]; more synapses per neuron[131,132]; and larger synaptic contacts[133] in complex-environment rats. The number of synapses in rats living in enriched environments is elevated by approximately 20% to 25% within superficial layers of the visual cortex.[132] The visual cortex also shows physiological alterations, which indicates that neuronal firing in animals housed in enriched environments is enhanced in comparison with that in animals housed in standard cages.[134] Very comparable anatomical data and concomitant electrophysiological alterations have been reported in cats given complex experience.[135,136]

The effects of environmental complexity have many different dimensions. The enriched environment's effects on brain structure cannot be attributed to general metabolic, hormonal, or stress differences across the different rearing conditions.[137] Thus, the structural brain changes may be specifically the result of altered neuronal activity and information storage. Young rats living in enriched environments have been shown to add new capillaries to the visual cortex, presumably in support of increased metabolic activity,[138] and increased capillary branching alters perfusion capacity.[139] Rats reared in a complex environment tend to have slower growth of skeleton and internal organs,[137] as well as altered immune system responsiveness.[140] Evidence that male and female rats have different responses to the complex environment in both the visual cortex and the hippocampus suggests that sex hormones have a modulatory role in the brain effects in the enriched and individual environments, at least in early postnatal development.[141] Multiple brain regions have shown evidence of structural change in animals in enriched environments, including the temporal cortex,[142] the striatum,[143] the hippocampus,[141] the superior colliculus,[144] and cerebellum.[101,145] Mice reared in a complex environment generate more neurons in the dentate gyrus than do those in the other conditions.[146] Investigators have detected significant changes in rat cortical thickness and dendritic branching after just 4 days of enrichment.[147] These effects are not limited to young animals, inasmuch as changes in neuronal dendrites and synapses in adult rats placed in the complex environment are substantial, although less so than those found in rats reared from weaning in enriched environments.[148,149]

Structural Effects of Learning

Although a variety of activities occur in an enriched environment, learning is clearly an important one. If learning in the enriched environment results in structural brain changes, then similar changes would be expected in animals in response to a variety of training procedures. Such studies have indeed demonstrated that major brain structure changes occur during learning. These changes have been found in the specific brain regions apparently involved in the learning. For example, training in complex mazes necessitating visuospatial memory has been found to result in increased dendritic arbors of the visual cortex in adult rats.[150] When split-brain procedures were performed and unilateral occluders placed on one eye, dendrites of neurons in the monocular cortex mediating vision in the unoccluded eye showed greater growth than in the visually inexperienced hemisphere of the visual cortex.[151]

Training animals on motor learning tasks results in site-specific neuronal changes. Rats extensively trained to use one forelimb to reach through a tube to receive highly attractive food showed dendritic growth within the region of the cortex involved in forelimb function,[152] in comparison with controls. When allowed to use only one forelimb for reaching, the dendritic arborizations of rats within the cortex opposite the trained forelimb were significantly increased in relation to the cortex opposite the untrained forelimb. Furthermore, reach training selectively alters only certain subpopulations of neurons; for example, layer II/III pyramidal neurons showed forked apical shafts.[153] Reach training may produce similar results in developing animals as well. Rat pups trained to reach with one forelimb over 9 days, beginning at weaning, exhibited increased cortical thickness in the hemisphere opposite the trained limb, in comparison to the nontrained limb.[154] A review and meta-analysis of more than 100 studies concluded that the neocortex tends to respond to learning with synaptogenesis, whereas the hippocampal formation tends to alter the structure of existing synapses, in accord with the roles of these two structures in persisting memory.[155]

A critical question is whether these training-induced brain changes result from special processes specifically involved in brain information storage or are simply an effect of increased activity within the affected brain systems; that is, do these changes reflect some generally trophic nature of experience, comparable to muscle hypertrophy with exercise, or do they correspond to changes in the brain's "wiring diagram" that actually subserve memory? A motor learning paradigm in which rats are required to master several new complex motor coordination tasks ("acrobatic" rats) addressed this question. These animals showed increased numbers of synapses per Purkinje neuron within the cerebellum, in comparison with inactive controls.[156] In contrast, animals exhibiting greater amounts of motor activity in running wheels or treadmills in which little information was learned[156] or yoked-control animals that made an equivalent amount of movement in a simple straight alley[157] did not show significant alterations in synaptic connections in the cerebellum. Thus, learning, and not simply the repetitive use of synapses that may occur during dull physical exercise, is selectively associated with synaptogenesis in the cerebellum. Subsequent research has reached a similar conclusion for synaptic changes in the motor cortex that arise after learning, in the same behavioral paradigm.[158]

Interestingly, the exercising animals did show some structural changes: The increase in density of capillaries in the involved region of cerebellum corresponded to expectations for new blood vessel development to support increased metabolic demand.[156] This indicates that the brain can independently generate adaptive changes in different cellular components. When metabolic "stamina" is required, vasculature is added. When motor skills need to be learned or refined, new synapses modify neural organization. In the enriched environment, both exercise and learning effects appear to be combined.

Cerebellar synaptic changes are accompanied by functional changes in electrophysiological recording. Stimulation of parallel fibers, constituting the primary excitatory input to Purkinje cells and accounting for the bulk of the added synapses, evoked larger postsynaptic changes in acrobatic rats than in motor activity controls,[159] which indicates that the training-induced synapses are functional. This effect probably also reflects increased parallel fiber input to inhibitory neurons, also evident in morphological changes of the acrobatic rats.[160]

We describe one example of neural plasticity and therapeutic training in an animal model of a clinical disorder, because the literature is quite extensive: There is increasing evidence that the postnatal environment strongly influences the outcome of prenatal exposure to alcohol in fetal alcohol syndrome and exposure.[161] Animal models of this important developmental disorder have been carefully developed.[162] Hannigan and colleagues[163] found that raising rats in a complex environment greatly attenuated the behavioral effects of prenatal exposure to low to moderate levels of alcohol. Animals with fetal alcohol syndrome that were raised from weaning in isolation showed ataxia and impairments in learning spatial tests. These alcohol-induced effects were largely absent in rats with fetal alcohol syndrome raised in a complex environment. Although the investigators found no indication of rehabilitation effects on hippocampal structure, a program of forced motor skill training (similar to the "acrobatic" training described previously) nearly eliminated motor dysfunction in rats with fetal alcohol exposure and substantially increased synapse number in their cerebellar cortex.[164-166] The intervention did not reverse the substantial loss of neurons in the cerebellum resulting from alcohol treatment, but the new synapses appeared to support enhanced motor performance. This work suggests that intervention focused on the skills that have been lost as a result of CNS damage can have potentially important therapeutic effects.

EVIDENCE FOR HUMAN NEURAL PLASTICITY

Because of ethical and technical limitations, it is quite difficult to demonstrate that the human brain has neural plasticity processes similar to those for other species described previously. In view of the massive amount of information that humans incorporate (e.g., consider language learning alone) and the fact that this material can be retained for decades without rehearsal, we surmise that information seemingly must be stored as lasting, structural neural changes. Although current evidence cannot be used to directly describe any changes in synaptic strength or number, human neural plasticity can be described in terms of experience-expectant and experience-dependent processes.

One kind of human experience-expectant process sensitive to selective deprivation involves perceptual mismatch from both eyes, such as when one eye deviates outward (strabismus) during early development. As in the cat and monkey studies described earlier, if the two eyes are sending competing and conflicting signals to the visual cortex during the sensitive period, the brain effectively "shuts down," or becomes insensitive to input from, the nondominant eye. In humans, the resulting perceptual disorder, amblyopia (or "lazy eye"), results in clear perceptual deficits if surgery does not correct this visual misalignment during the critical period. The strabismus-related perceptual

deficit was the first and still best-established example of human neural plasticity.[167] Technological methods, such as positron-emission tomography, has demonstrated that patients with uncorrected strabismus use different areas of the visual cortex for visual processing than do normal controls.[168] Although the timing, regulation, and structural changes of this sensitive period need further study, the early evidence suggests a clear parallel to the described studies of kittens with selective deprivation of vision.

Another developmental process with innate roots but nonetheless quite dependent on early experience is language acquisition.[169] Although the question of whether language has an innate deep structure is still debated, it is clear that children rapidly acquire an enormous amount of vocabulary, grammar, and related information. For middle-income American families, the rate of vocabulary acquisition is directly related to the amount of verbal stimulation that the mother provides.[170] There is apparently a sensitive period for acquiring the ability to discriminate speech contrasts. For example, Kuhl[171] reported that before about 6 months of life, infants from English-speaking homes are able to discriminate speech contrasts from a variety of languages, including Thai, Czech, and Swedish, much the way native adult speakers are able to. However, sometime between ages 6 and 12 months, this ability is gradually lost. After this age, infants become more like adults who are most proficient in discriminating the speech contrasts from their native language,[171] possibly paralleling synapse elimination as described by Huttenlocher.[50] Early exposure to the native language can be interpreted as a "neural commitment" of the brain's resources to the acoustic properties of the native language, in such a way that this dedication of resources interferes with any subsequent foreign language learning. Evidence for this commitment can be observed in both behavioral changes and in imaging data, such as magnetoencephalography.[172]

There exists some preliminary evidence that humans can alter brain function with extensive training, corresponding to the experience-dependent processes described previously. For example, using functional magnetic resonance imaging (fMRI) to measure regional blood flow in the brain, Karni and associates[173] demonstrated increased cortical involvement after training subjects in a finger-tapping sequence. Elbert and colleagues[174] showed substantial expansion of cortical involvement associated with the amount of training to play the violin. No one has yet shown directly that humans produce new synapses with this type of learning, but the fMRI changes are what would be expected if synaptogenesis were occurring in an experience-dependent process. Similarly, researchers have found that brain myelination patterns differ in musicians, depending on the ages during which training occurred[175]; this again emphasizes that plasticity extends beyond neurons and their synapses to glia as partners. Another provocative finding involved the relatively enlarged posterior hippocampi of London taxi drivers, who were required to encode massive amounts of spatial information for their occupation. Although synaptogenesis cannot be demonstrated directly, it is one of very few examples of structural plasticity in healthy humans.[176] An indirect line of evidence indicated that healthy, well-educated subjects had greater dendritic branching of large pyramidal neurons in the language cortex than did less well-educated subjects,[177] which is consistent with storage of education information in the neuropil. However, cause and effect remain obscure in this intriguing study.

Impressive findings of cortical reorganization after peripheral injury in adult humans correspond well to the previously described findings in nonhuman primates.[178] For example, Ramachandran and coworkers[179] examined adults who had experienced various forms of amputation, such as the forearm. One such individual experienced sensation in the limb that had, in fact, been amputated (i.e., "phantom limb phenomenon"). Ramachandran and coworkers then examined sensitivity to tactile stimulation along the regions of the face known to innervate the somatosensory cortex adjacent to the area previously innervated by the missing limb. When this region of the face was lightly stimulated, the patient reported sensation in both the face and the missing limb. Ramachandran and coworkers were eventually able to determine the degree to which the cortical surface had been reorganized to subsume the area previously occupied by the missing limb. Brain reorganization after trauma appears to be very complex, and this subject is beyond the scope of this chapter. In addition to developmental changes in the ability of adjacent tissue to reorganize,[180] the patient's learning of new behaviors is also an important component of neurobehavioral recovery.[181]

CLINICAL APPLICATIONS

The principles of neural plasticity reviewed in this chapter are important for understanding both pathogenesis and potential treatments in developmental and behavioral pediatrics. Clearly, some children have early-onset genetic or acquired brain pathology, and these structural problems cause them to interact differently with both subsequent experience and neural plasticity processes. Other children have either deficient or maladaptive experience; therefore, their subsequent neural development is affected by deprivation or trauma. A dynamic systems perspective builds upon complex interactions between brain structure and experience during development, in such a way that the culture, the family, and the child all make contributions to obtaining and organizing experience.

Gene-driven processes are important in constructing a brain that is enormously complex before any effects of experience. Much has been learned about the genetic and molecular basis of histogenesis, migration, and differentiation. These complex brain structures are the foundation upon which any subsequent modification by experience is made. If a child is born with a different brain, his or her experience of the world may be dramatically different. For example, if an infant with cerebral palsy is unable to control eye and hand movements smoothly, then processes involving coordinated information from both sources will be disrupted. Even if the subsequent experience-expectant and experience-dependent processes are functionally unimpaired, the experience itself is distorted by the disorder and will not be appropriately used. Many of the most common disorders of developmental and behavioral pediatrics (e.g., autism, ADHD, mental retardation, epilepsy, and learning disabilities) originate in both neurodevelopmental alteration and distorted experience. One widely applied clinical implication is that children whose experience is distorted or impoverished by neuropathology can benefit from corrective or enabling technology to restore the quality of experience. For example, the mandate to provide hearing- or vision-impaired children with corrective devices as early as possible may be conceptualized as important in restoring the quality of their experience. Similarly, computer technology enhances the experience of children with motor problems by enabling them to better control their actions and to greatly improve their communication.[182] In summary, the environment of children with disorders of brain development must be adapted to their needs; otherwise, their experience will be further distorted or impoverished, and development will go astray. As the understanding of neurodevelopmental disorders grows, the ability to provide evidence-based treatments to correct drifting developmental trajectories will also improve.

Some children with normal brains at birth may suffer from the effects of impoverishment or the poor quality of information during early development. As previously described, the effect of uncorrected, conflicting visual input caused by early strabismus is functional blindness in one eye. Similarly, the amount of verbal experience provided by a child's mother can significantly determine the child's vocabulary. Children's brain development can probably be substantially influenced by the quality and the amount of their experience. Finally, the child's early emotional relationship with a caregiver is probably important in fostering subsequent, healthy emotional development. For example, a child's attachment to a primary caretaker is known to develop over the first 2 years of life and, perhaps most critically, between 6 and 18 months of life. Failure to develop healthy attachment relationships may ultimately prove maladaptive to both the emotional and cognitive domains (e.g., securely attached children tend to be better at problem solving than are insecurely attached children). The vulnerability of the circuits that are critically involved in emotion, emotion regulation, and memory (e.g., corticolimbic) is the likely basis for the existence of this sensitive period. Collectively, these observations support efforts to enrich experience for young children (e.g., the Head Start program). This argument is probably strongest with regard to cognitive development, but it probably also extends to other important aspects of development, such as social abilities or attachment. We suspect that neural plasticity underlies the lasting and profound effects of early experience on emotional regulation and social behavior, so that humans have a sensitive period for emotional and social development.[183] It is thus important that researchers determine what brain regions may use associated experience-expectant processes and early experience to shape the brain. This knowledge may guide clinical efforts to redirect brain development in a more timely or focused manner. Advocacy and support for such interventions mandate evidence of their effectiveness.

A corollary of early and intensive intervention is that clinicians should not allow children to languish with active symptoms of their disorder. Delays in intervention may "waste" a sensitive period, making subsequent clinical intervention much more difficult and possibly leading to relatively irreversible pathol-

ogy. In addition, both experience-expectant and experience-dependent mechanisms may continue to operate in various pathological states, and a child with "pathological" experience in these circumstances may very well acquire neuropathology instead of functional connections. Consider what may happen to a child's brain structure after years of experience with auditory hallucinations, drug abuse, depression, or violence. The human brain has delayed prefrontal cortical development to adolescence, making young people prone to forms of executive function problems and emotional instability and leaving this important brain region vulnerable to damage from alcohol and drugs.[184] Exposure to addictive substances can result in lasting brain changes in cortical and subcortical systems, affecting hedonic drive, developing cognitive systems, and emotional regulation.[185] The effects of trauma on the developing brain are very complex. For example, Pollak and colleagues[186] demonstrated that children exposed to early violence had lasting changes in their emotional system, arousal responses, and their perception of negative expressions, as if they approached the world differently than did children who had not been abused; this finding emphasizes the importance of avoiding the consequences of negative experiences during development.

Considerable work remains to be done in neuroscience, developmental psychology, and the affiliated clinical disciplines, because interactions between children, altered brain structure, and the environment are very complex.[187] One example among many gene-environment interactions is the specific interaction of an adverse childhood environment with the genotype for low monoamine oxidase A activity, which results in an increased risk for conduct disorder in children[188] (Fig. 4-2). In addition to the genetic factors, prenatal exposure to smoking or alcohol

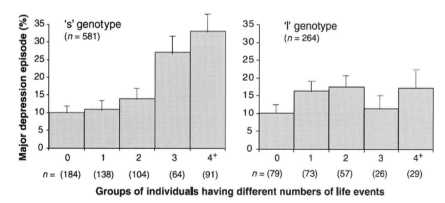

FIGURE 4-2 An interaction of genes and environment in human psychopathology. The figure shows individuals at age 26 with either one or two copies of the serotonin transporter (5HTT) short allele (left) and individuals homozygous for the 5HTT long allele (right). Data analysis found that subjects with more adverse life events were more likely to meet criteria for major depression, i.e., they were more vulnerable. (From Caspi A, Sugden K, Moffitt TE, Taylor A, Craig IW, Harrington H, McClay J, Mill J, Martin J, Braithwaite A, Poulton R. Influence of life stress on depression: Moderation by a polymorphism in the 5-HTT gene. Science, 301:386-389, 2003.)

increases the risk of a complex neurodevelopmental disorder such as ADHD.[189] Troubled or mentally ill parents serve as proximal mediators between children and the environment and can thus place a burden on children's mental health.[190] On the other hand, children with ADHD can present with such a burden of illness for parents that divorce is a common outcome.[191] Developmental-behavioral pediatricians are well aware of the complexity of these interactions, because they work closely with families, social institutions, and their developing patients.

On a positive note, children, like many organisms, are resilient and can thrive in a wide variety of environments. We suggest that children are actively involved in obtaining and structuring developmentally appropriate experience. One well-known aspect of this self-structuring of experience is play, a developmental process used by many mammalian species to improve skills and learn socialization. Just as Winnicott[192] proposed that a "good enough mother" can often suffice for normal emotional development, we suggest that many children can extract what they need from a "good enough environment." Clearly, parents play an important role in facilitating a child's experience, and their role should be considered extensively in studies of what might constitute a "good enough environment." Society and clinicians often need only to provide "just enough" of what children require to recover and resume a healthier trajectory.[193] The self-correcting and self-organizing properties of brain development may be among the most impressive themes of this chapter.

REFERENCES

1. Black JE, Greenough WT: Induction of pattern in neural structure by experience: Implications for cognitive development. In Lamb ME, Brown AL, Rogoff B, eds: Advances in Developmental Psychology, vol 4. Hillsdale, NJ: Erlbaum, 1986, pp 1-50.
2. Greenough WT, Black JE: Induction of brain structure by experience: Substrates for cognitive development. In Gunnar M, Nelson CA, eds: Behavioral Developmental Neuroscience. Minnesota Symposia on Child Psychology, vol 24. Hillsdale, NJ: Erlbaum, 1992, pp 155-200.
3. Black JE, Jones TA, Nelson CA, et al: Neural plasticity. In Alessi N, ed: The Handbook of Child and Adolescent Psychiatry, Volume 4: Varieties of Development, Section I: Developmental Neuroscience. New York: Wiley, 1998, pp 31-53.
4. Waddington CH: Concepts of development. In Tobach E, Aronson LR, Shaw E, eds: The Biopsychology of Development. New York: Academic Press, 1971, pp 17-23.
5. Chaudhari N, Hahn WE: Genetic expression in the developing brain. Science 220:924-928, 1983.
6. Milner RJ, Sutcliffe JG: Gene expression in rat brain. Nucleic Acids Res 11:5497-5520, 1983.
7. Gyllensten L, Malmfors T: Myelinization of the optic nerve and its dependence on visual function—A quantitative investigation in mice. J Embryol Exp Morphol 11:255-266, 1963.
8. Demerens C, Stankoff B, Logak M, et al: Induction of myelination in the central nervous system by electrical activity. Proc Natl Acad Sci U S A 93:9887-9892, 1996.
9. Barres BA, Raff MC: Proliferation of oligodendrocyte precursor cells depends on electrical activity in axons. Nature 361:258-260, 1993.
10. Uesaka N, Hirai S, Maruyama T, et al: Activity dependence of cortical axon branch formation: A morphological and electrophysiological study using organotypic slice cultures. J Neurosci 25:1-9, 2005.
11. Hawrylak N, Greenough WT: Monocular deprivation alters the morphology of glial fibrillary acidic protein-immunoreactive astrocytes in the rat visual cortex. Brain Res 683:187-199, 1995.
12. Jessell TM, Sanes JR: Development. The decade of the developing brain. Curr Opin Neurobiol 10:599-611, 2000.
13. Wilson SI, Edlund T: Neural induction: Toward a unifying mechanism. Nat Neurosci 4(Suppl):1161-1168, 2001.
14. Smith JL, Schoenwolf GC: Neurulation: Coming to closure. Trends Neurosci 20:510-517, 1997.
15. Rakic P: A Small step for the cell, a giant leap for mankind: A hypothesis of neocortical expansion during evolution. Trends Neurosci 18:383-388, 1995.
16. Wilson SW, Rubenstein JL: Induction and dorsoventral patterning of the telencephalon. Neuron 28:641-651, 2000.
17. Evans PD, Anderson JR, Vallender EJ, et al: Adaptive evolution of ASPM, a major determinant of cerebral cortical size in humans. Hum Mol Genet 13:489-494, 2004.
18. Sidman R, Rakic P: Development of the human central nervous system. In Haymaker W, Adams RD, eds: Histology and Histopathology of the Nervous System. Springfield, IL: CC Thomas, 1982, pp 3-143.
19. Marin O, Rubenstein JL: A long, remarkable journey: Tangential migration in the telencephalon. Nat Rev Neurosci 2:780-790, 2001.
20. Caviness VS Jr, Takahashi T, Nowakowski RS: Numbers, time and neocortical neuronogenesis: A general developmental and evolutionary model. Trends Neurosci 18:379-383, 1995.
21. Sidman RL, Rakic P: Neuronal migration, with special reference to developing human brain: A review. Brain Res 62:1-35, 1973.
22. Brazel CY, Romanko MJ, Rothstein RP, et al: Roles of the mammalian subventricular zone in brain development. Prog Neurobiol 69:49-69, 2003.
23. Rakic P: Neuronal migration and contact guidance in the primate telencephalon. Postgrad Med J 54(Suppl 1):25-40, 1978.

24. Rakic P: Mode of cell migration to the superficial layers of fetal monkey neocortex. J Comp Neurol 145:61-83, 1972.

25. Rakic P: Neurons in rhesus monkey visual cortex: Systematic relation between time of origin and eventual disposition. Science 183:425-427, 1974.

26. Lemke G: Glial control of neuronal development. Annu Rev Neurosci 24:87-105, 2001.

27. McGee AW, Yang Y, Fischer QS, et al: Experience-driven plasticity of visual cortex limited by myelin and Nogo receptor. Science 309:2222-2226, 2005.

28. Justice NJ, Jan YN: Variations on the Notch pathway in neural development. Curr Opin Neurobiol 12:64-70, 2002.

29. Gaiano N, Fishell G: The role of Notch in promoting glial and neural stem cell fates. Annu Rev Neurosci 25:471-490, 2002.

30. Bertrand N, Castro DS, Guillemot F: Proneural genes and the specification of neural cell types. Nat Rev Neurosci 3:517-530, 2002.

31. Rice DS, Curran T: Role of the Reelin signaling pathway in central nervous system development. Annu Rev Neurosci 24:1005-1039, 2001.

32. Eastwood SL, Harrison PJ: Interstitial white matter neurons express less Reelin and are abnormally distributed in schizophrenia: Towards an integration of molecular and morphologic aspects of the neurodevelopmental hypothesis. Mol Psychiatry 8:769, 821-831, 2003.

33. Gleeson JG, Walsh CA: Neuronal migration disorders: From genetic diseases to developmental mechanisms. Trends Neurosci 23:352-359, 2000.

34. Meng H, Smith SD, Hager K, et al: DCDC2 is associated with reading disability and modulates neuronal development in the brain. Proc Natl Acad Sci U S A 102:17053-17058, 2005.

35. Tessier-Lavigne M, Goodman CS: The molecular biology of axon guidance. Science 274:1123-1133, 1996.

36. Grunwald IC, Klein R. Axon guidance: Receptor complexes and signaling mechanisms. Curr Opin Neurobiol 12:250-259, 2002.

37. Brose K, Tessier-Lavigne M: Slit proteins: Key regulators of axon guidance, axonal branching, and cell migration. Curr Opin Neurobiol 10:95-102, 2000.

38. Kullander K, Klein R: Mechanisms and functions of Eph and Ephrin signalling. Nat Rev Mol Cell Biol 3:475-486, 2002.

39. Sanes JR, Lichtman JW: Induction, assembly, maturation and maintenance of a postsynaptic apparatus. Nat Rev Neurosci 2:791-805, 2001.

40. Benson DL, Colman DR, Huntley GW: Molecules, maps and synapse specificity. Nat Rev Neurosci 2:899-909, 2001.

41. Jan YN, Jan LY: Dendrites. Genes Dev 15:2627-2641, 2001.

42. Fuster JM: The Prefrontal Cortex: Anatomy, Physiology, and Neuropsychology of the Frontal Lobe, 3rd ed. Philadelphia: Lippincott-Williams & Wilkins, 1997.

43. Cragg BG: The development of synapses in the visual system of the cat. J Comp Neurol 160:147-166, 1975.

44. Greenough WT, Chang F-LF: Plasticity of synapse structure and pattern in the cerebral cortex. In Peters A, Jones EG, eds: Cerebral Cortex, vol 7. New York: Plenum Press, 1988, pp 391-440.

45. Boothe RG, Greenough WT, Lund JS, et al: A quantitative investigation of spine and dendrite development of neurons in visual cortex (area 17) of Macaca nemestrina monkeys. J Comp Neurol 186:473-489, 1979.

46. Bourgeois JP, Goldman-Rakic PS, Rakic P: Synaptogenesis in the prefrontal cortex of rhesus monkeys. Cereb Cortex 4:78-96, 1994.

47. Conel JL: The Postnatal Development of the Human Cerebral Cortex, vols 1-8. Cambridge, MA: Harvard University Press, pp 1939-1967.

48. Huttenlocher PR, de Courten C: The development of synapses in striate cortex of man. Hum Neurobiol 6:1-9, 1987.

49. Huttenlocher PR: Synaptogenesis, synapse elimination, and neural plasticity in human cerebral cortex. In Nelson CA, ed: Minnesota Symposia on Child Psychology, Volume 27: Threats to Optimal Development: Integrating Biological, Psychological, and Social Risk Factors. Hillsdale, NJ: Erlbaum, 1994, pp 35-54.

50. Huttenlocher PR: Synaptic density in human frontal cortex—Developmental changes and effects of aging. Brain Res 163:195-205, 1979.

51. Giedd JN, Blumenthal J, Jeffries NO, et al: Brain development during childhood and adolescence: A longitudinal MRI study. Nat Neurosci 2:861-863, 1999.

52. Hebb DO: The Organization of Behavior; a Neuropsychological Theory. New York: Wiley, 1949.

53. Zablocka T, Zernicki B: Partition between stimuli slows down greatly discrimination learning in binocularly deprived cats. Behav Brain Res 36:13-19, 1990.

54. Riesen AH: Effects of visual deprivation on perceptual function and the neural substrate. In DeAjuriaguerra J, ed: Symposium Bel Air II, Desafferentation Experimentale Et Clinique. Geneva: George & Cie, 1965, pp 47-66.

55. Wiesel TN, Hubel DH: Comparison of the effects of unilateral and bilateral eye closure on cortical unit responses in kittens. J Neurophysiol 28:1029-1040, 1965.

56. Michalski A, Wrobel A: Correlated activity of lateral geniculate neurones in binocularly deprived cats. Acta Neurobiol Exp (Wars) 54:3-10, 1994.

57. Walk RD, Gibson EJ: A comparative and analytical study of visual depth perception. Psychol Monogr 75(15):1-44, 1961.

58. Crabtree JW, Riesen AH: Effects of the duration of dark rearing on visually guided behavior in the kitten. Dev Psychobiol 12:291-303, 1979.

59. Gabbott PL, Stewart MG: Quantitative morphological effects of dark-rearing and light exposure on the synaptic connectivity of layer 4 in the rat visual cortex (area 17). Exp Brain Res 68:103-114, 1987.

60. Coleman PD, Riesen AH: Environmental effects on cortical dendritic fields. I. Rearing in the dark. J Anat 102(Pt 3):363-374, 1968.

61. Valverde F: Rate and extent of recovery from dark rearing in the visual cortex of the mouse. Brain Res 33:1-11, 1971.

62. Marchand AR, Cremieux J, Amblard B: Early sensory determinants of locomotor speed in adult cats: II. Effects of strobe rearing on vestibular functions. Behav Brain Res 37:227-235, 1990.

63. Cynader M, Chernenko G: Abolition of direction selectivity in the visual cortex of the cat. Science 193:504-505, 1976.

64. Hein A, Held R, Gower EC: Development and segmentation of visually controlled movement by selective exposure during rearing. J Comp Physiol Psychol 73:181-187, 1970.

65. Hirsch HV, Spinelli DN: Visual experience modifies distribution of horizontally and vertically oriented receptive fields in cats. Science 168:869-871, 1970.

66. Sengpiel F, Stawinski P, Bonhoeffer T: Influence of experience on orientation maps in cat visual cortex. Nat Neurosci 2:727-732, 1999.

67. Corrigan JG, Carpenter DL: Early selective visual experience and pattern discrimination in hooded rats. Dev Psychobiol 12:67-72, 1979.

68. Pettigrew JD, Freeman RD: Visual experience without lines: Effect on developing cortical neurons. Science 182:599-601, 1973.

69. Coleman PD, Flood DG, Whitehead MC, et al: Spatial sampling by dendritic trees in visual cortex. Brain Res 214:1-21, 1981.

70. Tieman SB, Hirsch HV: Exposure to lines of only one orientation modifies dendritic morphology of cells in the visual cortex of the cat. J Comp Neurol 211:353-362, 1982.

71. Banks MS: Infant Refraction and Accommodation. Int Ophthalmol Clin 20:205-232, 1980.

72. LeVay S, Wiesel TN, Hubel DH: The development of ocular dominance columns in normal and visually deprived monkeys. J Comp Neurol 191:1-51, 1980.

73. Shatz CJ: Impulse activity and the patterning of connections during CNS development. Neuron 5:745-756, 1990.

74. Antonini A, Stryker MP: Rapid remodeling of axonal arbors in the visual cortex. Science 260:1819-1821, 1993.

75. Mower GD, Caplan CJ, Christen WG, et al: Dark rearing prolongs physiological but not anatomical plasticity of the cat visual cortex. J Comp Neurol 235:448-466, 1985.

76. Swindale NV: Role of visual experience in promoting segregation of eye dominance patches in the visual cortex of the cat. J Comp Neurol 267:472-488, 1988.

77. Blakemore C, Garey LJ, Vital-Durand F: The physiological effects of monocular deprivation and their reversal in the monkey's visual cortex. J Physiol 283:223-262, 1978.

78. Bowering ER, Maurer D, Lewis TL, et al: Sensitivity in the nasal and temporal hemifields in children treated for cataract. Invest Ophthalmol Vis Sci 34:3501-3509, 1993.

79. Hubel DH, Wiesel TN: The period of susceptibility to the physiological effects of unilateral eye closure in kittens. J Physiol 206:419-436, 1970.

80. Olson CR, Freeman RD: Monocular deprivation and recovery during sensitive period in kittens. J Neurophysiol 41:65-74, 1978.

81. Cynader M, Mitchell DE: Prolonged sensitivity to monocular deprivation in dark-reared cats. J Neurophysiol 43:1026-1040, 1980.

82. Fagiolini M, Fritschy JM, Low K, et al: Specific GABAA circuits for visual cortical plasticity. Science 303:1681-1683, 2004.

83. Fagiolini M, Hensch TK: Inhibitory threshold for critical-period activation in primary visual cortex. Nature 404:183-186, 2000.

84. Durand GM, Zukin RS: Developmental regulation of mRNAs encoding rat brain kainate/AMPA receptors: A Northern analysis study. J Neurochem 61:2239-2246, 1993.

85. Cao Z, Lickey ME, Liu L, et al: Postnatal development of Nr1, NR2A and NR2B immunoreactivity in the visual cortex of the rat. Brain Res 859:26-37, 2000.

86. Freund P, Schmidlin E, Wannier T, et al: Nogo-A–specific antibody treatment enhances sprouting and functional recovery after cervical lesion in adult primates. Nat Med 12:790-792, 2006 [erratum in Nat Med 12:1220, 2006].

87. Liebscher T, Schnell L, Schnell D, et al: Nogo-A antibody improves regeneration and locomotion of spinal cord–injured rats. Ann Neurol 58:706-719, 2005.

88. Taha S, Hanover JL, Silva AJ, et al: Autophosphorylation of αCaMKII is required for ocular dominance plasticity. Neuron 36:483-491, 2002.

89. Tropea D, Kreiman G, Lyckman A, et al: Gene expression changes and molecular pathways mediating activity-dependent plasticity in visual cortex. Nat Neurosci 9:660-668, 2006.

90. Woolsey TA, Van der Loos H: The structural organization of layer IV in the somatosensory region (SI) of mouse cerebral cortex. The description of a cortical field composed of discrete cytoarchitectonic units. Brain Res 17:205-242, 1970.

91. Glazewski S, Fox K: time course of experience-dependent synaptic potentiation and depression in barrel cortex of adolescent rats. J Neurophysiol 75:1714-1729, 1996.

92. Holtmaat A, Wilbretcht L, Knott GW, et al: Experience-dependent and cell-type–specific spine growth in the neocortex. Nature 441:979-983, 2006.

93. Zuo Y, Yang G, Kwon E, et al: Long-term sensory deprivation prevents dendritic spine loss in primary somatosensory cortex. Nature 436:261-265, 2005.

94. Horn G: Imprinting, learning, and memory. Behav Neurosci 100:825-832, 1986.

95. Patel SN, Rose SN, Stewart MG: Training induced dendritic spine density changes are specifically related to memory formation processes in the chick, *Gallus domesticus*. Brain Res 463:168-173, 1988.)

96. Sackett GP, Novak MSFX, Kroeker R: Early experience effects on adaptive behavior: Theory revisited. Ment Retard Dev Disabil Res Rev 5:30-40, 1999.

97. Harlow HF, Harlow MK: The affectional systems. In Schrier AM, Harlow HF, Stollnitz F, eds: Behavior of Non-Human Primates, vol 2. New York: Academic Press, 1965, pp 287-334.

98. Sackett GP: Prospects for research on schizophrenia. 3. Neurophysiology. Isolation-rearing in primates. Neurosci Res Progr Bull 10:388-392, 1972.

99. Bennett AJ, Lesch KP, Heils A, et al: Early experience and serotonin transporter gene variation interact to influence primate CNS function. Mol Psychiatry 7:118-122, 2002.

100. Struble RG, Riesen AH: Changes in cortical dendritic branching subsequent to partial social isolation in stumptailed monkeys. Dev Psychobiol 11:479-486, 1978.

101. Floeter MK, Greenough WT: Cerebellar plasticity: Modification of Purkinje cell structure by differential rearing in monkeys. Science 206:227-229, 1979.

102. Martin LJ, Spicer DM, Lewis MH, et al: Social deprivation of infant rhesus monkeys alters the chemoarchitecture of the brain: I. Subcortical regions. J Neurosci 11:3344-3358, 1991.

103. Baumgardner TL, Reiss AL, Freund LS, et al: Specification of the neurobehavioral phenotype in males with fragile X syndrome. Pediatrics 95:744-752, 1995.

104. Franke P, Maier W, Hautzinger M, et al: Fragile X carrier females: evidence for a distinct Psychopathological Phenotype? Am J Med Genet 64:334-339, 1996.

105. Kerby DS, Dawson BL: Autistic features, personality, and adaptive behavior in males with the fragile X syndrome and no autism. Am J Ment Retard 98:455-462, 1994.

106. Sobesky WE, Hull CE, Hagerman RJ: Symptoms of schizotypal personality disorder in fragile X women. J Am Acad Child Adolesc Psychiatry 33:247-255, 1994.

107. Hinton VJ, Brown WT, Wisniewski K, et al: Analysis of neocortex in three males with the fragile X syndrome. Am J Med Genet 41:289-294, 1991.

108. Comery TA, Harris JB, Willems PJ, et al: Abnormal dendritic spines in fragile X knockout mice: Maturation and pruning deficits. Proc Natl Acad Sci U S A 94:5401-5404, 1997.

109. Irwin SA, Patel B, Idupulapati M, et al: Abnormal dendritic spine characteristics in the temporal and visual cortices of patients with fragile-X syndrome: A quantitative examination. Am J Med Genet 98:161-167, 2001.

110. Irwin SA, Idupulapati M, Gilbert ME, et al: Dendritic spine and dendritic field characteristics of layer V pyramidal neurons in the visual cortex of fragile-X knockout mice. Am J Med Genet 111:140-146, 2002.

111. Galvez R, Greenough WT: Sequence of abnormal dendritic spine development in primary somatosensory cortex of a mouse model of the fragile X mental retar-

dation syndrome. Am J Med Genet A 135:155-160, 2005.

112. Galvez R, Gopal AR, Greenough WT: Somatosensory cortical barrel dendritic abnormalities in a mouse model of the fragile X mental retardation syndrome. Brain Res 971:83-89, 2003.

113. Galvez R, Smith RL, Greenough WT: Olfactory bulb mitral cell dendritic pruning abnormalities in a mouse model of the fragile-X mental retardation syndrome: Further support for FMRP's involvement in dendritic development. Brain Res Dev Brain Res 157:214-216, 2005.

114. Antar LN, Afroz R, Dictenberg JB, et al: Metabotropic glutamate receptor activation regulates fragile X mental retardation protein and Fmr1 mRNA localization differentially in dendrites and at synapses. J Neurosci 24:2648-2655, 2004.

115. Antar LN, Dictenberg JB, Plociniak M, et al: Localization of FMRP-associated mRNA granules and requirement of microtubules for activity-dependent trafficking in hippocampal neurons. Genes Brain Behav 4:350-359, 2005.

116. Bagni C, Greenough WT: From mRNP trafficking to spine dysmorphogenesis: The roots of fragile X syndrome. Nat Rev Neurosci 6:376-387, 2005.

117. Grossman AW, Elisseou NM, McKinney BC, et al: Hippocampal pyramidal cells in adult Fmr1 knockout mice exhibit an immature-appearing profile of dendritic spines. Brain Res 1084:158-164, 2006.

118. Brown V, Jin P, Ceman S, et al: Microarray identification of FMRP-associated brain mRNAs and altered mRNA translational profiles in fragile X syndrome. Cell 107:477-487, 2001.

119. Darnell JC, Jensen KB, Jin P, et al: Fragile X mental retardation protein targets G quartet mRNAs important for neuronal function.[Comment]. Cell 107:489-499, 2001.

120. Miyashiro KY, Beckel-Mitchener A, Purk TP, et al: RNA cargoes associating with FMRP reveal deficits in cellular functioning in Fmr1 null mice. Neuron 37:417-431, 2003.

121. El-Husseini AE, Schnell E, Chetkovich DM, et al: PSD-95 involvement in maturation of excitatory synapses. Science 290:1364-1368, 2000.

122. Chen X, Vinade L, Leapman RD, et al: Mass of the postsynaptic density and enumeration of three key molecules. Proc Natl Acad Sci U S A 102:11551-11556, 2005.

123. Gray NW, Weimer RM, Bureau I, et al: Rapid redistribution of synaptic PSD-95 in the neocortex in vivo. PLoS Biol 4:e370, 2006.

124. Bennett EL, Diamond MC, Krech D, et al: Chemical and anatomical plasticity brain. Science 146:610-619, 1964.

125. Ravizza RJ, Hershberger AC: The effect of prolonged motor restriction upon later behavior of the rat. Psychol Rec 16:73-80, 1966.

126. Thinus-Blanc C: Volume discrimination learning in golden hamsters: Effects of the structure of complex rearing cages. Dev Psychobiol 14:397-403, 1981.

127. Greenough WT, Wood WE, Madden TC: Possible memory storage differences among mice reared in environments varying in complexity. Behav Biol 7:717-722, 1972.

128. Juraska JM, Henderson C, Muller J: Differential rearing experience, gender, and radial maze performance. Dev Psychobiol 17:209-215, 1984.

129. Holloway RL Jr: Dendritic branching: Some preliminary results of training and complexity in rat visual cortex. Brain Res 2:393-396, 1966.

130. Volkmar FR, Greenough WT: Rearing complexity affects branching of dendrites in the visual cortex of the rat. Science 176:1445-1447, 1972.

131. Turner AM, Greenough WT: Synapses per neuron and synaptic dimensions in occipital cortex of rats reared in complex, social, or isolation housing. Acta Stereol 2(Suppl):239-244, 1983.

132. Turner AM, Greenough WT: Differential rearing effects on rat visual cortex synapses. I. Synaptic and neuronal density and synapses per neuron. Brain Res 329:195-203, 1985.

133. Sirevaag AM, Greenough WT: Differential rearing effects on rat visual cortex synapses. II. Synaptic morphometry. Brain Res 351:215-226, 1985.

134. Greenough WT, Wang X: Altered post-synaptic response in the visual cortex in vivo of rats reared in complex environments. Abstr Soc Neurosci 19(11):19, 164, 1993.

135. Beaulieu C, Colonnier M: Effect of the richness of the environment on the cat visual cortex. J Comp Neurol 266:478-494, 1987.

136. Beaulieu C, Cynader M: Effect of the richness of the environment on neurons in cat visual cortex. I. Receptive field properties. Brain Res Dev Brain Res 53:71-81, 1990.

137. Black JE, Sirevaag AM, Wallace CS, et al: Effects of complex experience on somatic growth and organ development in rats. Dev Psychobiol 22:727-752, 1989.

138. Black JE, Sirevaag AM, Greenough WT: Complex experience promotes capillary formation in young rat visual cortex. Neurosci Lett 83:351-355, 1987.

139. Swain RA, Harris AB, Wiener EC, et al: Prolonged exercise induces angiogenesis and increases cerebral blood volume in primary motor cortex of the rat. Neuroscience 117:1037-1046, 2003.

140. Kingston SG, Hoffman-Goetz L: Effect of environmental enrichment and housing density on immune system reactivity to acute exercise stress. Physiol Behav 60:145-150, 1996.

141. Juraska JM: Sex differences in dendritic response to differential experience in the rat visual cortex. Brain Res 295:27-34, 1984.

142. Greenough WT, Volkmar FR, Juraska JM: Effects of rearing complexity on dendritic branching in frontolateral and temporal cortex of the rat. Exp Neurol 41:371-378, 1973.

143. Comery TA, Shah R, Greenough WT: Differential rearing alters spine density on medium-sized spiny neurons in the rat corpus striatum: Evidence for association of morphological plasticity with early response gene expression. Neurobiol Learn Mem 63:217-219, 1995.

144. Fuchs JL, Montemayor M, Greenough WT: Effect of environmental complexity on size of the superior colliculus. Behav Neural Biol 54:198-203, 1990.

145. Pysh JJ, Weiss GM: Exercise during development induces an increase in Purkinje cell dendritic tree size. Science 206:230-232, 1979.

146. Kempermann G, Kuhn HG, Gage FH: More hippocampal neurons in adult mice living in an enriched environment. Nature 386:493-495, 1997.

147. Wallace CS, Kilman VL, Withers GS, et al: Increases in dendritic length in occipital cortex after 4 days of differential housing in weanling rats. Behav Neural Biol 58:64-68, 1992.

148. Green EJ, Greenough WT, Schlumpf BE: Effects of complex or isolated environments on cortical dendrites of middle-aged rats. Brain Res 264:233-240, 1983.

149. Juraska JM, Greenough WT, Elliott C, et al: Plasticity in adult rat visual cortex: An examination of several cell populations after differential rearing. Behav Neural Biol 29:157-167, 1980.

150. Greenough WT, Juraska JM, Volkmar FR: Maze training effects on dendritic branching in occipital cortex of adult rats. Behav Neural Biol 26:287-297, 1979.

151. Chang FL, Greenough WT: Lateralized effects of monocular training on dendritic branching in adult split-brain rats. Brain Res 232:283-292, 1982.

152. Greenough WT, Larson JR, Withers GS: Effects of unilateral and bilateral training in a reaching task on dendritic branching of neurons in the rat motor-sensory forelimb cortex. Behav Neural Biol 44:301-314, 1985.

153. Withers GS, Greenough WT: Reach training selectively alters dendritic branching in subpopulations of layer II-III pyramids in rat motor-somatosensory forelimb cortex. Neuropsychologia 27:61-69, 1989.

154. Diaz E, Pinto-Hamuy T, Fernandez V: Interhemispheric structural asymmetry induced by a lateralized reaching task in the rat motor cortex. Eur J Neurosci 6:1235-1238, 1994.

155. Marrone DF: Ultrastructural plasticity associated with hippocampal-dependent learning: A meta-analysis. Neurobiol Learn Mem 87:361-371, 2006.

156. Black JE, Isaacs KR, Anderson BJ, et al: Learning causes synaptogenesis, whereas motor activity causes angiogenesis, in cerebellar cortex of adult rats. Proc Natl Acad Sci U S A 87:5568-5572, 1990.

157. Kleim JA, Swain RA, Czerlanis CM, et al: Learning-dependent dendritic hypertrophy of cerebellar stellate cells: Plasticity of local circuit neurons. Neurobiol Learn Mem 67:29-33, 1997.

158. Kleim JA, Lussnig E, Schwarz ER, et al: Synaptogenesis and Fos expression in the motor cortex of the adult rat after motor skill learning. J Neurosci 16:4529-4535, 1996.

159. Bendre AA, Swain RS, Wheeler BC, et al: Augmentation of cerebellar responses to parallel fiber activation

following skilled motor acquisition in rats. Soc Neurosci Abstr 21:444, 1995.

160. Kleim JA, Swain RA, Armstrong KA, et al: Selective synaptic plasticity within the cerebellar cortex following complex motor skill learning. Neurobiol Learn Mem 69:274-289, 1998.

161. Brown RT, Coles CD, Smith IE, et al: Effects of prenatal alcohol exposure at school age. II. Attention and behavior. Neurotoxicol Teratol 13:369-376, 1991.

162. Gallo PV, Weinberg J: Neuromotor development and response inhibition following prenatal ethanol exposure. Neurobehav Toxicol Teratol 4:505-513, 1982.

163. Hannigan JH, Berman RF, Zajac CS: Environmental enrichment and the behavioral effects of prenatal exposure to alcohol in rats. Neurotoxicol Teratol 15:261-266, 1993.

164. Klintsova AY, Matthews JT, Goodlett CR, et al: Therapeutic motor training increases parallel fiber synapse number per Purkinje neuron in cerebellar cortex of rats given postnatal binge alcohol exposure: Preliminary report. Alcohol Clin Exp Res 21:1257-1263, 1997.

165. Klintsova AY, Cowell RM, Swain RA, et al: Therapeutic effects of complex motor training on motor performance deficits induced by neonatal binge-like alcohol exposure in rats. I. Behavioral results. Brain Res 800:48-61, 1998.

166. Klintsova AY, Scamra C, Hoffman M, et al: Therapeutic effects of complex motor training on motor performance deficits induced by neonatal binge-like alcohol exposure in rats: II. A quantitative stereological study of synaptic plasticity in female rat cerebellum. Brain Res 937:83-93, 2002.

167. Crawford ML, Harwerth RS, Smith EL, et al: Keeping an eye on the brain: The role of visual experience in monkeys and children. J Gen Psychol 120:7-19, 1993.

168. Demer JL: Positron emission tomographic studies of cortical function in human amblyopia. Neurosci Biobehav Rev 17:469-476, 1993.

169. Locke JL: Thirty years of research on developmental neurolinguistics. Pediatr Neurol 8:245-250, 1992.

170. Huttenlocher J, Haight W, Bryk A, et al: Early vocabulary growth: Relation to language input and gender. Dev Psychol 27:236-248, 1991.

171. Kuhl PK: Learning and representation in speech and language. Curr Opin Neurobiol 4:812-822, 1994.

172. Zhang Y, Kuhl PK, Imada T, et al: Effects of language experience: Neural commitment to language-specific auditory patterns. Neuroimage 26:703-720, 2005.

173. Karni A, Meyer G, Jezzard P, et al: Functional MRI evidence for adult motor cortex plasticity during motor skill learning. Nature 377:155-158, 1995.

174. Elbert T, Pantev C, Wienbruch C, et al: Increased cortical representation of the fingers of the left hand in string players. Science 270:305-307, 1995.

175. Bengtsson SL, Nagy Z, Skare S, et al: Extensive piano practicing has regionally specific effects on white matter development. Nat Neurosci 8:1148-1150, 2005.

176. Maguire EA, Gadian DG, Johnsrude IS, et al: Navigation-related structural change in the hippocampi of taxi drivers. Proc Natl Acad Sci U S A 97:4398-4403, 2000.

177. Jacobs B, Schall M, Scheibel AB: A quantitative dendritic analysis of Wernicke's area in humans. II. Gender, hemispheric, and environmental factors. J Comp Neurol 327:97-111, 1993.

178. Weinberger NM: Dynamic regulation of receptive fields and maps in the adult sensory cortex. Annu Rev Neurosci 18:129-158, 1995.

179. Ramachandran VS, Rogers-Ramachandran D, Stewart M: Perceptual correlates of massive cortical reorganization. Science 258:1159-1160, 1992.

180. Ward NS: Functional reorganization of the cerebral motor system after stroke. Curr Opin Neurol 17:725-730, 2004.

181. Nudo RJ: Adaptive plasticity in motor cortex: Implications for rehabilitation after brain injury. J Rehabil Med 41(Suppl):7-10, 2003.

182. Merzenich MM, Jenkins WM, Johnston P, et al: Temporal processing deficits of language-learning impaired children ameliorated by training. Science 271:77-81, 1996.

183. Hensch TK: Critical period regulation. Annu Rev Neurosci 27:549-579, 2004.

184. Spear LP: The adolescent brain and age-related behavioral manifestations. Neurosci Biobehav Rev 24:417-463, 2000.

185. Koob GF, Le Moal M: Plasticity of reward neurocircuitry and the "dark side" of drug addiction. Nat Neurosci 8:1442-1444, 2005.

186. Pollak SD, Vardi S, Putzer Bechner AM, et al: Physically abused children's regulation of attention in response to hostility. Child Dev 76:968-977, 2005.

187. Caspi A, Moffitt TE: Gene-environment interactions in psychiatry: Joining forces with neuroscience. Nat Rev Neurosci 7:583-590, 2006.

188. Foley DL, Eaves LJ, Wormley B, et al: Childhood adversity, monoamine oxidase a genotype, and risk for conduct disorder. Arch Gen Psychiatry 61:738-744, 2004.

189. Mick E, Biederman J, Faraone SV, et al: Case-control study of attention-deficit hyperactivity disorder and maternal smoking, alcohol use, and drug use during pregnancy. J Am Acad Child Adolesc Psychiatry 41:378-385, 2002.

190. Oyserman D, Bybee D, Mowbray C, et al: When mothers have serious mental health problems: parenting as a proximal mediator. J Adolesc 28:443-463, 2005.

191. Murphy KR, Barkley RA: Parents of children with attention-deficit/hyperactivity disorder: Psychological and attentional impairment. Am J Orthopsychiatry 66:93-102, 1996.

192. Winnicott DW. The family and Individual Development. London: Tavistock Press, 1965.

193. Hoghughi M, Speight AN: Good enough parenting for all children—A strategy for a healthier society. Arch Dis Child 78:293-296, 1998.

Family Context in Developmental-Behavioral Pediatrics

BARBARA H. FIESE ■ MARY SPAGNOLA ■ ROBIN S. EVERHART*

Children's health and development are a family affair. Whether it involves keeping scheduled appointments for a child's immunizations, managing feeding difficulties in a child with Down syndrome, or negotiating an adolescent's desire for autonomy, the daily life of the family is integrally intertwined with the health and well-being of children and adolescents. Family-level factors such as direct and open communication and availability of support have been found to be associated with a host of child health outcomes, including infant mortality,[1] lifetime hospitalizations,[2] and the likelihood of developing post-traumatic stress symptoms after the diagnosis of a life-threatening illness.[3] There are several ways to consider family contributions to children's development.

First, families are responsible for providing food, shelter, and stability for children. At its most basic level, the provision of basic resources means that the family holds the key to children's nutritional status and physical comfort. However, families do not always have complete control over available resources; parent's educational backgrounds, their economic circumstances, and characteristics of the neighborhood also have influences on children's health.[4] Thus, a consideration of family influences on children's health and development must also include the environments in which families live. Second, families are the holding place for children's emotional development. Children learn to trust others and regulate their emotions in the safe surroundings of their home before venturing out to school and other social environments. For some children, this is a relatively positive experience, and they come to school well equipped to meet academic and social challenges. For other children, inconsistent and erratic experiences in the home often leave them ill equipped to interact with others, which thus places them at risk for school failure, behavioral problems, and strained peer relationships.[5] In all cases, these experiences are mutually influential: Characteristics of the child influence the family, and the family influences the child's development. Third, family members create practices and hold beliefs that often extend across generations and are influenced by culture. Family life is organized in such a way that it builds on past experiences, which results in predictable routines and imparting of values through recounting personal experience. Many families benefit from their heritages and can use them as guides in meeting the challenges of raising their children. For some families, however, personal histories of neglect, substance abuse, and parental psychopathology interfere with the constructive transfer of generational knowledge and can place children at risk for poor health and development.[6-8]

These multilayered influences of the family on children's health and development make researchers' task somewhat daunting. Although it is beyond the scope of this chapter to examine every conceivable way that families could influence children, we do address how families are embedded in neighborhoods and cultures that affect their daily practices and beliefs. We also consider how multiple risk factors in the environment can act synergistically to make children vulnerable to a host of poor outcomes. It is the exception, not the rule, that maladaptive outcomes are the result of a single family factor. Rather, multiple aspects of a child's life such as temperament, economic resources of the family, and psychological functioning of the parent must be considered in order to understand adaptation of the child at any given time.

The empirical study of family influences on children's development is complicated at best. Identifying who is in the family; whether to rely on direct

*Preparation of this manuscript was supported, in part, by grants from the National Institutes of Health (R01 MH51771) to the first author and from the Administration for Children and Families to the first and second authors.

observation of family interactions or parent's report of family climate; how to resolve inconsistencies in reports by mother, father, child, and teacher about child behavior; and adaptation of techniques across cultures[9] are just a few of the thorny issues in the scientific study of families. In addition, the changing demography of American families includes increasing numbers of children who are being raised by parents of different ethnic backgrounds, in single-parent households, or in multiple households.[10] For the medical clinician, keeping track of all the layers of family life can seem like an overwhelming task, particularly in the short amount of time allocated for patient visits. Rather than ignore the apparent complexity of family life, in this chapter we offer some guidelines for the busy clinician to consider in his or her contact with children and their families. Because the importance of establishing partnerships with families is the cornerstone of pediatric practice,[11] a greater understanding of how families operate is in order.

In the past there was a tradition in developmental studies to equate poor child outcomes directly with poor parenting. Such terms as "refrigerator mothers" were coined to suggest that parents (most notably mothers) with cold and harsh parenting techniques were the sole progenitors of their children's ill health, mentally and physically.[12] Childhood schizophrenia was thought to develop from rejecting and harsh parenting styles. Pediatric asthma was thought to arise from overcontrolling and smothering parenting styles.[13] At the root of these notions was the assumption that parenting effects were always direct and unidimensional and that neither characteristics of the child nor the surrounding environment had much of an effect on development. Clearly, these notions are outdated because advances in behavior genetics suggest heritability quotients for such conditions as schizophrenia and that symptom severity in asthma is the result of complex interactions among environmental conditions, genetic factors, and family factors.[14] The point is that parents do not directly *cause* their child's poor health or maladaptive development; rather, children's health and well-being are embedded in a family context that is subject to a variety of influences, some of which we outline in this chapter.

For the clinician, families are important not only as sources of information about the child's condition but also because they are responsible for carrying out treatment recommendations. Biological interventions are successful only to the extent that parents are able to follow treatment recommendations. How family members deal with stress, availability of resources, and histories of psychiatric disturbance and abuse can affect treatment planning and the likelihood that interventions will be successful. In essence, many aspects of primary care for children with developmental disabilities and pediatric chronic illness must take into account how families support their child's health and well-being.

This chapter is structured in the following ways. First, we provide an overview of a theoretical framework that we believe can be of use for clinicians as they think about the complexities of family life. We first review the social-ecological model originally proposed by Bronfenbrenner.[15] This theoretical model is useful in that it allows clinicians to consider not only how the child is situated in the family but also how the family is influenced by the neighborhood in which it lives, the schools that are available to the child, and the culture with which the family most closely identifies. Second, we also consider that children and families change. They do so as part of a process whereby families influence the growth and development of their children and the characteristics of the child also influence how the family functions. This process has been labeled *transactional,* which suggests that development is characterized by a series of active exchanges between parents and children and that both child and parent contribute to a child's condition at any given point in time. Thus, we also outline the transactional model as originally proposed by Sameroff and colleagues.[16,17] Integrally linked to the social-ecological and transactional perspectives is the role that multiple risk factors play in development. Optimal and poor outcomes are rarely the result of a single factor; rather, the multiple influences of culture, economic resources, family support, and child characteristics cumulatively affect development over time. Thus, we consider the compound effect of environmental risks.

Third, we consider how families are organized systems. Although oftentimes family life seems chaotic and it is difficult to keep track of everyone's whereabouts, there are principles of order and balance that we can identify at the level of the family that have direct implications for the practice of developmental and behavioral pediatrics. We aim to translate some of these more esoteric principles into real-life examples that can be of use to the busy practitioner. Furthermore, there are elements of family organization that may protect children from environmental threats and reduce the likelihood that they will develop behavioral problems when exposed to multiple risk factors.

After this strong theoretical grounding in the social-ecological and transactional models and family systems principles, we review some of the literature that illustrates family effects on child health and well-being. Specifically, we examine family factors that promote adjustment in children with a chronic illness, parenting variables that can reduce the risks associated with poverty, and how cultural beliefs and practices enacted in the family context can influence child health and well-being. We conclude with recommendations for clinicians in their clinical decision-making process with families, as well as policy makers responsible for the health and well-being of children. Throughout the chapter, we use vignettes to illustrate our points and to elucidate these complex concepts. Consider the following scenario:

It is 7:00 a.m. on a school day; three children between the ages of 6 and 10 years sit huddled around the television set munching on sweetened cereal with their eyes transfixed by the latest cartoon images of genetically engineered creatures fighting to save their village from intruders. The children's mother rushes through the family room, charging them to "get a move on it" because she is late for work and they will miss the school bus. As the last child is about to leave the house, he screams, "What about my homework? We forgot to finish it last night." Exasperated, the mother pulls at the child, tells him to get in the car, and instructs him to finish it while she drives him to school.

What happens next? In order to answer this question, we would need to know more about this family, including how they handle the challenges of everyday life, how they communicate their needs to each other, how they resolve conflict, what beliefs they hold about academic achievement, and the availability of social support within and outside the immediate family, as well as their economic resources and their cultural values. For the pediatrician, it is also important to know whether the last child has a learning problem that prevented him from completing his homework, whether the child is overweight and should not have been eating the sweetened cereal in the first place, and what the parent's relationship with teachers is in the event that a treatment plan that connects home and school needs to be implemented. We offer this brief scenario to illustrate that underlying the commonplace events of family life are a host of complex dynamics that, together, constitute family influences on child health and development. In this chapter, we aim to unravel some of these complexities by highlighting how families organize their daily lives in their routine practices. We also describe how families create beliefs about relationships that guide their behavior with their children and how these beliefs may affect families' responses to health care professionals. The creation of these routines and beliefs do not happen in a vacuum. They are constantly shaped and altered by availability of economic resources, as well as rooted in cultural heritage. Thus, we also aim to examine how socioeconomic and cultural contexts interface with family practices and beliefs.

SOCIAL-ECOLOGICAL MODEL

Jamie is a 4-year-old boy in whom an autism spectrum disorder has been diagnosed. He is the youngest of five siblings. His parents are newly divorced, and his mother is primarily responsible for his care. They have moved to a neighborhood where the nearest school with early childhood services is 25 miles away. His mother must leave early for work in the morning and take him to the babysitter's house via public transportation. The most accessible public transportation to the babysitter's home is five blocks from the family's new home. The mother holds strong religious beliefs and regularly attends church services.

In this brief scenario, we have several elements of Bronfenbrenner's social-ecological model (Fig. 5-1). The child is at the center of the model. The child's development is proposed to be influenced by the persons most immediately around him. In this case, Jamie's development is affected primarily by his mother and siblings. The child's developmental status is influenced by how responsive his mother is to his needs, as well as by the support and opportunities provided by interactions with his siblings. However, the degree to which the mother is emotionally available to interact with the child in a warm and responsive way may be influenced by her relationship with her ex-husband. We know, for example, that marital conflict can have detrimental effects on children's development by disrupting effective parenting styles and setting the stage for poor emotion regulation by

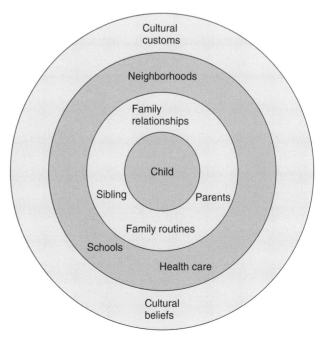

FIGURE 5-1 Social-ecological model.

children.[18] Thus, the environment closest to the child's daily experiences may have a direct influence on his development through exposure to supportive and warm interactions or through a home environment that is characterized by conflict and disruptions. These interactions do not operate in isolation but are influenced by the next level of Bronfenbrenner's model.

Once we move out of the immediate confines of the family home, we note that there are other influences on child development that can have profound effects on the development of children. This is the level most commonly encountered by pediatricians, inasmuch as how families interact with health care teams also affects how children cope with chronic illnesses.[19] In the preceding example, the likelihood that Jamie will develop to his fullest potential will depend not only on his family's best intentions but also on their ability to gain access to early childhood programs in their neighborhood. Transporting a 4-year-old child five blocks to the home of a babysitter, who must in turn put him on a bus for a long ride for a 3-hour early intervention program, represents a daily challenge. Even under the most optimal home conditions, this would be an added strain to the system that may compromise the child's developmental progress. Thus, the degree to which the resources available outside the home support, or derail, family investments can have a direct influence on child developmental outcomes.

There is a third level to the social-ecological model that can also influence child development. This layer of the social environment includes such factors as culture, social class, religion, and law. In the preceding example, the legal system has an indirect influence in that public laws guarantee access to public education for all children, regardless of developmental condition. However, as noted previously, gaining access to available education programs can be tempered by resources available in the neighborhood. Culture and religion can also influence child development indirectly. In the case of Jamie, we noted that his mother held strong religious beliefs. Religious beliefs may affect how parents cope with the daily care of children with special needs, so that practices endorsed by mandated programs must also coincide with deeply held doctrines.[20]

We offer this brief overview not as an exhaustive treatment of the literature that either supports or refutes the social-ecological model as it pertains to child development. Rather, we use it as a guide for considering the multiple influences on child development and families as a whole. Just as the existence of a chronic condition such as diabetes is likely the result of a host of factors, family effects on children's development are also multifaceted. Families are subject to influences beyond those that have a direct proximal

effect on children. Cultural mores, economic resources, and alterations in the life cycle indirectly influence child health and well-being by influencing how families regulate social interaction, allocate resources, and generate beliefs about relationships. The next section is a consideration of how children and families change over time and the process of development within the family context.

Transactional Model of Development

Joanna was born prematurely weighing 4½ pounds at birth. Joanna was discharged from the hospital 2 weeks after her mother was sent home. During those 2 weeks, her parents visited her daily but were very concerned about how fragile she appeared in the neonatal intensive care unit. Upon returning home, they attempted to keep noise at a minimum, thinking that reducing stimulation would soothe Joanna. However, she remained a fussy baby. Whenever her parents picked her up, she squirmed, and they would soon put her back in the crib. In comparison with her older brother, Joanna did not like to play teasing games such as "I'm going to get you" or "Peek-a-boo." For the most part, her parents left her to play by herself with stacking toys. Joanna was slow to talk, saying her first single words at 15 months. Once she reached preschool age, she received a diagnosis of a language delay from a speech pathologist.

Was the cause of Joanna's language delay her prematurity and low birth weight? It is known that premature children are at greater risk for developing language delays than are full-term infants.[21] Or was the cause of her language delay her fussiness and difficult temperament? Or being less favored than her older brother? Or being left alone? From a transactional perspective, all of these features may come into play when a child's developmental outcome at any given point in time is considered. In this case, the parents have reasonable concern about their vulnerable infant. Rather than being able to bring their infant directly home, they had to wait and ponder their daughter's health. Seeking information through the Internet or hospital personnel, they discovered that premature infants are sensitive to light and sound. In this case, Joanna's fussiness was interpreted by her parents as further indication of her need to have reduced exposure to stimulation, and thus they put her down in the crib frequently. There were fewer opportunities for social interaction and verbal play. This was interpreted as a temperamental difference or perhaps a gender difference in comparison to her brother. Without adequate opportunities for verbal play, Joanna did not develop an age-appropriate vocabulary; thus, her overall language abilities were delayed. This process is outlined in Figure 5-2.

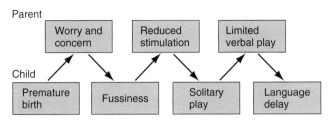

FIGURE 5-2 Transactional model depicting language delay in a premature infant.

The transactional model as proposed by Sameroff and colleagues[16,17,22] emphasizes the mutual effects of parent and caregiver, embedded and regulated by cultural mores. In this model, child outcome is predictable by neither the state of the child alone nor the environment in which he or she is being raised. Rather, it is a result of a series of transactions that evolve over time, with the child responding to and altering the environment. For pediatricians, this model is important because it gives due recognition to the child's effect on the environment, as well as to the environment's effect on the child. Pediatricians are frequently faced with situations in which parents feel ill equipped to deal with the challenges of parenting, assuming that childrearing is a one-dimensional task that should conform to a set of prescribed principles easily accessible through a book or the Internet. Typically, this naive view is quickly cast aside with the birth of a second child and parents realize that a one-size-fits-all approach to parenting is rarely successful. Thus, to be able to predict how families influence children, the investigator must also ask how children influence families and how this process develops over time. In addition to recognizing that parents and children mutually influence each other, the transactional model is also important in highlighting the multiply determined nature of risk in family environments.

Multiply Determined Nature of Risk in Family Environments

Jack is 12 years old and has a learning disability. His father has lost his job, and the family must move to a new town for the father to find employment. In their new neighborhood, Jack is befriended by a group of older boys who have been repeatedly in trouble with the law. Jack's mother feels lost in their new location and leaves her husband to live with her sister in a town 200 miles away. Jack is left to care for his three younger siblings. Jack's grades begin to slip, and he becomes truant from school.

In this brief scenario, we note several believable life circumstances. Any one of these conditions may be cause for concern and, with proper support, would be unlikely to cause a major disruption in the household or derail positive development. Having a learning disability does not cause a child to drop out of school, just as loss of a job does not necessarily lead to the breakup of a marriage. However, when there are multiple stressors in the family environment, there are increased risks for poor child outcomes. Across several investigations of different types of child outcomes, researchers have established that the absolute number of environmental risks that children are exposed to are what portend poorer outcomes. We highlight two of these programs of research that are of interest to pediatricians and illustrate the role that family context may play in exacerbating or reducing risk.

ADOLESCENT ACADEMIC ACHIEVEMENT AND PSYCHOLOGICAL ADJUSTMENT

In a large study of adolescents in Philadelphia, the relation between exposure to a variety of risk factors and both academic achievement and psychological adjustment was examined.[5] Using an ecological framework, the researchers identified six domains of risk: family process, parent characteristics, family structure, management of community (e.g., social networks), peers, and community (e.g., neighborhood). Adolescents were assigned risk scores for each domain. Lack of autonomy, low-level parent education, single marital status of parents, lack of informal networks, few prosocial peers, and low census tract socioeconomic status are examples of high risk in each of the domains. Increasing numbers of risk factors was associated with large declines in academic performance and psychological adjustment. Using an odds-ratio analysis, the authors compared the likelihood of poor outcomes in high-risk environments with those in low-risk environments. For academic performance, they found that a poor outcome increased from 7% in the low-risk group (three or fewer risk factors) to 45% in the high-risk group (eight or more risk factors)—an odds ratio of 6.7 to 1.

A similar pattern of effects was found in considering the promotive, or positive, contributions to child outcomes. Adolescents with more environmental resources fared better in terms of school performance and mental health than did those with fewer resources. Although this may make intuitive sense, it is important to emphasize that no single group of risk factors accounted for significant increases or decreases in adolescent outcomes. Rather, the cumulative set of environmental risks, including compromised parenting, lack of economic resources, and social isolation, was associated with poor outcomes for these adolescents.

Two factors that are repeatedly identified as contributors to children's well-being are parental income and marital status. Research on multiple risk factors highlights, in part, how income and marital status are embedded in larger social ecologies that act in concert with other risk and protective factors. This is important in consideration of family effects on child health and development, inasmuch as marital status and economic stability are commonly viewed as structural family variables essential for children's well-being. Whether a parent is married or holds a prestigious job is not the litmus test for positive family influence on child outcomes. In isolation, these structural variables are not informative about the larger social environment in which the child is being raised or the nature of family process in the home. For example, it is known that there are many types of single-parent families and that children of divorced parents do not necessarily develop mental health problems.[23]

How children fare during and after divorce is a topic of considerable concern to pediatricians. During the 1990s, more than 1 million children were involved in divorce every year.[24] In a meta-analysis of 67 studies conducted between 1990 and 1999, Amato[25] found that children of divorced parents scored significantly lower than did children with married parents on measures related to academic achievement, conduct, psychological adjustment, self-concept, and social relations. These differences were less pronounced in African-American children than in white children.[26] Marital discord appears to play an important role in how children are affected by parental divorce. Not only the presence or absence of discord but also how conflict unfolds during the dissolution of the marital relationship is important. When children have not been exposed to discord before the divorce, there are more long-term difficulties in adjustment, which suggests that there is an increase in conflict and stress after the divorce.[25] In contrast, when there are relatively high levels of conflict before the divorce, dissolution of the marriage can actually be a relief for the child, and there are fewer long-term effects on child adjustment. Thus, what results in poor adjustment in children is not divorce per se but exposure to marital conflict. Experimental studies have also documented that children's exposure to unresolved marital conflict, in particular, is more likely to result in emotional and behavioral disturbances than are marital disagreements that children witness as reaching some resolution.[18]

Only when investigators consider the social environments of the family, as a whole, can they begin to understand under what conditions structural variables such as marital status and employment will influence children's well-being. Next is a closer look at how the presence of multiple risk factors has been examined in the context of family poverty, an area of central concern for pediatricians.

MULTIPLE RISK FACTORS AND POVERTY

Children growing up in poverty are disproportionately affected by chronic health conditions, including asthma, obesity, and diabetes. Children growing up in poverty also show early signs of allostatic load and higher resting blood pressure, which suggests that they are at increased risk for developing other serious chronic health conditions.[27] In 2003, the poverty rate was highest for younger children; 20% of children between birth and the age of 5 years of age were being raised in households below the poverty line.[28] There are concerns that children exposed to poverty over long periods may be at increased risks for poor physical and social-emotional outcomes. Limited economic resources can have crushing effects on family life, not only through its effects on the provision of basic needs but also by its effects on relationships and parenting. For example, in studies of rural farm families in Iowa, it was found that the downward turn of economic circumstances preceded marital distress and led to increases in hostile and coercive interactions between parents and adolescents.[29] As noted previously, the compound effects of risk may influence child outcome; a similar picture holds true with regard to the effects of poverty on child health and well-being.

Evans[30] considered the physical and mental health of children raised in poor rural communities and the multiple environmental risks they were exposed to, including crowding, noise, housing problems, family separation, family turmoil, violence, single-parent status, and parent education level. In accordance with the previous reports on multiple risk factors in less economically disadvantaged families, increasing numbers of risk factors were associated with more child psychological distress and feelings of less self-worth. Furthermore, children exposed to more environmental risk factors also evidenced higher systolic blood pressure and elevated neuroendocrine stress reactivity. As Evans stated, "As childhood exposure to cumulative risk increased, overall wear and tear on the body was elevated." (p. 928).

Risk conditions are often compounded in nature and difficult to unravel. For example, the effects of family poverty on children's health depend on how long the poverty lasts and the child's age when the family is poor.[31] Single-parent status also cannot be viewed in isolation, because the number of adults in the household has been identified as a marker of socioeconomic status known to be associated with some child outcomes.[32] Perhaps one of the multiple-risk contexts that is most difficult to disentangle is that of the overlapping effects of economic conditions and ethnic background. In many empirically based studies of family effects on child development, poverty is confounded with minority status.[33] One exception is a study employing the National Longitudinal Survey of Youth. Bradley and colleagues examined nearly 30,000 home observations of young children diverse in economic and ethnic backgrounds.[34] Because of the relatively large sample size, the researchers were able to distinguish between poor and nonpoor European-American, African-American, and Hispanic-American families. In general, they found that poverty accounted for most, but not all, of the differences between the groups with regard to less stimulating home environments (availability of books, having parents read to the child, parent responsiveness). There were some differences, however, that were attributed to ethnic background when poverty status was controlled. For example, European-American mothers were more likely to display overt physical affection during the home observation than were African-American mothers. There were no ethnic group differences in the likelihood that mothers would talk to their infants or answer questions prompted by their elementary school–aged children. Thus, the distinguishing characteristics most often associated with poor outcomes for children, such as the lack of enriching home environments, were more closely associated with low income status than with ethnic background. Further efforts are warranted to separate the effects of poverty from the influence of ethnicity on child outcomes. The long-term effects of coping with discrimination may also affect parenting practices, particularly because these practices are evaluated by researchers within the dominant culture.[35] In this regard, it is also important to be cognizant of factors, such as race and economic background of the observer, that can influence evaluations of family process. We return to this point when we discuss family assessment.

We provide these examples of multiple risk factors to highlight the multifaceted context of family influences on child outcomes. It is not sufficient to note that children from poor families are at greater risk for developing certain physical and mental health problems than are their more economically advantaged peers. Nor is it sufficient to assert that children raised in warm and supportive households are less likely to develop mental health problems than are children raised in harsh and rejecting ones. The consequences for children's development are too far-reaching to expect that family influence would be simple and uniform. Therefore, a consideration of the family must likewise be sensitive to multiple avenues of effect while also accounting for the fact that there is diversity in the ways in which families go about the tasks of raising children. Thus far, we have presented a somewhat pessimistic view of family environmental

effects on child development. Just as there are multiple risk factors that can contribute to compromised outcomes for children, there are family-level factors that promote adaptation and adjustment even in the presence of known environmental risks. To understand how these positive factors may operate, we must first consider how families, as a whole, are organized to promote development.

FAMILIES AS ORGANIZED SYSTEMS

The alarm goes off at 6:00 a.m. David, the father, makes the coffee while Julie, his wife, makes lunch for the three children. Around the breakfast table, there is a quick check-in about everyone's day and reminders about who is going to pick up whom after band practice, the dentist, and dance lessons. The evening brings a recap of the day's events and a somewhat rushed dinner. During dinner, the youngest child describes being left out of an activity by her friends, the middle child brings up her daily request for a new puppy, and the oldest child (a teenager) is silent throughout much of the meal. At bedtime, the father finds out more about the youngest child's experience at school, the mother reaffirms that there will be no new puppies in the home, and, once the younger children are in bed, the teenager and mother review the study guide for his driver's license test. Husband and wife talk briefly about the failing health of his father and make plans to visit him in the extended-care facility over the weekend.

This is not an unlikely scenario that on the surface appears fairly mundane but may include several elements of healthy family functioning. Families are charged with a host of tasks to insure the health and well-being of their children. Families are responsible for providing structure and care in at least six domains: (1) physical development and health; (2) emotional development and well-being; (3) social development; (4) cognitive development; (5) moral and spiritual development; and (6) cultural and aesthetic development.[36] Each of these tasks can be considered as building on the other in a hierarchical manner; however, in day-to-day family life, they often overlap and are not clearly differentiated. In the example just provided, while the family is grabbing a quick breakfast before heading out the door for the day (and, it is hoped, fulfilling the nutritional needs of the children), they are also attending to their cultural and aesthetic development through the arrangement of after-school lessons. Families structure care and meet the developmental needs of their children through organized daily practices, as well as through beliefs that they carry about relationships. We now examine how daily practices, as reflected in family routines, and beliefs, as reflected in family narratives, are related to the health and well-being of developing children.

Family Routines and Healthy Development

In accordance with our focus on the multiply determined nature of child development, children's health is also considered part of a larger system of family functioning. When we think about family health, we think about what the family, as a group, must do to maintain the well-being of all its members, including establishing waking and sleeping cycles, establishing eating habits, responding to acute illness, coping with chronic illness, preventing disease, and communicating with health professionals. These activities, or practices, are often folded into the family's daily routines. Pediatricians are poignantly aware that for some chronic health conditions, family involvement in daily care is essential to good health but, at the same time, these management behaviors can be "tedious, repetitive, and invasive" (Fisher and Weihs,[37] p. 562). This repetitive nature of management activities sets the stage for creating routines that provide predictability and order to family life. Conversely, the repetitive demands associated with good health care may also disrupt routines already in place and threaten family stability. We first define what we mean by *family routines* and then examine their relation to child health and well-being.

DEFINING ROUTINES

There is a personalized nature to family routines that makes it somewhat difficult to provide a standard definition. What may be a routine for one family may be absent in another. For example, some families hold very high expectations for when everyone is to be home for dinner and have set rules for the expression of emotional displays, whereas other families have a more laissez faire attitude toward mealtime attendance and rarely remark when someone makes an angry outburst at the table.[38] Family routines tend to include some form of instrumental communication so that tasks get done, involve a momentary time commitment, and are repeated over time.[39] In terms of normative development, family routines such as dinnertime, weekend activities, and annual celebrations (e.g., birthday celebrations) tend to become more organized and predictable after the early stages of parenting an infant and into preschool and elementary school years.[40] The regularity of family routine events such as mealtimes have been found to be associated with reduced risk taking and good mental health in adolescents.[41,42] The sense of belong-

ing created during these gatherings has been found to be associated with self-esteem and relational well-being in adolescents and young adults.[40,43]

There are several aspects of family routines that serve to support or derail children's health. Family routines in relation to children's health can be examined along a dimension that ranges from discrete daily habits to a collective sense of belonging to a group that cares for and nurtures the individual. We now consider the effects of each aspect in turn.

HABITS

Habits are repetitive behaviors that individuals perform, often without conscious thought. Behavioral habits are automatic and typically involve a restricted range of behaviors. For example, some children may have developed a habit of snacking while sitting in front of the television set after school. A routine, on the other hand, involves a sequence of steps that are highly ordered.[44] For example, a child's morning routine may include a sequence of having breakfast, brushing teeth, checking the contents of a backpack, and playing catch with the dog before going to school. Healthy (or unhealthy) habits are often embedded in routines. Being in the habit of eating a nutritionally balanced meal may rely, in part, on shopping and cooking routines. For the most part, habits are rarely thought about, and pediatricians must ask repeatedly about parents' and children's daily routines to gather accurate information about healthy and unhealthy habits. It is not sufficient to ask whether a child eats a healthy diet, but it may be important to consider whether the diet is offered as part of a regularly organized routine.

Organized family routines may be part of good nutritional habits. For example, parents' report of the importance of family routines has been found to be associated with children's milk intake and likelihood of taking vitamins in low-income rural families.[45] During the preschool and early school years, if mealtime routines are rushed and interactions are marked by discouragements and conflict, then children are at greater risk for developing obesity.[46,47] Furthermore, if mealtime routines are regularly accompanied by television viewing rather than conversation, children consume 5% more of their calories from pizza, salty snacks, and soda and 5% less of their energy intake from fruits, vegetables, and juices than children from families with little or no television use during mealtimes.[48] Qualitative studies have noted that individual members can disrupt diabetes management by routinely eating late, regularly serving desserts, and making daily shopping trips to grocery stores that have few choices in the way of fresh fruits and vegetables.[49] Grocery shopping routines may also be affected by larger ecologies as lower income neighborhoods are often noted for grocery stores that do not have a full array of fresh produce. Thus, family routines may contribute to children's health through establishing good nutritional habits and providing regular rather than erratic opportunities to be fed.

ADHERENCE

Adherence to pediatric medical regimens is notoriously poor. According to most surveys, families fail to follow medical advice more than half the time.[50] It is unlikely that all cases of medical nonadherence are caused by lack of knowledge or a failure to fully understand doctor's orders.[51] Patients often remark that they fail to follow prescribed orders not because they want to but because they just could not find the time or because other responsibilities got in the way. There is no question that family life is busy and there are multiple demands on everyone's time. Whether it is juggling home and work, squeezing in one more extracurricular activity, or just trying to get everyone fed during the week, the addition of a medical regimen to family responsibilities can seem overwhelming. One way that some families can adapt to the challenges of medical management is through the organization of their daily routines.

Many treatment guidelines for chronic health conditions suggest folding disease management into daily routines. The management of pediatric asthma is one such condition. Current practice guidelines[14] emphasize the importance of daily and regular monitoring of asthma symptoms and detailed action plans in the event of an attack. Many of the recommendations are framed as part of the family's daily or weekly routines such as vacuuming the house once a week, monthly cleaning of duct systems, and daily monitoring of peak flows. Accordingly, asthma management becomes part of ongoing family life, and families who are more capable of the organization of family routines are expected to have more effective management strategies.

In a survey of 133 families with a child who had asthma, it was found that parents who identified regular routines associated with taking and filling prescriptions had children who took their medications on a more regular basis, both according to parents' report and according to computerized readings taken on the children's inhalers.[52] Furthermore, when there were regular medication routines in the home, parents had less trouble reminding their children to take their medications, and overall their children rarely or never forgot to take their medications. Because nonadherence to pediatric regimens is quite high[53] and parents find themselves in the role of perpetual nagger, the establishment of regular routines may be one way to alleviate distress and promote health in children with chronic conditions. Future

research appears warranted in order to consider whether interventions aimed at structuring family routines may positively affect disease management and increase medical adherence.

PARENTAL COMPETENCE

The establishment of daily habits and maintenance of medical regimens through family routines addresses how families organize behaviors that promote health and well-being. Families are also responsible for providing an environment in which individuals can gain a sense of personal efficacy and feel that they belong to a group that cares for and nurtures them. The repetition of routines over time and the creation of family rituals may afford such connections.

Family routines may also be important in promoting parental competence and establishing caregiving practices associated with children's health and well-being. There is some evidence to suggest that experience with childcare routines before the birth of the first child is positively related to feelings of parental competence.[54] However, in addition to parent skill set, the child contributes to these feelings, as was identified in the transactional model. Infant rhythmicity (e.g., regularity with which infants go to sleep at night) has been found to be associated with regularity of family routines, which, in turn, were associated with parental competence.[55] The relation between caregiving competence and family routines during the early stages of parenting is probably the result of a series of transactions. When there is a good match between infant and parent behavioral style, it may be easier to engage the child in family routines. Routines become relatively stable, and the infant is easier to soothe, more amenable to scheduled naps, and less likely to wake in the night. This predictability, in turn, may reduce parental uncertainty and concern and increase feelings of competence. As parents engage in more rewarding daily caregiving activities, they become more confident in their abilities, and the routines themselves become more familiar and easier to carry out; for example, the difference between diapering an infant for the first versus the thousandth time is remarkable. The transactional process of one evolving caregiving routine is presented in Figure 5-3.

BELONGING VERSUS BURDEN

As the family practices its routines over time, individual members come to expect certain events to happen on a regular basis and form memories about these collective gatherings. For some, family is seen as a group that is a source of support, and repeat gatherings are eagerly anticipated. For others, family is seen as a group unworthy of trust, and collective gatherings are avoided. We have found that families

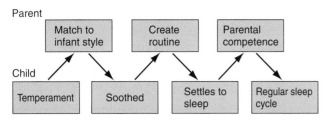

FIGURE 5-3 Transactional model depicting establishment of sleep patterns.

who ascribe positive meaning to repeated routine gatherings such as dinnertime, weekends, and special celebrations feel more connected as a group and consider these events as special times rather than times to be endured.[39] These feelings of belonging created during family routine gatherings are also associated with the health and well-being of children and adolescents. For example, children with chronic health conditions who report more connections during their family routines are less likely to report anxiety-related symptoms such as worry and somatic complaints.[56] Furthermore, adolescents raised in caregiving environments with high-risk characteristics such as parental alcoholism are less likely to develop substance abuse problems and mental health problems when they report a sense of belonging created during family routines.[57]

In contrast to eagerly anticipating family events are feelings of being burdened and overwhelmed by the daily demands of family life. Feelings of burden can be particularly poignant in caring for a child with a chronic illness. Chronic illnesses can affect family life in notable ways, including added financial burden,[58] and can place strains on marital relationships.[59]

Burden of care specifically associated with daily routine management may be related to quality of life for caregiver and child. In the previously mentioned study of 133 families with asthma, an element of daily care labeled *routine burden* was identified.[52] Routine burden was defined as daily care seen as a chore with little emotional investment in caring for the child with the chronic illness. For both the caregiver and the child, when daily routines were considered more of a burden, quality of life was compromised. Caregivers reported that they were more emotionally bothered by their child's health condition and their daily activities were affected more when there was more routine burden. Likewise, children reported that they were bothered more by their health symptoms, worried more, and were more frustrated by their health symptoms when their caregivers reported more routine burden. Routine burden was associated with functional disease severity, so that parents of children who required more care also believed that

management was a chore. However, even when investigators controlled for disease severity, parents who perceived asthma care as a burden also reported poorer quality of life, as did their children.

CHAOS

It is possible to consider that the absence of routines is expressed as chaos. Chaotic home environments can be characterized by unpredictability, overcrowding, and noisy conditions.[60] These types of conditions are more likely to exist in low-income environments and in neighborhoods perceived as dangerous and isolated. Research has indicated that the presence of chaos in the home, rather than poverty alone, mediates the effects of poverty on childhood psychological distress.[61] Furthermore, children raised in chaotic environments have more difficulties reading social cues, and their parents use less effective discipline strategies.[62] Thus, children exposed to chaotic environments lacking in predictable routines may also be exposed to other risks known to be associated with poor outcomes such as poverty, overcrowding, and dangerous neighborhoods. Again, we emphasize that family factors rarely, if ever, operate in isolation.

SUMMARY

One way to consider families as organized systems is to examine their daily practices. Families are faced with multiple challenges in keeping the group together; they must balance the needs of individuals who differ in age and personality, connect the family to institutions outside the home, and provide some regularity and predictability to daily life. At its most basic level, individuals create daily habits that become parts of the family's routine practices. These routines are associated with family health in areas such as nutrition, establishment of wake and sleep cycles, and exercise. The establishment and maintenance of routines may enhance adherence to medical regimens. Families who have had experience generating such practices should be better equipped to fold disease management into their daily lives. We return to this point when we discuss models of family intervention useful for pediatricians. The repetition of family routines over time may lead to feelings of efficacy and competence, particularly for parents. Success in caregiving routines may reduce the stresses and uncertainties that accompany being a new parent, which, in turn, may affect children's well-being in a transactional manner by increasing parents' sense of personal efficacy. Parents who feel more efficacious are also more likely to interact in positive and sensitive ways that promote child well-being.[63]

When family routines are repeated over time and family gatherings are anticipated as welcomed events, individual members create memories that include a sense of belonging. This connectedness to the family, as a group, is associated with general health and relational well-being for adolescents and young adults and may reduce some of the mental health risks associated with chronic illness. The converse is also true: If the repetition of family routines over time results in feelings of dread and distance from the group, then there are concomitant effects on the health and well-being of child and parent.

Family routine life can also be disrupted to the degree that there is little order and predictability and children are raised in primarily chaotic environments. A chaotic home life is probably associated with a number of other environmental risks, including overcrowding and ineffective discipline strategies. The daily practices of family life may be important for pediatricians to understand in considering the likelihood that treatment recommendations will be followed, a point to which we return later. There is also another level to family life that affects child well-being: the construction of beliefs about relationships. We now discuss how families impart values about relationships through the stories that they tell and how individuals construct beliefs about family relationships that affect health and well-being.

Family Stories of Health and Well-Being

Well, we more or less suspected that she had asthma for a while. And I guess you know I noticed more that she complained about feeling tight in her chest or whatever, and she was doing some wheezing. But I come from a family where my mother was a hypochondriac. I know from my own experience that kids make up stuff when they don't want to go to school. I just chose to ignore it. One night she was upset about something. I think we had an argument or something and she was crying. It was late at night. It was 10:00 at night, and I was very angry with her, and she was complaining about this tightness in her chest and she needed to get to the doctor, and of course I thought it was a way to get my attention, and I was ignoring her, but she kept insisting, so, as angry as I was, I loaded her into the car in the middle of the night [and] we went to the emergency room.

—Story told by parent of 9-year-old with asthma

This is an excerpt of an interview conducted with a parent about the effect of a chronic illness on family life. There are several elements of this example that reflect the parents' beliefs about relationships and illustrate how these beliefs influence behavior and ultimately affect the child's health. Before examining the elements of the story that may be important for clinicians' understanding of family process, we consider why family stories may reflect beliefs and values pertinent to children's health and well-being.

Family stories deal with how the family makes sense of its world, expresses rules of interaction, and creates beliefs about relationships.[64] When family members are asked to talk about a personal experience, they must interpret what happened to them in a way that reflects how they work together (or do not), how they ascribe meaning to difficult and challenging situations, and how they relate to the social world. Pediatricians are quite familiar with family narratives, inasmuch as each patient visit presents an opportunity to listen to stories of health as well as illness.[65]

For families, stories are used to impart values and to socialize children into the mores of the culture. For example, the thematic content of family stories told to children has been found to differ according to whether they are told to girls or boys and whether they are told by mothers or fathers.[66] This is important to pediatricians because mothers and fathers recount experiences of illnesses and trauma in different ways, as do boys and girls. For example, after treatment in the emergency department, mothers and daughters are more likely to recall details of the accident in a cohesive and integrated manner than are fathers or sons.[67] Thus, pediatricians must consider the source of the narrative, not only the content.

Family stories intersect in the social-ecological model by reflecting cultural values and mores in such a way that the types of stories told differ across societies. For example, European-American and Chinese parents reminisce and tell stories about the past in different ways. European-American parents are more likely to focus on everyday events and to highlight practical problem solving, whereas Chinese parents are more likely to use stories to solve interpersonal conflicts and promote social harmony.[68] The point is that the family environment is rich with narratives of personal experience that guide behavior and is influenced by larger social ecologies. We now discuss the key elements of family narratives that may be related to children's health and well-being.

NARRATIVE COHERENCE

Coherence refers to how well an individual is able to construct and organize a story. Coherence is seen as an integration of different aspects of an experience that provides a sense of unity and purpose and is essential in constructing a personal life story.[69] The elements of coherence include being able to tell a story that is succinct and yet including enough details to make it intelligible to the listener, having a logical flow, matching affect with content, and in some instances providing multiple perspectives.[70] There has been increasing interest in using personal narratives, or stories, as a means to educate physicians, as well as to connect patients to physicians in the healing process.[71,72] Stories that are coherent and well orga- nized are likely to be better understood and easier to incorporate into a therapeutic context than are ones that are disjointed and lack a clear sense of order. The small but burgeoning literature discussed next links the study of family narratives, specifically that of coherence, and health and well-being.

If the coherence of family narratives is to be associ- ated with child outcomes, it must be demonstrated that it varies systematically under high-risk condi- tions and that it is related to markers of family func- tioning. There is preliminary evidence that this is the case. Dickstein and colleagues found that parents with major affective disorders such as depression recount family experiences in a less coherent manner and that current depressive symptoms exacerbate this effect.[73] There is also evidence to suggest that families who recount experiences associated with chronic illness less coherently also report poorer family func- tioning overall.[74] Furthermore, when the narratives were less coherent, families had more difficulty engag- ing with the interviewer. Why might these findings be important for children and for pediatricians? First, consider their potential link to children's outcomes.

There is a relatively strong empirical base linking coherence of narratives told about attachment rela- tionships and the mental health and well-being of children, adolescents, and young adults.[75,76] When parents and children are able to create coherent accounts of their caregiving relationships, they tend to be secure in their attachments and mentally healthy in the long run. A similar pattern is emerging in the case of family relationships. When individuals talk about family relationships in a coherent manner, family functioning appears to be more well regulated, providing a potentially more supportive environment for children. Why might these findings be important for pediatricians? During the course of a routine patient visit, families present a wealth of information, often in narrative, or story form. Families who have difficulties getting their points across to the pediatri- cian and creating a coherent account of personal events may be presenting similar images to their chil- dren. We have been particularly struck by the relation between coherence and family problem solving. Fami- lies who have difficulties engaging with interviewers and creating coherent accounts of chronic illness also express difficulties in family problem solving and communication.[74] This combination may present added risks for children, who rely on their parents for clear and direct communication and effective problem solving. A cautionary note: This is a nascent line of research, and we also recognize that a transactional process is probably in place in which health care pro- fessionals probably influence the types and forms of information that families are willing to communi-

cate.[77] We also recognize that reliably detecting the relative coherence of a family narrative is beyond the reach of routine pediatric practice. Most systems for evaluating narrative coherence are fairly complex and involve lengthy training.[78,79] Furthermore, it is not clear whether the stresses associated with a doctor's visit may affect coherence in ways unrelated to psy- chological functioning.

Whereas the coherence of family narratives may be somewhat difficult to directly assess during a routine patient visit, the ways in which relationships are depicted are more accessible. Relationship beliefs are also an important part of family narratives and have been found to be related to children's health and well- being, and they are discussed next.

RELATIONSHIP BELIEFS

Families create beliefs about relationships that vary along the dimension of trust, reliability, and safety.[70] Relationships can be seen as sources of reward and worthy of trust or viewed as potential sources of harm and unreliable. Family narratives frequently depict the degree to which relationships are seen as some- thing that can be mastered and rewarding or as over- whelming and confusing. In the case of the latter, statements are often made that reflect dissatisfaction and disappointment in relationships. Also, statements are made whereby relationships are seen as opportu- nities for experiencing appreciation and pleasure. As families are built around mutuality in relationships, the degree to which they are satisfactory and reward- ing should bear concordance with children's health and well-being.

Just as there are different conditions in which nar- rative coherence systematically varied, there are dis- tinctions among family narratives about relationships in relation to children's outcomes. Two types of out- comes are particularly pertinent for pediatricians: children's behavior problems and health care utiliza- tion. There have been a few studies that have linked depictions of family relationships in stories to chil- dren's behavior problems. Parents who recount family experiences as including rejecting and unrewarding relationships tend to have children with more prob- lematic behaviors according to self-report measures.[80] Furthermore, when parents tell stories that include depictions of family relationships that are unreliable and unsatisfactory, there are increased levels of nega- tive affect when the family is gathered as a whole during routine mealtimes.[73,80] Children's stories of family experiences reflect a similar pattern. Children who have experienced abuse and neglect depict family relationships as less rewarding in stories about family events.[81,82] Interestingly, children enrolled in an attachment-based therapeutic intervention changed their representations of family relationships, depicting caregivers as more trustworthy in the narratives after intervention than did children in the comparison group.[82] Thus, the portrayal of relationships in family narratives reflects parents and children's interpretation of the trustworthiness of others, which, in turn, may be related to social interaction and the regulation of behavior.[75] There is also some evidence that narratives hold promise in understanding how families utilize health care services.

When asked to talk about the effects of an illness on daily life, family members typically have little trouble generating a story. However, there is no single way in which families meet the challenge of organizing their lives or responding to normative or nonnormative events, as already noted. The same holds true in considering how families recount strategies of care revealed in narratives. Families can rally around the care of an individual in a variety of ways.[83] For some families, everyone is involved, and there is a team-based strategy so that multiple members of the family are "on the lookout" for the identified patient. This may mean being available to pick up prescriptions from the pharmacist, translating doctor's orders into a native language, or reading a book out loud when a sibling does not feel well. For other families, there is one expert in the family who takes charge whenever someone is ill or whenever there is a chronic health condition. Sometimes this person takes on the role across generations, so that he or she is responsible for the care not only of offspring but also of older parents. In a third type of family management style, few roles are assigned, and there is little planning around emergencies and crises. Typically in these families, anxiety calls the family to action. These management strategies can be depicted in narratives and reflect beliefs about family relationships. In the first case, team-based strategies revolve around assumptions that family relationships are reliable and multiple members of the family can be called on at a moment's notice. In the second case, relationships in general may be rewarding, but roles are assigned in such a way that there is a clear leader and authority in the family. In the third case, either relationships are seen as a bother and unreliable, or worry and anxiety predominate to the extent that relationships are precarious. When interviews about coping with a chronic illness were categorized by these management strategies, it was found that families that use either the family partnership or the expert-based approach were more likely to adhere to the prescribed medical regimen than were those who used more anxiety-based coping strategies.[83] Furthermore, families that depicted their management strategies in the interviews as more reactive and relationships as less satisfactory were more likely to use the emergency room for care 1 year after the interview.

SUMMARY

There are several points to be made about family narratives that are important for pediatricians. First, family narratives are accessible to pediatricians and can be used as part of their routine practice. Families naturally tell stories, and children's socialization is affected, in part, by the types of personal stories that they hear at home. The types of stories that parents tell the pediatrician may provide a window into family process, as well as provide clues as to the type of messages that children are receiving at home. Second, in order for family narratives to have the most powerful effect, they should be coherent. If the pediatrician is having a difficult time following the family's account of a personal experience, then the health care professional has to question whether the information is being gathered in a way that makes sense to the family and, if so, the likelihood that that the child receives information in the home in similar ways. Children who are exposed to less coherent accounts of personal experiences may also be exposed to family environments in which communication is less direct and problem solving is compromised. Third, narrative accounts of family experiences reflect beliefs about relationships and how the family works together (or does not) as a group. For some families, providing an opportunity to tell their story is an enriching experience and sheds light on the multiple resources that are at hand. For other families, recounting personal experiences is an occasion to unload grievances about unsatisfactory relationships. This is not idle chatter, inasmuch as there are real consequences for behavior and health care. In the example of the 9-year-old with asthma, the parent's narrative focused on the bother and intrusion that the child's chronic health condition had caused the family. It should come as no surprise that this case is illustrative of a management style associated with poor medical adherence and high emergency room use. Thus, good listening skills and sensitivity to multilayered aspects of family narratives may be of benefit to the busy pediatrician.

Thus far, we have considered the family as an organized system that maintains itself as a group through organized routines and reaffirms its beliefs about the importance of relationships through accounts of personal experiences. These are family-level processes that come to form the family code. The family code is created to regulate child development, extending across generations, and involves the coordinated efforts of two or more people.[17] Embedded within the family code are parent-child interaction patterns that can facilitate the smooth operation of daily life, as well as foster achievement of developmental tasks. We now briefly review some of the essential ingredients of family interaction that serve to support healthy development.

Family Interaction and Healthy Development

A family of five sits around the dinner table talking about the events of the day. The mother comments that "Grammy" enjoyed her birthday card, at which point the middle child chimes in with a chorus of "Happy Birthday to You." The father asks the oldest child whether she liked the special treat he packed for her lunch. To which she responds, "Thanks, Dad!" The youngest child demonstrates her skills in using both hands with her "big girl" cup. There is a brief discussion about the new configuration of the dining room table. The older children and parents agree that they like the new arrangement, but the youngest child, 3 years of age, states adamantly that she does not like it. The rest of the family laughs, and the father remarks: "She is just expressing her opinion."
—*Example taken from Syracuse Mealtime Observation*

Family interaction can be evaluated along a variety of dimensions. Some of the more common domains are warmth, control, support, communication, problem solving, criticism, and affect.[84] In this snippet of a mealtime observation, the family balances the need to maintain the group as a whole with expressions of independence. For most families, this balance is struck relatively effortlessly with good humor and warmth. A chorus of "Happy Birthday to You" to the grandmother, even in her absence, does not disrupt the flow of the meal, and individual desires are respected. In other families, however, expressions of autonomy may be met with harsh control, and negative affect predominates. Considerable effort has been directed toward identifying patterns of interaction associated with more optimal outcomes for children with chronic illness and children at risk for developing health problems.

Children with a chronic illness are at greater risk than children without a chronic illness for developing behavior problems or a psychiatric disorder, such as depression or anxiety. In fact, epidemiological surveys have revealed that children with a chronic illness are twice as likely to develop a diagnosable behavioral or psychiatric disorder.[85] The causal mechanism for why children with a chronic illness are more at risk than their healthy counterparts is not known. Early speculations suggested that certain patterns of family interaction were more prevalent in families with a chronic illness and that these interaction patterns led to and sustained the disease state.[86] On the basis primarily of clinical observations, the most common pattern was considered to consist of parental overinvolvement, overprotection, poor conflict resolution, and a primary focus on the child with the illness to the neglect of the marriage and other family members' needs. This pattern has not been borne out in the empirical literature and fails to take into account the shifting nature of illness and its effect on family dynamics.[87]

Researchers have begun to examine how family interaction patterns may be part of a transactional process between characteristics of the child, health status, and caregiving. Researchers theorize that children may have a limited range of cognitive or emotional skills for coping with their disease or that the increase of environmental stressors, such as medication regimens and missed school days, may contribute to adjustment difficulties.[88,89] The increase of disease-specific responsibilities places greater burden on the family as a whole, with the potential risk for increased conflict among family members and impaired levels of family functioning. A child may resent such conflict or family changes and externalize his or her resentment in the form of behavioral problems.[89]

Family conflict, observed either directly or through self-report, appears to disrupt effective disease management strategies and to adversely affect child health and well-being. Highly conflict-ridden family relationships can compromise communication, supervision, and division of responsibilities.[90] It is likely that family conflict affects child outcomes through alterations in daily health practices, inasmuch as poor adherence to medical regimens has been found to be associated with family conflict.[91,92] Furthermore, family conflict has been associated with poor glycemic control in children with diabetes.[93] Family conflict may also be an indicator that the family as a group has not been able to adjust to the child's illness, which in turn can lead to emotional distress for parent and child alike.[94] Whereas the research linking family conflict and children's health under chronic conditions appears to be mediated by disruptions in medical adherence, other investigators have examined how exposure to family conflict may result in compromised health by reducing children's ability to respond to stress.

In summarizing the literature on high-risk family environments, Repetti and colleagues[27] reported that family conflict is associated with higher rates of reported physical symptoms and lower attainment of developmentally expected weights and heights. They suggested that family conflict may lead to increased stress reactivity and allostatic load in children in high-risk environments. This argument is consistent with the research that we reviewed on multiple risk factor effects under poverty conditions. Indeed, the profile of extensive conflict, poor emotional and social support, and children's heightened stress reactivity is consonant with the multidetermined model outlined previously. Thus, lower levels of family conflict may be one more element in the larger picture of family health.

Family conflict has received the most attention in the empirical literature perhaps because it is relatively easy to identify from video recordings. It may also be the case that negative interactions have a more toxic effect and that a modest amount of negativity can lead to poorer outcomes. According to family systems principles, there are other aspects of family interaction that should also contribute to healthy family functioning. These include direct and clear forms of communication, effective problem solving, responding to the emotional needs of others, showing genuine concern about the activities and interests of others, and supporting autonomy.[95] To date, most researchers have reported on the overall general functioning of the family as it relates to child and family adjustment to such conditions as pediatric cancer,[96] maternal depression,[7] cystic fibrosis,[97] and asthma.[98] There is some evidence to suggest, however, that effective problem solving and direct forms of communication are associated with healthier outcomes for children with chronic illnesses. For example, adherence to dietary restrictions for children with cystic fibrosis is related to more positive forms of communication and problem solving observed directly during mealtime interactions and during structured laboratory interaction tasks.[99,100] A similar pattern has been noted for families and children with diabetes.[101,102]

SUMMARY

Families vary considerably in how they interact with their children. Under optimal conditions, family members feel supported through warm and responsive interactions that also indicate respect for independence and autonomy. Family life would not be typical if there were not conflict of some sort, however. All families experience disagreements, whether it is over bringing home a new puppy or choice of peer group; these squabbles are part of family life. However, it is how disagreements are resolved, not necessarily the actual outcome, that portends good or poor functioning. Longitudinal evidence suggests that sustained and unresolved conflict in the home can compromise children's health through increased stress reactivity, disruptions in health management, and increased behavior problems. Over time, conflictive family interactions reduce opportunities for effective problem solving, and spiraling negativity may threaten the integrity of the family as a whole. For the busy pediatrician, it is important to recognize that persistent patterns of negativity and conflict in the family may reduce the likelihood that treatment regimens will be followed. There is a cause for optimism, however: The results from family-based intervention programs suggest that problem solving, communication, and positive parenting can ameliorate risks and lead to more optimal outcomes for children. We return to this point in our discussion of family-based interventions.

Thus far, we have considered variations in family process along the dimensions of family practices and beliefs as reflected in the construction of routines and representation of relationships expressed through family narratives. We have examined these variations in the context of environmental risks and family response to chronic illnesses. Another important source of variation in family process is the effects of culture on daily practices and regulation of beliefs. We now consider some of the general ways in which culture may intersect with family process and influence child health and development.

CULTURAL VARIATIONS IN FAMILY CONTEXT

Cultures, in general, are organized around a set of principles that guide individuals' behavior in such a way that they are consistent with the mores of the larger society. Cultures vary in terms of the relative values given to individual strivings for autonomy and independence versus placing the needs of the group before the needs of the individual.[103] In relation to these values of individualism and collectivism, there are variations in terms of deference to authority and what "counts" as a personal transgression. In some cultures, for example, a child is more likely to get into trouble or be disciplined for something that would cause shame to the family; in other cultures, punishment is doled out for not understanding how personal actions reflect flaws in an individual's character.[104] This point is important for pediatricians, because issues of discipline and parental control are embedded in both a cultural and a family context.

These values are transmitted, in part, through the organization of daily family life. The study of everyday tasks and situations is not only embedded in culture but is also at the very heart of how behavior is shaped by society.[105,106] By focusing on how families in different cultures carry out daily routines such as household chores, investigators are able to get a glimpse at what is culturally relevant and how roles are assigned to facilitate socialization. Thus, we consider how the practice of family routines in different cultural contexts is related to children's health and well-being.

When investigators consider cultural variations, they are also interested in situations in which there is a mismatch between the predominant society and families or between parents and children. A mismatch in values presents an added tension for individuals and family members, potentially compromising health and well-being. One such situation is a mismatch of values between generations during the process of immigration. A breakdown or deterioration of routines and rituals may indicate difficulties making the transition from one culture to another. Replacing old rituals with new ones, on the other hand, may also be an indication of adaptation to a new cultural environment. This is not an "either-or" process, inasmuch as current conceptualizations of the acculturation process suggest that there are family-level advantages to retaining connections to the country of origin, as well as incorporating aspects, such as language, of the newly adopted country into everyday practices.[107,108]

Recent census data document that 20% of children in the United States have immigrant parents and that 25% of children in low-income families are of immigrant status (www.census.gov). With immigration comes a blending of beliefs that regulates family interactions with health care professionals, as well as with each other. Therefore, we also consider briefly how cultural beliefs interface with family process and influence children's health and well-being. It is beyond the scope of this chapter to cover the multitude of ways that culture and family processes transact to affect children's development. Thus, we structure our discussion around three topics: family routine practices in Latino families, beliefs about autonomy in immigrant Chinese families, and disease management strategies in African American families. Although these may appear as disjointed topics, we have selected them to highlight how cultural values intersect with domains of family life that we have previously discussed.

Variations in Family Practices: Mealtime Routines in Latino Families

Ana, a young mother from Puerto Rico living in Boston, feeds her 13-month-old daughter while holding her in her lap. The toddler sits calmly waiting for the next spoonful of soup. Her next-door neighbor, who is a descendant of several generations of Irish Catholics, is chatting at the table while her toddler of 13 months roams around the kitchen. She feeds her daughter bites of a peanut butter and jelly sandwich as she moves from one part of the room to the next.

Here we see two approaches to feeding a toddler that may be rooted in cultural values of what is considered good conduct. Latino and Anglo individuals have been described as differing in the extent to which they hold values and meaning systems that are congruent with sociocentrism or individualism.[109-111] *Sociocentrism* refers to an emphasis on the relationship between the individual and the group and subordination of ones personal interest to that of the group, resulting in a construction of the self as fundamentally linked to others. Latino cultures have typically been identified in the research literature as sociocentric.[103] Within many Latino cultures, sociocentrism may be made evident through the importance placed on respect (*respeto*) and dignity (*dignidad*) in personal conduct. Both qualities are essential in the development of proper demeanor: knowing the level of decorum and courtesy that is required in a given situation.[112] With regard to child rearing, this does not necessarily mean that Latino parents want their children to always do what is best for the group at the expense of their own happiness; rather, it is through genuine care and not *malcriado* (being poorly brought up) that a person can bring respect and happiness to the family and to himself or herself. Traditional Puerto Rican culture, for example, has been described as emphasizing interpersonal obligations, personal dignity, and respect for others.[113] Puerto Rican mothers may believe that qualities such as *malcriado* and a lack of *dignidad* and *respeto* will give rise to a lack of acceptance from others in the community, which will reflect poorly on the family and the child, eventually leading to unhappiness for the child. In sum, the goal in traditional Latino cultures is to raise a child to become *una persona de provecho*—a person who is worthy of trust and is useful to the community.[112]

Harwood and Miller[110] found that Anglo mothers were more likely than Puerto Rican mothers to stress the importance of an infant's ability to cope autonomously with the stress of being left alone. In a series of studies, Harwood and Miller examined Anglo and Puerto Rican mothers' preferences for behavior in their children. Puerto Rican mothers were more concerned about their children's ability to maintain proper respect and dignity and were more likely to focus on their children's ability to remain calm and good-natured, and to be physically close with their mothers, whereas Anglo mothers reported that they preferred infants who were able to manage autonomously.[110] In a follow-up study, Harwood[109] interviewed mothers about what they valued in children and found evidence that Anglo mothers placed greater importance on personal development and self-control. Harwood's studies provide evidence for the existence of culturally defined values in the meanings that mothers may give to child behavior. Specifically, Anglo mothers placed more importance on personal competencies, and Puerto Rican mothers placed more importance on whether the infants were able to maintain proper demeanor and physical closeness.[109]

These beliefs and values may be expressed in the practice of mealtime routines. Latina (specifically Puerto Rican) mothers were less likely then Anglo mothers to encourage their children to feed themselves.[111] In addition, the strategies that parents used to teach their children to feed themselves differed. Latina mothers were more likely to guide their children in getting food from the plate into the mouth and/or holding their children in their lap while they ate, rather than seat them in a high chair. Although these are relatively simple examples, they highlight how repetitive socialization practices are embedded in cultural values. How might pediatricians encounter the effects of these cultural practices and belief systems? One way is through the parents' tolerance for and understanding of disruptive behaviors.

Families socialize their children in accordance with the values held by the culture as to what is acceptable and unacceptable behavior. As noted, in some Latino cultures, there are values held for self-control and personal demeanor that reflect the family's stature. In interviews of Latina mothers whose children were seen by professionals for disruptive behaviors, three personality characteristics of the children were identified as salient: *inteligente, malcriado,* and *de carácter fuerte.*[114] Children who were referred for disruptive behaviors by their teachers were seen as intelligent (*inteligente*) by their mothers, which suggests that misbehavior must be the result of giftedness or clever mischief. One half of the mothers interviewed mentioned their children's bad manners (*malcriado*); however, of those who alluded to their children's rude conduct, some did so as a means to disconfirm the trait and expressed concern that others would think of their child as spoiled. Mothers also described their children as possessing a willful temperament (*de carácter fuerte*). In contrast to *malcriado, de carácter fuerte* is seen as something that can be ultimately controlled, although not permanently altered. Together, this triad of characteristics provides the parents with an explanatory set of beliefs to account for disruptive behaviors that are inconsistent with the cultural values of good conduct.

Just as a cultural perspective may affect how misbehavior is understood, it can also affect how developmental milestones are interpreted. In consideration of whether a child is disabled or capable of performing the routine activities of daily living, it is also important to consider the degree to which the family and culture supports independence and autonomy. There may be significant cultural variations in the expected norms of activities of daily living for children with disabilities. For example, Latino parents, caregivers, teachers, and therapists expect children with disabilities to be dependent on their parents for many daily skills until much later than would be expected on tests with norms for white U.S. mainland residents.[115] This pattern holds true for their nondisabled peers and is attributed to the interdependence between parents and children and cultural values of *anonar* (pampering or nurturing) and *sobre protective* (over-protectiveness). Thus, parents may report the achievement of developmental milestones at a rate that would be cause for concern by the pediatrician and yet are within a range considered normative in a given culture.

We provide these examples of feeding practices, attributions of disruptive behavior, and achievement of developmental milestones to illustrate how cultural values are part of family life. Although something as commonplace as the choice to feed a toddler in a high chair or allowing the child to carry a peanut butter and jelly sandwich throughout the house may seem to be an inconsequential act, these are decisions rooted in cultural values. The consequences of cultural variations in family daily practices can be more substantial when there is a mismatch between values held within the family and expectations of conduct held by members of social institutions such as health care providers or schools. As in the examples provided here, Latino families may not allow their children to engage in independent activities of daily living (such as self-bathing), not because of skill deficiencies but because the parents consider it their familial duty to protect and nurture their children by performing these jobs as part of their role as good parents. Without this cultural perspective on family responsibility, the pediatrician may garner a misperception about the child's abilities to achieve developmental milestones. Mismatches in values can also occur within families, particularly when one generation is raised with different values than the older generation. We now consider how immigration may affect parent-child relationships and the health and well-being of adolescents.

Immigration and the Balance of Family Obligations

Susan, 16 years old, is the eldest daughter of Chinese immigrant parents. She is very active in her high school drama club, spending long hours at practice after school. She is also responsible for the care of her two younger siblings on the weekends while her parents work in the family business. Susan's friends persistently request that she spend more time with them on the weekends; she politely refuses.

The unanswered question to this scenario is whether Susan is relatively happy or distressed by not spending time with her peers. For native-born American teenagers, spending time with peers is considered part of the natural progression of moving out of the home and becoming more autonomous. For some adolescents of immigrant families, however, staying close to home is considered part of being a good son or daughter. Whether this causes distress may depend on the relationship between parent and adolescent and beliefs that the adolescent holds about family obligations. Chinese adolescents report, on average, two family obligation activities per day and spend slightly more than one hour each day assisting and being with their families.[116] Overall, girls spend more time and carry out more family obligations than do boys. Socializing with peers is negatively related to family obligations on any given day. However, the amount of time spent in family obligations does not necessarily lead to greater conflict or personal distress for these adolescents. These youths appear to expect to balance family and social obligations and make deliberate decisions to spend time with their families. Rather than leading to a sense of alienation from peers, these daily practices may reinforce cultural beliefs and provide a sense of identity. "Family obligations may provide the children from immigrant families with a sense of identity and purpose in an American society that, at times, has been accused of emphasizing individualism at the cost of heightened adolescent alienation" (Fuligini et al,[116] p. 311). Thus, obligation to the family is balanced with spending time with peers and does not necessarily create personal distress. Yet to be answered, however, is whether this balanced perspective weakens with subsequent generations as extended engagement with popular culture may create increased opportunities to weigh obligations to peers over those to parents.

A third area to consider is how ethnic and cultural variations influence family practices that can affect disease management. Although the research literature is somewhat sparse, there are some promising findings that may be of use to pediatricians.

Ethnic Variations in Family Management Practices

A central concern for pediatricians working with families who have a child with a chronic illness is the transfer of responsibility of disease management from parent to child. The decision to transfer responsibility can be influenced by cultural standards, or beliefs, that regulate how the family interacts with health care providers and with each other. One area that has received some attention is the division of responsibility in African-American families for asthma management tasks. Although our discussion is focused on pediatric asthma, many of the findings are pertinent to how cultural beliefs may intersect with family decision making and provider relationships.

A first step in considering how parents transfer responsibility of management practices is to identify beliefs that the family may hold about the condition that may act as a barrier to good health. In interviews with African-American parents of children with asthma, it was found that a more holistic approach to managing asthma that included both the child's mental and physical well-being was desirable.[117] Many parents reported that they modified the physician's treatment plan to include nonmedicinal alternatives for their children's symptoms and held strong personal beliefs against the use of medications. Thus, when it is time to transfer the responsibility of disease management to children, clinicians must consider how beliefs about medication are also being parlayed.

An additional point to consider is that transfer of responsibility may not necessarily be from one caregiver to the child, inasmuch as two or more caregivers are frequently involved in disease management in urban and African-American families.[118] Having multiple family members involved in asthma care extends into the patient's adolescent years.[119] Multiple family members and extended kin networks can serve as sources of support. It is also important, however, to carefully consider whether availability of support translates into clear assignment of responsibility. In interviews with adolescents and their parents, Walders and colleagues found that African-American parents overestimated the amount of responsibility that adolescents were taking for their asthma care.[119] As the authors pointed out, the wide array of family structures can be simultaneously a source of support and a source of confusion when it comes to assigning responsibility. Pediatricians are in the unique position to address transfer of responsibility with their patients over time while being sensitive to how variations in family structure and cultural beliefs may regulate this process.

Summary

Although there is little disagreement that changes in population demographics mandates broader conceptualizations of cultural influences on health,[120] the empirical base linking cultural variations in family practices and children's health is somewhat limited. There is a growing literature that documents cultural and ethnic variations in family routines and beliefs associated with child outcomes. It is important to emphasize that there is considerable heterogeneity within a given culture and that we have made only generalizations. Furthermore, the effects of economic stability and resources on immigration cannot be ignored and in all likelihood play a significant role in the understanding of how cultural variations in family context contribute to children's health.[121,122]

The challenges of working with children and their families are many. Thus far, we have considered how children are raised in families that are influenced by a multitude of factors, including culture, neighborhoods, and economic resources. When children experience distress, it is probably the result of a complex transaction that has evolved over time. To adequately assist families in need, interventions must also take into account the complex nature of child development. This does not necessarily mean that all aspects of family life need be changed at any given point in time. We now examine briefly some of the family-based models of intervention that are consistent with the principles that we have outlined thus far and are accessible to pediatricians.

FAMILY-BASED INTERVENTIONS

It is beyond the scope of this chapter to provide a comprehensive review of all the intervention programs available to families. The interested reader is referred to reviews and collected volumes for more thorough discussions of the topic.[123-127] There is growing empirical evidence that targeting the whole family as a method of treatment for disease-specific issues is effective. For example, in intervention studies aimed at improving disease management in insulin-dependent diabetes, families who participated in Behavioral Family Systems Therapy, in comparison with families who received educational forms of intervention, showed higher rates of improvement in parent-adolescent relations and lower rates of diabetes-specific conflict.[128] In a review of interventions for survivors of childhood cancer and their families, Kazak and associates[129] summarized empirical evidence for interventions from four categories specific to pediatric oncology: understanding procedural pain, realizing long-term consequences, appreciating distress at diagnosis and over time, and recognizing the importance of social relationships. Kazak and associates pointed to the importance of developing interventions that target families on the basis of a particular set of risk factors, of designing more empirical interventions for families experiencing disease relapse, and of striving to develop interventions that are effective for ethnically diverse families. Current thinking in family-based interventions for pediatric conditions is that a one-size-fits-all strategy is unlikely to be effective.[130] Because families are developmentally complex systems that routinely undergo change, as we have outlined, it is unreasonable to expect that a uniform strategy aimed at altering family level behaviors would be advantageous across all families

and all situations. Thus, in this section, we consider several approaches that may be appropriate for families at a given time. We place these strategies in the transactional model previously discussed. Using a decision tree, we outline different strategies that can be implemented by drawing on the existing strengths and resources of the family and tied into previously established forms of intervention such as interaction guidance, behavior management, and relationship building techniques.

Transactional Model of Intervention

Louisa is 4 years old and has suffered from chronic respiratory infections and allergies since she was an infant. After a recent hospitalization, she received a diagnosis of moderately severe asthma and has been prescribed a daily controller medication, as well as a short course of steroid treatment, to get her asthma symptoms under control. Her mother has become quite upset over the recent hospitalization and found it difficult to visit her in the hospital. Her father tends to be the "level-headed" member of the family and has taken over responsibilities for Louisa's medication regimen. Louisa has developed night terrors and wakes frequently in the night and can be calmed only by her mother, who worried that Louisa would die in the middle of the night from an asthma attack. Parents and children are seen in the pediatrician's office, tired, stressed, and at their wits' end as to how to manage all the new demands of asthma and still get a good night's sleep.

In this scenario, we see a transaction unfolding in which the child's symptoms have disrupted the daily routines of family life. According to the principles of the transactional model, behavior can change at multiple points, whereby the child's condition affects the organization of the family and the family's behavior affects the well-being of the child. Interventions that capitalize on the strengths of the system at a given time and minimize the need to alter the system as a whole—a timely and expensive endeavor—can be targeted. Sameroff[131] proposed that there are at least three categories of intervention that can be implemented to effect change in either the child or parent: remediation, redefinition, and re-education. *Remediation* efforts are aimed at changing the way the child behaves toward the parent. For example, providing Louisa with a controller medication should reduce her symptoms, which, in turn, should reduce her mother's worry about her condition. *Redefinition* changes the way the parent interprets the child's behavior. In Louisa's case, interventions aimed at helping her family understand her respiratory symptoms as part of a chronic illness rather than a recurring cold may change the ways in which they respond to her symptoms. *Re-education* efforts are aimed at changing the way the parent acts with the child through increased knowledge. In the case of Louisa, education efforts aimed at following an action plan and reducing exposure to environmental toxins would reduce Louisa's symptoms. To these three *R*s of intervention, Fiese and Wamboldt[132] added a fourth type of intervention often warranted in health care settings: realignment. *Realignment* is called for when family members disagree about a course of action and daily practices have been disrupted to the extent that the health and well-being of the child are compromised. In Louisa's case, if the parents disagreed on her diagnosis of asthma, then there would be serious consequences as to whether they would agree on a plan of action if she had another asthma attack. These four *R*s of intervention are now examined in the framework of family routines and a clinical decision-making process that is accessible to pediatricians.

CLINICAL DECISION MAKING APPLIED TO MEDICAL ADHERENCE

We have already discussed the roles that family routines and daily practices may play in the health and well-being of children. We now incorporate these practices into the clinical decision-making process as a guide for pediatricians when working with families who are expected to follow a daily treatment protocol to maintain the health and well-being of their children. We chart this process as part of a decision tree, although we also recognize that there are instances in which family circumstances warrant more than one type of intervention (Fig. 5-4).

The first step of the process involves educating the family about the treatment protocol. This may include review of treatment plans, dietary guidelines, or timing and dosage levels of prescribed medications. Most clinicians would agree that educating patients about treatment protocols is not an easy matter; it takes considerable care and must be reinforced over multiple points of contact and, perhaps, through multiple medias. For families that are relatively well organized, have a good sense of their daily habits, and are able to make alterations in their daily practices with minimal disruptions, there may be little need for additional assistance, and the pediatrician monitors adherence through standard practice procedures. However, in cases in which there are difficulties in following the prescribed treatment protocols, it may be beneficial to evaluate the family's daily routines.

First, is this a family in which routines are present and the family is relatively adept at carrying out the routines of daily living but there has been a disruption in some arenas because of the illness? In Louisa's case, it appears that the family is relatively well organized and that the father has taken over the role as medication manager. This is an adaptive response that

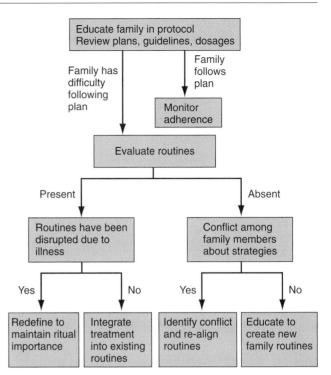

FIGURE 5-4 *Clinical decision tree.*

under most circumstances should lead to better medication adherence. However, her nighttime awakenings are of concern. On questioning the family about their daily routines, it may be the case that Louisa's previously established nighttime ritual of reading a book with her mother was replaced with her father's attention to taking medication, which turns into an evening routine. A redefinition of bedtime routines would be indicated, in which the book reading ritual would be reinstated to soothe Louisa to sleep.

For other families, there may be minimal disruptions to their routines, and they are able to fold treatment recommendations into existing routines. For example, a common recommendation for children with asthma is to place their medication next to their toothbrush as a reminder to take their medication. This of course is under the assumption that a child has the habit of brushing his or her teeth twice a day. If this is the case, further remediation is unlikely.

The second alternative in evaluating routines is cases in which families do not have routines in place. In these situations, it is important to consider whether there is conflict among family members about strategies for implementing treatment recommendations. As previously noted, conflict can have a detrimental effect on children's health. Family members can also disagree about the relative value of particular disease management routines and the relative importance of attending to specific aspects of an individual's prescribed protocol. We noted, for example, in families with a diabetic member that routinely eating late or serving sweet desserts can counteract the individual's good intentions. It is important to identify the source of conflict around implementing the routine. Sometimes these conflicts can be rooted in myths and misperceptions about the prescribed protocol: for example, not wanting to take daily prescribed medications for fear that the child will become "hooked on other drugs." There are other instances in which there are disagreements that are rooted in marital conflicts. Under these circumstances, it is important to separate marital conflict and discord from managing daily routines. This is particularly germane in the case of divorced and separated families in which children are living in two households and there may be two sets of rules and routines. It is important to come to an agreement about consistency in routines (e.g., bedtime, mealtime, medication use) so that the child is protected from the harmful effects of conflictive households.

There are also developmental characteristics to take into consideration in evaluating family conflict about routines. Adolescence is a time of transition for the entire family. For adolescents with a chronic health condition, this is a time when responsibility of disease management is transferred from the parent to the adolescent. This is a prime opportunity to identify healthy routines that can be under the adolescent's control. Indeed, astute clinicians have taken this transfer-of-responsibility notion as a central aspect of family-based interventions with adolescents. Anderson and her colleagues developed a brief intervention aimed at reducing conflict between adolescents and their parents over diabetes management.[133] Pediatricians may find it useful to discuss transfer of responsibility with adolescents and their parents in the context of other transitions that are occurring in the routine life of the family, such as curfews, after-school activities, and part-time employment.

The last form of routine intervention is reeducation. This type of intervention is called for when the family has been provided the basic information about the treatment protocol, there is an absence of conflict about how to carry out the protocol, but there is no previous experience in creating or sustaining regular routines. This type of intervention may be the most challenging to implement and maintain. For these families, it is important to first identify the physical settings in which the routines can occur and the time at which they can occur and then apply principles of parent management training.[134] Although there is a long tradition in implementing home-based interventions,[135] we want to emphasize the sensitive nature of creating family routines where there were previously none. The question that needs to be addressed

concerns what led to the impoverishment of family routines. For some families, a history of abuse and neglect provides little in the way of comfort when members are gathered together as a group. For other families, a chaotic home environment may have been the result of parental psychopathology and unstable economic resources, which led to unpredictable daily patterns of caregiving. Again, we highlight that family life is determined by multiple factors and that the presence or absence of family routines is likewise determined. We present these four forms of intervention as a heuristic for the busy pediatrician. Future research efforts are warranted to determine whether this approach to clinical decision making and the concomitant interventions qualify as empirically supported forms of intervention. However, the four *R*s of intervention are theoretically grounded and based on preexisting forms of intervention that have been proved effective in other domains such as home-based educational interventions.[135] What is unique to this format is a systematic consideration of family-level functioning in determining which form of intervention may be more appropriate at a given time.

We have used adherence to medical regimens as an example for this decision-making process and implementing routine-based interventions. Home- and routine-based interventions are also used frequently to address problem behaviors in children with developmental disabilities. Folding an intervention into everyday family household practices such as mealtime, playtime, and bedtime may be positively viewed by family members because they are less likely to be viewed as "one more thing" to be added on to an already busy day and may thus promote stronger family investment in the treatment protocol.[136] Interventions such as positive behavioral support[137] and routine-based intervention[138] are examples of programs that encourage families to identify specific daily routines as settings for behavioral interventions. These interventions enlist parents as the therapist and are tailored to fit the rhythms of a particular family. Results from these programs are promising in reducing problematic and disruptive child behaviors and are positively viewed by parents.

Family-Based Coping Interventions

The transactional model of interventions is useful for identifying points of entry to effect change with the aim to get the child and family back on track toward healthy development. There are other instances, however, in which the family may require assistance in coping with traumatic events and warrant interventions aimed not so much at changing the family's routines as at addressing the family's belief systems. One area that has received some attention in this regard is aiding families in coping with childhood cancer.

Most survivors of childhood cancer and their families do well after treatment; however there is a significant proportion of adolescents and their parents who report reexperiencing aspects of the illness that can be considered traumatic and stressful.[139] To address these symptoms, a family-based treatment program has been developed to assist adolescents and their families in coping with surviving cancer.[140,141] Families participate in a day-long discussion with other families who have been similarly affected by childhood cancer. The group discussion focuses on beliefs that survivors and their family members have about cancer with the ultimate aims of reducing stress and altering misperceptions. Findings from these interventions suggest that the intervention is successful in reducing adolescents' symptoms of post-traumatic stress and that there are positive benefits to family members. Although there is some evidence that the most stressed of family members may not be willing to participate in an all-day discussion format, Kazak and associates developed video formats that may be more accessible and show promising results in relieving stress in families with newly diagnosed cancer.[129]

Other examples of brief family-based interventions include targeting how parents and children interact with each other to promote better outcomes. As previously noted, family conflict can have detrimental effects on a variety of child health and behavioral outcomes. Some of these family-based interventions focus specifically on increasing positive forms of social interaction such as responsiveness, sensitivity, and warmth.[142,143] These interventions are often employed with families with young infants and toddlers, who are at risk for developing developmental and behavioral problems as a result of birth complications or environmental stress.

Other family-based interventions also attend to interaction patterns as part of the larger multisystemic influences on child and adolescent health. Most notably, Henggeler developed a multisystemic therapy model that includes an intensive home-based family therapy component to improve adherence to diabetic regimens.[144] Therapists' focuses include improving problem-solving skills, reducing conflict, and identifying monitoring strategies. Although labor intensive, this form of intervention has been shown effective in reducing health care costs.[145]

Summary

In view of the complexity of family effects on child development, family-based interventions are likewise multifaceted. Too often, when considering how best

to assist families in distress, clinicians become overwhelmed with the complexity of the situation and are left with little guidance as to how to begin addressing the problem. We have provided a set of decision rules that may assist pediatricians in working their way through the web of family influence on changing child behavior. It is unlikely that all forms of effective family-based interventions will fit neatly into a managed care environment or conform to common notions of what constitutes psychological interventions. Because families are composed of different numbers of members, who play different roles and are changing with time, it is unreasonable to expect that a one-size-fits-all approach to helping families will be effective.[130] In some cases, interventions must be implemented in the family's home at a time that is convenient for the family. In other cases, a videotape of other family members' experience with a particular condition may be as effective as gathering together a support group. In other instances, pediatricians and psychologists may need to work directly with a family who has been unresponsive to other forms of intervention.[146] Pediatricians are often in the position to refer families for evaluations conducted by social workers, psychologists, and psychiatrists. Although it is beyond the scope of this chapter to provide a comprehensive review of how families are likely to be assessed by these professionals, we provide a brief overview of some of the more commonly used instruments to familiarize the busy practitioner.

FAMILY ASSESSMENT

When families are referred for an evaluation to be conducted by a mental health professional, there are three primary ways to collect information: direct observation, structured interviews, and self-report questionnaires. Each method has its own strengths and limitations. We provide a few examples within each domain of evaluation.

Direct Observation

Skilled family clinicians make use of the power of observation to detect problematic patterns of interaction. Oftentimes aligned with different schools of family therapy, observation of how the family interacts as a group informs the clinician about such factors as balance of power in the family, expression of rules, gender roles, and tolerance for autonomy.[147] In clinical settings, these observations are usually conducted in conjunction with a family interview. In research settings, semistructured tasks are frequently used. A common strategy is to use a "revealed differences" task with couples or parent and child. In these instances, the individuals independently complete a questionnaire or checklist about family life. The researcher identifies one or two points over which the individuals disagree the most and then reveals the differences and ask the dyad to come to some resolution within a given period of time. The rationale behind such a task is that, by forcing the dyad to discuss an area of disagreement, the observer can detect problem solving and conflict resolution skills. An alternative to this approach is to select issues identified by the family as conflictive and instruct them to discuss the issue for 10 minutes.[148] Direct observation of whole family functioning has also been applied to group interactions such as mealtimes. The McMaster Mealtime Interaction Coding System[149] was devised to capture how family members interact during a routine mealtime. It includes seven scales (task accomplishment, communication, affect management, interpersonal involvement, behavior control, roles, and overall family functioning) that have been found to distinguish families who are functioning well from those who evidence problems in a variety of conditions, including parental psychiatric disturbances,[7] cystic fibrosis,[100] and asthma.[150] These coding systems are valuable research tools that allow for a careful examination of the types of family behaviors that are associated with more optimal functioning for children being raised under a variety of risk conditions. However, because of the dependence on video recordings and time involved in learning how to use these systems, they are unwieldy for pediatric practice. Another cautionary note is warranted because family interaction patterns may vary systematically by ethnic background.[9,35] Thus, it is important to consider the cultural context in which the observations are being conducted and in which the observers are operating.

Structured Interviews

Structured family interviews are used primarily for diagnostic purposes and typically last 1 to several hours. The McMaster Structured Interview of Family Functioning[95] focuses on six domains of family functioning: problem solving, communication, roles, affective responsiveness, affective involvement, and behavior control. Family members are asked to respond to a series of questions about daily life, such as how they solve problems around finances, leisure time, and relationships with in-laws. The interviews are rated along the McMaster Clinical Rating Scale,[95] in which a clinical cutoff score is used to distinguish families who are considered healthy from those experiencing psychological distress. The McMaster Clinical Rating Scale has proved reliable in distinguishing parents with a psychiatric disorder from those not

currently experiencing symptoms[7] and useful in assessing relative strengths in families who have a child who has experienced traumatic brain injury.[151]

Disease-specific interviews have also been developed. The Diabetes Social Support Interview[152] assesses children's perceived support from family and friends as it pertains specifically to diabetes care. Children are asked about how much help they receive from their family in such areas as insulin shots, as well as emotional support. Interrater reliability is reported to be acceptable,[153] and interview scores have been found to be related to concurrent disease states.[152] These types of interviews may be useful for pediatricians in assessing the degree to which family members support children's disease management activities.

Self-Report Questionnaires

Although it is unlikely that the busy pediatrician will have time to administer lengthy questionnaires to family members, there are some questionnaires that can be adapted for use in daily practice. The Family Adaptation, Partnership Growth, Affection, and Resolve Scale (Family APGAR)[154] is a brief five-item questionnaire that identifies a family member's level of satisfaction with family functioning. Examples of items include "I am satisfied that I can turn to my family for help when something is troubling me" and "I am satisfied with the way my family and I share time together." The Family APGAR has been found to have reasonable content validity and adequate test-retest reliability and useful in primary care settings.[155] Although the Family APGAR is not a direct measure of family functioning, its results indicate how satisfied the individual is with the way the family is working.[156]

The McMaster Family Assessment Device (FAD)[157] is a 60-item self-report questionnaire administered to adults. The FAD includes six subscales: Problem Solving, Communication, Roles, Affective Responsiveness, Affective Involvement, and Behavior Control. A General Functioning Score may also be derived. Test-retest reliability over a 1-week period ranged from 0.66 to 0.76. The FAD has been found to distinguish between clinical and nonclinical groups and is not related to measures of social desirability. Specifically for children, elevated scores (indicating poorer functioning) on the FAD have been associated with medication nonadherence in cases of asthma.[91] Higher FAD scores were also found in children with recurrent abdominal pain and with frequent headaches than in a healthy control group of children.[158]

We have highlighted a few of the more commonly used family assessment techniques. Our listing is not in any way exhaustive. However, it should provide the pediatrician with a flavor of what types of assessment are available when the pediatrician makes a referral or considers a more extensive evaluation of a particular family.

FUTURE DIRECTIONS IN FAMILY RESEARCH AND INTERVENTIONS

There has been a growing appreciation for the pivotal role that families play in the health and well-being of their children. Although this appreciation is somewhat intuitive, methodological and clinical interventions have not kept pace with theoretical advances. We have outlined some of the reasons for the relatively slow pace in advancing family research, including but not limited to the complexity of family systems, the multiply determined nature of risk, and the cultural influences on individual development. Future efforts are warranted to take this complexity into consideration when researchers tackle the thorny issues of how families come to affect children's development. This will call for a sophisticated research agenda that cuts across traditional disciplinary lines and incorporates multiple levels of analysis. The authors of the white paper report on early childhood development, *From Neurons to Neighborhoods,* persuasively argued that development can be understood only through an integration of knowledge gleaned from the behavioral, brain, social, economic, and political sciences.[159] A similar effort is warranted when investigators consider future directions in understanding the role that families play in promoting children's health. This will call for multiple levels of analysis, including the effects of physiology on social interactions and the manner in which family beliefs may alter disease status, for example. Multiple levels of analysis calls for strategies in which researchers consider variability within families across different classes of variables (e.g., physiology, mental health, physical health symptoms, cognitive functioning, family process), as well as variability across time.[160] For example, future efforts may be directed at asking questions such as how changes in the physical health of the child affect family beliefs about their own ability to change daily health habits. The shifting cultural landscape of contemporary families mandate sensitivity to variability rooted in traditions and beliefs that may extend across generations and geographic boundaries. Likewise, family-based interventions must also take into account family-level variability, including but not limited to availability of economic resources, ages of children, and ethnic background. These parameters are not just census markers but may be important moderators and mediators of treatment effectiveness. A family strength-based resilience approach may provide pediatricians

with the opportunity to identify which family-level factors are more likely to promote adjustment and reduce risk in their patients.[161] In this regard, interventions are aimed at restoring overall family health, not just addressing symptoms in the individual patient. The challenge for pediatricians is to effectively identify strategies and modalities that will fit for a particular family within a given developmental period. These decisions do not operate in a vacuum; they are also affected by the policies that are in place that support child and family health. We close with a brief note about public policy in the interest of child and family health.

CHILD AND FAMILY HEALTH: POLICY PRIORITIES

Clearly, it is beyond the charge or scope of this chapter to address how public policy affects children's health. However, we firmly believe that families make significant contributions to the health and well-being of children and that public policy should support and not get in the way of the best intentions of parents. Addressing policy issues is necessarily a question of costs, benefits, and how to effect change for the common good.[162] How might our understanding of the multifaceted role of the family inform public policy? First, there are many types of family structures, and family form does not dictate child health and well-being. Thus, policies that favor one family structure over another will probably not benefit children in any appreciable way and will probably harm a significant portion of children. Second, families need time to be together in order to foster more optimal outcomes for their children. It not desirable to implement heavy-handed policies that dictate the amount of time families should spend together. Again, we emphasize the personal nature of family time. However, when inflexible work policies make it difficult for families to adjust to the needs of their children, their children's health is often compromised. Parents often have to make the difficult choice between staying home with an ill child and going to work. These are not decisions that are in the best interest of the family. Third, the maintenance of children's health is more than just having access to care: It is also the family's ability to garner resources for transportation and following medical advice. Better support in terms of education, transportation, and support aimed at the entire family will probably reduce health care costs in the cases of chronic childhood illnesses.

Families are remarkably resilient. They are faced with multiple challenges every day, such as organizing daily life, making sure the emotional needs of each member are met, keeping conflict in check, and doing so within the boundaries of cultural mores. When a family walks into a pediatrician's office, the members bring a set of beliefs and catalog of practices that will influence how they respond to the simple question "How are you feeling today?" We hope that this brief tour of the family context of child health and well-being provides the pediatrician with an appreciation of how densely packed the answer to this question may be.

REFERENCES

1. Heaton TB, Forste R, Hoffman JP, et al: Cross-national variation in family influences in child health. Social Science Med 60:97-108, 2005.
2. Chen E, Bloomberg GR, Fisher EB, et al: Predictors of repeat hospitalization in children with asthma: The role of psychosocial and socioenvironmental factors. Health Psychol 22:12-18, 2003.
3. Kazak AE, Barakat LP, Meeske K, et al: Posttraumatic stress, family functioning, and social support in survivors of childhood leukemia and their mothers and fathers. J Consult Clin Psychol 65:120-129, 1997.
4. Case A, Lubotsky D, Paxson C: Economic status and health in childhood: The origins of the gradient. Am Econ Rev 92:1308-1334, 2002.
5. Furstenberg FF, Cook TD, Eccles J, et al: Managing to Make It: Urban Families and Adolescent Success. Chicago: University of Chicago Press, 1999.
6. Cowan PA, Cohn DA, Cowan CP, et al: Parents' attachment histories and children's externalizing and internalizing behaviors: Exploring family systems models of linkages. J Consult Clin Psychol 64:53-63, 1996.
7. Dickstein S, Seifer R, Hayden LC, et al: Levels of family assessment: II. Impact of maternal psychopathology on family functioning. J Fam Psychol 12:23-40, 1998.
8. Main M, Goldwyn R: Predicting rejection of her infant from mother's representation of her own experience: Implications for the abused-abusing intergenerational cycle. Child Abuse Negl 8:203-217, 1984.
9. Gonzales NA, Cauce AM, Mason CA: Interobserver agreement in the assessment of parental behavior and parent-adolescent conflict: African American mothers, daughters, and independent observers. Child Dev 67:1483-1498, 1996.
10. Teachman JD, Tedrow LM, Crowder KD: The changing demography of America's families. J Marriage Fam. 62:1234-1246, 2000.
11. Schor EL, American Academy of Pediatrics Task Force on the Family: Family pediatrics: Report of the Task Force on the Family. Pediatrics 111(suppl):1541-1571, 2003.
12. Lidz T, Cornelison A, Fleck S, et al: The intrafamilial environment of schizophrenic patients: II. Marital schism and marital skew. Am J Psychiatry 114:241-248, 1957.
13. Purcell K, Brady K, Chai H, et al: The effect on asthma in children of experimental separation from the family. Psychosom Med 31:144-164, 1969.
14. National Institutes of Health: Guidelines for the Diagnosis and Management of Asthma (NIH Publication No. 97-4051). Washington, DC: National Institutes of Health, 1997.
15. Bronfenbrenner U: The Ecology of Human Development. Cambridge, MA: Harvard University Press, 1979.
16. Sameroff AJ, Chandler MJ: Reproductive risk and the continuum of caretaking causality. In Horowitz FD, Hetherington M, Scarr-Salapetek S, et al, eds: Review of Child Development Research, vol 4. Chicago: Chicago University Press, 1975, pp 187-244.
17. Sameroff AJ, Fiese BH: Transactional regulation: The developmental ecology of early intervention. In Meisels SJ, Shonkoff JP, eds: Early Intervention: A Handbook of Theory, Practice, and Analysis. New York: Cambridge University Press, 2000, pp 3-19.
18. Cummings EM, Davies PT, Campbell SB: Developmental Psychopathology and Family Process. New York: Guilford, 2000.
19. Kazak AE, Rourke MT, Crump TA: Families and other systems in pediatric psychology. In Roberts MC, ed: Handbook of Pediatric Psychology. New York: Guilford, 2003, pp 159-175.
20. Marks LD, Dollahite DC: Religion, relationships, and responsible fathering in Latter-Day Saint families of children with special needs. J Soc Pers Relat 18:625-650, 2001.
21. Brooks-Gunn J, Klebanov P, Liaw F, et al: Enhancing the development of low birth weight, premature infants: Changes in cognition and behavior over the first three years. Child Dev 64:736-753, 1993.
22. Sameroff AJ: General systems theories and developmental psychopathology. In Cicchetti D, Cohen D, eds: Handbook of Developmental Psychopathology, vol 1. New York: Wiley, 1995, pp 659-695.
23. Hetherington EM, Kelly J: For Better or for Worse: Divorce Reconsidered. New York: Norton, 2002.
24. U.S. Bureau of the Census: Statistical Abstract of the United States 1999. Washington, DC: U.S. Government Printing Office, 1999.
25. Amato PR: Children of divorce in the 1990s: An update of the Amato and Keith (1991) meta-analysis. J Fam Psychol 15:355-370, 2001.
26. Hetherington EM, Stanley-Hagan M: The adjustment of children with divorced parents: A risk and resiliency perspective. J Child Psychol Psychiatry 40:129-140, 1999.
27. Repetti RL, Taylor SE, Seeman TE: Risky families: Family social environments and the mental and physical health of offspring. Psychol Bull 128:330-366, 2002.
28. U.S. Bureau of the Census: Current Population Survey, 1981 to 2004 Annual Social and Economic Supplements. Washington, DC: U.S. Government Printing Office, 2004.

29. Conger RD, Ge X, Elder GH, et al: Economic stress, coercive family process, and developmental problems of adolescents. Child Dev 65:541-561, 1994.

30. Evans GW: A multimethodological analysis of cumulative risk and allostatic load among rural children. Dev Psychol 39:924-933, 2003.

31. Duncan GJ, Brooks-Gunn J: Consequences of Growing up Poor. New York: Russell Sage Foundation, 1997.

32. Bradley RH, Corwyn RF: Socioeconomic status and child development. Annu Rev Psychol 53:371-399, 2002.

33. Huston AC, McLoyd VC, Garcia Coll C: Children and poverty: Issues in contemporary research. Child Dev 65:275-282, 1994.

34. Bradley RH, Corwyn RF, McAdoo HP, et al: The home environments of children in the United States part I: Variations by age, ethnicity, and poverty status. Child Dev 72:1844-1867, 2001.

35. McAdoo HP: Ethnic Families: Strength in Diversity. Newbury Park, CA: Sage Publications, 1993.

36. Landesman S, Jaccard J, Gunderson V: The family environment: The combined influence of family behavior, goals, strategies, resources, and individual experiences. *In* Lewis M, Feinman S, eds: Social Influences and Socialization in Infancy. New York: Plenum Press, 1991, pp 63-96.

37. Fisher L, Weihs KL: Can addressing family relationships improve outcomes in chronic disease? J Fam Pract 49:561-566, 2000.

38. Fiese BH, Foley KP, Spagnola M: Routine and ritual elements in family mealtimes: Contexts for child well-being and family identity. New Dir Child Adolesc Dev Spring(111):67-89.

39. Fiese BH, Tomcho T, Douglas M, et al: Fifty years of research on naturally occurring rituals: Cause for celebration? J Fam Psychol 16:381-390, 2002.

40. Fiese BH, Hooker KA, Kotary L, et al: Family rituals in the early stages of parenthood. J Marriage Fam 57:633-642, 1993.

41. Compan E, Moreno J, Ruiz MT, et al: Doing things together: Adolescent health and family rituals. J Epidemiol Community Health 56:89-94, 2002.

42. Eisenberg ME, Olson RE, Neumark-Sztainer D, et al: Correlations between family meals and psychosocial well-being among adolescents. Arch Pediatr Adolesc Med 158:792-796, 2004.

43. Fiese BH: Dimensions of family rituals across two generations: Relation to adolescent identity. Fam Process 31:151-162, 1992.

44. Clark FA: The concept of habit and routine: A preliminary theoretical synthesis. Occup Ther J Res 20:123S-137S, 2000.

45. Lee EJ, Murry VM, Brody G, et al: Maternal resources, parenting, and dietary patterns among rural African American children in single-parent families. Public Health Nurs 19:104-111, 2002.

46. Drucker RR, Hammer LD, Agras WS, et al: Can mothers influence their child's eating behavior? Dev Behav Pediatr 20:88-92, 1999.

47. Johnson SL, Birch LL: Parents' and children's adiposity and eating style. Pediatrics 94:653-661, 1994.

48. Coon KA, Goldberg J, Rogers BL, et al: Relationships between use of television during meals and children's food consumption patterns. Pediatrics 107(1):E7, 2001.

49. Gerstle JF, Varenne H, Contento I: Post-diagnosis family adaptation influences glycemic control in women with type 2 diabetes mellitus. J Am Diet Assoc 101:918-922, 2001.

50. Rapoff MA: Adherence to Pediatric Medical Regimens. New York: Kluwer Academic, 1999.

51. Drotar D: Promoting Adherence to Medical Treatment in Childhood Chronic Illness: Concepts, Methods, and Interventions. Mahwah, NJ: Erlbaum, 2000.

52. Fiese BH, Wamboldt FS, Anbar RD: Family asthma management routines: Connections to medical adherence and quality of life. J Pediatr 146:171-176, 2005.

53. Bender B, Milgrom H, Rand C: Nonadherence in asthmatic patients: Is there a solution to the problem? Ann Allergy Asthma Immunol 79:177-186, 1997.

54. Porter CL, Hsu H: First-time mothers' perceptions of efficacy during the transition to motherhood: Links to infant temperament. J Fam Psychol 17:54-64, 2003.

55. Sprunger LW, Boyce WT, Gaines JA: Family-infant congruence: Routines and rhythmicity in family adaptations to a young infant. Child Dev 56:564-572, 1985.

56. Markson S, Fiese BH: Family rituals as a protective factor against anxiety for children with asthma. J Pediatr Psychol 25:471-479, 2000.

57. Fiese BH: Family rituals in alcoholic and nonalcoholic households: Relation to adolescent health symptomatology and problematic drinking. Fam Relat 42:187-192, 1993.

58. Stein REK, Jessop DJ: The Impact on Family Scale revisited: Further psychometric data. J Dev Behav Pediatr 24:9-16, 2003.

59. Quittner AL, Espelage DL, Opipari LC, et al: Role strain in couples with and without a child with a chronic illness: Associations with marital satisfaction, intimacy, and daily mood. Health Psychol 17:112-124, 1998.

60. Evans GW: The environment of childhood poverty. Am Psychol 59:77-92, 2004.

61. Evans GW, Gonnella C, Marcynyszyn LA, et al: The role of chaos and poverty and children's socioemotional adjustment. Psychol Sci 16:560-565, 2005.

62. Dumas JE, Nissley J, Nordstrom A, et al: Home chaos: Sociodemographic, parenting, interactional, and child correlates. J Clin Child Adolesc Psychol 34:93-104, 2005.

63. Brody GH, Flor DL: Maternal psychological functioning, family processes, and child adjustment in rural, single-parent, African American families. Dev Psychol 33:1000-1011, 1997.

64. Fiese BH, Sameroff AJ, Grotevant HD, et al: The Stories that Families Tell: Narrative Coherence, Narrative Interaction, and Relationship Beliefs. Monographs of the Society for Research in Child Development, vol 64 (2), serial no. 257. Malden, MA: Blackwell Publishers, 1999, pp 1-36.

65. Brody H: Stories of Sickness. New Haven, CT: Yale University Press, 1987.

66. Fiese BH, Bickham NL: Pincurling grandpa's hair in the comfy chair: Parents' stories of growing up and potential links to socialization in the preschool years. *In* Pratt MW, Fiese BH, eds: Family Stories across Time and Generations. Mahwah, NJ: Erlbaum, 2004, pp 259-278.

67. Peterson JL, Peterson M: The Sleep Fairy. Omaha, NE: Behave'n Kids Press, 2003.

68. Wang Q: The cultural context of parent-child reminiscing: A functional analysis. *In* Pratt MW, Fiese BH, eds: Family Stories and the Life Course: Across Time and Generations. Mahwah, NJ: Erlbaum, 2004, pp 279-301.

69. McAdams DP: The psychology of life stories. Rev Gen Psychol 5:100-122, 2001.

70. Fiese BH, Sameroff AJ: The family narrative consortium: A multidimensional approach to narratives. *In* Fiese BH, Sameroff AJ, Grotevant HD, et al, eds: The Stories that Families Tell: Narrative Coherence, Narrative Interaction, and Relationship Beliefs. Monographs of the Society for Research in Child Development, vol 64 (2), serial no. 257. Malden, MA: Blackwell Publishers, 1999, pp 1-36.

71. Coles R: The Call of Stories. Boston: Houghton Mifflin, 1989.

72. Remen RN: Kitchen Table Wisdom. New York: Riverhead Books, 1996.

73. Dickstein S, St. Andre M, Sameroff AJ, et al: Maternal depression, family functioning, and child outcomes: A narrative assessment. *In* Fiese BH, Sameroff AJ, Grotevant HD, et al, eds: The Stories that Families Tell: Narrative Coherence, Narrative Interaction, and Relationship Beliefs. Monographs of the Society for Research in Child Development, vol 64 (2), serial no. 257. Malden, MA: Blackwell Publishers, 1999, pp 84-104.

74. Fiese BH, Wamboldt FS: Coherent accounts of coping with a chronic illness: Convergences and divergences in family measurement using a narrative analysis. Fam Process 42:3-15, 2003.

75. Carlson EA, Sroufe LA, Egeland B: The construction of experience: A longitudinal study of representation and behavior. Child Dev 75:66-83, 2004.

76. van Ijzendoorn MH, Bakersmans-Kranenburg MJ: Attachment representations in mothers, fathers, adolescents and clinical groups: A meta-analytic search for normative data. J Consult Clin Psychol 64:8-21, 1996.

77. DiMatteo MR: The role of effective communication with children and their families in fostering adherence to pediatric regimens. Patient Educ Couns 55:339-344, 2004.

78. Fiese BH, Spagnola M: Narratives in and about family relationships: An examination of coding schemes and guide for family researchers. J Fam Psychol 19:51-61, 2005.

79. Pratt MW, Fiese BH: Families, stories and the life course: An ecological context. *In* Pratt MW, Fiese BH,

eds: Family Stories across Time and Generations. Mahwah, NJ: Erlbaum, 2004, pp 1-26.

80. Fiese BH, Marjinsky KAT: Dinnertime stories: Connecting relationship beliefs and child behavior. *In* Fiese BH, Sameroff AJ, Grotevant HD, et al, eds: The Stories that Families Tell: Narrative Coherence, Narrative Interaction, and Relationship Beliefs. Monographs of the Society for Research in Child Development, vol 64 (2), serial no. 257. Malden, MA: Blackwell Publishers, 1999, pp 52-68.

81. Toth SL, Cicchetti D, Macfie J, et al: Representations of self and other in the narratives of neglected, physically abused, and sexually abused preschoolers. Dev Psychopathol 9:781-796, 1997.

82. Toth SL, Cicchetti D, Macfie J, et al: Narrative representations of caregivers and self in maltreated preschoolers. Attach Hum Dev 2:271-305, 2000.

83. Fiese BH, Wamboldt FS: Tales of pediatric asthma management: Family based strategies related to medical adherence and health care utilization. J Pediatr 143:457-462, 2003.

84. Markman HJ, Notarious CI: Coding marital and family interaction: Current status. *In* Jacob T, ed: Family Interaction and Psychopathology. New York: Plenum Press, 1987, pp 329-390.

85. Cohen MS: Families coping with childhood chronic illness: A research review. Fam Syst Health 17:149-164, 1999.

86. Minuchin S: Families and Family Therapy. Cambridge, MA: Harvard University Press, 1974.

87. Wood BL: Beyond the "psychosomatic family": A biobehavioral family model of pediatric illness. Fam Process 32:261-278, 1993.

88. Kaugars AS, Klinnert MD, Bender BG: Family influences on pediatric asthma. J Pediatr Psychol 29:475-491, 2004.

89. McQuaid EL: Behavioral adjustment in children with asthma: A meta-analysis. J Dev Behav Pediatr 22:430-439, 2001.

90. Schobinger R, Florin I, Reichbauer M, et al: Childhood asthma: Mothers' affective attitude, mother-child interaction, and children's compliance with medical requirements. J Psychosom Res 37:697-707, 1993.

91. Bender BG, Milgrom H, Rand C, et al: Psychological factors associated with medication nonadherence in asthmatic children. J Asthma 35:347-353, 1998.

92. Christiannse ME, Lavigne JC, Lerner CV: Psychosocial aspects of compliance in children and adolescents with asthma. Dev Behav Pediatr 10:75-80, 1989.

93. Jacobson AM, Hauser ST, Lavori P, et al: Family environment and glycemic control: A four-year prospective study of children and adolescents with insulin dependent diabetes mellitus. Psychosom Med 56:401-409, 1994.

94. Drotar D: Relating parent and family to the psychological adjustment of children with chronic health conditions: What have we learned? What do we need to know? J Pediatr Psychol 22:149-165, 1997.

95. Epstein NB, Ryan CE, Bishop DS, et al: The McMaster model: A view of healthy family functioning. *In* Walsh

F, ed: Normal Family Processes, 3rd ed. New York: Guilford, 2003, pp 581-607.

96. Kazak AE, McClure KS, Alderfer MA, et al: Cancer-related parental beliefs: The Family Illness Beliefs Inventory (FIBI). J Pediatr Psychol 29:531-542, 2004.

97. Stark LJ, Jelalian E, Powers SW, et al: Parent and child mealtime behavior in families of children with cystic fibrosis. J Pediatr 136:195-200, 2000.

98. Bihun JT, Wamboldt MZ, Gavin LA, et al: Can the Family Assessment Device (FAD) be used with children? Fam Process 41:723-731, 2002.

99. DeLambo KE, Ievers-Landis CE, Drotar D, et al: The association of observed family relationship quality and problem-solving skills with treatment adherence in older children and adolescents with cystic fibrosis. J Pediatr Psychol 29:343-354, 2004.

100. Speith LE, Stark LJ, Mitchell MJ, et al: Observational assessment of family functioning at mealtime in preschool children with cystic fibrosis. J Fam Psychol 26:215-224, 2001.

101. Hauser ST, Jacobson AM, Lavori P, et al: Adherence among children and adolescents with insulin-dependent diabetes mellitus over a four-year longitudinal follow-up: II. Immediate and long-term linkages with the family milieu. J Pediatr Psychol 15:527-542, 1990.

102. Wysocki T, Miller KM, Greco P, et al: Behavior therapy for families of adolescents with diabetes: Effects on directly observed family interactions. Behav Ther 30:507-525, 1999.

103. Markus HR, Kitayama S: A collective fear of the collective: Implications for selves and theories of selves. Pers Soc Psychol Bull 20:568-579, 1994.

104. Miller PJ, Wiley AR, Fung H, et al: Personal storytelling as a medium of socialization in Chinese and American families. Child Dev 68:557-568, 1997.

105. Goodnow J: Adding culture to studies of development: Toward changes in procedure and theory. Hum Dev 45:237-245, 2002.

106. Weisner TS: Ecocultural understanding of children's developmental pathways. Hum Dev 45:275-281, 2002.

107. Falicov CJ: Immigrant family processes. *In* Walsh F, ed: Normal Family Processes, 3rd ed. New York: Guilford, 2003, pp 280-300.

108. Gonzales NA, Knight GP, Birman D, et al: Acculturation and enculturation among Latino youth. *In* Maton KI, Schellenbach CJ, Leadbeater BJ, et al, eds: Investing in Children, Youth, Families, and Communities: Strengths-Based Research and Policy. Washington, DC: American Psychological Association, 2004, pp 285-302.

109. Harwood RL: The influence of culturally derived values of Anglo and Puerto Rican mothers' perceptions of attachment behaviors. Child Dev 63:822-839, 1992.

110. Harwood RL, Miller JG: Perceptions of attachment behavior: A comparison of Anglo and Puerto Rican mothers. Merrill Palmer Q 37:583-599, 1991.

111. Schultze PA, Harwood RL, Schoelmerich A: Feeding practices and expectations among middle-class Anglo

and Puerto Rican mothers of 12-month old infants. J Cross Cult Psychol 32:397-406, 2001.

112. Harwood RL, Miller JG, Irizarry NL: Culture and Attachment: Perceptions of the Child in Context. New York: Guilford, 1995.

113. Triandis HC, Marin G, Lisansky J, et al: *Simpatia* as a cultural script of Hispanics. J Pers Soc Psychol 47:1363-1375, 1984.

114. Arcia E, Fernandez MC, Jaquez M: Latina mothers' characterizations of their young children with disruptive behaviors. J Child Fam Stud 14:111-125, 2005.

115. Gannotti ME, Handwerker WP: Puerto Rican understanding of child disability: Methods for the cultural validation of standardized measures of child health. Soc Sci Med 55:2093-2105, 2002.

116. Fuligini AJ, Yip T, Tseng V: The impact of family obligation on the daily activities and psychological well-being of Chinese American adolescents. Child Dev 73:302-314, 2002.

117. Mansour ME, Lanphear BP, DeWitt TG: Barriers to asthma care in urban children: Parent perspectives. Pediatrics 106:512-519, 2000.

118. Wade SL, Islam S, Holden G, et al: Division of responsibility for asthma management tasks between caregivers and children in the inner city. Dev Behav Pediatr 20:93-98, 1999.

119. Walders N, Drotar D, Kercsmar C: The allocation of family responsibility for asthma management tasks in African-American adolescents. J Asthma 37:89-99, 2000.

120. Yali AM, Revenson TA: How changes in population demographics will impact health psychology: Incorporating a broader notion of cultural competence in the field. Health Psychol 23:147-155, 2004.

121. Beiser M, Hou F, Hyman I, et al: Poverty, family process, and mental health of immigrant children in Canada. Am J Public Health 92:220-227, 2002.

122. Parke RD, Coltrane S, Duffy S, et al: Economic stress, parenting, and child adjustment in Mexican American and European American families. Child Dev 75:1632-1656, 2004.

123. Drotar D: Psychological Interventions in Childhood Chronic Illness. Washington, DC: American Psychological Association, 2006.

124. Pinsof WM, Lebow JL, eds: Family Psychology: The Art of the Science. Oxford, UK: Oxford University Press, 2005.

125. Power TJ, DuPaul GJ, Shapiro ES, et al: Promoting Children's Health: Integrating School, Family, and Community. New York: Guilford, 2003.

126. Kazak AE, Simms S, Rourke MT: Family systems practice in pediatric psychology. J Pediatr Psychol 27:133-144, 2002.

127. Mikesell DH, McDaniel SH, eds: Integrating Family Therapy: Handbook of Family Psychology and Systems Theory. Washington, DC: American Psychological Association, 1995.

128. Wysocki T, Harris MA, Greco P, et al: Randomized, controlled trial of behavior therapy for families of adolescents with insulin-dependent diabetes mellitus. J Pediatr Psychol 25:23-33, 2000.

129. Kazak AE, Simms S, Alderfer MA, et al: Feasibility and preliminary outcomes from a pilot study of a brief psychological intervention for families of children newly diagnosed with cancer. J Pediatr Psychol 30:644-655, 2005.

130. Drotar D: Commentary: Involving families in psychological interventions in pediatric psychology: Critical needs and dilemmas. J Pediatr Psychol 30:689-693, 2005.

131. Sameroff AJ: The social context of development. *In* Eisenberg N, ed: Contemporary Topics in Developmental Psychology. New York: Wiley, 1987, pp 273-291.

132. Fiese BH, Wamboldt FS: Family routines, rituals, and asthma management: A proposal for family based strategies to increase treatment adherence. Fam Syst Health 18:405-418, 2001.

133. Anderson B, Brackett J, Ho J, et al: An intervention to promote family teamwork in diabetes management tasks. *In* Drotar D, ed: Promoting Adherence to Medical Treatment and Chronic Childhood Illness. Mahwah, NJ: Erlbaum, 2000, pp 347-365.

134. Lucyshyn JM, Kayser AT, Irvin LK, et al: Functional assessment and positive behavior support at home with families: Defining effective and contextually appropriate behavior support plans. *In* Lucyshyn JM, Dunlap G, eds: Families and Positive Behavior Support: Addressing Problem Behavior in Family Contexts. Baltimore, MD: Paul H. Brookes, 2002, pp 97-132.

135. Olds DL: Prenatal and infancy home visiting by nurses: From randomized trials to community replication. Prev Sci 3:153-172, 2002.

136. Rosenthal CJ, Marshall VW: Generational transmission of family ritual. Am Behav Sci 31:669-684, 1988.

137. Buschbacher P, Fox L, Clarke S: Recapturing desired family routines: A parent-professional behavioral collaboration. Res Pract Persons Severe Disabl 29:25-39, 2004.

138. Woods J, Goldstein H: When the toddler takes over: Changing challenging routines into conduits for communication. Focus Autism Other Dev Disabl 18:176-181, 2003.

139. Kazak AE, Alderfer MA, Rourke MT, et al: Posttraumatic stress disorder (PTSD) and posttraumatic stress symptoms (PTSS) in families of adolescent childhood cancer survivors. J Pediatr Psychol 29:211-219, 2004.

140. Kazak AE, Alderfer MA, Streisand R, et al: Treatment of posttraumatic stress symptoms in adolescent survivors of childhood cancer and their families: A randomized clinical trial. J Fam Psychol 18:493-504, 2004.

141. Kazak AE, Simms S, Barakat L, et al: Surviving Cancer Competently Intervention Program (SCCIP): A cognitive-behavioral and family therapy intervention for adolescent survivors of childhood cancer and their families. Fam Process 38:175-191, 1999.

142. Browne JV, Talmi A: Family-based intervention to enhance infant-parent relationships in the neonatal intensive care unit. J Pediatr Psychol 30:667-677, 2005.

143. McDonough SC: Interaction guidance: Understanding and treating early infant-caregiver relationship disturbances. *In* Zeenah CH, ed: Handbook of Infant Mental Health. New York: Guilford, 1993, pp 414-426.

144. Henggeler SW: Multisystemic therapy: An overview of clinical procedures, outcomes, and policy implications. Child Psychol Psychiatry Rev 4:2-10, 1999.

145. Ellis DA, Naar-King S, Frey M, et al: Multisystemic treatment of poorly controlled type I diabetes: Effects on medical resource utilization. J Pediatr Psychol 30:656-666, 2005.

146. McDaniel SH, Campbell TL, Hepworth J, et al, eds: Family-Oriented Primary Care, 2nd ed. New York: Springer, 2005.

147. Kerig P, Lindahl K, eds: Family Observational Coding Systems: Resources for Systemic Research. Mahwah, NJ: Erlbaum, 2001.

148. Holmbeck GN, Coakley RM, Hommeyer JS, et al: Observed and perceived dyadic and systemic functioning in families of preadolescents with spina bifida. J Pediatr Psychol 27:177-189, 2002.

149. Dickstein S, Hayden LC, Schiller M, et al: Providence Family Study Mealtime Family Interaction Coding System. Adapted from the McMaster Clinical Rating Scale. East Providence, RI: E. P. Bradley Hospital, 1994.

150. Jacobs MP, Fiese BH: Family mealtime interactions and overweight children with asthma: Potential for compounded risks? J Pediatr Psychol 32:64-68, 2007.

151. Barney MC, Max JE: The McMaster family assessment device and clinical rating scale: Questionnaire vs. interview in childhood traumatic brain injury. Brain Inj 19:801-809, 2005.

152. LaGreca AM, Auslander WF, Greco P, et al: I get by with a little help from my family and friends: Adolescents' support for diabetes care. J Pediatr Psychol 20:449-476, 1995.

153. Schroff Pendley J, Kasmen LJ, Miller DL, et al: Peer and family support in children and adolescents with type 1 diabetes. J Pediatr Psychol 27:429-438, 2002.

154. Smilkstein G: The Family APGAR: A proposal for family function test and its use by physicians. J Fam Pract 6:1231-1239, 1978.

155. Palermo TM, Childs G, Burgess ES, et al: Functional limitations of school-aged children seen in primary care. Child Care Health Dev 28:379-389, 2002.

156. Jellinek MS, Murphy JM, Robinson J, et al: Pediatric Symptom Checklist: Screening school-age children for psychosocial dysfunction. J Pediatr 112:201-209, 1988.

157. Epstein NB, Baldwin LM, Bishop DS: The McMaster Family Assessment Device. J Marital Fam Ther 9:171-180, 1983.

158. Liakopoulou-Karis M, Alifieraki T, Protagora D, et al: Recurrent abdominal pain and headache: Psychopathology, life events, and family functioning. Eur Child Adolesc Psychiatry 11:115-122, 2002.

159. Shonkoff JP, Phillips DA, eds: From Neurons to Neighborhoods: The Science of Early Childhood Development. Washington, DC: National Academies Press, 2000.

160. Cicchetti D, Dawson G: Editorial: Multiple levels of analysis. Dev Psychopathol 14:417-420, 2002.

161. Walsh F: A family resilience framework: Innovative practice applications. Fam Relat 51:130-137, 2002.

162. Huston AC: Connecting the science of child development to public policy. SRCD Public Policy Rep 19(4):3-7, 2005.

Diagnostic Classification Systems

MARK L. WOLRAICH ▪ DENNIS D. DROTAR

Diagnostic classification systems (DCSs) for children's developmental and behavioral problems are important in clinical care, teaching, consultation, and research in the field of developmental-behavioral pediatrics. In order to conduct diagnosis and treatment planning, teaching, and research, clinicians with an interest in developmental and behavioral problems need to understand DCSs that are appropriate for children and adolescents. As specialists, developmental-behavioral pediatricians are called on to conduct comprehensive diagnosis and treatment planning for children and adolescents who present with a wide range of behavioral and developmental problems.[1] Reimbursement for clinical practice is also tied to specific codes that are used for purposes of diagnostic classification.[2] Clinicians with expertise in developmental and behavioral problems are also called on to teach pediatricians and members of other professional disciplines to diagnose and manage these problems.[3] Finally, research on the diagnosis and treatment of children with developmental and behavioral problems requires knowledge of the reliability and validity of DCSs.

The purpose of this chapter is to summarize the state of the art with regard to diagnostic classification of children and adolescents with behavioral and emotional problems. We consider challenges in diagnosis, history of classification of mental disorders, systems for classification, and future research directions.

CHALLENGES OF DIAGNOSIS IN DEVELOPMENTAL AND BEHAVIORAL PEDIATRICS

Practitioners, consultants, teachers, and researchers with involvement in developmental and behavioral problems may be interested in any number of questions that relate to various functions of a DCS. Relevant clinical questions include the following: How well does a DCS capture the range of symptoms and

functional problems of children and adolescents that are seen in practice? How does a DCS facilitate treatment planning for children and adolescents who are seen in practice and facilitate communication and consultation with parents, providers, and systems of care?

Clinicians are also interested in how DCSs can facilitate the teaching and training of pediatricians and other professionals to diagnose and manage clinical problems. Relevant research questions include the interrater reliability and validity of the DCS, stability of diagnosis and prognosis over time, and the functional significance or validity of the diagnostic criteria.[4]

The complexity of the diagnosis and treatment of developmental and behavioral problems in children and adolescents presents significant challenges for any DCS. For example, children and adolescents present to clinical attention with an extraordinary number of developmental and behavioral problems that involve a wide range of symptoms that can affect functioning in different domains. The expression and severity of problems and symptoms vary dramatically as a function of the child's age, as do normative developmental expectations for behaviors and symptoms.[5] Moreover, the functional consequences of specific behavioral and developmental problems and diagnoses also vary widely in ways that may or may not be captured by a DCS.[6] Finally, available scientific data concerning the validity of specific diagnostic categories also vary with DCSs and specific conditions.

SYSTEMS FOR DIAGNOSTIC CLASSIFICATION OF DEVELOPMENTAL AND BEHAVIOR PROBLEMS

A number of alternative DCSs can be used by clinicians with an interest in developmental and behavioral problems of children and adolescents to diagnose and treat these problems. We now describe several diagnostic classifications and their potential relevance to practice, teaching, and research.

Diagnostic and Statistical Manual of Mental Disorders, Fourth Edition (DSM-IV)

HISTORY

In the United States, the initial interest in developing a classification of disorders started in the 1800s in order to collect statistical information. In 1840, this consisted of recording the category of idiocy or insanity. By 1880, the census distinguished between mania, melancholia, monomania, paresis, dementia, dipsomania, and epilepsy. In 1917, the American Medico-Psychological Association (a forerunner of the American Psychiatric Association [APA]) adopted a plan to collect uniform information across mental hospitals. The APA subsequently collaborated with the New York Academy of Medicine to develop a nationally acceptable nomenclature that was incorporated into the first edition of the American Medical Association's *Standard Classified Nomenclature of Disease*. Later, a broader nomenclature was developed by the U.S. Army in order to better incorporate the outpatient presentations of veterans of World War II. At around the same time, the World Health Organization published the sixth edition of its International Classification of Diseases (ICD-6), which for the first time included a mental disorders section that included psychoses (10 categories); psychoneuroses (9 categories); and disorders of character, behavior, and intelligence (7 categories).

The APA published a variation of the ICD-6 mental disorders categories in 1952, as the first edition of the *Diagnostic Statistical Manual of Mental Disorders (DSM)*, and it was first revised in 1967.[7] Both of these editions were influenced predominantly by a psychoanalytic approach, and the term *reaction* was used for many of the disorders, more so in the first edition. For example, in 1967, what is now defined as attention-deficit/hyperactivity disorder (ADHD) was still labeled *hyperkinetic reaction of childhood*. The classificatory structure was organized with two poles: psychosis on the severe end, characterized by a disconnection with reality and typically manifested by hallucinations, delusions, and illogical thinking, and neurosis at the mild end, characterized by distortions of reality and typically manifested by anxiety and depression.

In 1980, when the *DSM* was revised to the third edition,[8] the psychodynamic view was discarded, and a biomedical model became the principal approach. The system included explicit diagnostic criteria and a multiaxial system. The revised system tried to make a clear distinction between normal and abnormal. The revision of the third edition, *DSM-III-R*,[9] was published in 1987 and was based on additional research and consensus. It was subsequently revised again in 1994 as the fourth edition (*DSM-IV*),[10] in part to develop compatibility between the *DSM* system and the tenth edition of the International Classification of Diseases (ICD-10).[11] Additional revisions in the text were published in 2000 without any substantial changes in the disorder characteristics (*DSM-IV-TR*).[12]

ORGANIZATIONAL PLAN

The *DSM-IV* system has become the most well established and widely used of diagnostic classification systems in clinical practice with children with behavioral disorders. The *DSM-IV* system is divided into five axes to provide for the assessment of multiple domains of information. These axes are described as follows.

Axis I: Clinical Disorders and Other Conditions

The first axis consists of most of clinical mental disorders and other conditions that may be a focus of clinical attention. They are grouped into 16 major diagnostic classes. The first section is devoted to disorders usually first diagnosed in infancy, childhood, and adolescence (Table 6-1). Communication Disorders; Pervasive Developmental Disorders; Attention-Deficit and Disruptive Behavior Disorders; Feeding and Eating Disorders of Infancy or Early Childhood; Tic Disorders; Elimination Disorders; and Other Disorders of Infancy, Childhood, or Adolescence. However, some individuals with disorders that may be diagnosed during childhood (e.g., ADHD) may not present for clinical attention until adulthood. Moreover, it is not uncommon for the age at onset of many disorders in other sections (e.g., Major Depressive Disorder) to begin during childhood or adolescence. Significant controversy has arisen about when bipolar disorders are likely to manifest.[13] Other diagnoses that are not specific to children but are applicable for children and adolescents include Anxiety, Mood Disorders, Eating Disorders, Somatoform Disorders, and Substance Use Disorders.

Axis II: Personality Disorders and Mental Retardation

Axis II, which includes Personality Disorders and Mental Retardation, is a carryover from the psychoanalytic concept separating permanent brain conditions from those caused by adverse childhood experiences. However, these distinctions have become much less clear with the subsequent finding of evidence of the importance of biological and genetic factors in the etiology of mental disorders and the contributions of environmental factors to Axis II as

TABLE 6-1 ■ *DSM-IV* Axis I Disorders	
Disorders Usually First Diagnosed in Infancy, Childhood, or Adolescence	Transient Tic Disorder
	Tic Disorder NOS
Learning Disorders	
Reading Disorder	*Elimination Disorders*
Mathematics Disorder	Encopresis
Disorder of Written Expression	With Constipation and Overflow Incontinence
Learning Disorder NOS	Without Constipation and Overflow Incontinence
	Enuresis (Not Due to a General Medical Condition)
Motor Skills Disorder	
Developmental Coordination Disorder	*Other Disorders of Infancy, Childhood, or Adolescence*
	Separation Anxiety Disorder
Communication Disorders	Selective Mutism
Expressive Language Disorder	Reactive Attachment Disorder
Mixed Receptive-Expressive Language Disorder	Stereotypic Movement Disorder
Phonological Disorder	*Specify if:* With Self-Injurious Behavior Disorder of Infancy,
Stuttering	Childhood
Communication Disorder NOS	
	Delirium, Dementia, and Other Cognitive Disorders
Pervasive Developmental Disorders	
Autistic Disorder	**Mental Disorders Due to a General Medical Condition not Otherwise Classified**
Rett Disorder	
Childhood Disintegrative Disorder	**Substance-Related Disorders**
Asperger Disorder	
Pervasive Developmental Disorder NOS	**Schizophrenia and Other Psychotic Disorders**
Attention-Deficit and Disruptive Behavior Disorders	**Mood Disorders**
Attention-Deficit/Hyperactivity Disorder	Major Depressive Disorder
Predominantly Inattentive Type	Dysthymic Disorder
Predominantly Hyperactive-Impulsive Type	Bipolar Disorder
Attention-Deficit/ Hyperactivity Disorder NOS	
Conduct Disorder	**Anxiety Disorder**
Childhood-Onset Type	*Eating Disorders*
Adolescent-Onset Type	Anorexia Nervosa
Unspecified Onset	Bulimia Nervosa
Oppositional Defiant Disorder	Eating Disorder NOS
Disruptive Behavior Disorder NOS	*Somatoform Disorders*
Feeding and Eating Disorders of Infancy or Early Childhood	Somatization Disorder
Pica	Undifferentiated Somatoform Disorder
Rumination Disorder	Conversion Disorder
Feeding Disorder of Infancy or Early Childhood	Pain Disorder
	Hypochondrosis
Tic Disorders	Body Dysmorphic Disorder
Tourette Disorder	Somatoform Disorder NOS
Chronic Motor or Vocal Tic Disorder	Substance Use Disorder
	Mental Retardation?

DSM-IV, Diagnostic and Statistical Manual of Mental Disorders, Fourth Edition (American Psychiatric Association); NOS, not otherwise specified.

well as physical (Axis III) conditions. For instance, Autism Disorder is in Axis I even though it has much in common with Mental Retardation.

Axis III: General Medical Conditions

Axis III includes general medical conditions that may be relevant for the understanding and management of the child's behavioral and developmental problems.

Axis IV: Psychosocial and Environmental Problems

Axis IV includes psychosocial and environmental factors that may be important in the initiation or exacerbation of the disorder.

Axis V: Global Assessment of Functioning

Axis V is used to report the clinician's ratings of the child's overall level of impairment. For this purpose, the Global Assessment of Functioning Scale is used. Scores on this scale range from 1 to 100; a low score is indicative of greater impairment, and a high score is indicative of mild, transient, or absence of significant impairment.

ADDITIONAL INFORMATION

The *DSM-IV* manual also includes the following areas of additional information that may be important to diagnostic and treatment planning: (1) *variations in the presentation of the disorder* that are attributable to cultural setting, developmental stage (e.g., infancy, childhood, adolescence, adulthood, late life), or gender (e.g., sex ratio); (2) *prevalence,* which includes data on point and lifetime prevalence, incidence, and lifetime risk as available for different settings; (3) *course,* which consists of typical lifetime patterns of presentation and evolution of the disorder: age at onset and mode of onset (e.g., abrupt or insidious) of the disorder; episodic versus continuous course; single versus recurrent episodes; and duration and progression (e.g., the general trend of the disorder over time); (4) *familial pattern* (e.g., data on the frequency of the disorder among first-degree biological relatives and family members in comparison with the general population); and (5) *differential diagnosis.*

CLINICAL USE AND LIMITATIONS

The *DSM* system has become the standard for diagnosing mental disorders. It provides criteria for establishing diagnoses of mental disorders in the United States and other countries. The criteria are widely accepted for both research and clinical purposes, and both structured interviews and rating scales have been developed on the basis of this system. Third-party payers have used the system as their basis for reimbursement, and federal and state agencies use the diagnostic categories for providing services and funding research.

Despite its broad utility, however, the *DSM* is by no means a perfect system from a scientific and clinical standpoint in the field of developmental-behavioral pediatrics. Limitations of this system include the fact that it is not developmentally based and provides only a dichotomy of disorders, being present or absent, rather than a continuum. Moreover, the same diagnostic criteria are required for all patients regardless of age. In addition, the *DSM* system addresses developmental issues inconsistently. For example, in conditions such as mental retardation or learning disabilities, the testing process to establish the diagnosis provides for the variations anticipated for age. On the other hand, conditions such as ADHD or major depressive disorder require the same number of behavioral manifestations regardless of age. Developmental changes can be used to define the appropriate manifestation or frequency of particular behaviors, but developmental criteria remain loosely defined and therefore very subjective.

A critical assumption in the *DSM* system is that an individual's symptoms either meet the criteria for a particular disorder or fall within a normal range. However, many of the characteristics of the disorders may be present in varying degrees along a spectrum. This situation can be present in children who manifest behaviors severe enough to cause problems for the child but not severe enough to be characterized as a disorder. Children in this situation have been referred to as having a "subthreshhold" condition. Children with subthreshhold conditions have tended to be much more of a focus in primary care settings than in the mental health service sector.

The occurrence of behavioral symptoms along a spectrum leads to much subjectivity in defining the boundaries of many disorders. The difficulty has been most prominent for ADHD, resulting in concerns about how many children receive a diagnosis of this condition[14] and wide variations in the prevalence rates of how many children are being treated for the condition.[15]

International Classification of Diseases, 10th Edition (ICD-10)

HISTORY

A unified classification of diseases started in 1853 at the First International Statistical Congress. The Bertillon Classification of Causes of Death was a synthesis of English, German, and Swiss classifications that was general accepted internationally at the end of the 19th century and was accepted by the American, Canadian, and Mexican organizations in 1898. In 1929, a Mixed Commission made up of representatives of the International Statistical Institute and the Health Organization of the League of Nations developed the Fourth Revision of the International List of Causes of Death; this was revised as the fifth edition in 1938. A recognition that morbidity needed to be included started in the earlier 1900s, so that the fourth revision included further subdivisions to reflect morbid conditions that were not causes of death. The sixth edition, titled *International Classification of Diseases,* was entrusted to the Interim Commission of the World Health Organization in 1948.

In the early 1960s, the Mental Health Program of the World Health Organization worked to improve the diagnosis and classification of mental disorders. These activities resulted in major revisions in the mental disorders, classified in the eighth edition. In both the eighth and ninth revisions, like *DSM-II,* the system contained the divisions between neurotic and psychotic disorders. However, the 10th edition (ICD-10), published in 1992,[11] took a more atheoretical approach, similar to that of *DSM-IV.* The number of categories expanded from 30 in ICD-9 to 100 in ICD-10.

ORGANIZATIONAL PLAN

The mental disorders in ICD-10 are divided into ten categories: organic, including symptomatic, mental disorders (F00-09); mental and behavioral disorders caused by psychoactive substance use (F10-19);

schizophrenia, schizotypal, and delusional disorders (F20-29); mood (affective) disorders (F30-39); neurotic, stress-related, and somatoform disorders (F40-49); behavioral syndromes associated with physiological disturbances and physical factors (F50-59); disorders of adult personality and behavior (F60-69); mental retardation (F70-79); disorders of

psychological development (F80-89); and behavioral and emotional disorders with the onset usually occurring in childhood and adolescence (F90-98). The behavioral and emotional disorders with onset usually occurring in childhood and adolescence and the disorders of psychological development are presented in Table 6-2.

TABLE 6-2 ■ ICD-10: Behavioral and Emotional Disorders with Onset Usually Occurring in Childhood and Adolescence and Disorders of Psychological Development

Behavioral and Emotional Disorders with Onset Usually Occurring in Childhood and Adolescence

Hyperkinetic Disorders

Disturbances of activity and attention
Hyperkinetic conduct disorder
Other hyperkinetic disorders
Hyperkinetic disorder, unspecified

Conduct Disorders

Conduct disorder confined to the family context
Unsocialized conduct disorder
Socialized conduct disorder
Oppositional defiant disorder
Other conduct disorders
Conduct disorder, unspecified

Mixed Disorders of Conduct and Emotions

Depressive conduct disorder
Other mixed disorders of conduct and emotions
Mixed disorder of conduct and emotions, unspecified

Emotional Disorders with Onset Specific to Childhood

Separation anxiety disorder of childhood
Phobic anxiety disorder of childhood
Social anxiety disorder of childhood
Sibling rivalry disorder
Other childhood emotional disorders
Childhood emotional disorder, unspecified

Disorders of Social Functioning with Onset Specific to Childhood and Adolescence

Elective mutism
Reactive attachment disorder of childhood
Disinhibited attachment disorder of childhood
Other childhood disorders of social functioning
Childhood disorders of social functioning, unspecified

Tic Disorders

Transient tic disorder
Chronic motor or vocal tic disorder
Combined vocal and multiple motor tic disorder [Tourette syndrome]
Other tic disorders
Tic disorder, unspecified

Other Behavioral and Emotional Disorders with Onset Usually Occurring in Childhood and Adolescence

Nonorganic enuresis
Nonorganic encopresis

Feeding disorder of infancy and childhood
Pica of infancy and childhood
Stereotyped movement disorders
Stuttering [stammering]
Cluttering
Other specified behavioral and emotional disorders with onset usually occurring in childhood and adolescence
Unspecified behavioral and emotional disorders with onset usually occurring in childhood and adolescence

Disorders of Psychological Development

Specific Developmental Disorders of Speech and Language

Specific speech articulation disorder
Expressive language disorder
Receptive language disorder
Acquired aphasia with epilepsy [Landau-Kleffner syndrome]
Other developmental disorders of speech and language
Developmental disorders of speech and language, unspecified

Specific Developmental Disorders of Scholastic Skills

Specific reading disorder
Specific spelling disorder
Specific disorder of arithmetical skills
Mixed disorder of scholastic skills
Other developmental disorders of scholastic skills
Developmental disorders of scholastic skills, unspecified

Specific Developmental Disorder of Motor Function

Mixed Specific Developmental Disorders

Pervasive Developmental Disorders

Childhood autism
Atypical autism
Rett syndrome
Other childhood disintegrative disorders
Overactive disorder associated with mental retardation and stereotyped movements
Asperger syndrome
Other pervasive developmental disorders
Pervasive developmental disorder, unspecified

Other Disorders of Psychological Development

Unspecified Disorders of Psychological Development

ICD-10, International Classification of Diseases, Tenth Edition (World Health Organization).

Diagnostic and Statistical Manual for Primary Care (DSM-PC), Child and Adolescent Version

HISTORY

For many years, pediatricians were concerned that the *DSM-IV* was of limited the primary care setting for several critical reasons: (1) lack of a spectrum that characterizes issues at less than a disorder level; (2) limited developmental perspective; and (3) limited characterization of environmental factors of importance for prevention. On the basis of these concerns, there was an interest to develop a modified system that would address these deficiencies. The development process started in 1989 under the auspices of the National Institute of Mental Health, which sponsored two meetings between representatives of the four primary care disciplines of internal medicine, family practice, pediatrics, and obstetrics/gynecology and representatives from the APA who were responsible for the *DSM-IV.* Participants at those meetings concluded that primary care clinicians did not find the *DSM* system useful for their purposes and formulated the recommendation to develop a more user-friendly system for primary care clinicians.

For adult mental disorders, the APA assumed responsibility for the system development with consultants from the primary care participants at the meetings. To address the need for a more extensive, child-oriented system, the American Academy of Pediatrics took the lead by forming a task force. From the outset, the process was a collaborative effort among the American Academy of Pediatrics, the APA, and the American Psychological Association (primarily through the Society for Pediatric Psychology). Other organizations also participated, including the Society for Developmental and Behavioral Pediatrics, the American Academy of Child and Adolescent Psychiatry, the American Academy of Family Physicians, the Canadian Pediatric Society, the Zero to Three/National Center for Clinical Infant Programs, the Maternal and Child Health Bureau, and the National Institute of Mental Health. Funding was obtained from the Robert Wood Johnson Foundation, the Maternal and Child Health Bureau, and the American Academy of Pediatrics Friends of Children Fund.

The intent of the *DSM-PC Child and Adolescent Version* was to develop a system that would help primary care clinicians better identify psychosocial issues and conditions affecting their patients, so that they could provide interventions when appropriate and make referrals to mental health clinicians where needed. The development of a common language between general medical and mental health clinicians was essential in this process. At the outset of the project, several assumptions and directives concerning the construction of the system were made:

- Children demonstrate symptoms that vary along a continuum from normal variations to mental disorders, and this continuum can be subgrouped into normal developmental variations, problems, and disorders.
- Environment has an important effect on the mental health of children, and if stressful situations are addressed, more severe mental health problems can be prevented.
- Children vary in how they respond to situations, depending on their age and development.
- A useful system must remain compatible with existing systems, especially the *DSM-IV.*
- The system must be clear, concise, and user friendly for primary care physicians.
- The system must be based on objective information as much as possible, with consensus when this is not possible, and organized so that it can be verified or revised by subsequent research.

The project brought together experts from pediatrics, psychiatry, and psychology to develop the system. There were seven working groups. Each was chaired by a pediatrician and consisted of two additional pediatricians, one of whom was always a primary care physician; two child psychiatrists; and two child psychologists. An important part of the process was the collaborative dialog that developed in each of the working groups. This allowed the final system to have a broader perspective than occurs within any one discipline. After completion, the *DSM-PC* was reviewed by 171 professionals from the fields of primary care pediatrics, developmental-behavioral pediatrics, child psychiatry, child psychology, and child neurology.

ORGANIZATIONAL PLAN

The manual is divided into two major sections. The first section addresses the issue of a child's environment, and the second section discusses a child's manifestations of behavior. The *preamble* to the child's environment "Situations Section" is provided to help the clinician describe and consider the effect of situations that present in practice and affect a child's mental health. It also helps the clinician determine the potential consequences of an adverse situation and identify factors that may make a child more vulnerable or resilient and thus lessen or heighten the situation's effect. The preamble is followed by *a list of potentially adverse situations grouped by their nature,* in which more common and/or well-researched situations are more specifically defined (Table 6-3). To help clinicians evaluate the effects of stressors,

CHAPTER 6   Diagnostic Classification Systems   **115**

TABLE 6-3 ■ *DSM-PC* Classification of Situations

Challenges to Primary Support Group

Challenges to Attachment Relationship
Death of a Parent or Other Family Member
Marital Discord/Divorce
Domestic Violence
Other Family Relationship Problems
Parent-Child Separation

Changes in Caregiving

Foster Care/Adoption/Institutional Care
Substance Abusing Parents
Physical Abuse/Sexual Abuse
Quality of Nurture Problem
Neglect
Mental Disorder of Parent
Physical Illness of Parent
Physical Illness of Sibling
Mental or Behavioral Disorder of Sibling

Other Functional Change in Family

Addition of a Sibling
Change in Parental Caregiver

Community or Social Challenges

Acculturation
Social Discrimination and/or Family Isolation
Religious or Spiritual Problem

Educational Challenges

Illiteracy of Parent
Inadequate School Facilities
Discord with Peers/Teachers

Parent or Adolescent Occupational Challenges

Unemployment
Loss of Job
Adverse Effect of Work Environment

Housing Challenges

Homelessness
Inadequate Housing
Unsafe Neighborhood
Dislocation

Economic Challenges

Poverty/Inadequate Financial Status

Inadequate Access to Health and/or Mental Health Services

Legal System or Crime Problem

Crime Problem of Parent
Juvenile Crime Problem

Other Environmental Situations

Natural Disaster
Witness of Violence

Health-Related Situations

Chronic Health Conditions
Acute Health Conditions

DSM-PC, Diagnostic and Statistical Manual for Primary Care (American Psychiatric Association).

information concerning key *risk* and *protective factors* is provided. To help clinicians assess the effects of situations on the behavior of children, a table summarizes the common behavioral responses to stressful events for children of varying ages.

The second major section describes *child manifestations,* organized into behavioral clusters (Table 6-4). Because clinicians are usually first presented with concerns raised by children or their parents, an *index of presenting complaints* is also included. The clusters are also presented as an algorithm to facilitate the clinician's ability to form a differential diagnosis. The design of each cluster was developed to help the primary care clinician evaluate (1) the spectrum of the child's symptoms, (2) common developmental presentations, and (3) the differential diagnosis.

The *DSM-PC* classification system is based on the assumption that most behavioral manifestations reflect a spectrum from normal to disordered behavior. Accordingly, each cluster has three categories: developmental variations, problems, and disorders.

1. *Developmental variations* are behaviors that parents may raise as a concern with the primary care clinician but that are within the range of expected behaviors for the age of the child. The clinician can best address these variations by reassuring the parents that they are appropriate behaviors. The code provided for this, V65.49, is a nonspecific counseling code in the *International Classification of Diseases, Ninth Revision, Clinical Modification (ICD-9-CM)*.

2. *Problems* reflect behavioral manifestations that are serious enough to disrupt the child's functioning with peers, in school, and/or in the family but do not involve sufficient severity or impairment to warrant the diagnosis of a mental disorder. In many cases, these problems may be treated with short-term counseling, frequently provided by the primary care clinician. However, some of the problems are referred to mental health practitioners for assessment and intervention. If a specific V code is available, it is used; otherwise, a general ICD-9-CM problem (V) code is utilized.

TABLE 6-4 ■ *DSM-PC:* Classification of Child Manifestations

Developmental Competency

Cognitive/Adaptive Skills (Mental Retardation)
Academic Skills
Motor Development
Speech and Language

Impulsive/Hyperactive or Inattentive Behaviors

Hyperactive/Impulsive Behaviors
Inattentive Behaviors

Negative/Antisocial Behaviors

Negative Emotional Behaviors
Aggressive/Oppositional Behaviors
Secretive Antisocial Behaviors

Substance Use/Abuse

Emotions and Moods

Anxious Symptoms
Sadness and Related Symptoms
Ritualistic, Obsessive, Compulsive Symptoms
Suicidal Thoughts or Behaviors

Somatic and Sleep Behaviors

Pain/Somatic Complaints
Excessive Daytime Sleepiness
Sleeplessness
Nocturnal Arousals

Feeding, Eating, Elimination Behaviors

Soiling Problems
Day/Nighttime Wetting Problems
Purging/Binge Eating
Dieting/Body Image Problems
Irregular Feeding Behaviors

Illness-Related Behaviors

Psychological Factors Affecting Medical Condition

Sexual Behaviors

Gender Identity Issues
Sexual Development Behaviors

Atypical Behaviors

Repetitive Behavioral Patterns
Social Interaction Behaviors
Bizarre Behaviors

DSM-PC, Diagnostic and Statistical Manual of Primary Care (American Psychiatric Association).

3. *Disorders* are those defined in *DSM-IV.* Detailed criteria are provided in each cluster or, if a disorder is less likely to be diagnosed by primary care clinicians, are summarized in the clusters to provide the clinician with enough information to identify the disorder and the specific detailed criteria are provided in the appendix. All disorder codes are based on the *DSM-IV.*

The clusters also provide information about any expected differences in presentation that are based on age. Four age periods are defined: infancy (birth to 2 years of age), early childhood (3 to 5 years of age), middle childhood (6 to 12 years of age), and adolescence (13 years of age or older).

DIFFERENTIAL DIAGNOSIS

The clusters also help the clinician develop a differential diagnosis. This component follows the spectrum component and is divided into two sections: *alternative causes* and *comorbid and associated conditions.* The differential diagnosis component begins with phenomena that could be alternative causes for the behaviors and is divided into three parts. The first part lists *general medical conditions* that could cause the child's behavioral manifestations. The second part lists *substances, legal and illegal,* that may cause the behavioral manifestations. The third part lists *other mental disorders* that may manifest with similar behavioral symptoms and that, if present, should be coded in place of the disorder in the cluster. The *comorbid section* is organized similarly to the alternative causes section with only two parts: *other mental disorders* and *general medical conditions* that commonly co-occur with the disorder.

SEVERITY

Severity is somewhat addressed in the spectrum section of the child manifestations, because the decision about behavioral symptoms reflecting variation, problem, or disorder is a severity judgment. In addition, the system provides clinicians with general guidelines to characterize their patient's overall functioning, describes the key elements that should help determine the severity of a child's condition (*symptoms, functioning, burden, suffering,* and *risk/protective factors*), and suggests using the three categories *mild, moderate,* and *severe* to describe the severity.

HOW IS THE *DSM-PC* CURRENTLY BEING USED IN PRACTICE?

How the *DSM-PC* is currently being used in a range of settings is an important issue. To provide some preliminary information on this topic, Drotar and associates[16] surveyed two groups, each of whom would be expected to be more knowledgeable about the *DSM-PC* and more likely to use it than the average group of professionals: (1) the Ohio Chapter of the Society for Developmental and Behavioral Pediatrics (an interdisciplinary group of pediatricians, psychologists, and social workers) and (2) an interdisciplinary group consisting of the faculty trainers for *DSM-PC.* Professionals who reported using the *DSM-PC* were also asked to describe the advantages and disadvantages of the instrument. Most respondents believed that an advantage of the *DSM-PC* was its conceptualization of behavioral problems and the environmental contexts. Others reported that the developmental spectrum and the age-appropriate examples of symptom presentations were very useful and that the continuum of symptom severity and ability to label subsyndromal conditions was also an advantage. The primary disadvantage involved problems with reimbursement from third-party payers. Other disadvantages were lack of specificity or clarity of concepts outlined and an absence of guides to facilitate its use.[16]

CLINICAL APPLICATION: AN EXAMPLE FROM A PRIMARY CARE PRACTICE SETTING

To address the need for clinical application of the *DSM-PC*, Sturner and Howard[17] developed a computerized version of a parent inventory known as the Child Health and Development Interactive System (CHADIS). In the inventory, parents are asked to identify their level of concern (very, somewhat, or not at all concerned) among a list of general concerns derived from the "presenting complaint" section of the *DSM-PC* Child Manifestations section. If more than one concern is identified, the parent is asked to prioritize among them. The parent is then prompted to respond to an algorithm of questions related to the identified chief complaint. The parent continues through the series of questions until (1) criteria for a diagnostic level are not achieved or (2) all the questions necessary to make a *DSM-PC* diagnosis have been reached. A pilot and feasibility study conducted with 27 children from a pediatric practice indicated positive parental reactions to participating in visits in which the CHADIS application of the *DSM-PC* was used.[17] In several studies, Sturner and colleagues described the utility of the CHADIS system in identifying children in primary care who have *DSM-PC* diagnoses.[18-20]

Sturner and colleagues[18] described the kinds of mental health problems documented by pediatricians during the course of child health supervision and the *DSM-PC* diagnoses made for the same children by the CHADIS. A convenience sample of inner-city children was seen by pediatricians for child health visits in two university-affiliated community pediatric clinics. After each visit, CHADIS/*DSM-PC* was administered to the child's caregiver. Mental health diagnostic information documented on the clinic's standard encounter forms was noted by two reliable coders. *DSM-PC* diagnoses were obtained from the CHADIS/*DSM-PC*. CHADIS/*DSM-PC* identified a "disorder" diagnosis in 27%, a "problem" in 28%, "developmental variation" in 21%, and no diagnosis for 23%. Pediatricians used a *DSM-IV* disorder label for 13% and informal diagnostic labels for another 10%.

INTERDISCIPLINARY USE

The *DSM-PC* can be a very useful tool for training psychologists and mental health professionals to understand the full range of clinical problems and environmental stressors among children when providing consultation to primary care physicians.[4,21] Because the *DSM-PC* emphasizes the concept of a continuum of behavioral problems, it can be used to teach undergraduate and graduate students concepts of child development and developmental psychopathology.[5]

USE IN TARGETING AND MONITORING INTERDISCIPLINARY COMMUNITY-BASED PREVENTIVE INTERVENTION FOR CHILDREN AT RISK

Because the *DSM-PC* contains nontechnical language and is not limited to profession-specific, diagnostic classification language such as that in the *DSM-IV*, it may be useful to a broad range of professional service providers for organizing and targeting interventions for children at risk of emotional disturbance or with early signs of emotional disturbance.

The *DSM-PC* also provides a method for community-based service providers to categorize the types of environmental situations or stressors that might be expected to affect treatment planning and prognosis for at-risk children.[16] For example, some children may receive early intervention services in response to specific environmental stressors (e.g., domestic violence or problems in caregiving) that are readily categorized by the *DSM-PC*.

RESEARCH

To our knowledge, Sturner and colleagues[19] presented the first data on the validation of the *DSM-PC*, by using the previously described CHADIS/*DSM-PC*. Caregivers of children completed the CHADIS/*DSM-PC* and were assessed for *DSM* disorders through a computerized parent version of the Diagnostic Interview for Children and Adults (DICA),[22] measures of child behavioral symptoms,[23] and competencies.[24]

No child with a diagnosis of *DSM-PC* Developmental Variation was found to have a disorder according to the DICA, and only two children in the problem category were shown to have a disorder on the DICA. Only one child who received no *DSM-PC* diagnosis was shown to have a DICA disorder. These results also supported the *DSM-PC*'s theoretical definitions for both Developmental Variations and Problems. For example, when parents raised concerns about behaviors that fall into the developmental variation category, the child's behaviors were within the range of expected behaviors for the age and rarely warranted a diagnosis of mental disorder. This finding provides empirical support for the clinical utility of the developmental variations category.

Sturner and colleagues[20] also described, on the basis of *DSM-PC* categories, the 1-year stability of children's mental health status and morbidity in preschool- and school-aged children seen for health supervision visits at one of two Baltimore City clinics. Total scores used to represent mental health status (1 for each variation, 2 for each problem, 3 for each disorder) demonstrated excellent stability, as shown by a correlation of 0.69. Children with *DSM-PC* category diagnoses continued to show similar levels of morbidity 1 year later, whereas most children who received a diagnosis of a disorder persisted with the disorder. Moreover, most children who received an initial diagnosis of a problem either sustained the problem diagnosis or worsened. The Problem category demonstrated a positive predictive value of 0.71 for Problem or Disorder categories 1 year later, which provided evidence for the predictive utility of the *DSM-PC* categories.

The research conducted by Sturner and colleagues concerning the clinical application and validity of the *DSM-PC* represents an important beginning concerning empirical validation of the *DSM-PC*. However, findings should be interpreted with caution because they have not yet been published in the peer-reviewed literature. For this reason, research on the *DSM-PC* needs to be extended by other investigators in other settings.

Diagnostic Classification of Mental Health and Developmental Disorders of Infancy and Early Childhood: Zero to Three (DC:03 and DC:03R)

HISTORY

Infants and young children present a particular challenge for diagnostic classification because of the rapid developmental change and fluidity of change during this developmental period. The DC:03 was developed to categorize the developmental and mental health problems of infants and young children for purposes of diagnosis and treatment planning by a wide range of practitioners. Expert, consensus-based categorizations of mental health and developmental disorders in the early years of life were developed by the Multidisciplinary Diagnostic Classification Task Force established by the Zero to Three National Center for Infants, Toddlers, and Families. This task force recognized that many infants and young children presented in practice situations with problems that could not be readily classified within the *DSM-IV*. The DC:03 was intended to complement and extend the *DSM-IV* as an

initial guide for clinicians and researchers to facilitate clinical diagnosis, treatment planning, and research.[25]

The revision of the DC:03, the DC:03R, was developed on the basis of clinical experience and the findings of the Task Force on Research Diagnostic Criteria: Infancy and Preschool.[26,27] The DC:03R provides clearer, more operational criteria than the original version as shown in Table 6-5.

ORGANIZATIONAL PLAN

The DC:03R proposes a multiaxial classification system that included five axes, described as follows.

Axis I: Clinical Disorders

This axis includes the following categories: Posttraumatic Stress Disorder; Deprivation/Maltreatment

---

TABLE 6-5 ■ DC:03R Axis I Disorders

Post-traumatic Stress Disorder
Deprivation/Maltreatment Disorder
Disorders of Affect
Prolonged Bereavement/Grief Reaction
Anxiety Disorders of Infancy and Early Childhood
  Separation Anxiety Disorder
  Specific Phobia
  Social Anxiety Disorder (Social Phobia)
  Generalized Anxiety Disorder
  Anxiety Disorder NOS
Depression of Infancy and Early Childhood
  Type I: Major Depression
  Type II: Depressive Disorder NOS
Mixed Disorder of Emotional Expressiveness
Adjustment Disorder
Regulation Disorders of Sensory Processing
Hypersensitive
  Type A: Fearful/Cautious
  Type B: Negative Defiant
Hyposensitive/Underresponsive
Sensory Stimulation–Seeking/Impulsive
Sleep Behavior Disorder
Sleep-Onset Disorder (Protodyssomnia)
Night-Waking Disorder (Protodyssomnia)
Feeding Behavior Disorder
  Feeding Disorder of State Regulation
  Feeding Disorder of Caregiver-Infant Reciprocity
  Infantile Anorexia
  Sensory Food Aversions
  Feeding Disorder Associated with Concurrent Medical
    Condition
  Feeding Disorder Associated with Insults to the
    Gastrointestinal Tract
Disorders of Relating and Communicating
Multisystem Development Disorder (MSDD)
Other Disorders (*DSM-IV-TR* or ICD 10)

DC:03R, Diagnostic Classification of Mental Health and Developmental Disorders of Infancy and Early Childhood: Zero to Three revision (Zero to Three Revision Task Force); *DSM-IV-TR, Diagnostic and Statistical Manual of Mental Disorders, Fourth Edition, Text Revision;* ICD-10, International Classification of Diseases, Tenth Edition; NOS, not otherwise specified.

Disorder; Disorders of Affect; Prolonged Bereavement/Grief Reaction; Anxiety Disorders of Infancy and Early Childhood; Depression of Infancy and Early Childhood; Mixed Disorder of Emotional Expressiveness; Adjustment Disorder; Regulation Disorders of Sensory Processing; Hypersensitive; Hyposensitive/Underresponsive; Sensory Stimulation–Seeking/Impulsive; Sleep Behavior Disorder; Sleep-Onset Disorder (Protodyssomnia) and Night-Waking Disorder (Protodyssomnia); Feeding Behavior Disorder; Disorders of Relating and Communication; Multisystem Developmental Disorder; and Other Disorders.

Axis II: Relationship Classification

Axis II characterizes the functional level of the relationships and interactions of infants and young children and their parents' level of distress and conflict, adaptive flexibility, and the effect of the relationship on the child's parents and family. Two instruments, the Parent-Infant Relationship Global Assessment Scale and the Relationships Problems Checklist, provide a guide to evaluating relationships.

Axis III: Medical and Developmental Disorders and Conditions

Axis III describes physical (including medical and neurological), mental health, and/or developmental diagnoses established from other diagnostic and classification systems, such as the *DSM-IV* and the ICD-9 or ICD-10, and from specific classifications used by speech/language pathologists, occupational therapists, physical therapists, and special educators, and the *DSM-PC*.

Axis IV: Psychosocial Stressors

Axis IV describes the nature and severity of psychosocial stress that are influencing disorders in infancy and early childhood. A specific instrument, the Psychological and Environmental Stressor Checklist,[26] provides a framework for identifying (1) the multiple sources of stress experienced by individual effects on the young child and the family and (2) the duration and effect of stressors.

Axis V: Emotional and Social Functioning

The fifth axis reflects the infant or young child's emotional and social functioning in the context of interaction with caregivers and in relation to expectable patterns of development. Relevant dimensions of emotional and social functioning in the DC:03R include the following: (1) Attention and Regulation; (2) Forming Relationships, Mutual Engagement; (3) Intentional Two-way Communication; (4) Complex Gestures and Problem Solving; (5) Use of Symbols to communicate; and (6) Connecting Symbols Logically.

For each of these, the clinician may rate the child's functioning on the 6-point Capacities for Emotional and Social Functioning Rating Scale.[26]

Appendix

The final section of DC:03R includes an appendix that presents an approach for prioritizing diagnostic classifications and planning interventions.

CLINICAL APPLICATION AND RESEARCH

Despite these potential advantages, the DC:03 has not been used extensively by either pediatricians or developmental-behavioral pediatricians in practice, in comparison with either the *DSM-IV* or the *DSM-PC*. Research on either the DC:03 or DC:03R has been very limited. Frankel and associates'[27] chart reviews of children aged newborn to 58 months described the range and frequency of presenting symptoms, relationships between symptoms and diagnoses, and comparisons of the DC:03 and *DSM-IV*. Presenting symptoms were categorized into five groups: (1) Sleep Disturbances; (2) Oppositional and Disruptive Behaviors; (3) Speech and Language/Cognitive Delays; (4) Anxiety and Fears; and (5) Relationship Problems. Findings demonstrated interrater reliability for diagnoses with the use of both diagnostic systems, evidence of diagnostic validity through regression analyses, and good concordance for diagnoses in which the *DSM-IV* and DC:03 overlap.[27]

International Classification of Functioning, Disability, and Health for Children and Youth (ICF-CY)

ORGANIZATIONAL PLAN

Available DCSs focus primarily on the categorizations of symptoms rather than on children's functioning. To address the need to describe child and adolescent functioning with a common nomenclature, the International Classification of Functioning, Disability, and Health (ICF) was developed for clinical practice, research, and policy development across disciplines and service systems.[28] Key dimensions of this system include (1) impairments in body functions and in structured activities; (2) activity limitations; and (3) participation, defined as involvement in a life situation. In addition, the system describes environmental factors (e.g., the physical, social, and attitudinal settings in which individuals conduct their lives) and personal factors that affect functioning. A version of the ICF for children and youths (ICF-CY) has been developed.[29] The ICF-CY includes more than 100 functional impairments and relevant codes that are applicable to *DSM-IV, DSM-PC* diagnostic categories,

TABLE 6-6 ■ Example of Dimensions and Codes from the ICF-CY for Attention-Deficit/Hyperactivity Disorder

Impairment	Activities	Participation	Environment
Attention	Focusing	Excluded from social activities	Access to health care
Impulse control	Carrying out multiple tasks	Poor grades	Medication
			Classroom

Adapted from Lollar and Simeonsson, 2005.
ICF-CY, International Classification of Functioning, Disability, and Health for Children and Youth (World Health Organization Work Group).

and the DC:03R. An example of the relevant dimensions and codes that are applicable to one disorder (ADHD) is shown in Table 6-6.

APPLICATIONS OF CLINICAL CARE, RESEARCH, AND POLICY

Lollar and Simeonsson[30] discussed potential applications of the ICF-CY for developmental and behavioral problems in clinical care in describing activity limitations and access to care, for policy to define gaps in service, and for research concerning the functioning of children and adolescents and training.

One of the most important potential clinical applications of the ICF involves the facilitation of a common language and framework for professionals about impairment in functioning, diagnosis and treatment planning, and changes in these parameters.[31] This common language facilitates professionals' abilities to understand aspects of functional status or dysfunction in diagnosis and management of developmental and behavioral problems. For example, with ADHD, medication treatment might focus on addressing the child's impairment in attention. In contrast, a psychologist's behavioral intervention might focus on control of behavior and social relations. The ICF-CY system also provides a language for parents and various professional disciplines with which to communicate about goals for intervention and response to intervention.

Other potential clinical applications of the ICF-CY include identification of activity limitations associated with specific conditions (e.g., difficulty carrying out multiple tasks in association with ADHD). Another example is identification of specific environmental factors (e.g., access to medical treatment) that can help or hinder necessary treatment (e.g., medication) that may be necessary to reduce functional impairments associated with conditions such as ADHD.

Finally, the ICF-CY system also can be used to describe and manage the variations in the functioning of children with specific diagnoses. This is important in view of the considerable variation in the functional status of children who have specific behavioral and/or developmental disorders[6] and the fact that such variation is often the focus of clinical atten-

tion. The clinical importance of functional status also highlights the need to better use measures of functioning[31] in clinical practice. Finally, like the *DSM-PC*, the ICF-CY highlights the importance of including environmental factors in diagnosis and treatment planning.

Despite limited research on the ICF-CY system, emerging developments and opportunities[32] include measures of critical dimensions that focus on school participation[33] and assessment of activity limitations. For example, Fedeyko and Lollar[34] used the ICF-CY to organize prevalence rates of activity limitations from the National Health Interview Survey, 1994-1995. Learning limitations were found to have the highest prevalence (9.4%) among children 5 to 17 years of age, followed by communication (4.8%) and behavior limitations (4.6%). Field trials are under way in the United States, Europe, Africa, Asia, and Latin America to complete age-specific assessments of functional codes among different age groups (0 to 3, 4 to 6, 7 to 12, and 13 to 18).[30]

Perhaps the most important future applications of the ICF-CY focus on policy. The ICF-CY provides a common language with which to describe interdisciplinary clinical care and research on functional differences in children and adolescents across a range of settings.[35] In addition, the ICF-CY can facilitate health care practitioners', teachers', and therapists' communications about children's functional status in response to psychological and medical interventions.[30] The ICF-CY is a method that can be used to facilitate interdisciplinary care, research, and training[31] across a wide range of different populations of children with behavioral and developmental disorders, impairments that result from these disorders, and settings in which these disorders are treated.

For all the diagnoses of mental disorders, impairment is part of the diagnostic criteria. In addition, the *DSM-PC* categories of problems and normal variations are defined by the extent of impairment. For this reason, the application of the ICF-CY provides an opportunity to define the metric by which the extent of impairment can be measured across different DCSs. It provides a construct on which a generalizable system of measurement of functional impairment can be developed. To accomplish this goal, measures must be developed and applied to specific chronic conditions,[35] and modifications of the ICF-CY must be made in order to consider variations in the developmental levels of children and adolescents.

FUTURE RESEARCH DIRECTIONS IN CLASSIFICATION SYSTEMS

The future research related to DCS falls into one of two categories. The first category is research to document the validity and reliability of the systems. This issue is particularly important for the *DSM-PC*, DC:03, and the ICF-CY, for which new categories not defined previously were created. Studies need to include reliability, as well as concurrent and predictive validity. Some of the studies can be conducted globally for the overall system (e.g., Sturner et al[20]). However, some of the needed research should focus on specific diagnostic categories.

The second category of research entails determining the utility of the DCS and how it can be disseminated into practice settings. One of the most important research directions is for greater description of the use of DCSs by developmental-behavioral pediatricians in practice settings. Moreover, it would be important to compare the clinical utility of the DCSs for various clinical problems. For example, the *DSM-PC* appears to provide a tool for descriptive research concerning the incidence and prevalence of problems seen by primary care physicians, including problems that are at subthreshhold level for a diagnosis according to the *DSM-PC*, whereas the DC:03 better categorizes the relationship issues between parent and child. It will be useful to determine the barriers to their use, as well as determine effective methods to increase their use. The relationship between the conditions and the function assessment systems such as the ICF-CY is needed, as well as further definition and application of how a system of functional classification relates to the diagnosis of behavioral and developmental conditions.

REFERENCES

1. Wolraich ML: Diagnostic and Statistical Manual for Primary Care (DSM-PC) Child and Adolescent Version: Design, intent, and hopes for the future. J Dev Behav Pediatr 18:171-172; 1997.
2. Rappo PD: Use of DSM-PC and implications for reimbursement. J Dev Behav Pediatr 18:175-177, 1997.
3. Coury DL, Berger SP, Stancin T, et al: Curricular guidelines for residency training in developmental-behavioral pediatrics. J Dev Behav Pediatr 20(2 Suppl): S1-S28, 1999.
4. Drotar D: The Diagnostic and Statistical Manual for Primary Care (DSM-PC), Child and Adolescent Version: What pediatric psychologists need to know. J Pediatr Psychol 24:369-380, 1999.
5. Sroufe LA, Rutter MC: The domain of developmental psychopathology. Child Dev 55:17-29, 1984.
6. Kazdin AE: Evidence-based assessment for children and adolescents: Issues in management development and clinical application. J Clin Child Adolesc Psychol 34:548-558, 2005.
7. American Psychiatric Association: Diagnostic and Statistical Manual for Mental Disorders, 2nd ed. Washington, DC: American Psychiatric Association, 1967.
8. American Psychiatric Association: Diagnostic and Statistical Manual for Mental Disorders, 3rd ed. Washington, DC: American Psychiatric Association, 1980.
9. American Psychiatric Association: Diagnostic and Statistical Manual of Mental Disorders, 3rd ed., Revised. Washington, DC: American Psychiatric Association, 1987.
10. American Psychiatric Association: Diagnostic and Statistical Manual of Mental Disorders, 4th ed. Washington, DC: American Psychiatric Association, 1994.
11. World Health Organization: The ICD-10 Classification of Mental and Behavioural Disorders. Geneva: World Health Organization, 1992.
12. American Psychiatric Association: Diagnostic and Statistical Manual of Mental Disorders, 4th ed, Text Revision. Washington, DC: American Psychiatric Association, 2000.
13. Biederman J, Mick E, Faraone SV, et al: Current concepts in the validity, diagnosis and treatment of paediatric bipolar disorder. Int J Neuropsychopharmacol 6:293-300, 2003.
14. Diller LH: The run on Ritalin: Attention deficit disorder and stimulant treatment in the 1990s. Hastings Cent Rep 26(2):12-18, 1996.
15. LeFever G, Dawson KV, Morrow AL: The extent of drug therapy for attention deficit–hyperactivity disorder among children in public schools. Am J Public Health 89:1359-1364, 1999.
16. Drotar D, Sturner R, Nobile C: Diagnosing and managing behavioral and developmental problems in primary care: Applications of the DSM-PC. *In*: Wildman BG, Stancin T, eds: Treating Children's Psychosocial Problems in Primary Care. Greenwich, CT: Information Age Publishing, 2004, pp 191-224.
17. Sturner RA, Howard BJ, eds: The Child Health and Development System. Millersville, MD: Center for Promotion of Child Development through Primary Care, 2000.
18. Sturner R, Morrel T, Howard BJ: Mental health diagnoses among children being seen for child health supervision visits: Typical practice and DSM-PC diagnoses (Abstract in Pediatric Residence 441). Pediatric Academic Society, 2004.
19. Sturner R, Howard BJ, Morrel T, et al: Validation of a Computerized Parent Questionnaire for Identifying Child Mental Health Disorders and Implementing

DSM-PC (Report 3801). Presented at the Pediatric Academic Society Meeting, San Francisco, 2003.

20. Sturner R, Morrel T, Howard BJ: DSM-PC diagnoses predict psychiatric morbidity one year later. Pediatric Academic Society 57:2711, 2005.

21. Drotar D: Consulting with Pediatricians: Psychological Perspectives. New York: Plenum Press, 1995.

22. Reich W: Diagnostic Interview with Children and Adolescents (DICA). J Am Acad Child Adolesc Psychiatry 39:59-66, 2000.

23. Achenbach TM, Rescorla LA: Manual for the ASEBA School-Age Forms & Profiles. Burlington, VT: University of Vermont, Research Center for Children, Youth, & Families, 2001.

24. Goodman R: The Strengths and Difficulties Questionnaire: A research note. J Child Psychol Psychiatry 38:581-586, 1997.

25. Diagnostic Classification 0-3: Diagnostic Classification of Mental Health and Developmental Disorders of Infancy and Early Childhood. Washington, DC: Zero to Three, National Center for Infant Programs, 1994.

26. Zero to Three: Diagnostic Classification of Mental Health and Developmental Disorders of Infancy and Early Childhood. Washington, DC: Zero to Three Press, 2005.

27. Frankel KA, Boyum LA, Harmon RJ: Diagnoses and presenting symptoms in an infant psychiatry clinic: Comparison of two diagnostic systems. J Am Acad Child Adolesc Psychiatry 43:578-587, 2004.

28. World Health Organization: International Classification of Functioning, Disability and Health: ICF. Geneva, Switzerland: World Health Organization, 2001.

29. World Health Organization: ICF Child-Youth Adaptation. Geneva, Switzerland: World Health Organization, 2004.

30. Lollar DJ, Simeonsson RJ: Diagnosis to function: Classification for children and youths. J Dev Behav Pediatr 26:323-330, 2002.

31. Lollar DJ, Simeonsson RJ, Nanda U: Measures of outcomes for children and youth. Arch Phys Med Rehabil 81(12 Suppl 2):S46-S52, 2000.

32. Simeonsson RJ, Leonardi M, Lollar D, et al: Applying the International Classification of Functioning, Disability, and Health to measure childhood disability. Disabil Rehabil 25:602-610, 2003.

33. Simeonsson RJ, Carlson D, Huntington GS, et al: Students with disabilities: A national survey. Disabil Rehabil 23:49-63, 2001.

34. Fedeyko HJ, Lollar DJ: Classifying disability data: A fresh integrative perspective. *In* Altman BM, Barnartt SN, Hendershot GE, et al, eds: Using Survey Data to Study Disability: Results from the National Health Interview Survey on Disability Research in Social Science and Disability. Oxford, UK: Elsevier, 2003, pp 55-72.

35. Cieza A, Brockow T, Ewert T, et al: Linking health status measurements to the International Classification of Functioning, Disability, and Health. J Rehabil Med 34:205-210, 2004.

Screening and Assessment Tools

7A.
Measurement and Psychometric Considerations

GLEN P. AYLWARD ■ TERRY STANCIN

In a general pediatric population, practitioners can expect 8% of their patients to experience significant developmental or behavioral problems between the ages of 24 and 72 months, this rate increasing to 12% to 25% during the first 18 years.[1,2] Therefore, consideration and interpretation of tests and rating scales are part of the clinician's day-to-day experience, regardless of whether the choice is made to administer evaluations or review test or rating scale data obtained by other professionals.

This chapter is an introduction to the section on assessment and tools. It contains topics such as: discussion of descriptive statistics (e.g., mean, median, mode), distributions of scores and standard deviations, transformation of scores (percentiles, z-scores, T-scores), psychometric concerns (sensitivity, specificity, positive and negative predictive values), test characteristics (reliability, validity), and age and grade equivalents. Many of these topics are also elaborated in greater detail in subsequent chapters of this text. A more thorough discussion of psychological assessment methods can be found in Sattler's text.[3]

Developmental and psychological evaluations usually include measurement of a child's development, behavior, cognitive abilities, or levels of achievement. Comprehensive child assessments involve a multistage process that incorporates planning, collecting data, evaluating results, formulating hypotheses, developing recommendations, and conducting follow-up evaluations.[3] Test data provide samples of behavior, with scores representing measurements of inferred attributes or skills. These scores are *relative* and not *absolute* measures, and rating scales and test instruments are typically used to compare a child to a standardized, reference group of other children. Approximately 5% of the general population obtains scores that fall outside the range of "normal." However, the range of normal is descriptive, not diagnostic: it describes problem-free individuals, but does not provide a diagnosis for them.[3] No test is without error, and scores may fall outside the range of normal simply as a result of chance variation or issues such as refusal to take a test. Three major sources of variation that may affect test data include characteristics of a given test, the range of variation among normal children, and the range of variation among children who have compromised functioning.

Selection of which test to use depends on the referral questions posed, as well as time and cost constraints. Testing results vary in terms of levels of detail, complexity, and definitiveness of findings. The first level of testing is screening, the results of which are suggestive. The second level is administration of more formal tests designed to assess development, cognition, achievement, language, motor, adaptive, or similar functions, the results being indicative. The third tier involves administration of test batteries to assess various areas and abilities; these results are assumed to be definitive. This third tier typically includes a combination of formal tests or test batteries, history, interview, rating scales, and observations. The primary goal of more detailed testing is to delineate patterns of strengths and weaknesses so as to provide a diagnosis and guidance for intervention and placement purposes. Results gain meaning through comparison with norms. A caveat is that tests differ markedly in their degree of accuracy.

In general, regardless of whether a measurement tool is designed to be used as an assessment or a screening instrument, the normative sample on which the test is based is critical. Test norms that are to be applied nationally should be representative of the general population. Demographics must proportionately reflect characteristics of the population as a whole, taking into account factors such as region (e.g., West, Midwest, South, Northeast), ethnicity, socioeconomic status, and urban/rural setting. If a test is developed with a nonrepresentative population, characteristics of that specific sample may bias norms and preclude appropriate application to other populations. Adequate numbers of children need to be included at each age across the age span evaluated by a given test so as to enhance stability of test scores. Equal numbers of boys and girls should be included. Clinical groups should also be included for comparison purposes. Convenience samples, or those obtained from one geographic location are not appropriate for development of test norms.

Tests generally need to be reduced and refined by eliminating psychometrically poor items during the development phase. Conventional item analysis is one such approach and involves evaluation of an item difficulty statistic (percentage of correct responses) and patterns of responses. The use of item discrimination indexes (item-total correlations) and item validity (discrimination between normative and special groups, by T-tests or chi square analyses) is routine. More recent tests such as the Bayley Scales of Infant and Toddler Development–Third Edition (BSID-III)[4] or the Stanford-Binet V[5] employ inferential norming[6] or item response theory.[7] Item response theory analyses involve difficulty calibrations for dichotomous items and step differences for polychotomous items, the goal being a smooth progression of difficulty across each subtest (e.g., as in the Rasch probabilistic model[8]). Item bias and fairness analysis are also components; this procedure is called differential item functioning.[9] See Roid[5] or Bayley[4] for a more detailed description of these procedures.

STANDARDIZED ASSESSMENTS

Standardized norm-referenced assessments (SNRAs) are the tests most typically administered to infants, children, and adolescents. The most parsimonious definition of SNRAs is that they compare an individual child's performance on a set of tasks presented in a specific manner with the performance of children in a reference group. This comparison is typically made on some standard metric or scale (e.g., scaled score).[10] Although there may be some allowance for flexibility in rate and order of administration procedures (particularly in the case of infants), administration rules are precisely defined. The basis for comparison of scores is that tasks are presented in the same manner across testings, and there are existing data that represent how similar children have performed on these tasks. However, if this format is modified, additional variability is added, precluding

accurate comparison of the child's data and those of the normative group.

A major issue facing users of SNRAs is identification of the question to be answered from the results of testing. One of two contrasting questions is probably the reason for testing: (1) How does this child compare with his or her referent group? or (2) What are the limits of the child's abilities, regardless of comparison to a referent group? SNRAs are suited to answer the first question. Examiners can subsequently test limits or alter procedures to clarify clinical issues such as strengths and weaknesses after the standard administration is completed. However, these data, although clinically useful, should not be incorporated into the determination of the test score because of the reasons cited previously. Also, no single SNRA in isolation can provide all the answers regarding a child's development or cognitive status; rather, it is a component of the overall evaluation.

Use of SNRAs is not universally endorsed, particularly with regard to infant assessment, because of concerns regarding one-time testing in an unfamiliar environment, different objectives for testing, and linkage to intervention, instead of diagnosis. Therefore, emphasis is placed on alternative assessments that rely on *criterion-referenced* and *curriculum-based* approaches. In actuality, curriculum-based assessment is a type of a criterion-referenced tool. These assessments can help to answer the second question posed previously and could also better delineate the child's strengths. Both provide an absolute criterion against which a child's performance can be evaluated. In criterion-referenced tests, the score a child obtains on a measurement of a specific area of development reflects the proportion of skills the child has mastered in that particular area (e.g., colors, numbers, letters, shapes). For example, in the Bracken Basic Concepts Scale—Revised,[11] in addition to norm-referenced scores, examiners can also determine the percentage of mastery of skills in the six areas included in the School Readiness Composite. More specifically, in the colors subtest, the child is asked to point to colors named by the examiner. This raw score can be converted to a percentage of mastery, which is computed regardless of age. Similarly, other skills such as knowledge of numbers and counting or letters can be gauged. In curriculum-based evaluations, the emphasis is on specific objectives that are to be achieved, the potential goal being intervention planning.[12,13] The Assessment, Evaluation, and Programming System for Infants and Children[14] and the Carolina Curricula for Infants and Toddlers with Special Needs[15] are examples of curriculum-based assessments. Therefore, SNRAs, criterion-referenced tests, and curriculum-based tests each have a role, depending on the intended purpose of the evaluation.

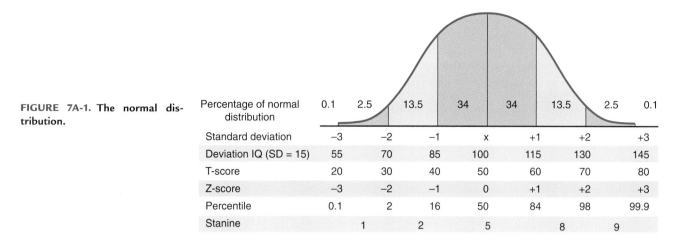

FIGURE 7A-1. The normal distribution.

Percentage of normal distribution	0.1	2.5	13.5	34	34	13.5	2.5	0.1
Standard deviation	−3	−2	−1	x	+1	+2	+3
Deviation IQ (SD = 15)	55	70	85	100	115	130	145
T-score	20	30	40	50	60	70	80
Z-score	−3	−2	−1	0	+1	+2	+3
Percentile	0.1	2	16	50	84	98	99.9
Stanine		1	2	5		8	9

PRIMER OF TERMINOLOGY USED TO DETECT DYSFUNCTION

The *normal range* is a statistically defined range of developmental characteristics or test scores measured by a specific method. Figure 7A-1 depicts a normal distribution or bell-shaped curve. This concept is critical in the development of test norms and provides a basis for the following discussion.

Descriptive Statistics

The *mean (M)* is a measure of central tendency and is the average score in a distribution. Because it can be affected by variations caused by extreme scores, the mean can be misleading in scores obtained from a highly variable sample. In Figure 7A-1, the mean score is 100.

The *mode,* also a measure of central tendency, is the most frequent or common score in a distribution.

The *median* is defined as the middle score that divides a distribution in half when all the scores have been arranged in order of increasing magnitude. It is the point above and below which 50% of the scores fall. This measure is not affected by extreme scores and therefore is useful in a highly variable sample. In the case of an even number of data points in a distribution, the median is considered to be halfway between two middle scores. Noteworthy is the fact that in the normal distribution depicted in Figure 7A-1, the mean, mode, and median are equal (all scores = 100), and the distribution is unimodal.

The *range* is a measure of dispersion that reflects the difference between the lowest and highest scores in a distribution (highest score − the lowest score +1). However, the range does not provide information about data found between two extreme values in the test distribution, and it can be misleading when the clinician is dealing with skewed data. In this situation, the *interquartile range* may be more useful: The distribution of scores is divided into four equal parts, and the difference between the score that marks the 75th percentile (third quartile) and the score that marks the 25th percentile (first quartile) is the interquartile range.[16]

The *standard deviation (SD)* is a measure of variability that indicates the extent to which scores deviate from the mean. The standard deviation is the average of individual deviations from the mean in a specified distribution of test scores. The greater the standard deviation, the more variability is found in test scores. In Figure 7A-1, *SD* = 15 (the typical standard deviation in norm-referenced tests). In a normal distribution, the scores of 68% of the children taking a test will fall between +1 and −1 standard deviation (square root of the variance). In general, most intelligence and developmental tests that employ deviation quotients have a mean of 100 and a standard deviation of 15. Scaled scores, such as those found in the Wechsler tests, have a mean of 10 and a standard deviation of 3 (7 to 13 being the average range). If a child's score falls less than 2 standard deviations below average on an intelligence test (i.e., IQ < 70), he or she may be considered to have a cognitive-adaptive disability (if adaptive behaviors are also impaired).

Skewness refers to test scores that are not normally distributed. If, for example, an IQ test is administered to an indigent population, the likelihood that more children will score below average is increased. This is a *positively skewed* distribution (the tail of the distribution approaches high or positive scores, i.e. the right portion of the *x*-axis). Here, the mode is a lower score than the median, which, in turn is lower than the mean. Probabilities based on a normal distribution will yield an underestimate of the scores at the lower end and an overestimate of the scores at the higher end. Conversely, if the test is administered to children of high socioeconomic status, the distribution might be *negatively skewed,* which means that most children will do well (the tail of the distribution trails toward lower scores or the left portion of the *x*-axis). In negatively skewed distributions, the value of the median < mean < mode scores at the lower end will be overestimated, and those at the upper end will be underestimated. Skewness has significant ramifications in interpretation of test scores. In fact, the meaning of a score in a distribution depends on the mean, standard deviation, and the shape of the distribution.

Kurtosis reflects the shape of the distribution in terms of height or flatness. A flat distribution, in which more scores are found at the ends of the distribution and fewer in the middle, is *platykurtic,* in comparison with the normal distribution. Conversely, if the peak is higher than the normal distribution, scores do not spread out and instead are compressed and cluster around the mean. This is called a *leptokurtic* distribution.

Transformations of Raw Scores

LINEAR TRANSFORMATIONS

Linear transformations provide information regarding a child's standing in comparison to group means. The *z-score* is a standard score (standardization being the process of converting each raw score in a distribution into a z-score: raw score – the mean of the distribution, divided by the standard deviation of the distribution) that corresponds to a standard deviation; that is, a z-score of +1 is 1 standard deviation above average and a z-score of −1 is 1 standard deviation below average. The mean equals a z-score of 0; therefore scores between z-scores of −1 and +1 are in the average range. Stated differently, if a child receives a z-score of +1, he or she obtained a score higher than those of 84% of the population (see Fig. 7A-1).

The *T-score* is another linear transformation and can be considered a z-score $\times$ 10 + 50. The mean T-score is 50, and the standard deviation is 10. Therefore a z-score of 1 equals a T-score of 60. T-scores are often found in psychopathology-related test instruments such as the Minnesota Multiphasic Personality Inventory–A, the Conners rating scales, or the Child Behavior Checklist, on which T-scores of 70 or greater are considered to be clinically relevant (approximately the 98th percentile); these cutoffs are depicted in many scoring forms.

AREA TRANSFORMATIONS

A *percentile* (the technical slang is "centile") tells the practitioner how an individual child's performance compares to a specified norm group. If a percentile score is 50, half of the children tested will score above this, and half will score below. A score that is 1 standard deviation below average is at approximately the 16th percentile; a score 1 standard deviation above

average is at the 84th percentile. Clinicians must be aware that small differences in scores in the center of the distribution produce substantial differences in percentile ranks, whereas greater raw score differences in outliers do not have as much of an effect on percentile scores. Oftentimes, the third percentile is considered to be a clinical cutoff (e.g., in the case of the infant born small for gestational age). *Deciles* are bands of percentiles that are 10 percentile ranks in width (each decile contains 10% of the normative group). *Quartiles* are percentile bands that are 25 percentile ranks in width; each quartile contains 25% of the normative group. Percentiles require the fewest assumptions for accurate interpretation and can be applied to virtually any shape of distribution. This metric is most readily understood by parents and professionals and is recommended as the preferred way to describe how a child's score compares within a group of scores. For example, a Wechsler Intelligence Scale for Children–Fourth Edition (WISC-IV) Full Scale IQ score of 70 indicates that fewer than 3% of children of a similar age score lower on that measure of intelligence; conversely, more than 97% of children taking the test have a higher score.

The *stanine* is short for *standard nine,* and this metric divides a distribution into nine parts. The mean = 5, and the SD = 2, with the third to seventh stanine being considered the average range. Approximately 20% of children score in the fifth stanine, 17% each in the fourth and sixth stanines, and 12% each in the third and seventh stanines (78% in total). Stanines are frequently encountered with group administered tests such as the Iowa Tests of Basic Skills, the Metropolitan Achievement Tests, or the Stanford Achievement Tests. The interrelatedness of these scores is depicted in Figure 7A-1.

PSYCHOMETRIC CONCERNS

Appropriate interpretation of test data necessitates consideration of other important test characteristics. As mentioned previously, when a child's norm-referenced test results are interpreted, the extent to which the child's characteristics are represented in the normative sample from which scores were derived is a critical concern. Moreover, caution is recommended when test results for children from cultural and ethnic minorities drive academic or clinical decisions, unless there is adequate representation of this diversity in standardization samples and validation studies.

Sensitivity and Specificity

Frequently, interpretation of test results must take into account how well the instrument performs with set cutoff scores. *Sensitivity* is a measure of the proportion of children with a specific problem who are positively identified by a test, with a specific cutoff score. Children who have a disorder but are not identified by the test are considered to have false-negative scores. In developmental/behavioral pediatrics, the "gold standard" (criterion used to determine the presence of a given problem) often is not definitive but rather is a reference standard. Comparison with an imperfect "gold standard" may lead to erroneous conclusions that a screening test is inaccurate. As a result, sensitivity may be better conceptualized as copositivity. Desired sensitivity rates are 70% to 80%, and sensitivity is the true positive rate of a test.

Specificity is a measure of the proportion of children who actually are normal and who also are correctly determined by a given test to not have a problem. Children who are normal but who are incorrectly determined by a test cutoff score to be delayed or learning disabled are considered to have false-positive scores. Specificity is the true negative rate of a test. Again, in cases such as developmental screening, the presence of a reference (and not "gold") standard makes the term *conegativity* more appropriate. A specificity rate of 70% to 80% is desirable. However, in the case of screening, it is better to have a higher sensitivity rate, perhaps at the cost of lowered specificity, so as to enhance identification of infants and children who might be at risk.

Cutoff scores can be adjusted to enhance sensitivity. By making criteria more inclusive, fewer children with true abnormalities will be missed; however, a more restrictive cutoff will also increase the probability of false-positive findings (overidentifying "normal" children as being abnormal). Conversely, if the cutoff score is made more exclusive to enhance specificity, the number of normal children inaccurately identified as abnormal is decreased, but some of those who are truly abnormal will be erroneously called normal (false-negative findings). Sensitivity and specificity are described in Figure 7A-2.

Positive predictive value refers to the proportion of children with a positive test result who actually are delayed or learning disabled. This reflects the probability of having a problem when the test result is positive. The lower the prevalence of a disorder, the lower is the positive predictive value. Sensitivity may be a better measure in low-prevalence problems. In developmental screening, positive predictive values often are in the range of 30% to 50%.

Negative predictive value refers to the proportion of children with a negative test result who indeed do not have developmental delays or learning problems. It is the probability of not having the disorder when the test result is negative. This value is influenced by the frequency or prevalence of a problem; in low-prevalence problems, specificity may be a better measure.

Gold (Reference) Standard—Outcome Measure			
	Delayed (+)	Normal (−)	
Screening Test Delayed (+)	**A.** Children with delays who were identified by screening test (*True positives*) N = 70	**B.** Normal children identified as being delayed by screening test (*False positives*) N = 20	N = 90
Screening Test Normal (−)	**C.** Children with delays who were not identified on the test (*False negatives*) N = 30	**D.** Normal children who were found to be "normal" on screening test (*True negatives*) N = 80	N = 110
	100	100	200

Sensitivity = A/A + C(70/70 + 30 = 0.70)
Specificity = D/B + D(80/20 + 80 = 0.80)
PPV = A/A + B(70/70 + 20 = 0.78)
NPV = D/C + D(80/30 + 80 = 0.73)
False positive rate = B/B + D(20/20 + 80 = 20%)
False negative rate = C/A + C(30/70 + 30 = 30%)

FIGURE 7A-2. Example highlighting sensitivity and specificity.

Frequency of a Disorder/Problem

Prevalence rate refers to the number of children in the population with a disorder, in relation to the total number of children in the population, measured at a given time. The *incidence rate* indicates the risk of developing a disorder: namely, new cases of a problem that develop over a period of time. The relationship between incidence and prevalence can best be illustrated by the following: prevalence rate = the incidence rate × the duration of the disorder. In essence, the predictive value of screening takes into account sensitivity and specificity of the screening procedure and the prevalence of the disorder.

Base rate is the naturally occurring rate of a given disorder. For example, the base rate of learning disabilities would be much higher in children referred to a learning and attention disorders clinic than in the general population. If a screening instrument were used to detect learning disabilities for this group, sensitivity and specificity values would differ from those found in the general pediatric population. For example, in the follow-up of low-birth-weight infants, the base rate for major handicaps (moderate to severe mental retardation; cerebral palsy; epilepsy; deafness or blindness) is 15%; therefore, in 85% of this population, the findings would be true negative. Low base rates increase the possibility of false-positive results. High base rates do not leave much room for improvement in terms of locating true-positive scores and result in an increase in false-negative findings. Tests can be most helpful in decision making when the base rate is in the vicinity of 0.50. Therefore, particularly in the case of screening, the relatively low base rates of developmental problems in very young children may increase the probability of false positive findings. However, in such situations, this scenario is more desirable than the converse: false negative findings.

Relative risk provides an alternative strategy for evaluating test accuracy.[17,18] This approach involves use of the likelihood ratio, which indicates the increased probability that the child will display a developmental problem, if the results of an earlier screening test were abnormal or suspect. This approach recognizes that not all children at early risk will later manifest a developmental problem, but there is a greater likelihood that they will. If a problem or disorder is rare, relative risk and odds ratios are nearly equal.

Test Characteristics

RELIABILITY

Measurement is the ability to assign numbers to individuals in systematic ways as a means of inferring properties of these individuals. *Reliability* refers to consistency or accuracy in measurement. Reliability focuses on how much error is involved in measurement or how much an obtained score varies from the "true score." An observed test score = true score + measurement error. *Internal consistency* is a measure of whether all components of a test evaluate a cohesive construct or set of constructs (e.g., verbal ability or visual-motor skills). Stated differently, high internal consistency means that all items are highly intercorrelated. This is measured with Cronbach's alpha, split-half reliability, or the Kuder-Richardson reliability estimate. Cronbach's alpha is used to evaluate how individual items relate to the test as a whole (intercorrelation among items); split-half reliability relates half of the test items to the remaining half, often by an odd-even split; and the Kuder-Richardson reliability estimate is used for dichotomous (i.e., "yes"/"no") items. *Test-retest reliability* is particularly pertinent in developmental and psychological testing because it takes into account the "true score" and error, addressing whether the same score would be obtained if a specific test were readministered. The length of time between the two administrations of the test is critical in regard to this measurement; that is, the sooner the test is readministered, the greater the reliability estimate is. In general, test-retest correlations of 0.70 are considered moderate, 0.80 moderate to high, and 0.90, high (scores >0.85 are desirable, although explicit, evidence-based criteria have not been defined yet). Tests with more items tend to have higher reliability, because of the likelihood of a greater variance

in scores. *Interrater reliability* refers to how well independent examiners agree on results of a test. *Alternate forms* involve use of parallel tests, so as to prevent carryover (score inflation) if the parallel test is administered soon after the first. For example, the Peabody Picture Vocabulary Test–III has two forms, as does the Wide Range Achievement Test–4.

Reliability is affected by test length (longer tests are more reliable), test-retest interval (longer interval lessens reliability), variability of scores (greater variance increases reliability estimate), guessing (increased guessing decreases reliability), variations in test situation, and practice effects.[3]

VALIDITY

Validity refers to whether a test measures what it is supposed to measure for a specific purpose. A test may be valid for some uses and not others. For example, the Peabody Picture Vocabulary Test–III may be a valid measure of receptive vocabulary, but it is not a valid measure of overall cognitive ability or even overall language ability. It is important to keep in mind that test validation is context specific. In order to determine whether an assessment method is "psychometrically sound" or "valid," the clinician must consider how it is being used. For example, an intelligence test may be a valid method for determining a child's cognitive abilities but may have limited validity for treatment design and planning (see previous discussion of SNRAs). Similarly, a test may have demonstrated evidence as a valid measure of severity of general anxiety but not of phobias; a certain behavior rating scale may be valid as a measure of current clinical symptoms but may not have validity for treatment planning or for predicting outcomes. Thus, the *purpose* of the assessment needs to be considered in order to properly evaluate the psychometric characteristics of an assessment method.

Content validity determines whether the items in the test are representative of the domain the test purports to measure: that is, whether the test does cover the material it is supposed to cover. *Construct validity* concerns whether the test measures a particular psychological construct or trait (e.g., intelligence). *Criterion-related validity* involves the current relationship between test scores and some criterion, such as results of another test. Criterion-related validity can be *concurrent* (convergent) or *predictive*. In both instances, the results of a test under consideration are compared to an established reference standard to determine whether findings are comparable. In concurrent validity, the two tests (e.g., a screen such as the Bayley Infant Neurodevelopmental Screener and a "reference standard" such as the BSID-II) are administered at the same time, and the results are correlated. With predictive validity, a screening test might be given at one time, followed by administration of the reference standard at a later date (e.g., the BSID-II is given to children aged 36 months, and the Wechsler Preschool and Primary Scales of Intelligence–III at age $4\frac{1}{2}$ years). *Discriminant validity* shows how well a screening test detects a specific type of problem. For example, autism might be the condition of concern, and a screening test such as the Modified Checklist for Autism in Toddlers (M-CHAT) is used to distinguish children with this disorder from those with mental retardation without autism. *Face validity* involves whether the test appears to measure what it is supposed to measure. Test-related factors (examiner-examinee rapport, handicaps, motivation), criterion-related factors, or intervening events could affect validity.

With regard to the interrelatedness among reliability and validity, reliability essentially sets the upper limit of a test's validity, and reliability is a necessary but not sufficient condition for valid measurement. A specific test can be reliable, but it may be invalid when used to evaluate a function that it was not designed to measure. However, if a test is not reliable, it cannot be valid. Stated differently, all valid tests are reliable, unreliable tests are not valid, and reliable tests may or may not be valid.[19]

Practitioners should also be cognizant of the fact that testing can involve a speed test, in which items are relatively easy but there is a specific time limit and it is difficult to answer all of the items. The infamous 2-minute math test is an example. A power test involves progressively more difficult items, this difficulty being determined by the limits of a child's knowledge base.

Age and Grade Equivalents

Age- and *grade-equivalent* scores are based on raw scores and portray the average age or grade placement of children who obtained a particular raw score. Although these metrics are useful in explaining results to parents and make conceptual sense, age- and grade-equivalent scores are uneven units of measurement. For example, a six-month difference in performance at the age of 2 years is much more significant than a 6-month lag at age 8 years. Moreover, a 9-year-old with an age equivalent of 7 years is quite different from a 4-year-old functioning at a 7-year age equivalent, or an average 7-year-old. These measures lack precision, and in some test manuals, the same standard scores can produce somewhat different age/grade equivalents. Both metrics assume that growth is consistent throughout the school year and tend to exaggerate small differences in performance. These measures also vary from test to test. Furthermore, with achievement testing, it is necessary to know whether age or grade norms were used to obtain standard scores. For example, if age norms are used and the child had been retained in grade, he or she would be at a significant disadvantage because he or she would not have been exposed to the more advanced material. Conversely, if a child failed second grade and is being tested in early fall while repeating second grade, he or she may receive inflated scores if grade norms are used.

The *IQ/DQ ratio* (developmental quotient) is computed as mental age (obtained by the use of a test score) ÷ the child's chronologic age and then multiplied by 100. Although *developmental age* refers to a level of functioning, DQ reflects the rate of development.[19] IQ/DQ ratio scores are not comparable at different age levels because the standard deviation (variance) of the ratio does not remain constant. As a result, interpretation is difficult, and these scores generally are not used very much in contemporary standardized testing. Instead, the *deviation IQ/DQ* is employed. The deviation IQ is a method of estimation that allows comparability of scores across ages and is used with most major psychological and developmental test instruments. The deviation IQ/DQ is norm referenced and normally distributed, with the same standard deviation; typically, $M = 100$ and $SD = 15$. Therefore, a deviation IQ of 85 obtained at age 6 should have the same meaning as a score of 85 obtained at age 9.

The *standard error of measurement (SEM)* is an estimate of the error factor in a test that is the result of sampling or test characteristics, taking into account the mean, standard deviation, and size of the sample. The larger the standard error of measurement, the greater the uncertainty associated with a given child's score. The *SEM* is produced by multiplying the standard deviation of the test by the square root of (1− the reliability coefficient of the test). In 95% of cases, the interval of approximately two times (1.96) the *SEM* above or below a child's score would contain the "true" score: a 95% confidence interval. Stated differently, a 95% confidence interval indicates that if a test is given 100 times with different samples, scores will fall in this interval 95% of the time. In a 90% confidence interval, an interval of 1.64× the *SEM* above and below a child's score would contain the "true" score. Such estimates are important in test-retest situations or in the case of a child who does not receive services because of missing a cutoff score by only a few points (e.g., a WISC-IV Full Scale IQ score of 72).

A final concern is the *Flynn effect,*[20] in which test norms increase approximately 0.3 to 0.5 points per year, which is equivalent to a 3- to 5-point increment per decade. This finding has ramifications in comparisons of scores obtained on earlier versions of tests to more contemporary scores (e.g., WISC-Revised to the WISC–Third Edition or WISC-IV; BSID to BSID-II; Stanford-Binet form LM to the 5th edition). Caution is warranted when the practitioner attributes a decline in scores to a loss of cognitive ability, because in actuality this decline may be attributable to the fact that a newer test has mean scores that are considerably lower than those of an earlier version of the test (e.g., 5-8 points).[20] This issue would also have ramifications for children whose IQ score on an older version of a test is in the low 70s but decreases to below the cutoff for mild mental retardation on a newer version.

Although some practitioners may administer tests, all have occasion to respond to inquiries from parents about their child's test performance or diagnosis derived from testing. The physician's role includes explaining test results to parents, acknowledging parental concerns and advocating for the child, providing additional evaluation, or referring to other professionals.[21]

REFERENCES

1. Costello EJ, Edelbrock C, Costello AJ, et al: Psychopathology in pediatric primary care: The new hidden morbidity. Pediatrics 82:415-424, 1988.
2. Lavigne JV, Binns HJ, Christoffel KK, et al: Behavioral and emotional problems among preschool children in pediatric primary care: Prevalence and pediatricians' recognition. Pediatrics 91:649-657, 1993.
3. Sattler JM: Assessment of Children, 4th ed. San Diego: Jerome M. Sattler, 2001.
4. Bayley N: Bayley Scales of Infant and Toddler Development, Third Edition: Technical Manual. San Antonio, TX: PsychCorp, 2005.
5. Roid GH: Stanford-Binet Intelligence Scales for Early Childhood, Fifth Edition: Manual. Itasca, IL: Riverside, 2005.
6. Wilkins C, Rolfhus E, Weiss L, et al: A Simulation Study Comparing Inferential and Traditional Norming with Small Sample Sizes. Paper presented at annual meeting of the American Educational Research Association, Montreal, Canada, 2005.
7. Wright BD, Linacre JM: WINSTEPS: Rasch Analysis for All Two-Facet Models. Chicago: MESA, 1999.
8. Rasch G: Probabilistic Models for Some Intelligence and Attainment Tests. Chicago: University of Chicago Press, 1980.
9. Dorans NJ, Holland PW: DIF detection and description: Mantel-Haenszel and standardization. In Holland PW, Wainer H, eds: Differential Item Functioning. Mahwah, NJ: Erlbaum, 1993, pp 35-66.
10. Gyurke JS, Aylward GP: Issues in the use of norm-referenced assessments with at-risk infants. Child Youth Fam Q 15:6-8, 1992.
11. Bracken BA: Bracken Basic Concepts Scale—Revised. San Antonio, TX: The Psychological Corporation, 1998.
12. Greenspan SI, Meisels SJ: Toward a new vision for the developmental assessment of infants and young children. In Meisels SJ, Fenichel E, eds: New Visions for the Developmental Assessment of Infants and Young Children. Washington, DC: Zero to Three: National Center for Infants Toddlers and Families, 1996, pp 11-26.
13. Meisels S: Charting the continuum of assessment and intervention. In Meisels SJ, Fenichel E, eds: New Visions for the Developmental Assessment of Infants and Young Children. Washington, DC: Zero to Three: National Center for Infants Toddlers and Families, 1996, pp 27-52.
14. Bricker D: Assessment, Evaluation and Programming System for Infants and Children, Volume 1: AEPS Measurement for Birth to Three Years. Baltimore: Paul H. Brookes, 1993.
15. Johnson-Martin N, Jens K, Attermeir S, et al: The Carolina Curriculum, 2nd ed. Baltimore: Paul H. Brookes, 1991.
16. Urdan T: Statistics in Plain English. Mahwah, NJ: Erlbaum, 2001.
17. Frankenburg WK, Chen J, Thornton SM: Common pitfalls in the evaluation of developmental screening tests. J Pediatr 113:1110-1113, 1988.
18. Frankenburg WK: Preventing developmental delays: Is developmental screening sufficient? Pediatrics 93:586-593, 1994.
19. Salvia J, Ysseldyke JE: Assessment, 8th ed. New York: Houghton Mifflin, 2001.
20. Flynn JR: Searching for justice. The discovery of IQ gains over time. Am Psychol 54:5-20, 1999.
21. Aylward GP: Practitioner's Guide to Developmental and Psychological Testing. New York: Plenum Medical, 1994.

7B.
Surveillance and Screening for Development and Behavior

FRANCES P. GLASCOE
PAUL H. DWORKIN

More than three decades have elapsed since the identification of developmental, behavior, and psychosocial problems as the so-called "new morbidity" of pediatric practice.[1] During the ensuing years, profound societal change, with public policy mandates for deinstitutionalization and mainstreaming, has further influenced the composition of pediatric practice. Studies have documented the high prevalence of developmental and behavioral issues within the practice setting, including disorders of high prevalence and lower severity such as specific learning disability, attention-deficit/hyperactivity disorder, and speech and language impairment, as well as problems of higher severity and lower prevalence such as mental retardation, autism, cerebral palsy, hearing impairment, and serious emotional disturbance.[2]

The critical influence of the early childhood years on later school success and the well-documented benefits of early intervention provide a strong rational for the early detection of children at risk for adverse developmental and behavioral outcomes. Neurobiological, behavioral, and social science research findings from the 1990s, the so-called decade of the brain, have emphasized the importance of experience on early brain development and on subsequent development and behavior and the extent to which the less differentiated brain of the younger child is particularly amenable to intervention.[3]

In this chapter, we highlight links between early detection and early intervention. Much has been written on this topic and the American Academy of pediatrics has recently revised its policy statement on developmental screening. The new statement includes expert opinion on how to provide quality developmental surveillance (the process of incorporating medical/developmental history, knowledge of the family, parents' concerns, screening test results, and clinical observation) in order to make informed decisions about any needed referrals. Thus, this chapter offers a review of evidence and challenges in surveillance and screening, reconciles both approaches, includes a list of quality screening measures, describes effective early identification initiatives, and provides suggestions for enhancing the well-child visits to facilitate early detection of developmental and behavioral problems.

BACKGROUND

Early identification and intervention affords the opportunity to avert the inevitable secondary problems with loss of self-esteem and self-confidence that result from years of struggle with developmental dysfunction. Federal legislation, the Individuals with Disabilities Education Act (IDEA) of 2004, and related state legislation mandate early detection and intervention for children with developmental and behavioral disabilities. Surveys indicate that parents have strong interest in promoting children's optimal development.[4,5]

Perhaps the most compelling rationale for early detection is the effectiveness of early intervention. Researchers have documented the benefits of early intervention in children with mental retardation and

physical handicaps, particularly when improved family functioning is a measured outcome.[6] More recently, the benefits of early intervention for children at environmental risk has also been demonstrated. For example, enrollment and participation of disadvantaged children in Head Start programs contribute to a decreased likelihood of grade repetition, less need for special education services, and fewer school dropouts.[7] Detection is also supported by the clearer delineation of adverse influences on children's development. For example, the effect of such diverse factors as low-level lead exposure and adverse parent-infant interaction on child development has implications for early identification.

By virtue of their access to young children and their families, child health providers are particularly well positioned to participate in early identification of children at risk for adverse outcomes through ongoing monitoring of development and behavior. Clinicians' knowledge of medical and genetic factors also facilitates early identification of conditions associated with developmental problems. Furthermore, through their relationships with children and their families, pediatricians and other child health providers are familiar with the social and familial factors that place children at environmental risk. Professional guidelines emphasize the importance of early detection by child health providers. The American Academy of Pediatrics' Committee on Children with Disabilities; Medicaid's Early Periodic Screening, Diagnosis, and Treatment (EPSDT) program; and *Bright Futures* (guidelines for health supervision of infants, children, and adolescents developed by the American Academy of Pediatrics and the Maternal and Child Health Bureau) all encourage the effective monitoring of children's development and behavior and the prompt identification of children at risk for adverse outcomes.[8,9] The emphasis on the primary care practice as a comprehensive medical home for all children also supports the office as the ideal medical setting for developmental and behavioral monitoring.[10]

Despite this strong rationale, results of surveys of parents and child health providers demonstrate that current practices widely vary and suggest the need to strengthen developmental monitoring and early detection. Only about half of parents of children aged between 10 and 35 months recall their children's ever having received structured developmental assessments from their child health providers.[11] Parents also report gaps in the discussion of development and related issues with pediatric providers.[12] Most pediatricians employ informal, nonvalidated approaches to developmental screening and assessment. The majority of pediatricians do not incorporate within their practice such tools as those recommended by *Bright Futures* to aid in early detection.[13]

Not surprisingly, the early detection of children at risk for adverse developmental and behavioral outcomes has proved elusive. Fewer than 30% of children with such disabilities as mental retardation, speech and language impairments, learning disabilities, and serious emotional/behavioral disturbances are identified before school entry.[13] This lack of detection precludes the opportunity and benefits of timely, early intervention. Although nearly half of parents have some concerns for their child's development or behavior, such concerns are infrequently elicited by child health providers.[14]

Multiple factors have been cited as barriers to effective developmental monitoring. Child health providers report inadequate time during the office visit to deliver developmental services, including monitoring and early detection. A professionally administered developmental test (e.g., the Denver-II) cannot be adequately performed in a child health supervision visit that lasts, on average, less than 20 minutes and in which other content must be delivered. Other recognized barriers include the inadequate training of child health providers and ineffective administrative and clinical practices, including staffing and record keeping. Despite the assigning of a value to the billing code for developmental screening (96110) by the Centers for Medicare and Medicaid Services, reimbursement for developmental services in general and for developmental monitoring specifically by third-party payers remains inadequate. Health care organizations do not measure or prioritize the developmental content of child health supervision services. Furthermore, even if at-risk children are identified, the linkage of such children and their families to developmentally enhancing programs and services is often inefficient and challenging.

DEVELOPMENTAL SURVEILLANCE

Currently, child health providers employ a variety of techniques to monitor children's development and behavior. History taking during a health supervision visit typically includes a review of age-appropriate developmental milestones. Unfortunately, recall of such milestones is notoriously unreliable and typically reflects parents' prior conceptions of children's development.[15] Although the accuracy in determining the age of performing certain tasks is certainly improved by the use of diaries and records, the wide range of normal acquisition for such milestones limits their value in assessing children's developmental progress. Child health providers may also question parents as to their predictions for their child's development. Predictions (typically elicited with questions

such as "when your child becomes an adult, do you think he or she will be above average, average, or below average?") are also unhelpful in developmental monitoring, because parents are likely to expect average functioning for children with delays and predict overachievement for children developing at an average pace, a phenomenon dubbed the *presidential syndrome*.[15]

During the physical examination, child health providers may interact with children by using an informal collection of age-appropriate tasks. The lack of a standardized approach to measuring developmental progress makes interpretation of children's performance on such tasks difficult. The reliance of child health providers on "clinical judgment," based on subjective impressions during the performance of the history and physical examination, are also fraught with hazard. Such impressions are unduly influenced by the extent to which a child is verbal and sociable in a setting that may be frightening, an effect likely to restrict affect and deter spontaneous demonstrations of pragmatic language skills. Studies have documented the poor correlation between provider's subjective impressions of children's development and the results of formal assessments. Clinical judgment identifies fewer than 30% of children with developmental disabilities.[15] The reliance on subjective impressions undoubtedly contributes to the late identification of children with such developmental issues as mild mental retardation.

According to research findings and expert opinion, surveillance and screening constitute the optimal approach to developmental monitoring.[16] As originally described by British investigators, surveillance encompasses all activities relating to the detection of developmental problems and the promotion of development through anticipatory guidance during primary care.[17] Developmental surveillance is a flexible, longitudinal, continuous process in which knowledgeable professionals perform skilled observations during child health care.[17] Although surveillance is most typically performed during health supervision visits, clinicians may perform *opportunistic surveillance* during sick visits by exploring the child's understanding of illness and treatment.[18a]

The emphasis of developmental surveillance is on skillfully observing children and identifying parental concerns. Components include eliciting and attending to parents' opinions and concerns, obtaining a relevant developmental history, skillfully and accurately observing children's development and parent-child interaction, and sharing opinions and soliciting input from other professionals (e.g., visiting nurse, child care provider, preschool and school teacher), particularly when concerns arise. Developmental history should include an exploration of both risk and protective factors, including environmental, genetic, biological, social, and demographic influences, and observations of the child should include a careful physical and neurological examination. Surveillance stresses the importance of viewing the child within the context of overall well-being and circumstance.[17]

The most critical component of surveillance is eliciting and attending to parents' opinions and concerns. Research has elucidated the value of information available from parents. Although there are several ways to obtain quality information, research on parents' concerns is voluminous. Concerns are particularly important indicators of developmental problems, particularly for speech and language function, fine motor skills, and general functioning (e.g., "He's just slow").[15,18] Although concerns about self-help skills, gross motor skills, and behavior are less sensitive indicators of developmental functioning, such opinions should serve as clinical "red flags," mandating closer clinical assessment and developmental promotion.[15,18] The manner in which parental concerns are elicited is important. Asking parents whether they have worries about their children's development is unlikely to be useful, because they may be reluctant to acknowledge fears and interpret "development" as merely reflecting physical growth. In contrast, asking parents whether they have any concerns about the way their child is behaving, learning, and developing, followed by more specific inquiry about functioning in specific developmental domains, is more likely to yield valid and clinically useful responses.[18,19] Clinicians must be mindful of the complex relationship between concerns and disability (some concerns are predictors of developmental status only at certain ages), the critical importance of eliciting concerns rather than relying on parents to volunteer, and the value of an evidence-based approach to interpreting concerns.[18,21]

Parents' estimations are also accurate indicators of developmental status. For example, a study conducted in primary care demonstrated the extent to which parents' estimates of cognitive, motor, self-help, and academic skills correlate with findings on developmental assessments.[22] Parental responses to the question, "Compared with other children, how old would you say your child now acts?" are important indicators of developmental delay, although such questions are more challenging for parents than elicitations of concerns.[22]

In contrast to the limitations of parents' recall of developmental milestones, contemporaneous descriptions of children's current skills and achievements are useful indicators of developmental status. Similar to the solicitation of parental concerns, the format of questions eliciting parental report is important. Rec-ognition questions such as "Does your child use any of the following words?" are more likely to yield helpful information than are such identification questions as "What words does your child say?" that rely on parents' spontaneous recall and report. Parental report is likely to yield higher estimates of children's functioning than is professional assessment. This discrepancy is less likely to result from parental inaccuracy or exaggeration than from parents' reports on newly emerging skills that are inconsistency demonstrated in the familiar and supportive home environment.

Parents' opinions and concerns must be considered within the context of cultural influences. Parents' appraisals and descriptions are influenced by expectations for children's normal development, and such expectations vary among different ethnic groups. For example, in a study of Latino (primarily Puerto Rican), African American, and European American mothers, Puerto Rican mothers expected personal and social milestones to be normally achieved at a later age than did the other groups, whereas first steps and toilet training were expected at an older age by European American mothers.[23] Such differences were often explained by underlying cultural beliefs, values, and childrearing practices. For example, the older age for achievement of self-help skills is consistent with the Puerto Rican concept of *familismo* and its emphasis on caring for children.

USE OF SCREENING TOOLS

The effectiveness of developmental surveillance is enhanced by incorporating valid measures of parents' appraisals and descriptions of children's development and skilled professional observations. The process is enhanced by the periodic use of evidence-based screening tools (meaning that measures are repeatedly administered over time), including parent-completed questionnaires and professionally administered tests. Screening tools that elicit information from parents may be used on a routine basis to supplement data gathering during health supervision visits, may be used periodically at select ages (e.g., 9, 18, and 24 months), or may be used in a targeted manner to further explore the significance of parental concerns. Similarly, professionally administered screening tests may be administered periodically to help ensure that children do not elude early identification, or they may be used when concerns arise (so-called second-stage screening) or when parents are not able to provide information.

Table 7B-1 includes descriptions of screening tools that are highly accurate: that is, based on nationally representative samples, fulfilling psychometric

TABLE 7B-1 ■ Developmental, Mental Health/Behavioral and Academic Screens

Screen	Age Range/Time Frame	Description	Scoring	Accuracy	Notes
		Developmental-Behavioral Screens Relying on Information from Parents			
Infant-Toddler Checklist for Language and Communication (ITC) (1998) Paul H. Brookes Publishing, Inc., P.O. Box 10624, Baltimore, MD 21285; Phone: 1-800-638-3775; *http://www.pbrookes.com/* Part of Communication and Symbolic Behavior Scales Developmental Profile ($99.95 with CD-ROM)	6-24 months	Parents complete the ITC's 24 multiple-choice questions in English. Reading level is 6th grade. Based on screening for delays in language and social-emotional development as the first evident symptom that a child is not developing typically. Does not screen for motor milestones. Optional CD-ROM copyrighted but remains free for use at the Brookes Web site.	Cut-off scores at 1.25 standard deviations below in four domains. facilitates factor scoring. The Checklist is	Sensitivity: 78% Specificity: 84% Information about accuracy across age ranges is not available.	
Parents' Evaluations of Developmental Status (PEDS) (2007) Ellsworth & Vandermeer Press, Ltd., P.O. Box 68164, Nashville, TN 37206; Phone: 615-226-4460; Fax: 615-227-0411; *http://www.pedstest.com* $30.00 PEDS is also available online together with the Modified Checklist of Autism in Toddlers for electronic records, individual parents, and computer-assisted telephone interviews.	Birth to 8 years/ 2-5 minutes	10 questions eliciting parents' concerns in English, Spanish, Vietnamese, Thai, Indonesian, Hmung, Somali, etc. Written at the 5th grade level. Determines when to refer, provide a second screen, educate patient/parents, or carefully monitor development, behavior/emotional, and academic progress. Provides longitudinal surveillance and triage. Web site has downloadable training materials. Computer-assisted telephone interview versions are available.	Identifies children as being at low, moderate, or high risk for various kinds of disabilities and delays.	Sensitivity ranges from 74% to 79% and specificity ranges from 70% to 80% across age levels.	
PEDS: Developmental Milestones (PEDS:DM) (2007) Ellsworth & Vandermeer Press, Ltd., P.O. Box 68164, Nashville, TN 37206; Phone: 615-226-4460; Fax: 615-227-0411; *http://www.pedstest.com* $275.00 Available electronically through *pedssupport@forepath.org*	0-95 months/ 3-6 minutes	The PEDS:DM is a laminated book consisting of 6-8 items, one per domain (fine and gross motor, receptive and expressive language, self-help, academics, and social-emotional), across each age level (spanning the well-visit schedule). Can be administered by parent report or by direct elicitation. Helps comply with AAP policy when used together with PEDS.	Cutoffs tied to performance above and below the 16th percentile for each item and its domain. An assessment level version for NICU follow-up and early intervention, also provides age-equivalent scores and percentage of delay.	Sensitivity (0.75-0.87) and specificity (0.71-0.88) to performance in each domain. Sensitivity (0.70-0.94) and specificity (0.77-0.93) across age levels	

Behavioral/Emotional Screens Relying on Information from Parents

Tool	Age/Time	Description	Scoring	Psychometrics
Ages & Stages Questionnaires: Social-Emotional (ASQ:SE) (2004) Paul H. Brookes, Publishers, P.O. Box 10624, Baltimore, MD 21285; Phone: 1-800-638-3775; http://www.pbrookes.com/ (likely to be online soon) $125.00	6-60 months/ 10-15 minutes	Designed to supplement the ASQ, the ASQ:SE consists of 30 item forms (4-5 pages long) for each of 8 visits between 6 and 60 months. Items focus on self-regulation, compliance, communication, adaptive functioning, autonomy, affect, and interaction with people.	Single cutoff scores when a referral is needed.	Sensitivity ranged from 71%-85%. Specificity from 90% to 98%.
Brief-Infant-Toddler Social-Emotional Assessment (BITSEA) (2005) Harcourt Assessment, Inc., 19500 Bulverde Road, San Antonio, TX 78259; Phone: 1-800-211-8378; www.harcourtassessment.com $99.00	12-36 months/ 5-7 minutes	42 item parent-report measure for identifying social-emotional/behavioral problems and delays in competence. Items were drawn from the assessment level measure, the ITSEA. Written at the 4th-6th grade level. Available in Spanish, French, Dutch, Hebrew.	Cut-points based on child age and sex show presence/absence of problems and competence.	Sensitivity (80%-85%) in detecting children with social-emotional/behavioral problems and specificity 75% to 80%.
Eyberg Child Behavior Inventory/Sutter-Eyberg Student Behavior Inventory. (ECBI/SESBI) (1999) Psychological Assessment Resources, P.O. Box 998, Odessa, FL 33556; Phone: 1-800-331-8378; http://www.parinc.com/ $120.00	2-16 years of age/ 5-9 minutes	The ECBI/SESBI consists of 36-38 short statements of common behavior problems. More than 16 suggests referral for behavioral interventions. Fewer than 16 enables the measure to function as a problems list for planning in-office counseling and selecting handouts. The tools are helpful in monitoring behavioral progress.	Single refer/nonrefer score for externalizing problems—conduct, attention, aggression, etc.	Sensitivity 80%, specificity 86% to disruptive behavior problems.
Ages and Stages Questionnaire (formerly Infant Monitoring System) (2004) Paul H. Brookes Publishing, Inc., PO Box 10624, Baltimore, MD 21285; Phone: 1-800-638-3775; http://www.pbrookes.com/ $190.00	4-60 months/ 10-15 minutes	Parents indicate children's developmental skills on 25-35 items (4-5 pages) using a different form for each well visit. Reading level varies across items from 3rd to 12th grade. Can be used in mass mail-outs for child-find programs. In English, Spanish, French.	Single pass/fail score for developmental status.	Sensitivity ranged from 70% to 90% at all ages except the 4 month level. Specificity ranged from 76% to 91%.

Developmental Screens (Relying on Directly Eliciting Skills from Children)

Tool	Age/Time	Description	Scoring	Psychometrics
Bayley Infant Neurodevelopmental Screen (BINS) (1995) The Psychological Corporation, 555 Academic Court, San Antonio, TX 78204; Phone: 1-800-228-0752; http://www.psychcorp.com $265.00	3-24 months/ 10-15 minutes	Uses 10-13 directly elicited items per 3-6 month age range to assess neurological processes (reflexes and tone); neurodevelopmental skills (movement and symmetry) and developmental accomplishments (object permanence, imitation, and language).	Categorizes via cutscores, performance into low, moderate, or high risk in each domain.	Specificity and sensitivity are 75% to 86% across ages.

TABLE 7B-1 ■ Developmental, Mental Health/Behavioral and Academic Screens—cont'd

Developmental-Behavioral Screens Relying on Information from Parents

Screen	Age Range/ Time Frame	Description	Scoring	Accuracy	Notes
Battelle Developmental Inventory Screening Test-II (BDIST)–2 (2006) Riverside Publishing Company, 8420 Bryn Mawr Avenue, Chicago, IL 60631; Phone: 1-800-323-9540; *www.riversidepublishing.com* $239.00	0-95 months/ 10-30 minutes	Items (20 per domain) use a combination of direct assessment, observation, and parental interview. A high level of examiner skill is required. Well standardized and validated. Scoring software including a PDA application is available. English and Spanish.	Age equivalents and cutoffs at 1.0, 1.5, and 2.0 SDs below the mean in each of 5 domains.	Sensitivity (72% to 93%) to various disabilities; specificity (79% to 88%). Accuracy information across age ranges is not available.	
Brigance Screens-II (2005) Curriculum Associates, Inc., 153 Rangeway Road, N. Billerica, MA 01862; Phone: 1-800-225-0248; *http://www.curriculumassociates.com/* $501.00	0-90 months/ 10-15 minutes	Nine separate forms, one for each 12 month age range. Taps speech-language, motor, readiness, and general knowledge at younger ages and also reading and math at older ages. Uses direct elicitation and observation. In the 0-2 year age range, can be administered by parent report.	Cutoff, quotients, percentiles, age equivalent scores in various domains and overall.	Sensitivity and specificity to giftedness and to developmental and academic problems are 70% to 82% across ages.	
Capute Scales: Cognitive Adaptive Test/Clinical Linguistic Auditory Milestone Scale (CAT/CLAMS) (2005) Paul H. Brookes, Publishers, PO Box 10624, Baltimore, MD 21285; Phone: 1-800-638-3775; *http://www.pbrookes.com/* $350.00	0-36 months/ 6-20 minutes	Measures visual-motor, expressive, and receptive language development. Also available in Spanish and Russian.	Developmental age levels and quotients.	Sensitivity: 0.21-0.67 in low risk population. Sensitivity: 0.05-0.88 in high risk populations. Specificity: 0.95-1.00 in low risk population. Specificity: 0.82-0.98 in high risk populations).	Standardized on a small, nonrepresentative sample. Validated against the Bayley Scales of Infant Development, largely on clinic-referred rather than general pediatric samples.
Denver-II (1992) Developmental Learning Materials, Inc., P.O. Box 371075, Denver, CO 80237-5075; Phone: (800) 419-4729; *www.denverii.com* $90.00	Birth to 6 years of age/ 10-20 minutes	Has four factors: personal-social, language, fine-motor-adaptive, and gross motor. Also available in Spanish. A derivative measure, the Denver Prescreening Questionnaire (PDQ-II), is administered by parental report and used to indicate need to administer the Denver-II. Training videos are available for rent or purchase ($410). Publisher also offers a training institute ($395).	Produces four scores: abnormal, suspect, pass, untestable.	With suspect scores grouped with passing scores: Sensitivity: 56% Specificity: 80% With suspect scores grouped with abnormal scores: Sensitivity: 83% Specificity: 43%	Standardized in Colorado. Not validated by the authors. High reliability suggests grouping suspect with abnormal scores is the better of the two accuracy indices.

Measure	Age/Time	Description	Scoring/Cutoffs	Accuracy	Cost/Comments
Developmental Indicators for the Assessment of Learning (DIAL-III) (1998) American Guidance Service Inc., 4201 Woodland Road, Circle Pines, MN 55014; Phone: (800) 627-7271; *http://www.agsnet.com* $469.00	3-0 to 6-11 years/ 20-30 minutes	Views performance in five domains: motor, concepts, language, self-help, and social. Scoring software is available in both English and Spanish. Has training materials and administration video available as well as parent-education guides. SPEED-DIAL (3 of the 5 subtests) takes 10-20 minutes.	Offers five cutoff options (from 1.0 SDs to 2.0 SDs below the mean) for each domain. Percentiles optional.	Sensitivity/ specificity: 50%-60% (no information on accuracy across age ranges).	Very small sample in accuracy studies with no information on which cutoffs were used.
Early Screening Inventory-Revised (ESI-R) (1993) Pearson Education, One Lake Street, Upper Saddle River, NJ 07458; Phone: 201-236-7000; *http://phcatalog.pearson.com* $237.50	3-0 to 6-0 years/ 15-20 minutes	120 items, tapping performance in three areas: visual-motor, language/cognitive, gross-motor. Onsite training and tapes are available from the publisher.	Cutoffs indicating when to refer or rescreen.	Sensitivity = 92%-93% Specificity = 80% Computed on performance below/above the 6th percentile.	Validation and accuracy indices computed against the 1974 McCarthy Scales (normed on an upper SES sample).
Family Screens					
Family Psychosocial Screening (1996) Kemper KJ, Kelleher KJ: Family psychosocial screening: instruments and techniques. Ambul Child Health 4:325-339, 1996 The measures are included in the article and downloadable at *http://www.pedstest.com*	Screens parents for risk factors	A two-page clinic intake form that identifies psychosocial risk factors including: (1) a four item measure of parental history of physical abuse as a child; (2) a six item measure of parental substance abuse; and (3) a three item measure of maternal depression.	Refer/nonrefer scores for each risk factor. Also has guides to referring and resource lists.		About 15 minutes (if interview needed) Materials ≈$.20 Admin. ≈$4.20 Total ≈$4.40
Academic Screens					
Comprehensive Inventory of Basic Skills-Revised Screener (CIBS-R Screener) (1985) Curriculum Associates, Inc., 153 Rangeway Road, N. Billerica, MA 01862; Phone: 1-800-225-0248; *http://www.curriculumassociates.com* $224.00/	1st-6th grade	Administration involves one or more of three subtests (reading comprehension, math computation, and sentence writing). Timing performance also enables an assessment of information processing skills, especially rate.	Computerized or hand-scoring produces percentiles, quotients, cutoffs.	70% to 80% accuracy across all grades.	Takes 10-15 minutes Materials≈$.53 Admin.≈$10.15 Total ≈ $10.68
Safety Word Inventory and Literacy Screener (SWILS) (2002) Glascoe FP: Clinical Pediatrics. Items courtesy of Curriculum Associates, Inc. The SWILS can be freely downloaded at: *http://www.pedstest.com/*	6-14 years	Children are asked to read 29 common safety words (e.g., High Voltage, Wait, Poison) aloud. The number of correctly read words is compared to a cutoff score. Results predict performance in math, written language, and a range of reading skills. Test content may serve as a springboard to injury prevention counseling.	Single cutoff score indicating the need for a referral.	78% to 84% sensitivity and specificity across all ages.	About 7 minutes (if interview needed) Materials ≈$.30 Admin. ≈$2.38 Total ≈$2.68

TABLE 7B-1 ■ Developmental, Mental Health/Behavioral and Academic Screens—cont'd

Screen	Age Range/Time Frame	Developmental-Behavioral Screens Relying on Information from Parents			
		Description	Scoring	Accuracy	Notes
Narrow-Band Screens for Autism and ADHD					
Connors Rating Scale-Revised (CRS-R) (1997) Multi-Health Systems, Inc., P.O. Box 950, North Tonawanda, NY 14120-0950; Phone: 1-800-456-3003 or 1-416-492-2627; Fax: 1-888-540-4484 or 1-416-492-3343; http://www.mhs.com/ $193.00	3 to 17 years	Although the CRS-R can screen for a range of problems, several subscales specific to ADHD are included: DSM-IV symptom subscales (Inattentive, Hyperactive/Impulsive, and Total); Global Indices (GI) (Restless-Impulsive, Emotional Lability, and Total), and an ADHD Index. The GI is useful for treatment monitoring. Also available in French.	Cutoff tied to the 93rd percentile for each factor.	Sensitivity: 78% to 92% Specificity: 84% to 94%	About 20 minutes Materials ≈$.2.25 Admin. ≈$20.15 Total ≈$22.40
Modified Checklist for Autism in Toddlers (M-CHAT) (1997) Free download at the First Signs Web site: http://www.firstsigns.org/downloads/m-chat.PDF ($0.00) Online for parents and EMRS at www.forepath.org ($1.00)	18-60 months	Parent report of 23 questions modified for American usage at 4th-6th grade reading level. Available in English and Spanish. Uses telephone follow-up for concerns. The M-CHAT is copyrighted but remains free for use on the First Signs Web site.	Cutoff based on 2 of 3 critical items or any 3 from checklist.	Initial study shows sensitivity at 90%; specificity at 99%. Future studies are needed for a full picture. Promising tool.	About 5 minutes Print Materials ≈$.10 Admin. ≈$.88 Total ≈$.98

Compiled by Frances Page Glascoe, PhD, Adjunct Professor of Pediatrics (Frances.P.Glascoe@Vanderbilt.edu). Copyright 2006, Glascoe FP: Collaborating with Parents. Nashville: Ellsworth & Vandermeer, 2006.

Numerous broad-band screening measures (meaning that multiple domains are measured) are listed. Several narrow-band tools essential for primary care (e.g., for ADHD and autism spectrum disorder) are listed at the end. The left column provides publication information and the cost of purchasing a specimen set. The "Description" column offers information on what the instrument measures, what factor or subtests are included, and administration methods. The "Scoring" column shows how scores were produced. The "Accuracy" column shows the percentage of patients with and without problems identified correctly. Ideally, sensitivity should be at least 70%, meaning that the majority of children with disabilities are correctly detected in a one-time administration. Specificity, correct detection of children without disabilities, should also be at least 70%. All measures, except where noted (see "Notes" column), were developed on nationally representative samples (meaning a group with geographic and sociodemographic characteristics proportional to those found in the U.S. Census, including correct proportions of children with disabilities), have high levels of reliability (interrater, test-retest, internal consistency), and have been validated against a range of criterion measures in general pediatric samples (because broadband screens must prove that they have validity across a range of developmental domains and because calculation of sensitivity and specificity on referred populations is likely to be inflated).

AAP, American Academy of Pediatrics; ADHD, attention-deficit/hyperactivity disorder; DSM-IV, Diagnostic and Statistical Manual of Mental Disorders, Fourth Edition (American Psychiatric Association, 1994); NICU, neonatal intensive care unit; PDA, personal digital assistant; SD, standard deviation.

criteria (see Chapter 7A), and having both sensitivity and specificity of at least 70% to 80%. Two types of tools are presented: those relying on information from parents and those requiring direct elicitation of children's skills. The latter are useful in practices with staff (e.g., nurses, pediatric nurse practitioners) who have the time and skill to administer relatively detailed screens. Such measures are also useful in early intervention programs. Information is included on purchasing, cost, time to administer, scores produced, and age ranges of the children tested.

COMBINING SCREENING AND SURVEILLANCE

We now present an algorithm for combining surveillance and screening into an effective, evidence-based process for detecting and addressing developmental and behavioral issues. The American Academy of Pediatrics recently revised its policy statement on early detection.[8] We include the elements of the statement, as follows.

1. Review the patient's chart for medical risk factors. Take note of such potentially teratogenic exposures as radiation or medications, infectious illnesses, fever, addictive substances, and trauma, and review results of neonatal screens, including phenylketonuria, hypothyroidism, and other metabolic conditions. Also consider the perinatal history, including birth weight, gestational age, Apgar scores, and any medical complications. In addition, postnatal medical factors to be considered include chronic respiratory or allergic illness, recurrent otitis, head trauma, and sleep problems, including symptoms of obstructive sleep apnea.

2. Identify psychosocial risk factors. Common risk factors for developmental and behavioral problems include parents with less than a high school education, parental mental health or substance abuse problems, four or more children in the home, single-parent family, poverty, frequent household moves, limited social support, parental history of abuse as a child, and ethnic minority status. Four or more risk factors are associated with developmental performance that is well below average, which, in turn, has an adverse effect on future success in school.[24] The presence of multiple risk factors suggests the need for enrichment or remedial programs, regardless of screening results. Examples include Head Start, after-school tutoring, parenting training, social work services, mentoring, quality child care, and summer school. A measure such as the Family Psychosocial Screen (available at *www.pedstest.com*) is often helpful for identifying psychosocial risk factors and can be used as a standard intake form for new patients.

3. Elicit parents' concerns and observations. Careful attention to wording is essential. Although facilitating conversations with parents can be informally accomplished, several helpful sources suggest well-worded questions. For example, *Bright Futures* contains useful trigger questions. A parent-completed measure, the Parents' Evaluation of Developmental Status questionnaire (see Table 7B-1), has empirically tested wording and weighs the types of concerns parents raise, assigns levels of risk, and identifies optimal responses to concerns.

4. Conduct a physical examination. Examination should include attention to growth parameters, head shape and circumference, facial and other body dysmorphology, eye findings (e.g., cataracts in various inborn errors of metabolism), vascular markings, and signs of neurocutaneous disorders (e.g., café-au-lait spots in neurofibromatosis, hypopigmented macules in tuberous sclerosis). Vision and hearing screening are essential.

5. Administer/score developmental screening tests. Use of parent report measures, completed before the visit or in the waiting/examination room, reduces the amount of time needed for screening. Positive results may be followed by additional screening of social-emotional functioning (e.g., Ages & Stages Questionnaires: Social-Emotional and the Modified Checklist for Autism in Toddlers; see Table 7B-1) to better identify the areas of delay and types of services needed. Note that the AAP's new statement recommends use of an autism specific screen like the M-CHAT at both 18 and 24 months, regardless of performance on broad-band tools like PEDS or the ASQ.

6. Provide additional medical screens when developmental-behavioral screens are positive. When indicated, common health-related causes for delays and disorders should include screens for iron deficiency and lead toxicity. Unless suggested by parental report (e.g., seizure activity) or clinical findings (e.g., microcephaly, expanding head circumference), neurophysiological (e.g., electroencephalogram) and neuroimaging (e.g., computed tomographic scan, magnetic resonance imaging) studies are not routinely indicated. Developmental delay may suggest the need for metabolic screening for ammonia, organic, and amino acids (or referral for such screens). A progressive loss of milestones suggests the possible need to screen for human immunodeficiency virus (HIV).

7. Explain results to parents. When parents' concerns have been elicited, the process of explaining findings can begin with a simple affirmation of parents' observations. It is important to present results in

person and to maintain a positive outlook about available services and their potential to improve outcome. Because screening/surveillance activities are not diagnostic in nature, the clinician should avoid diagnostic labels in favor of euphemisms, such as "developmental delay," "behind other children," and "having difficulties with. . . ." When a parent reports conflicting perceptions within the family about the possibility of problems, the clinician should offer to explain findings to other family members. Asking parents whether they know other families with children who have developmental-behavioral differences may be helpful in clarifying discussions.

8. If indicated, make referrals for subspecialty medical services. When medical factors are identified, an appropriate response is referral for further evaluation.

9. Seek nonmedical interventions. Nonmedical interventions need not await a complete diagnosis. All children with apparent delays or disorders should be referred promptly to appropriate programs and services. Public programs, including those mandated by such legislation as the IDEA, should be available through community-based agencies or the public schools without cost to the family and generally provide a range of high-quality therapies and evaluations, including speech-language, physical, and occupational therapy; assistive technology evaluations; and behavioral interventions. Most IDEA programs do not provide a detailed diagnosis but rather define functional skills and deficits. As a consequence, a referral may also need to be made to a multidisciplinary diagnostic service. Because such centers typically have long waiting lists and because a final diagnosis is not necessary for initiating intervention, it is best to make such referrals concurrent with a referral to an IDEA program. Other services should be sought (e.g., Head Start, after school tutoring, quality daycare, parent training) for children with psychosocial risk factors who do not fulfill specific eligibility requirements for early intervention or special education. Referral letters to programs and services should include suggestions for the types of evaluations needed (e.g., speech-language therapy, occupational and physical therapy, social-emotional assessment, intelligence testing, academics). Programs offered through IDEA often require documentation of hearing and vision status. Some programs require the completion of specific referral forms. Parental consent should be obtained for sharing information, including copies of subsequent evaluations.

10. Offer developmental promotion. Regardless of whether a child has developmental problems, parents need advice and encouragement on promoting optimal development, particularly in domains associated with school success: language, academic/preacademic skills, and cognition. Clinicians may provide patient education materials, lists of informative and factual Web sites, lists of parent training services, and contacts for social support programs. Group discussions for parents on developmental topics are another potential strategy but require careful planning and organization. Developmental promotion is assisted by a well-organized system for filing and retrieving parent-focused materials (see *www.dbpeds.org* for materials and links).

11. Establish a medical home. For children with developmental-behavioral problems and/or complex health care needs, primary care contact and perspectives are of critical importance to promote optimal health and development. The American Academy of Pediatrics National Center of Medical Home Initiatives for Children with Special Needs *(www.medicalhomeinfo.org)* provides an essential guide for organizing practices to ensure continuity of care, manage multiple referrals and comprehensive records, coordinate appointments, and communicate with various providers.

SYSTEMWIDE APPROACHES TO SURVEILLANCE AND SCREENING

State wide and countywide efforts to enhance collaboration among medical and nonmedical providers offer some of the most promising evidence for the effectiveness of surveillance and screening. Documented outcomes include large increases in screening rates during EPSDT visits;[25] a fourfold increase in early intervention enrollment, resulting in a match between the prevalence of disabilities and receipt of services[26]; a 75% increase in identification of children from birth to age 3 with autism spectrum disorder[27]; improvement in reimbursement for screening[28]; and, interestingly, increased attendance at well-child visits when parents' concerns are elicited and addressed.[25]

Among the numerous initiatives—national, international, and regional—we selected a few to highlight because they employed varied models and gathered outcome data to support their successes (and challenges).

The Assuring Better Child Health and Development (ABCD) Program

Created by The Commonwealth Fund, the ABCD Program has identified policy strategies for state Medicaid agencies to strengthen the delivery and financing of early childhood services for low-income families. The emphasis is on assisting participating states in developing care models that promote healthy development, including the mental development of young children. Models include developmental screening, referral, service coordination, and educational materials and resources for families and clinical providers. The program has resulted in improvements in screening, surveillance, and assessment. Most notably, work in North Carolina facilitated a 75% increase in screening, increased enrollment rates in early intervention from 2.6% to 8% (in line with the Centers for Disease Control and Prevention's prevalence projections), while simultaneously lowering referral age[26] *(http://www.nashp.org; http://www.cdc.gov/ncbdd/child/interventions.htm).*

Help Me Grow

A program of the Connecticut Children's Trust Fund, Help Me Grow links children and families to community programs and services by using a comprehensive statewide network. Components of the program include the training of child health providers in effective developmental surveillance; the creation of a triage, referral, and case management system that facilitates access for children and families to services through Child Development Infoline; the development and maintenance of a computerized inventory of regional services that address developmental and behavioral needs of children and their families; and data gathering to systematically document capacity issues and gaps in services. The program has increased identification rates of at-risk children by child health providers and increased referral rates of such children to programs and services. For example, chart reviews conducted in participating practices noted an increase in documented developmental or behavioral concerns from 9% before training to 18% after training. Furthermore, training resulted in significant differences in referral rates for certain conditions. Behavioral conditions were involved in 4% of referrals from trained practices, in comparison with 1% from untrained practices. Four percent of referrals from trained practices were for parental support and guidance, in comparison with fewer than 1% from untrained practices[29] *(http://www.infoline.org/Programs/helpmegrow.asp).*

Promoting Resources in Developmental Education (PRIDE)

This program is a 3-year project funded by the Duke Endowment through a partnership of the Children's Hospital, the Center for Developmental Services (a colocation of agencies serving children with developmental disorders), the regional office of the state's early intervention system (BabyNet), the local school district's Childfind and Parents-as-Teachers programs, and a parent-to-parent mentoring program for parents of children with special health care needs. The goal of PRIDE is earlier identification and intervention for children in Greenville County, South Carolina with developmental delays and improved support for their parents.

The program has targeted key players in the lives of infants and toddlers as follows: *Parents* sign up around the time of their child's birth to receive milestone cards every 3 to 6 months during the first 3 years that describe the key developmental attainments, activities to promote development at that age, and red flags for potential developmental problems. Parents are instructed to discuss any concerns with their physician. *Primary care physicians* are provided with information and tools (the Parents Evaluation of Developmental Status questionnaire) to improve their system of developmental screening. A nurse practitioner employed by PRIDE as the "physician office liaison" works closely with practices, initially by setting up lunch meetings with physicians and staff that are also attended by the PRIDE developmental-behavioral pediatrician. With the agreement of the physicians, the liaison then assists the office staff in implementing the system and provides a "Resource Guide" with information on local developmental services and forms to facilitate referrals. *Child care providers* have the opportunity to attend educational sessions (for credit hours) in which they learn about child development, signs of developmental problems, and services that are available for these children. The training sessions are provided in collaboration with local programs that promote higher quality child care and early education (Success By 6 and First Steps), and the attendees receive "toolkits" with information on the topics discussed. Initial results of the program indicate success; 16 of 17 local pediatric practices (which previously had no standardized system of developmental screening) now utilize the Parents Evaluation of Developmental Status questionnaire. Over the first 18 months of the program, referrals to early intervention have increased almost 100% and referrals to the school's Childfind program by 30%. Other service providers have seen increases in new referrals of up to 30%. The average age at referral to early intervention has also dropped slightly.

Not surprisingly, increasing rates of referral raised the likelihood of even longer waiting lists for tertiary-level developmental-behavioral pediatric evaluations. To address this challenge, the PRIDE staff sought funding from The Commonwealth Fund to study the feasibility and cost effectiveness of a model of "mid-level" developmental-behavioral pediatrics assessment (as a step between telephone triage/record review and comprehensive diagnostic evaluation) for children younger than 6 years.[30]

First Signs

This national and international training effort is devoted to early detection of children with disabilities, with a particular focus on autism spectrum disorders. This detection is accomplished through a mix of print materials and broadcast press, direct mail, public service announcements, presentations (to medical and nonmedical professionals), a richly informative website *(www.firstsigns.org)*, and detailed program evaluation. Although First Signs initiatives have been conducted in several states, including New Jersey, Alabama, Delaware, and Pennsylvania, the Minnesota campaign is highlighted here because of that state's assistance in program evaluation. Minnesota is divided into discrete service regions. Centralized train-the-trainers forums were conducted to prepare 130 professionals as outreach trainers. These individuals were from all regions of the state, and most were early interventionists, family therapists, and other nonmedical service providers. They then provided more than 165 workshops to 686 medical providers, to whom they offered individualized training tailored for health care clinics, as well as training for more than 3000 early childhood specialists. First Signs Screening Kits (which include video, information about and in some cases copies of appropriate screening tools, wall charts and parent handouts on warning signs) were distributed to more than 900 practitioners and clinics. In addition, public service announcements were aired across the state in collaboration with the Autism Society of Minnesota. Within 12 months, there was a 75% increase in the number of young children identified in the 0- to 2-year age group and an overall increase of 23% in detection of autism spectrum disorders among all children aged 0 to 21 years in that same period. The state has now expanded the initiative to include childcare providers and is educating them about red flags and warning signs. In addition, physicians with the Minnesota Chapter of the American Academy of Pediatrics Committee for Children with Disabilities have begun incorporating First Signs information into physician training program at the University of Minnesota.[27]

Blue Cross/Blue Shield of Tennessee

Blue Cross/Blue Shield of Tennessee requested that child health providers use standardized, validated screening at all EPSDT visits. To facilitate compliance, Blue Cross/Blue Shield of Tennessee piloted a program in 34 high-volume, Medicaid-managed care practices. Outreach nurses, called *regional clinical network analysts*, trained providers on site how to administer, score, interpret, and submit reimbursement for the Parents' Evaluation of Developmental Status

questionnaire (the standardized developmental-behavioral surveillance and screening instrument that elicits parents' concerns about their children). After training, screening rates increased from 0% to 43.5% during the pilot phase. At the same time, the practices experienced a 16% increase in attendance at scheduled well-child visits, which suggests that focusing on parents' concerns may increase their adherence to visit schedules. Blue Cross/Blue Shield of Tennessee, together with the Tennessee Chapter of the American Academy of Pediatrics, is now providing training across the state.[25] More information can be found through the Center for Health Care Strategies, "Best Clinical and Administrative Practices for State-wide" developmental and behavioral screening initiatives as established by the Center for Health Care Strategies [http://www.chcs.org/]

Healthy Steps for Young Children

This a national initiative improves traditional pediatric care with the assistance of an in-office child development specialist, whose duties include expanded discussions of preventive issues during well-child and home visits, staffing a telephone information line, disseminating patient education materials, and networking with community resources and parent support groups. Now in its 12th year, Healthy Steps followed its original cohort of 3737 intervention and comparison families from 15 pediatric practices in varied settings. In comparison with controls, Healthy Steps families received significantly more preventive and developmental services, were less likely to be dissatisfied with their pediatric primary care, and had improved parenting skills in many areas, including adherence to health visits, nutritional practices, developmental stimulation, appropriate disciplinary techniques, and correct sleeping position. In practices serving families with incomes below $20,000, use of telephone information lines increased from 37% before the intervention to 87% after; office visits with someone who teaches parents about child development increased from 39% to 88%; and home visits increased from 30% to 92%. Low-income families receiving Healthy Steps services were as likely as high-income parents to adhere to age-appropriate well-child visits at 1, 2, 4, 12, 18, and 24 months.[31,32] One program evaluation suggests that Healthy Steps offers a benefit comparable with that of Head Start at about one-tenth the cost,[33] although this claim is somewhat premature because Head Start data now extend to more than 35 years of follow-up research with a proven return rate of $17.00 for each $1.00 spent on early intervention, with savings realized through reductions in teen pregnancy, increases in high school graduation and employment rates, and decreased adjudication and violent crime.[7] Nevertheless, Healthy Steps is extremely promising and inexpensive and includes a strong evaluation component that will answer questions about its long-term effect.

CONCLUSION

In summary, both expert opinion and research evidence support surveillance and screening as the optimal clinical practice for monitoring children's development and behavior, promoting optimal development, and effectively identifying children at risk for delays. The effectiveness of surveillance is enhanced by incorporating valid measures of parents' appraisals and descriptions of children's development and behavior and skilled professional observations. Developmental monitoring should combine surveillance at all health supervision visits with the periodic use of evidence-based screening tools, including parent-completed questionnaires and professionally administered tests.

To be effective, identification must lead to intervention through referral to appropriate programs and services. Surveillance and screening activities must ensure access to medical evaluations, developmental assessments, and intervention programs. Ultimately, collaboration among health care providers, parents, and early intervention and other social service providers is crucial for effectively addressing the challenges of detection and timely enrollment in early intervention programs and services.

Establishing effective surveillance and screening in primary care is nevertheless challenging.[13] Effective initiatives consistently offer training to providers, office staff, and nonmedical professionals. Implementation details are numerous (e.g., incorporation into existing office workflow, ordering and managing screening materials, gathering and organizing lists of referral resources and patient education handouts, identifying measures that work well with available personnel, and determining how best to communicate with nonmedical providers).[18,18a,26,34] Ultimately, helping health care providers recognize the need to adopt effective detection methods is the critical first step.

DIRECTIONS FOR FURTHER RESEARCH

Although much is known about the accuracy of screening tools, studies are needed to determine their accuracy when used repeatedly (given that screening

measures both overrefer and underrefer to some extent). Other rich topics of inquiry include the following: How do surveillance methods enhance development and early detection, and which specific techniques most enhance decision making? Does improved reimbursement have a positive effect on provider behavior? How can surveillance and screening be incorporated into electronic health records? In the absence of regional and state initiatives, can primary care professionals engage in effective self-study and thus positive practice change? What teaching methods and content best help residents master efficient surveillance and screening techniques that work well in primary care? Perhaps the most critical area in need of further inquiry is determining the longitudinal outcomes of families and children when surveillance and screening are used together.

REFERENCES

1. Haggerty RJ, Roughman KJ, Pless IB: Child Health and the Community. New York: Wiley, 1975.
2. Dobos AE, Dworkin PH, Bernstein BA: Pediatricians' approaches to developmental problems: Has the gap been narrowed? J Dev Behav Pediatr 15:34-38, 1994.
3. Institute of Medicine: From Neurons to Neighborhoods: The Science of Early Childhood Development. Washington, DC: National Academies Press, 2000.
4. Blumberg SJ, Halfon N, Olson LM: The national survey of early childhood health. Pediatrics 113:1899-1906, 2004.
5. Young KT, Davis K, Schoen C, et al: Listening to parents. A national survey of parents with young children. Arch Pediatr Adolesc Med 152:255-262, 1998.
6. Shonkoff JP, Hauser-Cram P: Early intervention for disabled infants and their families: a quantitative analysis. Pediatrics 80:650-658, 1987.
7. Shonkoff JP, Meisels SJ: Handbook of Early Childhood Intervention, 2nd ed. New York: Cambridge University Press, 2000.
8. American Academy of Pediatrics, Council on Children with Disabilities: Identifying infants and young children with developmental disorders in the medical home: An algorithm for developmental surveillance and screening. Pediatrics 118:403-420, 2006.
9. Green M, Palfrey JS, eds: Bright Futures: Guidelines for Health Supervision of Infants, Children, and Adolescents, 2nd ed. Arlington, VA: National Center for Education in Maternal and Child Health, 2002.
10. American Academy of Pediatrics, Medical Home Initiatives for Children with Special Needs Project Advisory Committee: The medical home. Pediatrics 110:184-186, 2002.
11. Halfon N, Regalado M, Sareen H, et al: Assessing development in the pediatric office. Pediatrics 113:1926-1933, 2004.
12. Bethell C, Reuland CHP, Halfon N, et al: Measuring the quality of preventive and developmental services for

young children: National estimates and patterns of clinicians' performance. Pediatrics 113:1973-1983, 2004.

13. Silverstein M, Sand N, Glascoe FP, et al: Pediatricians' reported practices regarding developmental screening: Do guidelines work? And do they help? Pediatrics 116:174-179, 2005.

14. Inkelas M, Glascoe FP, Regalado M, et al: National Patterns and Disparities in Parent Concerns about Child Development. Paper presented at the annual meeting of the Pediatric Academic Societies, Baltimore, 2002.

15. Glascoe FP, Dworkin PH. The role of parents in the detection of developmental and behavioral problems. Pediatrics 95:829-836, 1995.

16. Regalado M, Halfon N: Primary care services promoting optimal child development from birth to age 3 years: review of the literature. Arch Pediatr Adolesc Med 12:1311-1322, 2001.

17. Dworkin PH: British and American recommendations for developmental monitoring: The role of surveillance. Pediatrics 84:1000-1010, 1989.

18. Glascoe FP: Collaborating with Parents: Using Parents' Evaluations of Developmental Status to Detect and Address Developmental and Behavioral Problems. Nashville: Ellsworth & Vandermeer, 1998.

18a. Houston HL, Davis RH: Opportunistic surveillance of child development in primary care: is it feasible? (Comparative Study Journal Article) J R Coll Gen Pract 35(271):77-79, 1985.

19. Glascoe FP: Toward a model for an evidenced-based approach to developmental/behavioral surveillance, promotion and patient education. Ambul Child Health 5:197-208, 1999.

20. Rydz D, Shevell MI, Majnemer A, et al: Developmental screening. Child Neurol 20:4-21, 2005.

21. Glascoe FP: Do parents' discuss concerns about children's development with health care providers? Ambul Child Health 2:349-356, 1997.

22. Glascoe FP, Sandler H: The value of parents' age estimates of children's development. J Pediatr 127:831-835, 1995.

23. Pachter LM, Dworkin PH: Maternal expectations about normal child development in four cultural groups. Arch Pediatr Adolesc Med 151:1144-1150, 1997.

24. Glascoe FP: Are over-referrals on developmental screening tests really a problem? Arch Pediatr Adolesc Med 155:54-59, 2001.

25. Smith PK: BCAP Toolkit: Enhancing Child Development Services in Medicaid Managed Care. Center for Health Care Strategies, 2005. (Available at: http://www.chcs.org/; accessed 10/13/06.)

26. Pinto-Martin J, Dunkle M, Earls M, et al: Developmental stages of developmental screening: Steps to implementation of a successful program . Am J Public Health 95:6-10, 2005.

27. Glascoe FP, Sievers P, Wiseman N: First Signs Model Program makes great strides in early detection in Minnesota: Clinicians and educators play major role in increased screenings. American Academy of Pediatrics' Section on Developmental and Behavioral Pediatrics Newsletter. August, 2004. (Available at: www.dbpeds.org; accessed 10/13/06.)

28. Inkelas M, Regalado H, Halfon N: Strategies for integrating developmental services and promoting medical homes. National Center for Infant and Early Childhood Health Policy, 2005. (Available at: http://www.healthychild.ucla.edu; accessed 10/13/06.)

29. McKay K: Evaluating model programs to support dissemination. An evaluation of strengthening the developmental surveillance and referral practices of child health providers. J Dev Behav Pediatr 27(1 Suppl):S26-S29, 2006.

30. Kelly D: PRIDE. American Academy of Pediatrics' Section on Developmental and Behavioral Pediatrics Newsletter. March, 2006 (Available at: www.dbpeds.org; accessed 10/13/06.)

31. McLearn KT, Strobino DM, Hughart N, et al: Narrowing the income gaps in preventive care for young children: Families in Healthy Steps. J Urban Health 81:206-221, 2004.

32. McLearn KT, Strobino DM, Minkovitz CS, et al: Developmental services in primary care for low-income children: Clinicians' perceptions of the Healthy Steps for Young Children Program. J Urban Health 81:556-567, 2004.

33. Zuckerman B, Parker S, Kaplan-Sanoff M, et al: Healthy Steps: A case study of innovation in pediatric practice. Pediatrics 114:820-826, 2004.

34. Hampshire A, Blair M, Crown N, et al: Assessing the quality of child health surveillance in primary care. A pilot study in one health district. Child Health Care Dev 28:239-249, 2002.

7C.
Assessment of Development and Behavior

TERRY STANCIN ■ GLEN P. AYLWARD

"Assessment is a means to an end, not an end in itself.
—Jerome M. Sattler, 2001

Assessment of child development and behavior involves a process in which information is gathered about a child so that judgments can be made. This process generally includes a multistage approach, designed to gain sufficient understanding of a child so that informed decisions can be made.[1] In contrast to psychological testing (which includes the administration of tests), assessment is the process in which data from clinical sources and tools (including history, interviews, observations, formal and informal tests), preferably obtained from multiple perspectives, are interpreted and integrated into relevant clinical decisions.

Developmental and behavioral assessments may be conducted for several purposes.[1,2] *Screening* involves procedures to identify children who are at risk for a particular problem and for whom there are available effective interventions. *Diagnosis and case formulation* procedures help determine the nature, severity, and causes of presenting concerns and often result in classification or a label. *Prognosis and prediction* methods result in generating recommendations for possible outcomes. *Treatment design and planning* assessment strategies aid in selecting and implementing interventions to address concerns. *Treatment monitoring* methods track changes in symptoms and functioning targeted by interventions. Finally, *treatment evaluation* procedures help investigators examine consumer satisfaction and the effectiveness of interventions.

The purpose of this chapter is to describe methods and tools for assessing children's development and behavior. In accordance with current discussions within the child psychology literature,[2] we advocate the development of integrated evidence-based assessment strategies for childhood problems with emphasis placed on research concerning the reliability, validity, and clinical utility of commonly used measures in assessment and treatment planning of developmental and behavioral problems (i.e., what methods have been shown to be useful and valid for what purpose). We describe general information about clinical interviewing and observational methods required to conduct comprehensive child assessments (for more extensive discussions, see McConaughy[3]). To help guide the pediatric practitioner's and researcher's appropriate use of assessment results, we provide information on the range of methods used for assessing developmental abilities, intelligence and cognitive abilities, behavioral and emotional functioning, and specialized testing, including neuropsychological

testing and measures of functional outcome. However, we do not attempt to address the complex manner in which information, obtained from different assessment data sources, is weighted and synthesized in the formulation of clinical judgments. The discussions of assessment tools is not meant to be all-inclusive—there are literally thousands of developmental and behavioral assessment measures in the literature—nor an endorsement of one instrument over others. Rather, it is a sampling the array of instruments available to clinicians and researchers (Table 7C-1). We present implications and recommendations for future research concerning measures of psychological assessment as they pertain to the field of developmental behavioral pediatrics.

CASE ILLUSTRATIONS

The following case examples are referred to throughout the discussion of assessment methods:

- Case 1: Jane is a 21-month-old (corrected age) girl who was born at 27 weeks' gestation, with a birth weight of 850 g, having a grade III intraventricular hemorrhage, bronchopulmonary dysplasia, and hyperbilirubinemia. Her young, single mother resides in low-income housing and may have used cocaine during pregnancy. Her score on the revised Bayley Scales of Infant Development (BSID-II) Mental Developmental Index (MDI) was 90 at age 12 months (corrected age). Her developmental status is being evaluated at a high-risk infant follow-up clinic at this time to determine need for early intervention services.
- Case 2: Rachel is a 15-year-old girl with mild cerebral palsy with no identified learning disorders who

TABLE 7C-1 ■ Illustrative Behavioral and Developmental Assessment Methods		
Method	**Applications**	**Illustrative Methods**
Structured/semistructured interviews	Diagnostic assessments	Diagnostic Interview for Children–IV (DISC-IV)[8]
		Diagnostic Interview for Children and Adolescents (DICA-IV)[9]
	Assessment and treatment planning	Comprehensive Assessment to Intervention System (CAIS)[7]
		Child and Adolescent Psychiatric Assessment (CAPA)[12]
		Semistructured Parent Interview (SPI)[3]
		Semistructured Clinical Interview for Children and Adolescents (SCICA)[10]
Standardized cognitive methods	Developmental assessments	Manual of Developmental Diagnosis[32]
		Cattell Infant Intelligence Scale[31]
		Bayley Scales of Infant and Toddler Development–Third Edition (BSID-III)[27]
		Battelle Developmental Inventory–Second Edition (BDI-2)[39]
		Mullen Scales of Early Learning (MSEL)[41]
		Differential Ability Scales (DAS)[43]
		McCarthy Scales of Children's Abilities (MSCA)[44]

TABLE 7C-1 ■ Illustrative Behavioral and Developmental Assessment Methods—cont'd

Method	Applications	Illustrative Methods
	Intelligence assessment	Kaufman Brief Intelligence Test, Second Edition (KBIT-2)[45] Stanford-Binet Intelligence Scale–Fifth Edition[26] Stanford-Binet Intelligence Scales for Early Childhood–5 (SB-5)[46] Kaufman Assessment Battery for Children–Second Edition (KABC-II)[47] Wechsler Preschool and Primary Scale of Intelligence–Third Edition (WPPSI-III)[48] Wechsler Intelligence Scale for Children–Fourth Edition (WISC-IV)[49] Wechsler Abbreviated Scale of Intelligence (WASI)[50]
	Achievement	Kaufman Test of Educational Achievement-II (KTEA-II)[52] Peabody Individual Achievement Test–Revised (PIAT-R)[53] Peabody Individual Achievement Test–Normative Update[54] Wechsler Individual Achievement Test-II (WIAT-II)[55] Wide Range Achievement Test–3 (WRAT-3)[56] Woodcock-Johnson III Tests of Achievement (WJ III)[58]
	Neuropsychological assessments	Children's Memory Scale (CMS)[60] NEPSY—A Developmental Neuropsychological Assessment (NEPSY)[61] Behavior Rating Inventory of Executive Function (BRIEF)[62] Wide Range Assessment of Memory and Learning (WRAML; 2nd edition: WRAML-2)[63,64]
Global behavior rating scales	Broad measures of pathology	Achenbach System of Empirically Based Assessment (ASEBA)[11,67-71] Caregiver completed: Child Behavior Checklist (CBCL/$1^1/_2$-5, CBCL/6-18) Teacher Report Form Youth Self-Report Form Behavior Assessment System for Children–Second Edition (BASC-2)[75] Parent Rating Scales Teacher Rating Scales Self-Report of Personality Infant-Toddler Social-Emotional Assessment Scale (ITSEA)[76] Minnesota Multiphasic Personality Inventory–Adolescent (MMPI-A)[78]
Peer reports	Broad measure of pathology	Peer-Report Measure of Internalizing and Externalizing Behavior (PMIEB)[81]
Observational coding methods	Assessment of parent child interactions	Dyadic Parent-Child Interaction Coding System (DPICS)[83]
Problem-specific questionnaires and rating scales	Depression	Children's Depression Inventory (CDI)[87] Mood and Feeling Questionnaire (MFQ)[88] Reynolds Child Depression Scale (RCDS)[89] Reynolds Adolescent Depression Scale (RADS)[90] Children's Depression Rating Scale Revised (CDRS-R)[91] Preschool Feelings Checklist[92]
	Anxiety	Multidimensional Anxiety Scale for Children (MASC)[94] Social Phobia and Anxiety Inventory for Children (SPAI-C)[95] Social Anxiety Scale for Children (SAS-C)[96] and Social Anxiety Scale for Adolescents (SAS-A)[97] Revised Children's Manifest Anxiety Scale (RCMAS)[98]
	Attention-deficit/hyperactivity disorder (ADHD)	ADHD Rating Scale-IV[99] Vanderbilt ADHD Diagnostic Parent Rating Scales[100]
	Autism spectrum disorders	Autism Diagnostic Interview-Revised (ADI-R)[106] Autism Diagnostic Observation Schedule (ADOS)[107] Social Communication Questionnaire (SCQ)[108] Childhood Autism Rating Scale (CARS)[110]
Family assessment methods	Parent and family assessment	Parenting Stress Index (PSI) 3rd ed[113]
Functional outcome methods	Global functioning	Children's Global Assessment Scale (CGAS)[115] Child and Adolescent Functional Assessment Scale (CAFAS)[116]
	Adaptive behavior	Vineland Adaptive Behavior Scales (Vineland-II)[117]
	Health-related quality of life	PedsQL 4.0[118]

presents with depressed mood and falling grades in her ninth grade placement. Academic strengths have been language arts, but she has always been weak in math. Historically she has been a B and C student, but in her freshman year, she is in danger of failing math. Rachel complains about trouble getting work done this year, especially in algebra. Her mother is puzzled that Rachel has requested counseling.

■ Case 3: Jose is a 9-year-old third grader referred to the Developmental-Behavioral Pediatrics Clinic because of the following problems: poor academic performance, disruptive behavior, and trouble getting along with peers. His first language is Spanish, but he is considered fluent in English. He was born in Puerto Rico, and his parents do not speak or read English. A note from his teacher indicates concerns that Jose has a short attention span and fails to complete many assignments.

"WHAT MEASURE SHOULD I USE?"

Kazdin[4] noted that in clinical situations, this question suggests a misunderstanding of the assessment process, because it is unlikely that any one measure or method can suitably capture child functioning. Although some measures have been shown to be perform better than others, a single "gold standard" tool does not exist for assessing most aspects of children's functioning. Valid child assessment often requires data from multiple sources, including interviews, direct observations, standardized parents' and teachers' rating scales, self-reports, background questionnaires, and standardized tests. Multiple methods are needed not only to evaluate different facets of problems but also because of the high rate of comorbidity in children with developmental and behavioral conditions. In clinical settings, methods should be tailored to address the specific referral questions and assessment goals; therefore, preordained "assessment batteries" should be avoided. Moreover, clinical assessments often have multiple goals, such both diagnosis and treatment planning. Diagnostic methods, shown to be evidenced-based (e.g., structured diagnostic interviews or rating scales), are often not helpful in treatment planning, whereas a functional analysis of impairment (i.e., identification of environmental contexts and socially valid target behaviors) are more useful.[5] Different methods of data collection yield different information, and one is not inherently better than the other; each method contributes unique elements. Moreover, assessments must adopt a framework that maintains a correct developmental perspective, including use of methods and procedures that fit a child's developmental stage.

INTERVIEWS

Clinical assessment interviews are face-to-face interactions with bidirectional influence for the purpose of planning, implementing, or evaluating treatment.[3] The interview is a fundamental technique for gathering assessment data for clinical purposes and is considered by many clinicians to be an essential component. Interviews provide respondents the opportunity to offer personal reflections of concerns and historical events. Thoughts, feelings, and other private experiences are conveyed in conversation that is not readily obtainable in any other format. The interview often serves a dual purpose. Not only does a clinical interview provide valuable assessment data, but it also is probably the first opportunity for a clinician to begin to build a positive therapeutic relationship that is the foundation for effective behavioral change. In practice, most clinical assessment interviews use unstructured or semistructured formats in order to obtain detailed information about a particular presenting problem. Greater flexibility in interview formats is often desirable when the clinical goals include not just reaching a diagnosis but also establishing a therapeutic relationship with a family and developing a treatment plan.

An effective clinical interview needs to establish a condition of trust and rapport so that the interviewee can feel comfortable in divulging personal information.[6] It is important to outline the purpose and nature of the interview at the outset and to discuss issues and limits of confidentiality. Effective interviewing requires listening skills, strategic use of open-ended and direct questions, and verbal and nonverbal empathic communications. The clinician needs to offer careful statements that reflect, paraphrase, reframe, summarize, and restate to verify accurate interpretation of client statements.[6] At the same time, the clinician is gathering verbal and nonverbal information conveyed by the client. Most interviewers take notes during interviews.

Most clinical assessments of children begin with a parent interview, the content of which depends on its purpose. Interviewing in the context of a developmental-behavioral problem usually focuses on identification and analysis of parental concerns so that an intervention plan can be developed and implemented. Psychosocial interviews typically elicit parent perceptions about the specific nature of the problem (including antecedents and consequences of the problem), family relations and home situation, social and school functioning, developmental history, and medical history. A practical interview format that is well suited for primary care settings is the Comprehensive Assessment to Intervention System, developed by Schroeder and Gordon.[7] This behaviorally oriented format clusters information in six areas for quick response: referral question, social context of question, general information about the child's development and family, specifics of the concern and functional analysis of behavior, effects of the problem, and areas for intervention. Schroeder and Gordon used this system both in their telephone call-in service and in their pediatric psychology office practices.

Child interviews are generally viewed as an essential component of clinical assessments and can be conducted with children as young as age 3 years.[3] Child clinical interviews are useful for establishing rapport, learning the child's perspective of functioning, selecting targets for interventions, identification of the child's strengths and competencies, and assessing the child's view of intervention options. Moreover, child interviews offer an opportunity to observe the child's behavior, affect, and interaction style directly. However, competent interviewing of children and adolescents interviews requires considerable skills and knowledge of development. For example, preschool children often respond better in interviews that the interviewer conducts while sitting at the child's level on the floor or at a small table and with toys, puppets, and manipulative items. School-age children may end communication if they feel barraged by too many direct questions, especially if asked "why" about motives, or if questions are abstract or rhetorical. Adolescent interviews may require additional attention to matters of confidentiality, trust, and respect.

Interviews of children and adolescents may include a brief observational, descriptive report of clinician impressions, summarized as a behavioral observations or a mental status examination. Key areas of psychological functioning are examined, including general appearance and behavior (physical appearance, nonverbal behaviors, attitudes), emotional expression (mood and affect), characteristics of speech and language, form (how thoughts are organized) and content (e.g., delusions, obsessions, suicidal/homicidal ideation) of thought, perceptual disturbances (e.g., hallucinations, dissociation), cognition (orientations, attention, memory), and judgment and insight (developmentally appropriate).

Structured and Semistructured Diagnostic Interviews

Assessment data obtained from unstructured clinical interviews tend to vary considerably and are largely interviewer dependent. As a result, unstructured interviews have particularly poor reliability and validity. When the primary assessment goal is to provide a diagnosis or a specific judgment with high inter-assessor reliability, as would be desired in research studies on specific psychiatric diagnoses, standardized, structured psychiatric interviews are often preferable. Structured interviews contain specific, predetermined questions with a format designed to elicit information efficiently and thoroughly. Key questions are followed by specified branch questions with restricted, closed ("yes"/"no") or brief responses.

An example of a structured interview is the National Institute of Mental Health Diagnostic Interview for Children–IV.[8] This instrument is a highly structured interview with nearly 3000 questions designed to assess more than 30, psychiatric disorders and symptoms listed in the American Psychiatric Association's *Diagnostic and Statistical Manual of Mental Disorders, Fourth Edition (DSM-IV)*[8a] in children and adolescents aged 9 to 17 years. Parent and child versions in English and Spanish are available, and lay interviewers can administer it for epidemiological research. The Diagnostic Interview for Children and Adolescents[9] is another structured diagnostic interview for children ages 6 to 17. This instrument consists of nearly 1600 questions that address 28 *DSM-IV* diagnoses relevant to children. Interrater reliability estimates of individual diagnoses range from poor to good, and diagnoses are moderately correlated with clinicians' diagnoses and self-rated measures.

Structured interviews result in higher interrater (or interobserver) reliability because there is little opportunity for the interviewer to influence the content of data collected. Although sometimes considered to be the "gold standard" for psychiatric diagnostic and epidemiological research, standardized interviews are not impervious to reporter bias. In addition, structured diagnostic interviews tend to rely on *DSM-IV* symptoms which may not be developmentally appropriate, particularly for very young children. Moreover, structured diagnostic interviews may take 1 to 3 hours to complete, which renders them impractical for most clinical settings, especially because they typically do not assess background and family factors that are necessary for developing and implementing an intervention plan.

Semistructured interviews combine aspects of traditional and behavioral interviewing techniques. Specific topic areas and questions are presented, but, in contrast to structured interviews, more detailed responses are encouraged. Semistructured formats also support use of empathic communication described previously (e.g., reflecting, paraphrasing). For example, the Semistructured Parent Interview[3] contains sample questions organized around six topic areas: concerns about the child (open ended), behavioral or emotional problems (eliciting elaboration to begin a functional analysis of behavior), social functioning, school functioning, medical and developmental history, and family relations and home situations. Like other semistructured formats, the Semistructured Parent Interview encourages parent interviews built around a series of open-ended questions to introduce a topic, followed by more focused questions about specific areas of concern.

The Semistructured Clinical Interview for Children and Adolescents (SCICA)[10] is an interview designed for children aged 6 to 16. It is part of the Achenbach System of Empirically Based Assessment (ASEBA)[11] and was designed to be used separately or in conjunction with other ASEBA instruments (e.g., Child Behavior Checklist [CBCL], Teacher Report Form). The SCICA contains a protocol of questions and procedures assessing children's functioning across six broad areas: (1) activities, school, and job; (2) friends; (3) family relations; (4) fantasies; (5) self-perception and feelings; and (6) problems with parent/teacher. There are additional optional sections pertaining to achievement tests, screening for motor problem, and adolescent topics (e.g., somatic complaints, alcohol and drug abuse, trouble with the law). Interview information (observations and self-report) are scored on standardized rating forms and aggregated into quantitative syndrome scales and *DSM-IV*–oriented scales. Test-retest, interrater, and internal consistency evaluations indicate excellent to moderate estimates of reliability. Accumulating evidence for validity of the SCICA includes content validity, as well as criterion-related validity (ability to differentiate matched samples of referred and nonreferred children).

The Child and Adolescent Psychiatric Assessment[12] is another semistructured diagnostic interview for children and adolescents aged 9 to 17. One interesting feature of this instrument is the inclusion of sections assessing functional impairment in a number of areas (e.g., family, peers, school, and leisure activities), family factors, and life events.

Motivational Interviewing

Motivational interviewing is an empirically supported interviewing approach gaining considerable attention in medical and mental health settings. More than an assessment strategy, motivational interviewing is a brief, client-centered directive intervention designed to enhance intrinsic motivation for behavior change through the exploration and reduction of patient ambivalence.[13] Based on a number of social and behavioral principles, including decisional balance, self-perception theory, and the transtheoretical model of change,[14] motivational interviewing combines rogerian and strategic techniques into a directive and yet patient-centered and collaborative encounter. Assess-

ment from a motivational interviewing perspective involves addressing the patient's ambivalence about making a change in behavior, exploring the negative and positive aspects of this choice, and discussing the relationship between the proposed behavior change (e.g., compliance with mediations) and personal values (e.g., health). This information is elicited in an empathic, accepting, and nonjudgmental manner and is used by the patient to select goals and create a collaborative plan for change with the provider.

The effectiveness of motivational interviewing with children and young adolescents has not been established. However, there is emerging evidence of its utility with adolescents and young adults, particularly in the areas of risk behavior, program retention, and substance abuse.[15,16]

TESTING METHODS: DEVELOPMENTAL AND COGNITIVE

Infancy and Early Childhood

Since the 1980s, there has been increased interest in the developmental evaluation of infants and young children.[17,18] This began with the 1986 Education of the Handicapped Act Amendments (Public Law 99-457) and continues with the Individuals with Disabilities Education Improvement Act of 2004 (Public Law 108-446), a revision of the Individuals with Disabilities Education Act (IDEA). These laws involve provision of early intervention services and early childhood education programs for children from birth through 5 years of age. Developmental evaluation is necessary to determine whether children qualify for such intervention services. Part C of the IDEA revision (Section 632) delineates five major areas of development: cognitive, communication, physical, social-emotional, and adaptive. However, definitions of delay vary, criteria being set on a state by state basis. These can included a 25% delay in functioning in comparison with same-aged peers, 1.5 to 2.0 standard deviations below average in one or more areas of development, or performance on a level that is a specific number of months below a given child's chronological age. However, pressure to quantify development has caused professionals working with infants and young children to attribute a degree of preciseness to developmental screening and assessment that is neither realistic nor attainable. Additional problems include test administration by examiners who are not adequately trained and use of instruments that have varying degrees of psychometric rigor.[19] Nonetheless, developmental evaluation is critical, because timely identification of children with developmental problems affords the opportunity for early intervention, which enhances skill acquisition or prevents additional deterioration.

Again, choice of the type of developmental assessment that is administered is driven by the purposes of the evaluation: for example, determination of eligibility for early intervention or early childhood education services, documentation of developmental change after provision of intervention, evaluation of children who are at risk for developmental problems because of established biomedical or environmental issues, documentation of recovery of function, or prediction of later outcome. Assessment of infants and young children is in many ways unique, because it occurs against a backdrop of qualitative and quantitative developmental, behavioral, and structural changes, the velocity of change being greater during infancy and early childhood than at any other time. The rapidly expanding behavioral repertoire of the infant and young child and the corresponding divergence of cognitive, motor, and neurological functions pose distinct evaluation challenges.[18,19]

Another significant testing concern in this age range is test refusal.[20] Test refusal, where a child either declines to respond to any items, or eventually stops responding when items become increasingly difficult, occurs in 15% to 18% of preschoolers.[21-24] Occasional refusals occur in 41% of young children. In addition to the immediate ramifications problematic test-taking behaviors have on actual test scores, there is evidence that early high rates of refusals are associated with similar behaviors at later ages, and with lower intelligence, visual perceptual, neuropsychological, or behavioral scores in middle childhood.[22-25] Non-compliance has been reported to occur in verbal production tasks, gross motor activities, or toward the end of the testing session, and it occurs more in children born at biologic risk or those from lower socioeconomic households. Children who refuse any aspect of testing differ from those who refuse some items, or who are compliant and cooperative to a certain point and then refuse more difficult items. This situation prompted inclusion of the Test Observation Checklist (TOC) in the Stanford-Binet Scales for Early Childhood, 5th Edition (SB5).[26]

A distinction is often made between developmental tests and intelligence tests,[27] and both are used in the age range under discussion. The assessment of intelligence originated from the need to determine which children would be able to learn in a classroom and which would be mentally deficient. In fact, this was the original purpose of the Binet test. Intelligence tests have become more psychometrically sophisticated but still assess different facets of primary cognitive abilities such as reasoning, knowledge, quantitative reasoning, visual-spatial processing, and working memory. In contrast, the purpose of early developmental measures such as the Bayley Scales of Infant Development (BSID)[28] or the Gesell Developmental Schedules[29] was to be diagnostic of developmental delays, providing a benchmark of developmental acquisitions (or lack thereof) in comparison to same-aged peers. Nonetheless, this distinction is often blurred, perhaps because there is no specific age at which a child shifts from "development" to "intelligence" (although the culmination of the infancy period is often indicated), nor is there a clear-cut transformation from a delay to a deficit. Developmental tests also tend to include motor and social-adaptive skills. Both tests of development and intelligence are driven by the theoretical model of the test developer and the constructs measured by the test. Those that assess the former are considered more dynamic or fluid; those that assess intelligence are more consistent and predictive. Herein, we discuss both developmental and intelligence tests that are used in children in this age level.

Developmental Assessment Instruments

GESELL DEVELOPMENTAL SCHEDULES/ CATTELL INFANT INTELLIGENCE TEST

The Gesell Developmental Schedules[29,30] and the Cattell Infant Intelligence Test[31] are the oldest developmental test instruments and exemplify the blurring of developmental and intelligence testing boundaries. The most recent version of the former is Knobloch and associates' *Manual of Developmental Diagnosis* (for children aged 1 week to 36 months).[32] Gesell specified key ages at which major developmental acquisitions occur: 4, 16, 28, and 40 weeks and 12, 18, 36, and 48 months. Gross motor, fine motor, adaptive, language, and personal-social areas are assessed, with 1 to 12 items at each age. A developmental quotient is computed for each area with the formula maturity age level/chronological age ×100. The Cattell test is essentially an upward extension of the Gesell schedule over the first 21 months and a downward extension of early versions of the Stanford-Binet tests from age 22 months and older (the Cattell age range is 2 to 36 months). A major drawback of both instruments is the limited standardization sample size (e.g., 107 for the Gesell schedule, 274 for the Cattell test). As a result, neither is used frequently at this time, although the Cattell test does yield so-called IQ scores below 50 (the floor of the BSID).

BAYLEY SCALES OF INFANT DEVELOPMENT[27,28,33]

The original BSID[28] evolved from versions administered to infants enrolled in the National Collaborative Perinatal Project. It was the reference standard for the assessment of infant development, administered to infants 2-30 months of age. The BSID was theoretically eclectic and borrowed from different areas of research and test instruments. It contained three components—the MDI, the Psychomotor Developmental Index (PDI), and the Infant Behavior Record ($M = 100$, $SD = 16$)—and was applicable for children aged 2 to 30 months. The BSID subsequently was revised as the BSID-II,[33] this partly because of the upward drift of approximately 11 points on the MDI and 10 points on the PDI, reflecting the Flynn effect[34] ($M = 100$, $SD = 15$). As a result, the BSID-II scores were 12 points lower on the MDI and 10 points lower on the PDI in comparison with the original BSID.[35] The Behavior Rating Scale was developed to enable assessment of state, reactions to the environment, motivation, and interaction with people. The age range for the BSID-II was expanded to 1 to 42 months. Unfortunately, this instrument had 22 item sets and basal and ceiling rules that differed from the original BSID. These rules were controversial in that if correction is used to determine the item set to begin administration, or if an earlier item set is employed because of developmental problems, scores tend to be somewhat lower, because the child is not automatically given credit for passing the lower item set. It was also criticized because it did not provide area scores compatible with IDEA requirements such as cognitive, motor communication, and social and adaptive function.[35]

For the newest version of the BSID, the Bayley Scales of Infant and Toddler Development–Third Edition (BSID-III),[27] norms were based on responses of 1700 children. The BSID-III assesses development (at ages 1 to 42 months) across five domains: cognitive, language, motor, social-emotional, and adaptive. Like its predecessors, the BSID-III is a power test. Assessment of the first three domains is accomplished by item administration, whereas the latter two are evaluated by means of caregiver's responses to a questionnaire. A Behavior Observation Inventory is completed by both the examiner and the caregiver. The Language scale includes a Receptive Communication and an Expressive Communication scaled score; the Motor Scales includes a Fine Motor and a Gross Motor score. The BSID-III Social-Emotional Scale is an adaptation of the Greenspan Social-Emotional Growth Chart: A Screening Questionnaire for Infants and Young Children.[36] The Adaptive Behavior Scale is composed of items from the Parent/Primary Caregiver Form of the Adaptive Behavior Assessment System–Second Edition;[37] it measures areas such as communication, community use, health and safety, leisure, self-care, self-direction, functional preacademic performance, home living, and social and motor skills and yields a General Adaptive Composite score.

Scaled scores ($M = 10$, $SD = 3$), composite scores ($M = 100$, $SD = 15$), percentile ranks, and growth scores are provided, as are confidence intervals for the scales and age-equivalent scores for subtests. Growth scores are new and, with caution, are used to plot the child's growth over time for each subtest in a longitudinal manner. This metric is calculated on the basis of the subtest total raw score and ranges from 200 to 800 ($M = 500$, $SD = 100$). As in the original BSID, there are basal rules (passing the first three items at the appropriate age starting point) and a ceiling or discontinue rules (a score of 0 for five consecutive items).

The correlation between the BSID-III Language Composite and the BSID-II MDI is 0.71; that between the Motor Composite and the BSID-II PDI is 0.60; and that between the Cognitive Composite and the BSID-II MDI is 0.60. The moderate correlation between the older PDI and MDI and their BSID-III counterparts underscores the significant differences between the old and new BSIDs. However, in contrast to the expected Flynn effect (see Chapter 7A and Flynn[34]), the BSID-III Cognitive and Motor composite scores are approximately 7 points *higher* than the corresponding BSID-II MDI and PDI. This phenomenon has also been reported with the Peabody Picture Vocabulary Test–Third Edition,[38] and the Battelle Developmental Inventory–Second Edition[39] (Box 7C-1).

BATTELLE DEVELOPMENTAL INVENTORY–SECOND EDITION (BDI-2)[39]

The norms of the BDI-2 were based on the performances of 2500 children, and this instrument is applicable to children from birth through age 7 years 11 months. Data are collected through a structured test format, parent interviews, and observations of the child. The scoring system is based on a 3-point scale: 2 if the response met a specified criteria, 1 if the child attempted a task but it was incomplete (emerging skill), and 0 if the response was incorrect or absent. The original Battelle Developmental Inventory[40] and the BDI-2 were developed on the basis of milestones: that is, development reflects the child's attainment of critical skills or behaviors. Five domains are assessed: (1) The *Adaptive Domain,* which contains the Self-Care (e.g., eating, dressing toileting) and Personal Responsibility subdomains (initiate play, carry out tasks, avoid dangers); (2) the *Personal-Social Domain,* which contains the Adult Interaction (e.g., identifies familiar people), Peer Interaction (shares toys, plays cooperatively) and Self-Concept and Social Role subdomains (express emotions, aware of gender differences); (3) the *Communication Domain,* which contains the Receptive Communication and Expressive Communication subdomains; (4) the *Motor Domain,* which contains

---

BOX 7C-1

CASE 1: DEVELOPMENTAL ASSESSMENT DISCUSSION

The toddler in Case 1 was given a developmental assessment that included the BSID-III. Results are shown in the table below.

BSID-III Scale	Standard Score	Percentile	95% Confidence Interval
Cognitive	9		
Cognitive composite	95	37	87-103
Receptive communication	9		
Expressive communication	8		
Language composite	91	27	84-99
Fine motor	7		
Gross motor	6		
Motor composite	79	16	73-88
Social-emotional	8		
Social-emotional composite	90	25	83-99
General Adaptive Composite (GAC)	81	18	76-86

BSID, Bayley Scales of Infant Development.

BSID-III results indicate that the child had average cognitive abilities, low-average language skills, borderline motor abilities (Gross Motor worse than Fine Motor scores), low-average social-emotional functioning, and borderline adaptive skills. Her low average language may be influenced by the nonoptimal environment; the motor deficits are most likely attributable to the grade III bleed. The Cognitive composite score is 5 points higher than the previous BSID-II MDI score that the child had received at age 1; this is in contrast to the Flynn effect (whereby scores generally increase 0.5 points per year) but is within the 7-point increment that is found when the BSID-II and BSID-III scores are compared (BSID-III scores are somewhat higher than BSID-II scores). On the basis of these data, early intervention services geared toward language and adaptive skills are recommended. Moreover, the motor deficits will require occupational and physical therapy services.

---

the Gross Motor, Fine Motor, and Perceptual Motor subdomains (stacks cubes puts small object in bottle); and (5) the *Cognitive Domain,* which contains Attention and Memory (follows auditory and visual stimuli), Reasoning and Academic Skills (names colors, uses simple logic), and Perception and Concepts subdomains (compares objects, puzzles, group-

ing). The BDI-2 *full assessment* incorporates all five domains, whereas the *screening test* includes two items at each of 10 age levels for each of the five domains. A developmental quotient is produced for each domain and for a total BDI-2 Composite score ($M = 100$, $SD = 15$); scaled scores are applied to the subdomains ($M = 10$, $SD = 3$). Noteworthy is the fact that these are normalized standard scores and not ratio scores. Percentiles, age-equivalent scores, and confidence intervals are provided; the domain developmental quotients are the most reliable scores. The correlation between the original Battelle Developmental Inventory and the BDI-2 total developmental quotient is 0.78; the total BDI-2 score is 1.1 points higher than that of the original Battelle Developmental Inventory, with domain differences ranging from 1.4 to 2.8 points. Again, this is in contrast to the Flynn effect.

MULLEN SCALES OF EARLY LEARNING (MSEL)[41]

The MSEL assess the learning abilities and patterns in various developmental domains in children 2 to $5\frac{1}{2}$ years of age. Particular emphasis is placed on differentiation of visual and auditory learning, thereby enabling measurement of unevenness in learning. The MSEL differentiates receptive or expressive problems in the visual or auditory domain through four scales: Visual Receptive Organization, Visual Expressive Organization, Language Receptive Organization, and Language Expressive Organization. At the receptive level, processing that involves one modality (visual or auditory) is defined as *intrasensory reception;* processing that involves two modalities (auditory and visual) is termed *intersensory reception.* This design provides assessment of visual, auditory, and auditory/visual reception and of visual-motor and verbal expression. The MSEL AGS Edition[42] combines the Infant MSEL and Preschool MSEL and is applicable to children from birth to age 68 months. A gross motor scale is also included (T-scores, Early Learning Composite [$M = 100$, $SD = 15$]). The Early Learning Composite has a correlation of 0.70 with the BSID MDI.

DIFFERENTIAL ABILITY SCALES[43]

The Differential Ability Scales is applicable to children aged $2\frac{1}{2}$ to 17 years but is most useful in the range from age $2\frac{1}{2}$ to 7 years. Many clinicians consider the Differential Ability Scales an intelligence test, although it yields a range of scores for developed abilities and not an IQ score; it is rich in developmental information of a cognitive nature. On the basis of reasoning and conceptual abilities, a composite score, the General Conceptual Ability score ($M = 100$, $SD = 15$; range, 45 to 165), is derived. Subtest ability scores have a mean of 50 and a standard deviation of 10 (T-scores). In addition, verbal ability and nonverbal ability cluster scores are produced for upper preschool-age children ($3\frac{1}{2}$ years and older). For ages 2 years 6 months to 3 years 5 months, four core tests constitute the General Conceptual Ability composite (block building, picture similarities, naming vocabulary, and verbal comprehension), and there are two supplementary tests (recall of digits, recognition of pictures). For ages 3 years 6 months to 5 years 11 months, six core tests are included in the General Conceptual Ability composite (copying, pattern construction, and early number concepts in addition to verbal comprehension, picture completion, and naming vocabulary; block building is now optional). The test is unique in that it incorporates a developmental and an educational perspective, and each subtest is homogeneous and can be interpreted in terms of content.

McCARTHY SCALES OF CHILDREN'S ABILITIES (MSCA)[44]

The MSCA essentially bridges developmental and IQ tests.[17] It is most useful in the 3- to 5-year age range (age range, $2\frac{1}{2}$ to $8\frac{1}{2}$ years). Some clinicians would question viewing the MSCA as a developmental test; however the term *IQ* was avoided initially, with the test considered to measure the child's ability to integrate accumulated knowledge and adapt it to the tasks of the scales. Eighteen tests in total are divided into Verbal (five tests), Perceptual-Performance (seven tests), Quantitative (three), Memory (four tests), and Motor (five) categories. Several tests are found on two scales. The Verbal, Perceptual-Performance, and Quantitative scales are combined to yield the General Cognitive Index ($M = 100$, $SD = 16$; 50 is the lowest score). The mean scale standard score (T-score) for each of the five scales is 50 ($SD = 10$). The MSCA is attractive because in enables production of a profile of functioning (with age-equivalent scores) and it includes motor abilities; conversely, the test was devised in 1972, and hence there is inflation of scores vis-à-vis the Flynn effect (i.e., increments in test norms over time result in lower scores on newer tests than those obtained on measures with older norms; see Chapter 7A for a discussion of the Flynn effect[34]). Short forms of the MSCA are available, but these are not useful in the younger age ranges.[17]

Intelligence Assessment Instruments

KAUFMAN BRIEF INTELLIGENCE TEST, SECOND EDITION (KBIT-2)[45]

The KBIT-2 was released 14 years after the original Kaufman Brief Intelligence Test and is applicable for ages 4 to 90 years. It is particularly useful as an estimate of IQ, for screening, and in time-limited situations. The test produces Verbal, Non-verbal, and Composite IQ scores ($M = 100$, $SD = 15$), as well as 90% confidence intervals, age-equivalent scores, and scaled scores for two of the three subtests. The Verbal scale consists of two subtests: Verbal Knowledge (60 items measuring both receptive vocabulary and range of general information; child points to the picture matching the word or question) and Riddles (48 items measuring verbal comprehension, reasoning, vocabulary knowledge, and deductive reasoning, based on two or three clues). The Riddles subtest replaces the Definitions from the original Kaufman Brief Intelligence Test, thereby circumventing reading. Matrices is the nonverbal scale (46 items with meaningful stimuli [people, objects] and abstract stimuli [designs, symbols]). Discrepancies between Verbal and Nonverbal scores are of interest. The KBIT-2 Verbal score is approximately 1 point lower than that of the original Kaufman Brief Intelligence Test, the KBIT-2 Non-verbal score is 3 points lower, and the KBIT-2 Composite is, on average, 2 points lower. The KBIT-2 composite score is typically within 2 points of the Wechsler Intelligence Scale for Children–Fourth Edition (WISC-IV), composite score, and correlations with the Verbal Comprehension Index, Perceptual Reasoning Index, and the Full Scale IQ (FSIQ) are 0.79, 0.56, and 0.77, respectively.

STANFORD-BINET INTELLIGENCE SCALES, FIFTH EDITION/STANFORD-BINET INTELLIGENCE SCALES FOR EARLY CHILDHOOD–5 (EARLY SB5)[26,46]

The 10 subtests of the Early SB5 are drawn from the SB5, and the norms are derived from approximately 1660 children aged 7 years 3 months or younger. The test is applicable from age 2 to $7\frac{1}{4}$ years (the SB5 extends to adulthood). The 10 subtests constitute the FSIQ, and various combinations of these subtests constitute other scales. An Abbreviated Battery IQ scale consists of two routing subtests: Object Series/Matrices and Vocabulary. Routing subtests enable the examiner to know the level at which to begin subsequent subtests. The Nonverbal IQ scale consists of five subtests measuring the factors of nonverbal fluid reasoning, knowledge, quantitative reasoning, visual-spatial processing, and working memory. The Verbal IQ scale is composed of five subtests measuring verbal ability domains in the same five factor areas as for the Nonverbal IQ scale. The Early SB5 also includes the Test Observation Checklist. The test differs markedly from the fourth edition of the Stanford-Binet Intelligence Tests. Nonverbal IQ, Verbal IQ, and FSIQ scores are obtained ($M = 100$, $SD = 15$), as are total factor index scores (sum of verbal and nonverbal scaled scores) for fluid reasoning, knowledge, quantitative reasoning, visual-spatial processing, and working memory; scaled scores ($M = 10$, $SD = 3$) can be computed for each of the nonverbal and verbal domains. Optional change-sensitive scores and age-equivalent scores are also computed. The SB5 FSIQ is approximately 3.5 points lower than the that of the fourth edition. The SB5 FSIQ is approximately 5 points lower than the FSIQ for the Wechsler Intelligence Scale for Children–Third Edition (WISC-III).

KAUFMAN ASSESSMENT BATTERY FOR CHILDREN–SECOND EDITION[47]

This battery, with norms based on scores from 3025 children, is applicable in children aged 3 to 18 years (the original Kaufman Assessment Battery for Children ceiling was 12) and contains 18 core and supplementary subtests (the number of core and supplementary tests administered varies, depending on age). It is similar to the original battery in that there is a simultaneous and sequential processing approach, vis-à-vis the Luria neuropsychological model. However, the test also uses the Cattell-Horn-Carroll abilities model that includes fluid crystallized intelligence. As a result, interpretation is based on the model that is selected; the number of scales produced is also model-dependent. The five areas assessed include (1) simultaneous processing (eight subtests; e.g., triangles, face recognition, pattern reasoning, block counting, gestalt closure), (2) sequential processing (word order, number recall, hand movements), (3) planning (a new scale applicable for ages 7 to 18; includes pattern reasoning, story completion), (4) learning (four subtests, e.g., Atlantis, Rebus), and (5) knowledge (optional and only for the Cattell-Horn-Carroll model; includes riddles, verbal knowledge, and expressive vocabulary, some of which were previously achievement tests).

For subjects at age 3 years, a Mental Processing Index (from the Luria model) and a Fluid Crystallized Index (FCI-from the Cattell-Horn-Carroll model) are derived. For children by age 7 years, the full array of scores can be derived; this includes the Mental Processing Index, a Global Score, a Fluid-Crystallized Index, and a Nonverbal Index (four or five subtests, depending on age, and including language-reduced instructions and nonverbal responses). The number of core subtests for the Cattell-Horn-Carroll mode is 7 to 10, depending on age, and the number of core subtests for the Luria approach is 5 to 8. Subtest scale scores have a mean of 10 ($SD = 3$); the index score mean is 100 ($SD = 15$). As with the SB5 and WISC-IV, intraindividual differences can be computed.

WECHSLER PRESCHOOL AND PRIMARY SCALE OF INTELLIGENCE–THIRD EDITION (WPPSI-III)[48]

Whereas the Wechsler Preschool and Primary Scale of Intelligence–Revised was a downward extension of the Wechsler Intelligence Scale for Children, this is not the case with the WPPSI-III. The current version, with norms based on scores of 1700 children, contains 14 subtests (7 new, 7 revised) and has two age ranges: from 2 years 6 months to 3 years 11 months and from 4 years 0 months to 7 years 3 months. In the first age range, FSIQ, Verbal IQ, and Performance IQ scores are obtained, through four core subtests. Seven core subtests are applicable to the second age range. Supplemental and optional subtests are used to obtain a General Language Composite in the younger children and a Processing Speed Quotient in the older children. Inclusion of the Picture Concepts, Matrix Reasoning, and Word Reasoning subtests allows for better assessment of fluid reasoning. For IQ and composite scores, $M = 100$ and $SD = 15$; for scaled scores, $M = 10$, $SD = 3$. Children tested with the WISC-III and the WPPSI-III at overlapping ages had a WISC-III FSIQ score that was, on average, 4.9 points higher than the WPPSI-III FSIQ score; correlations with the BSID-II MDI score were 0.80; those with the Differential Ability Scales General Conceptual Ability composite were 0.87. As in many of the newer IQ tests, various composite scores allow for testing of more specific cognitive abilities and better interpretation of findings.

WECHSLER INTELLIGENCE SCALE FOR CHILDREN–FOURTH EDITION[49]

The WISC-IV, with norms based on responses from 2200 children, is applicable to ages 6 years 0 months to 16 years 11 months, and contains 15 subtests (10 core, 5 supplementary). The Verbal IQ and Performance IQ scores of the WISC-III are no longer used. Gone also are the Picture Arrangement, Object Assembly, and Mazes subtests from the WISC-III, to decrease the emphasis on performance time. Instead, the WISC-IV contains a Verbal Comprehension Index (Similarities, Vocabulary, Comprehension, Information,* and Word Reasoning*), a Perceptual Reasoning Index (Block Design, Picture Concepts, Matrix Reasoning, Picture Completion*), a Working Memory Index (Digit Span, Letter-Number Sequencing, Arithmetic*), and a Processing Speed Index (Coding, Symbol Search, Cancellation*). In addition to these four index scales, a measure of general intellectual function (FSIQ) is produced. The more narrow domains and emphasis on fluid reasoning reflect contemporary thinking with regard to intelligence per se. For index and FSIQ scores, $M = 100$ and $SD = 15$; the mean scaled score is 10 ($SD = 3$). The WISC-IV is highly correlated with WISC-III indexes ($rs = 0.72$ to 0.89). The FSIQ score is approximately 2.5 points less than that of its predecessor; the Verbal Comprehension Index score is 2.4 points less than the WISC-III Verbal IQ score; the Perceptual Reasoning Index score

*Supplementary tests.

is 3.4 points less than the Performance IQ score; the Working Memory Index score is 1.5 points lower than the Freedom from Distractibility Index score; and the Processing Speed Index score is 5.5 points lower than its WISC-III counterpart. In comparison with the Wechsler Abbreviated Scale of Intelligence (WASI) (described next), the WISC-IV FSIQ score is 3.4 points lower, the Verbal Comprehension Index score is 3.5 points lower than the WASI Verbal IQ, and the Perceptual Reasoning Index score is 2.6 points lower. A General Ability Index (containing three verbal comprehension and three perceptual reasoning subtests), can be computed; this is less sensitive to the influence of working memory and processing speed and therefore is useful with children who have learning disabilities or attention-deficit/hyperactivity disorder (ADHD) (Box 7C-2).

WECHSLER ABBREVIATED SCALE OF INTELLIGENCE[50]

The WASI is applicable to ages 6 years 0 months through 89 years. Verbal IQ, Performance IQ, and either FSIQ-4 (with four subtests) or FSIQ-2 (two subtests) scores are obtained. Although subtests are similar to those found in other Wechsler scales, the actual items differ. Subtests include Vocabulary, Matrices, Block Design, and Similarities (the first two are used to compute the FSIQ-2). T-scores are used for subtests ($M = 10$, $SD = 5$). The WASI is very useful in both clinical and research settings, because of its reduced administration time. The downside is a reduction in the amount of information obtained, particularly in terms of more specific indexes of cognitive abilities. The scores are generally a few points higher than those of more detailed tests, but they still are comparable; the correlation between the FSIQ-2 and WISC-IV FSIQ scores is 0.86; between the FSIQ-4 and WISC-IV scores, 0.83 (comparable with the correlation among the WISC-III and WISC-IV FSIQ scores). Very small differences are noted on the subtest level.

Achievement Testing

Use of individually-administered achievement tests has increased dramatically since the introduction of Public Law 94-142 (Education of All Handicapped Children Act), and these tests continue to be a critical component in the evaluation of children with academic difficulties under the IDEA revision of 2004. The major reason is that achievement tests enable the delineation of aptitude-achievement discrepancies, a hotly debated requirement for establishment of a learning disability (versus response to treatment intervention). It is assumed that such tests identify children who need special instructional assistance; help recognize the nature of a child's difficulties/

deficiencies, thereby clarifying the nature of the learning problem; and assist in planning, instruction, and intervention. Unfortunately, achievement tests do not adequately meet these needs. In general, standard scores (with percentiles) are the most precise metric; age- and grade-equivalent scores are least useful. With regard to the Wechsler tests, the Verbal IQ (or Verbal Comprehension Index) and FSIQ are most highly correlated with achievement, particularly reading; the Performance IQ (Perceptual Reasoning Index), with mathematics.[51] Achievement tests differ in terms of content and type of response required (e.g., multiple choice vs. recall of information), and these differences sometimes cause one test to produce lower scores than another.

KAUFMAN TEST OF EDUCATIONAL ACHIEVEMENT–II[52]

This test is available in two formats: the Comprehensive form (with parallel forms A and B) and the Brief form. The mean score is 100 ($SD = 15$). Noteworthy is the fact that this test's norms were based on the scores of the same population as for the Kaufman Assessment Battery for Children–Second Edition. The Comprehensive form, applicable from ages 4 years 6 months to 25, assesses reading (letter/word recognition, comprehension), math (computation, concepts and application), written language (spelling, written expression), and oral language (listening comprehension and written expression). Several reading-related skill areas are also assessed (e.g., phonological awareness). The Brief form (for ages 4 years 6 months to 90 years) measures reading (word recognition and comprehension), math computation and application problems, and written expression (written language and spelling) and yields a battery composite score as well. Age- and grade-equivalent scores are provided. The test differs significantly from the original Kaufman Test of Educational Achievement and from the version with normative data update.

PEABODY INDIVIDUAL ACHIEVEMENT TEST–REVISED–NORMATIVE UPDATE[53,54]

This test is applicable for kindergarten through grade 12 (ages 5 to 19). It differs from others in that spelling and math are presented in a multiple-choice format and in other subtests such as reading comprehension, the student selects a picture that best illustrates the sentence that was read. The test includes scores for general information, reading recognition, reading comprehension, total reading, math, spelling, written expression, written language, and the total test. The normative update version is the same test, with updated norms. Some clinicians argue that the multiple-choice format may yield higher test scores because of the recognition, as opposed to recall, format.

BOX 7C-2

CASE 2: COGNITIVE ASSESSMENT DISCUSSION

Because of concerns related to academic ability and performance, Rachel was administered the WISC-IV. These results revealed that Rachel's cognitive abilities have developed very unevenly (probably in relation to underlying cerebral palsy). Her verbal comprehension abilities are within the high average range and represent a significant strength for her. Significant weaknesses are perceptual reasoning and processing speed, which are in the borderline range of functioning. Tasks that required abstract perceptual reasoning were particularly difficult for her. Despite cognitive weaknesses, Rachel's cluster scores on the Woodcock-Johnson III Tests of Achievement were all in the average range or better. This suggests that she has been able to use her verbal abilities to compensate for weaknesses in other areas. However, she has struggled in some academic subject areas, especially algebra, as the content has become more abstract.

Cognitive Assessment Results

WISC-IV	Subtest	Index	Subtest Index	Percentile	Description
Verbal Comprehension		114		82	High average
	Similarities		12		
	Vocabulary		13		
	Comprehension		13		
Perceptual Reasoning		75		5	Borderline
	Block Design		4		
	Picture Concepts		9		
	Matrix Reasoning		5		
	Picture Completion		7		
Working Memory		97		42	Average
	Digit Span		8		
	Letter-Numbering Sequencing		11		
	Arithmetic		10		
Processing Speed		70		2	Borderline
	Coding		4		
	Symbol Search		5		
	Cancellation		2		
Full Scale IQ		88		21	Low average

WISC-IV, Wechsler Intelligence Scale for Children–Fourth Edition.

Academic Achievement Assessment Results on the Woodcock-Johnson III Tests of Achievement, Form B (Actual Grade: 9)

Cluster	Standard Score	Grade Equivalent
Oral Language	113	13.3
Total Achievement	103	10.4
Broad Reading	106	11.0
Broad Math	93	7.9
Broad Written Language	108	12.9
Math Calculation Skills	97	8.9
Written Expression	101	9.9
Academic Skills	106	11.5
Academic Fluency	104	10.9
Academic Applications	94	8.0
Academic Knowledge	110	13.9

WECHSLER INDIVIDUAL ACHIEVEMENT TEST–II[55]

This test is applicable for prekindergarten through college (ages 4 to 85). This is an updated form of the original Wechsler Individual Achievement Test. There are four composite scores: (1) Reading (word reading, pseudoword decoding, reading comprehension); (2) Mathematics (numerical operations, math reasoning); (3) Written Language (spelling, written expression); and (4) Oral Language (listening comprehension, oral expression). Standard scores ($M = 100$, $SD = 15$), age- or grade-equivalent scores, and quartile scores are reported. Reading rate can also be assessed, and the test form includes qualitative observational descriptions for various subtests. The test is linked to Wechsler IQ tests, and aptitude/achievement discrepancy tables are included.

WIDE RANGE ACHIEVEMENT TEST–3[56]

This is the seventh edition of the Wide Range Achievement Test and is applicable for ages 5 to 75 years. There are two equivalent forms (Blue, Tan) and each contains reading (read letters, pronounce words), spelling (write letters, words from dictation) and arithmetic (40 computation problems) tests. The test is based on norms by age and not grade. Critics of this test argue that it is outdated and provides very gross estimates of academic achievement because it contains few items within each content area; conversely, it is easy and quick to administer. An Expanded Version is also available[57] that contains a group (G) form with reading/reading comprehension, math, and nonverbal reasoning (some tests are multiple choice), and an individual (I) form that assesses reading, mathematics, listening comprehension, oral expression, and written language. The Expanded Version group form is applicable to grades 2 to 12; the Individual form, to ages 5 to 24.

WOODCOCK-JOHNSON III TESTS OF ACHIEVEMENT (WJ III)[58]

The WJ III has two parallel forms (A and B) that are divided into a standard battery (12 subtests) and an extended battery (10 tests); therefore, there are 22 subtests in all. The latter provides the opportunity for more in-depth diagnostic evaluation of specific academic functions (e.g., word attack, oral comprehension). The WJ III contains a reading cluster, an oral language cluster, a math cluster, a written language cluster, and an academic knowledge cluster. Clusters are designed to correspond with IDEA areas. The standard battery provides 10 cluster scores, and the extended battery provides an additional 9 cluster scores. Broad reading, broad math, and broad written language are often used to provide an overview of the child's achievement. The WJ III is used by many school systems. Of note is the fact that the WJ III Tests of Achievement norms were based on the scores of the same population as those of the WJ III Tests of Cognitive Abilities and are designed to be used in combination. Standard scores ($M = 100$, $SD = 15$), percentile scores, and age- and grade-equivalent scores are the most helpful metrics. Computer scoring is necessary.

Neuropsychological Testing

There are three approaches to neuropsychological testing of children, and all involve the assessment of brain-behavior relationships. The first approach entails modification of traditional neuropsychological batteries such as the Halstead-Reitan Neuropsychological Battery or the Luria-Nebraska Neuropsychological Battery, to form corresponding children's batteries.[59] The second approach involves interpretation of standard tests such as those measuring intelligence, with the use of a neuropsychological "mind-set." In this case, results from standardized tests are tied into neuropsychological constructs and functions (e.g., the Kaufman Assessment Battery for Children–Second Edition). The third approach includes tests or rating scales designed to assess specific areas of neuropsychological function. Neuropsychological testing generally is more specific in terms of pinpointing strengths and deficits, and the results more precisely describe brain-behavior relationships. Neuropsychological testing may elucidate more subtle problems that contribute to cognitive, academic, or social difficulties; these problems may not be apparent from results of more routine measures used to detect learning disabilities. Noteworthy is the fact that standard intellectual assessment is typically part of a neuropsychological workup. Selected tests from this third approach are discussed as follows.

CHILDREN'S MEMORY SCALE[60]

The Children's Memory Scale assesses learning and memory function with nine subtests. There are two levels: one for ages 5 to 8 years and one for ages 9 to 16 years. The Children's Memory Scale includes three domains: Auditory/Verbal, Visual/Nonverbal, and Attention/Concentration, each with two core and one supplemental test. The first two domains have an immediate-memory component and a delayed-memory component (tested 30 minutes later). Eight index scores are produced: verbal immediate, verbal delayed, delayed recognition, learning visual immediate, visual delayed, attention/concentration, and general memory (global memory function). Core subtests include: Stories, Word Pairs, Dot Locations, Faces, Numbers, and Sequences. Word Lists, Family Pictures, and Picture Locations are the supplementary tests. The general memory score is moderately correlated with IQ scores.

NEPSY–A DEVELOPMENTAL NEUROPSYCHOLOGICAL ASSESSMENT (NEPSY)[61]

The NEPSY is based on Luria's theoretical model,[59] is applicable for ages 3 to 12 years, and consists of 27 subtests that encompass five domains: (1) Attention and Executive Functions (e.g., Tower test, Auditory Attention and Response Set, Visual Attention); (2) Language (Speeded Naming, Comprehension of Instructions, Phonological Processing); (3) Sensorimotor Functions (e.g., Fingertip Tapping, Visuomotor Precision); (4) Visuospatial Functions (Design Copying, Arrows, Block Construction); and (5) Learning and Memory (e.g., Memory for Faces, Names, Sentence Repetition). There is an 18-subtest core assessment. In general, each domain contains five to six subtests. Subtest scaled scores are obtained ($M = 10$, $SD = 3$), and these can be combined into summary domain scores ($M = 100$, $SD = 15$). Correlations with the Children's Memory Scale range from 0.36 to 0.60.

BEHAVIOR RATING INVENTORY OF EXECUTIVE FUNCTION (BRIEF)[62]

Executive function is an umbrella construct that refers to interrelated neuropsychological functions that are responsible for purposeful, problem-solving, goal-directed behavior. Executive function is involved in guiding, directing, regulating, and managing cognitive, behavioral, and emotional functions. The BRIEF measures executive function in an ecological manner: namely, it is a questionnaire given to parents and/or teachers, thereby assessing executive function in home and school environments. The BRIEF is applicable for school-aged children (5 to 18 years), although a preschool version is also available (BRIEF-P). In addition, a BRIEF-SR (self-report) version has become available for ages 11 to 18 years, requiring a fifth grade reading level. Each version consists of 86 items scored "never" (1), "sometimes" (2), or "often" (3). There are eight clinical scales: Inhibit (controlling impulses, modifying behavior), Shift (cognitive flexibility, transitioning), Emotional Control (emotional modulation), Initiate (beginning a task/activity, independently generating ideas), Working Memory (holding information in mind, persistence), Plan/Organize (anticipating future events, setting goals), Organization of Materials (workspace, play areas, orderliness), and Monitor (work checking, keeping track of how behaviors affect others). The first three scales combine to form the Behavioral Regulation Index; the remaining five constitute the Metacognition Index. The Global Executive Composite is computed from the combination of the Behavioral

Regulation Index and Metacognition Index. There are also two validity scales, the Inconsistency and Negativity scales, that assist in detecting response biases. T-scores and percentiles are computed from raw scores and can be graphed on the reverse side of the scoring summary sheet. T-scores higher than 65 (1.5 standard deviations above average) are considered to have reached a clinical threshold. There are different norms for boys and girls. The BRIEF is particularly useful in evaluating children with ADHD, traumatic brain injury, autism spectrum disorders (ASDs), and learning disorders and those who experience cognitive, behavioral, or academic problems and whose initial test results are inconclusive.

WIDE RANGE ASSESSMENT OF MEMORY AND LEARNING (WRAML)/WIDE RANGE ASSESSMENT OF MEMORY AND LEARNING–2 (WRAML-2)[63,64]

The WRAML (ages 5-17) and WRAML-2 (ages 5-90) are designed to test visual and verbal memory. The WRAML-2 contains six core subtests (the WRAML has nine): Story Memory, Verbal Learning, Design Memory, Picture Memory, Finger Windows, and Number/Letter Memory. Verbal Memory Index (Story Memory, Verbal Learning), Visual Memory Index (Design Memory, Picture Memory) and Attention/Concentration (Finger Windows, Number/Letter Memory) summary scores are obtained ($M = 100$, $SD = 15$). There are optional Sentence Memory, Sound-Symbol, Verbal Working Memory, and Symbolic Memory subtests. Delayed recall and recognition memory can also be assessed. A General Memory Index is computed from the core subtests. Scores on Memory Screening, consisting of the first four core subtests (taking 20 minutes), correlate highly with those of the General Memory Index ($r = 0.91$). In contrast to the WRAML, there is no Learning Index in the WRAML-2. The WRAML-2 also allows assessment of primary/recency effects, immediate/delayed recall, rote versus meaningful information, visual/verbal differences, working memory, short-term memory, sustained attention, and recognition versus retrieval memory. This test is useful in evaluation of children with learning disorders, those suspected of having verbal processing problems, and those suspected of having ADHD.

TESTING METHODS: BEHAVIORAL AND EMOTIONAL

Assessment of social, emotional, and behavioral adjustment of children typically begins with a parent or caregiver interview regarding the nature, severity, and frequency of concerns. Most child assessment techniques rely on caregiver reports because it is presumed that adults who interact daily with a child are the most knowledgeable informants about a child's functioning. School-aged children and adolescents should also have the opportunity to provide their own perceptions and information about their symptoms. Younger children (younger than 10 years) can provide assessment information, but their self-descriptions tend to be less reliable; therefore, direct and multiple observations and interviews may be necessary.

A criticism of reliance on caregiver reports in child assessments is that they are subject to reporter bias. However, all reports are subject to "bias," including those from the child, parents, clinicians, teachers, and other observers. All reports are to some extent limited (or "biased") by the perspectives, knowledge, recall, and candor of the informants. Because there is no unbiased "gold standard" source of data about children's problems, data from multiple sources are always needed. Regardless of the child's age, behavioral and emotional assessment strategies almost always should include information obtained from multiple sources, including parents, teachers, and the child, as well as by direct observation of the child. Data from multiple informants with different perspectives provide critical information about how the child functions in different settings such as at home, at school, and with friends. Even when there is discrepant information obtained from caregivers (as is often true), multiple vantage points are useful in determining the scope and functional effect of behavior problems.[65]

Assessment of child and adolescent emotional and behavioral problems is further complicated because of the high rate of comorbidity, heterogeneity, and severity of concerns. Children referred for assessments often meet diagnostic criteria for multiple disorders or display symptoms associated with multiple disorders. Thus, it is often important to assess not only a referred problem but also a broad range of social, emotional, and behavioral domains. For example, in their review of evidence-based assessment of conduct problems, McMahon and Frick[66] concluded that because of the high rate of comorbid disorders (e.g., ADHD, depressive and anxiety disorders, substance use problems, language impairment, and learning difficulties), initial assessments of youth with conduct problems should include broadband measures to screen for all conditions, followed by disorder-specific scales, interview strategies, and standardized testing of conduct and comorbid disorders.

Behavioral Rating Scales

Behavior rating scales are an extremely useful and efficient method for obtaining data on child function-

ing. Most rating scales use a standard questionnaire, checklist, or Likert-response format for surveying areas of interest and usually are completed by caregivers without much assistance. Rating scales include brief screening measures that assess global, broad-based measures, and problem-specific scales.

Broad-based behavioral assessment instruments assess multiple dimensions of behavior in children. Most are empirically developed taxonomies that are symptom driven and do not necessarily correspond to specific diagnostic schemas. On rating scales, informants rate the child on a broad range of social competencies and problematic behaviors. Results produce empirically derived factor scores on broad dimensions (e.g., internalizing and externalizing problems) and specific symptom areas (e.g., depression or aggressiveness) based on age and gender norms. Parent, teacher, and self-report forms are available for cross-informant comparisons. Rating scales yield very useful information about a child's functioning in comparison with children of the same age and gender, and generally are viewed as necessary components of most child assessments.

ACHENBACH SYSTEM OF EMPIRICALLY BASED ASSESSMENT/CHILD BEHAVIOR CHECKLIST[11,67-71]

The CBCL was one of the first broad-based rating scales of behavior in children to be developed, and it continues to be the most widely used method for behavioral assessments in children. Achenbach began work on what would become the CBCL in the 1960s in an effort to differentiate child and adolescent psychopathology.[68] At that time, the *DSM* provided just two categories for childhood disorders: Adjustment Reaction of Childhood and Schizophrenic Reaction, Childhood Type. Achenbach and collaborators applied an empirically based approach to child psychopathology much like what was used in the development of the Minnesota Multiphasic Personality Inventory. This approach involved recording problems for large samples of children and adolescents, performing multivariate statistical analyses to identify syndromes of problems that co-occur, using reports to assess competencies and adaptive functioning, and constructing age- and gender-specific profiles of scales on which to display individuals' scores.[11] These taxonomic procedures revealed that most behavior problems in children could be broadly divided into "internalizing" and "externalizing" conditions. This pioneering work had enormous influence on clinical and research assessment practices and established the empirical foundation for contemporary conceptualizations of child psychopathology.

The CBCL was published first in 1983 as a measure of behavior problems in children aged 4 to 18 years.

Currently, there are ASEBA materials for ages $1\frac{1}{2}$ to older than 90 years. There are forms for preschoolers ($1\frac{1}{2}$ to 5 years, parent and teacher/daycare versions)[69] and school-aged children (parent, teacher versions for children aged 6 to 18 years and youth self-report for ages 11 to 18 years),[67] as well as for adults (18 to 59 years)[70] and older adults (60 to older than 90 years)[71] (both with caregiver and self-report formats). For each problem listed, informants provide ratings on the following scale: 0 = "not true," 1 = "somewhat or sometimes true," and 2 = "very true or often true." Hand-scored and computer-scored profiles are available, as are Spanish-language forms.

The Child Behavior Checklist for Ages $1\frac{1}{2}$-5 (CBCL/$1\frac{1}{2}$-5) obtains parents' ratings of 99 problem items along with descriptions of concerns and competencies. Scales are based on parent ratings of 1728 preschool children; norms are based on a national sample of 700 children. Raw scores can be translated into standard T-scores, yielding interpretative information on three summary scales (Internalizing, Externalizing, and Total Problems), as well as on clinical syndromes scales (Emotionally Reactive, Anxious/Depressed, Somatic Complaints, Withdrawn, Attention Problems & Aggressive Behavior, and Sleep Problems). A Language Development Survey is included to screen for language delays. *DSM*-oriented scales pertaining to affective problems, anxiety problems, pervasive developmental problems, attention-deficit/hyperactivity problems, and oppositional defiant problems are now available.

The Child Behavior Checklist for Ages 6-18 (CBCL/6-18) similarly obtains reports from parents, close relatives, and/or guardians regarding school-aged children's competencies and behavioral/emo-tional problems. The competency scale includes 20 items about a child's activities, social relations, and school performance. Specific behavioral and emotional problems are described in 118 items that are rated along the 0-to-2 scale described previously, along with two open-ended items for reporting additional problems. A scoring profile provides raw scores, T-scores, and percentiles for three competence scales (Activities, Social, and School); Total Competence; eight cross-informant (clinical scale) syndromes; and Internalizing, Externalizing, and Total Problems (broad scales). The eight clinical scales scored from the CBCL/6-18 Teacher Report Form and Youth Self-Report are Aggressive Behavior; Anxious/Depressed; Attention Problems; Rule-Breaking Behavior; Social Problems; Somatic Complaints; Thought Problems; and Withdrawn/Depressed. Now available are also six *DSM*-oriented scales associated with affective problems, anxiety problems, somatic problems, attention-deficit/hyperactivity problems, oppositional defiant problems, and conduct problems. The school-age scales are based on new factor analyses of parents' ratings of nearly 5000 clinically referred children, and norms are based on results from a nationally representative sample of 1753 children aged 6 to 18 years[11] (Box 7C-3).

ASEBA materials are backed by extensive research in their development and have been used in more than 6000 studies pertaining to a broad range of behavioral health topics. There is strong support for its use with multidimensional child assessments in pediatric settings, (e.g., Mash and Hunsley[2]; Riekert et al,[72] Stancin and Palermo[73]), although criticisms have been raised about the validity of the CBCL for populations of chronically ill children.[74]

BOX 7C-3

CASE 2: BEHAVIORAL AND EMOTIONAL ASSESSMENT DISCUSSION

The behavior problem profiles obtained on the CBCL/6-18 and the Youth Self-Report for Rachel are shown in the following two illustrations. On the CBCL problem scales (completed by her mother), Rachel's Total Problems, Internalizing, and Externalizing scores and syndrome scales were all in the normal ranges for girls aged 12 to 18. Similarly, a teacher completed a Teacher Report Form, and results were all within the normal range. However, on the Youth Self-Report problem scales, Rachel reported more problems than are typically reported by teenage girls, particularly withdrawn behavior, somatic complaints, problems of anxiety or depression, problems in social relationships, thought problems, attention problems, and problems of an aggressive nature. Rachel's responses on the Minnesota Multipha-sic Personality Inventory–Adolescent indicated that she was experiencing high levels of general distress. Elevations on clinical scales 2,3,7,8,0 suggested that she may have felt anxious, lonely, and pessimistic much of the time and may have felt isolated from others and inferior. In other words, Rachel reported having high levels of internalizing symptoms, as well as difficulties managing social relationships and aggression. Cross-informant comparisons indicate that adults in Rachel's life were not aware of the level of her internal distress. Discrepancies between Rachel's self-report of symptoms and the ratings by her mother became a springboard for validating Rachel's need for mental health attention and led to better communication within the family.

BOX 7C-3

CASE 2: BEHAVIORAL AND EMOTIONAL ASSESSMENT DISCUSSION—cont'd

ID:
Name: Rachel (none)

Gender: Female
Age: 15

Date Filled: 01/03/2006
Birth Date: 10/01/1990

Clinician:
Agency:
Verified: Yes

Informant: Jane Doe
Relationship: Biological Mother

CBCL/6-18—Syndrome Scale Scores for Girls 12-18

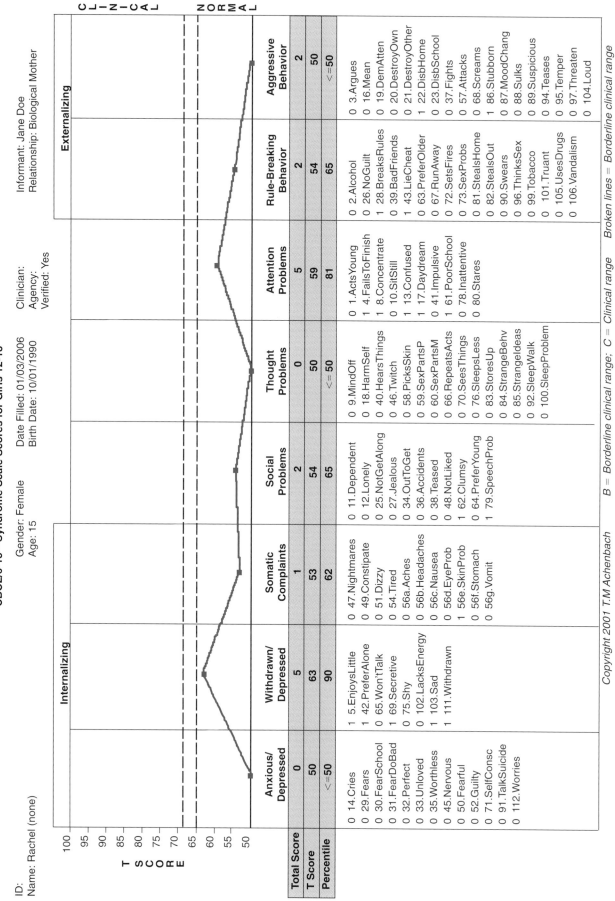

	Anxious/Depressed	Withdrawn/Depressed	Somatic Complaints	Social Problems	Thought Problems	Attention Problems	Rule-Breaking Behavior	Aggressive Behavior
Total Score	0	5	1	2	0	5	2	2
T Score	50	63	53	54	50	59	54	50
Percentile	<=50	90	62	65	<=50	81	65	<=50

Anxious/Depressed
0 14.Cries
0 29.Fears
0 30.FearSchool
0 31.FearDoBad
0 32.Perfect
0 33.Unloved
0 35.Worthless
0 45.Nervous
0 50.Fearful
0 52.Guilty
0 71.SelfConsc
0 91.TalkSuicide
0 112.Worries

Withdrawn/Depressed
1 5.EnjoysLittle
1 42.PreferAlone
0 65.Won'tTalk
1 69.Secretive
0 75.Shy
0 102.LacksEnergy
1 103.Sad
1 111.Withdrawn

Somatic Complaints
0 47.Nightmares
0 49.Constipate
0 51.Dizzy
0 54.Tired
0 56a.Aches
0 56b.Headaches
0 56c.Nausea
0 56d.EyeProb
1 56e.SkinProb
0 56f.Stomach
0 56g.Vomit

Social Problems
0 11.Dependent
0 12.Lonely
0 25.NotGetAlong
0 27.Jealous
0 34.OutToGet
0 36.Accidents
0 38.Teased
0 48.NotLiked
1 62.Clumsy
0 64.PreferYoung
1 79.SpeechProb

Thought Problems
0 9.MindOff
0 18.HarmSelf
0 40.HearsThings
0 46.Twitch
0 58.PicksSkin
0 59.SexPartsP
0 60.SexPartsM
0 66.RepeatsActs
0 70.SeesThings
0 76.SleepsLess
0 83.StoresUp
0 84.StrangeBehv
0 85.StrangeIdeas
0 92.SleepWalk
0 100.SleepProblem

Attention Problems
0 1.ActsYoung
1 4.FailsToFinish
1 8.Concentrate
0 10.SitStill
1 13.Confused
1 17.Daydream
0 41.Impulsive
1 61.PoorSchool
0 78.Inattentive
0 80.Stares

Rule-Breaking Behavior
0 2.Alcohol
0 26.NoGuilt
1 28.BreaksRules
0 39.BadFriends
1 43.LieCheat
0 63.PreferOlder
0 67.RunAway
0 72.SetsFires
0 73.SexProbs
0 81.StealsHome
0 82.StealsOut
0 90.Swears
0 96.ThinksSex
0 99.Tobacco
0 101.Truant
0 105.UsesDrugs
0 106.Vandalism

Aggressive Behavior
0 3.Argues
0 16.Mean
0 19.DemAtten
0 20.DestroyOwn
0 21.DestroyOther
1 22.DisbHome
0 23.DisbSchool
0 37.Fights
0 57.Attacks
0 68.Screams
1 86.Stubborn
0 87.MoodChang
0 88.Sulks
0 89.Suspicious
0 94.Teases
0 95.Temper
0 97.Threaten
0 104.Loud

Internalizing

Externalizing

Copyright 2001 T.M Achenbach   B = Borderline clinical range;   C = Clinical range   Broken lines = Borderline clinical range

BOX 7C-3

CASE 2: BEHAVIORAL AND EMOTIONAL ASSESSMENT DISCUSSION—cont'd

CBCL/6-18—Internalizing, Externalizing, Total Problems, Other Problems for Girls 12-18

ID:
Name: Rachel (none)

Gender: Female
Age: 15

Date Filled: 01/03/2006
Birth Date: 10/01/1990

Clinician:
Agency:

Informant: Jane Doe
Relationship: Biological Mother

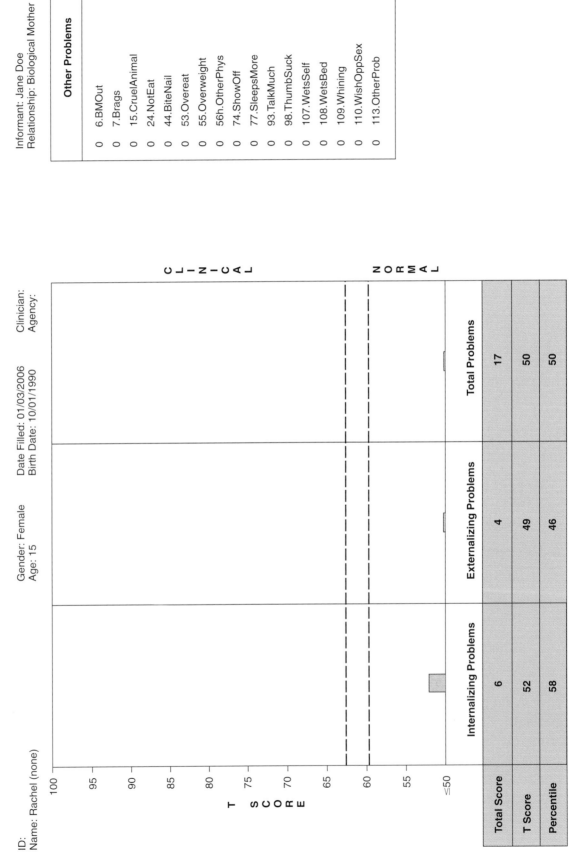

Other Problems	
0	6.BMOut
0	7.Brags
0	15.CruelAnimal
0	24.NotEat
0	44.BiteNail
0	53.Overeat
0	55.Overweight
0	56h.OtherPhys
0	74.ShowOff
0	77.SleepsMore
0	93.TalkMuch
0	98.ThumbSuck
0	107.WetsSelf
0	108.WetsBed
0	109.Whining
0	110.WishOppSex
0	113.OtherProb

	Internalizing Problems	Externalizing Problems	Total Problems
Total Score	6	4	17
T Score	52	49	50
Percentile	58	46	50

B = Borderline clinical range; C = Clinical range   *Broken lines = Borderline clinical range*

ID:
Name: Rachel (none)

Gender: Female
Age: 15

Date Filled: 01/03/2006
Birth Date: 10/01/1990

Clinician:
Agency:

Informant: Jane Doe
Relationship: Biological Mother

CBCL/6-18—DSM-Oriented Scales for Girls 12-18

C L I N I C A L

N O R M A L

	Affective Problems	Anxiety Problems	Somatic Problems	Attention Deficit/ Hyperactivity Problems	Oppositional Defiant Problems	Conduct Problems
Total Score	2	0	1	2	2	2
T Score	54	50	54	52	52	55
Percentile	65	<=50	65	58	58	69

Affective Problems	Anxiety Problems	Somatic Problems	Attention Deficit/ Hyperactivity Problems	Oppositional Defiant Problems	Conduct Problems
1 5.EnjoysLittle	0 11.Dependent	0 56a.Aches	1 4.FailsToFinish	0 3.Argues	0 15.CruelAnimal
0 14.Cries	0 29.Fears	0 56b.Headaches	1 8.Concentrate	1 22.DisbHome	0 16.Mean
0 18.HarmSelf	0 30.FearSchool	0 56c.Nausea	0 10.SitStill	0 23.DisbSchool	0 21.DestroyOther
0 24.NotEat	0 45.Nervous	0 56d.EyeProb	0 41.Impulsive	1 86.Stubborn	0 26.NoGuilt
0 35.Worthless	0 50.Fearful	1 56e.SkinProb	0 78.Inattentive	0 95.Temper	1 28.BreaksRules
0 52.Guilty	0 112.Worries	0 56f.Stomach	0 93.TalkMuch		0 37.Fights
0 54.Tired		0 56g.Vomit	0 104.Loud		0 39.BadFriends
0 76.SleepsLess					1 43.LieCheat
0 77.SleepsMore					0 57.Attacks
0 91.TalkSuicide					0 67.RunAway
0 100.SleepProb					0 72.SetsFires
0 102.Underactiv					0 81.StealsHome
1 103.Sad					0 82.StealsOut
					0 90.Swears
					0 97.Threaten
					0 101.Truant
					0 106.Vandalism

B = Bord rline clinical range; C = Clinical range

Broken lines = Borderline clinical range

T SCORE: 100 95 90 85 80 75 70 65 60 55 50

BOX 7C-3

CASE 2: BEHAVIORAL AND EMOTIONAL ASSESSMENT DISCUSSION—cont'd

YSR/11-18—Syndrome Scale Scores for Girls

ID:
Name: Rachel (none)

Gender: Female
Age: 15

Date Filled: 01/03/2006
Birth Date: 10/01/1990

Clinician:
Agency:
Verified: Yes

Informant: Self
Relationship: Self

CLINICAL   NORMAL

Internalizing   **Externalizing**

	Withdrawn	Somatic Complaints	Anxious/ Depressed	Social Problems	Thought Problems	Attention Problems	Delinquent Behavior	Aggressive Behavior
Total Score	12	13	27	12	8	16	5	17
T Score	85-C	79-C	88-C	85-C	69-B	90-C	62	67-B
Percentile	>98	>98	>98	>98	97	>98	89	96

Withdrawn	Somatic Complaints	Anxious/ Depressed	Social Problems	Thought Problems	Attention Problems	Delinquent Behavior	Aggressive Behavior
2 42.PreferAlone	1 51.Dizzy	2 12.Lonely	0 1.ActsYoung	2 9.MindOff	0 1.ActsYoung	2 26.NoGuilt	2 3.Argues
1 65.Won'tTalk	2 54.Tired	2 14.Cries	2 11.Dependent	1 40.HearsThings	2 8.Concentrate	0 39.BadCompany	0 7.Brags
2 69.Secretive	2 56a.Aches	0 18.HarmSelf*	2 25.NotGetAlong	0 66.RepeatsActs	2 10.SitStill	0 43.LieCheat	2 16.Mean
1 75.Shy	2 56b.Headaches	2 31.FearDoBad	1 38.Teased	1 70.SeesThings	2 13.Confused	0 63.PreferOlder	0 19.DemAtten
2 102.Underactive	2 56c.Nausea	2 32.Perfect	2 48.NotLiked	0 83.StoresUp*	2 17.Daydream	1 67.RunAway	0 20.DestroyOwn
2 103.Sad	0 56d.EyeProb	2 33.Unloved	2 62.Clumsy	2 84.StrangeBehav	2 41.Impulsive	1 72.SetsFires	0 21.DestroyOther
2 111.Withdrawn	2 56e.SkinProb	2 34.OutToGet	1 64.PreferYoung	2 85.StrangeIdeas	2 45.Nervous	0 81.StealsHome	0 23.DisobeySchl
	2 56f.Stomach	2 35.Worthless	2 111.Withdrawn*		2 61.PoorSchool	0 82.StealsOther	1 27.Jealous
	0 56g.Vomit	2 45.Nervous			2 62.Clumsy	1 90.Swears	2 37.Fights
		2 50.Fearful				0 101.Truant	1 57.Attacks
		0 52.Guilty				0 105.AlcDrugs	1 68.Screams
		2 71.SelfConsc					0 74.ShowOff
		2 89.Suspicious					1 86.Stubborn
		1 91.ThinkSuic*					2 87.MoodChang
		2 103.Sad					1 93.TalkMuch
		2 112.Worries					0 94.Teases
							2 95.Temper
							1 97.Threaten
							1 104.Loud

B = Borderline clinical range;   C = Clinical range   Broken lines = Borderline clinical range   *Not on CBCL or TRF construct

YSR/11-18—Internalizing, Externalizing, Total Problems, Other Problems, Profile ICCs, Clinical T Scores for Girls

ID:
Name: Rachel (none)

Gender: Female
Age:15

Date Filled: 01/03/2006
Birth Date: 10/01/1990

Clinician:
Agency:

Informant: Self
Relationship: Self

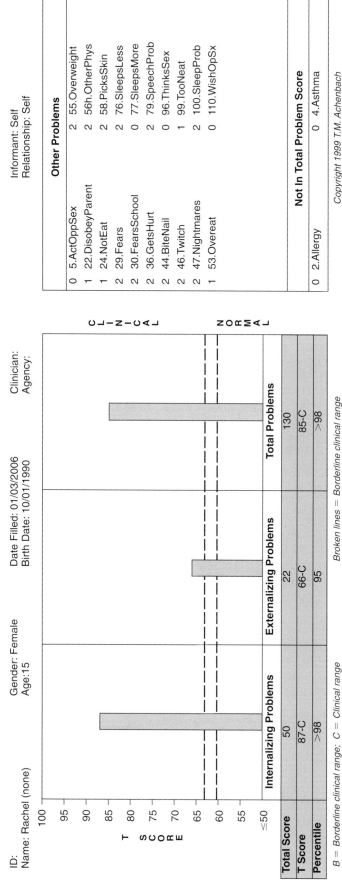

Other Problems

0	5.ActOppSex	2	55.Overweight
1	22.DisobeyParent	2	56h.OtherPhys
1	24.NotEat	2	58.PicksSkin
2	29.Fears	2	76.SleepsLess
2	30.FearsSchool	0	77.SleepsMore
2	36.GetsHurt	2	79.SpeechProb
2	44.BiteNail	0	96.ThinksSex
2	46.Twitch	1	99.TooNeat
2	47.Nightmares	2	100.SleepProb
1	53.Overeat	0	110.WishOpSx

Not In Total Problem Score

0	2.Allergy	0	4.Asthma

Copyright 1999 T.M. Achenbach
ADM Version 4

	Internalizing Problems	Externalizing Problems	Total Problems
Total Score	50	22	130
T Score	87-C	66-C	85-C
Percentile	>98	95	>98

B = Borderline clinical range; C = Clinical range   *Broken lines = Borderline clinical range*

Cross-Informant Profile Types

	Intraclass Corr.(ICC)	Significant Similarity*
Withdrawn	−0.474	No
Somatic Complaints	−0.663	No
Social Problems	−0.036	No
Delinquent-Aggressive	−0.878	No

Profile Types Specific to YSR

	Intraclass Corr.(ICC)	Significant Similarity*
YSR Social	−0.588	No
Delinquent	−0.869	No

*Intraclass correlations >0.444 indicate statistically significant similarity between a child's profile and previously identified profile types.

	Withdrawn	Somatic Complaints	Anxious/ Depressed	Social Problems	Thought Problems	Attention Problems	Delinquent Behavior	Aggressive Behavior
T scores based on clinical sample	73	71	71	75	62	74	48	56

Copyright by T. M. Achenbach. Reproduced with permission.

BEHAVIOR ASSESSMENT SYSTEM FOR CHILDREN–SECOND EDITION (BASC-2)[75]

The BASC-2 is another broad, multidimensional rating scale system designed to measure behavior and emotions of children and adolescents. It includes a Parent Rating Scale, a Teacher Rating Scale, and a Self-Report of Personality. Norms are provided for ages 2 years 0 months through 21 years 11 months (Teacher Rating Scale and Parent Rating Scale) and 8 years 0 months through college age (Self-Report of Personality). T-scores and percentiles for a general population and clinical populations are available for interpretation. Computer scoring and Spanish language forms are available. The Parent Rating Scale requires approximately a fourth grade reading level; forms pertaining to three age levels—preschool (ages 2 to 5), child (ages 6 to 11), and adolescent (ages 12 to 21)—measure adaptive and problem behaviors in the community and home setting. The Parent Rating Scale contains 134 to 160 items and entails use of a four-choice response format. Clinical scales include Aggression, Anxiety, Attention Problems, Atypicality, Conduct Problems, Depression, Hyperactivity, Somatization, and Withdrawal. Adaptive scales include Activities of Daily Living, Adaptability, Functional Communication, Leadership, and Social Skills. The Teacher Rating Scale similarly measures adaptive and problem behaviors in the preschool or school setting. An additional clinical domain in the Teacher Rating Scale is Learning Problems; Study Skills are measured on the Adaptive Scales. The Self-Report of Personality provides insight into a child's or adolescent's thoughts and feelings, including scales such as Anxiety, Attention Problems, Sense of Inadequacy, Social Stress, Interpersonal Relations, and Self Esteem (among others). One strong advantage of the BASC-2 over other rating scales is the inclusion of validity and response set indexes that may be used to judge the quality of responses.

INFANT-TODDLER SOCIAL-EMOTIONAL ASSESSMENT SCALE (ITSEA)[76]

The ITSEA provides a comprehensive analysis of emerging social-emotional development of infants and toddlers aged 12 to 36 months. It includes parallel parent and child care provider forms that contains 166 items focusing on behavioral and emotional problems and competencies. A national normative sample consisted of 600 children, with clinical groups that included children with autism, language delays, prematurity, and other disorders. English and Spanish forms are available with computer or hand scoring that yield T-scores for 4 broad domains, 17 specific subscales, and 3 index scores. An interesting feature of the ITSEA is its companion measure, the Brief Infant-Toddler Social-Emotional Assessment Scale.[77]

This measure contains 42 items, is completed by a parent or caregiver, and can be used first to screen for possible concerns and then followed with the ITSEA for more comprehensive evaluation.

MINNESOTA MULTIPHASIC PERSONALITY INVENTORY–ADOLESCENT (MMPI-A)[78]

Although it is not a behavior rating scale per se, the MMPI-A is a self-report questionnaire that yields indices pertaining to the nature and severity of symptoms in relation to peers with psychiatric disorders. Norms are based on a nationally representative sample of more than 1600 male and female adolescents in the United States. The MMPI-A scoring yields T-scores for 7 validity scales, 10 clinical scales, 15 content scales, and other supplementary scales and indices. The MMPI-A is a lengthy measure (478 true/false items) that requires at least a sixth grade reading level; therefore, some adolescents find it to be difficult to complete. However, a shortened 350-item version yielding basic results can be administered to save administration time.

Projective Techniques

Projective assessment techniques encourage a respondent to "project" issues, concerns, and perceptions onto ambiguous stimuli such as an inkblot or a picture. The basic premise is that when the child is faced with an ambiguous stimulus or one requiring perceptual organization, underlying psychological issues affecting the child will influence interpretation of these stimuli. The most commonly used projective techniques with children include use of child human figure or family drawings, storytelling responses to pictures or photographs, and reactions to Rorschach inkblots. Once the mainstay of personality assessment, projective assessment techniques have fallen out of favor in the era of evidence-based assessment techniques. However, some techniques continue to have clinical utility and validity with specific assessment purposes. They can provide clues that subsequently can be pursued with interviews and other techniques. For example, family drawings can be a helpful source of qualitative information about a child's view of family relations, especially with younger children with more limited verbal expressions. Responses to incomplete sentences, story cards, and "3 wishes" ("if you could have 3 wishes, what would they be?") can reveal insights into a child's internal representations of relationships. In addition, the Rorschach has been shown to be a valid method for examining perceptual accuracy in youth with possible thought disorders when used with validated scoring systems such as John E. Exner's system for scoring the Rorschach test.[79]

Assessing Peer Relationships

Peer perspectives contain unique and important information about children but are usually missing in multi-informant clinical assessments. Peers play critical social roles in children's lives and have access to information that adults may not have and that children may be reluctant to self-report. For example, social acceptance within a peer group is an important aspect of a child's functional status, but it can be difficult to assess accurately by interview or parent report. Sociometric assessments that use peer nomination methods have been developed as a systematic way of gathering information about the extent to which a child is accepted or rejected within a peer group.[80] Strategies may involve asking children by interview or on paper to nominate three classmates with whom they most like to play (positive nominations/peer acceptance) and three classmates with whom they would least like to play (negative nominations/peer rejection). An alternative method is for children to rate how much they like to play with each classmate, for example, on a scale from 1 ("I don't like to") to 5 ("I like to a lot"). Using various statistical classification schemes, children can be considered to be popular, accepted, rejected, neglected, or controversial.

Peer nomination assessment instruments have been used to measure specific domains of child functioning besides peer acceptance. Techniques often involve presenting children in a classroom with a list of behavioral descriptions and asking them to select which of their peers best match each descriptor. Peer nomination approaches with acceptable reliability and validity have been developed to obtain peer ratings for a number of specific behavioral or emotional problem domains in children, such as ADHD symptoms, aggression and withdrawal, and depression.[81]

The Peer-report Measure of Internalizing and Externalizing Behavior[81] was developed to assess a broad range of peer-reported externalizing and internalizing child psychopathology. As with other peer-nomination inventories, students are provided with classroom roster sheets that contain listings of all of the children in the classroom. Then, they are asked to select up to three classmates (either gender) who best fit the description read to them (e.g., "worry about things a lot" or "get mad and lose their temper"). Preliminary reports suggest that this measure demonstrates adequate reliability and validity as a broad measure of psychopathology.

Peer nomination procedures may be useful for psychosocial screening in the classroom, evaluating the effectiveness of mental health interventions on social behaviors in school settings, and conducting research on a range of child social behaviors. However, for clinical purposes, it may difficult (and impractical) to obtain peer ratings of an individual child. For this reason, parent, teacher, and rating scales of behavior in children can be used to as a more practical alternative for multi-informant assessments of peer relationships and functioning. For example, the ASEBA scales (e.g., the CBCL Teacher Report Form) include positive peer relationship items on the competence scales and a social problems scale highlighting peer difficulties on the problem scales.

Testing for Specific Problems

PARENT-CHILD INTERACTIONS

Parent-child interaction problems contribute significantly to the origin and maintenance of a wide range of behavior problems in children. Therefore, treatment of children in mental health settings, especially children with negative, externalizing behaviors, often focuses on promoting optimal parenting styles and parent-child interactions. For these reasons, assessment of parent-child interactions is essential when treatment interventions are planned for children with a wide range of behavioral problems.[82]

Parent-child interactions may be assessed through observation, Q-sorts (cards with descriptive labels are "sorted" into piles as to how well they pertain to a child), or rating scales. Qualitative assessments through observations may be conducted in vivo or by using videotape recordings of parent-child interactions. The Dyadic Parent-Child Interaction Coding System[83] is widely used in clinical and research settings to code direct observations in a standardized laboratory setting. Observations (through a one-way mirror or videotape) are made during three standard parent-child interaction settings: child-led play, parent-led play, and cleaning up. Parent and child verbalizations and physical behaviors are coded along 25 categories. Reliability and validity studies provide good support for use of the Dyadic Parent-Child Interaction Coding System to evaluate baseline and post treatment behaviors, as well as to measure ongoing treatment progress.[83] In addition to this structured method of observation, it is sometimes useful to observe parent-child interactions in more naturalistic settings.[84]

The classic research method for assessing the quality of parent-child relationships is the laboratory Strange Situation Paradigm developed by Ainsworth (described by Shaddy and Colombo[85]). Strength and quality of an infant's attachment to a caregiver are assessed by placing the child in situations in which he or she is alone with the caregiver, separated from caregiver and introduced to a stranger, and then reunited with the caregiver. The infant can be classified as securely attached, ambivalent/resistant, avoidant, or disorganized on basis of reactions in those situations.

Information about parent-child interactions in clinical settings can be obtained from sorting techniques and rating scales. The Attachment Q-Set (as described by Querido and Eyberg)[82] is a measure of a child's attachment related behaviors. Parents sort 90 behavioral dimensions of security, dependency, and sociability into piles according to the extent to which they describe the child. Results of the Q-set are related to results obtained by exposing infants to the Strange Situation Paradigm. In addition, there are a variety of measures by which to assess various dimensions of parent-child relationships and interactions through the use of rating scales and checklists.[82]

DEPRESSION

Self-report questionnaires and rating scales are usually preferred over parent or teacher rating scales for screening depression in children and teens and for monitoring symptoms during treatment. However, they tend to have limited sensitivity and specificity and therefore should be used cautiously.[86] Moreover, they can be influenced by respondent bias if the child does not want to divulge information. The most widely used depression rating scale for children and adolescents is the Children's Depression Inventory.[87] This instrument includes 27 items covering a range of depressive symptoms and associated features and it can be used in youth ages 7-17. Research on the Children's Depression Inventory has generally shown it to have good internal consistency, test-retest reliability, and sensitivity to change, but the evidence for discriminant validity is more limited.[86]

The Mood and Feeling Questionnaire[88] is a 32-item measure of depression (and there is an even briefer 13-item version) that has been shown to have good estimates of reliability, discriminant validity, and sensitivity to change for children aged 8 to 18 years.[86] The Reynolds Child Depression Scale[89] and the Reynolds Adolescent Depression Scale[90] are 30-item scales for youth aged 8 to 12 and 13 to 18. These scales have also been shown to be internally consistent and stable, although there is more limited evidence of discriminant validity and sensitivity to change.[86]

The Children's Depression Rating Scale[91] is an interesting hybrid measure that combines separately obtained responses from a child and an informant along with the clinician's behavioral observations. Seventeen items assess cognitive, somatic, affective, and psychomotor symptoms; cutoff scores provide estimates of level of depression. Moderate reliability, convergent validity, and sensitivity to treatment have been demonstrated, but, as with most measures of depression, it does not distinguish between depression and anxiety very well.[86]

Assessment of depression in infants and preschool children is very challenging because of the difficulty of eliciting self-report information in a reliable or valid manner. Caregiver reports obtained with broadband measures (such as the CBCL/1½-5 or Teacher Report Form 1-5) may be a useful alternative or adjunctive tool. A new parent report screening measure of preschool depression is the Preschool Feelings Checklist.[92] This 20-item checklist of depressive symptoms in young children was shown to have high internal consistency and to be correlated highly with the Diagnostic Interview for Children–IV and the CBCL on a sample of 174 preschool children from a primary care setting. Moreover, preliminary study suggested that it had acceptable sensitivity and specificity when a cutoff score of 3 was used.[92]

ANXIETY

Screening for anxiety disorders is most often done with rating scales, although data supporting their use are sparse, and several scales have been shown to measure different anxiety constructs.[93] The Multidimensional Anxiety Scale for Children[94] is a youth self-report rating scale that assesses anxiety in four domains: physical symptoms, social anxiety, harm avoidance, and separation/panic. Children aged 8 to 19 are asked to rate how true 39 items are for them. Internal consistency reliability coefficients of subscales and total scores range from 0.74 to 0.90, although interrater reliability is lower (0.34 to 0.93). The Multidimensional Anxiety Scale for Children has some support for use as a screener for anxiety disorders, as does the Social Phobia and Anxiety Inventory for Children,[95] the Social Anxiety Scale for Children[96] and the Social Anxiety Scale for Adolescents.[97] The Revised Children's Manifest Anxiety Scale,[98] although widely used, does not appear to discriminate between children with anxiety disorders and those with other psychiatric conditions and therefore should be used cautiously as a screening or diagnostic tool.[93] However, it does appear to be sensitive to change and therefore may be a useful tool for monitoring treatment effects.

ATTENTION-DEFICIT/ HYPERACTIVITY DISORDER

ADHD is one of the most common childhood mental health disorders and a frequent diagnostic consideration in developmental-behavioral pediatric settings. Despite the vast literature on ADHD psychopathology and treatment, considerably less research has been directed toward determining best assessment practices.[5] The most efficient empirically based assessment methods for diagnosing ADHD are parent and teacher symptom rating scales based on *DSM-IV* criteria (e.g., the ADHD Rating Scale[99] or the Vanderbilt ADHD Diagnostic Scales[100]) or derived from a rational or empirical basis (e.g., BASC or CBCL).[101] Broadband rating scales (such as the BASC or CBCL) were not recommended for diagnosing ADHD in the American Academy of Pediatrics Diagnostic Guidelines[102] because broad domain factors (e.g., externalizing) do not discriminate children referred for ADHD from non-referred peers.[103,104] However, a more recent review[5] challenged this recommendation, concluding that the Attention Problems subscales within the CBCL and BASC do accurately identify children with ADHD. Because of their ability to identify other comorbid conditions and impairments, broadband measures (which also have advantages of extensive normative information across gender and developmental ages) are probably more efficient than *DSM-IV*–based rating scales for diagnosing ADHD.[5]

As with any disorder, ADHD should not be diagnosed with symptom rating scales alone. Clinical interviews and other sources of data are needed to establish pertinent history, to rule out other disorders that may better account for symptoms (e.g., autism, low intellectual functioning, post-traumatic stress disorder, adjustment problems), and to assess comorbid conditions. Interestingly, *DSM*-based structured interviews have not been shown to add incremental validity to parent and teacher rating scales.[5] Behavioral observation assessment procedures have been shown to be empirically valid in numerous studies but practically impossible in most clinical settings, although parent and teacher proxy observational measures have been developed.[5] Measures of child functioning and impairment in key domains including peer relationships, family relationships, and academic settings, should be included in an ADHD assessment and are likely to be more useful for treatment purposes than are global ratings of impairment. Moreover, assessment of ADHD needs to emphasize situational contexts and socially valid target behaviors (i.e., functional analysis of behavior) necessary for treatment planning (Box 7C-4).

AUTISM SPECTRUM DISORDERS

Empirically based procedures for assessing ASDs have emerged since the 1990s, greatly improving the accuracy and validity of the diagnoses and the ability to plan and evaluate interventions. Ozonoff and associates[105] summarized the current state of the art with regard to assessment of ASDs and recommended a core assessment battery that includes collecting diagnostic information from parents and by direct observation along with standardized measures of intelligence, language, and adaptive behavior. One ASD-specific measure is the Autism Diagnostic Interview–Revised,[106] a comprehensive, semistructured

---

BOX 7C-4

CASE 3: BEHAVIORAL ASSESSMENT RESULTS

Jose is reported to have a short attention span and to display social and academic impairment. Parent and teacher CBCL measures were obtained to broadly examine the nature and severity of behavior problems (the Spanish version was administered to parents). Clinically significant scores were on the following parent and teacher subscales: Social Problems, Attention Problems, and Aggressive Behavior. Scores on the Teacher Report Form Attention Problems subscales were further clinically significant for Inattention (98th percentile) and Hyperactivity-Impulsivity (97th percentile). Scores on the Vanderbilt ADHD Diagnostic Scales, used to collect information about the presence of *DSM-IV* symptoms, showed that Jose's mother and teacher considered him to display symptoms associated with ADHD, combined type. Maternal reports on the Vanderbilt scales were considered cautiously because of possible language and cultural differences from the normative sample. Clinical interviews and academic screening to rule out communication problems and learning disorders led to diagnoses of ADHD and Oppositional Defiant Disorder. Idiographic measures of daily behavior problems targeted out-of-seat behaviors during instruction, schoolwork completion, and peer aggression for behavioral interventions. A treatment plan was developed to include a trial of stimulant medication, home and classroom behavioral interventions, parent training in behavior management skills, and a social skills group.

---

diagnostic parent interview that elicits current behavior and developmental history. It yields three algorithm scores measuring social difficulties, communication deficits, and repetitive behaviors; these scores have been shown to distinguish children with autism from children with other developmental delays. I is very labor intensive in terms of training (3 days) and administration time (3 hours) and therefore has been used more in research than in clinical settings.[105]

The Autism Diagnostic Observation Schedule (ADOS)[107] is a widely used semistructured, interactive assessment of ASD symptoms. It includes four graded modules and can be used with a broad range of patients from the very young and nonverbal to high-functioning, verbal adults. Modules 1 and 2, geared toward developmentally younger children, assess social interest, joint attention, communication behaviors, symbolic play, and atypical behaviors. Modules 3 and 4 assess higher level functioning individuals, with a focus on conversational reciprocity, empathy, insight into social relationships, and special interests. Administration time is typically less than an hour. For either pair of modules there are empirically derived cutoff scores for autistic disorder and for broader ASDs (such as Asperger syndrome). Studies on the psychometric properties of the Autism Diagnostic Observation Schedule indicate excellent reliability (interrater, internal consistency, and test-retest reliability) for each module, as well as excellent diagnostic validity.[105]

A parent-report alternative to the Autism Diagnostic Interview–Revised for children older than 4 years is the Social Communication Questionnaire.[108] This instrument has a lifetime-behavior version helpful for diagnostic purposes, as well as a current-behavior version that can be used for evaluating a person's change over time.[105] Currently, the widely popular Gilliam Autism Rating Scale[109] has not been subjected to sufficient psychometric study to recommend its use.[105] Several parent report measures have been developed to help diagnose other ASD disorders (e.g., Asperger syndrome), but at present, there is not sufficient empirical study to recommend their use. A clinically practical method of direct observation for children older than 24 months is the Childhood Autism Rating Scale.[110] Little training is necessary to rate 15 items on a 7-point scale (from "typical" to "severely deviant"); the results yield a composite score that is correlated highly with that of the Autism Diagnostic Interview–Revised (although it may over-identify children with mental retardation as having ASD).

Family Assessment

Evaluations in developmental and behavioral pediatrics often include a family assessment in order to understand the interpersonal dynamics of the family system.[111] Using an *unstructured interview format,* a clinician may inquire about family structure, roles, and functioning and explore each family member's perception of a presenting issue or problem. This assessment approach is often useful in family therapy sessions. *Structured interviews* may be employed to ensure that specific areas or topics are covered. *Genograms* are graphic representations of families that begin with a family tree and may include additional details about family structure, cohesiveness or conflicts, timelines of events, and family patterns (e.g., domestic violence, substance abuse, divorce, suicides, health conditions, presence of behavioral disorder). Formal, validated *observational approaches* to family assessment typically involved trained observers who coded ratings during live or videotaped observations of family interactions and are mostly confined to research settings.

There are many *family self-report questionnaires* targeting different aspects of functioning that may be useful in family assessments, especially in research settings.[112] Although questionnaires have psychometric appeal, they carry biases of the individual completing them, which is counter to the spirit of family assessment. Moreover, questionnaires may have limited utility when specific treatment recommendations are developed in clinical settings for a particular family's set of concerns.[111] A popular example of a parent report family questionnaire with research and clinical applications is the Parenting Stress Index.[113] This index consists of 120 items about child characteristics, parent personality, and situational variables, and it yields a Total Stress Score, as well as scale scores for child and parent characteristics. It has been translated and validated for use with a variety of international populations and has been shown to be useful in a clinical contexts.

Functional Outcomes

Measures of global functioning are typically ratings of a clinician's judgment about a child or adolescent's overall functioning in day-to-day activities at school, at home, and in the community.[114] Measures of global functioning are useful for identifying need for treatment, as well as for monitoring treatment effects and predicting treatment outcome. The importance of global functioning is reflected in the placement of the Global Assessment of Functioning—which stipulates that impairment in one of more areas of functioning is necessary in order to meet criteria for a diagnosis—as Axis V on the *DSM-IV.* The Global Assessment of Functioning is a scale of a mental health continuum from 1 to 100 with 10 anchor descriptions; higher scores reflect better functioning. For example, a score between 31 and 40 would be given for a child with major functional impairment in several areas (frequently beats up younger children, is unruly at home, and is failing in school); a score between 61 and 70 is given to a child with mild symptoms (mild depressed mood) or some difficulties in functioning (disruptive in school) but who generally functions fairly well and who has good social relationships. Shaffer and colleagues modified the anchors of the Global Assessment of Functioning to pertain better to youth, creating the Children's Global Assessment Scale (CGAS).[115] This instrument yields one score and has been used in a large number of psychiatric outcome studies, especially medication-related research.[111]

A widely used measure of functioning is the Child and Adolescent Functional Assessment Scale.[116] This measure is a clinician-rated instrument consisting of behavioral descriptions (e.g., is expelled from school, bullies peers) grouped into levels of impairment for each of five domains: role performance (school/work, home, community), behavior toward others, moods/self-harm, substance use, and thinking. The Child and Adolescent Functional Assessment Scale has been shown to have considerable criterion-related and predictive validity and is widely used to evaluate outcome in clinical settings and in clinical research.[111]

Adaptive functioning measures such as the Vineland Adaptive Behavior Scales[117] are used to assess personal and social skills needed for everyday living and are especially useful for identifying children with mental retardation, developmental delays, and pervasive developmental disorders. The Vineland scales include survey interview and parent/caregiver rating forms that yield domain and adaptive behavior composite standard scores ($M = 100$, $SD = 15$), percentile ranks, adaptive levels, and age-equivalent scores for individuals from birth to age 90 years. Domains assessed include Communication, Daily Living Skills, Socialization, Motor Skills, and an optional Maladaptive Behavior Index.

Health-related quality-of-life (HRQOL) measures have been developed to evaluate functional outcomes in clinical and health services research. HRQOL measures differ from more traditional measures of health status and physical functioning by also assessing broader psychosocial dimensions such as emotional, behavioral, and social functioning. The Pediatric Quality of Life Inventory (PedsQL 4.0)[118] is an example of an HRQOL measure that has been developed and validated for use in pediatric settings. The PedsQL 4.0 Generic Core Scales assess physical, emotional, social, and school functioning with child self-report (ages 5 to 18) and parallel parent proxy-report formats (for children aged 2 to 18 years). Physical Health and Psychosocial Health summary scores are transformed to a scale of 0 to 100 in which higher scores reflect better health-related quality of life. The PedsQL 4.0 had excellent internal consistency reliability in a large pediatric sample, distinguished healthy children from those with chronic health conditions, and was related to other indicators of health status.[118]

SUMMARY AND IMPLICATIONS FOR CLINICAL CARE

Interviews, psychological tests, rating scales, and other measurement strategies are central in the comprehensive assessment of behavior and development of children. Use of assessment techniques in the cases featured in this chapter highlight the contributions of multi-informant, multimethod evidence-based approaches to the clinical care of children

referred for developmental and behavioral services. As a result of the comprehensive evaluation, the teenager in Case 2 (Rachel) received a diagnosis of Major Depression, single episode, along with Cognitive Disorder not otherwise specified. Treatment recommendations included individual cognitive behavior therapy to focus on adaptive coping, a trial of antidepressive medication, family education, and educational adjustments to allow her to have more time to complete school work. She opted to continue to take advanced language courses but enrolled in slower paced math courses. Interventions were very successful; subsequent assessments were used to verify treatment effects.

A psychological evaluation is complete when assessment data have been organized, synthesized, integrated, and presented, usually in the form of a written report.[1,17] Reports are usually independent documents written with an intended audience in mind. They should include assessment findings, such as relevant history, current problems, assets, and limitations, as well as behavioral observations and test interpretations. A typical report includes the following sections or elements: identifying information, reason for referral, sources of assessment information (including tests administered if any), behavioral observations, results and impressions, recommendations, and summary.

A major concern in developmental and behavioral assessment has been the misuse of test data.[1] For example, deviations from standardized procedures in test administration, disrespect for copyrights, use of tests for purposes without adequate research support, interpretation of results without taking into account appropriate norms or reference groups, and use of a single test score for making decisions about a child are among more common problems with test use. Led by a consortium of professional associations (including the American Educational Research Association, the American Psychological Association, and the National Council on Measurement in Education), the Joint Committee on Testing Practices has ongoing workgroups charged with improving quality of test use. Several documents have been created to guide professionals who might develop or use educational or psychological tests, including *Standards for Educational and Psychological Testing*[119] and the *Code of Fair Testing Practices in Education (Revised)*.[120]

Another important clinical issue pertains to what qualifications are necessary for psychological test administrators. Although a thorough review of these issues is beyond the scope of this chapter, the Joint Committee on Testing Practices has developed guidelines that address this issue.[121,122] Most discussions about user qualifications emphasize knowledge and skills necessary to administer and interpret tests in the context in which a particular measure is being used, as opposed to a particular professional degree or license. Some instruments can be administered with relatively little training in psychometric issues (e.g., clinical rating scales such as the Vanderbilt ADHD Diagnostic Scales), whereas other instruments require extensive training and supervised experience (e.g., individually administered ability tests such as the BSID or Wechsler tests). To be qualified to administer most of the instruments discussed in this chapter, a test user should have extensive knowledge and skills related to psychometrics and measurement, selection of appropriate tests, test administration, and other variables that influence test data. Such knowledge and skills generally require advanced graduate level coursework in psychology and supervised clinical experience. Psychologists (among others) are generally those who are qualified to use psychological tests properly.

Proper use of tests in clinical assessments require high level skills and professional judgments in order to make valid interpretation of scores and data collected from multiple sources, with the use of proper test selection, administration, and scoring procedures.[122] When selecting methods, the clinician evaluates whether the construction, administration procedures, scoring, and interpretation of the methods under consideration match the current assessment need, knowing that mismatches may invalidate test interpretation. Instrument selection also is influenced by practical considerations such as training, familiarity, personal preference, and availability of test materials. Cost considerations may also factor into instrument selection. Test development can be very costly, especially if normative samples are broadly developed. Therefore, it may not be financially feasible to purchase test materials for all clinical assessments.

We wish to emphasize the importance of adhering to standardized administration procedures in using psychological tests. Valid interpretation of measurement results cannot be made if there are deviations in administration or scoring procedures. For example, interpretations based on test procedures that have been altered or shortened for convenience or other reasons without accompanying psychometric study are not valid or clinically sound. Likewise, interpretation of assessment results should never rely solely on test scores.[1] Clinical judgments should be made by integrating assessment and observational data, taking into consideration whether results are congruent with other pieces of information, discrepancies from different sources, and factors affecting the reliability and validity of results (e.g., motivation of child, language barriers).

Use of standardized ability, achievement, and behavioral tests has come under attack since the 1980s. Critics have argued that intelligence and achievement tests used to allocate limited educational resources penalize children whose family, cultural, and socioeconomic status are different from middle-class European American children.[1] Specifically, it has been argued that intelligence and achievement tests are culturally biased and thus harmful to African American children and other ethnic minorities. Other experts have been critical of test use to label children or have argued that norm-referenced tests are imperfect in what they measure and therefore have little or no utility in the classroom. Dialog on these criticisms has led to improved test practices, including more representative normative groups, increased availability of tests in languages other than English, increased awareness of cultural factors among clinicians administering and interpreting tests, and use of criterion- or curriculum-based assessments.

Computers are playing more of a role in clinical assessments. They can facilitate administration and scoring of some tests and interview methods, recording of observational data, preparation of reports, and transmittal of assessment information.[1] For example, the CBCL's computer scoring program yields several score profiles, including useful cross-informant comparisons along with a narrative report.[67] Computer-administered assessment methods have several advantages, including eliminating human clinicians' biases, calculation errors, and memory difficulties. Computers will probably be used more extensively in the future to assist in selecting assessment instruments, making diagnoses, designing interventions, and monitoring treatment effects. However, it unlikely that computers will supplant the clinician, who will still be needed to integrate computer-generated results into meaningful recommendations. In fact, there are potential dangers of using computer-generated reports, and knowledgeable professionals understand that these reports should be used cautiously when being incorporated into assessment reports.

SUMMARY AND IMPLICATIONS FOR RESEARCH

Selecting the right measure for a specific research or clinical purpose can be a daunting prospect. It is important to recognize that developmental and behavioral measures are not limited to published tests and that literally thousands of unpublished, noncommercial inventories, checklists, scales, and other instruments exist in the behavioral sciences literature. To avoid the time-consuming task re-creating instruments, researchers are urged to investigate what existing measures are available to suit a particular need. The American Psychological Association Web site *(http://www.apa.org/science/faq-findtests.html)* provides helpful information about locating both published and unpublished test instruments. For example, the PsycINFO database (usually available at a local library) is an excellent source of information on the very latest behavioral science research, including testing. In addition, the *Buros Mental Measurements Yearbooks*[123] have provided consumer-oriented, critical test reviews since 1938 and can provide evaluative information for informed test selection. The Buros Center for Testing also offers online reviews and information about nearly 4000 measures at *www.unl.edu/buros*. Fortunately, most commercially available tests can be located and purchased easily by accessing Web sites on the Internet.

Practitioners may be tempted to use measures developed as research tools for clinical purposes. This is unwise and may represent a misuse of an instrument. Measures shown to be "reliable and valid" for a research study application may have little evidence of validity for a particular child in a clinical context. For example, a measure of family dysfunction that predicts symptom improvement in group comparisons may have little applicability in clinical settings. Often, the length of the research instrument and/or the scoring procedures precludes clinical use.

Unfortunately, there are as yet no clear guidelines or criteria with which to evaluate measures or to decide what measures are better than others.[4] However, with psychometric study and refinement, many research tools can become important clinical measures with evidence to support their use.

Assessment in developmental-behavioral pediatrics is continually evolving in response to new research and clinical problems. This chapter highlights some of the emerging assessment trends being studied such as development of empirically based assessment procedures, expansion of measures appropriate for ethnic minorities and culturally diverse populations (especially children with limited English proficiency), and use of computer-assisted technologies. Internet and Web-based assessment applications are of particular interest, but they also raise concerns about threatened test security, psychometric integrity, and ethical and legal ramifications.[124]

In conclusion, tests and other assessment instruments provide valuable data. Clinicians must consider the levels of assessment involved in obtaining these data: (1) refinement of questions to be answered, (2) selection of appropriate tests to answer questions posed, (3) proper administration and scoring, (4) interpretation, and (5) synthesis with other information and observations. The art of assessment resides in how these findings are integrated and interpreted, so as to develop diagnostic hypotheses and recommendations for intervention. Thus, although knowledge about tests is important, ultimately it is the clinician who is the most important component of the evaluation process.

REFERENCES

1. Sattler JM: Assessment of Children: Cognitive Applications, 4th ed. San Diego: Jerome M. Sattler, 2001.
2. Mash EJ, Hunsley J: Evidence-based assessment of child and adolescent disorders: Issues and challenges. J Clin Child Adolesc Psychol 34:362-379, 2005.
3. McConaughy SH: Clinical Interviews for Children and Adolescents: Assessment to Intervention. New York: Guilford, 2005.
4. Kazdin AE: Evidence-based assessment for child and adolescents: Issues in measurement development and clinical applications. J Clin Child Adolesc Psychol 34: 548-558, 2005.
5. Pelham WE, Fabiano GA, Massetti GM: Evidence-based assessment of attention deficit hyperactivity disorder in children and adolescents. J Clin Child Adolesc Psychol 34:449-476, 2005.
6. Spence SH: Interviewing. *In* Ollendick TH, Schroeder CS, eds: Encyclopedia of Clinical Child and Pediatric Psychology. New York: Kluwer Academic/Plenum, 2003, pp 324-326.
7. Schroeder CS, Gordon BN: Assessment and Treatment of Childhood Problems: A Clinician's Guide, 2nd ed. New York: Guilford, 2002.
8. Shaffer D, Fisher P, Lucas CP, et al: NIMH Diagnostic Interview for Children–IV (NIMH DISC-IV): Description, differences from previous versions, and reliability of some common diagnoses. J Am Acad Child Adolesc Psychiatry 39:28-38, 2000.
8a. American Psychiatric Association: Diagnostic and Statistical Manual of Mental Disorders, 4th ed. Washington, DC: American Psychiatric Association, 1994.
9. Reich W: Diagnostic Interview for Children and Adolescents (DICA). J Am Acad Child Adolesc Psychiatry 39:59-66, 2000.
10. McConaughy SH, Achenbach TM: Manual for the Semistructured Clinical Interview for Children and Adolescents, 2nd ed. Burlington: University of Vermont, Research Center for Children, Youth, & Families, 2001.
11. Achenbach TM: ASEBA: Achenbach System of Empirically Based Assessment, 2005. (Available at: http://www.aseba.org/aboutus/aboutus.html; accessed 10/18/06.)
12. Angold A, Prendergast M, Cox A, et al: The Child and Adolescent Psychiatric Assessment (CAPA). Psychol Med 25:739-753, 1995.
13. Miller WR, Rollnick S: Motivational Interviewing: Preparing People to Change, 2nd ed. New York: Guilford, 2002.
14. DiClemente CC, Prochaska JO: Toward a comprehensive, transtheoretical model of change: Stages of change and addictive behaviors. *In* Miller WR, Heather

N, eds: Treating Addictive Behaviors, 2nd ed. New York: Plenum Press, 1998, pp 3-24.

15. Baer JS, Peterson PL: Motivational interviewing with adolescents and young adults. In Miller WR, Rollnick SR, eds: Motivational Interviewing: Preparing People to Change, 2nd ed. New York: Guilford, 2002, pp 320-332.

16. Sindelar HA, Abrantes AM, Hart C, et al: Motivational interviewing in pediatric practice. Curr Prob Pediatr Adolesc Health Care 34:322-339, 2004.

17. Aylward GP: Practitioner's Guide to Developmental and Psychological Testing. New York: Plenum Medical, 1994.

18. Aylward GP: Infant and Early Childhood Neuropsychology. New York: Plenum Press, 1997.

19. Aylward GP: Measures of infant and early childhood development. In Goldstein G, Beers SR, eds: Comprehensive Handbook of Psychological Assessment, vol 1. Hoboken, NJ: Wiley, 2004, pp 87-97.

20. Aylward GP, Carson AD: Use of the Test Observation Checklist with the Stanford-Binet Intelligence Scales for Early Childhood, Fifth Edition (Early SB5). Presented at the National meeting of the National Association of School Psychologists, Atlanta, GA, April 1, 2005.

21. Bishop D, Butterworth GE: A longitudinal study using the WPPSI and WISC-R with an English sample. Br J Educ Psychol 49:156-168, 1979.

22. Mantynen H, Poikkeus AM, Ahonen T, et al: Clinical significance of test refusal among young children. Child Neuropsychol 7:241-250, 2001.

23. Ounsted M, Cockburn J, Moar VA: Developmental assessment at four years: Are there any differences between children who do, or do not, cooperate? Arch Dis Child 58:286-289, 1983.

24. Wolcaldo C, Rieger I: Very preterm children who do not cooperate with assessments at three years of age: Skill differences at five years. J Dev Behav Pediatr 21:107-113, 2000.

25. Langkamp DL, Brazy JE: Risk for later school problems in preterm children who do not cooperate for preschool developmental testing. J Pediatr 135:756-760, 1999.

26. Roid G: Stanford-Binet Intelligence Scales for Early Childhood. Itasca, IL: Riverside, 2005.

27. Bayley N: Bayley Scales of Infant and Toddler Development. San Antonio, TX: The Psychological Corporation, 2006.

28. Bayley N: Bayley Scales of Infant Development. San Antonio, TX: The Psychological Corporation, 1969.

29. Gesell AL, Halverson HM, Amatruda CS: The First Five Years of Life: A Guide to the Study of the Preschool Child, From the Yale Clinic of Child Development. New York: Harper, 1940.

30. Gesell A: The Mental Growth of the Preschool Child. New York: Macmillan, 1925.

31. Cattell P: Cattell Infant Intelligence Scale. New York: The Psychological Corporation, 1940.

32. Knobloch H, Stevens F, Malone AE: Manual of Developmental Diagnosis. New York: Harper & Row, 1980.

33. Bayley N: Bayley Scales of Infant Development–II. San Antonio, TX: The Psychological Corporation, 1993.

34. Flynn JR: Searching for justice. The discovery of IQ gains over time. Am Psychol 54:5-20, 1999.

35. Black M, Matula K: Essentials of Bayley Scales of Infant Development–II Assessment. New York: Wiley, 2000.

36. Greenspan SI: Greenspan Social-Emotional Growth Chart: A Screening Questionnaire for Infants and Young Children. San Antonio, TX: Harcourt Assessment, 2004.

37. Harrison PL, Oakland T: Adaptive Behavior Assessment System, 2nd ed. San Antonio, TX: The Psychological Corporation, 2003.

38. Dunn LM, Dunn LM: The Peabody Picture Vocabulary Test–III. Circle Pines, MN: American Guidance Service, 1997.

39. Newborg J: Battelle Developmental Inventory–Second Edition. Itasca, IL: Riverside, 2005.

40. Newborg J, Stock JR, Wnek L, et al: The Battelle Developmental Inventory. Itasca, IL: Riverside, 1994.

41. Mullen EM: Mullen Scales of Early Learning. Circle Pines, MN: American Guidance Service, 1984.

42. Mullen EM: Mullen Scales of Early Learning: AGS Edition. Circle Pines, MN: American Guidance Service, 1995.

43. Elliott CD: Differential Ability Scales. San Antonio, TX: The Psychological Corporation, 1990.

44. McCarthy DA: McCarthy Scales of Children's Abilities. New York: The Psychological Corporation, 1972.

45. Kaufman AS, Kaufman NL: Kaufman Brief Intelligence Test, Second Edition. Circle Pines, MN: American Guidance Service, 2004.

46. Roid G: The Stanford-Binet Intelligence Scale–Fifth Edition. Itasca, IL: Riverside, 2003.

47. Kaufman AS, Kaufman NL: Kaufman Assessment Battery for Children–Second Edition. Circle Pines, MN: American Guidance Service, 2004.

48. Wechsler D: Wechsler Preschool and Primary Scale of Intelligence–Third Edition. San Antonio, TX: The Psychological Corporation, 2002.

49. Wechsler D: Wechsler Intelligence Scale for Children–Fourth Edition. San Antonio, TX: The Psychological Corporation, 2003.

50. Wechsler D: The WASI: Wechsler Abbreviated Scale of Intelligence. San Antonio, TX: The Psychological Corporation, 1999.

51. Ramsay MC, Reynolds CR: Relations between intelligence and achievement tests. In Goldstein G, Beers SR, eds: Comprehensive Handbook of Psychological Assessment, vol 1. Hoboken, NJ: Wiley, 2004, pp 25-50.

52. Kaufman AS, Kaufman NL: Kaufman Test of Educational Achievement, 2nd ed. Circle Pines, MN: American Guidance Service, 2004.

53. Markwardt EC: Peabody Individual Achievement Test–Revised. Circle Pines, MN: American Guidance Service, 1989.

54. Markwardt EC: Peabody Individual Achievement Test–Normative Update. Circle Pines, MN: American Guidance Service, 1998.

55. Wechsler D: The Wechsler Individual Achievement Test, 2nd ed. San Antonio, TX: The Psychological Corporation, 2001.

56. Wilkerson G: Wide Range Achievement Test, 3rd ed. Wilmington, DE: Wide Range, Inc., 1993.

57. Robertson GJ: Wide Range Achievement Test–Expanded Version. Odessa, FL: Psychological Assessment Resources, 2002.

58. Woodcock RW, McGrew KS, Mather N: Woodcock-Johnson III. Tests of Achievement. Itasca, IL: Riverside, 2001.

59. Leark RA: The Luria-Nebraska Neuropsychological Battery–Children's Revision. *In* Goldstein G, Beers SR, eds: Comprehensive Handbook of Psychological Assessment, vol 1. Hoboken, NJ: Wiley, 2004, pp 147-156.

60. Cohen M: Children's Memory Scale. San Antonio, TX: The Psychological Corporation, 1997.

61. Korkman M, Kirk U, Kemp SL: NEPSY—A Developmental Neuropsychological Assessment. San Antonio, TX: The Psychological Corporation, 1998.

62. Gioia GA, Isquith PK, Guy SC, et al: Behavior Rating Inventory of Executive Function (BRIEF). Odessa, FL: Psychological Assessment Resources, 2000.

63. Sheslow D, Adams W: The Wide Range Assessment of Memory and Learning. Wilmington, DE: Jastak Associates, 1990.

64. Sheslow D, Adams W: Wide Range Assessment of Memory and Learning, 2nd ed. Odessa, FL: Psychological Assessment Resources, 2003.

65. Achenbach TM, McConaughy SH, Howell CT: Child/adolescent behavioral and emotional problems: Implications of cross-informant correlations for situational specificity. Psychol Bull 101:213-232, 1987.

66. McMahon RJ, Frick PJ: Evidence-based assessment of conduct problems in children and adolescents. J Clin Child Adolesc Psychol 34:477-505, 2005.

67. Achenbach TM, Rescorla LA: Manual for ASEBA School-Age Forms & Profiles. Burlington: University of Vermont, Research Center for Children, Youth, & Families, 2001.

68. Achenbach TM: The classification of children's psychiatric symptoms: A factor-analytic study. Psychol Monogr 80(No. 615), 1966.

69. Achenbach TM, Rescorla LA: Manual for ASEBA Preschool Forms & Profiles. Burlington: University of Vermont, Research Center for Children, Youth, & Families, 2000.

70. Achenbach TM, Rescorla LA: Manual for ASEBA Adult Forms & Profiles. Burlington: University of Vermont, Research Center for Children, Youth, & Families, 2003.

71. Achenbach TM, Newhouse PA, Rescorla LA: Manual for ASEBA Older Adult Forms & Profiles. Burlington: University of Vermont, Research Center for Children, Youth, & Families, 2004.

72. Riekert KA, Stancin T, Palermo TM, et al: A psychological behavioral screening service: Use, feasibility, and impact in a primary care setting. J Pediatr Psychol 24:405-414, 1999.

73. Stancin T, Palermo TM: A review of behavioral screening practices in pediatric settings: Do they pass the test? J Dev Behav Pediatr 18:183-194, 1997.

74. Perrin EC, Stein REK, Drotar D: Cautions in using the Child Behavior Checklist: Observations based on research about children with a chronic illness. J Pediatr Psychol 16:411-421, 1991.

75. Reynolds CR, Kamphaus RW: Behavior Assessment System for Children–Second Edition (BASC-2) Manual. Circle Pines, MN: AGS Publishing, 2006.

76. Carter A, Briggs-Gowan M: Infant Toddler Social Emotional Assessment (ITSEA). San Antonio, TX: Harcourt Assessment, 2006.

77. Carter A, Briggs-Gowan M: Brief Infant Toddler Social Emotional Assessment (BITSEA). San Antonio, TX: Harcourt Assessment, 2006.

78. Butcher JN, Williams CL: Minnesota Multiphasic Personality Inventory–Adolescent (MMPI-A) Manual. Minneapolis, MN: University of Minnesota Press, 1992.

79. Society for Personality Assessment: The status of the Rorschach in clinical and forensic practice: An official statement by the Board of Trustees of the Society for Personality Assessment. J Pers Assess 85:219-237, 2005.

80. Morris TL: Sociometric assessment. *In* Ollendick TH, Schroeder CS, eds: Encyclopedia of Clinical Child and Pediatric Psychology. New York: Kluwer Academic/Plenum, 2003, pp 632-634.

81. Weiss B, Harris V, Catron B: Development and initial validation of the Peer-Report Measure of Internalizing and Externalizing Behavior. J Abnorm Child Psychol 30:285-294, 2002.

82. Querido JG, Eyberg SH: Assessment of parent-child interactions. *In* Ollendick TH, Schroeder CS, eds: Encyclopedia of Clinical Child and Pediatric Psychology. New York: Kluwer Academic/Plenum, 2003, pp 40-41.

83. Eyberg SM, Nelson MMcD, Duke M, et al: Manual for the Dyadic Parent-Child Interaction Coding System Third Edition, 2005. (Available at: *http://www.phhp. ufl.edu/~seyberg/PCITWEB2004/Measures/DPICS%20III %20final%20draft.pdf;* accessed 10/18/06.)

84. White S: Parent training: Use of videotaped interactions. Presented at the Great Lakes Society of Pediatric Psychology Conference, Cleveland, OH, March 20, 2000.

85. Shaddy DJ, Colombo J: Attachment. *In* Ollendick TH, Schroeder CS, eds: Encyclopedia of Clinical Child and Pediatric Psychology. New York: Kluwer Academic/Plenum, 2003, pp 43-44.

86. Klein DN, Dougherty LR, Olino TM: Toward guidelines for evidence-based assessment of depression in children and adolescents. J Clin Child Adolesc Psychol 34:412-432, 2005.

87. Kovacs M: Children's Depression Inventory (CDI) Manual. North Tonawanda, NY: Multi-Health Systems, 1992.

88. Angold A, Costello EJ, Messer SC, et al: Development of a short questionnaire for use in epidemiological studies of depression in children and adolescents. Int J Methods Psychiatric Res 25:237-249, 1995.

89. Reynolds WM: Reynolds Child Depression Scale: Professional Manual. Odessa, FL: Psychological Assessment Resources, 1989.

90. Reynolds WM: Reynolds Adolescent Depression Scale: Professional Manual. Odessa, FL: Psychological Assessment Resources, 1987.

91. Poznanski EO, Mokros HB: Children's Depression Rating Scale–Revised (CDRS-R). Los Angeles: Western Psychological Services, 1999.

92. Luby JL, Heffelfinger A, Koenig-McNaught AL, et al: The Preschool Feelings Checklist: A brief and sensitive measure for depression in young children. J Am Acad Child Adolesc Psychiatry 43:708-717, 2004.

93. Silverman WK, Ollendick TH: Evidence-based assessment of anxiety and its disorders in children and adolescents. J Clin Child Adolesc Psychol 34:380-411, 2005.

94. March JS, Parker JDA, Sullivan K, et al: The Multidimensional Anxiety Scale for Children (MASC): Factor structure, reliability, and validity. J Am Acad Child Adolesc Psychiatry 36:554-565, 1997.

95. Beidel DC, Turner SM, Morris TL: A new inventory to assess childhood social anxiety and phobia: The Social Phobia and Anxiety Inventory for Children. Psychol Assess 7:73-79, 1995.

96. La Greca AM, Stone WL: Social Anxiety Scale for Children–Revised: Factor structure and concurrent validity. J Clin Child Psychol 22:7-27, 1993.

97. La Greca AM, Lopez N: Social anxiety among adolescents: Linkages with peer relations and friendships. J Abnorm Child Psychol 26:83-94, 1998.

98. Reynolds CR, Richmond BO: Revised Children's Manifest Anxiety Scale: Manual. Los Angeles: Western Psychological Services, 1985.

99. DuPaul GJ, Power TJ, Anastopoulos AD, et al: ADHD Rating Scale-IV—Checklists, Norms, and Clinical Interpretations. New York; Guildford, 1998.

100. Wolraich ML, Lambert W, Doffing MA, et al: Psychometric properties of the Vanderbilt ADHD Diagnostic Parent Rating Scale in a referred population. J Pediatr Psychol 28:559-567, 2003.

101. Collett BR, Ohan JL, Myers KM: Ten-Year Review of Rating Scales. V: Scales Assessing Attention-Deficit/Hyperactivity Disorder. J Am Acad Child Adolesc Psychiatry 42:1015-1037, 2003.

102. American Academy of Pediatrics: Diagnosis and evaluation of the child with attention-deficit/hyperactivity disorder. Pediatrics 105:1158-1170, 2000.

103. Brown RT, Freeman WS, Perrin JM, et al: Prevalence and assessment of attention-deficit/hyperactivity disorder in primary care settings. Pediatrics 107:e43, 2001. (Available at: http://pediatrics.org/cgi/content/full/107/3/e43; accessed 10/18/06).

104. Dulcan M: Practice parameters for the assessment and treatment of children, adolescents, adults with attention-deficit/hyperactivity disorder. American Academy of Child and Adolescent Psychiatry. J Am Acad Child Adolesc Psychiatry 36(10 Suppl):85S-121S, 1997.

105. Ozonoff S, Goodlin-Jones BL, Solomon M: Evidence-based assessment of autism spectrum disorders in children and adolescents. J Clin Child Adolesc Psychol 34:523-540, 2005.

106. Rutter M, LeCouteur A, Lord C: Autism Diagnostic Interview–Revised Manual. Los Angeles: Western Psychological Services, 2003.

107. Lord C, Rutter M, DiLavore PC, et al: Autism Diagnostic Observation Schedule Manual. Los Angeles: Western Psychological Services, 2002.

108. Rutter M, Bailey A, Berument SK, et al: Social Communication Questionnaire (SCQ) Manual. Los Angeles: Western Psychological Services, 2003.

109. Gilliam JE: Gilliam Autism Rating Scale. Austin, TX: PRO-ED, 1995.

110. Schopler E, Reichler R, Renner B: Childhood Autism Rating Scale (CARS). Los Angeles: Western Psychological Services, 1988.

111. Kazak A: Family assessment. *In* Ollendick TH, Schroeder CS, eds: Encyclopedia of Clinical Child and Pediatric Psychology. New York: Kluwer Academic/Plenum, 2003, pp 231-232.

112. Touliatos J, Straus M, Perlmutter B: Handbook of family measurement techniques. Thousand Oaks, CA: Sage Publications, 2000.

113. Abidin RR: Parenting Stress Index, 3rd Edition Manual. Lutz, FL: Psychological Assessment Resources, 1995.

114. Hodges K: Assessment of global functioning. *In* Ollendick TH, Schroeder CS, eds: Encyclopedia of Clinical Child and Pediatric Psychology. New York: Kluwer Academic/Plenum, 2003, pp 38-40.

115. Shaffer DM, Gould S, Brasic J, et al: A Children's Global Assessment Scale (CGAS). Arch Gen Psychiatry 40:1228-1231, 1983.

116. Hodges K: Child and Adolescent Functional Assessment Scale (CAFAS). *In* Marnish ME, ed: The Use of Psychological Testing for Treatment Planning and Outcomes Assessment, 2nd ed. Mahwah, NJ: Erlbaum, 1999, pp 631-664.

117. Sparrow SS, Cicchetti DV, Balla DA: Vineland Adaptive Behavior Scales, 2nd ed. Circle Pines, MN: AGS Publishing, 2006.

118. Varni JW, Burwinkle TM, Seid M, et al: The PedsQL™ 4.0 as a pediatric population health measure: feasibility, reliability, and validity. Ambul Pediatr 3:329-341, 2003.

119. American Educational Research Association, American Psychological Association, National Council on Measurement in Education: The Standards for Educational and Psychological Testing. Washington, DC: AERA Publications, 1999. (Available at: *http://www.apa.org/science/standards.html;* accessed 10/18/06.)

120. Joint Committee on Testing Practices: Code of Fair Testing Practices in Education (Revised). Educational Measurement: Issues and Practice 2:23-26, 2005.

121. Eyde LD, Moreland KL, Robertson GJ: Test User Qualifications: A Data-Based Approach to Promoting Good

Test Use. Washington, DC: American Psychological Association, 1988.

122. Turner SM, DeMers ST, Fox HR, et al: APA's guidelines for test user qualifications: An executive summary. American Psychologist 56:1099-1113, 2001.

123. Spies RA, Plake BS, eds: The Sixteenth Mental Measurements Yearbook. Lincoln: University of Nebraska Press, 2005.

124. Naglieri J, Drasgow F, Schmit M, et al: Psychological testing on the Internet: new problems, old issues . Am Psychol 59:150-162, 2004.

7D.
Assessment of Language and Speech

HEIDI M. FELDMAN ■ CHERYL MESSICK

The development of language represents an important accomplishment for young children, allowing them to participate fully in the human community. Language learning progresses rapidly in the toddler and preschool era. At age 1 year, typically developing children are just beginning to understand and produce words. By age 4 to 5 years, they can participate actively in conversations and construct long and complex discussions. The process of language learning proceeds in a predictable and orderly manner for the majority of children. However, the pace is slow and the pattern disordered for many children. The overall prevalence of language disorders at school entry has been estimated at approximately 7%,[1] and the overall prevalence of speech disorders, at nearly 4%.[2] In view of the pivotal role of language and speech in learning, communication, and social relationships, and because of the high prevalence of disorders, screening for language delays and disorders is appropriate for all children and comprehensive assessments of language and speech is appropriate for those at high risk for delays or disorders.

Language is conceptualized as being composed of receptive and expressive domains and as having multiple components within those domains. These subcomponents are usually coordinated in normal functioning. However, in disorders, one or more subcomponents may become deficient or abnormal. Similarly, speech is composed of multiple, independent features. Assessment strategies and tools for language and speech at any age are designed to assay skills in several components. Assessment strategies and tools for language and speech in children are also based on the normal progression of milestones throughout early childhood and on evidence of substantial delay or difference. Accordingly, this chapter begins with definitions of language, speech, and the subcomponents. It proceeds to a review of the course of language development in children from birth to school age and a description of individual variations within the normal range. Next follows a discussion of the approaches to assessing language in infants, toddlers, and young preschoolers. The approaches for young children are contrasted with the approaches for school-aged children and adolescents. Finally, tables of measures that can be used across the age range for assessments of language and speech are included.

BASIC DEFINITIONS

Language is the main medium through which humans share ideas, thoughts, emotions, and beliefs. Unlike other methods of communication, language is symbolic; meaning is conveyed by arbitrary signs. Cries and giggles are signs that arise as reflexive responses or as emissions from the emotional or motivational state that they represent. Therefore, cries and giggles are communicative but not language. In contrast, words and sentences are arbitrary and therefore can vary from language to language. A dog can be labeled *perro* in Spanish, *chien* in French, and so forth. Language is also rule-governed. In English, for example, the order of words in a sentence cannot be significantly altered without changing meaning or rendering the sequence ungrammatical. For example, "Bill kissed Sue" has a different meaning than "Sue kissed Bill." Moreover, "See the dog" is a grammatical sentence, but "dog the see" is not. These features of language—the use of symbols in a systematic manner to convey meanings—provide people with the ability to create and understand an infinite number of messages.

Language is distinct from speech. *Speech* refers specifically to articulation of sounds and syllables created by the complex interaction of the respiratory system, the larynx, the pharynx, the mouth structures, and the nose. Sign languages also meet the definition of language but entail the configuration and movement of hands, arms, facial muscles, and body to articulate meaning. Similarly, written languages convey meaning through the use of arbitrary symbols on a page. It is possible to have a speech disorder without a language disorder and the converse. However, children may exhibit disorders in speech and language concurrently. In this chapter, discussion focuses on the assessment of verbal language and speech.

TABLE 7D-1 ■ Domains and Components of Language and Speech

Term	Definition	Example
Language		
Receptive language	Ability to understand another's language	A father says, "Where are my shoes?" and the child points under the chair to the father's sneakers.
Expressive language	Ability to produce language	A father says, "Where are my shoes?" and the child responds, "Under the chair."
Phoneme	The smallest units of the sound system that change meaning of a word	/b/ and /p/ are different phonemes, and their use results in different words, as in *bat* and *pat*.
Morpheme	The smallest unit of meaning in language	The plural /s/ is a morpheme; when added to the word *book,* it conveys a different meaning: *books.*
Syntax	The set of rules for combining morphemes and words into sentences	"The boy ate his supper" follows English syntax. "Ate the boy supper the" does not follow English syntax.
Semantics	The meaning of words and sentences	Vocabulary, categorization of meanings, and sentence structures all contribute to semantics.
Pragmatics	Social aspects or actual use of language	Pragmatic behaviors focus on discourse rules, presuppositional behavior, and communicative functions.
Speech		
Intelligibility	The ability of speech to be understood	Speech sound errors, rate of speech, familiarity with the speaker and message, and background noise are some of the factors that may decrease intelligibility.
Fluency	The forward flow of speech	Dysfluency may involve pausing or repetition of sounds, words, and phrases
Stuttering	Repetitions of consonant sounds, prolongation of vowel sounds, or other forms of fragmentation, blockage, or dyscoordination of the forward flow of speech	An example of stuttering is the following: "W-w-would you give m-m-m-eeeee the m-m-milk." Stuttering is often accompanied by secondary behaviors, such as head movements or facial expressions that appear designed to permit forward flow.
Voice and resonance	Qualities of speech based on the passage of air through the larynx, mouth, and nose	Hoarseness may be caused by laryngeal inflammation or nodules. Hyporesonance may be caused by adenoidal hypertrophy. Hypernasality may be due to velopharyngeal insufficiency.

For purposes of understanding mature language use, language is subdivided into several components. Table 7D-1 lists some of the terms used to describe components of language and their definitions. In terms of language, an important division is between receptive and expressive language. *Receptive language* refers to the ability to understand or comprehend another person's language. *Expressive language* refers to the ability to produce language. Receptive language typically begins to develop before expressive language. The two components typically progress in relative synchrony. In some toddlers, however, the ability to produce language lags significantly behind the ability to understand language. Older children may show uneven skills in their abilities to understand and produce, with either domain more advanced than the other. Therefore, comprehensive assessments of language usually include separate evaluations of receptive language or comprehension and expressive language or production. Some standardized measures include separate subtests for comprehension and production. Some measures focus on one or the other component.

Language is also subdivided into subsystems or components, in large part on the basis of the size of units. Comprehensive assessments evaluate multiple subsystems of language in terms of both comprehension and production.

- *Phonemes* are the smallest units in the sound system of a language that serve to change the meaning of a word. For example, in English *bat, pat, bit,* and *bid* are all recognized as different words. Therefore, the single sounds that differentiates among them—/b/, /p/, /a/, /i/, /t/, and /d/—all represent different phonemes in English. The phonological system of a language is composed of the inventory of phonemes and the rules by which phonemes can interact with each other. For example, if a new word in English were needed, the sounds represented by /i/ and /b/ could be combined to create the word *ib,* but the sounds /b/ and /d/ could not be combined because that combination violates the phonological rules of English.
- *Morphemes* are considered the smallest unit of meaning in oral and written language. Words are

free-standing morphemes that are the meaningful building blocks of larger units, such as sentences. Meaningful parts of words, such as the plural "-s" or past tense "-ed" markers are bound morphemes, which, when attached to another morpheme, alter the meaning of the word. In English, there are relatively few bound morphemes, but in other languages, such as Hebrew and Italian, there are many morphemes that can be attached to other morphemes and change the meaning of words.

- *Syntax* comprises the rules for combining morphemes and words into organized and meaningful sentences. In English, most sentences begin with a noun phrase, such as "The boy," followed by a verb phrase, such as "gave the girl a red book." In addition, the adjective *red* should come before the noun *book*, but that arrangement is reversed in some languages. In other languages, such as Italian and German, the syntactic rules require a different arrangement of words: for example, the adjective occurring after the noun it describes, and the verb appearing at the end of the sentence rather than in the middle.

- *Semantics* refers to the meaning of words and sentences. The number of words that a child produces and understands can be considered one element of the child's semantic knowledge. The meaning of sentences is described in such terms as *agents* and *actions,* as distinct from syntax in which sentences may be described in terms of noun and verb phrases. In the sentence "The boy gave the girl a red book," the *boy* is the agent, *gave* is the action, and the *girl* is the recipient or dative. Semantics also includes meaning at concrete and abstract levels, word definitions, and word categories such as synonyms and antonyms. During school age, semantic skills that are learned include knowledge of metaphorical language as in idioms, proverbs, and similes.

- *Pragmatics* refers to social aspects or actual use of language. Pragmatic skills address three broad areas of using language: discourse rules, communicative functions, and presuppositional skills. Examples of discourse rules include features such as appropriate use of intonation and tone of voice, as well as the inclusion of politeness markers in communication. Discourse guidelines also consider the ability to initiate, respond, maintain topics, and appropriately take turns. Discourse rules also cover aspects such as varying the language used in relation to different environments and social interactions. Children vary the style and tone of voice when asking an adult for a favor in comparison with asking a peer. Communicative functions examine the purpose behind a communication act (e.g., requesting, commenting, protesting). Presuppositional skills address the ability to provide a listener with appropriate background information. For example, once a speaker realizes that his or her listeners do not know that "Bob" is his or her cousin, the speaker needs to tell listeners who he is, to increase their understanding of the message.

Several aspects of verbal production are considered parts of speech. Table 7D-1 includes definitions and examples of these components. Speech includes the accuracy of speech sound production. Assessments of speech typically include analysis of the types of speech sound errors. Estimates of intelligibility are used to describe the functional consequences of speech sound errors. Another component of speech production is fluency, defined as the forward flow of speech. Stuttering is a type of dysfluency, characterized by repetition or prolongation of sounds and other fragmentation of the sounds, often accompanied by a sense of effort and by secondary behavioral characteristics that the speaker uses to attempt to reinitiate forward flow of speech. Voice and resonance also affect speech. The flow of air through the vocal cords into the nose and mouth affect the quality of speech. Voice disorders include hoarseness, which may be caused by temporary inflammation of the larynx or by nodules from vocal abuse. Resonance disorders include hyponasality, which is a reduction in the usual amount of air through the nose and may be caused by adenoidal hypertrophy, and hypernasality, which results from excessive air through the nose and may be secondary to a cleft palate.

TYPICAL LANGUAGE DEVELOPMENT

Infancy

Newborns demonstrate the basic building blocks for language development through social interactions with adults. They show preferences for looking at the human face over other visual stimuli and for looking at the eyes and the mouth over other body parts. They also show preferences for listening to the human voice over other auditory stimuli. As newborns, they prefer to listen to their mother's voice over the voice of an unfamiliar woman.[3,4] Some evaluations of newborns include these prerequisites for language in their assessment.

Experimental studies show that infants have fundamental abilities for perceiving, discriminating, and learning speech sounds. At very young ages, they are able to differentiate, for example, between two similar sounds (e.g., /ba/ vs. /pa/).[5] During infancy, they can also detect and use the statistical properties of sound co-occurrences in continuous streams of speech to group syllables into wordlike units.[6] These nonspecific perceptual mechanisms are probably extremely important in helping children to parse the sound stream and begin to comprehend language.[7,8] At the time of this writing, these abilities have been demonstrated in research studies but have not yet been integrated into language assessments.

The language that babies hear from the adults in their environment refines these innate mechanisms. By the time that they are about 9 months of age, children show greater precision in differentiating the phonemes of the native language than phonemes from other languages.[7,9] For example, all infants less than 6 months of age can differentiate between the sounds /r/ and /l/. However, by the time they reach 9 months of age, Japanese infants no longer make that distinction because /r/ and /l/ are not separate phonemes in Japanese[7] while English or American infants still can make the distinction. Although infants as a group show these early abilities in speech perception, it is not clear whether individual differences in the nature or timing of how children process the speech stream are predictive of later functioning. Therefore, clinical assessments of infants currently do not include these types of measures of speech perception.

Table 7D-2 summarizes key milestones in language and speech. All of these milestones should be considered approximations, in view of the wide range of normal. Delays in one or more specific behaviors may or may not prove clinically significant, depending on such variables as risk factors, patterns of development, severity, and the rate of progress in other developmental areas.

In terms of receptive language skills, a few milestones are worth highlighting because either they play a key role in screening tests and assessments of early communication or because they may be demonstrable in a health supervision clinical visit with a child and parent. In terms of receptive language, by about 6 months of age, babies often demonstrate recognition of their own names, either by pausing in their activity when they hear their names or even by looking toward a speaker. By 9 months of age, they typically participate in some social routines, linking appropriate actions with commands, such as "Wave bye-bye," or responding with arms raised to "Would you like me to pick you up?" At around 12 months of age, they show understanding of simple words, responding appropriately to questions, such as "Where's mama?" or commands, such as "Show me the ball."

In terms of expressive language skills, children begin to produce voluntary vocalizations by about 2 to 3 months of age. The first form of sound production is called *cooing,* which is composed of musical vowel-like sounds and occasional /k/- and /g/-like consonants. Shortly after producing such coos in isolation, infants demonstrate the ability to take turns, by vocalizing and cooing responsively with other people in their environment while maintaining eye contact. These patterns constitute the initial phases of communication and establish the patterns for later conversational exchanges. At approximately 6 months of age, children produce more differentiated vocal productions with the addition of consonant sounds. Sounds are produced in syllable chains referred to as *babbling.* Initially the babble is simple repetition of a single syllable, such as "bababa," and as the child gets older, it becomes a chain of different syllables, such as "dabigu." By 12 months of age, some children add sentence-like intonation patterns to the babbling. At this point, the output is referred to as *jargon.* Around the same time, children also begin to produce their first words.

Second Year of Life

In the first half of the second year, receptive language skills progress from understanding single words to simple commands. Toddlers demonstrate the ability to follow common routines, such as "Let's go bye-bye" or "Time for bath" and then simple commands that make arbitrary connections, such as "kiss the pencil." In the second half of the second year, they are able to identify body parts, and as they approach age 2 years, they begin to follow two-part instructions (e.g., "Get the ball and give it to Daddy").

The pace of expressive language skills is initially slow. After the first words appear, at approximately 12 months of life, vocabulary initially grows at a rate of about 5 to 10 words each month, with some words entering and then disappearing from the repertoire. The early vocabulary generally includes more nouns than verbs.[10] Early words may be immature in terms of their sound patterns, restricted to simple combinations of consonants and vowels, such as "baba" for bottle or "wawa" for water. The meaning of early vocabulary words may be quite different from mature meanings. Children may apply a word very selectively, such as the word *dog* only for the family's pet or relatively indiscriminately, such as the word *dog* for any four-legged animal, including cows and cats.

In the second half of the first year, many children developing typically undergo a rapid change in the rate of word learning.[11,12] This spurt usually occurs after a child has at least 35 to 50 different words in his or her vocabulary. The vocabulary grows at a rate of 4 or 5 words a day. At about that time, two-word phrases emerge. Thus, by 2 years of age, children typically can say about 100 words and some two-word phrases. Children use their language to talk about things in the here and now. From that point on, language development proceeds rapidly.

TABLE 7D-2 ■ Developmental Milestones in Receptive and Expressive Language

Age Range	Receptive	Expressive
0-1 months	Startles or widens eyes to sound	Cries
2-4 months	Quiets to voice, blinks eyes to sound	Makes musical sounds, called *cooing* Coos in reciprocal exchanges
5-7 months	Turns head toward sound Looks and responds to own name	Babbles Repeats self-initiated sounds
8-10 months	Links actions to words, responding with raised arms when a parent says "up" or waves when person says "wave bye-bye" Looks at the direction of a point Stops action when hears "no"	Says *mama* or *dada* indiscriminately Points at interesting objects or events
11-14 months	Listens selectively to familiar words Indicates understanding of single words Respond to simple questions such as "Where's mama?" Follows simple commands, such as "Show me the ball"	Uses symbolic gestures Repeats parent-initiated sounds Babbles with intonation patterns of sentences, called *jargon* Uses a few words, such as names, *mama* or *dada* specifically, or animal noises
15-18 months	Points to three body parts (eyes, nose, mouth) Understands up to 50 words Recognizes common objects by name (dog, cat, bottle, ball, book) Follows one-step commands accompanied by gesture ("Give me the doll," "Hug your bear," "Open your mouth")	Uses words to express needs Learns at least 20 words Uses words inconsistently and mixed with jargon, echolalia, or both
19 months- 2 years	Points to pictures when asked, "Show me" Understands *in, on,* and *under* Begins to distinguish *you* from *me* Can formulate negative judgments (a pear is not a cookie)	Says 50 words Uses telegraphic two-word sentences ("Go bye-bye," "Up daddy," "Want cookie")
25-30 months	Follows two-step commands Can identify objects by use	Uses jargon and echolalia infrequently Generates average sentence of $2\frac{1}{2}$ words Learns adjectives and adverbs Begins to ask questions with *what* or *who* Asks adults to repeat actions ("Do it again")
3 years	Knows several colors Knows what people do when they are hungry, thirsty, or sleepy Is aware of past and future Understands *today* and *not today*	Uses pronouns and plurals Can tell stories that begin to be understood Uses negative ("I can't," "I won't") Verbalizes toilet needs Can state full name, age, and gender Creates sentences of 3 to 4 words Asks *why*
$3\frac{1}{2}$ years	Can answer such questions as "Do you have a doggie?"; "Which is the boy?"; and "What toys do you have?" Understands *little, funny,* and *secret*	Can relate experiences in sequential order Says a nursery rhyme Asks permission
4 years	Understands *same* versus *different* Follows three-step commands Completes opposite analogies ("A brother is a boy, a sister is a. . . .") Understands why people have houses, stoves, and umbrellas	Tells a story Uses past tense Counts to 3 Names primary colors Enjoys rhyming nonsense words Enjoys exaggerations
5 years	Understands what people do with eyes and ears Understands differences in texture (hard, soft, smooth) Understands *if, when,* and *why* Identifies words in terms of use Begins to understand *left* and *right*	Indicates "I don't know" Indicates *funny* and *surprise* Can define in terms of use Asks definition of specific words Makes serious inquiries ("How does this work?" and "What does it mean?") Uses mature sentence structure and form, including complex sentences

Unfamiliar listeners may have some difficulty in understanding children younger than age 2 years. The children often show phonetic variability in the production of consonants and multiple processes that simplify speech sounds. It is generally stated that only about half of what 2-year-olds say is intelligible to strangers, although accurate estimation during conversation is quite challenging. By age 2 years, children typically master consonants created at the front of the mouth, including /b/, /p/, /m/, and /w/, and sometimes the sounds produced when the tongue is placed behind the teeth, including /t/, /d/, and /n/. At this age, children use /w/ for many sounds they cannot produce accurately. Their speech is also rendered less intelligible because they reduce consonant clusters to a single sound, such as *top* for *stop*, and they leave off the ends of words or other sounds ("da" for *dog;* "nana" for *banana*).

Preschool Period

By age 3 years, children understand much of what is said to them, commensurate with their cognitive abilities. For example, they learn to recognize colors and can respond appropriately to questions, such as "What do we do when we are hungry?" They can also appreciate what a parent means when he or she says, "We will go to the park today" versus when he or she answers, "Not today" to a question about going to the park. Preschoolers gradually begin to answer different types of questions, including *which, what,* and *when* questions.

In expressive language, they gradually include pronouns, increase the number of verbs and adjectives, and introduce abstract vocabulary items, such as color, quantity, and size terms. Children acquire a variety of grammatical morphemes, including plural marker "-s," possessive marker "-'s," and the "-ing" attached to verbs to convey an ongoing action (e.g., *jumping; eating*). Their syntactic skills expand to include the ability to ask questions and create negative sentences. They build sentences of increasing length and, although still immature in the mastery of syntax, begin to produce sentences with increasing grammatical complexity, including compound sentences with independent and dependent clauses (e.g., "that the one that jump").

A child's phonological system develops as well during the preschool period, and so an increasing proportion of his or her sentences become fully intelligible. On the third birthday, a child's speech is typically intelligible to unfamiliar adults approximately 75% of the time. However, at this age, it is common for children to experience dysfluency in their speech. Often they repeat entire words or phrases, such as, "I want, I want, I want an apple." The impression on

adults is that this developmental dysfluency represents poor coordination of language, speech, and thought. For most children, the dysfluency gradually disappears between ages 4 and 5 years. Characteristics of clinically significant stuttering are as follows: repetition of initial sounds, prolongation of sounds, the need for effort to speak, appearance of secondary behavioral characteristics such as grimacing or repetitive movements, or the child's feelings of inadequacy or embarrassment.

By ages 3 to 4 years, preschoolers begin to participate in conversations, with gradual mastery of pragmatic skills. The also begin to talk about past events and tell short stories, although their initial efforts may be marked by considerable disorganization. However, by ages 4 to 5 years, they connect sentences to describe sequences or scenes or to tell stories in a logical or chronological way. These multiple sentence productions are called *narratives*. They also improve conversational abilities, which allows for longer dialogs. By this age, children are able to converse easily on a variety of topics with familiar as well as unfamiliar listeners. They also show expertise in concepts and vocabulary according to their individual interests (e.g., names of different types of dinosaurs).

School Age through Adulthood

The fundamentals of language are established by school age. At kindergarten entry, typically developing children can understand and produce complex sentences. Language sophistication is typically commensurate with cognitive abilities. Because children have facility with understanding and creating at least simple sentences, individual differences in language and speech abilities may be difficult to detect in routine conversation. It may not be apparent, even to parents and teachers, that children's lack of compliance is related to poor comprehension of what they have been told. Thus, in the late preschool period and at school age, systematic evaluation, with standardized assessment measures, should form the basis of evaluation, rather than informal observational techniques.

By school age, most speech sounds are mature, although some sounds may still be underdeveloped. These include /sh/, /th/, /s/, /z/, /l/, and /r/ and consonant blends such as /sp/, /tr/, and /bl/. Such errors however should not affect intelligibility significantly. By 8 years of age, children should articulate all sounds of the English language correctly in spontaneous conversation.

INDIVIDUAL VARIATIONS IN SPEECH AND LANGUAGE DEVELOPMENT

Patterns of early language development vary among children.[13] Understanding these variations are important for interpretation of assessment data. Some children early on build a vocabulary of object names and use language to talk about the items around them. These children typically pass through the stages described previously, with a clear one-word phase followed by telegraphic two-word sentences (e.g., "Mommy sock" or "baby eat"). Other children learn social expressions, such as "Thank you" or "Give it to me," and use language to express needs or to interact with others. It appears that these children may not understand the components within these rehearsed forms. Their vocabulary of single nouns may be limited, and their speech often includes a lot of jargon. Their progression through the stages described previously may also vary. These early stylistic differences do not seem predictive of major differences in later development and may reflect individual strategies or style, although children who use language to refer to objects come from families with higher levels of education.[13]

The rate of language learning also varies among children. One important factor that has been shown to be predictive of the rate of vocabulary and syntactic development is the amount of child-directed language in the environment.[14,15] Descriptive studies have demonstrated that, on average, parents in the lower socioeconomic strata provide less child-directed language than do parents in the middle socioeconomic class.[16] Children from the lower socioeconomic classes are more likely to show slower language development, reduced vocabulary, and a higher prevalence of language delays than are children from the middle socioeconomic classes.[17] It is important to consider the environmental input of children when the results of language assessments are interpreted. There is no professional consensus about whether and when these early delays constitute an actual language disorder; however, prognosis for spontaneous improvement is affected by the severity of the gap between a child's development and that of peers and by delays across multiple components of language.

Another factor associated with delayed and disordered development is a family history of speech/language or learning difficulties in a first-degree relative. These findings suggest that there are both environmental and biological contributors to the rate and pattern of language development.[18] It is useful to know the family history in interpreting the assessment results of children who have minor delays in language or speech. In addition, for some assessment purposes, evaluation of parental input along with the child's language may provide insights into the causes of developmental deficits.

It is difficult to predict which "late talkers"—that is, children who show initial delays—are destined to develop language disorders. Careful analysis of their language production has not yielded valid prediction. Two features of the child's development that have been associated with resolution of the delays are good receptive language skills and mature symbolic play skills.[19] For this reason, assessment of language in young children should include an evaluation of their play. In addition, the range of communicative functions and social skills that children show may be very indicative of the nature of a language disorder. Mature communication entails using language for varied purposes, including expressing wants and needs, greeting others, describing objects or actions, and answering questions. Communicative and social functioning may be assessed in some evaluation protocols. Finally, the more components of language affected, and the greater the severity of deficit, the higher the likelihood that the child will have long-term communication deficits. A thorough speech/language evaluation therefore requires the assessment of multiple components of language. It includes standardized measures and analysis of spontaneous communication behaviors.

ASSESSMENTS

Purposes of Assessment

There is no single procedure or scheme for the assessment of language and speech in all children. Assessment procedures vary as a function of the age, cognitive level, and social characteristics of the children. In addition, the purpose of evaluation must be considered in the selection of assessment procedures.

Screening is appropriate to establish whether asymptomatic children are at high risk for language or speech impairment. Screening is appropriate for language and speech disorders because the conditions are prevalent and early treatment can reduce the severity of the resulting condition. Screening instruments must be inexpensive to administer because they are designed to be used with large populations. They must also have good sensitivity and specificity, or accuracy in prediction, so that only children at the highest risk of disorder are required to go through a full assessment. In most cases, screening of infants and toddlers relies heavily on parent report because direct assessment of children at young ages is time consuming and nonetheless may not produce representative samples of what the child can do.

Diagnostic testing establishes the clinical status of the child in terms of language abilities and performance. Comprehensive diagnostic testing requires characterization of multiple aspects of language and speech skills. In infants, toddlers, and young preschoolers, the purpose of assessment is often to identify children with delays and disorders who could benefit from early intervention services. The earlier such children can be identified, the more likely they are to benefit from treatment. These diagnostic assessments may also be useful for designing intervention strategies and targets, as well as to monitor the effectiveness of treatment.

In older preschool- and school-aged children, the purpose of assessment is often to explain academic, social, or communication difficulties and to identify children in need of therapeutic and support services. Early speech and language delays are often associated with later reading and spelling problems.[20,21] Speech and language assessment are also important for children who have behavior difficulties, because comprehension deficits may be one factor contributing to behavior disorders. Again, such evaluations may establish the nature of intervention or specific target outcomes. As children get older, assessments are more likely to provide insights into the prognosis for future functioning. At all ages, language and speech assessment are prerequisites for planning treatments and monitoring progress.

Assessing Language in Infants, Toddlers, and Preschoolers

Accurate assessment of infants and toddlers is very challenging. First, the behaviors of interest occur infrequently and unpredictably in young children who are just learning language. Second, young children may have difficulty cooperating for formal assessment procedures. Infants and toddlers are more likely to demonstrate their emerging skills in interactions with parents and other familiar adults rather than with strangers. Third, the attention span of young children is short. Finally, infants and toddlers are not used to remaining seated and following the adult lead in interactions. For all of these reasons, informal observational studies, parent interview tools, and/or natural assessments play an important role in the evaluation of young children. Formal assessments become more central to evaluation as the child reaches preschool age and beyond.

OBSERVATIONAL AND INTERVIEW ASSESSMENT STRATEGIES

Parent diaries have made an important contribution to the initial understanding of the course of language development in young children.[22] The advantage of the diary method, particularly in the hands of parents who are linguists, is that it can be a comprehensive report of verbal output. Creative strategies can be employed to assess the level of comprehension, as well as production. Of course, it is impractical for average parents to keep a comprehensive diary for clinical assessments. Each alternative method requires some degree of sampling from the rich array of child capacities.

An authentic informal approach to language assessment is language sampling. For toddlers, this method typically involves the analysis of parent-child (or clinician-child) conversations. Children and their communicative partners are typically observed as they play with a set of toys, either the child's own or a standardized collection. A sample of at least 50 to 100 utterances is obtained. Experienced speech and language pathologists are able to transcribe and then analyze the conversation with young children in real time, identifying patterns that are used frequently. One major advantage of language sampling is that it assesses functional communication in a naturalistic setting. Another advantage is that multiple components of language, such as vocabulary, syntax, and pragmatics, can be assessed concurrently. Many formal assessment tools do not have strategies for assessing pragmatics, and therefore conversational analysis or language sampling is often a secondary procedure in a comprehensive assessment. Speech sounds in context can also be assessed simultaneously. Formal tests often assess speech sounds in single words rather than in continuous speech. A third advantage is that parental language can be assessed at the same time as child language; this provides the clinician with insight into the quality of the language environment. Often for more detail or for research purposes, the conversation is videotaped and/or audiotaped for later transcription and analysis. If the transcript is prepared as a computer file and transcribed according to a few basic conventions, two prominent programs now available can analyze multiple features of the child's language, as well as the parental language input. Child Language Data Exchange System is publicly available *(http://childes. psy.cmu.edu).*[23] Systematic Analysis of Language Transcripts (SALT) software is commercially available *(http://www.languageanalysislab.com/).*[24] In addition, an automated method to analyze speech sounds is called Programs to Examine Phonetic and Phonological Evaluation Records (PEPPER) *(http://www. waisman.wisc.edu/phonology/project/project.htm)* is also available.[24]

Analysis of parent-child conversation has several limitations in clinical practice. It may require substantial time to transcribe and analyze the conversation. Except for a few measures, such as the mean length of utterances (average sentence length), grammatical morpheme usage, and syntactic complexity,[25] there are no norms for the child's output. Interpretations about the child's level of functioning are based on the types of sentence patterns used, in comparison to the expectations for the child's age. Parents who themselves are not highly communicative may not elicit a representative sample of the child's full capacities. Finally, the method does not directly assess comprehension. In many situations, the advantages of this approach outweigh the limitations. This approach is very useful to monitor progress over time in individual children.

Parent report inventories circumvent some of the challenges of conversational analysis. The inventories tap into a parent's extensive knowledge and frequent observations of their child's abilities. To improve reliability and validity, these inventories concern current abilities rather than past skills or age at acquisition and rely heavily on a recognition rather than recall format. The MacArthur-Bates Communicative Development Inventory (CDI)[11] *(http://www.brookes publishing.com/store/books/fenson-cdi/index.htm)* is designed for children 8 to 30 months of age. The version for children 8 to 16 months of age prompts parents to indicate, from a list of more than 400 words, the number of words understood and produced and also asks parents about specific symbolic gestures and actions that the child performs. The version for children aged 16 to 30 months asks parents to indicate, from a list of almost 700, the words the child produces and also to assess early grammatical development. A shorter version of this inventory is now available. The Language Development Survey (LDS) *(http://www. aseba.org/research/language.html)* assesses vocabulary development in children 18 to 35 months of age.[26] It uses a similar format, with a vocabulary list of 310 words selected on the basis of diary studies. It includes questions about the average length of the child's phrases. Both of these parent report inventories have been shown to have good to excellent reliability and concurrent validity in relation to direct assessments and analysis of conversational samples. Predictive validity is only fair.[27] Specificity of the inventory is higher than sensitivity, which indicates that many children with early delays catch up to within the normal range at older ages.

Parent interview tools provide an alternative method of language assessment. The Receptive-Expressive Emergent Language Test–Third Edition, published by PRO-ED, is designed for infants to 3-year-olds.[27a] The test has two subtests, Receptive Language and Expressive Language, and a new supplementary subtest, Inventory of Vocabulary Words. Parent interviews are also useful in screening tests of

language abilities in infants and toddlers because the relevant data can be collected efficiently. An example is the Pediatric Evaluation of Developmental Status, which asks parents questions and scores their responses in reference to the child's age.[28] This parent report screening tool has comparable sensitivity and specificity as screening tests that assess the child directly.

Direct child observation is another strategy of evaluation for young children. For example, with the Communication and Symbolic Behavior Scales, clinicians evaluate the communication skills of children by observing their play in structured and unstructured situations and their interactions with adults.[29] It is recommended as a tool to use for children with disorders in the autism spectrum (see Chapter 13). On the basis of these observations, the professional administering the test rates the child on multiple scales organized into clusters, such as communicative functions and social-affective signaling. These ratings are converted to standard norm-referenced scores. The Autism Diagnostic Observation Schedule combines parent interview with professional observations of social and communicative behaviors under structured situations.[30] A cutoff score distinguishes children who meet the criteria for autism from children with normal development or other disorders. Finally, the combination of parent interview and direct observation constitutes other language and communication screening tests, such as the Early Language Milestone test,[31] a test that is used as a screening instrument in some pediatric practices.

FORMAL ASSESSMENTS

Individually administered formal assessments of young children can be subdivided into two categories: norm-referenced and criterion-referenced tests. Norm-referenced tests have standardized procedures for administering and scoring the items. Raw scores are converted to age-adjusted standard scores that allow a designated child's results to be compared with those children of the same age. Norm-referenced tests of language development that are used to assess infants, toddlers, and preschoolers are listed in Table 7D-3.

Such tools are often used to qualify a child for early intervention services. In addition, norm-referenced tests are good for comparing the level of language skills to the level of cognitive or motor abilities.

Criterion-referenced tests measure what skills the child has mastered from a set of skills in the usual sequence of development or from a curriculum used to treat children who are delayed in development. Administration of items is flexible and can be adjusted if, for example, children have sensory or motor impairment. Multiple sources of data, including indi-

TABLE 7D-3 ■ **Norm-Referenced Tests for the Assessment for Infants, Toddlers, and Preschoolers**

Assessment Tool	Publisher, Date	Age Rang (Years)	Features
Clinical Evaluation of Language Fundamentals: Preschool (CELF-P)	The Psychological Corporation, 1992	3.0-6.11	Assesses expressive and receptive skills Total language and subscale scores
Kaufman Survey of Early Academic and Language Skills (K-SEALS)	American Guidance Service, 1993	3.0-6.11	Screens speech, language, and preacademic skills Generates scaled scores
Mullen Scales of Early Learning	American Guidance Service, 1993	0-5.8	Includes broad array of abilities
Preschool Language Scale: Fourth Edition (PLS-4)	The Psychological Corporation, 2002	0-6.11	Assesses auditory comprehension and expressive communication Three supplemental tests Generates total score plus separate subscale scores
Receptive-Expressive Emergent Language Test (REEL-3)	PRO-ED, 2003	0-3.0	Assesses comprehension and expressive communication through parent interview and observation format
Sequenced Inventory of Communication Development: Revised (SICD-R)	University of Washington Press, 1984	0.4-4.0	Assesses expressive and receptive skills and areas in need of further assessment Generates age-equivalent score
Test of Early Language Development: Third Edition (TELD-3)	PRO-ED, 1999	2.0-7.11	Assesses receptive and expressive language, syntax, and semantics Generates scaled scores plus subtest scores

TABLE 7D-4 ■ **Criterion-Referenced Assessments for Infants, Toddlers, and Preschoolers**

Assessment Tool	Publisher, Date	Age Range (Years)	Features
Battelle Developmental Inventory–2	Riverside Publishing, 2005	0-7.11	Allows multiple assessment methods Provides scaled scores and age-equivalent scores
Brigance Diagnostic Inventory of Early Development: Revised Edition	Curriculum Associates, 1991	0-6.11	Generates a developmental quotient and developmental age
Developmental Assessment of Young Children	PRO-ED, 1998	0-5.0	Allows multiple assessment methods Provides scaled scores and age-equivalent scores
Diagnostic Evaluation of Language Variance (DELV)	Harcourt, 2003	4.0-9.0	Appropriate for children who speak nonstandard English Integrates assessment of phonology, semantics, syntax, and pragmatics
Hawaii Early Learning Profile: Birth to Three	VORT Corporation, 1994	0-3.0	Allows multiple assessment methods Generates age-equivalent score
Rossetti Infant-Toddler Language Scale	Lingui Systems, Inc., 1990	0-3.0	Assesses interaction-attachment, gesture, play, comprehension and expression

vidually administered test items, parent reports, and casual professional observations, can all be used to determine whether a child should be given credit for any given item. Criterion-referenced measurement emphasizes the specific behaviors that have been mastered, rather than the relative standing of the child in reference to the group. A listing of representative criterion-referenced tests can be found in Table 7D-4.

An advantage of criterion-referenced tests, particularly for young children, is that they can be used to simultaneously assess children and plan educational or therapeutic interventions. For this reason, these measures are often used in federally funded early intervention programs to qualify children for services and generate the Individualized Family Service Plans. Most of these tests are comprehensive and include one or more sections on communication or language. Many criterion-referenced tests generate age-equivalent scores or developmental quotients, rather than or in addition to scaled scores.

Assessing Language in Older Preschool- and School-Aged Children

As children grow older, their language and speech skills become increasingly differentiated. Assessment of language and speech skills often requires either a comprehensive test or multiple measures to survey the full array of language components. Formal norm-referenced measures play an increasingly prominent role, although informal assessment continues to provide interesting insights into functional communication, as well as speech patterns.

COMPREHENSIVE FORMAL MEASURES

In assessing speech and language skills in children in the late preschool- or school-age period, speech and language pathologists frequently choose a comprehensive formal measure that surveys a variety of language components. These tests usually assess receptive and expressive skills in separate subtests. They typically generate subscale scores, as well as a composite score. It is essential to evaluate the pattern of subtest scores, as well as the composite, to determine whether a child's disorder is general or specific. A representative list of comprehensive language measures is found in Table 7D-5. Note that the age ranges for the tests and the types of subtests vary across instruments. The choice of an instrument from this list is often related to the purpose of the evaluation.

FORMAL MEASURES OF LANGUAGE COMPONENTS AND SPEECH

In many situations, a single comprehensive measure fails to provide the necessary information for understanding a child's profile of strengths and weaknesses in language and speech. In these circumstances, speech and language pathologists design an assessment protocol, often choosing one or more formal measures for specific language components to supplement the comprehensive tests or to test specific hypotheses about a child's profile. For example, a child's scores on a receptive vocabulary test may be depressed because the child impulsively pointed at a picture after presentation of the stimulus before carefully considering all options. In such a case, the comparison of receptive and expressive vocabulary may be informative. If the child's performance on one domain of language is particularly weak on a comprehensive test, validation with a second measure might be advisable. Table 7D-6 lists some of the measures that assess specific components of language.

In addition to measures of oral language, the speech and language pathologist may also be called upon to provide measures of preliteracy and literacy skills. Children with deficits in language or speech are at high risk for deficits in reading and writing skills. In preschool children, formal measures of prereading

TABLE 7D-5 ■ Comprehensive Norm-Referenced Tests of Language Abilities for School-Aged Children and Adolescents			
Assessment Tool	**Publisher, Date**	**Age Range (Years)**	**Features**
Clinical Evaluation of Language Fundamentals: Fourth Edition	Psychological Corporation, 2003	5.0-21.0	Assesses language content, structure, and memory Generates total language and subtest scores
Comprehensive Assessment of Spoken Language	American Guidance Service, 1999	3.0-21.0	Measures comprehension, expression, and retrieval Generates scaled scores for total and supplemental indices
Language Processing Test: Revised	Lingui Systems, Inc., 1995	5.0-11.11	Assesses ability to process, organize, and attach meaning to sound
Oral and Written Language Scales (OWLS)	American Guidance Service, 1995	3.0-21.0	Assesses listening comprehension, oral expression, and written expression Composite and Listening comprehension scores
Test of Adolescent Language: Third Edition (TOAL-3)	PRO-ED, 1994	12.0-24.11	Assesses verbal language, reading and written language Generates composite and subscale scores
Test of Language Development–Intermediate: Third Edition (TOLD-I:3)	PRO-ED, 1997	8.0-12.11	Assesses spoken language, semantics, syntax, listening, and speaking Generates quotients for each section
Test of Language Development–Primary: Third Edition (TOLD-P:3)	PRO-ED, 1997	4.0-8.11	Assesses listening, organizing, speaking, semantics, syntax, and spoken language Generates scaled score for each section

TABLE 7D-6 ■ Tests to Assess Specific Subcomponents of Language

Assessment Tool	Publisher, Date	Age Range (Years)	Features
Expressive One Word Vocabulary Test (EOWVT)	Academic Therapy Publications, 2000	2.0-12.1	Primarily assesses words but may provide information on other components Provides scaled scores
Listening Skills Test (LIST)	The Psychological Corporation, 2001	3.0-11.0	Assesses ability to make decisions about verbal language Provides total score
Peabody Picture Vocabulary Test: Third Edition (PPVT-III)	American Guidance Service, 1997	2.5-adulthood	Primarily assesses single-word vocabulary by pointing, but may provide information on attention
Receptive One-Word Vocabulary Test: 2000	Academic Therapy Publications, 2000	2.0-18.11	Single-word vocabulary comprehension Provides scaled score
Structured Photographic Expressive Language Test: Third Edition (SPELT-3)	Janelle Publications, 2003	4.0-9.11	Assesses morphology and syntax Generates scaled score
Test for Auditory Comprehension of Language: Third Edition (TACL-3)	PRO-ED, 1999	3.0-9.11	Assesses understanding of vocabulary, grammar, and sentence structure Generates total composite score
Test of Pragmatic Language (TOPL)	PRO-ED, 1992	5.0-13.11	Assesses appropriateness of pragmatic and social skills Generates composite score

TABLE 7D-7 ■ Individually Administered Speech Assessment Tools

Assessment Tool	Publisher, Date	Age Range (Years)	Features
Arizona Articulation Proficiency Scale: Third Edition	Western Psychological Services, 2000	1.5-18.0	Generates age-equivalent, intelligibility, and severity ratings
Goldman-Fristoe Test of Articulation: Second Edition	American Guidance Service, 2000	2.0-20.0	Three subtests: Sounds-in-Words, Sounds-in-Sentences, Stimulability Generates age- and grade-equivalent scores, gender-specific norms
Khan-Lewis Phonological Analysis: Second Edition	American Guidance Service, 2002	2.0-21.0	To analyze speech sound errors, this is used with the Goldman Fristoe test Generates standard score, age- and grade-equivalent scores, and percentage of occurrence
Photo Articulation Test: Third Edition	PRO-ED, 1997	3.0-8.11	Generates standard, age-, and grade-equivalent scores
Stuttering Severity Instrument for Children and Adults: Third Edition	PRO-ED, 1994	2.10-adulthood	Provides frequency and duration scores, physical concomitants, total score Mean scaled score and descriptive severity level
Voice Assessment Protocol for Children and Adults	PRO-ED, 1997	4.0-18.0	Evaluates pitch, loudness, quality, breath features, rate, and rhythm Generates scaled score for pitch

and prewriting skills, tools such as the Test of Early Reading Abilities provide measures of whether the child is acquiring the foundation for beginning to acquire reading skills. In school-aged children, reading and writing skills can be assessed by standardized tools such as the Woodcock-Johnson battery or the Test of Written Language.

Because a child's skills in language and speech may be completely different, it is usually appropriate to include specific procedures to assess speech in a comprehensive evaluation of a young child. Several tests are available to assess speech sound development. A representative list of such tests is included in Table 7D-7. In school-aged students who may exhibit articulation difficulties on a small subset of sounds, measures from conversational samples may be used, rather than testing from single-word articulation tests.

INFORMAL ASSESSMENTS

Informal assessment strategies continue to play an important role in the evaluation of school-aged children. Informal assessments are sometimes the best strategy for evaluating pragmatic skills, such as topic maintenance, speech acts, and sensitivity to the needs of a listener. They may also serve to demonstrate how a child integrates knowledge and skills at the level of words and sentences into connected discourse, such as in telling or retelling stories, relating the sequence of a day or daily activity, or describing a complex picture. Finally, direct observations or parent-child, clinician-child, or peer-peer interaction may be used to generate a speech/language sample. The advantage of using observations is that formal tests tend to evaluate only speech sounds in individual words. Observations of speech in conversation and narratives allow the clinician to determine whether sounds that are intelligible in individual words remain interpretable in connected discourse.

CONCLUSIONS AND EMERGING ISSUES

Evaluation of language and speech in young children is an essential component of developmental assessments because language and speech play a vital role in multiple functional domains, including learning, communication, controlling behavior, and interacting with others; because developmental delays and disorders in these domains are highly prevalent; and because early treatment is effective at reducing long-term adverse outcomes. Screening assessments for language and speech should be part of routine health supervision in children up to school age. Screening measures tend to rely on or incorporate parental reports of the child's communication. These reports tend to be comparable to observational measures. Comprehensive assessments of speech and language by a speech and language pathologist should be completed when parents, physicians, or educators have concerns about a child or when a child does not pass a screening test. Observational or interview procedures are important in the assessment of young children, because children may have difficulty in cooperating with formal procedures. Comprehensive assessments of school-aged children must include formal techniques because children may have adequate conversational skills that mask difficulties in comprehension or production. Comprehensive assess-

ments must address multiple components of communication, including comprehension and production of language and speech. In assessments of language, clinicians should consider strengths and weaknesses in the various subcomponents, including vocabulary, syntax, and pragmatics. Assessments of speech should include evaluation of sounds in single words and in connected discourse and should also address the issues of fluency, voice, and resonance, when appropriate. In addition, level of speech intelligibility in conversation should be addressed. When these elements are included in the assessment, the nature of the child's communication deficits can be understood, appropriate diagnostic workups conducted, and suitable interventions initiated.

Research to evaluate and demonstrate the reliability and validity of measures to assess speech and language functioning and disorders in children is still needed. Some measures in common use have limited reliability and validity. Many of the measures do not have norms for subgroups within the populations, such as children from low socioeconomic status, children from racial and ethnic minorities, and bilingual children. There is a stunning lack of appropriate instruments for assessing speech and language in many subgroups defined in terms of language, dialect, or cultural characteristics.

Research is also needed to determine whether speech and language assessment instruments in current use are appropriate for assessment of children with different disorders, such as hearing impairment, cognitive impairments, and autism. Such research would require testing the measures on large and representative samples of these subgroups. It would also require establishing the reliability and validity of instruments for the subpopulations and not just for the total normative sample.

A major issue in language and speech assessments at present is that current evaluations of children, particularly at the youngest ages, have limited predictive validity with regard to language or speech skills at older ages.[27] Specificity of these early assessments is considerably higher than sensitivity. Determining the developmental skills in which early delays confer the highest risk for language or speech disorder would allow early intervention to be appropriately targeted to the neediest children. Similarly, identifying the aspects of language or speech most predictive of later reading disorders is a prerequisite for early intervention for reading.

Finally, research has uncovered at least some mechanisms with which infants detect and analyze the speech stream. However, individual differences in the adequacy or use of these mechanisms have not yet been described. Assessment of differences in these very basic mechanisms may identify children at risk for language and speech disorders at much younger ages than is currently possible. Further research into the nature of these mechanisms may also reveal strategies for early treatment.

REFERENCES

1. Tomblin JB, Records NL, Buckwalter P, et al: Prevalence of specific language impairment in kindergarten children. J Speech Lang Hear Res 40:1245-1260, 1997.
2. Shriberg LD, Tomblin J, McSweeny JL: Prevalence of speech delay in 6-year-old children and comorbidity with language impairment. J Speech Lang Hear Res 42:1461-1481, 1999.
3. DeCasper A, Fifer W: Of human bonding: Newborns prefer their mothers' voices. Science 208:1174-1176, 1980.
4. Eisenberg R: Auditory competence in early life: The roots of communicative-behavior. Baltimore, MD: University Park Press, 1976.
5. Eimas PD, Siqueland ER, Jusczyk P, et al: Speech perception in infants. Science 171:303-306, 1971.
6. Saffran JR, Aslin RN, Newport EL: Statistical learning by 8-month-old infants. Science 274:1926-1928, 1996.
7. Kuhl PK: Early language acquisition: Cracking the speech code. Nat Rev Neurosci 5:831-843, 2004.
8. Saffran JR: Musical learning and language development. Ann N Y Acad Sci 999:397-401, 2003.
9. Werker JF, Tees RC: Cross-language speech perception: Evidence for perceptual reorganization during the first year of life. Infant Behav Dev 7:49-63, 1984.
10. Gentner D: On relational meaning: The acquisition of verb meaning. Child Dev 49:988-998, 1978.
11. Fenson L, Dale PS, Reznick J, et al: Variability in early communicative development. Monogr Soc Res Child Dev 59:1-173, 1994.
12. Houston-Price C, Plunkett K, Harris P: "Word-learning wizardry" at 1;6. J Child Lang 32:175-189, 2005.
13. Bates E, Marchman VA, Thal D, et al: Developmental and stylistic variation in the composition of early vocabulary. J Child Lang 21:85-123, 1994.
14. Huttenlocher J: Language input and language growth. Prev Med 27:195-199, 1998.
15. Huttenlocher J, Vasilyeva M, Cymerman E, et al: Language input and child syntax. Cognit Psychol 45:337-374, 2002.
16. Hart B, Risley TR: Meaningful Differences in the Everyday Experience of Young American Children. Baltimore: Paul H. Brookes, 1995.
17. Dollaghan CA, Campbell TF, Paradise JL, et al: Maternal education and measures of early speech and language. J Speech Lang Hear Res 42:1432-1443, 1999.
18. Campbell TF, Dollaghan CA, Rockette HE, et al: Risk factors for speech delay of unknown origin in 3-year-old children. Child Dev 74:346-357, 2003.
19. Thal DJ: Language and cognition in normal and late-talking toddlers. Top Lang Disord 11(4):33-42, 1991.
20. Tomblin J, Zhang X, Buckwalter P, et al: The association of reading disability, behavioral disorders, and language impairment among second-grade children. J Child Psychol Psychiatry 41:473-482, 2000.
21. Catts HW, Fey ME, Tomblin J, et al: A longitudinal investigation of reading outcomes in children with language impairments. J Speech Lang Hear Res 45:1142-1157, 2002.
22. Brown RW: A First Language: The Early Stages. Cambridge, MA: Harvard University Press, 1973.
23. Sagae K, MacWhinney B, Lavie A: Automatic parsing of parental verbal input. Behav Res Methods Instrum Comput 36:113-126, 2004.
24. Weston A, Shriberg L, Miller J: Analysis of language-speech samples with SALT and PEPPER. J Speech Hear Res 32:755-766, 1989.
25. Miller J, Chapman R: The relation between age and mean length of utterance in morphemes. J Speech Hear Res 24:154-161, 1981.
26. Rescorla L, Achenbach TM: Use of the language development survey (LDS) in a national probability sample of children 18 to 35 months old. J Speech Lang Hear Res 45:733-743, 2002.
27. Feldman HM, Dale PS, Campbell TF, et al: Concurrent and predictive validity of parent reports of child language at ages 2 and 3 years. Child Dev 76:856-868, 2005.
27a. Bzoch KR, League R, Brown VL: 2003 Receptive-Expressive Emergent Language Test. Austin, TX: Pro-Ed.
28. Glascoe F: Parents' Evaluation of Developmental Status. Nashville, TN: Ellsworth & Vandermeer, 2005.
29. Wetherby AM, Prizant BM: Communication and Symbolic Behavior Scales: Developmental Profile, 1st normed ed. Baltimore: Paul H. Brookes, 2002.
30. Lord C, Risi S, Lambrecht L, et al: The Autism Diagnostic Observation Schedule–Generic: A standard measure of social and communication deficits associated with the spectrum of autism. J Autism Dev Disord 30:205-223, 2000.
31. Coplan J, Gleason JR, Ryan R, et al: Validation of an early language milestone scale in a high-risk population. Pediatrics 70:677-683, 1982.

7E.
Assessment of Motor Skills

MARIA A. JONES
IRENE R. MCEWEN
LYNN M. JEFFRIES

Motor disorders in children are associated with a number of conditions that vary widely in age at manifestation, the type and severity of the motor deficits, and prognosis.[1] Arthrogryposis, developmental coordination disorder, Down syndrome, cerebral palsy, meningomyelocele, muscular dystrophy, osteogenesis imperfecta, spinal muscular atrophy, and traumatic brain injury are some of the diagnoses in children who have motor disorders.

Assessment of motor skills is a process of gathering and synthesizing information to describe and understand motor skills, through such means as interviews, observations, questionnaires, and formal assessment tools.[1] Information obtained through assessment can be useful for such purposes as diagnosing conditions associated with disordered movement, documenting eligibility for services available for children with developmental delays and disabilities, planning intervention to remediate or compensate for motor deficits, and evaluating change in motor skills over time.

Many professionals have interest and expertise in motor skill assessment. Child development specialists, educators, neuropsychologists, occupational therapists, pediatricians, and physical therapists are some of the potential team members in assessment and intervention for children with conditions that affect their motor skills. To promote a shared understanding of motor skill assessment, the purposes of this chapter are (1) to describe a common framework for assessment of motor skills in children, with emphasis on the focus of the assessment and its purpose; (2) to review general considerations for measurement of motor skills; and (3) to summarize formal tools that are commonly used for assessment of motor skills of neonates and infants, preschool-aged children, school-aged children, and adolescents.

FOCUS OF MOTOR SKILLS ASSESSMENT

The World Health Organization's International Classification of Functioning, Disability and Health (ICF)[2] provides a useful framework for deciding which aspect of motor skills to measure when planning an assessment (also see Chapter 6). The ICF is a biopsychosocial model in which health and disability are viewed

as the result of the interaction between a health condition (disease, disorder, or injury) and contextual factors, including those related to the person and those related to the environment. A health condition can be classified by three interrelated domains: body structures and functions, activities, and participation. Examples of body structures are brain formation, bone density, and muscle composition. Strength, balance, and coordination are examples of body functions. Activities are specific tasks or actions, such as walking, running, and climbing, which when combined contribute to participation in home, school, community, and other situations of life. Figure 7E-1 shows the ICF classification system and the definitions and interrelations of the components. Figure 7E-2 illustrates an application of the ICF framework for a child with Down syndrome.

The ICF framework is helpful for deciding what to assess to answer specific questions related to a child's motor skills.[3] If parents were concerned, for example, about why their young child is not yet sitting, use of a tool that assessed the child's body functions and structures, such as strength and postural reactions would be appropriate. (Table 7E-1 contains definitions of some terms used in motor assessment.) A test designed to measure the child's ability to sit (activity) would elicit results that confirm or contradict the parent's observations but would not provide information about possible limitations in body functions and structures that prevented the child from sitting. If parents were seeking early intervention services under the Individuals with Disabilities Education Improvement Act,[4] then a tool that included measured activities would be most helpful for determining the child's eligibility for services on the basis of delayed motor skills in comparison to typical peers. Measurement of activity and participation would be required if a child with motor deficits entered first grade in a new school and the parents and school team members questioned the child's ability to func-

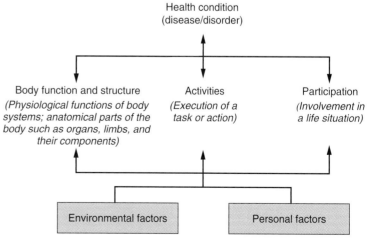

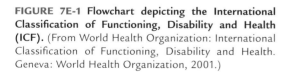

FIGURE 7E-1 Flowchart depicting the International Classification of Functioning, Disability and Health (ICF). (From World Health Organization: International Classification of Functioning, Disability and Health. Geneva: World Health Organization, 2001.)

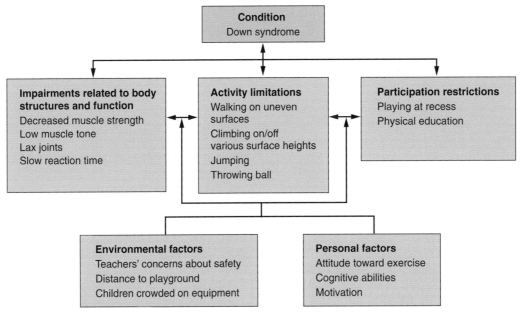

FIGURE 7E-2 Flowchart illustrating the Application of the International Classification of Functioning, Disability and Health to a child with Down syndrome who wants to participate in recess and physical education.

TABLE 7E-1 ■ Motor Assessment Terms

Term	Definition
Automatic reactions or movements	Coordinated patterns of movement that occur in response to a stimulus, such as reactions that maintain balance (equilibrium reactions) or align the head and body (righting reactions); may include primitive reflexes, described at end of table.[76]
Developmental motor skills	Observable milestones of typical children that represent progress toward achieving upright posture, mobility, and manipulation.[73]
Functional motor skills	Self-chosen, self-directed motor skills that are meaningful for the child and family.[77]
Fine motor skills	Skills that involve the small muscles of the body, especially in eye-hand coordination tasks, to make small, precise movements.
Gross motor skills	Skills or movement, such as jumping, that involve the large muscles of the body.
Muscle tone	Tension or stiffness of muscles at rest; resistance to quick passive movement. Stiffness may be abnormally high (hypertonia), low (hypotonia), or fluctuating. Muscle tone varies with position and activity. The relationship of passive stiffness at rest to active movement is unclear.[76]
Postural control or reactions	Regulation of the body's position in space for stability and orientation. *Stability* (or balance) maintains or regains the position of the body over the base of support. *Orientation* aligns the body parts, in relation to one another, so that they are appropriate for the movement or task being accomplished.[78]
Primary, early, or primitive reflexes	Coordinated patterns of movement demonstrated spontaneously by normally developing infants that may also be elicited by external stimuli. Examples include the rooting, Moro, and asymmetrical tonic neck reflexes.[79]

tion in the school environment and wanted to identify supports that the child might need or goals for intervention.

The ICF is similar to the older frameworks that the World Health Organization and other groups have developed, but more positive terminology is used to focus on "components of health" (World Health Organization,[2] p 4) rather than on the consequences of disease. The overall purpose of the ICF is to provide a common language and framework for describing health and health-related status.[2,3]

Because many factors are related to children's performance of motor skills, a number of tests and measures exist for assessment of the dimensions of the ICF, particularly body structure and function and activity. When clinicians decide on a tool to use, the purpose for the assessment is another important consideration.

PURPOSES OF MOTOR ASSESSMENT

Kirshner and Guyatt[5] described three purposes for clinical measurement: discrimination, prediction, and evaluation. These purposes provide a framework to use in conjunction with ICF domain for identifying appropriate tools for measurement of children's motor skills. Discriminative measures identify children with and without a particular characteristic or with varying degrees of a characteristic,[6] such as delayed gross motor skills, impaired balance, or superior manual dexterity. Discriminative measures can be norm referenced or criterion referenced. In norm-referenced tests, a child's motor skills are compared with those of typical children of the same age, and scores indicate how the child's skills compare within the normal distribution of scores of typical children.[7] Criterion-referenced tests can be used to assess such body structures and functions as postural control and reactions, but they also are used to measure performance of activities such as the ability to kneel, drink from a cup, or open a locker. Although criterion-referenced tests often are constructed to allow comparison of a child's development or performance with estimates of development or performance of typical children, nor-

mative data obtained from measurement research are not available.[8]

Predictive measures are used for screening and diagnostic purposes to identify which children have or are likely to have a particular condition or status in the future.[5] Testing of infants who are at risk for abnormal motor development, for example, is an attempt to predict which infants will be later receive diagnoses of conditions such as cerebral palsy. Early identification can lead to intervention aimed at preventing or ameliorating the effects of the condition.

Evaluative measures are used to assess change over time or as a result of intervention.[5,6] Good evaluative measures are responsive to change that occurs, whether in body structures and functions, activity, or participation. Although measuring change in body structures and function can be appropriate, evaluation of change also should include measurement of activities and participation that are meaningful to the child and family.[6]

Most tests and measures for assessment of motor skills are useful for only one or two purposes. Norm-referenced developmental tests, for example, often are not good predictors of infant's motor performance at later ages.[9] Other assessments effectively identify children with delayed motor development but are not useful for evaluation of change as a result of intervention. Selection of tools that match the purpose of the assessment is key to obtaining useful test results. Table 7E-2 lists commonly used motor assessment

TABLE 7E-2 ■ Common Motor Assessment Tools			
Test Name	Type of Test, Most Useful Purpose	Age for Testing	ICF Dimension
Alberta Infant Motor Scale (AIMS)[9]	Discriminative, norm-referenced Evaluative for infants with delayed, but not abnormal movement Predictive	0-18 months	Body structure and function: postural control Activity: motor performance
Assessment of Preterm Infant Behavior (APIB)[20]	Discriminative, norm-referenced	Preterm to full-term infants	Body structure and function: physiological/ autonomic system reactions, attention, state and motor organization, self-regulation
Battelle Developmental Inventory–2nd ed. (BDI-2)[31]	Discriminative, norm-referenced	0-7.11 years	Activity: cognitive, communication, social-emotional, motor, and adaptive skills
Bayley Scales of Infant and Toddler Development–Third Edition (BSID-III)[32]	Discriminative, norm-referenced	1-42 months	Activity: cognitive, motor, language, social-emotional, adaptive behavior
Birth to Three Assessment[33]	Discriminative, criterion-referenced	0-36 months	Activity: gross motor, fine motor, language, personal-social skills; nonverbal thinking
Bleck's Locomotor Prognosis in Cerebral Palsy[48]	Predictive of ambulation in children with cerebral palsy at 7 years of age	12 months and older	Body structure and function: postural reactions and reflexes

TABLE 7E-2 ■ Common Motor Assessment Tools—cont'd

Test Name	Type of Test, Most Useful Purpose	Age for Testing	ICF Dimension
Bruininks-Oseretsky Test of Motor Proficiency, 2nd ed. (BOT-2)[42]	Discriminative, norm-referenced	4-21 years	Body structure and function: balance and coordination Activity: gross and fine motor performance
Canadian Occupational Performance Measure, 4th ed[67]	Discriminative Evaluative	Any	Any
Children's Handwriting Evaluation Scale for Manuscript Writing (CHES)[59]	Discriminative	Grades 1-2	Activity: manuscript handwriting performance
Diagnosis and Remediation of Handwriting Problems[62]	Discriminative, criterion-referenced	Grade 3+	Activity: handwriting performance
Early Learning Accomplishment Profile (E-LAP)[34]	Discriminative, criterion-referenced	0-36 months	Activity: gross motor, fine motor, cognitive, language, self-help, social-emotional development
Evaluation Tool of Children's Handwriting (ETCH)[63]	Discriminative, criterion-referenced	Grades 1-2	Activity: handwriting performance
General Movements[29]	Discriminative, criterion-referenced	Preterm to 4 months	Body structure and function: general movement of trunk and extremities
Gross Motor Function Measure (GMFM)[45]	Discriminative, criterion-referenced Evaluative	Any age	Activity: lying and rolling, sitting, crawling, kneeling, standing, walking, running, and jumping
Hawaii Early Learning Profile[35]	Discriminative, curriculum-referenced	0-6 years	Activity: cognition, language, motor, fine motor, social, self-help skills
Infant Neurobiological International Battery (INFANIB)[21]	Discriminative, criterion-referenced Predictive	0-18 months	Body structure and function: postural control, muscle tone, vestibular function
Minnesota Handwriting Test[61]	Discriminative, norm-referenced	Grades 1-2	Activity: manuscript handwriting performance
Movement Assessment Battery for Children (Movement ABC)[55]	Discriminative, norm-referenced	4-12 years	Activity: Manual dexterity, balance, ball handling, visual-motor skills
Neonatal Behavioral Assessment Scale[18]	Discriminative, criterion-referenced	Full-term infants	Body structure and function: oral-motor, muscle tone, vestibular function
Neonatal Individualized Developmental Care and Assessment Program (NIDCAP)[17]	Discriminative, criterion-referenced	Preterm–4 weeks	Body structure and function: autonomic and motor organization, attention
Newborn Behavioral Observation system[19]	Discriminative, criterion-referenced	Birth–2 months	Body structure and function: physiological, motor, state organization
Peabody Developmental Motor Scales, 2nd ed. (PDMS-2)[30]	Discriminative, norm- and criterion-referenced	0-5 years	Activity: gross motor and find motor skills
Pediatric Evaluation of Disability Inventory (PEDI)[44]	Discriminative, norm- and criterion-referenced Evaluative	6 months–7$\frac{1}{2}$ years functional level	Activity and participation: self-care, mobility, social function
School Function Assessment (SFA)[66]	Discriminative, criterion-referenced Evaluative	Kindergarten–sixth grade	Participation, task supports, activity performance (physical tasks, cognitive/behavioral tasks)
Test of Infant Motor Performance (TIMP)[23]	Discriminative, norm-referenced Predictive	32 weeks' gestation to 4 months post term	Body function/structure and activity: postural control; ability to orient and stabilize head in space and in response to stimulation; selective control of distal movements; antigravity control of trunk and extremities
Test of Legible Handwriting[60]	Discriminative	7-18.5 years	Activity: handwriting performance

ICF, International Classification of Functioning, Disability, and Health.

tools, their most useful purposes, and the dimensions of the ICF that they measure.

GENERAL CONSIDERATIONS FOR ASSESSMENT OF MOTOR SKILLS

When deciding among tools to assess children's motor skills, examiners should identify the ICF dimension of interest, the purpose of the assessment, the psychometric properties of the tests, and the age group for which the tests were developed. Psychometric properties, such as reliability and validity, are important for controlling measurement error and ensuring that the measurements will be useful. Because reliability of measurements is population specific, reporting of reliability coefficients in a text such as this could be misleading without a full description of the characteristics of the study participants and the examiners.[8] For diagnostic tests, sensitivity and specificity are important, and responsiveness is important for evaluative tests. Psychometric properties of tests often are provided in test manuals and in reports of research conducted after the tests were published.

Examiners also need to be consistent with test administration and knowledgeable in interpreting the results. The results of repeated testing and observation of motor skills in the environment where they will be used will provide information to guide and modify intervention. However, intervention should not be driven by items failed on motor assessments; rather, they should focus on activities that children and their families identify as meaningful and that children perform in everyday environments.[10] The questions to be answered often are different for children of different ages, and many tools are age specific. In the following sections, we describe considerations for motor skills assessment of children in four age groups and describe some of the tools available for assessment of each group.

MOTOR ASSESSMENT OF INFANTS AND TODDLERS

Motor development in typical infants and toddlers is predictable and shifts from reflexive to purposeful movement, leading to the ability to move against gravity, transition in and out of different body positions, and explore the environment by crawling, walking, and climbing.[9] For infants born prematurely and for infants and toddlers who are not achieving typical motor milestones, discriminative measures to identify delays in motor development and the reasons

for the delays are important, as are measures that are predictive of future diagnoses, such as cerebral palsy.[11] Motor assessment of infants often focuses on body structures and function, such as muscle tone and reflexes,[12] as well as neuromotor development, postural reactions, and fine and gross motor skills (see Table 7E-2).[13] For infants born prematurely or with other risk factors, periodic monitoring beyond the neonatal period is important; the assessment of motor skills is a component of the monitoring process.[14] Repeated assessment is recommended for early identification of infants with motor dysfunction or delay and to predict which infants may later receive diagnoses of conditions not evident at birth or shortly thereafter.[15,16]

Tool That Focus Specifically on Motor-Related Function

The Neonatal Individualized Developmental Care and Assessment Program[17] is a comprehensive criterion-referenced assessment for preterm or full-term infants up to 4 weeks' post-term age. It involves a systematic observation of the infant's autonomic, motor, and attention responses during caregiving routines and discriminates infants with difficulty in the three areas. It is a total program that encompasses both the assessment and related caregiving recommendations. Other neonatal assessments that focus on the motor, behavioral, and physiological function of infants born at term or before term include the Neonatal Behavioral Assessment Scale,[18] the Newborn Behavioral Observations system,[19] and the Assessment of Preterm Infants' Behavior.[20]

The Infant Neurobiological International Battery (INFANIB)[21] is a criterion-referenced tool used to assess neuromotor status of infants from birth to age 18 months who were born prematurely. In addition to the test's discriminating between normal and abnormal development, an infant's scores on spasticity and head and trunk subscales at 6 months of age are highly predictive of cerebral palsy at 12 months (86.8% for spasticity and 87.1% for head and trunk subscales).[22]

The Test of Infant Motor Performance[23] assesses motor development of infants from 32 weeks after conception through 4 months' post-term age. The test discriminates infants at risk for motor dysfunction from typically developing infants[24] and had 0.92 sensitivity for identifying infants at age 3 months with delayed performance on the Alberta Infant Motor Scale (AIMS)[1] at 12 months of age.[25] The test also is one of the best predictors of a later diagnosis of cerebral palsy. Of infants whose motor performance was delayed at 3 months according to their Test of Infant

Motor Performance scores, 75% received a diagnosis of cerebral palsy by preschool age.[11]

The AIMS is a norm-referenced discriminative measure of the infant's gross motor development from 40 weeks after conception to independent walking. The AIMS differentiates infants' motor development as normal, at risk, and abnormal. A score at the 10th percentile or below at age 4 months (sensitivity, 0.77; specificity, 0.82) or at the 5th percentile or below at age 8 months (sensitivity, 0.86; specificity, 0.93) is predictive of motor delay at 18 months of age.[26]

The general movements assessment[27] also is a discriminative measure with predictive validity. Examiners observe the quality of infants' gross movements at variable speeds and amplitudes and then classify the movements as normal or abnormal. When infants show abnormal general movements at 2 and 4 months after term, the test is predictive of cerebral palsy, with accuracy of 0.85 to 0.98.[28,29]

As infants develop and motor delays are suspected, motor assessment often focuses on early identification to determine whether infants meet eligibility criteria for early intervention services under the Individuals with Disabilities Education Improvement Act.[4] Criteria vary from state to state; however, most are based on presence of a qualifying condition, such as Down syndrome, or on a documented development delay. A tool that is widely used to identify and document motor delays is the Peabody Developmental Motor Scales,[30] a norm-referenced discriminative test of gross and fine motor development for children from birth to age 72 months.

Comprehensive Developmental Assessment Tools That Include Motor Development

Most other assessments used for early identification are comprehensive criterion-referenced or norm-referenced tools that assess infants' and toddlers' development in several areas, such as motor, cognitive, social-emotional, communication, and adaptive development. Frequently used norm-referenced tests include the Battelle Developmental Inventory[31] and the Bayley Scales of Infant and Toddler Development.[32] Examples of criterion-referenced tests include the Birth to Three Assessment,[33] the Early Learning Accomplishment Profile,[34] and the Hawaii Early Learning Profile.[35] Although discriminative tools for infants and toddlers measure skills that might be meaningful for evaluation of change in some individual children, they are not useful as evaluative measures for most children with motor impairments. The most useful individual evaluative measure is often to determine whether a child achieves mean-

ingful, measurable goals identified by the family and other team members.[10]

MOTOR ASSESSMENT OF PRESCHOOL-AGED CHILDREN

Motor development of preschool-aged children is characterized by active movement throughout their environments and continued refinement of skills previously acquired.[36] In the preschool years, motor skills become particularly important for social interaction and play. Children with motor impairments that limit their ability to explore and interact with their environment are at risk for delayed development in cognitive, communication, and social domains.[37-39] Because most children with moderate to severe motor impairments have been identified as having delayed motor development or have a medical diagnosis by this age, norm-referenced discriminative measures are rarely useful, but other types of discriminative measures can be helpful for measurement of motor-related dimensions within ICF, such as range-of-motion (body functions/structures); mobility, and self-help skills (activities); and the child's ability to participate within family routines and community settings (participation).

For all preschool-aged children with delayed motor development, measurement of the effect of motor skills on functioning is more important than simply documenting a motor delay.[10] The ability of a child to function in age-appropriate daily activities of the family and community[40] also needs to be assessed, and interventions must be provided to remediate when possible or to compensate when children are unlikely to achieve necessary motor skills. Observation of motor skills in the environments in which children use them usually yields the most useful information for intervention planning.[41]

Tools That Measure Motor Skills

In children with mild motor disorders or with acquired or progressive conditions, such as Duchene muscular dystrophy, a motor delay might first be identified during the preschool years. The Peabody Developmental Motor Scales,[30] a norm-referenced tool commonly used to assess infants' fine and gross motor development, also is widely used for children of preschool age. The Bayley Scales of Infant and Toddler Development[32] is appropriate for children up to 42 months of age, and motor skills of children as young as 4 years can be assessed with the Bruininks-Oseretsky Test of Motor Proficiency (BOT-2).[42]

Few tools have been developed to assess the motor capabilities of children with disabilities or change in those capabilities. A systematic review of motor assessments used with children with cerebral palsy[43] concluded that only two measures are responsive to change: the Pediatric Evaluation of Disability Inventory (PEDI)[44] and the Gross Motor Function Measure (GMFM).[45]

The PEDI is a discriminative and evaluative tool designed to measure the self-care, mobility, and social function of children with disabilities. It measures not only function (activity) in each of the areas but also the amount of caregiver assistance and modifications needed in daily self-care, mobility, and social activities (participation). The items on the PEDI cover key functional skills achieved by typical children aged 6 months through $7^1/_2$ years. Although the PEDI's normative standard scores can be used to compare the development of children with disabilities at age $7^1/_2$ years and younger with the development of typically developing children, the authors used Rasch analysis, which "statistically manipulates ordinal data to create a linear measure on an interval scale" (Portney and Watkins,[8] p 305) to calculate scaled scores that allow comparison of the development of children with disabilities with their own development over time. This approach is often preferable because a child's development, no matter how slow, will show increasing scores over time rather than decreasing scores in comparison with typical children of the same age whose development is more rapid.

The GMFM[45] is another discriminative and evaluative tool, which was developed to measure motor skills of children with cerebral palsy. In contrast to the PEDI, which measures functional skills, the GMFM is a criterion-referenced measure of basic gross motor abilities in five dimensions: lying and rolling; sitting; crawling and kneeling; standing; and walking, running, and jumping. Typically developing children accomplish all of these activities by 5 years of age.

The GMFM is in two versions: the original GMFM with 88 items (GMFM-88) and the newer version with 66 items (GMFM-66). Rasch analysis was used to identify the 66 items that make up a interval scale, which improved the scoring over that of the original GMFM ordinal scale.[46] Both the GMFM-88 and the GMFM-66 have been shown to be responsive to change in basic gross motor abilities children with cerebral palsy,[45,46] and the GMFM-88 has been shown to be responsive to change in children with Down syndrome.[47]

Tools That Are Predictive of Motor Skills

Many parents of preschool-aged children have one question related to motor development: "Will my child walk?" For children with cerebral palsy, the

---

TABLE 7E-3 ■ Prognosis for Ambulation of Children with Cerebral Palsy, Based on Postural Reactions and Primitive Reflexes[48]

When the child is at least 12 months old, score one point for each of the following primitive reflexes if obligatory:
    Asymmetrical tonic neck reflex
    Symmetrical tonic neck reflex
    Moro
    Neck righting
    Extensor thrust

Score one point for each of the following postural reactions if absent:
    Foot placement
    Parachute

Prognosis for ambulation:
    0 points = good
    1 point = guarded
    2+ points = poor

From Rothstein JM, Roy SH, Wolf SL: Rehabilitation Specialist's Handbook, 3rd ed. Philadelphia: FA Davis, 2005, p 577.

TABLE 7E-4 ■ Prognosis for Ambulation of Children with Cerebral Palsy, Based on Gross Motor Skills[49]

Gross Motor Skill	Age (Months)	Prognosis
Head control	<9	Good
	9-19	Guarded
	>20	Poor
Sitting	<24	Good
	24-35	Guarded
	>36	Poor
Crawling	<0	Good
	30-61	Guarded
	>61	Poor

From: Rothstein JM, Roy SH, Wolf SL: Rehabilitation Specialist's Handbook, 3rd ed. Philadelphia: FA Davis, 2005, p 577.

---

question often can be answered with relative certainty by the time a child is 3 years old—and often before. In the 1970s, Bleck[48] predicted ambulation of children with cerebral palsy at 7 years of age on the basis of postural reactions and primitive reflexes at 12 months of age or older (Table 7E-3), with sensitivity of 0.98 and specificity of 0.84.[45] Other investigators[49] have predicted ambulation on the basis of age at achievement of gross motor skills (Table 7E-4).

Researchers[50] also have developed motor development curves for children with cerebral palsy on the basis of GMFM-66 scores and the severity of disability by using the Gross Motor Function Classification System.[51] The motor development curves predict the rates and limits of development of children with cerebral palsy at each of the five levels of this classification system, as measured by the GMFM-66. Researchers also have predicted gross motor function growth curves for children with Down syndrome on the basis of GMFM scores and the children's severity of motor impairment.[52]

MOTOR ASSESSMENT OF SCHOOL-AGED CHILDREN

As the demands of the environment increase and children are required to perform more complex motor tasks, such as writing and physical education activities, parents and teachers may become concerned about uncoordinated movements in children not previously identified as having motor deficits. Uncoordinated movements are characterized by inconsistency in performance, asymmetry, loss of balance, falling, slow reaction and movement timing, decreased muscle force, and poor motor planning.[53] Children who consistently show uncoordinated movements may have a developmental coordination disorder or other developmental disability that was not apparent until the child reached school age.

If children have not previously been identified as having difficulty with motor skills, norm-referenced discriminative tools can be useful for comparing a child's performance with typical children of the same age and for identifying strengths and deficits in components of motor skills, such as balance, coordination, and visual-motor skills. Norm-referenced tools usually are not helpful for school-aged children whose motor disorders were previously identified, but tools that help identify functional deficits and that evaluate change over time can be useful. Observation in children's own environments often is the most valuable method for identifying the effects of motor disorders on activities and participation and for identifying potential goals of intervention.[10] The previously described methods for predicting motor development of preschool-aged children with cerebral palsy and Down syndrome continue to be useful for predicting motor skills in some school-aged children.

Tools That Measure Developmental Motor Skills

A motor-related condition that often is identified during the school years is developmental coordination disorder, which affects movement in the absence of identified neurological dysfunction.[54] Two norm-referenced tests that commonly are used to help identify children with developmental coordination disorder are the BOT-2[42] and the Movement Assessment Battery for Children (M-ABC).[55] The BOT-2 assesses fine motor skills, gross motor skills, balance, and coordination and can be used with persons aged 4 to 21 years. The M-ABC also includes items that

assess manual dexterity, balance, ball handling, and visual motor skills. The M-ABC can be used with children aged 4 to 12 years. Although these tests are often used, authors have expressed concern about the potential lack of agreement between the tests in identifying children with developmental coordination disorder.[53,56]

Both the BOT-2 and the M-ABC have components that address fine motor skills, but neither specifically addresses the development of handwriting, which is a common reason that school-aged children are referred for motor assessments.[57,58] Frequently used tools for assessing handwriting include the Children's Handwriting Evaluation Scale for Manuscript Writing,[59] the Test of Legible Handwriting,[60] the Minnesota Handwriting Test,[61] Diagnosis and Remediation of Handwriting Problems,[62] and the Evaluation Tool of Children's Handwriting.[63] Although these and other tools for assessing handwriting are used, the identification of the reason for handwriting problems can be difficult because a child's motor and visual perceptual abilities, as well as orthographic, spelling, and written language processing, all contribute to writing success.[64,65]

Tools That Measure Motor-Related Functional Skills

Another frequent purpose of motor assessment of school-aged children is to measure the effects of motor skills on children's ability to function within the school environment. This is similar to assessing preschool-aged children with motor delays, in which the focus of assessment shifts from identifying the presence of motor delays or evaluating the effects of intervention aimed at improving developmental motor skills in isolation to measuring functional changes within the activities and participation levels of the ICF framework. The use of assessment tools designed to measure functional changes over time is important for identifying and measuring individually meaningful goals and planning intervention.

The PEDI[44] continues to be appropriate for assessing change in function and caregiver assistance over time for school-aged children. Tools such as the School Function Assessment (SFA)[66] and the Canadian Occupational Performance Measure (COPM)[67] also can be useful for these purposes. The SFA includes items that address the activity and participation levels of the ICF framework. The SFA is intended to determine the child's current level of participation and performance in elementary school activities and to document the supports a child needs to participate and perform in those activities. The SFA can be completed by one or more school professionals who have observed the child during typical school activities and routines. One weakness of the SFA is that it takes about 1.5 hours to complete the assessment.

The COPM was designed to identify goals of intervention and to measure outcomes. It has been widely used in adult rehabilitation to detect change in a person's self-perception of performance over time[68]; however, its use for children with disabilities and their families is increasing.[69] Authors of the COPM recognize the limitations with using the COPM with children younger than 8 years because of the difficulty with the self-assessment necessary to complete the COPM, but they reported that research is under way to develop a different method for accessing young children's goals and priorities.

MOTOR ASSESSMENT OF ADOLESCENTS

Adolescence is a time of increased independence, beginning separation from family, and physical body changes. More complex motor skills develop and often are practiced through participation in sports and involvement in community activities.[36] Adolescence also is a time when risk of injury increases, and the incidence of traumatic brain injury, which can have a range of motor and behavioral consequences,[70] is particularly high between the ages of 15 to 19 years.[71]

For adolescents with relatively high levels of motor function, the BOT-2,[42] for which normative data up to age 21 are available, could be a useful discriminative measure. Depending on the purpose for the assessment, tools used with school-aged children also may be appropriate for adolescents with motor disorders. For those functioning at less than a 7-year age level, the PEDI[44] could be useful for identifying mobility and self-care skills that are lacking and for measuring change in those skills over time if intervention is determined to be appropriate. The COPM is a particularly valuable measure for helping adolescents identify meaningful motor-related goals and to rate their perceptions of changes and satisfaction with the goals over time.[64]

RECOMMENDATIONS FOR THE FUTURE

Although many tools have been developed to assess children's motor skills and their underlying components, most are discriminative tools that assess the body function and activities domains of the ICF. Few tools are available to measure motor-related participation, and, except for the individual-specific COPM,[67] those that do exist are most appropriate for children of elementary school age or younger. Development of new tools to measure broader aspects of motor-related participation for children of all ages would not only enable researchers to identify participation limitations that might be ameliorable but, if developed as discriminative and evaluative measures, would also allow measurement of change in participation over time or with intervention.[72] Psychometrically sound measures of participation also would be useful for aggregating data for program evaluation purposes.

Research to determine minimal clinically important change in scores on evaluative tools is important for understanding the relevance of change in individual children and for program evaluation.[73,74] Development of computer-adapted testing to minimize the number of test items that need to be administered would reduce the time required for assessment.[75] New tools also are needed to help predict motor disorders other than cerebral palsy in young infants and to help predict the likely limits of development in children with a variety of conditions associated with motor disorders.

REFERENCES

1. Tupper DE, Sondell SK: Motor disorders and neuropsychological development. *In* Dewey D, Tuper DE, eds: Developmental Motor Disorders: A Neuropsychological Perspective. New York: Guilford, 2004, pp 3-25.
2. World Health Organization: International Classification of Functioning, Disability and Health. Geneva: World Health Organization, 2001.
3. Lollar DJ, Simeonsson RJ: Diagnosis to function: classification for children and youths. J Dev Behav Pediatr 26:323-330, 2005.
4. Individuals with Disabilities Education Improvement Act of 2004 (Public Law 108-446), 20 U.S.C. 1400.
5. Kirshner B, Guyatt B: A methodological framework for assessing health and disease. J Chron Dis 38:27-36, 1985.
6. Rosenbaum PL: Clinically based outcomes for children with cerebral palsy: Issues in the measurement of function. *In* Sussmann M, ed: The Diplegic Child. Parkridge, IL: American Academy of Orthopaedic Surgeons, 1992, pp 125-132.
7. Long T, Toscano K: Handbook of Pediatric Physical Therapy, 2nd ed. Philadelphia: Lippincott Williams & Wilkins, 2002.
8. Portney LG, Watkins MP: Foundations of Clinical Research: Applications to Practice. 2nd ed. Upper Saddle River, NJ: Prentice-Hall Health, 2000.
9. Piper MC, Darrah J: Motor Assessment of the Developing Infant. Philadelphia: WB Saunders, 1994.
10. Harris SR, McEwen IR: Assessing motor skills. *In* McLean M, Bailey DB Jr, Wolery M, eds: Assessing

Infants and Preschoolers with Special Needs, 2nd ed. Englewood Cliffs, NJ: Prentice-Hall, 1996, pp 305-333.

11. Kolobe THA, Bulanda M, Susman L: Predictive validity of the Test of Infant Motor Performance at pre-school age. Phys Ther 84:1144-1156, 2004.

12. Andre-Thomas CY, Saint-Anne Dargassies S: The Neurological Examination of Infants. Little Club Clinics in Developmental Medicine, No. 1. London: National Spastics Society, 1960.

13. Case-Smith J, Bigsby R: Motor assessment. *In* Singer LT, Aeskind PS, eds: Biobehavioral Assessment of Infants. New York: Guilford, 2001, pp 423-442.

14. Allen MC, Alexander GR: Using motor milestones as a multistep process to screen preterm infants for cerebral palsy. Dev Med Child Neurol 39:12-16, 1997.

15. Escobar GJ, Littenberg B, Pettiti DB: Outcome among surviving very low birthweight infants: A meta-analysis. Arch Dis Child 66:204-211, 1991.

16. Ferrari F, Cioni G, Prechtl HFR: Qualitative changes of general movements in preterm infants with brain lesions. Early Hum Dev 23:193-231, 1990.

17. Als H: Program Guide: Newborn Individualized Developmental Care and Assessment Program (NIDCAP): An Education and Training Program for Health Care Professionals. Boston: Children's Medical Center Corporation, 1986.

18. Brazelton TB: The Neonatal Behavioral Assessment Scale. Philadelphia: JB Lippincott, 1984.

19. Nugent JK, Keefer C, O'Brien S, et al: The Newborn Behavioral Observations system. Boston: Brazelton Institute, 2005.

20. Als H, Lester BM, Tronick EZ, et al: Toward a research instrument for the Assessment of Preterm Infants' Behavior (APIB). *In* Fitzgerald H, Lester B, Yogman M, eds: Theory and Research in Behavioral Pediatrics, vol 1. New York: Plenum Press, 1982, pp 35-63.

21. Ellison PH: INFANIB. A Reliable Method for the Neuromotor Assessment of Infants. Tucson, AZ: Therapy Skill Builders, 1994.

22. Stavrakas PA, Kemmer-Gacura GE, Engelke SC, et al: Predictive validity of the Infant Neurological International Battery. Dev Med Child Neurol Suppl 64:35-36, 1991.

23. Campbell SK, Kolobe THA, Osten ET, et al: Construct validity of the Test of Infant Motor Performance. Phys Ther 75:585-596, 1995.

24. Campbell SK, Hecker D: Validity of the Test of Infant Motor Performance for discriminating among infants with varying risk for poor motor outcome. J Pediatr 139:546-551, 2001.

25. Campbell SK, Kolobe THA, Wright BD, et al: Validity of the Test of Infant Motor Performance for prediction of 6-, 9-, and 12-month scores on the Alberta Infant Motor Scales. Dev Med Child Neurol, 44:263-272, 2002.

26. Darrah J, Piper MC, Watt MJ: Assessment of gross motor skills of at-risk infants: Predictive validity of the Alberta Infant Motor Scale. Dev Med Child Neurol 40:485-491, 1998.

27. Prechtl HFR: Qualitative changes of spontaneous movements in fetus and preterm infant are a marker of neurological dysfunction. Early Hum Dev 23:151-158, 1990.

28. Hadders-Algra M, Groothuis AMC: Quality of general movements in infancy is related to the development of neurological dysfunction, attention deficit hyperactivity disorder and aggressive behavior. Dev Med Child Neurol 41:381-391, 1999.

29. Prechtl HFR, Einspieler C, Cioni G, et al: An early marker of neurological deficits after prenatal brain lesions. Lancet 349:1361-1363, 1997.

30. Folio MR, Fewell RR: Peabody Developmental Motor Scales, 2nd ed. Austin, TX: PRO-ED, 2000.

31. Newborg J: Battelle Developmental Inventory–2nd ed. Itasca, IL: Riverside, 2005.

32. Bayley N: Bayley Scales of Infant and Toddler Development–Third Edition. San Antonio, TX: The Psychological Corporation, 2005.

33. Ammer JJ, Bangs TE: Birth to Three Assessment and Intervention System. Austin, TX: PRO-ED, 2000.

34. Glover ME, Preminger JL, Sanford AR: Early Learning Accomplishment Profile. Lewisville, NC: Kaplan Early Learning Company, 2002.

35. Parks S: Hawaii Early Learning Profile. Palo Alta, CA: Vort Corporation, 2004.

36. Cech DJ, Martin ST: Functional Movement Development across the Lifespan, 2nd ed. Philadelphia: WB Saunders, 2002.

37. Hays RM: Childhood motor impairments: Clinical overview and scope of the problem. *In* Jaffee KM, ed: Childhood Powered Mobility: Developmental, Technical and Clinical Perspectives. Washington, DC: Rehabilitation Engineering and Assistive Technology Society of North America, 1987, pp 1-10.

38. Tefft D, Guerette P, Furumasu J: Cognitive predictors of young children's readiness for powered mobility. Dev Med Child Neurol 41:665-670, 1999.

39. Kermoian, R: Locomotion experience and psychological development in infancy. *In* Furumasu J, ed: Pediatric Powered Mobility: Developmental Perspectives, Technical Issues, Clinical Approaches. Arlington, VA: Rehabilitation Engineering and Assistive Technology Society of North America, 1997, pp 7-21.

40. Miller LJ, Robinson C: Strategies for meaningful assessment of infants and toddlers with significant physical and sensory disabilities. *In* Meisels SJ, Fenichel E, eds: New Visions for the Developmental Assessment of Infants and Young Children. Washington, DC: Zero to Three, 1996, pp 313-329.

41. McEwen IR, Hansen LH: Children with cognitive impairments. *In* Campbell SK, Vander Linden DW, Palisano RJ, eds: Physical Therapy for Children, 3rd ed. Philadelphia: WB Saunders, 2006, pp 591-624.

42. Bruininks RH, Bruininks BD: Bruininks-Oserestsky Test of Motor Proficiency, 2nd ed. Circle Pines, MN: American Guidance Service Publishing, 2005.

43. Ketelaar M, Vermeer A, Helders PJ: Functional motor abilities of children with cerebral palsy: A systematic literature review of assessment measures. Clin Rehabil 12:369-380, 1998.

44. Hayley SM, Coster WJ, Ludlow LH, et al: Pediatric Evaluation of Disability Inventory. Development, Standardization and Administration Manual. Boston: Health and Disability Research Institute, 1992.

45. Russell DJ, Rosenbaum PL, Avery LM, et al: Gross Motor Function Measure (GMFM-66 & GMFM-88) User's Manual. London: Mac Keith Press, 2002.

46. Russell DJ, Russell DJ, Avery LM, et al: Improved scaling of the Gross Motor Function Measure for children with cerebral palsy: Evidence of reliability and validity. Phys Ther 80:873-885, 2000.

47. Russell D, Palisano R, Walter S, et al: Evaluating motor function in children with Down syndrome: Validity of the GMFM. Dev Med Child Neurol 40:693-701, 1998.

48. Bleck EE: Locomotor prognosis in cerebral palsy. Dev Med Child Neurol 17:18-25, 1975.

49. Campos du Paz A, Burnett S, Braga L: Walking prognosis in cerebral palsy. Dev Med Child Neurol 36:130-134, 1994.

50. Rosenbaum PL, Walter SD, Hanna SE, et al: Prognosis for gross motor function in cerebral palsy: Creation of motor development curves. JAMA 288:1357-1363, 2002.

51. Palisano RJ, Rosenbaum P, Walter S, et al: Development and reliability of a system to classify gross motor function in children with cerebral palsy. Dev Med Child Neurol 39:214-223, 1997.

52. Palisano RJ, Walter SD, Russell DJ, et al: Gross motor function of children with Down syndrome: Creation of motor growth curves. Arch Phys Med Rehabil 82:494-500, 2001.

53. Barnhart RC, Davenport MJ, Epps SB, et al: Developmental coordination disorder. Phys Ther 83:722-731, 2003.

54. Dewey D, Wilson BN: Developmental coordination disorder: What is it? Phys Occup Ther Pediatr 20(2-3):5-27, 2001.

55. Henderson SE, Sugden DA: Movement Assessment Battery for Children. San Antonio, TX: The Psychological Corporation, 1992.

56. Crawford SG, Wilson BN, Dewey D: Identifying developmental coordination disorder: Consistency between tests. Phys Occup Ther Pediatr 20(2-3):29-50, 2001.

57. Cermak SA: Fine motor functions and handwriting. In Fisher AG, Murray EA, Bundy A, eds: Sensory Integration: Theory and Practice. Philadelphia: FA Davis, 1991, pp 166-170.

58. Missiuna C: Strategies for success: Working with children with developmental coordination disorder. Phys Occup Ther Pediatr 20(2-3):1-4, 2001.

59. Phelps J, Stempel L: Children's Handwriting Evaluation Scale for Manuscript Writing. Dallas: Texas Scottish Rite Hospital for Crippled Children, 1987.

60. Larsen S, Hammill D: Test of Legible Handwriting. Austin, TX: PRO-ED, 1989.

61. Reisman JE: Development and reliability of the research version of the Minnesota Handwriting Test. Phys Occup Ther Pediatr 13(2):41-55, 1993.

62. Stott DH, Moyes FA, Henderson SE: Diagnosis and Remediation of Handwriting Problems. Cardiff, UK: Drake Educational Associates, 1985.

63. Amundson SJ: Evaluation Tool of Children's Handwriting. Homer, AK: OT Kids, 1995.

64. Adams MJ: Beginning to Read: Thinking and Learning about Print. Cambridge, MA: MIT Press, 1990.

65. Feder KP, Majnemer A: Children's handwriting evaluation tools and their psychometric properties. Phys Occup Ther Pediatr 23(3):65-84, 2003.

66. Coster W, Deeney T, Haltiwanger J, et al: School Function Assessment Materials. San Antonio, TX: The Psychological Corporation, 1998.

67. Law M, Baptiste S, Carswell A, et al: Canadian Occupational Performance Measure. 4th ed. Ottawa, ON: CAOT Publications ACE, 2005.

68. Atwal A, Owen S, Davies R: Struggling for occupational satisfaction: Older people in care homes. Br J Occup Ther 66:118-124, 2003.

69. Law M, Darrah J, Pollock N, et al: Family-centered functional therapy for children with cerebral palsy: An emerging practice model. Phys Occup Ther Pediatr 18(1):83-102, 1998.

70. Dewey D, Bottos S, Tupper DE: Acquired childhood conditions with associated motor impairments. In Dewey D, Tuper DE, eds: Developmental Motor Disorders: A Neuropsychological Perspective. New York: Guilford, 2004, pp 169-196.

71. Langlois JA, Rutland-Brown W, Thomas KE: Traumatic brain injury in the United States: Emergency department visits, hospitalizations, and deaths. Atlanta, GA: Centers for Disease Control and Prevention, National Center for Injury Prevention and Control, 2004.

72. Wright FV, Boschen K, Jutai J: Exploring the comparative responsiveness of a core set of outcome measures in a school-based conductive education programme. Child Care Health Dev 31:291-302, 2005.

73. Beaton DE, Boers M, Wells GA: Many faces of The Minimal Clinically Important Difference (MCID): A literature review and directions for future research. Curr Opin Rheumatol 14:109-114, 2002.

74. Iyer LV, Haley SM, Watkins MP, et al: Establishing minimal clinically important differences for scores on the Pediatric Evaluation Of Disability Inventory for inpatient rehabilitation. Phys Ther 83:888-898, 2003.

75. Haley SM, Raczek AE, Coster WJ, et al: Assessing mobility in children using a computer adaptive testing version of the Pediatric Evaluation Of Disability Inventory. Arch Phys Med Rehabil 86:932-939, 2005.

76. Palisano RJ: Neuromotor and developmental assessment. In Wilhelm IJ, ed: Physical Therapy Assessment in Early Infancy. New York: Churchill Livingstone, 1993, pp 173-224.

77. Campbell SK: The child's development of functional movement. In Campbell SK, Vander Linden DW, Palisano RJ, eds: Physical Therapy for Children, 3rd ed. Philadelphia: WB Saunders, 2006, pp 33-76.

78. Shumway-Cook A, Woollacott M: Theoretical issues in assessing postural control. In Wilhelm IJ, ed: Physical Therapy Assessment in Early Infancy, New York: Churchill Livingstone, 1993, pp 161-171.

79. Crutchfield CA, Barnes MR: Motor Control and Motor Learning in Rehabilitation. Atlanta, GA: Stokesville, 1993.

Treatment and Management

8A.
The Interdisciplinary Team Approach

ROSE ANN (ROZ) PARRISH
SONYA OPPENHEIMER

In this chapter, we discuss the interdisciplinary team approach within health care and the field of developmental disabilities. We cover such topics as the history of interdisciplinary teams, including history in the field of developmental disabilities; the definition of a team; models of teamwork; factors that contribute to or present a challenge to interdisciplinary team collaboration; conceptual models used to evaluate interdisciplinary teams; and a review of the research on interdisciplinary teams. In referring to "disciplines," we imply that the family is a discipline that has a specific body of knowledge to contribute as a member of the interdisciplinary team. Also, the term *health care* in the context of the interdisciplinary team approach does not mean solely medical care focusing on biological factors; it also includes behavioral factors, as well as physical and social environmental factors.[1]

HISTORY

Isolated models of interdisciplinary health care teams, as defined as professionals from two or more disciplines working together, have existed in the United States since the beginning of the 20th century. Complex social issues related to the effects of industrialization (e.g., poverty, overcrowded housing, child labor) began to come to attention in the early 1900s, and there was a recognition among some professionals that health care involved joining "medical care with social fact."[2] The first publication in the United States to introduce the concept of interdisciplinary care is attributed to Richard Cabot of Massachusetts General Hospital; in 1915, he wrote about the value of ". . . teamwork of the doctor, educator and social worker in the clinical efficiency."[3]

With World War I, and to a greater extent with World War II, rehabilitation teams emerged to address the needs of veterans. After World War II, there was a rapid expansion of knowledge in medicine, an increase in accompanying technology, and the emergence of new specialties.[4] Simultaneously in the 1940s, a new body of knowledge known as *group dynamics* was emerging from the fields of social psychology, sociology, and anthropology.[5] In the mid-1940s, knowledge from the fields of group dynamics, social psychology, and educational psychology were melded to develop the unstructured Training Group (T-Group) as an intensive learning experience in small-group behavior.[6]

In the early 1960s, issues related to poverty became a major national focus, and the concept of "comprehensive care" provided by interdisciplinary teams evolved as a means of addressing both social and medical needs of the individual.[4] Demonstration team–managed neighborhood health centers were established in underserved areas to provide comprehensive care, which included medical, social, and vocational services. These types of clinics rapidly expanded during the 1970s to more than 850 by 1980.[7] At the same time, knowledge in the field of group dynamics/theory was expanding to such areas as the integration of personal learning and planned action for social improvement, phases of group development, communication in groups, and conditions that encourage group participation.[5]

In the equal rights climate of the 1960s, there emerged a professional interdisciplinary movement that embraced the team concept as an approach to improve health care delivery. The team concept was also viewed by some professionals as a means of achieving a greater equality in status of certain disciplines, which in turn would lead to improved health care delivery.[4,8] For example, in 1971, Madeleine Leininger[9] stated the following in an article about interdisciplinary education: "... in our future conceptualizations of health education and service models, there is a need to consider ways to reduce and redistribute physician power so that other health disciplines and consumers can share in his power, decision-making, and the control of health matters and resources" (p 789).

The 1970s marked the integration of group theory principles into examining interdisciplinary health care teams.[9-12] Also, aging of the population became of concern, and interdisciplinary teams began to increase within the field of geriatrics. During this period, the Department of Veterans Affairs implemented the Interdisciplinary Team Training in Geriatrics program, a clinically based educational program for both staff and students. The program eventually expanded beyond geriatrics and became the Interprofessional Team Training and Development Program.[13] In the 1980s, the Bureau of Health Professions also began awarding Geriatric Education Center and Rural Health initiative grants to universities to teach collaborative teamwork practices to professionals in medical and health-related fields for working in the area of geriatrics and to students working in rural areas.

The 1990s were a time of changes in the health care environment, with increased reliance on primary care, disease prevention, evidence-based practice, and cost containment. Health care organizations incorporated organizational and management theory into their operations and adopted concepts of total quality management, total quality improvement, and continuous quality improvement.[14] "Team" became a buzz word, and self-directed work groups emerged to address issues related to reducing costs and increasing productivity. In 1995, the Pew Health Professions Commission issued *Critical Challenges: Revitalizing the Health Professions for the Twenty-First Century.*[15] This report presented a comprehensive analysis of the trends and strategies for successful outcomes in health care. One of the Commission's recommendations for the future was team training and cross-professional education for all health professionals. In relation to this recommendation, the Commission expressed concern that model experiments involving team training and cross-professional education had stopped; the Commission urged that they be "rekindled" through "more sharing of clinical resources, more cross-teaching by professional faculties, more exploration of the various roles played by professionals and the active modeling of effective team integration in the delivery of efficient, high quality care" (p 22).

The beginning of the 21st century is an era in which teamwork is becoming a norm within health care organizations. With the Institute of Medicine's 1999 report, *To Err is Human: Building a Safer Health System,*[16] teamwork became to be viewed as crucial for ensuring patient safety, and a variety of medical team training programs began to emerge.[17] After publication of the report, the Agency for Healthcare Research and Quality commissioned an evidence-based literature review regarding safety improvement, which included a review of Crew Resource Management (CRM) and its application to medicine.[18] CRM, an approach to safety training focusing on effective team management, was developed by experts in aviation to improve the operation of flight crews and was beginning to be applied to high-stress decision-making health care environments such as the operating room, the labor and delivery suite, and the emergency room. Although additional evidence-base studies were indicated, it was concluded that CRM had tremendous potential applications in the health care field.[18] By 2005, a variety of CRM-based medical training programs had been developed with the goal of reducing the number of medical errors through the application of teamwork skills training. A formal review of six of these medical training programs was commissioned by the Agency for Healthcare Research and Quality as part of a report on what federally funded programs had accomplished in understanding medical errors and implementing programs to improve patient safety over the 5 years since *To Err is Human* was published.[17] Among the recommendations that resulted from the review was the recommendation that "the health care community develop a standard set of generic teamwork-related knowledge, skill and attitude competencies" (p 263).

As the team concept was gaining momentum in the actual delivery of health care, it was also gaining momentum in relation to the educational preparation of health care professionals. The 2001 Institute of Medicine report *Crossing the Quality Chasm: A New Health System for the 21st Century*[19] expressed concern that although health professionals were asked to work in interdisciplinary teams, they did not receive education together or receive training to develop team skills. A recommendation of *Crossing the Quality Chasm* was that a multidisciplinary summit of leaders within the health professions be held to identify strategies for restructuring educational programs. The summit was convened in 2002, and recommendations were issued in the 2003 report *Health Professions Education: A Bridge to Quality.*[20] Resulting was an overarching vision for clinical education in the health professions: "All health professions should be educated to deliver patient-centered care as members of an interdisciplinary team, emphasizing evidence-based practice, quality improvement approaches, and informatics" (p 3). To achieve this vision, five core competencies for the areas identified were proposed as competencies that all clinical health professions should possess.

The challenge ahead will be for the traditionally autonomous health professions to agree that these core competencies should indeed become part of the curricula for all clinical health professions.

HISTORY WITH REGARD TO CHILDREN WITH DEVELOPMENTAL DISABILITIES

The Children's Bureau, established in 1912, was the first government agency to focus on providing services to all children, including children with mental retardation and disabilities. In 1954, the Children's Bureau awarded a project grant to the Children's Hospital in Los Angeles to establish an interdisciplinary diagnostic clinic for children with mental retardation. By 1956, the Children's Bureau had 36 demonstration projects to provide services to children with mental retardation, develop new methods of service delivery, and provide training for professional workers.[21]

With the 1960s, there emerged an emphasis on focusing not only on the treatment of a specific disability but also on the child who happened to have the disability and on his or her family.[22] Inspired by personal experience, President John F. Kennedy created a President's Panel on Mental Retardation in 1961 to advise him on how the federal government could best meet the needs of children with mental retardation and of their families. In 1962, the Panel issued a report that included recommendations for more comprehensive and improved clinical services, as well as efforts to overcome serious problems of personnel in the field.[23] Legislation signed into law by President Kennedy in 1963 and funding provided by Amendments to Title V of the Social Security Act is administered by the Health Resources and Services Administration of the Public Health Service Department of Health and Human Service and legislates maternal and child health programs. In 1965 led to the development of University Affiliated Facilities (UAFs) in medical centers to provide both comprehensive interdisciplinary services to children with mental retardation and interdisciplinary training in the evaluation and management of children with mental retardation. This was considered a major breakthrough to systematically address personnel needs for children with mental retardation. It was the first time that the Congress and the Executive Branch recognized the need for federal funds to assist in establishing a national network of interdisciplinary training programs centered on models of service.[24] However during this period, the interdisciplinary team approach to service and training did not go without criticism on a variety of grounds. Many of the critics believed that the expense of the interdisci-plinary approach was not warranted; that there was an excessive duplication in the evaluation; and poor team dynamics resulted from conflicts among disciplines, personal frictions, defense of territory, or domination by one discipline or team member.[25]

Legislation in 1972 expanded the service and training roles of UAFs to include both children with mental retardation and those with other developmental disabilities. The number of UAFs continued to grow, and by the mid-1970s, there were about 40 in 30 states. In 1976, a UAF Long Range Planning Task Force was established to reassess the original UAF concept and make recommendations as to their future direction and role. Their reassessment indicated that, overall, the original UAF concept was sound and experience had proved that the program concept was effective in meeting a significant social need.[24] On the basis of the review, the Task Force made a number of recommendations to modernize and extend the program to serve individuals, both children and adults, with developmental disabilities in all states. The Task Force also reaffirmed the importance of training, both pre-service and in-service, as a role of the UAFs and endorsed a definition of interdisciplinary training, which had been developed by UAF training directors:

> *Interdisciplinary training means an integrated educational process involving the interdependent contributions of the several relevant disciplines to enhance professional growth as it relates to training, service and research. This process promotes development and use of a basic language, a core body of knowledge, relevant skills and the understanding of the attitudes, values and methods of the participating disciplines.*
>
> —*UAF Long Range Planning Task Force,[24] p 11*

The reader is referred to the UAF Long Range Planning Task Force report *The Role of Higher Education in Mental Retardation and Developmental Disabilities.*[24] The values and concepts related to interdisciplinary training and service described are as important today as they were in 1976.

The funding for the programs came from two sources the Administration for Developmental Disabilities and the Maternal and Child Health Bureau. The Maternal and Child Health Bureau programs maintained a stronger child and health focus than did those funded by the Administration for Developmental Disabilities. These programs became the Leadership Education in NeuroDevelopment and Related Disabilities (LEND). The LEND programs were developed by the Maternal and Child Health Bureau to improve the health status of infants, children, and adolescents with or at risk for neurodevelopmental and related disabilities and the health status of their families. This is accomplished through the training of professionals for leadership roles in the provision of health and related care, continuing education, technical assistance, research, and consultation.

Interdisciplinary training is the hallmark of LEND programs. Faculty and trainees represent 11 core academic disciplines: audiology, health administration, nursing, nutrition, occupational therapy, pediatrics, pediatric dentistry, physical therapy, psychology, social work, and speech and language pathology. Many LENDs have additional disciplines, including assistive technology, genetics, rehabilitation, and psychiatry. All LEND programs include parents and families as paid staff, faculty, consultants, and/or trainees.

LEND programs operate within a university system, usually as part of a University Center for Excellence in Developmental Disabilities or other larger entity, and have collaborative arrangements with local university hospitals and/or health care centers. The LEND curriculum includes graduate education at the master's, doctoral, and postdoctoral levels, with an emphasis on developing a knowledge and experience base that includes (1) neurodevelopmental and related disabilities, (2) family-centered, culturally competent care, and (3) interdisciplinary and leadership skills. Traineeships include classroom course work, leadership development, clinical skills building, mentoring, research, and outreach to the community through clinics, continuing education, consultation, and technical assistance. Currently, there are 35 LEND programs in 29 states. With roots in the 1950s efforts of the Children's Bureau (now the Maternal and Child Health Bureau) to identify children with disabilities as a Title V program priority, they have a long history of training leaders, providing interdisciplinary care and complimenting the work of Title V programs in their regions.

The 1970s also marked the expansion of interdisciplinary teams in education with the 1975 passage of the Education for All Handicapped Children Act (Public Law 94-142). The Act mandated that public school districts develop interdisciplinary teams as the core of the decision-making process in special education for children with disabilities. The team process was to encompass both assessments and program planning and to include both professionals and the family. Because the legislation did not provide specific guidelines as to how these teams were to be developed, which professionals should be on the team, or how they should make decisions, enormous variability resulted in the way different states developed the teams and processes to respond to the federal requirement. In the 1980s, a national concern arose for young children and their families, resulting in the Education of the Handicapped Act Amendments of 1986 (Public Law 99-457), which extended special education services to children 3 to 6 years of age and

encouraged the provision of family-centered interdisciplinary early intervention services for children from birth to 3 years of age.

WHAT IS A TEAM?

There are multiple definitions of what a team is; many of the definitions are based on different theoretical frames of reference. One definition, based on organizational design theory, that is frequently cited is that a "team" is a small number of people with complementary skills who are committed to a common purpose, performance goals, and approach for which they hold themselves mutually accountable.[26] The four elements of this definition are as follows:

1. A small number of people: There is no universal agreement as to what a small number of people is, but often no more than 7 to 10 is considered optimal.[27,28] The size of the group becomes important because teams need to work together in some manner to accomplish their work. Research regarding health care teams has indicated that as the group size increases, team cooperation and team member participation decrease.[29,30] In addition, the larger the size of a team, the more difficult it is for all team members to meet together at the same time, and the amount of time needed increases if all members are to be involved in decision making.

2. Complementary skills: The required complementary skills include technical or functional skills, problem-solving and decision-making skills, and interpersonal skills.[31] This does not mean that each individual has all the required skills initially, but they must have the potential to develop all the skills if the team is to succeed. For example, someone can have excellent technical/functional skills in his or her discipline, but if he or she does not also have, or have the potential to develop, the interpersonal skills to interact with the team, the work of the team will be adversely affected. The involvement of multiple disciplines with the complementary knowledge and skills needed to provide comprehensive care is the foundation for the interdisciplinary team approach.

3. Commitment to a common purpose: Katzenbach and Smith[31] viewed this as the essence of a team, and without it, they become a powerful unit of collective performance. This common purpose is then translated into specific performance goals that facilitate communication and help the team keep track of progress and hold itself accountable. Commitment to a common purpose is also cited in health care team literature as one of the essential aspects of successful team functioning.[32-35]

4. Mutual accountability: For a team to be successful, teams need to hold themselves accountable for the team's performance, both as individuals and as a team. In health care team literature, this is frequently referred to as *shared responsibility* and is considered essential for interdisciplinary team decision making.[36-39]

Although the term *team* is often used interchangeably with *workgroup,* it is viewed as different in several ways. Katzenbach and Smith[31] identified both collective performance and mutual responsibility as two major ways in which teams differ from workgroups. In their view, a workgroup's performance is a function of what its members do as individuals, and responsibility for performance is solely at the individual level. Drinka[40] distinguished between the two on the basis of three factors present in health care teams, but not workgroups, that can negatively affect group process: presence of autonomous disciplines who are used to doing things independently of other disciplines; the ongoing nature of health care teams rather than being time-limited, as workgroups are; and the continual entering and leaving of members as a result of high staff turnover.

MODELS OF TEAMWORK

The composition, organization, and functioning of health care teams varies widely among institutions, medical specialties, and type of services offered.[41] Many teams include a number of loosely associated personnel or a smaller number of highly interdependent professionals. Multiple terms are used in an attempt to describe the different models of current health care teams, including *unidisciplinary, intradisciplinary, cross-disciplinary, multidisciplinary, interdisciplinary, intraprofessional,* and *transdisciplinary.* The most common terms, often used interchangeably, are *multidisciplinary, interdisciplinary,* and *transdisicplinary.* All three models are based on the recognition that no one discipline has the breadth of knowledge and skills that are necessary to provide quality health care.

Unidisciplinary

This term in the past has not been included as a model of teamwork, because it was traditionally used to refer to one professional working independently in his or her specialty. Historically, in terms of the interdisciplinary approach, it also implied a professional who perceived himself or herself as have the knowledge and skills needed to identify and address all areas related to his or her field of focus. The well-known fable of "The Blind Men and the Elephant" has often been used as a metaphor in describing unidisciplinary functioning. Just as each man who was blind determined what the elephant was like on the basis of the individual part the man touched, each discipline perceives the individual in a unique, valid way and yet risks remaining "blind" to the total individual. With the emergence of single-discipline group practices, the term is also used at times to refer to two of more professionals in a discipline who share the same professional skills and training, have a common language, and function in a group.[42] As a result of increased specialization within medicine, *unidisciplinary,* or what sometimes is referred to as *intradisciplinary,* has been used to describe a team of professionals in a discipline who have additional professional skills and training in varying specialty areas and, although they share some common language, have developed a language specific to their specialty. An example of a unidisciplinary team would be a pediatric urologist, a pediatric neurologist, and a pediatric orthopedist who communicate with each other and share information in the provision of care to an individual child.

Multidisciplinary

This team is sometimes used to refer to an intradisciplinary team but in most instances is used to refer to a team that is composed of two or more disciplines. The features most often identified in relationship to the multidisciplinary team are as follows:

1. *Assessments* are conducted independently by the individual disciplines according to traditional concepts of disciplinary roles.[38,42-45]
2. *Communication* is limited or lacking.[37,38,46] The mode of communication may be solely through individual written reports, which are collected by one team member, usually the physician, who then synthesizes the information and recommendations.[43,47] Some multidisciplinary teams may also hold team meetings as a forum for communication through information sharing.[43-45]
3. *Intervention plans* are developed independently by the individual disciplines.[38,42,44]
4. *Delivery of services* is provided independently by the individual disciplines.[38,42,44,45]

Some authorities also equate the multidisciplinary team model with "The Blind Men and the Elephant" in that each discipline "feels" or focuses on its own area. The difference with the multidisciplinary team is that there is some form of communication about the information that was obtained that potentially contributes to decision making with regard to the "whole." There is, as a result, less chance for one person's mistakes or biases to determine the course of events.[43] However, the model can result in simply piecing information together on the basis of the individual discipline results, especially if the model is implemented without the opportunity for interaction between team members at a team meeting.[38]

Interdisciplinary

This term is increasingly being used interchangeably with *interprofessional,* which is widely used in health care team publications from the United Kingdom and Canada. The features most frequently identified in relationship to interdisciplinary teams are as follows:

1. *Assessments* are conducted by independently by the individual disciplines according to traditional concepts of disciplinary roles.[38,42-45]
2. *Communication* is through both written reports and team meetings that serve as a forum for information sharing, collaborative decision making, and planning among team members.[43,44,46,47]
3. *Intervention plans* are developed in collaboration with other disciplines into a unified plan of care.[38,43,44]
4. *Delivery of services* is provided independently by the agreed-upon disciplines.[38,47]

One of the strengths of the interdisciplinary model is the integration of the individual contributions of team members to address a common set of issues or problems.[37,45-47] Another strength is the collaborative decision making that occurs to establish a holistic plan of care or recommendations.[37,45,47] Over time, the team members also develop a "common language" that facilitates communication and collaborative decision making.[36,37] The interdisciplinary team model, however, also presents several challenges, which are discussed separately.

Transdisciplinary

The features most frequently identified in relationship to transdisciplinary teams are as follows:

1. *Assessments* are conducted by one or more team members who share, or transfer, knowledge and skills across traditional disciplinary boundaries.[43,44] At times these assessments, especially in the area of early intervention, may be referred to as *arena assessments,* in which one team member conducts the assessment while other team members, including the parent or parents, observe.[43]
2. *Communication* involves highly coordinated efforts for team members to interact with one another during the assessment and intervention processes.[43]

3. *Intervention plans* are developed collaboratively among team members.[43]
4. *Delivery of services* is provided by one or two team members who share, or transfer, knowledge and skills across traditional disciplinary boundaries while consulting with the other team members.[38,43]

Strengths of the transdisciplinary model include a high degree of interaction and coordination; increased agreement among team members about the acceptability of recommendations; enhanced opportunities for team members to learn from one another; decreased fragmentation of services; and increased continuity and consistency of services.[43] Also, in the area of early intervention, limiting the number of people who come in contact with a very young child prevents duplication of services and unnecessary intrusion into family activities and routines.[44] Although the high degree of interaction and coordination is a strength, it is also a potential challenge in that the required degree of role sharing and transfer may lead to role ambiguity, role conflict, and role release to the extent of loss of professional identity.[43]

Transdisciplinary has also been used to refer to teams of multiskilled health practitioners who are trained to provide a wide range of services in a specific field, such as geriatrics, apart from training in a traditional discipline.[38] This approach to the provision of health care has also been referred to as a *pandisciplinary* model, in which a single new discipline's role spans all areas of competence relevant to a specific field.[42] Unfortunately, in many ways, the pandisciplinary model brings teamwork full circle back to an unidisciplinary approach in which practitioners from one discipline assume that they have all the knowledge and skills needed to provide services in a particular field.

Each model of teamwork described has its strengths and challenges. Some professionals advocate one model over, implying that the particular model is better than others. It is more constructive to think of the models as points along a continuum of approaches, all of which have the common goal of providing high-quality services to children with developmental disabilities and to their families. Different programs serving children with developmental disabilities and their families use different models along this continuum to reach the common goal. For a program that provides ongoing services to a large number of children with medically complex health needs that necessitate the involvement of multiple medical specialties, the multidisciplinary team model may be the only feasible model. However, in a program that provides diagnostic and treatment services for children of varying ages with a broad range of developmental disabilities, the interdisciplinary team approach may be the model by which services are provided for older children, and the transdiciplinary model, by which services are provided for very young children and their families.

In the interdisciplinary and transdisciplinary model, and frequently in the multidisciplinary model, decision making involves face-to-face interaction. A new type of team, the virtual team, is emerging in the health care field. Virtual teams have been used in business for some time and consist of geographically or organizationally dispersed members who use technologies to perform team tasks.[48] Rather than communication during face-to-face meetings, communication and decision making are accomplished through such technologies as email or video teleconferencing. Within health care, with the increasing demands for productivity and changing reimbursement, traditional models of teamwork may no longer be as functional as they once were and may be replaced by virtual teams.[49,50] According to a developing body of knowledge about virtual teams, virtual teams apparently go through the same stages of team development and confront the same interpersonal process issues that exist in teams that meet face to face.[51,52]

FACTORS THAT CONTRIBUTE TO INTERDISCIPLINARY TEAM COLLABORATION

As discussed under the definition of a team, three important factors are complementary skills (discipline skills, problem-solving and decision-making skills, and interpersonal skills), commitment to a common purpose, and mutual accountability. Closely related to these factors are the concepts of shared leadership roles and shared power.[31,33,37,39] *Shared leadership* means that each team member, depending on the situation, assumes the role of either team leader or team member.[53] Historically, interdisciplinary teams tended to have one member who was designated the team leader upon whom the onus was placed for the success or failure of the team. A large body of literature emerged addressing leadership roles and styles of successful and unsuccessful team leaders. Slowly the responsibility for success or failure of interdisciplinary teams in achieving their goals shifted also to team members, and literature focusing on the attributes and behaviors of effective team members began to emerge.[38] As the concept of shared leadership evolved, the concept of shared power among team members, regardless of educational or professional preparation, also evolved.[39] Power and status within the interdisciplinary team was historically accorded to the physician, who usually was also the team leader.[9,37,54] However, other hierarchies also exist not only between other disciplines but also within disciplines, on the basis of educational preparation (e.g., doctoral, master's, bachelor's degrees).[37,55] Shared power is viewed as a means to bestow each team member equal status within the interdisciplinary team. This concept is especially important if family members are truly to be members of the interdisciplinary team.

Among the additional factors that have been identified as contributing to interdisciplinary team collaboration are individual or personal attributes. Simply placing someone in a team will not make him or her an effective team member. The reality is that some people are egocentric and do not have the collective orientation to be team members.[56] Some of the individual attributes identified as enhancing interdisciplinary team function are flexibility and adaptability[31,34] and the abilities to view diverse perspectives as learning opportunities, to engage in critical thinking, and to synthesize information adaptability.[57]

Another factor that is frequently mentioned as contributing to interdisciplinary team collaboration is the development of "common language" among the team members. Individual disciplines speak different languages that contain very discipline-specific terminology, jargon, and acronyms,[37] which become even more difficult to understand the more specialized a discipline becomes.[58] The process of developing a common language takes time and evolves from communication and learning that occurs as the team works together. It involves recognizing that, for disciplinary knowledge explicit and accessible to other disciplines, it must be translated into a language that other people will understand.[36] However, members of other disciplines must be comfortable enough within the team to ask for clarification when they do not understand members of another discipline. Another problem of "common language" that often takes a longer time to surface occurs when two or more disciplines use a common term and thus think they are communicating, when in reality they are not because they define the term differently in subtle ways.

Just as members of different disciplines speak different languages, they differ in other ways. It has been suggested that viewing disciplines as culturally diverse groups will result in a better understanding of and respect for the diverse perspectives of the disciplines.[57,59] Some of the ways in which disciplines, like cultures, may differ are in their theoretical orientation and assumptions (e.g., biomedical, behavioral, and biopsychosocial)[37,60]; their mode of thinking (e.g., divergent/inductive vs. convergent/deductive)[55,61]; and values (e.g., saving life vs. quality of life).[60,61] Also involved is developing an understanding of such areas as the education, levels of practice, areas of expertise, and roles of the individual disciplines.[37,42,62] By learning about one another, team members not only develop a better general understanding of one another but are able to identify the specific roles and responsibilities of individual team members, how they interface with each other, and where their disciplines overlap.[42,60]

FACTORS THAT PRESENT CHALLENGES FOR INTERDISCIPLINARY TEAM COLLABORATION

Many of the factors discussed previously, if not present, present challenges for interdisciplinary team collaboration. Even if those factors are present, however, others may become a challenge if not addressed in constructive ways. An example is role overlap. Interdisciplinary team members may learn about one another to the degree that they are able to identify the areas in which two or more disciplines share expertise. However, if they are not able to trust other team members enough to relinquish that role when appropriate to the situation or common goal, interdisciplinary team collaboration is negatively affected. Two additional factors that have the potential to contribute to interdisciplinary team collaboration are organizational structure and interdisciplinary education. These factors, however, currently represent major challenges for interdisciplinary team collaboration.

The organizational structures in which interdisciplinary teams operate are vital to their survival and significantly affect their performance.[39,63-65] In an era in which teamwork is becoming a norm within health care organizations, there is concern that many health care organizations may not be ready or able to support interdisciplinary teams as the norm in service provision.[35,66] The interdisciplinary approach requires an organizational structure that values the interdisciplinary team approach and is able to support the approach fiscally. Increased emphases on fee-generating services and productivity are already having affecting the provision of interdisciplinary team services in organizations in which this approach to service provision has been used, especially in which health care team services cannot also be covered by facility charges.[67] The fee-for-service structure and current reimbursement policies are real barriers to the interdisciplinary team approach[68] and are being questioned if the team model, although based on "best practices," is financially viable.[67] Settings in which the interdisciplinary approach is used to serve children with developmental disabilities and their families are facing the same emphases on fee-generating services and productivity as are other settings that provide services through the interdisciplinary approach. The issue of reimbursement for services has created the hierarchy of disciplines that can generate fees and disciplines that cannot; those that cannot are at risk of no longer being included in the provision of services to the degree they once were. Also, one of the advantages of the interdisciplinary team approach has been the team meetings, which provide team members the opportunity to learn from one another, share information, and participate in collaborative decision making and planning. Current payment policies, however, do not cover the time involved in team meetings.[68] As a result, some settings that had been based on an interdisciplinary team model of services have had to retrench to the multidisciplinary model.

A second challenge to the interdisciplinary team collaboration is the current status of interdisciplinary education. Although interdisciplinary training has been promoted in areas such as developmental disabilities, geriatrics, rehabilitation, and primary care for underserved populations since the 1960s, it has never been widely incorporated into disciplinary training. Disciplinary education is viewed as a means of socializing a student to his or her future roles within the discipline. This role socialization has often been considered a major barrier to interdisciplinary teamwork because it is conducted in isolation from other disciplines.[9,35,42,54,58,63] Not only is it conducted in isolation but also students are not necessarily rewarded for looking beyond their discipline for knowledge. Frequently, students are awarded grades on written assignments on the basis of their knowledge of disciplinary literature rather than their ability to integrate congruent or noncongruent knowledge from other disciplines into their assignment.

Ducanis and Golin[63] identified three elements of interdisciplinary or team training: cognitive information, affective and experiential learning, and clinical competence. Within universities, there have been isolated models of interdisciplinary training that have especially addressed the areas of cognitive information and experiential learning, but for the most part they have not been widely incorporated.[15,19] As with the implementation of the interdisciplinary team approach within health care organizations, interdisciplinary education requires a university structure that values the interdisciplinary education and is willing to support the approach fiscally.[42,54] In addition, universities have been challenged with integrating additional emerging discipline-specific knowledge areas into already crowded curricula; when faced with this situation, faculty members are more likely to support discipline-specific knowledge than interdisciplinary knowledge.[54]

CONCEPTUAL MODELS USED TO EVALUATE INTERDISCIPLINARY TEAMS

Multiple conceptual models have been used to study and evaluate interdisciplinary teams. In some models, originating from group process theory, teams are viewed as evolving through various developmental stages. One of these models was developed by Drinka[40] and identifies the stages as forming, "norming," confronting, performing and leaving. Another model, developed by Lowe and Herranen,[69] identifies the stages as becoming acquainted, trial and error, collective indecision, crisis, resolution, and team maintenance. One of the differences in the models is that the first model recognizes that team membership does not remain constant and, as team members leave and new team members enter, there is an effect on team performance. In additional models, teams are viewed in terms of group problem solving as an indicator of group effectiveness,[62,70] the social climate of the groups,[71] group interactions and relational norms,[65] or role behavior and conflict.[54]

As organizational theory began to be applied to interdisciplinary teams, models were developed in which teams were also viewed in terms of processes in different areas. In one model, teams are viewed in terms of the areas of establishing trust, developing common beliefs and attitudes, empowering team members, having effectively managed team meetings, and providing feedback about team functioning.[33] Other models integrate multiple theoretical perspectives into the model. For example, a model developed by Bronstein[34] focuses on team processes in the areas of interdependence, newly created professional activities, flexibility, collective ownership of goals, and reflection on process. All these models focus on team process as indicators of team performance, with the assumption that an effectively functioning interdisciplinary team will provide quality services. However, it has been suggested that process measures really do not reflect team outcome and are important primarily for team training purposes when the intent is to identify performance issues and provide feedback to assist the individual in improving his or her behavior.[35]

REVIEW OF THE RESEARCH ON INTERDISCIPLINARY TEAMS

Several articles have included extensive reviews of the literature regarding interdisciplinary team care. The majority of these reviews concluded that there is little evidence of the effectiveness of interdisciplinary teams.[45,53,60,68,72,73] These reviews of the literature also indicated the following:

1. Opinions differ as to whether the lack of evidence of the effectiveness of the interdisciplinary team is attributable to limited emphasis on outcomes[60,68,72,73] or process.[45,53]
2. For the most part, the effectiveness of the interdisciplinary team approach has been based on assumption.[68,73,74]
3. There are few clear theory-based conceptual models of the interdisciplinary team approach.[60,73]
4. The terms *multidisciplinary* and *interdisciplinary* were seldom defined and were frequently used interchangeably.[45,73]
5. The barriers to the interdisciplinary team approach were discussed equally as often as, if not more frequently than, the benefits of the interdisciplinary team approach.[73,74]

Interestingly, the implementation of the interdisciplinary team approach on the basis of assumption is not unique in relation to the team approach. An example is the CRM approach to teamwork skills training, which serves as the basis for a variety of medical training programs focusing on reducing medical errors. The CRM has been used since 1980 to improve the operation of flight crews, despite the lack of definitive evidence that CRM decreases aviation errors.[18] In addition, despite years of research regarding team performance in the military and corporate world, very little is known about the factors of that determine effective team performance.[56]

Schofield and Amodeo[73] conducted an extensive review of the literature related to interdisciplinary teams in health care and human services settings. Not only did they conclude that there is limited evidence regarding the effectiveness of interdisciplinary teams, but the review also provided information regarding the fields from which the articles originated and the types of articles that have been written about interdisciplinary teams. From abstracts, Schofield and Amodeo identified 224 articles that potentially focused on the interdisciplinary approach to the provision of services. The majority of articles were in the fields of rehabilitation, geriatrics, health services, and mental health services; fewer than 25 articles were found in the field of developmental disabilities. After they eliminated articles that used the terms *multidisciplinary* or *interdisciplinary* without additional explanation, there were 138 potentially useful articles. Of theses articles:

1. Fifty-five were descriptive articles that discussed the concept of the interdisciplinary team, or some aspect of it, in a general way on the basis of observation or past experience.

2. Fifty-one were process-focused articles that described the process of the interdisciplinary team but whose authors did not use any formal research measures.
3. Twenty-one articles were empirically based in that some research or quantitative measure was used and the focus of the study was on the interdisciplinary team.
4. Eleven articles were outcome-based articles in that the authors used formal research methods and examined the effect of the interdisciplinary team on an external outcome.

Although concluding that there is little evidence regarding the effectiveness of interdisciplinary teams, the authors of these literature reviews acknowledged that research regarding interdisciplinary teams is complex and presents several challenges.[68,72,74] For one thing, no two teams appear to be alike. The structure of interdisciplinary teams varies greatly between settings and, at times, within settings in terms of structure (e.g., composition of disciplines and number of team members).[68] In addition, interdisciplinary teams function in clinical settings in which it is more difficult to use rigorous research designs.[72] Third, the concept of the interdisciplinary team is to use the knowledge and skills of a number of disciplines to address a range of needs rather than an outcome in one area. As a result, the outcome of interdisciplinary team care becomes multidimensional and is more difficult to measure.[72]

Today there is an emphasis on cost containment, productivity, and evidence-based practice. If the interdisciplinary team approach is to survive this era, the approach based on assumption can no longer be justified. Research regarding the effectiveness of the interdisciplinary team approach needs to be better conceptualized, employ more sophisticated research designs when possible, and focus on both process and outcome.[35,73] Studies must also clearly define what is meant when the terms *multidisciplinary* and *interdisciplinary* are used[73] and must capture individual and team-level performance.[35] Some of the specific challenging questions for future research include the following:[68]

What are the costs and costs benefits of teams?
Under what conditions are teams cost effective or not cost effective?
Are teams more effective for certain populations (e.g., patients with chronic conditions; those needing preventive care or long-term care) than other populations?
Do less costly multidisciplinary teams achieve the same outcomes as interdisciplinary teams, and is one team model (multidisciplinary or interdisciplinary) more effective for certain populations?

REFERENCES

1. U.S. Department of Health and Human Services: Healthy People 20010, 2nd ed. Washington, DC: U.S. Government Printing Office, 2000.
2. Brown TM: An historical view of health care teams. *In* Agich GJ, ed: Responsibility in Health Care. Dordrecht, Holland: D. Reidel, 1982, pp 3-21.
3. Cabot R: Social Service and the Art of Healing. New York: Moffat, Yard & Company, 1915.
4. Keith RA: The comprehensive treatment in rehabilitation. Arch Phys Med Rehabil 72:269-274, 1991.
5. Royer JA: Historical overview: Group dynamics and health care teams. *In* Baldwin DC, Rowley BD, eds: Interdisciplinary Health Team Training. Lexington: University of Kentucky, Center for Interdisciplinary Education in Allied Health, 1982, pp 12-28.
6. Benne KD, Bradford L, Gibb J, et al: The Laboratory Method of Changing and Learning. Palo Alto, CA: Science and Behavior Books, 1975.
7. Lefkowitz B: The health center story: Forty years of commitment. J Ambul Care Manage 28:295-303, 2005.
8. Purtilo RG: Interdisciplinary health care teams and health care reform. J Law Med Ethics 22:121-126, 1994.
9. Leininger M: This I believe . . . about interdisciplinary education for the future. Nurs Outlook. 19:787-791, 1971.
10. Wise H, Beckard R, Rubin I, et al: Making Health Teams Work. Cambridge, MA: Ballinger, 1973.
11. Wise H, Rubin I, Beckard R: Making health teams work. Am J Dis Child 127:537-542, 1974.
12. Kane RA: The interprofessional team as a small group. Soc Work Health Care 1(1):19-31, 1975.
13. Reuben DB, Levy-Storms L, Yee MN, et al: Disciplinary split: A treat to geriatrics interdisciplinary team training. J Am Geriatr Soc 52:1000-1006, 2004.
14. Drinka TJK: Applying learning from self-directed work teams in business to curriculum development for interdisciplinary geriatric teams. Educ Geront 22:433-450, 1996.
15. Pew Health Professions Commission: Critical Challenges: Revitalizing the Health Professions for the Twenty-First Century. Berkeley, CA: University of California at Berkeley, Center for Health Professions, 1995.
16. Institute of Medicine: To Err Is Human: Building a Safer Health System. Washington, DC: National Academies Press, 2000.
17. Baker DP, Gustafson S, Beaubien JM, et al: Medical team training programs in health care. *In* Advances in Patient Safety: From Research to Implementation. Volume 4: Programs, Tools, and Products (AHRQ Publication No. 050021 [4]). Rockville, MD: Agency for Healthcare Research and Quality, 2005, pp 253-267. (Available at: *http://www.ahrq.gov/qual/advances*; accessed 10/23/06.)
18. Pizzi L, Goldfarb NI, Nash DB: Crew resource management and its application in medicine. *In Making Health Care Safer: A Critical Analysis of Patient Safety*

Practices. Evidence Report/Technology Assessment: Number 43 (AHRQ Publication No. 01-E058). Rockville, MD: Agency for Healthcare Research and Quality, 2001, pp 501-509. (Available at: *http://www.ahrq.gov/clinic/ptsafety;* accessed 10/23/06, Chapter 44.)

19. Institute of Medicine: Crossing the Quality Chasm: A New Health System for the 21st Century. Washington, DC: National Academies Press, 2001.

20. Institute of Medicine: Health Professions Education: A Bridge to Quality. Washington, DC: National Academies Press, 2003.

21. Peppe KK, Sherman RG: Nursing in mental retardation: Historical perspective. *In* Curry JB, Peppe KK, eds: Mental Retardation: Nursing Approaches to Care. St. Louis: CV Mosby, 1978, pp 3-18.

22. Sheridan MD: The Handicapped Child and His Home. London: National Children's Home, 1965.

23. The President's Panel on Mental Retardation: A Proposed Program for National Action to Combat Mental Retardation. Washington, DC: Superintendent of Documents, 1962.

24. UAF Long Range Planning Task Force: The Role of Higher Education in Mental Retardation and Other Developmental Disabilities. Washington, DC: Department of Health, Education and Welfare, 1976.

25. Chamberlin HR: The interdisciplinary team: Contributions by allied medical and nonmedical disciplines. *In* Gabel S, Erickson MT, eds: Child Development and Developmental Disabilities. Boston: Little, Brown, 1980, pp 435-470.

26. Katzenbach JR, Smith DK: The Wisdom of Teams. Boston: Harvard Business School Press, 1993.

27. Cowell J, Michaelson J: Flawless teams. Executive Excellence 17(3):11, 2000.

28. Hrickiewicz M: What makes teams successful? Health Facil Manage 14(3):4, 2001.

29. Stahelski AJ, Tsukuda RA: Predictors of cooperation in health care teams. Small Group Res 21:220-233, 1990.

30. Poulton BC, West MA: The determinants of effectiveness in primary health care teams. J Interprof Care 13:7-18, 1999.

31. Katzenbach JR, Smith DK: The discipline of teams. Harv Bus Rev 71(2):111-120, 1993.

32. Sands RG, Stafford RG, McClelland M: "I beg to differ": Conflict in the interdisciplinary team. Soc Work Health Care 14(3):55-72, 1990.

33. Dukewits P, Gowan, L: Creating successful collaborative teams. J Staff Dev 17(4):12-16, 1996.

34. Bronstein LR: A model for interdisciplinary collaboration. Soc Work 48(3):113-116, 2003.

35. Baker DP, Salas E, King H, et al: The role of teamwork in the professional education of physicians: Current status and assessment recommendations. J Qual Patient Safety 31:185-202, 2005.

36. De Wachter M: Interdisciplinary teamwork. J Med Ethics 2:52-57, 1976.

37. Pearson PH: The interdisciplinary team process, or the professionals' Tower of Babel. Dev Med Child Neurol 25:390-397, 1983.

38. Frattali CM: Professional Collaboration: A Team Approach to Health Care. Clinical Series No. 11. Rockville, MD: National Student Speech Language Hearing Association, 1993.

39. Orchard CA, Curran V, Kabene S: Creating a culture for interdisciplinary collaborative professional practice. Med Educ Online 10:11, 2005. (Available at: *http://www.med-ed-online.org;* accessed 10/24/06.)

40. Drinka TJ: Interdisciplinary geriatric teams: Approaches to conflict as indicators of potential to model teamwork. Educ Gerontol 20:87-103, 1994.

41. Ellingston LL: Communication, collaboration, and teamwork among health care professionals. Commun Res Trends 21(3):3-21, 2002.

42. Satin DG: A conceptual framework for working relationships among disciplines and the place of interdisciplinary education and practice: Clarifying muddy waters. Gerontol Geriatr Educ 14(3):3-24, 1994.

43. McCollum JA, Hughes M: Staffing patterns and team models in infancy programs. *In* Jordan JB, ed: Early Childhood Education: Birth to Three. Reston, VA: Council for Exceptional Children, 1988, pp 130-146.

44. Briggs MH: Team decision-making for early intervention. Infant Toddler Interv Transdiscip J 1(1):1-9, 1991.

45. Wiecha J, Pollard T: The interdisciplinary eHealth team: Chronic care for the future. J Med Internet Res 6(3):e22, 2004. (Available at: http://www.jmir.org/2004/e22/; accessed 10/24/06.)

46. Meeth LR: Interdisciplinary studies: A matter of definition. CHANGE 10(7):10, 1978.

47. Hall P, Weaver L: Interdisciplinary education and teamwork: A long and winding road. Med Educ 35:867-875, 2001.

48. Maruping LM, Agarwal R: Managing team interpersonal process through technology: A task-technology fit perspective. J Appl Psychol 89:975-990, 2004.

49. Cole KD: Organizational structure, team process, and future directions of interprofessional health care teams. Gerontol Geriatr Educ 24(2):35-49, 2003.

50. Rothschild SK, Lapidos S: Virtual integrated practice: Integrating teams and technology to manage chronic disease in primary care. J Med Syst 27(1):85-93, 2003.

51. Vroman K, Kovacich J: Computer-mediated interdisciplinary teams: Theory and reality. J Interprof Care 16:159-170, 2002.

52. Furst S, Reeves M, Rosen B, et al: Managing the life of virtual teams. Acad Manage Exec 18(2):6-20, 2004.

53. McCallin A: Interdisciplinary team leadership: A revisionist approach for an old problem? J Nurs Manage 11:364-370, 2003.

54. Aaronson WE: Interdisciplinary health team role taking as a function of health professional education. Gerontol Geriatr Educ 12(1):97-110, 1991.

55. Drinka TJK: From double jeopardy to double indemnity: Subtleties of teaching interdisciplinary geriatrics. Educ Gerontol 28:433-449, 2002.

56. Driskell JE: Collective behavior and team performance. Hum Factors 34:277-288, 1992.

57. Vincenti VB: Family and consumer sciences university faculty perceptions of interdisciplinary work. Fam Consum Sci Res J 34(1):81-104, 2005.

58. Garner HG: Challenges and opportunities of teamwork. *In* Orelove FP, Garner HG, eds: Teamwork: Parents and Professionals Speak for Themselves. Washington, DC: Child Welfare League of America, 1998, pp 11-29.

59. Clark P: Values in health care professional socialization: Implications for geriatric education in interdisciplinary teamwork. Gerontologist 37:441-451, 1997.

60. Simpson G, Rabin D, Schmitt M, et al: Interprofessional health care practice: Recommendations of the National Academies of Practice expert panel on health care in the 21st century. Issues Interdiscip Care: Natl Acad Pract Forum 3(1):5-19, 2001.

61. Qualls SH, Czirr R: Geriatric health teams: Classifying models of professional and team functioning. Gerontologist 28:372-376, 1988.

62. Christensen C, Larson JR: Collaborative medical decision making. Med Decis Mak 13(4):339-346, 1993.

63. Ducanis AJ, Golin AK: The Interdisciplinary Health Care Team: A Handbook. Germantown, MD: Aspen, 1979.

64. Butterill D, O'Hanlon J, Book H: When the system is the problem, don't blame the patient: Problems inherent in the interdisciplinary inpatient team. Can J Psychiatry 37:168-172, 1992.

65. Amundson SJ: The impact of relational norms on the effectiveness of health and service teams. Health Care Manag (Frederick) 24:216-224, 2005.

66. Cashman SB, Reidy P, Cody K, et al: Developing and measuring progress toward collaborative, integrated, interdisciplinary health care teams. J Interprof Care 18:183-196, 2004.

67. Melzer SM, Richards GE, Covington MW: Reimbursement and costs of pediatric ambulatory diabetes care by using the resource-based relative value scale: Is multidisciplinary care financially viable? Pediatr Diabetes 5:133-142, 2004.

68. Cooper BS, Fishman E: The Interdisciplinary Team in the Management of Chronic Conditions: Has Its Time Come? Baltimore: John Hopkins University, Partners for Solutions, 2003.

69. Lowe JI, Herranen M: Understanding teamwork: Another look at the concepts. Soc Work Health Care 7(2):1-11, 1981.

70. Whorley LW: Evaluating health care team performance: Assessment of joint problem-solving action. Health Care Superv 14(4):71-76, 1996.

71. Brock D, Barker C: Group environment and group interaction in psychiatric assessment meetings. Int J Soc Psychiatry 36:111-120, 1990.

72. Schmitt MH, Farrell MP, Heinemann GD: Conceptual and methodological problems in studying the effects of interdisciplinary geriatric teams. Gerontologist 28:753-764, 1988.

73. Schofield RF, Amodeo M: Interdisciplinary teams in health care and human service settings: Are they effective? Health Soc Work 24:210-219, 1999.

74. Opie A: Thinking teams thinking clients: Issues of discourse and representation in the work of health care teams. Sociol Health Illness 19:259-280, 1997.

8B.
Family-Centered Care and the Medical Home

LAURA MCGUINN ■ LOUIS WORLEY

Family-centered care is a term widely used to describe a philosophy of health care service delivery for children and their families. Despite this, confusion persists about what the concept means and how to apply it when working with patients and families; therefore, the purpose in this chapter is to assist child health practitioners to understand family-centered care and the related idea of the "medical home."

Societal changes have affected the relationship between families, children, and pediatricians.[1,2] Technological advances, the growing prevalence of chronic disease in children, increasing empowerment of patients as consumers, and public access to information once available only through professionals, as well as the decreasing frequency of longitudinal patient-physician relationships, have affected the capability of the existing health care system to meet the needs of children and their families. If primary authority for clinical decision making in behalf of children is delegated to the pediatrician on the basis of professional expertise, there is a risk of minimizing the family's lived experience; therefore, from many perspectives, traditional roles are no longer preferred. Instead, many families and pediatricians desire a relationship in which the contributions of each is valued. These role changes, along with acknowledgement that the health care system is failing to produce desired outcomes despite dramatically spiraling costs, urge redesign.[3] Efforts to improve the quality of health care have focused on transforming biomedically dominated care processes to those guided by patients' and families' unique needs and values. In this chapter, we address relationship-focused quality improvement strategies by exploring the concept of family-centered care, examining selected evidence linking family-centered care to outcomes for children and families, discussing how family-centered care is applied in the medical home model within pediatric primary health care settings, and suggesting future directions in family-centered care practices and research.

HISTORICAL FOUNDATIONS OF THE FAMILY-CENTERED CARE CONCEPT

Family-centered care is one of several terms referring to a patient-centric view of the patient-physician relationship, and this concept is a relatively recent social movement. Although the concept began gaining momentum largely through the advocacy led by parents of children with special health care needs (CSHCN) in the 1980s, aspects of its underlying principles can be found in philosophical writings on the patient-physician relationship from ancient through contemporary times.[3-5] Through the years, the concept has been discussed under the guise of different labels, including *client-centered therapy*,[6] *patient-centered care*,[4,7] and *relationship-centered care*.[8] The common theme is that successful caregiving requires not only accurately diagnosing disease but also valuing the importance of human interactions in health care experiences and the legitimacy of the patient's beliefs and preferences. Patient centeredness is frequently described by contrasting it to physician or system centeredness; the difficulty in attaining the required paradigm shift is highlighted by comparison to the inversion of thinking necessary to view the sun rather than the earth as the center of the universe.[9] In a system-centered model, care processes are structured to facilitate the function of health care professionals to serve patients; patients must adapt to the constraints of the system. When a patient-centered model is used, the opposite is true: The system accommodates the individual. In pediatrics, patient-centered care is typically referred to as *family-centered care* to acknowledge that children's well-being is inextricably linked to that of their families. A family-centered approach requires recognition that families have the most expertise about their child and, therefore, that they have the right and the responsibility to collaborate in medical decision making in behalf of their child.[9,10] The following sections highlight some of the historical forces that have shaped the concept of family-centered care, including policy changes affecting family presence during hospitalizations, epidemiological changes in children's health, broadening views of health determinants, and growing numbers of families raising CSHCN. Theoretical benefits of family-centered care, as well as empirical evidence regarding the efficacy of its use, are examined later in the chapter.

Changes in Hospital Policies Affecting Families Rights and Responsibilities

Even until the late 1950s, most medical professionals believed that visits from parents to their hospitalized children would inhibit effective care. Observations that children cried more in the presence of a parent or became distressed when their parent left led physicians and nurses to interpret parental visits as harmful for children.[11] As a result, parents were regularly excluded from partnership in medical decision making

about their children. By the 1970s, because of accumulating evidence that episodes of separation from their parents had the potential to harm children's psychological well-being,[12-14] U.S. hospital policies began allowing parents to stay with their children during admissions.[15] Newborns began rooming in with their mothers instead of group nurseries, and fathers were permitted in the delivery room to support mothers during labor.[16] The restrictive hospital policies before the 1970s that curtailed the family's ability to comfort a hospitalized child (or other family member) provide an example of strategies that maintained institutional and staff control and exemplify system-centered models of health care delivery.

Epidemiological Changes in Children's Health and Broadening Views of Health Determinants

In the 1970s, health services researchers brought attention to the growing prevalence of children's psychosocial difficulties. Haggerty and colleagues called this growing challenge "the new morbidity" in their 1975 publication, *Child Health and the Community*,[17] and conceptualized the interdependence of the family, the community, and children's health. The authors asserted that for pediatricians to remain relevant to the well-being of children, pediatric training and practice would have to shift from focusing solely on the individual child to examining broader contextual aspects, including the family. The shift in thinking that Haggerty and colleagues' work prompted, together with the rising tide of consumerism, undoubtedly fostered child health professionals to begin exploring the value of encouraging parents to be partners in medical decision making.

Further support for the importance of the family to children's health came in 1977 in Engel's classic article presenting the biopsychosocial medical model.[18] His argument for a new paradigm of medical thinking that moved beyond a solely biomedical view to one that incorporated the inseparability of social and psychological influences on human health lent further support to Haggerty and colleagues' argument that pediatricians needed to shift their focus beyond the child to the family context in order to foster children's health.

Children with Special Health Care Needs and Their Families

Increasing recognition of the growing proportion of CSHCN and the ability of the U.S. health care system to successfully meet their needs spurred public organizers and government policy makers to improve the lives of these children and their families. In the U.S., key agencies that pioneered the CSHCN and family-centered care movement included the Maternal and Child Health Bureau (MCHB), the Association for the Care of Children's Health (ACCH), Association of University Centers of Excellence in Disabilities, and the American Academy of Pediatrics (AAP). As a division of the Health Resources and Services Administration of the U.S. federal government's Department of Health and Human Services, MCHB has long been charged with improving all children's, women's, and families' health and is the designated organization that allocates funds from the federal Social Security Title V Act. ACCH, a now-defunct public organization originally formed in the 1960s, advocated along with MCHB for children's health care system improvements. In the 1980s and 1990s, both organizations, along with the AAP and Association of University Centers of Excellence in Disabilities, were instrumental in broadening the conceptualization of children's chronic disabling health conditions beyond one divided into specific disease categories to a more general category labeled *children with special health care needs,* defined as:

> *Those children who have or are at increased risk for a chronic physical, developmental, behavioral, or emotional condition and who also require health care-related services of a type or amount beyond that required by children generally.*[19]

Former Surgeon General C. Everett Koop's 1987 Conference on Children with Special Health Care Needs disseminated the first widely acknowledged definition of family-centered care in the United States.[20] This definition, formulated before the conference by parents, professionals, and policy makers active in the ACCH and MCHB, was published as a monograph, "Family-centered Care for Children with Special Health Care Needs," that came to be commonly known as "Big Red" because of the red color of the cover.[21] The ACCH made further refinements of the "Big Red" definition in 1994,[9] which resulted in the key principles of family-centered care listed in Table 8B-1.[22] Although the ACCH eventually disbanded, the Institute for Family-Centered Care, established in 1992, assumed the role that ACCH played and continues to disseminate information to promote the practice of family-centered care through annual conferences, information publications, guidelines for hospitals, and consultations to individual health organizations.[23] MCHB also continues to include family-centered care into its improvement mandates for CSHCN:

> *The overall national agenda is to provide and promote family-centered, community-based, coordinated care for CSHCN and to facilitate the development of community-based systems of services for such children and their families.*[24]

TABLE 8B-1 ■ Key Elements of Family-Centered Care
Incorporating into policy and practice the recognition that **the family is the constant** in the child's life, while the service systems and personnel within those systems fluctuate.
Facilitating **family/professional collaboration** at all levels of hospital, home, and community care—care of an individual child; program development, implementation, evaluation and evolution; and policy formation.
Exchanging complete and unbiased information between families and professionals in a supportive manner at all times.
Incorporating into policy and practice the **recognition and honoring of cultural diversity,** strengths, and individuality within and across all families, including ethnic, racial, spiritual, social, economic, educational, and geographic diversity.
Recognizing and **respecting different methods of coping** and implementing comprehensive policies and programs that provide developmental, educational, emotional, environmental, and financial **supports to meet the diverse needs of families.**
Encouraging and facilitating **parent-to-parent support.**
Ensuring that **hospital, home, and community service and support systems** for children needing specialized health and developmental care and their families are **flexible, accessible, and comprehensive** in responding to diverse family-identified needs.
Appreciating families as families and **children as children,** recognizing that they possess a wide range of strengths, concerns, emotions, and aspirations beyond their need for specialized health and developmental services and support.

From Shelton TL, Stepanek JS: The key elements of family-centered care. *In* Family-Centered Care for Children Needing Specialized Health and Developmental Services, 3rd ed. Bethesda, MD: Association for the Care of Children's Health, 1994, p vii.

The concept of family-centered care has undergone further refinements by researchers interested in early intervention services for CSHCN. Dunst and colleagues found that early intervention professionals and programs employing an empowering or enabling help-giving relationship model more effectively achieve desirable child and family outcomes. The work of Dunst and colleagues has focused on outcomes, including family self-determination, decision-making capability, control, and self-efficacy and has precipitated a deeper understanding of the family-centered concept.[25] They have extended the notion of family-centered care from one of simply incorporating parents in the delivery of health care to their children to the broader ideals of family-empowerment and marshalling community supports that are individualized by child and family need instead of imposing help from menu-driven service systems. Family empowerment has been explained as follows: "Family empowerment refers to families acquiring the capacity to exercise power. It makes them not just into actors, but into agents capable of shaping the conditions in which they live as they would want to shape them."[26] Dunst and colleagues proposed employing a conceptual framework of help-giving relationships that empowers families by promoting family competency to identify and manage their child's needs. Their model of empowerment requires specific conditions for both families and professionals. They require that families have (1) an increased understanding of their child's needs, (2) the ability to deploy competencies to meet those needs, and (3) self-efficacy (a belief that they are capable) to do so.[27] Among the conditions for help givers in their model are that professionals (1) have a proactive stance (help givers believe help seekers are already competent or have the capacity to become competent), (2) create opportunities for competence to be displayed (help givers provide enabling experiences to help seekers), and (3) allow help seekers to use their competencies to access resources and attribute success to their own actions, not the professional's. In essence, Dunst and colleagues suggested that viewing the relationship from a strengths-based perspective rather than a deficit one is a more effective way to achieve desired outcomes for CSHCN and their families.

The multidisciplinary research group at McMaster University in Ontario, Canada also has done extensive work on refining the concept of family-centered care as it relates to CSHCN (note that they use the word *service* in place of the word *care*). In a summary of the theoretic and research literature,[28] Rosenbaum attempted to organize the sometimes disparate meanings of family-centered service by dividing the concept into a three-level framework consisting of (1) basic premises or assumptions, (2) guiding principles, and (3) elements or key service provider behaviors. The basic premises are beliefs, values, and ideals about families and together form the backbone of the concept of family-centered service. Each premise has several guiding principles directed to professionals to help them ground their interactions with families. The elements are specific provider behaviors that follow from the assumptions and guiding principles. The addition of the key elements was an attempt to approach a definition that included measurable behaviors. Their conceptualization is summarized in Table 8B-2.

SELECTED RESEARCH EVIDENCE REGARDING FAMILY-CENTERED CARE

Summary of Evidence

Our discussion to this point has focused on the development of the concept of family-centered care. Now we turn to an examination of the empirical evidence

---

TABLE 8B-2 ■ Premises, Principles, and Elements of Family-Centered Service

Premises (Basic Assumptions)

Parents know their children best and want the best for their children.	Families are different and unique.	Optimal child functioning occurs within a supportive family and community context. The child is affected by the stress and coping family members.

Guiding Principles ("Should" Statements)

Each family member should have the opportunity to decide the level of involvement they wish in decision-making for their child.	Each family and family member should be treated with respect (as individuals).	The needs of all family members should be considered.
Parents should have the ultimate responsibility for the care of their children.		The involvement of all family members should be supported and encouraged.

Elements (Key Service Provider Behaviors)

Service Provider Behaviors	Service Provider Behaviors	Service Provider Behaviors
To encourage parent decision-making	To respect families	To consider psychosocial needs of all members
To assist in identifying strengths	To support families	To encourage participation by all members
To provide information	To listen	To respect coping styles
To assist in identifying needs	To provide individualized service	To encourage use of community supports
To collaborate with parents	To accept diversity	To build on strengths
To provide accessible services	To believe and trust parents	
To share information about the child	To communicate clearly	

Adapted from Rosenbaum P: Family-Centered Service. Phys Occup Ther Pediatr 18(1):1-20, 1998.

regarding this process of care. At first glance, in view of the convincing arguments of the many stakeholders interested in disseminating family-centered care improvements throughout the health care system, the reader might conclude that shifting existing care processes to those that are more family-centered is the most desirable method to successfully support families as they adapt to raising a child with special health care needs. However, before widespread dissemination of any improvement strategy, it is desirable to explore the intervention for the possibility of lack of desired benefit or even potential to harm.[29] In addition, understanding how organizational structure affects patient outcomes is important but suffers from a lack of available methods of studying this aspect of care.[30] Furthermore, despite the existing literature on family-centered and patient-centered care, commentaries and qualitative studies continue to point out that parents and professionals have limited or conflicting ideas about the meaning and scope of these concepts.[31-34]

Before discussing the research regarding family-centered care interventions and outcomes, an example involving the "Mr. Yuk" sticker in the childhood poisoning prevention campaign illustrates the importance of empirical evaluation of interventions. "Mr. Yuk," created by the Pittsburgh Poison Center at the Children's Hospital of Pittsburgh in 1971, was based on a logical assumption that applying these bright green stickers with a scowling face to bottles of medicines and other potentially toxic substances would help discourage children from ingesting the contents. Distributing these stickers to parents of young children became routine practice in most ambulatory child health care settings after clinicians incorporated the expert recommendation to do so. However, at least two studies[35,36] done in the 1980s long after the intervention was entrenched suggested that "Mr. Yuk" stickers do not effectively keep toddlers away from potential poisons and may even attract children to them. One of the studies did note, however, that the stickers might work for older children or as part of a larger poisoning prevention campaign, highlighting the importance of tailoring interventions.[36]

Research linking family-centered care to desired outcomes is available but challenging to summarize as a whole because of the heterogeneity of the definitions of the concept, study populations, focus of investigation, and methodological quality across studies. Furthermore, a complete review of the existing literature on family-centered care is beyond the scope of this chapter. With these limitations in mind, we have chosen to explore several articles linking family-centered care and outcomes and summarized several other articles according to quality of study methodology in Table 8B-3. Evidence is listed alphabetically by

author's names in columns based on the commonly used categorization scheme that organizes studies according to strength of the methodological quality.[37] Class I evidence is considered the strongest for drawing valid conclusions between interventions and outcomes and results from randomized controlled trials. Class II evidence is second most powerful and includes nonrandomized trials, before-and-after evaluations, and studies in which participants serve as their own controls. Class III evidence refers to cross-sectional and case-control designs. Class IV evidence, derived from the weakest study designs, pertains to descriptive studies, case reports, and expert opinion. Note that classes III and IV evidence hold value in that they provide starting points for further study and suggested practices in the absence of higher classes of data.

Selected Class I Evidence Regarding Family-Centered Care and Outcomes

Randomized controlled trials of components of family-centered care summarized in the two left columns of Table 8B-3 are described in further detail. Ireys and colleagues evaluated the effect of referral to parent-to-parent support for mothers caring for children with chronic illness and found that mothers in the intervention group had lower anxiety levels, as measured by the Beck Depression Inventory and the Psychiatric Symptom Index.[38] Stein and Jessop showed that in a longitudinal family-centered support program for families of CSHCN (the Pediatric Ambulatory Care Treatment Study), the group receiving intervention showed greater satisfaction with care, improvements in children's psychological adjustment, and fewer psychiatric symptoms for mothers.[39] In Australia, Sanders demonstrated in multiple studies the effectiveness of a family-centered parenting intervention, the Positive Parenting Program (Triple-P) for problematic child behaviors.[39a] Another study done in Sweden with children with newly diagnosed insulin-dependent diabetes mellitus showed associations between outpatient family-centered care processes and parent-reported improvement in family climate but failed to show a relationship to children's glycemic control or rate of readmission.[40] The last report mentioned in the randomized controlled trials in Table 8B-3 is a summary of class I studies that failed to show a simple link between care processes and child outcomes.[41] Instead, the authors argued that only if interventions addressed maternal responsiveness were they successful in improving children's developmental outcomes.

Using the three-level framework conceptualization of family-centered care noted in Table 8B-2, research-

TABLE 8B-3 ■ Selected Evidence on the Relationship of Family Centered Care with Child and Family Outcomes

Class I Studies with + Family and/or Child Outcomes	Class I Studies Linking FCC to + Family Outcomes but No Link to Child Outcomes	Class III Studies	Class IV Studies
Ireys et al[38] Randomized controlled trial (RCT) of Parent-to-Parent community support intervention—intervention linked with maternal anxiety	**Forsander et al[40]** RCT of outpatient family-support program for children with newly diagnosed insulin dependent diabetes mellitus versus inpatient treatment showed parent-reported improvement in family climate but NO relationship to glycemic control or rate of readmission	**Dempsey & Dunst[63]** Parent survey—Early Intervention providers use of empowering help-giving linked with parents' report of sense of control	**Lubetsky et al[64]** Case study of FCC approach associated with better outcome in a child with multiple chronic needs and behavioral problems
Stein and Jessop[39] RCT of FCC—intervention linked with families satisfaction with care, improvements in children's psychological adjustment, and ↓ psychiatric symptoms for mothers **Sanders[39a]** Review of RCTs of Triple P family-centered parenting intervention—intervention linked with improved parent self-efficacy and child behavior	**Mahoney et al[41]** Summary of 4 longitudinal RCTs and secondary analysis of data—FCC process alone does not improve child developmental outcomes, changes in maternal responsiveness are necessary	**King et al[42,44]** Service providers respect for families and including families in decision making linked with satisfaction and improved parent and child psychosocial well-being **Korsch et al[65]** Pediatricians' communication style linked with parents' satisfaction **Wasserman et al.[66]** Pediatrician's encouragement, reassurance, and empathy linked with mothers' satisfaction with clinicians, changes in concerns, perceptions of their infants, and self-confidence **Wissow et al.[67]** Pediatricians' interviewing style linked with increased likelihood of mothers' to discuss behavioral and emotional symptoms	

ers in the Ontario group documented an association between family-centered care for CSHCN and their families in Canadian children's rehabilitation centers and outcomes such as parent satisfaction with services,[42,43] as well as improved parent and child psychosocial well-being.[44] In these and other studies listed in Table 8B-3 in the two right columns, the investigators used methods that make it difficult to draw firm conclusions between family-centered care and outcomes. Furthermore, criticisms of using satisfaction and psychosocial well-being as outcomes are derived from the bias presumed inherent in subjective data and the observation that the measurement of traits is more psychometrically reliable than

the measurement of states (i.e., satisfaction). In a summary of selected evidence, Rosenbaum found five randomized controlled trials evaluating family-centered care and provided a summary of other pertinent publications, most of who authors had used methods in the class II to class IV categories.[28] Shields and associates published a Cochrane Colloquium review protocol for meta-analysis of family-centered care for hospitalized children in 2003 (updated in 2004) but have not begun collecting studies based on the protocol.[45] We were not able to find any other publications of controlled trials or meta-analyses pertaining to family-centered care, despite an extensive search.

Other Selected Evidence Regarding Receipt of Family-Centered Care and CSHCN

MCHB, in collaboration with the National Center for Health Statistics of the Centers for Disease Control and Prevention, surveyed a nationally representative sample of more than 100,000 households across the country to measure the health and well-being of U.S. children.[46,47] The National Survey of Children's Health (NSCH), administered to families by telephone, included more than 38,000 families across the United States that had at least one child with special health care need and included questions to measure the six core outcomes listed in Table 8B-4. To assess the progress in achieving their national agenda for CSHCN, the survey included questions regarding families' perceptions that their care was family-centered. Prevalence estimates from this study showed that 12.8% of children (9.3 million) younger than 18 years need a special health care issue to be addressed. Approximately one third of the families surveyed indicated that they were dissatisfied by the lack of critical elements of family centeredness. Questions regarding family centeredness emphasized the extent to which care provided by the child's physicians and nurses focused on the family's needs and not simply the child's medical condition. Areas addressed included whether the professional (1) met information needs, (2) made the parent feel like a partner, (3) was sensitive to family values and culture, (4) spent enough time, and (5) listened to family concerns. One third of the families reported being *usually or always dissatisfied* with at least one family-centered aspect of their child's care. Furthermore, families of such children living in poverty and from minority groups were

more likely to be dissatisfied with these aspects of care. Although the data were based on self-report and collected cross-sectionally, which precluded causal conclusions, this study provides an important starting point from which to design more in-depth evaluations of family-centered aspects of the health care system and family health care provider interactions.

THE MEDICAL HOME

We now turn to a discussion of how the family-centered care concept is applied in the "medical home" model within pediatric primary health care settings. We trace the AAP's history of the concept and current models of medical home promotion and implementation at both the state and individual practice levels.

History and Definition of the Medical Home Concept

The AAP has called for children to have a "medical home" since the 1960s.[48] The original 1967 AAP definition referred to a single location of all medical information about a patient, especially children with chronic disease or disabling conditions.[49] The idea evolved over the next 35 years to the current one, which emphasizes a concept broader than the notion of a single location. Now the medical home is conceptualized as a quality approach to providing cost-effective primary health care services in which families, health care providers, and related professionals work as partners to identify and access medical and nonmedical services to help children and their families achieve their maximum potential. In 2002, the AAP published a more definitive operational definition clarifying specific activities within each of seven medical home domains: accessible, *family-centered*, continuous, comprehensive, coordinated, compassionate, and culturally effective (see Appendix, Chapter 8B for a more complete description of the domains).[50-52] Despite progress in clarifying the concept, significant challenges to establishing medical homes for all children remain; an important one is the lack of an adequate reimbursement structure for physicians' services provided in a medical home. The next section describes a model that has been used to study the implementation of the medical home concept.

Efforts to Promote the Medical Home Concept

The MCHB funded the National Initiative for Children's Healthcare Quality (NICHQ) to conduct mul-

---

TABLE 8B-4 ■ **Maternal and Child Health Bureau Core Outcomes for CSHCN**

All CSHCN will receive coordinated, ongoing comprehensive care in a medical home.

All families of CHSCN will have adequate public and/or private health insurance to pay for the services they need.

All children will be screened early and continuously for special health care needs.

Services for CHSCN and their families will be organized in ways that families can easily use them.

All families of CHSCN will **partner in decision-making** at all levels, and will be satisfied with the services they receive.

All youth with SHCN will receive the services necessary to make appropriate transitions to adult health care, work, and independence.

From McPherson M, Weissman G, Strickland BB, et al: Implementing community-based systems of services for children and youths with special health care needs: How well are we doing? Pediatrics 113:1538-1544, 2004.
CSHCN, children with special health care needs.

tistate learning collaboratives to help disseminate the medical home concept throughout the United States.[52] NICHQ staff and faculty, state Title V leaders, and private practices constituted two consecutive 15-month Medical Home Learning Collaboratives, the first occurring in 2003 to 2004 and the second in 2004 to 2005. The first collaborative included 30 practices in 12 states: Colorado, Connecticut, Florida, Louisiana, Michigan, New York, North Carolina, Ohio, Oklahoma, Utah, Virginia, and Wisconsin. The second consisted of nine states and multiple practices in the District of Columbia, Illinois, Maine, Maryland, Minnesota, Pennsylvania, Texas, Vermont, and West Virginia. The Learning Collaboratives studied the recommended best practices for making changes to enhance care for CSHCN. They employed NICHQ's framework for improvement, which is based on a synthesis of models from the Institute for Healthcare Improvement's Breakthrough Series Model,[53] the Model for Improvement,[54-56] and the Chronic Care Model.[57] NICHQ's model for improvement highlights the need for four key components of practice Microsystems: a clinical information system, effective decision support, a well-designed delivery system emphasizing planned care, and expert support for both family and developmentally appropriate child self-management. The model, schematically represented in Figure 8B-1, also highlights the key role of organizational leadership and the importance of linking health services and community resources.[58] The second collaborative used process information regarding what did or did not work from the first learning experience and assessed resulting outcomes occurring as a result of incorporating medical home principles in primary care practices.

Select Evidence Regarding Elements of the Medical Home and Outcomes

Documented outcomes from the second NICHQ Medical Home Learning Collaborative included an increase in implementation of medical home concepts in the practices, an improvement in participation of parents in their children's care, a decrease in unplanned hospitalization rates for CSHCN, a reduction in emergency department visits, decreases in numbers of missed school and work days, and an increase in capability of Title V organizations to implement, spread, and sustain medical home concepts within practices. A report on the implementation process and outcomes can be accessed at NICHQ's Web site.[58]

A descriptive study with a screening tool to identify CSHCN[59] in primary care settings revealed that the screener has the potential to identify a vulnerable group of children who need comprehensive and coordinated care. An example study of care coordination's effect on outcomes demonstrated that care coordination was accepted by families and resulted in increased services, but the authors were not able to link the process of coordinating care with the outcomes.[60]

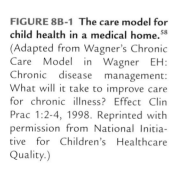

FIGURE 8B-1 **The care model for child health in a medical home.**[58] (Adapted from Wagner's Chronic Care Model in Wagner EH: Chronic disease management: What will it take to improve care for chronic illness? Effect Clin Prac 1:2-4, 1998. Reprinted with permission from National Initiative for Children's Healthcare Quality.)

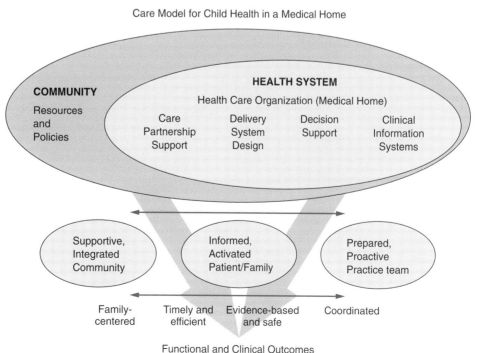

Practical Suggestions for Practitioners Wishing to Implement a Medical Home

NICHQ, the AAP National Center for Medical Home Initiatives for Children with Special Health Care Needs (*http://www.medicalhomeinfo.org/*), and the Center for Medical Home Improvement (*http://www. medicalhomeimprovement.org/*) have a wealth of information available for practitioners interested in implementing components of a medical home in their practice or who desire to advocate at a systems level for children with special health care needs. NICHQ has organized specific suggestions by area of focus, including community, health care organization, care partnership support, delivery system design, decision support, and clinical information systems, and these suggestions are listed in Table 8B-5. The AAP National Center for Medical Home Initiatives and Georgetown University collaborated on a report outlining specific

methods for creating improvements in communication between primary care practitioners and subspecialists.[61] The report contains practical suggestions and non-copyrighted form templates (a medical home-based care plan; an emergency information form for a child with special health care needs; a family-centered health care plan; a referral fax-back form; and examples of disease-specific forms, such as an action asthma plan) that practitioners can use to implement components of the medical home in their practices. In additiony, example templates for cataloguing resources and for tracking referral responses are included in Appendix, Chapter 8B.

Practitioners who have implemented quality improvements in their practices indicate that working with other practitioners who are similarly interested is a key to their success.[62] They also typically identify individual practice staff members who will help outline the existing workflow and who will be responsible for delegated tasks (e.g., deciding who will distribute forms to families, where families will complete them—at home, in the office waiting room, in the physician office exam room, over the Web—and who will ensure that forms are replenished). Creating (and documenting) a standardized approach to information flow provides a way for all office staff to remain invested in the process and facilitates orientation for new employees.

TABLE 8B-5 ■ Ideas for Improvement in Care for CSHCN Found on the NICHQ Web Site	
Community	Identify and meet with key community partners; learn their responsibilities and roles
	Catalogue community resources and contact persons for referrals
Health Care Organization	Gain commitment of health care system's senior leadership to have quality standards in place for meeting the needs of CSHCN and their families
	Establish a plan to maximize reimbursement for medical home visits
Care Partnership Support	Engage parents as partners at practice level
	Develop a care planning process and plan with families
Delivery System Design	Develop a strategy and identify specific roles for care coordination and communication at practice level
	Use planned encounters
Decision Support	Co-manage care with specialists and choose information exchange method (fax-back, email, Web-based system)
	Select and use evidence-based practice guidelines
Clinical Information System	Identify, categorize complexity, and create a registry of CSHCN (retrospectively, use flu-list, diagnostic lists, and memory; prospectively, use the CSHCN screener, definition, and computer flags, or other systematic reminders)
	Use the registry to enroll identified CSHCN, for visit reminders, to support care planning processes, and to monitor clinical needs

From Medical Home Initiatives for Children with Special Needs Project Advisory Committee: The medical home. Pediatrics 110:184-186, 2002. CSHCN, children with special health care needs; NICHQ, National Initiative for Children's Healthcare Quality.

Example of Use of the "Plan, Do, Study, Act" Method of Quality Improvement

Using the "plan, do, study, act" method of improvement that originated within the business field[55,55a,56] allows practitioners to identify a specific problem area in need of improvement and create a new solution or process ("plan"), implement change on a small scale ("do"), measure the impact of implementing the change ("study") and permanently implement the change with modifications as necessary identified in the measurement process ("act"). For example, a practitioner may recognize that he or she is not routinely receiving feedback after referring a child for consultation and decide that he or she wants to prioritize improving the referral communication process:

Plan: The practitioner decides that he or she will create a tracking form for referrals (see Appendix, Chapter 8B for an example template) and delegates the responsibility for entering information on the sheet to the office referral manager, who shares the practitioner's concern about timely feedback. The practitioner and referral manager agree to try the new process with the next 10 children they see needing referrals.

Do: They pilot the tracking form for the next 10 referrals.

Study: Over the following month, the referral coordinator notes that 2 of the 10 referrals have not received a response and follows up with the referring practitioner or agency. In one case, the pediatric neurologist's note was dictated on a hospital system that did not usually work with this practitioner's office. In the other case, the referral manager discovered that the early intervention program did not routinely send information back to referring practitioners. In both cases, the practitioner and the referral coordinator work together to request changes in the communication processes and create a standard referral form with a section for the agency or provider to write in a short synopsis and fax it back.

Act: They decide to implement this tracking form over the next 6 months and reevaluate using another "plan, do, study, act" cycle every 2 months.

CONCLUSION

In this chapter, we have explored relationship-focused quality improvement strategies by tracing the development of the concept of family-centered care, examining selected evidence linking family-centered care to outcomes for children and families and presenting specific examples of implementing aspects of a medical home in pediatric primary health care settings. More evidence linking family-centered care processes to desired child and family outcomes is needed. Furthermore, studies assessing the effects of health care financing on individual practitioners' ability to provide high-quality care would also prompt clinicians to provide high-quality pediatric care that meets the needs of children and their families.

REFERENCES

1. Leslie L, Rappo P, Abelson H, et al: Final report of the FOPE II Pediatric Generalists of the Future Workgroup. Pediatrics 106 (suppl 5):1199-223, 2000.
2. Starr P: The social transformation of American medicine. New York: Basic Books, 1982.
3. Institute of Medicine Committee on Quality of Health Care in America: Crossing the Quality Chasm: A New Health System for the 21st Century. Washington, DC: National Academies Press, 2001.
4. Brown JB, Stewart M, Weston WW, et al: Introduction. *In* Stewart M, Brown JB, Weston WW, et al, eds: Patient-Centered Medicine: Transforming the Clinical Method, 2nd ed. Oxford, UK: Radcliffe Medical Press, 2003, pp 3-15.
5. McWhinney IR: The evolution of clinical method. *In* Stewart M, Brown JB, Weston WW, et al, eds: Patient-Centered Medicine: Transforming the Clinical Method, 2nd ed. Oxford, UK: Radcliffe Medical Press, 2003, pp 17-30.
6. Rogers CR: Significant aspects of client-centered therapy. Am Psychol 1:415-422, 1946.
7. Gerteis M, Edgman-Levitan S, Daley J: Through the Patient's Eyes. Understanding and Promoting Patient-Centered Care. San Francisco: Jossey-Bass, 1993.
8. Tresolini CP, the Pew-Fetzer Task Force: Health Professions Education and Relationship-Centered Care. San Francisco: Pew Health Professions Commission, 1994.
9. Shelton TL, Stepanek JS: Family-Centered Care for Children Needing Specialized Health and Developmental Services, 3rd ed. Bethesda, MD: Association for the Care of Children's Health, 1994, pp 1-120.
10. Hostler SL: Family centered care. Pediatr Clin North Am 38:1545-1560, 1991.
11. Johnson BH: The changing role of families in health care. Child Health Care 19:234-241, 1990.
12. Spitz RA: Hospitalism, an inquiry into the genesis of psychiatric conditions in early childhood. Psychoanal Study Child 1(53):74-82, 1945.
13. Bowlby J: Maternal care and mental health. Bull World Health Organ 3:355-533, 1951.
14. Klaus MH, Kennell JH: Maternal-Infant Bonding: The Impact of Early Separation or Loss on Family Development. St. Louis: CV Mosby, 1976.
15. Seagull EAW: The child's rights as a medical patient. J Clin Child Psychol 7:202-205, 1978.
16. Tanner JL: Training for family-oriented pediatric care. Issues and options. Pediatr Clin North Am 42:193-207, 1995.
17. Haggerty RJ, Roghmann KJ, Pless IB: Child Health and the Community. New York: Wiley, 1975.
18. Engel GL: The need for a new medical model: A challenge for biomedicine. Science 196:129-136, 1977.
19. McPherson M, Arango P, Fox H, et al: A new definition of children with special health care needs. Pediatrics 102:137-140, 1998.
20. Koop CE: Surgeon General's Report: Children with Special Health Care Needs. Rockville, MD: U.S. Department of Health and Human Services, 1987.
21. Shelton T, Jepson E, Johnson BH: Family-centered care for children with special health care needs. Washington, DC: Association for the Care of Children's Health, 1987.
22. Shelton TL, Stepanek JS: The key elements of family-centered care. *In* Family-Centered Care for Children Needing Specialized Health and Developmental Services, 3rd ed. Bethesda, MD: Association for the Care of Children's Health, 1994, p vii.
23. The Institute for Family Centered Care: About Us. (Available at: *http://www.familycenteredcare.org/about/index.html;* accessed 10/24/06.)
24. Maternal and Child Health Bureau: Achieving and Measuring Success: A National Agenda for Children with Special Health Care Needs 2006. (Available

at: *http://www.mchb.hrsa.gov/programs/specialneeds/
measuresuccess.htm;* accessed 10/24/06.)

25. Dunst CJ, Trivette CM, Deal AG: Enabling and empow-
ering families. *In* Dunst CJ, Trivette CM, Deal AG, eds:
Supporting and Strengthening Families: Methods,
Strategies, and Practices. Cambridge, MA: Brookline
Brooks, 1994.

26. Kordesh R: Irony and Hope in the Emerging Family
Policies: A Case for Family Empowerment Associations. University Park, PA: Pennsylvania State University, Institute for Policy Research and Evaluation,
1995.

27. Dunst CJ, Trivette CM, Davis M, et al: Effective Help-
Giving Practices. *In* Dunst CJ, Trivette CM, Deal AG,
eds: Supporting and Strengthening Families: Methods,
Strategies, and Practices. Cambridge, MA: Brookline
Books, 1994, pp 171-186.

28. Rosenbaum P: Family-Centred Service. Phys Occup
Ther Pediatr 18(1):1-20, 1998.

29. Donabedian A: The quality of care: How can it be
assessed? JAMA 260:1743-1748, 1988.

30. Aiken LH, Sochalski J, Lake ET: Studying outcomes of
organizational change in health services. Med Care
35(11 suppl):NS6-NS18, 1997.

31. Knafl K, Breitmayer B, Gallo A, et al: Parents' view of
health care providers: An exploration of the components of a positive working relationship. Child Health
Care 21(2):90, 1992.

32. Gillespie R, Florin D, Gillam S: How is patient-centred
care understood by the clinical, managerial and lay
stakeholders responsible for promoting this agenda?
Health Expect 7:142-148, 2004.

33. Blue-Banning M, Summers JA, Frankland HC, et al:
Dimensions of family and professional partnerships:
Constructive guidelines for collaboration. Except Child
70:167-184, 2004.

34. Loewy EH: In defense of paternalism. Theor Med
Bioeth 26:445-468, 2005.

35. Fergusson DM, Horwood LJ, Beautrais AL, et al: A
controlled field trial of a poisoning prevention method.
Pediatrics 69:515-520, 1982.

36. Vernberg K, Culver-Dickinson P, Spyker DA: The deter-
rent effect of poison-warning stickers. Am J Dis Child
138:1018-1020, 1984.

37. McKibbon A, Hunt D, Richardson WS, et al:
Introduction: The philosophy of evidence-based medi-
cine. *In* Guyatt G, Rennie D, eds: Users' Guides to the
Medical Literature: A Manual for Evidence-Based
Clinical Practice. Chicago: AMA Press, 2002,
pp 3-12.

38. Ireys HT, Chernoff R, DeVet KA, et al: Maternal
outcomes of a randomized controlled trial of a
community-based support program for families of children with chronic illnesses. Arch Pediatr Adolesc Med
155:771-777, 2001.

39. Stein RE, Jessop DJ: Does pediatric home care make a
difference for children with chronic illness? Findings
from the Pediatric Ambulatory Care Treatment Study.
Pediatrics 73:845-853, 1984.

39a. Sanders MR: Triple P—Positive Parenting Program:
Towards an empirically validated multilevel parenting

and family support strategy for the prevention of
behavior and emotional problems in children. Clin
Child Fam Psychol Rev 2(2):71-90, 1999.

40. Forsander GA, Sundelin J, Persson B: Influence of the
initial management regimen and family social situation on glycemic control and medical care in children
with type I diabetes mellitus. Acta Paediatr 89:1462-
1468, 2000.

41. Mahoney G, Boyce G, Fewell RR, et al: The relationship of parent-child interaction to the effectiveness of
early intervention services. Top Early Child Spec Educ
18(1):5, 1998.

42. King G, Cathers T, King S, et al: Major Elements of
parents' satisfaction and dissatisfaction with pediatric
rehabilitation services. Child Health Care 30:111-134,
2001.

43. Law M, Hanna S, King G, et al: Factors affecting
family-centred service delivery for children with
disabilities. Child Care Health Dev 29(5):357-366,
2003.

44. King G, King S, Rosenbaum P, et al: Family-centered
caregiving and well-being of parents of children with
disabilities: Linking process with outcome. J Pediatr
Psychol 24:41-53, 1999.

45. Shields L, Pratt J, Flenady VJ, et al: Family-centred
care for children in hospital [protocol]. Cochrane
Database Syst Rev (1):CD1-21, 2006.

46. van Dyck PC, Kogan M, McPherson MG, et al: Prevalence and characteristics of children with special health
care needs. Arch Pediatr Adolesc Med 158:884-890,
2004.

47. McPherson M, Weissman G, Strickland BB, et al:
Implementing community-based systems of services
for children and youths with special health care needs:
How well are we doing? Pediatrics 113:1538-1544,
2004.

48. Sia C, Tonniges TF, Osterhus E, et al: History of the
medical home concept. Pediatrics 113:1473-1478,
2004.

49. American Academy of Pediatrics Council on Pediatric
Practice: Pediatric Records and a "medical home." *In*
Standards of Child Care. Evanston, IL: American
Academy of Pediatrics, 1967, pp 77-79.

50. Committee on Children with Disabilities: Care Coor-
dination: Integrating Health and Related Systems of
Care for Children with Special Health Care Needs.
Pediatrics 104:978-981, 1999.

51. Council on Children with Disabilities: Care coordination in the medical home: Integrating health and
related systems of care for children with special health
care needs. Pediatrics 116:1238-1244, 2005.

52. Medical Home Initiatives for Children with Special
Needs Project Advisory Committee: The medical home.
Pediatrics 110:184-186, 2002.

53. National Initiative for Children's Healthcare Quality:
NICHQ Medical Home Learning Collaborative. (Available at: *http://www.nichq.org/NR/rdonlyres/83AFF39E-
BF99-40B3-8803-442623776043/0/MHLC_2_Final_Report_Final.
pdf;* accessed on April 2, 2006.)

54. Institute for Healthcare Improvement: The Breakthrough Series: Institute for Healthcare Improvement's

Collaborative Model for Achieving Breakthrough Improvement. (Available from: *http://www.ihi.org/NR/rdonlyres/BCA88D8F-35EE-4251-BB93-E2252619A06D/0/BreakthroughSeriesWhitePaper2003.pdf.;* accessed 10/24/06.)

55. Institute for Healthcare Improvement: Improvement Methods. (Available at: *http://www.ihi.org/IHI/Topics/Improvement/ImprovementMethods/HowToImprove/;* accessed 10/24/06.)

55a. Deming WE: The New Economics for Industry, Government, Education, 2nd ed. Cambridge, MA: MIT Press, 2000.

56. Langley GL, Nolan KM, Nolan TW, et al: The Improvement Guide: A Practical Approach to Enhancing Organizational Performance. San Francisco: Jossey-Bass, 1996.

57. Wagner EH: Chronic disease management: What will it take to improve care for chronic illness? Effect Clin Prac 1:2-4, 1998.

58. National Initiative for Children's Healthcare Quality: NICHQ Medical Home Learning Collaborative. (Available at: *http://www.nichq.org/NICHQ/Topics/Chronic Conditions/;* accessed 10/24/06.)

59. Farmer JE, Marien WE, Frasier L: Quality improvements in primary care for children with special health care needs: Use of a brief screening measure. Child Health Care 32:273-285, 2003.

60. Smith K, Layne M, Garell D: The impact of care coordination on children with special health care needs. Child Health Care 23:251, 1994.

61. Antonelli R, Stille C, Freeman L: Enhancing Collaboration between Primary and Subspecialty Care Providers for Children and Youth with Special Health Care Needs. Washington, DC: Georgetown University Center for Child and Human Development. (Available at: *http://gucchd.georgetown.edu/files/products_publications/PrimarySpecialityCollaboration.pdf;* accessed 10/24/06.)

62. Duncan P: 2006 Apr 30.

63. Dempsey I, Dunst CJ: Helpgiving styles and parent empowerment in families with a young child with a disability. J Intellect Dev Disabil 29:40-51, 2004.

64. Lubetsky MJ, Mueller L, Madden K, et al: Family-centered/interdisciplinary team approach to working with families of children who have mental retardation. Ment Retard 33:251-256, 1995.

65. Korsch BM, Gozzi EK, Francis V: Gaps in doctor-patient communication. 1. Doctor-patient interaction and patient satisfaction. Pediatrics 42:855-871, 1968.

66. Wasserman RC, Inui TS, Barriatua RD, et al: Pediatric clinicians' support for parents makes a difference: an outcome-based analysis of clinician-parent interaction. Pediatrics 74:1047-1053, 1984.

67. Wissow LS, Roter DL, Wilson ME. Pediatrician interview style and mothers' disclosure of psychosocial issues. Pediatrics 93:289-295, 1994.

68. Medical home helpful Web sites. Pediatrics 113(5):1548, 2004.

8C.
Psychopharmacological Management of Disorders of Development and Behavior

JEFFREY HUNT ■ SAURABH GUPTA

Prescriptions of psychotropic medications have dramatically increased since the mid-1990s.[1] This includes stimulants, antidepressants, and, more recently, mood stabilizers and atypical antipsychotic medications. Nonpsychiatric practitioners (pediatricians, family physicians) continue to prescribe the majority of psychotropic medications, often because of lack of available child psychiatry consultation.[2] One concern about this practice is that the evidence base for the clinical usefulness of these medications has not kept pace with practice patterns. In addition, training for primary care clinicians in the management of psychiatric disorders is scant, in spite of the fact that they are often responsible for that management.[3] This chapter focuses on general principles of psychotropic medication use, major categories of psychotropic medications, and their basic mechanisms of action. We review common indications and the evidence supporting that use. Finally, we describe the guidelines for medication use in general and in specific disorders, along with any controversies about their use.

GENERAL PRINCIPLES OF PSYCHOTROPIC MEDICATION USE IN CHILDREN AND ADOLESCENTS

Before medication management of children with behavioral disorders is instituted, a complete assessment must result in a diagnosis and a comprehensive treatment plan. Medications for behavior are rarely indicated as the sole modality for most children and adolescents. Parents or legal guardians need to be actively involved in the formation of this treatment plan and must give full informed consent for their child or adolescent to take medication. In addition, the clinicians prescribing the medication need to carefully assess the reliability of the individuals responsible for administering the medication.

Although it is essential to determine a diagnosis before medication is instituted, it is often the target symptoms that are responsive to medication. The symptoms should be of sufficient severity and interfere with the child's or adolescent's daily functioning within his or her family, peer group, and school. In addition, the clinician needs to be aware that certain target symptoms may originate from different causes, and the medication must address the underlying disorder. For example, treating the target symptom depression with antidepressant medications in a patient with bipolar disorder may exacerbate the depression, instead of reducing it.

All patients should have a physical examination soon before starting medications. This should include baseline temperature, pulse and respiratory rate, and blood pressure. Height and weight should be monitored at each visit and charted on a standardized growth chart. Baseline laboratory tests may also be indicated, depending on the medication to be started. The specific tests are discussed later under each category of medication. Electrocardiography and electroencephalography may be indicated for certain medications.

Careful monitoring of the efficacy of medications for behavioral disorders requires systematic review of the target symptoms over time. This can include narrative observations from parents and teachers. The use of rating scales for the particular target symptom can be very helpful.[67] Such rating scales can also be useful for monitoring side effects. Many such rating scales are proprietary and can be purchased; many are available online without charge.

In general, optimal treatment of childhood psychiatric disorders should include medication that has been well studied and has U.S. Food and Drug Administration (FDA) approval. However, for most disorders, with the exception of attention-deficit/hyperactivity disorder (ADHD), some anxiety disorders, and mood disorders, this is not the case. Many treatments include "off label" use of medications. Use of these medications is completely proper if rational scientific theory, expert medical opinion, or controlled clinical studies provide the basis for the proposed use.

Understanding the meaning of medications to the child and adolescent patients and their families is also important.[4] The clinician should explore parents' attitudes and expectations about medication before instituting a treatment. Children are often apprehensive about taking medications. This is often related to their developmental level of understanding. Adolescents may initially rebel against the idea of taking medications and also worry about the effects, both positive and negative, of medications.

MEDICATIONS FOR ATTENTION-DEFICIT/HYPERACTIVITY DISORDER

Stimulants

Stimulants remain the most commonly prescribed medication for behavioral disorders.[5] Psychostimu-lants are thought to exert their influence on the catecholamine system by reuptake inhibition, enhanced release, or both.[6] Amphetamines affect reuptake inhibition, enhanced release, and storage. Methylphenidate appears to work primarily through presynaptic reuptake inhibition of dopamine and norepinephrine.

The effectiveness of stimulants for the short-term treatment of ADHD is well documented.[6] By 1996, 161 randomized controlled trials had been published, including 5 in preschool-aged patients, 150 in school-aged patients, 7 in adolescents, and 9 in adults (American Academy of Child and Adolescent Psychiatry practice parameters, 2002[6]). The finding of improvement in the patients randomly assigned to receive stimulants was robust in comparison with the finding in patients assigned to receive placebo. Studies consistently noted a positive response for core ADHD symptoms, reduced aggression, and improved behavioral compliance. Methylphenidate is the best studied, but dextroamphetamine and amphetamines salts are also reported to be efficacious.[6] Stimulant medications are FDA approved for use with ADHD (minimum age of 3 for dextroamphetamine, minimum age of 6 for methylphenidate). Although the majority of the studies were short term, lasting less than 12 weeks, longer term trials of up to 24 months also revealed stable long-term improvements, as long as medication was taken.[7] Of interest is that during a naturalistic follow-up over 24 to 60 months, there appeared to be a gradual increase in noncompliance with treatment and fewer physician visits per year.[8]

GUIDELINES FOR USE

Once the diagnosis of ADHD is established according to accepted practice and baseline measures indicate that the severity of the disorder warrants a medication trial, clinicians must educate the parents or guardians and the patient about the treatment plan. At the first visit and all subsequent visits, the patient's height, weight, and vital signs should be documented.[6]

Multiple stimulant preparations are available. Newer longer acting preparations of methylphenidate and mixed salts of amphetamine have been shown to be effective.[9] There is limited evidence for choosing one stimulant over another. One study demonstrated that of a group of patients given both methylphenidate and dextroamphetamine, 40% responded to both, 26% responded best to methylphenidate, and 35% responded best to dextroamphetamine.[10] Clinicians often employ longer-acting preparations after establishing tolerability with immediate-release stimulants. Fewer total daily doses per day appear to improve adherence. In addition, longer acting preparations eliminate the need for school-time dosing. Many longer acting preparations have been introduced since the mid-1990s. Although all contain the same active drug, these formulations differ pharmacologically because of modified-release technology. Many of these take advantage of a bead drug release technology or, in the case of methylphenidate XR (Concerta), a novel, osmotically driven delivery system. In addition, a dermal administration system (Daytrana) has recently been approved. The dermal administration allows for a short-term presence of the one isomer of methylphenidate that is rapidly metabolized in its first pass through the liver, but it is not clear that this fact alters the effects of methylphenidate.

If possible, it is advisable to start a medication trial on a Saturday, so that parents or caregivers can observe the effect or side effects. For optimum effect, the child or adolescent should be seen regularly by the physician to review the effect of the dose trial; the physician should use global parent's or caregiver's report and patient's report, along with standard rating scales. The treatment of ADHD practice parameters from the American Academy of Child and Adolescent Psychiatry provides the reader with many other tips for initiation of stimulants.[6] The dose ranges of medication for ADHD are as listed in Table 8C-1.

Comorbid psychiatric disorders complicate the treatment of ADHD with stimulants. Anxiety occurs in 25% of clinic-referred patients with ADHD.[11] Results of a multisite study revealed that children with ADHD with and without anxiety responded similarly to methylphenidate on all study outcome domains.[6,12] Treatment of ADHD and comorbid tic disorders remains challenging. Results of randomized controlled studies by several groups have suggested that stimulants can be safely and effectively prescribed in ADHD patients with comorbid tic disorders.[13,14] Tics may emerge in 9% of children treated with stimulants but persist in fewer than 1%.[15] One study revealed that the combined use of methylphenidate and clonidine led to reduction in tic severity, reduc-

TABLE 8C-1 ■ Medicines Used Primarily for Attention-Deficit/Hyperactivity Disorder

Trade Name	Approved Age	Strengths Available	Starting Dosages and Maximum	Duration of Action
Amphetamine Preparations				
Adderall	>3 years	5, 7.5, 10, 12.5, 15, 20, 30 mg tablets	2.5-5 mg/day Max 40 mg/day	3-6 hours
Adderall XR	>3 years	5, 10, 15, 20, 25, 30 mg tablets	5-10 mg/day Max 30 mg/day	8-12 hours
Dexedrine	>3 years	5-mg tablet	2.5 mg/day Max 40 mg/day	3-6 hours
		5-, 10-, 15-mg spansule	5 mg/day Max 40 mg/day	
Methylphenidate				
Focalin	>6 years	2.5, 5, 10 mg tablets	2.5 mg b.i.d. Max 20 mg/day	3-5 hours
Focalin XR	>6 years	5, 10, 15, 20 mg capsule	5 mg/day Max 20 mg/day	8-12 hours
Ritalin	>6 years	5, 10, 20 mg tablets	5 mg/day Max 20 mg/day	2.5-4 hours
Ritalin SR	>6 years	20 mg tablet	20 mg/day Max 60 mg/day	≤8 hours
Ritalin LA	>6 years	20, 30, 40 mg capsule	20 mg/day Max 60 mg/day	10-12 hours
Methylin	>6 years	5, 10, 20 mg tablets	5 mg/day Max 60 mg/day	2.5-4 hours
Methylin ER	>6 years	10, 20 mg tablets	5 mg/day Max 60 mg/day	6-8 hours
Metadate ER	>6 years	10, 20 mg tablets	5 mg/day Max 60 mg/day	6-8 hours
Metadate CD	>6 years	10, 20, 30 mg capsule	10 mg/day Max 60 mg/day	8-12 hours
Concerta	>6 years	18, 27, 36, 54 mg tablets	18 mg/day Max 72 mg/day	10-12 hours
Norepinephrine Reuptake Inhibitor (Atomoxetine)				
Strattera	>6 years	10-, 18-, 25-, 40-, 60-mg capsule	0.5 mg/day Max 1.2 mg/kg/day	10-12 hours

Adapted from Physician's Desk Reference, 60th ed. Montvale, NJ: Thomson Healthcare, 2006.

tion in impulsivity, and improvement in attention.[16] Management of ADHD and comorbid mood disorders remains challenging and not well studied. ADHD often manifests with concurrent mood disorders (6% to 38% of patients).[7,17] Few studies have assessed treatment of comorbid ADHD and depression. In most, methylphenidate has been combined with a selective serotonin reuptake inhibitor (SSRI) with positive results.[18] There is a suggestion that stimulants can worsen moods in patients with bipolar disorder,[19] but this is not yet clear; the differential of juvenile mania and ADHD continues to be examined. Finally, studies of the treatment of ADHD and comorbid substance abuse suggest that stimulant medication have a protective effect against later substance abuse by adolescents.[20]

ADVERSE EFFECTS AND THEIR MANAGEMENT

The most frequent and troublesome immediate side effects include insomnia, anorexia, headache, irritability, weeping, tachycardia, and elevated blood pressure (Table 8C-2). Many of the symptoms diminish

TABLE 8C-2 ■ Management of Common Stimulant Side Effects

Adverse Effect	Management Strategies
Insomnia	Give medication early
	Prescribe short-acting meds
	Consider adjunctive meds
	Administer last dose no later than 3 p.m.
Decreased appetite/weight loss	Give with meals
	Offer bedtime snack
	Change preparation
Irritability	Consider medication "wearing off" effect
	Reduce dose
	Change to long-acting preparation
	Assess comorbidity
Rebound phenomena	Change to long-acting preparation
	Consider alternative treatments/adjuvants
	Overlap stimulant dosing
Headaches	Change medicine
	Consider alternative preparation
"Zombie-like" effect/behavioral toxicity	Lower dose
	Change stimulant
	Consider nonstimulant
Growth slowing	Use weekend/vacation drug holiday
	Lower dose
	Consider nonstimulant

Adapted from Greenhill LL, Pliszka S, Dulcan MK, et al: Practice parameters for the use of stimulant medications in the treatment of children, adolescents and adults. J Am Acad Child Adolesc Psychiatry 41(2 suppl):26S-49S, 2002.

over a period of weeks. The 2002 American Academy of Child and Adolescent Psychiatry practice parameters describe commonly employed methods of managing these side effects.[6] The effect of stimulants on long-term growth, particularly height, has been controversial. In the multisite study on treatment of ADHD, subjects at 24 months showed slower growth velocity than did nonmedicated children (about a half inch per year slower).[8] However, the children in the study were initially taller than average. It is unclear whether the medicated children catch up. Overall, children who stayed on stimulants did better globally, but the tradeoff might be the slight reduction in growth velocity.

CURRENT CONTROVERSIES

There continue to be concerns that stimulants are overprescribed. When the diagnosis is carefully established, according to some authors, undertreatment remains the major concern.[21] The treatment of preschoolers has increased, according to one survey, by 169%.[22] There has been only a small number of randomized controlled studies of stimulants in this population.[23] It appears that these medications are efficacious, but this age group is also more prone to side effects.[23] The long-term effect of stimulants also remains controversial. One of the longest running multisite studies has shown that the symptoms in patients who started taking stimulants were similar to those of patients who were unmedicated.[8] This appears to be mostly related to compliance with medication, and patients who continued to use stimulant medication maintained their global improvements. The significance of a concern related to cardiac and emotional side effects of a particular long-acting methylphenidate preparation is uncertain. There has also been concern about long-acting mixed salts of amphetamine. Carefully obtaining informed consent for all patients is prudent, and avoiding these medications in patients with structural cardiac disorders is recommended. One study revealed that children starting methylphenidate had white blood cell changes that increased the risk of cancer. The numbers of children studied were small, and previous animal studies and one surveillance study of cancer related to methylphenidate did not demonstrate the relationship. Further study is necessary to determine whether this finding is a concern.

Atomoxetine

Atomoxetine was the first nonstimulant medication approved for the treatment of ADHD. It is a highly selective norepinephrine reuptake inhibitor that may also have dopaminergic effects in the prefrontal cortex. Atomoxetine has FDA approval for the treatment of ADHD in children, adolescents, and adults. The drug manufacturer provides most of the evidence base for atomoxetine. Results of several large studies indicate it is significantly better than placebo across several measures.[24] It also appeared to be comparable in efficacy with methylphenidate in one study to date.[25]

For patients with an established diagnosis of ADHD, a baseline physical examination, including heart rate, blood pressure, height, and weight, should be documented. Starting doses for atomoxetine are 0.5 mg/kg/day in single or divided doses. Titration of the dose can be up to 1.8 mg/kg/day, although most studies have indicated that 1.2 mg/kg/day is adequate.

The most common side effects reported in children and adolescents include sedation, dizziness, change in appetite, and mood instability. Mood instability may be more common in patients who have a bipolar spectrum disorder along with comorbid ADHD. At the time of this writing, the FDA was also considering adding a "black box warning" because of a slight increase in suicidal behavior.[26] An independent review of this issue is lacking. Premarket studies documented a slight increase in blood pressure and pulse.[25] Drug interactions are also of concern, particularly with agents that are CYP2D6 inhibitors, such as fluoxetine or paroxetine. Two cases of hepatic toxicity have been reported, both of which resolved with stopping the medication. Seven cases of suicidal thoughts were found on reanalyses of the existing studies. It is important to monitor patients for suicidal tendencies.

α-Adrenergic Agents

α-Adrenergic medications such as clonidine and guanfacine are commonly prescribed for patients with ADHD who have comorbid tics, insomnia, or aggression. The α-adrenergic drugs affect central presynaptic and postsynaptic α_2-adrenergic receptors and mediate cognition and attention through norepinephrine.[27] Clonidine appears to have more potent mixed receptor effects than does guanfacine.[28] Possible indications for the α-adrenergic drugs include tic disorders, ADHD, sleep disturbances caused by stimulants, aggression, and hyperarousal from post-traumatic stress disorder.

There are few controlled studies of the α-adrenergic drugs.[29] The number of patients in each study is relatively small. One multisite study demonstrated effectiveness of clonidine and of clonidine plus methylphenidate for the treatment of tics and ADHD.[30] A similar study of guanfacine also demonstrated improvement in patients with ADHD and tics.

GUIDELINES FOR USE

Dosages of α-adrenergic drugs should be individualized and carefully monitored. Electrocardiography is recommended before these medications are initiated, in addition to a baseline physical examination with vital signs, height, and weight. For clonidine, the dose should be initiated at 0.025 mg twice a day and titrated slowly upward to a range of 0.1 mg three to four times a day (total daily dose, 0.15 to 0.4 mg). For guanfacine, the initial dose may start as low as 0.25 mg twice a day and may be titrated slowly to a range of 1.5 mg three times a day.

Common side effects for both agents include dry mouth, sedation, fatigue, dizziness, weakness, hypotension, and bradycardia. In addition, there are reports of depressive symptoms with clonidine.[31] When abrupt withdrawal of α adrenergics occurs, rebound hypertension may occur. Therefore, it is advisable to taper both medications gradually, at a rate of 0.05 mg every 3 to 5 days for clonidine and 0.5 mg every 3 to 5 days for guanfacine.

ANTIDEPRESSANTS

Antidepressants, particularly the SSRIs, are increasingly used worldwide in the pediatric population.[3] However, research regarding the efficacy and safety for children and adolescents has yielded mixed results and remains inadequate.

SSRIs increase the amount of serotonin in the synaptic cleft. Tricyclic antidepressants block the reuptake inactivation of serotonin and norepinephrine. Newer, so-called novel antidepressants affect serotonin, norepinephrine, and dopamine in varying ways. All of these immediate effects lead to subsequent changes at the level of neurotransmitters that reduce depressive symptoms.[32]

There are multiple indications for the use of antidepressants, some with FDA approval and some off label.[69,70] Table 8C-3 and Table 8C-4 outline these indications.

Selective Serotonin Reuptake Inhibitors

The evidence base for the treatment of depression in children and adolescents is improving.[33] The Treatment of Adolescent Depression Study clearly showed the benefit of both fluoxetine and the combination of fluoxetine and cognitive behavioral therapy.[34] In addition, the study demonstrated the reduction in suicidal behavior for the course of the study. Table 8C-3 lists the research base to date for the treatment of juvenile depression with antidepressants.

TABLE 8C-3 ■ Medications Studied in Treating Depression

Study	Medicine	Type of Study	Duration	N	Results
Emslie et al, 1997[68]	Fluoxetine	Double-blind, placebo control	8 weeks	64	Fluoxetine superior to placebo
Emslie et al, 2002[73]	Fluoxetine	Double-blind, placebo control	8 weeks	219	Fluoxetine superior to placebo
Keller et al, 2001[74]	Paroxetine, imipramine	Double-blind, placebo control	8 weeks	275	Paroxetine superior to imipramine and placebo
Wagner et al, 2001[75]	Citalopram	Double-blind, placebo control	8 weeks	174	Citalopram superior to placebo
Wagner et al, 2003[72]	Sertraline	Double-blind, placebo control	10 weeks	376	Sertraline superior to placebo
Emslie et al, 2002[73]	Nefazodone	Double-blind, placebo control	8 weeks	195	Not superior to placebo
Ryan, 2003[74]	Tricyclic antidepressants	Aggregate studies	8 weeks	500	Not superior to placebo
TADS[34]	Fluoxetine	Double-blind	12 weeks–1 year	439	Combined cognitive-behavioral therapy plus fluoxetine superior to placebo. Fluoxetine superior to placebo

TADS, Treatment for Adolescents with Depression.

TABLE 8C-4 ■ Indications for Commonly Used Antidepressants in Children and Adolescents

Drug	FDA-Approved Indications	Other Possible Indications	Dosage
Fluoxetine	Depression OCD	Anxiety disorder Behavior disorders in PDD/MR Mood symptoms in ADHD, conduct disorder, and OCD	5 mg/day to max 60 mg/day
Paroxetine	None	Depression OCD	10 mg/day to max 40 mg/day
Sertraline	OCD	Depression Selective mutism	12.5 mg/day to max 200 mg/day
Citalopram	None	MDD OCD PTSD	10 mg/day to max 40 mg/day
Escitalopram	None	No data	10 mg/day to max 20 mg/day
Bupropion	None	ADHD Depression	25 mg/day to max 300 mg/day
Venflaxine	None	Repetitive behaviors in autism ADHD	37.5 mg/day to 225 mg/day
Mirtazapine	None	MDD Irritability, anxiety, depression, insomnia	7.5 mg/day to 45 mg/day
Trazodone	None	Adjunctive treatment for insomnia	25 mg/day to 300 mg/day
Nefazodone	None	MDD	100 mg/day to 300 mg/day
Imipramine	OCD	Separation anxiety and school refusal Acute stress disorder	10-25 mg/day starting dose; may raise up to 200 mg/day
Amitriptyline	None	Headache/polyneuropathy	25 mg/day up to 150 mg/day
Clomipramine	OCD	Autism with anxiety Compulsive behaviors	10 mg/day to 200 mg/day
Desipramine	None	ADHD Anxiety	25-100 mg/day
Nortriptyline	None	No data	10 mg/day to 150 mg/day
Fluvoxamine	OCD	Social phobia Separation anxiety	25-50 mg/day initially to max 300 mg/day

Data from Emslie et al, 2004[38] and Thienemann, 2004.[58]
ADHD, attention-deficit/hyperactivity disorder; FDA, U.S. Food and Drug Administration; MDD, major depressive disorder; MR, mental retardation; OCD, obsessive-compulsive disorder; PDD, pervasive developmental disorder; PTSD, post-traumatic stress disorder.

OTHER INDICATIONS

At this time, the strongest evidence for efficacy with the SSRIs is with obsessive-compulsive disorder.[33] Five randomized, controlled trials have yielded results indicating positive response in comparison to placebo. Also, treatment of other mixed anxiety disorders with these medications is supported. Table 8C-4 lists evidence to date for use of antidepressants in a variety of psychiatric conditions.

Novel Antidepressants

This category includes venflaxine, bupropion, and mirtazapine. The evidence for the efficacy of these newer antidepressants for any condition is scant.[32] Several small studies of bupropion for ADHD that have yielded positive results.[35] One study yielded negative results for venlafaxine in major depression.[36] Two open label studies of juveniles with ADHD demonstrated some improvement on certain ADHD rating scales.[37] With regard to other novel antidepressants, there have been no randomized controlled trials, but there have been some open label trials for depression and insomnia.[38]

Tricyclic Antidepressants

Of the 13 studies of tricyclic antidepressants for major depression, none yielded positive findings.[33] Clomipramine has been well studied for obsessive-compulsive disorder, and three studies have yielded positive findings indicating its efficacy for obsessive-compulsive disorder. Imipramine has been established as an effective medication for enuresis. Imipramine, amitriptyline, and desipramine have all been found to be effective for ADHD.[39]

Guidelines for Use

The diagnosis of major depression or one of the anxiety disorders must be made through accepted assessment protocols. It is important to use available rating scales to establish the baseline of the mood or anxiety symptoms and then to enable the clinician to monitor the symptoms over time.

Once the decision is made, in collaboration with parents or guardians, to initiate a trial of an antidepressant, the clinician needs to review the current FDA warnings and guidelines for their use.[40] The black box warning describes the possible risk of increased suicidal behavior in patients who are taking antidepressants. In addition, the FDA has provided guidance to enhance the monitoring of patients who have begun taking antidepressants. The current recommendations are four weekly face-to-face contacts

for the first month, biweekly contacts for the second month, and another contact at 12 weeks. Subsequent frequency of follow-up is guided by clinical necessity. The American Academy of Child and Adolescent Psychiatry and the American Psychiatric Association have created a guide for clinicians and one for parents of children who are being treated with antidepressants.[41] The guide discusses the potential deleterious effect of the FDA warning on the treatment of depression in children and adolescents by primary care clinicians. The risk of untreated major depression leading to suicide clearly exceeds the relatively small risk of these medications for inducing suicidal behavior in juveniles. Without treatment, the consequences of depression are extremely serious.

The antidepressant drug of first choice is not clear. Fluoxetine is the only antidepressant approved by the FDA for treatment of depression in pediatric patients. Off-label prescribing of antidepressants is both common and consistent with clinical practice. Of the approximately 30% to 40% of children and adolescents who do not respond to an initial medication, a substantial number respond to an alternative.[41]

SSRIs, novel antidepressants, and tricyclic antidepressants should all be initiated at low dosages to avoid adverse effects. The dosages should be slowly titrated to monitor for adverse effects, particularly behavioral activation or manic symptoms. Family members should contact their clinician when any of the following emerge: patients express new or more frequent thoughts of wanting to die or hurt themselves; signs of increased anxiety/panic, agitation, aggression, or impulsivity; or evidence of involuntary restlessness, elation, or increased energy. Table 8C-4 lists dosage ranges.

When a patient begins taking tricyclic antidepressants, it is important to have a baseline medical workup, including blood pressure, heart rate, electrocardiography, liver function tests, and height and weight. It is also important to monitor serum levels of these medications to avoid toxicity. At each follow-up visit, vital signs, height, and weight must be documented. In addition, an electrocardiogram should be obtained after each dose increase to monitor for a prolonged QT interval. These medications are potentially dangerous in overdose; therefore, educating the family about these risks and prevention methods is important.

Adverse Effects

Table 8C-5 lists common side effects of antidepressants. Common adverse effects of the SSRIs include nausea, decreased appetite and weight loss, insomnia, sedation, sweating, and sexual dysfunction. More rare side effects include behavioral activation or manic

TABLE 8C-5 ■ Side Effects of Antidepressants

Drug	Gastrointestinal Symptoms	Agitation/Insomnia	Anticholinergic Effects	Sedation	Sexual Dysfunction
		Probability of Side Effects			
Citalopram	High	Low	None	Low	Very high
Escitalopram	Moderate	Low	None	Low	No data
Fluoxetine	High	Very high	None	None	Very high
Paroxetine	High	Low	Low	Low	Very high
Fluvoxamine	High	Low	None	Moderate	Very high
Sertraline	Very high	Moderate	None	Very low	Very high
Bupropion	Moderate	High	None	None	None
Bupropion SR	Moderate	Moderate	None	None	None
Trazodone	Moderate	None	Very low	Very high	None
Mirtazapine	Very low	None	None	High	None
Venflaxine	Very high	Moderate	None	Low	High
Nefazodone	Moderate	Very low	None	High	None
Tricyclic antidepressants	High	Low	High	High	Low

Data from Emslie G, Portteus A, Kumar E, et al: Antidepressants: SSRIs and novel atypical antidepressants—An update on psychopharmacology. *In* Steiner H, ed: Handbook of Mental Health Interventions in Children and Adolescents: An Integrated Developmental Approach. San Francisco: Jossey-Bass, 2004, pp 318-362.

symptoms, allergic reactions, and increased suicidal behavior.

Common adverse effects of tricyclic antidepressants include cardiac conduction delay, anticholinergic effects, behavioral activation or hypomania, sedation, increased appetite, and weight gain. Less common side effects include seizures, psychosis, hypertension, and, in extremely rare cases, sudden death.

Current Controversies

With the introduction of the FDA black box warning, there appears to be a trend of a reduced number of prescriptions of SSRIs and novel antidepressants. Primary care physicians and clinicians have become more anxious about prescribing these medications. It is clear, however, from worldwide research that introduction of these medications has led to reductions in suicide rates in countries in which the medications are prescribed.[42] The concern is that the black box warning will result in even more delay in appropriate treatment of major depression, which in turn could possibly result in more suicide deaths.

The efficacy of SSRIs for major depression appears to be emerging, despite some negative studies. More needs to be done in this area to ensure that these medications are clearly more efficacious than placebo. One of the challenges seems to be discriminating unipolar disorders from bipolar disorders. Apparently, up to 40% of patients who ultimately have bipolar disorder present first with a depressive episode.[43] It is clinically challenging to make this differentiation. However, antidepressants taken by patients with bipolar disorder can lead to exacerbation in mood symptoms.[44,45] More research needs to be done to help with this distinction. In general, clinicians need to be extremely vigilant when treating adolescents and children with antidepressants, especially in the first weeks after initiation of treatment.

ANTIPSYCHOTICS

Patients with psychotic symptoms were the intended users of antipsychotic agents, both typical and atypical. However, clinicians more widely prescribe these drugs for other indications such as aggressive behavior in juveniles, pervasive developmental disorders, severe ADHD, tic disorders, and certain mood disorders.[1]

Typical antipsychotics preferentially block dopamine D_2 receptors in the mesolimbic, mesocortical, and nigrostriatal areas. "Atypical "antipsychotics have a weaker affinity for dopamine D_2 receptors and varying affinity for other dopamine receptors. There also is a greater specificity for the mesocortical and mesolimbic areas. There is a stronger affinity for serotonergic receptors, which seems to result in differences in the side effect profile between the two groups, as well as enhanced efficacy for symptoms of schizophrenia.[46]

Common indications, both FDA approved and off label, are listed in Table 8C-6. Some of the typical agents are approved for use in psychosis in children and adolescents, severe behavior disorders, ADHD, and severe anxiety. Pimozide and haloperidol are

TABLE 8C-6 ■ Antipsychotics: Indications and Common Side Effects

Generic	Strengths Available	Dose Range	Indications	Side Effects
Olanzapine	2.5, 5, 7.5, 10, 15, 20 mg 5, 10, 15, 20 mg tablet disintegrating tablet	2.5-5 mg/day Max 20 mg/day	Schizophrenia Bipolar disorder	Weight gain Somnolence Hypotension
Risperidone	0.25-, 0.5-, 1-, 2-, 3-, 4-mg tab 1 mg/mL solution 0.5, 1, 2, 3, 4 disintegrating tablet 25, 37.5, 50 mg IM	0.125 mg/day to 6 mg/day Every 2 weeks depot injection	Bipolar disorder Autism Schizophrenia Tics Aggression	Extrapyramidal symptoms Weight gain Sedation Increased prolactin Hepatic changes
Quetiapine	25, 100, 200, 300 mg tabs 400 mg	25-400 mg/day	Schizophrenia Bipolar mania Bipolar depressed	Sedation Hypotension Altered liver function tests
Ziprasidone	20-, 40-, 60-, 80-mg caps	20-160 mg/day	Bipolar Disorder Schizophrenia	QTc prolongation Rash Somnolence Hypotension
Aripiprazole	5, 10, 15, 20, 30 mg tabs and disintegrating tabs IM 9.75 mg/1.3 ml	5 mg/day to 30 mg/day	Bipolar Disorder Schizophrenia	Activation Insomnia Somnolence
Clozapine	12.5, 25-50, 100-mg tabs 25, 50 disintegrating tablets	12.5-900 mg/day	Treatment resistant Schizophrenia Bipolar disorder	Agranulocytosis Lower seizure threshold Hypotension Anticholinergic effects Weight gain Sedation Drooling
Chlorpromazine	10-, 25-, 50-, 100-, 200-mg tabs 10/5 mL, 20/mL solution 25, 100 mg PR 25 mg/mL injection	50-500 mg/day	Schizophrenia Bipolar disorder Aggression	Anticholinergic effects Hypotension
Haloperidol	0.5-, 1-, 2-, 5-, 10-, 20-mg tab 2 mg/mL oral solution 5 mg/mL IM 50, 100 mg IM decanoate	0.5 mg/day to 15 mg/day Every 4 weeks	Psychosis Severe behavior Tourette syndrome Autism	Extrapyramidal symptoms
Loxapine	5, 10, 25, 50 mg capsules 12.5 mg IM	10-250 mg/day	Schizophrenia	Extrapyramidal symptoms Anticholinergic effects Sedation
Pimozide	1, 2 mg tabs	0.5-10 mg/day	Tourette syndrome	QTc prolongation Extrapyramidal symptoms

Data from McClellan and Werry, 2003,[33] and DeJong et al, 2004.[49]
PDD, pervasive developmental disorder; QTc, corrected QT interval.

approved for Tourette syndrome. The use of these medications for a variety of other disorders is supported by a limited evidence base. Research has documented the effectiveness of typical antipsychotics, such as haloperidol, in schizophrenia, autistic disorders, tic disorders, conduct disorder, and mental retardation.[33] Research has also demonstrated the effectiveness of atypical antipsychotics, such as risperidone, in tic disorders, conduct disorder, autism, and mental retardation.[33] To date, the best evidence for efficacy of these agents is with autism.[47] These agents have also been studied for the treatment of pediatric bipolar disorder.[1]

Guidelines for Use

In view of the limited evidence base just described, it is important to establish the specific diagnosis and target symptoms thought to be responsive to these agents.[48] Methods of tracking improvements need careful consideration. This may include rating scales, parents' and teachers' reports, patient's reports, and clinician's observation. Baseline medical evaluations for patients taking these medications include a recent physical examination, with documentation of height, weight (and body mass index), blood pressure, heart rate, temperature, and electrocardiographic measurements. A baseline investigation for abnormal involuntary movements should be conducted (with a standard measure), and any preexisting extrapyramidal symptoms should be documented. In addition, standard laboratory evaluation should include a comprehensive hepatic panel, fasting glucose measurement, fasting lipid profile, complete blood cell count with differential, and possibly prolactin level measurement. Other evaluations to consider include electroencephalography, especially if clozapine is being considered.

Because of the side effects of these medications, careful informed consent is required from both patient and parent or guardian. This discussion should include describing the off-label use of most of these agents. The dosage ranges for each agent are presented in Table 8C-6. The choice of agents is most often based on side effect profile. Lower initial dosing, until tolerance of the medication is established, is essential. Once the patient has started taking the medication, regular scheduled follow-up is imperative, and constant monitoring of the efficacy of the medication and side effects is necessary. Patients should be encouraged to maintain regular exercise and consider a nutrition consultation. After a period of 6 to 12 months of steady improvement in clinical symptoms, the clinician might consider reducing the dosage to find the lowest effective dosage.[49] For patients with conditions refractory to these agents, it is prudent to consider assessing for rarer central nervous system disorders.[48]

Adverse Effects

Table 8C-6 lists the common adverse effects of this category of medications. The most common concern with typical antipsychotics is the development of extrapyramidal symptoms such as dystonia, tremor, and other parkinsonian symptoms. In addition, these agents can induce involuntary and persistent dyskinetic movements and tardive dyskinesia. Atypical agents, in general, do not cause the same degree of extrapyramidal symptoms. The side effect of most concern in this category has been weight gain and the possible induction of type 2 diabetes.[50]

Current Controversies

Since the mid-1990s, clinicians have increased their prescribing of atypical antipsychotics for the multiple indications listed previously. The evidence base for use of these medications for most of the disorders is weak.[33] The significant weight gain documented with most of these agents is of great concern, and the risk of obesity is significantly elevated whenever these medications are initiated.[46] The long-term benefits of the medications need to be considered against these very serious medical complications.

MOOD STABILIZERS

Medications that treat at least one mood state of bipolar disorder without worsening the other mood state are called *mood stabilizers*.[51] This category includes lithium and many of the anticonvulsants. Although the atypical antipsychotics have properties of mood stabilization, they are not included in this category at this time.

The mechanism of action of lithium remains unknown. It appears to act through augmentation of the serotonergic system, affecting the second messenger system and upregulating a neuroprotective protein. It also may increase gray matter, as evidenced by neuroimaging.[52]

The mechanism of actions of anticonvulsants are also unknown; however, they appear to enhance γ-amino butyric acid (GABA) and decrease glutamate. These medications also increase neuroprotective factors.[53]

Common indications (i.e., with FDA approval) for lithium include treatment of bipolar disorder and acute mania in patients older than 12 years and prophylaxis for bipolar disorder in patients older than 12 years. Possible indications for lithium (i.e., off-label use) include treatment of acute mania in patients younger than 12 years of age, bipolar depression, and cyclothymia; augmentation of antidepressants in the treatment of refractory major depression and obsessive-compulsive disorder; and treatment of aggression and rage in patients with ADHD and conduct disorder.

There is no current FDA approval of anticonvulsants for behavioral disorders in children and adolescents. Possible indications include treatment of bipolar disorder, acute mania, and bipolar depression in children and adolescents; treatment of aggression and rage in conduct disorder; and treatment of chronic pain. Valproic acid and lamotrigine have FDA-approved indications in adults for the treatment of acute mania and bipolar depression.

Table 8C-7 lists the indications to date of mood stabilizers in the treatment of child and adolescent psychopathology.

Guidelines for Use

When mood stabilizers are used in the treatment of mania, depression, or aggression, it is crucial that the specific target symptoms be defined. Algorithms now exist for choosing medications for the treatment of juvenile bipolar disorder on the basis of the evidence and expert consensus.[54] Baseline rating scales for tracking mania, depression, or aggression are available.[55] In addition, longitudinal and prospective mood charting is very helpful in determining the effect of

TABLE 8C-7 ■ Mood Stabilizers in Children and Adolescents

Drug	Strengths	Dosage	Possible Indications	Common Side Effects
Divalproex	125-, 250-, 500-mg tabs 125-mg sprinkle caps 250-, 500-mg caps extended release	125-250 mg/day Titrate to max 60 mg/kg/day Serum level, 50-100 µg/mL	Bipolar disorder Conduct disorder	Gastrointestinal symptoms Sedation Weight gain
Lithium	150, 300-600 mg caps 450-mg cap 300, 450 extended release Liquid 5 mL = 300 mg	150-1800 mg/day Titrate clinically Serum levels to 1.2 mEq/L	Bipolar disorder Major depressive disorder Aggressive behaviors	Polyuria, polydipsia, tremors Hypothyroidism Gastrointestinal symptoms
Carbamazepine	100-mg chew tabs 200 mg tabs 100, 200, 300 mg extended tabs 100 mg/5 mL solution	100 mg b.i.d. to max 600/day depending on serum level 4-10 µg/mL serum level range	Bipolar disorder Aggression	Rash, nausea, dizziness Sedation Bone marrow suppression
Gabapentin	100-, 300-, 400-mg caps 600-, 800-mg tabs 250 mg/5 mL solution	10-15 mg/kg/day in divided doses t.i.d. Max 60 mg/kg/day Adults, up to 4800 mg/day	Mood instability	Somnolence Nystagmus Edema, fatigue
Lamotrigine	25, 100, 150, 200 mg tabs 2-, 5-, 25-mg chewable tabs	≥12 years: 12.5 mg/day to max 200 mg/day ≤12 years: 0.6 mg/kg/day to max 4.5 mg/kg/day	Bipolar depression	Somnolence, rash, vomiting, dizziness, ataxia
Oxcarbazepine	150-, 300-, 600-mg tabs 300 mg/5 mL solution	8-10 mg/kg/day, in b.i.d. doses, 900-1800 mg/day max	Bipolar mania	Somnolence Dizziness, nausea, fatigue Hyponatremia
Topiramate	25-, 50-, 100-, 200-mg tabs 15-, 25-mg caps	Initiate at 25 mg/day to max 400 mg/day 5-9 mg/kg/day recommended	Bipolar disorder	Somnolence, fatigue, decrease in weight, cognitive dulling

Data from Paruluri et al, 2005,[55] and Physician's Desk Reference, 60th ed. Montvale, NJ: Thomson Healthcare, 2006.

these medications on the targeted symptoms. Once the decision to prescribe these medications is made, the following should be completed: physical examination, vital sign measurements, height and weight measurements, and specific laboratory tests. For lithium, a complete blood cell count with differential; blood urea nitrogen, creatinine, and electrolyte measurements; thyroid profile; and pregnancy test are necessary. In addition, an electrocardiogram should be obtained; if clinically necessary, an electroencephalogram should also be obtained. For the anticonvulsants, all of these procedures should be completed, with the addition of a hepatic profile and lipid profile.

The dosing of these medications should conservatively follow the guideline of "start low and go slow." Children metabolize lithium and the anticonvulsants faster than adults do; however, there is great inter-individual variability. Lithium, valproate, and carbamazepine serum levels are helpful in determining the optimal dose. Although there is no evidence that a specific serum level must be achieved, these tests are helpful in avoiding toxicity. At each follow-up visit, blood pressure, heart rate, height, and weight should be documented. Serum levels of lithium and the anti-convulsants (if available) should be checked after each dose increase and, once steady state has been reached, every 3 to 4 months thereafter. Baseline laboratory test results should be checked more frequently during initiation and then every 3 to 4 months thereafter.

Adverse effects of lithium and the anticonvulsants are listed in Table 8C-7. It is also important to be wary of specific drug interactions.

Current Controversies

Increasingly, clinicians are prescribing mood stabilizers for many children and adolescents who have symptoms of mania but do not fulfill the diagnostic criteria for bipolar disorder.[55,56] Frequently, the main target symptom is irritability and rage. Although some studies have indicated the efficacy of these medications for this symptom, the risk of significant side effects must be considered. In addition, the frequency of treating patients with more than one medication for their emotional disorder is increasing. However, if the diagnosis of bipolar disorder is accurate, the risks of not aggressively treating these individuals include worsening or progressing of the condition.[55]

ANXIOLYTICS

The agents most commonly used for the short-term reduction of anxiety are the benzodiazepines. In children and adolescents, clinicians rarely prescribe them for the long-term management of anxiety. The mechanism of action of the benzodiazepines appears related to decreased neuronal excitability by affecting the GABA neurotransmitter system. Some of the benzodiazepines have FDA approval for the treatment of seizures, anxiety, and insomnia. Possible indications include short-term management of anxiety, acute agitation in adolescents, and alcohol withdrawal syndromes.

The evidence base for the usefulness of benzodiazepines for anxiety is limited.[33] There have been few randomized controlled trials.[57] In addition, there is a high placebo response rate, and the active medications are often not significantly better than placebo.

Other agents in the anxiolytic category include buspirone, antihistamines, and β blockers. Buspirone is a novel anxiolytic agent approved for use in adult anxiety syndromes. There is no FDA approval for children younger than 18 years. The mechanism of action is not clear, but buspirone appears to affect serotonin and dopamine neurotransmitters and is a partial α-adrenergic agonist. Its use includes treatment of pediatric anxiety conditions and aggression, ADHD, oppositional defiant disorder, and conduct disorder. There have been no controlled trials of this medication. If used, it is best to start at low doses and use two or three times per day. There are minimal reports of adverse effects. Mild sedation and, in rare cases, behavioral activation may occur.

Psychiatrists and pediatricians often use antihistamines for the management of agitation, insomnia, and extrapyramidal symptoms. In general, these medications block central histamine and have anticholinergic effects and some serotonergic effects. There is FDA approval for hydroxyzine for pediatric anxiety; there are no other approved uses for juvenile patients. The evidence base is limited to a few open label trials for anxiety and agitation. Diphenhydramine is most often used for the short-term management of anxiety or agitation. Dosages of 25 to 50 mg every 6 hours are common; the maximum dose is less than 5 mg/kg/day. Adverse effects include sedation, cognitive dulling, dizziness, anticholinergic effects, lowered seizure threshold, and tachycardia.

The use of β-blocking drugs in pediatric populations for anxiety and aggression is common, despite the lack of controlled studies and no FDA approval for psychiatric conditions. The mechanism of action includes the blockade of β-adrenergic receptors, centrally and peripherally. It appears the peripheral effects are more important for the reduction of anxiety and aggression. There are no firm guidelines about dosing. However, 20 mg to 120 mg in divided doses, with a maximum of 300 mg, has been reported for propranolol. There is no other information about other β blockers for the treatment of juvenile emotional disorder. Common adverse effects include bradycardia, lethargy, sexual side effects, depression, hypotension, and bronchoconstriction. These medications are contraindicated in patients with asthma, diabetes, hyperthyroidism, and depression and in pregnant patients.

Current Controversies

There is inadequate study of the long-term use of benzodiazepines in children and adolescents. The risk of dependence and abuse with these medications is high. There does seem to be a role for these medications in the short-term management of anxiety. Their role in reducing acute agitation in adolescents is not as clear. The induction of disinhibited behavior continues to be a reported concern, although this is not carefully documented in studies of these adolescents.[58]

RATIONAL POLYPHARMACY

Children and adolescents often have more than one psychiatric diagnosis; comorbidity is the rule, not the exception. In patients with multiple diagnoses or one diagnosis of a condition refractory to monotherapy, polypharmacy may be warranted. The mechanisms of actions of these combined treatments are not known. There are no current approved indications for combined agents. One report reviewed studies of rates of polypharmacy in the United States.[59] Psychiatric inpatient facilities have higher rates of polypharmacy prescriptions than do outpatient facilities and pediatric offices.[1,59] In all populations, stimulants plus another agent seem to be the most frequent form of polypharmacy.[1,59] In addition, there has been an increase in the rates of prescribing atypical antipsychotics.[1,59] The most significant concern with polypharmacy is the increased risk of adverse events. Drug-drug interactions are a particular concern.

Although there is some evidence for the efficacy for combined stimulant and α-adrenergic treatment of ADHD and tic disorders, research in this area is limited.[60] In addition, there are reports on the treatment of ADHD and depression with stimulants and SSRIs.[61]

Guidelines for Combining Psychotropic Medications

Clinicians should first clearly establish the diagnosis and target symptoms. Before patients begin taking each medication, clinicians should perform a baseline physical examination and appropriate laboratory evaluations. Assessing for drug-drug interactions, with computerized tools if available, is imperative. Before adding more medication, clinicians should determine that each medication in the regimen is beneficial. Discontinuing one medication before adding another should always be considered.

The rates of side effects increase with each additional medication. Until a systematic study of the safety and efficacy of concomitant medication is completed, a combined treatment regimen must be initiated with caution. The need to treat complex and poorly understood psychiatric disorders in children and adolescents must be balanced against the unknown risks of polypharmacy.

NONSTANDARD AND ALTERNATIVE THERAPIES

Alternative therapies, such as vitamins and herbal medications, are gaining increasing attention because of their widespread use. Despite the limited study of these agents, they continue to be of interest to parents of children with psychiatric disorders. Reviews have indicated that there is evidence for few of these agents of their effectiveness in children and adolescents.[62]

Omega-3 fatty acids have been studied in adults for mood disorders and in children and adolescents for ADHD. Preliminary investigations have generally not demonstrated any clear benefits.[33] However, further study of these agents may be useful.

Uses of melatonin, an exogenous hormone, include a variety of psychiatric disorders. Preliminary studies on a small number of subjects have suggested that melatonin may be appropriate treatment for a variety of sleep disorders. Children with development disabilities may be particularly responsive.[63] Doses of melatonin have varied from 1 to 3 mg/day. It generally appears to be safe. The most common side effects include nightmares, headaches, morning sedation, mild depression, and decreased libido.

Researchers of St. John's wort in adult depression have found effectiveness in mild to moderate, but not severe, depression.[64] To date, there are no published data concerning the use of St. John's wort in children and adolescents. Side effects with this agent are limited, with reports of fatigue, restlessness, and headache.

Numerous herbal medications and dietary supplements are available for use in the United States for a variety of unproven indications. In general, there are only studies in adults, which have provided few data on the effects of these treatments in children and adolescents. The products are not regulated and therefore may be impure, inconsistent in their potency, and expensive. Their use with prescribed medications can be dangerous, and clinicians must ask patients and their parents about their use.

FUTURE DIRECTIONS

The evidence base for pharmacological treatments for child psychiatric disorders is limited but improving. The importance of advancing knowledge is clear. One exhaustive epidemiological study documented the high rates of childhood psychiatric disorders.[65] Twenty percent of children and adolescents suffer from a significant emotional disorder. Half of all lifetime cases of emotional disorder begin by age 14, and 75%, by age 24. Of those ill children and adolescents, only about 30% receive treatment. Lack of access to care from qualified mental health professionals remains a large, unmet need. The projected need for child psychiatrists is not keeping up with the projected increase of at-risk children and adolescents. It is likely that nonpsychiatry clinicians, such as primary care physicians and nurse practitioners, will need to fill these gaps.[66] Currently, there is great variability between clinicians and between different communities with regard to standards of psychopharmacological care for children and adolescents. There is a clear need for more well-defined standards of care. Practice parameters currently exist but are based mainly on clinical opinion and limited research. One exciting research initiative is the Child and Adolescents Clinical Trials Network (CAPTN).[67] This is a nationwide collection of investigators representing the entire prescribing community, enrolling a few patients at each site, which leads to a large overall number. Multiple investigators will use this network for variety of psychopharmacological studies in children and adolescents. This network may be able to address the absence of long-term safety data for most psychotropic agents in use. In addition, the efficacy of polypharmacy should be studied.

The lack of safety and efficacy data for psychotropic medications should be a concern for clinicians, patients, and their families. With initiatives such as CAPTN, we are cautiously optimistic for the future of pediatric psychopharmacology.

REFERENCES

1. Jensen PS, Vinod SB, Vitiello B, et al: Psychoactive medication prescribing practices for U.S. children: Gaps between research and clinical practice. J Am Acad Child Adolesc Psychiatry 38:5, 1999.
2. Olfson M, Marcus SC, Weissman M, et al: National trends in the use of psychotropic medications by children. J Am Acad Child Adolesc Psychiatry 41:5, 2002.
3. Williams J, Klinepeten K, Palmes G, et al: Diagnosis and treatment of behavioral health disorders in pediatric practice. Pediatrics 114:601-606, 2005.
4. Rappaport N, Chubinski P: The meaning of psychotropic medications for children, adolescents and their families. J Am Acad Child Adolesc Psychiatry 39:9, 2000.
5. Safer DJ, Zito JM: Pharmacoepidemiology of psychotropic medications in youth. *In* Rosenberg D, Davanzo PA, Gershon S, et al, eds: Pharmacotherapy for Child and Adolescent Psychiatric Disorders. New York: Marcel Dekker, 2002, pp 23-50.
6. Greenhill LL, Pliszka S, Dulcan MK, et al: Practice parameters for the use of stimulant medications in the treatment of children, adolescents and adults. J Am Acad Child Adolesc Psychiatry 41(2 suppl):26S-49S, 2002.
7. A 14-month randomized clinical trial of treatment strategies for attention deficit hyperactivity disorder. The MTA Cooperative Group. Multimodal Treatment Study of Children with ADHD. Arch Gen Psychiatry 56:1073-1086, 1999.
8. MTA Cooperative Group, National Institute of Mental Health Multimodal Treatment Study of ADHD followup: 24-Month outcomes of treatment strategies for attention-deficit/hyperactivity disorder. Pediatrics 113: 754-761, 2004.
9. Biederman J, Spencer T, Wilen T: Evidence-based psychotherapy for attention-deficit hyperactivity disorder. Int J Neuropsychopharmacol 7:77-97, 2004.
10. Elia J, Borcheding B, Rapoport J, Keysor C: Methylphenidate and dextroamphetamine treatments of hyperactivity: Are there true non-responders? Psychiatry Res 36:141-155, 1991.
11. Biederman J, Newcorn J, Sprich S: Comorbidity of attention deficit hyperactivity disorder with conduct, depression, anxiety and other disorders. Am J Psychiatry. 148:564-577, 1991.
12. Diamond IR, Tannock R, Schachar RJ: Response to methylphenidate in children with ADHD and comorbid anxiety. J Am Acad Child Adolesc Psychiatry 38:402-409, 1999.
13. Castellanos FX, Giedd JN, Eliz J, et al: Controlled stimulant treatment of ADHD and comorbid Tourette's syndrome: Effects of stimulants and dose. J Am Acad Child Adolesc Psychiatry 36:589-596, 1997.
14. Law SF, Schachar RJ: Do typical clinical doses of methylphenidate cause tics in children treated for attention-deficit hyperactivity disorder? J Am Acad Child Adolesc Psychiatry 1997.
15. Liplin PH, Goldstein IJ, Adesman AR: Tics and dyskinesias associated with stimulant treatment in attention deficit hyperactivity disorder. Arch Pediatr Adolesc Med 148:859-861, 1994.
16. The Tourette's Syndrome Study Group: Treatment of ADHD in children with tics: A randomized controlled trial. Neurology 58:527-536, 2002.
17. Pliszka SR: Comorbidity of attention deficit hyperactivity disorder with psychiatric disorder: an overview. J Clin Psychiatry 59(suppl 7):50-58, 1998.
18. Findling RL: Open-label treatment of comorbid depression and attentional disorders with co-administration of serotonin reuptake inhibitors and psychostimulants in children, adolescents and adults: A case series. J Child Adolesc Psychopharmacol 3:1-10, 1996.
19. Biederman J, Klein RG, Pine DS, et al: Resolved mania is mistaken for ADHD in prepubetal children. J Am Acad Child Adolesc Psychiatry 37:1091-1096, 1998.
20. Wilens TE, Faraone SV, Biederman J, et al: Does stimulant therapy of attention-deficit/hyperactivity beget later subtance abuse? a meta-analytic review of the literature. Pediatrics 111:179-185, 2003.
21. Jensen, P, Kettle L, Roper MT, et al: Are stimulants overprescribed? Treatment of ADHD in four US communities. J Am Acad Child Adolesc Psychiatry 38:797-804, 1999.
22. Zito JM, Safer DJ, dosReis S, et al: Trends in prescribing of psychotropic medications to preschoolers. JAMA 283:1025-1030, 2000.
23. Firestone P, Musten LM, Pisterman S, et al: Short-term side effects of stimulant medications are increased in preschool children with attention-deficit/hyperactivity disorder: A double-blind, placebo-controlled study. J Child Adolesc Psychopharmacol 8:13-25, 1998.
24. Spencer T, Heiligenstein JH, Biederman J: Results from 2 proof-of-concept, placebo-controlled studies of atomoxetine in children with attention-deficit/hyperactivity disorder. J Clin Psychiatry 63:1140-1147, 2002.
25. Michelson D, Faries D, Wernike J: Atomoxetine in the treatment of children and adolescents with attention deficit/hyperactivity disorder: A randomized, placebo-controlled, dose response study. Pediatrics 108(5):E83, 2001.
26. U.S. Food and Drug Administration: Public Health Advisory on Atomoxetine. September 29, 2005. (Available at: *http://www.fda.gov/bbs/topics/news/2005/new01237.html;* accessed 10/27/06.)
27. Hunt RD, Capper L, O'Connell P: Clonidine in child and adolescent psychiatry. J Child Adolesc Psychopharmacol 1:87-101, 1990.
28. Arnstein AF, Steere JC, Hunt RD: The contribution of alpha 2–noradrenergic mechanisms of prefrontal cortical cognitive function. Potential significance for attention-deficit hyperactivity disorder. Arch Gen Psychiatry 53:448-455, 1996.
29. Joshi SV: Psychostimulant, atomoxetine, and alpha-agonists. *In* Steiner H, ed: Handbook of Mental Health Interventions in Children and Adolescents: An Integrated Developmental Approach. San Francisco: Jossey-Bass, 2004, pp 258-287.
30. Tourette's Syndrome Study Group: Treatment of ADHD in children with tics: A randomized controlled trial. Neurology 58:527-536, 2002.

31. Steingard R, Biederman J, Spenser T, et al: Comparison of clonidine response in the treatment of attention deficit hyperactivity disorder with and without comorbid tic disorders. J Am Acad Child Adolsc Psychiatry 32:350-353, 1993.

32. Emsle GJ, Walkup JT, Pliska SR: Non-tricyclic antidepressants: Current trends in children and adolescents. J Am Acad Child Adolesc Psychiatry 38:517-528, 1999.

33. McClellan JM, Werry JS: Evidence-based treatments in child and adolescent psychiatry: An inventory. J Am Acad Child Adolesc Psychiatry 42:12, 2003.

34. Treatment for Adolescents with Depression (TADS) Team: Fluoxetine, cognitive-behavioral therapy and their combination for adolescents with depression. JAMA 292:807-820, 2004.

35. Connors CK, Casat CD, Gualtieri CT, et al: Bupropion hydrochloride in attention deficit disorder with hyperactivity. J Am Acad Child Adolesc Psychiatry 35:1314-1321, 1996.

36. Mandoki M, Tapia MR, Tapia MA, et al: Venlafaxine in the treatment of children and adolescents with major depression. Psychopharmacol Bull 33:149-154, 1997.

37. Findling RL: Open label treatment of comorbid depression and attention deficit disorder. J Child Adolesc Psychopharmacol 6:165-175, 1996.

38. Emslie G, Portteus A, Kumar E, et al: Antidepressants: SSRIs and novel atypical antidepressants—An update on psychopharmacology. *In* Steiner H, ed: Handbook of Mental Health Interventions in Children and Adolescents: An Integrated Developmental Approach. San Francisco: Jossey-Bass, 2004, pp 318-362.

39. Geller B, Reising D, Leonard H, et al: Critical review of tricyclic antidepressant use in children and adolescents. J Am Acad Child Adolesc Psychiatry 38:513-516, 1999.

40. U.S. Food and Drug Administration: FDA Public Health Advisory: Suicidality in Children and Adolescents Being Treated with Antidepressant Medication, October 15, 2004. (Available at: *http://www.fda.gov/cder/drug/ antidepressants/SSRIPHA200410.htm;* accessed 10/27/06.)

41. American Psychiatric Association, American Academy of Child and Adolescent Psychiatry: The Use of Medication in Treating Childhood and Adolescent Depression: Information for Physicians, January 2005. (Available at: *http://www.parentsmedguide.org/physicansmedguide. pdf;* accessed 10/27/06.)

42. American College of Neuropsychopharmacology, Executive Summary Preliminary Report of the Task Force on SSRI and Suicidal Behavior in Youth. January, 2004.

43. Geller B, Fox LW, Clark KA: Ratio and predictors of prepubertal bipolarity during follow-up of 6- to 12-year-old depressed children. J Am Acad Child Adolesc Psychiatry 33:461-468, 1994.

44. Carlson GA: The bottom line. J Child Adolesc Psychopharmacol 13:115-118, 2003.

45. Biederman J, Mick E, Prince J, et al: Therapeutic dilemmas in the pharmacotherapy of bipolar depression in the young. J Child Adolesc Psychopharmacol 10:185-192, 2000.

46. Findling R, Schulz S, Reed M, et al: The antipsychotics. A pediatric perspective. Pediatric Clin North Am 45:1205-1232, 1998.

47. McCracken JT, McGough J, Shah B: Risperidone in children with autism and serious behavioral problems. N Engl J Med 347:314-321, 2002.

48. McClellan J, Werry J: Practice parameters for the assessment and treatment of children and adolescents with schizophrenia. J Am Acad Child Adolesc Psychiatry 40(7 suppl):4S-23S, 2001.

49. DeJong S, Ginliano A, Frazier J: Antipsychotic medication. *In* Steiner H, ed: Handbook of Mental Health Interventions in Children and Adolescents: An Integrated Developmental Approach. San Francisco: Jossey-Bass, 2004, pp 413-464.

50. Food and Drug Administration: Warning about hyperglycemia and atypical antipsychotic drugs. FDA Patient Safety News Show #28, June, 2004. (Available at: *http://www.accessdata.fda.gov/scripts/ cdrh/cfdocs/psn/printer.cfm?id=229;* accessed 10/27/06.)

51. Keck P, McElroy S: Redefining mood stabilization. J Affect Disord 73:163-169, 2003.

52. Moore G, Bebchuk J, Wilds I, et al: Lithium-induced increase in human brain grey matter. Lancet 356:1241-1242, 2000.

53. Manji H, Moore G, Chen G: Clinical and preclinical evidence for the neurotropic effects of mood stabilizers: Implications for the pathophysiology and treatment of manic-depressive illness. Biol Psychiatry 48:740-754, 2000.

54. Paruluri M, Henry D, Devieneni B, et al: A pharmacotherapy algorithm for stabilization and maintenance of pediatric bipolar disorder. J Am Acad Child Adolesc Psychiatry 43:859-867, 2004.

55. Paruluri M, Birmaher B, Naylor M: Pediatric bipolar disorder: A review of the past 10 years. J Am Acad Child Adolesc Psychiatry 44:846-871, 2005.

56. Carlson GA, Kelly KL: Mania symptoms in psychiatrically hospitalized children. What do they mean? J. Affect Disord 51:123-125, 1998.

57. Simeon J, Knott V, Thatte S, et al: Pharmacotherapy of childhood anxiety disorder. Clin Neuropharmacol 15:229-230, 1992.

58. Thienemann M: Medications for pediatric anxiety. *In* Steiner H, ed: Handbook of Mental Health Interventions in Children and Adolescents: An Integrated Developmental Approach. San Francisco: Jossey-Bass, 2004, pp 288-317.

59. Duffy F, Narrow W, Rae D, et al: Concomitant pharmacotherapy among youths treated in routine psychiatric practice. J Child Adolesc Psychopharmacol 15:12-25, 2005.

60. Wilens T, Spencer T, Swanson J, et al: Combining methylphenidate and clonidine: A clinically sound medication option. J Am Acad Child Adolesc Psychiatry 38:614-619, 1999.

61. Kratochvil C, Newcorn J, Arnold L, et al: Atomoxetine alone or combined with fluoxetine for treating ADHD

with comorbid depression or anxiety symptoms. J Am Acad Child Adolesc Psychiatry 44:915-924, 2005.

62. Rojas N, Chan E: Old and new controversies in the alternative treatment of attention-deficit hyperactivity disorder. Ment Retard Dev Disabil Res Rev 11:116-130, 2005.

63. Smits M, Nagtegaal E, Vander H, et al: Melatonin for chronic sleep onset insomnia in children—A randomized placebo-controlled trial. J Child Neurol 16:86-92, 2001.

64. Shatkin J, Davanzo P: Atypical and adjunctive agents. *In* Rosenberg D, Davanzo PA, Gershon S, et al, eds: Pharmacotherapy for Child and Adolescent Psychiatric Disorders. New York: Marcel Dekker, 2002, pp 597-634.

65. Kessler R, Berglund P, Dember O, et al: Lifetime prevalence and age-of-onset distributions of *DSM-IV* disorders in the national comorbidity survey replication. Arch Gen Psychiatry 62:593-602, 2005.

66. Satcher D: Surgeon General Agent—National Action Agenda for Children's Mental Health. January 2001.

67. March J: The Child and Adolescent Psychiatry Trials Network. Washington, DC: National Institute of Mental Health and American Academy of Child and Adolescent Psychiatry, 2005.

68. Emslie GJ, Rush AJ, Weinberg WA, et al: A double blend, randomized, placebo controlled trial of fluoxetine in children and adolescents with depression. Arch Gen Psychiatry 54:1031-1037, 1997.

69. Emslie GJ, Heilgenstein JH, Wagner KD, et al: Fluoxetine for acute treatment of depression in children and adolescents: A placebo controlled randomized clinical trial. J Am Acad Child Adolesc Psychiatry 41:1205-1214, 2002.

70. Keller MB, Ryan ND, Strober M, et al: Efficacy of paroxetine in the treatment of adolescent major depression: A randomized controlled trial. J Am Acad Child Adolesc Psychiatry 40:762-772, 2001.

71. Wagner KD, Robb AS, Findley R, et al: Citalopram treatment of pediatric depression: Results of a placebo controlled trial. Sponsored by Hirschfield RMA. Presented at American College of Neuropsychopharmacology, Waikoloa, HI, 2001.

72. Wagner KD, Wohlberg CJ: Efficacy and Safety of Sertraline in the Treatment of Pediatric Major Depressive Disorder (MDD). Presented at the 155th annual meeting of the American Psychiatric Association, Philadelphia, 2002.

73. Emslie GJ, Findling RL, Rynn MA, et al: Efficacy and safety of nefazodone in the treatment of adolescents with major depressive disorder. Presented at the 42rd annual meeting of the New Clinical Drug Evaluation Unit, Boca Raton, FL, 2002.

74. Ryan ND: Medication treatment for depression in children and adolescents. CNS Spectrums 8:283-287, 2003.

SUGGESTED READING

Birmaher B, Brent D, Benson R: Summary of the practice parameters for the assessment and treatment of children and adolescents with depressive disorder. American Academy of Child and Adolescent Psychiatry. J Am Acad Child Adolesc Psychiatry 37:1234-1238, 1998.

Bernstein G, Kinlan J: Practice parameters for the assessment and treatment of children and adolescents with anxiety disorders. J Am Acad Child Adolesc Psychiatry 36(suppl), 1997.

Myers K, Winters NC: Ten-year review of rating scales. II: Scales for internalizing disorders. J Child Adolesc Psychopharmacol 41:634-659, 2002.

8D.
Evidence-Based Psychological Interventions for Emotional and Behavioral Disorders

KRISTIN M. HAWLEY

AMANDA JENSEN-DOSS

Psychological interventions include a wide array of behavioral and psychotherapeutic treatments designed to reduce psychological distress and maladaptive behavior and to increase adaptive behavior, typically through counseling, support, interaction, or instruction. For younger children and adolescents (hereafter referred to collectively as *children* except when a distinction is necessary), such interventions are conducted with the children themselves, their parents, their teachers, and/or other significant persons in their lives. Psychological treatments have traditionally been administered largely by professionals with specialized therapy training (e.g., psychiatrists, psychologists, clinical social workers) who work in mental health or psychiatric settings (e.g., inpatient psychiatric hospitals, outpatient mental health clinics). Unfortunately, evidence suggests that only a small minority of the estimated 20% of children experiencing significant mental health problems ever receive such treatment.[1] Because of this, there is an increasing awareness that access to care can be improved if mental health screening, referral, and even service provision are integrated into settings in which children in need are most likely to be observed (e.g., schools, primary care practices). The objectives of this chapter are to provide a review of the empirical evidence supporting psychological interventions for emotional and behavioral disorders and to encourage informed referral and enhanced care for children seen in pediatric and primary care settings. The chapter begins with a brief introduction to the child psychological treatment literature as a whole and then describes the specific psychological interventions with the strongest evidence base for treating the most common emotional and behavioral problems experienced by children.

OVERVIEW OF PSYCHOLOGICAL INTERVENTION LITERATURE

There is a wealth of scientific literature supporting the efficacy of psychological treatments for mental health problems in children. More than 1500 trials have tested the effects of various psychological treatments for a broad range of childhood problems, including depression, anxiety, and disruptive behavior, and new trials begin each year.[2] One method usd to summarize this literature is meta-analysis, in which study results are converted to a common effect size metric in order to combine the results from a group of studies into a single comprehensive analysis. Several meta-analyses have been conducted on this burgeoning evidence base, each demonstrating that psychological treatment is, on average, more effective than no treatment, wait-list, and placebo conditions.[3-6] More specifically, the average effect sizes obtained in these meta-analyses were all at or above 0.71, which indicates that the average treated child showed better outcomes than did more than 75% of control children. Weisz and colleagues[6] also found that these positive treatment effects endure beyond the end of treatment, at least over the 6-month follow-up periods typically examined.

Because of the overall efficacy of psychological treatment, complementary efforts have focused on identifying which particular treatments for specific child problems have the strongest research support. Perhaps the most visible of these efforts have been those initiated by the American Psychological Association's Task Force on the Promotion and Dissemination of Psychological Procedures.[7-9] The purpose of the Task Force was to identify effective psychological treatments for mental disorders and psychological aspects of physical disorders and to regularly update and distribute this list to mental health providers and training programs. The Task Force outlined criteria for three distinct levels of empirical support: well-established treatments, probably efficacious treatments, and experimental treatments. Well-established treatments are those with the highest level of supportive evidence, including multiple randomized controlled trials or a large series of well-done single-case design studies demonstrating their efficacy. Well-established treatments must also be clearly described in treatment manuals, and their efficacy must have

been established by at least two unrelated investigative teams. Probably efficacious treatments are those supported by results of at least one randomized clinical trial or a small series of well-done single-case design studies, otherwise meeting the well-established criteria. Experimental treatments are those that have not received either level of support.

The original American Psychological Association Task Force reports[9,10] focused primarily on adult interventions, but they spawned similar efforts to identify efficacious psychological interventions for children. A special section of the *Journal of Clinical Child Psychology*[11] reported findings for well-established and probably efficacious interventions for depression,[12] phobia and anxiety disorders,[13] autism,[14] conduct disorders,[15] and attention-deficit/hyperactivity disorder (ADHD).[16] A series of articles published from 1999 to 2001 in the *Journal of Pediatric Psychology* reported findings for elimination conditions,[17,18] sleep problems,[19] feeding problems,[20] and obesity.[21] A number of other reviewers have followed suit, using varied criteria to identify the treatments with the most consistent support for ameliorating a variety of child mental health problems, including child abuse and neglect,[22] substance abuse,[23,24] and autism and pervasive developmental disorders.[25-27]

In this chapter, we provide a review of efficacious psychological treatments for the four most common classes of child emotional and behavioral disorders: (1) depression and mood; (2) anxiety and fears; (3) attention problems, impulsivity, and ADHD; and (4) conduct problems and disorders. Coverage of treatments for other childhood disorders is beyond the scope of this chapter, but interested readers are referred to the cited reviews for information regarding evidence-based psychological treatments. For information about pharmacological interventions, readers are referred to Chapter 8C.

Previous reviews of empirically supported (evidence-based) psychological interventions have been criticized for not applying clear standards for how to synthesize positive and negative findings[28] or, worse yet, for requiring only a minimum number of positive findings with no consideration of negative findings (e.g., Bickman[29]). In this chapter, we address these criticisms by including and evaluating both positive and negative findings. We briefly describe all available evidence for each problem and then provide greater detail for the psychological treatments with the most consistent empirical support. We also provide guidance for pediatricians and primary care physicians about factors to consider when making a referral for specialty mental health care. We focus on the treatments that (1) were examined in at least two separate randomized clinical trials and (2) showed an average unweighted effect size at or above 0.50 across all trials and across all outcome measures of the target problem (e.g., measures of anxiety for a study targeting anxiety). We chose an effect size of 0.50 because this is considered a medium effect and one that is large enough to be intuitively obvious; it indicates that the average treated child is better off after treatment than more than 69% of those who did not receive treatment (the control condition).[30]

To identify psychological treatments, we use data from an ongoing broad-based meta-analysis of the child treatment literature.[31] Here we briefly describe that search process, the inclusion criteria that we applied, and the coding system used to characterize the studies. For a more detailed description of these procedures, please see Weisz and associates.[2] We searched PsycINFO and Medline, standard computerized databases, for studies beginning in 1965 and continuing through December 2005, using key terms from previous meta-analyses.[5,6] We also surveyed published reviews and meta-analyses of the child psychotherapy literature,[3,32,33] followed reference trails of reviewed studies, and screened studies suggested by investigators in the field. This search led to a pool of more than 3000 published trials, of which 244 met our inclusion criteria.

To be included in this review, studies were required to be tests of *psychotherapy,* defined as any psychological or behavioral intervention designed to alleviate nonnormative psychological distress, reduce maladaptive behavior, or increase deficient adaptive behavior through counseling, interaction, a training program, or a predetermined treatment plan. We also required that studies (1) include comparison of psychotherapy to a control group (wait-list, placebo, or other procedure intended to control for the passage of time and/or receipt of attention), (2) involve random assignment of participants to conditions, (3) use a sample with a mean age between 4 and 18 years, (4) use participants selected for having psychological problems within depression, anxiety, ADHD, or conduct problem domains (i.e., prevention studies were not included), (5) include a post-treatment assessment of the psychological problem for which participants were selected and treated, and (6) have been subjected to peer review.

We identified 244 peer-reviewed randomized clinical trials published from 1963 to 2005. Of these, 20 were focused on depression or mood-related problems; 84 on anxiety or fears; 40 on ADHD and related problems of attention, hyperactivity, or impulsivity; and 100 on conduct-related problems and disorders. In 143 (58.6%) of the studies, the researchers compared the tested treatments with no treatment or wait-listed control conditions; of the remainder, 81 (33.2%) used attention/placebo control conditions

and 20 (8.2%) used standard case management, such as probation, inpatient, or ward milieu.

PSYCHOLOGICAL MANAGEMENT OF DEPRESSION

The mood disorders that affect children include major depressive disorder, dysthymic disorder, bipolar I and II disorders, and cyclothymic disorder. Rates tend to increase as children age, from about 1.7% among children to 5.6% or higher among adolescents.[34] Depression is associated with significant functional impairments and, often, physiological symptoms, such as psychomotor agitation or retardation and hypersomnia or insomnia. It also substantially increases the risk of suicide,[35] and thus it is an area for essential clinical attention. For a more thorough review of the prevalence and expression of mood disorders, see Chapter 18A.

In our review, we sought randomized clinical trials of psychological treatments for children with a diagnosed mood disorder or subclinical depressive symptoms. Reflecting the relatively recent recognition that children and adolescents can experience depression, the treatment studies here are both newer (1986 to 2005) and fewer (20 studies testing 29 treatment conditions) than the other problem areas we describe later. In 15 (75%) of these studies, investigators used a no-treatment or wait-list control condition; of the remainder, 4 (20%) used an attention control condition and 1 (5%) used a placebo control condition. Three types of psychological interventions have shown consistently positive effects across two or more controlled trials: relaxation training; cognitive-behavioral therapy (CBT), including child-focused CBT, child CBT plus parent CBT, and family-focused CBT; and interpersonal therapy (Table 8D-1). All targeted unipolar depression and related symptoms. Other interventions have not yet been examined in multiple studies (e.g., self-modeling of positive affect and attachment-based family therapy for unipolar depression; multifamily psychoeducation groups for bipolar disorder).

Relaxation Training

Relaxation training is a class of techniques that include slow, controlled breathing; deep muscle relaxation (wherein the major muscle groups are tensed and relaxed); and guided imagery (e.g., the child is encouraged to imagine a calm, soothing scene). It has been examined in two studies[36,37] for children with elevated levels of depressive symptoms; both studies showed significant decreases in depressive symptoms

TABLE 8D-1 ■ **Evidence-Based Psychological Treatments for Depression and Related Problems in Children**

Type of Intervention	No. Studies	Publication Dates	Ages	Gender	Race/Ethnicity	Symptom Severity
Child Focused						
Relaxation training	2	1986-1990	10-17	Both	White only	Elevated symptoms
Cognitive-behavioral therapy	15	1986-2004	7-18	Both	White, African American, Hispanic/Latino, Asian	Elevated symptoms, diagnosed disorder
Interpersonal therapy	2	1999	12-18	Both	Hispanic/Latino, non-Hispanic (not otherwise specified)	Diagnosed disorder
Multiple Systems Targeted						
Child and parent/family cognitive-behavioral therapy	3	1990-2002	9-18	Both	White, African American, Hispanic/Latino, Asian	Elevated symptoms, diagnosed disorder

in comparison to no treatment. Relaxation training has not yet been examined in children with diagnosed depressive disorders. Furthermore, these two studies included only white children. Thus, although such techniques may well be worthwhile for children experiencing mild to moderate levels of distress, it remains to be seen whether these techniques alone would suffice for those experiencing diagnosable levels of depression.

Cognitive-Behavioral Therapy

As shown in Table 8D-1, CBT has received the most research attention. CBT has been supported across numerous clinical trials, some targeting just the children for intervention and others targeting both the children and their parents. CBT has demonstrated positive effects across a wide range of ages, across diverse racial and ethnic groups, and both with children who demonstrate elevated levels of depression symptoms and with those who meet diagnostic criteria for major depressive disorder, dysthymic disorder, or depression not otherwise specified. It been administered successfully in both individual and group formats. In addition to showing beneficial effects when tested in research settings, CBT has also been used effectively in school settings.[36,38,39] It has also been examined as bibliotherapy (i.e., having children learn about the therapy components through reading, rather than interaction with a therapist) but with little success.[40] To date, the successful CBT trials have all involved mental health professionals as therapists, and most of the investigators provided them with additional training, supervision, and a manual to guide the intervention.

CBT treats depression by addressing emotional, behavioral, and cognitive skill deficits linked with the onset and maintenance of depression. Several differ-

ent CBT manuals have been examined. The Adolescent Coping with Depression Course developed by Clarke and colleagues[41,42] has been used successfully across the greatest number of trials. For children, manuals include Taking Action[43] and Primary and Secondary Control Enhancement Training.[44] The manuals for children and adolescents vary in developmental level, but they share many core components:

- Psychoeducation about the nature of depression and the treatment rationale.
- Affective education and mood monitoring (the child learns to recognize and label his or her own feelings and the feelings of others, and to monitor and chart his or her mood).
- Relaxation training (described previously).
- Pleasant activity scheduling (the child learns to increase pleasant activities and decrease unpleasant and solitary activities).
- Cognitive restructuring (the child learns to identify and challenge irrational, negative thoughts and replace them with realistic, positive thoughts).
- Thought stopping or interruption (the child learns to distract himself or herself to stop ruminating, or obsessively thinking, about depressing topics).
- Social skills and assertive communication (the child learns strategies to make friends, improve his or her social support system and resolve interpersonal conflicts).
- Problem solving skills (the child learns to generate and evaluate potential solutions to problems and to make plans to implement the chosen solution).
- Reinforcement and self-reinforcement (the child is rewarded, and learns to reward himself or herself, for a variety of behaviors, including increasing activity level, problem solving, and social interaction).

In CBT, parents are often involved in their child's treatment. Typically, parents are (1) informed of the skills their child is learning, (2) taught to reinforce their child's efforts and behavior changes, and (3) encouraged to communicate better with their child via negotiation and problem solving. In most programs, this parent involvement occurs when one or both parents join the child's session for a few minutes at the end of each appointment or, occasionally, attend an entire session together with the child or alone with the therapist. In other programs, parent involvement is more intense, including a series of parent or family sessions in addition to the sessions with the child. Two of the CBT studies actually tested the benefit of combined child CBT plus parent CBT versus child-focused CBT.[45,46] Neither study found the combined treatment significantly better than child-focused CBT.

Interpersonal Therapy for Adolescents

Interpersonal therapy has been examined in two studies, each focused on adolescents with a diagnosis of a depressive disorder.[47,48] Interpersonal therapy has been tested primarily with Hispanic adolescents, but non-Hispanic adolescents made up one third of the sample in the trial by Mufson and colleagues.[48] Mufson and colleagues also included adolescents with comorbid anxiety and were able to treat them successfully. Interpersonal therapy for adolescents has been administered only in an individual format. In both trials, mental health professionals were employed as therapists and were provided with additional training, supervision, and a manual to guide intervention.

Interpersonal therapy for adolescents is designed to reduce depressive symptoms by focusing on important interpersonal relationships, including the parent-child relationship, peer friendships, and romantic relationships. It stems from research indicating that significant interpersonal difficulties often both precipitate and maintain depression.[49-51] Some features of interpersonal therapy for adolescents are reminiscent of CBT, but the overarching focus is the interpersonal problem associated with the onset of depression. Interpersonal therapy includes the following:

1. Psychoeducation about the nature of depression and the treatment rationale.
2. Affective education and mood monitoring (described previously).
3. Attention to the primary interpersonal problem areas:
   a. Interpersonal conflicts (the adolescent develops problem-solving and conflict resolution skills).
   b. Interpersonal deficits (the adolescent improves deficits in social skills and broadens his or her social support system).
   c. Grief and loss (the adolescent is assisted in mourning, in reestablishing interests, and in increasing social contacts).
   d. Role transitions (the adolescent adjusts to his or her new developmental phase of life and adjusts relationships with parents and peers accordingly).
   e. Single-parent families (the adolescent accepts his or her new family situation and improves communication with parents).

Although interpersonal therapy is an adolescent-focused intervention, parents and other significant individuals in the adolescent's life are sometimes brought into treatment sessions to assist the adolescent in dealing with interpersonal problems that the adolescent may be experiencing with those individuals.

Summary and Recommendations

The evidence for the treatment of depression in children supports three psychological interventions: relaxation training, CBT, and interpersonal therapy. Of these, CBT currently has the most consistent evidence across a wide range of ages, ethnicities, and symptom severity levels. CBT has thus far been administered only by mental health professionals, the majority of whom received additional specialty training in those techniques. Therefore, we recommend referral to a child mental health provider specializing in CBT for depression. If trained providers are available, the clinician might consider referring Hispanic adolescents for interpersonal therapy, as this appears to be an effective treatment for that group, perhaps because of the fit between the principles of interpersonal therapy and the collectivist nature of Hispanic culture.[48]

PSYCHOLOGICAL MANAGEMENT OF ANXIETY AND FEARS

Anxiety disorders in children consist of anxiety that is excessive in its frequency, duration, and/or intensity so that it significantly interferes with functioning or causes distress. The anxiety disorders that affect children include separation anxiety disorder, generalized anxiety disorder, social phobia, specific phobia, panic disorder, agoraphobia, post-traumatic stress disorder, acute stress disorder, and obsessive-compulsive disorder. Estimates of the prevalence of anxiety disorders in childhood have varied widely, from 1.0% to 19.7%.[52-34] There is evidence that more than 30% of the children seen in primary care settings have anxiety symptoms associated with some level of impairment, and as much as 15% meet diagnostic criteria for an anxiety disorder.[54] For a more thorough review of the prevalence and expression of anxiety, see Chapter 18B.

We reviewed treatments for children with anxiety disorders and significant anxiety-related problems that did not meet full diagnostic criteria. We located randomized clinical trials in which psychological treatments for anxiety were examined, dating as early as 1967 and totaling 84 trials (testing 140 treatment conditions) by the end of 2005. In 52 (61.9%) of these studies, investigators used a no-treatment or wait-list control condition; of the remainder, 27 (32.1%) used an attention control condition, 1 (1.2%) used a placebo control condition, and 4 (4.8%) used standard case management, such as study skills training for children with test anxiety or incarceration. Several psychological interventions have shown positive effects across two or more controlled trials (Table 8D-2), including relaxation training, exposure, CBT, and client-centered therapy. Other interventions have not yet been examined in multiple studies (e.g., interventions targeting the parent only; insight-oriented therapies).

Relaxation Training

Relaxation training, including muscle relaxation and imagery, was examined in six studies, published between 1969 and 1996, for children with anxiety-related problems. Thus far, it has been examined only in children aged 7 to 18 with anxiety symptoms or fearful behavior but without a diagnosis of anxiety. Despite these early promising findings and the simplicity of the intervention, relaxation training has not been examined as a stand-alone intervention with children who have a diagnosed anxiety disorder. Instead, relaxation training has been integrated into both exposure-based therapies and CBT (see later discussion). In view of these findings, relaxation training may be a helpful intervention for children who show fearfulness and anxiety-related symptoms, but it is unclear whether relaxation alone would provide clinically significant benefit for children with a diagnosed anxiety disorder.

Exposure with Reinforcement, Relaxation, and/or Modeling

The majority of supported interventions involve controlled exposure to the feared object or situation

TABLE 8D-2 ■ Evidence-Based Psychological Treatments for Anxiety and Related Problems in Children						
Type of Intervention	No. Studies	Publication Dates	Ages	Gender	Race/Ethnicity	Symptom Severity
Child Focused						
Relaxation training	6	1969-1996	7-18	Both	White, African American	Elevated symptoms
Exposure with relaxation, reinforcement, and/or modeling	29	1967-2002	3-18	Both	White, African American, Asian	Elevated symptoms, diagnosed disorder
Cognitive-behavioral therapy	40	1974-2005	3-18	Both	White, African American, Hispanic/Latino, Asian, Native American	Elevated symptoms, diagnosed disorder
Client-centered therapy	5	1970-1999	3-16	Both	White, African American, Hispanic/Latino	Elevated symptoms
Family Focused						
Family behavioral therapy	4	1977-2004	6-17	Both	Unknown	Elevated symptoms, diagnosed disorder
Multiple Systems Targeted						
Child and parent/family cognitive-behavioral therapy	9	1967-2003	6-18	Both	White, African American, Hispanic/Latino, Asian	Elevated symptoms, diagnosed disorder
Child and parent/family cognitive-behavioral therapy and teacher consultation	2	1998-2000	5-17	Both	Unknown	Elevated symptoms, diagnosed disorder

(e.g., a specific object such as a spider or dog; public speaking; social interaction; separation from parents). Exposure has been tested as a stand-alone intervention in 29 studies; exposure is also a key component of CBT for anxiety (see later discussion). It has demonstrated positive effects across a wide range of ages, across diverse racial and ethnic groups, and both with children who show elevated levels of anxiety symptoms and those who meet diagnostic criteria for specific phobia[55-57] and post-traumatic stress disorder (see Table 8D-2).[58] One trial of exposure involved participants who had comorbid depression and enuresis and found that the presence or absense of comorbidity was unrelated to treatment outcomes.[55]

Exposure therapy has been administered successfully in both individual and group formats. In addition to producing beneficial effects when tested in research settings, it has also been used effectively in school settings[58-63] and, once, in a dental practice.[64] In one study, the investigators conducted exposure through videotaped modeling without the involvement of a therapist, but they achieved little success.[65] The majority of successful trials of exposure therapy have employed mental health professionals; however, researchers in one study of children with dental fears successfully trained dental students to implement the procedures.[64] In addition, most investigators have not reported extensive additional training, supervision, or manuals to guide intervention, but it is not clear from the published reports whether these efforts were unnecessary or simply not described.

Exposure is typically graduated, beginning with real or imagined situations that are minimally threatening and progressing to those that are maximally anxiety provoking. The therapist generally works with the child to develop a fear hierarchy, with the feared stimuli ordered from least to most anxiety provoking. Then, the child moves through the hierarchy in a graduated manner, with the therapist's assistance, so that each new exposure is challenging but not overwhelming. For a child with separation anxiety, for example, the initial exposure may entail being in a different room from the caregiver for a few minutes, working up to longer periods of time and greater distances, until the child is able to stay with a babysitter for a parent's evening out.

Exposure is often accompanied by relaxation training (19 studies), reinforcement or rewards (2 studies) and/or modeling (12 studies). (In total, there were more than 29 studies because some included more than one exposure condition.) Systematic desensitization combines graduated exposure with relaxation training so that the child uses relaxation skills in order to cope more easily with the real or imagined anxiety-provoking situation. Reinforced exposure entails rewarding the child with praise, a privilege or a desired prize on completion of each step in the exposure hierarchy. Modeling has also been combined with exposure with good effect. In this situation, the therapist, another child, or an actor in a video undergoes exposure to the feared situation or object so that the fearful child can observe the model and see that the model is unharmed. After the child observes the model, he or she is encouraged to imitate the model and thus undergo exposure himself or herself. Often, combinations of these techniques are employed (e.g., exposure with relaxation and reinforcement).

Cognitive-Behavioral Therapy

CBT has received the greatest empirical attention in treating anxiety-related problems and disorders. CBT has been supported in versions targeting just the child for intervention (40 studies) and in versions targeting both the child and his or her parent or parents together (4 studies) and separately (9 studies). Two studies also included a teacher consultation component.[66,67] This component has demonstrated positive effects across a wide range of ages, across diverse racial and ethnic groups, and both with children who show elevated levels of anxiety symptoms and with those who meet diagnostic criteria for social phobia,[55,68-70] generalized anxiety disorder,[70-77] separation anxiety,[71-77] post-traumatic stress disorder,[78] and obsessive-compulsive disorder.[79-81] Several trials have revealed positive treatment effects even when participants have comorbid conditions in addition to their anxiety.[55,67,68,72-74,76-82]

CBT for anxiety has been successfully administered in both individual and group contexts. In addition to showing beneficial effects in research settings, it has also been used effectively in jail[83] and school settings.[61,75,84-86] In the majority of successful trials of CBT, the investigators have employed mental health professionals; however, two groups successfully trained college students to implement the procedures.[87,88] The amount of additional specialty training and supervision has varied across studies, but in most, therapists were provided with a manual to guide intervention.

CBT for anxiety and CBT for depression share a focus on emotions, behaviors, and cognitions. However, exposure, which is not present in CBT for depression, is a core component of CBT for anxiety. Several different CBT manuals have been examined and shown success, including Coping Cat,[89,90] FRIENDS,[91-93] social effectiveness training,[94] and family anxiety management.[95]

CBT for child anxiety typically involves the following:

- Psychoeducation about the nature of anxiety and fear, and the treatment rationale.
- Affective education and monitoring (discussed previously).
- Relaxation training (discussed previously).
- Cognitive restructuring (discussed previously; in this situation, anxiety-provoking thoughts are targeted).
- Thought stopping or interruption (described previously; in this situation, anxious rumination is targeted).
- Fear hierarchy and planning for success (the child learns to generate a fear hierarchy to break down a big problem into smaller steps and to plan ahead for how he or she will successfully navigate anxiety-provoking situations).
- Exposure (described previously).
- Skill building (the child learns to improve skills that may contribute to his or her anxiety, such as social skills and problem-solving).
- Reinforcement and self-reinforcement (described previously; in this situation, the rewards are for using coping skills and engaging in feared activities).

As in CBT for child depression, parents of anxious children are often involved in their child's treatment. During occasional check-in or complete sessions, parents are educated about the treatment their child is receiving and are provided with the necessary skills to implement intervention components with their child at home. In 15 studies, parents were provided with a more extensive intervention. For example, in family anxiety management training,[95] parents are provided with a CBT program to help them deal with their own anxiety and to help them more effectively assist their child with the treatment program. The parents attend a group that covers essentially the same therapeutic content as in the child's sessions (described previously). In addition, parents are taught to act as role models to show their children how to manage anxiety successfully. They also learn to provide reinforcement to their child for completing exposures and engaging in feared activities outside of sessions. Finally, parents learn to discourage repeated displays of anxiety through planned selective ignoring (e.g., the parent intentionally fails to notice their child's whining or clinging, rather than responding by allowing the child to avoid a feared situation). Some of these studies directly tested the benefit of this additional parent involvement by comparing the effects of traditional child-focused CBT with child-focused CBT plus parent CBT. The results of these studies have been mixed, some indicating superior effects of combined treatments (e.g., Deblinger et al[78]) and others finding no differences (e.g., King et al[67] and Nauta et al[96]).

Client-Centered Therapy

Client-centered therapy has yielded positive effects across five studies. In client-centered therapy, children are encouraged to express themselves openly while the therapist listens supportively and encourages the children to accept their feelings and gain greater self-awareness. This therapy has been examined in both individual and group formats and has demonstrated efficacy across a wide range of ages. In one study of client-centered therapy for anxiety, involving African American and Hispanic children, investigators reported treatment effects that were smaller than in the studies including only white children. In addition, none of the studies involved participants with an anxiety disorder diagnosis, instead focusing on children with subclinical levels of anxiety, and none included children with comorbidity. Thus, it is not clear whether this intervention would be effective with children from minority groups or with those experiencing more severe anxiety.

Summary and Recommendations

The evidence for the treatment of anxiety and fears in children supports four psychological interventions: relaxation training, graduated exposure, CBT, and client-centered therapy. Of these, CBT and exposure-based interventions with reinforcement, relaxation, and modeling currently show the most consistent success across a wide range of ages, ethnicities, and symptom severity levels. Some investigators have successfully trained paraprofessionals to administer these treatments to children who have mild anxiety, but most have employed trained mental health professionals. Therefore, we recommend additional training for providers interested in implementing these procedures in their own practices. For children with moderate to severe levels of anxiety, we recommend referral to a child mental health provider who specializes in administering exposure-based interventions.

PSYCHOLOGICAL MANAGEMENT OF INATTENTION, IMPULSIVITY, AND HYPERACTIVITY

ADHD includes three types of difficulties: (1) inattention, characterized by difficulty sustaining attention in tasks or play activities; (2) hyperactivity, characterized by excessive energy; and (3) impulsivity, characterized by difficulty controlling one's actions, such as interrupting conversations or having difficulty waiting in line. Prevalence estimates of ADHD range from

0.9% to 8.0%.[34,52,97] For a more thorough review of ADHD, please see Chapter 16.

Our review included treatment studies of children meeting diagnostic criteria for ADHD and those experiencing attention, impulsivity, or hyperactivity problems that do not meet full criteria for ADHD diagnosis. We found a total of 40 randomized clinical trials for ADHD and related problems (testing 73 treatment conditions) dating as far back as 1968 and as recently as the end of 2005. In 27 (67.5%) of these studies, investigators used an attention control group; of the remainder, 13 (32.5%) used a no-treatment or wait-list control condition; studies lacking a control condition, such as the Multimodal Treatment Study of ADHD study, were not included. Several types of psychological interventions—including client-centered therapy; modeling (e.g., the child observes a model demonstrating how to approach tasks in a careful, deliberate manner); and cognitively and behaviorally oriented interventions targeting only the child, the parent, or the teacher—have been examined for children with ADHD, but most have failed to show substantial benefits. However, we found some support for child-focused relaxation training in children with ADHD-related symptoms. In addition, although child-focused CBT, behavioral parent training (BPT), and teacher-focused consultation and classroom management training did not meet our effect size cutoff when administered in isolation, their use in combination showed quite positive effects for children with ADHD (Table 8D-3).

Relaxation Training

Relaxation training, including controlled breathing and muscle relaxation, was tested in six studies for children with inattention, impulsivity, and/or hyperactivity. It has been successfully implemented in both individual and group formats and has been used with success in school settings.[98-101] Interestingly, despite the relative simplicity of these techniques, relaxation training for ADHD has been tested only with trained mental health professionals as therapists. Thus far, it has been examined only in children aged 6 to 12 who exhibited symptoms of inattention, impulsivity, and/or hyperactivity but who had no diagnosis of ADHD and no comorbid conditions. Furthermore, the studies are quite old in comparison with the rest of the evidence base (the newest one is dated 1984), and the samples are poorly described (e.g., no information is provided about the ethnicity of the clients). Thus, although relaxation training may be a worthwhile recommendation for children who show somewhat greater activity levels than others, it is unclear whether it would provide benefit for children with a diagnosis of ADHD.

Multimodal Cognitive and Behavioral Intervention

The most promising psychological intervention for children with ADHD is a combination of child-focused CBT, BPT, and/or teacher consultation or classroom management training (CMT). Some combination of these treatments has been tested in three trials: one trial involved CBT and CMT,[102] and two trials involved CBT and BPT.[103,104] These multitargeted interventions showed positive effects with both white and African American children between the ages of 7 and 13. They have been used successfully with children who had a diagnosis of ADHD, as well as undiagnosed hyperactivity problems. Furthermore, one trial successfully used this intervention with participants whose comorbid conditions included conduct disorder, oppositional defiant disorder, anxiety disorders, and dysthymic disorder.[104] In each trial, mental health professionals were employed as therapists and were provided with either ongoing supervision or a manual to guide intervention.

In these multitargeted interventions, the children are taught self-control skills while parents and

TABLE 8D-3 ■ Evidence-Based Psychological Treatments for Attention-Deficit/Hyperactivity Disorder and Related Problems in Children						
Type of Intervention	No. Studies	Publication Dates	Ages	Gender	Race/Ethnicity	Symptom Severity
Child Focused						
Relaxation training	6	1977-1984	6-12	Both	Unknown	Elevated symptoms
Multiple Systems Targeted						
Child and parent/ family cognitive-behavioral therapy and/or teacher consultation	3	1976-1997	7-13	Both	White, African American	Elevated symptoms, diagnosed disorder

teachers are taught behavioral child management skills. Child CBT generally focuses on teaching children how to use self-instruction to reduce impulsivity, increase reflection and control, and improve performance on tasks requiring concentration. BPT is aimed at helping parents create contingencies in the home that will make appropriate, on-task behavior more rewarding than less desirable behavior. Iindividual or group sessions with the parents focus on learning and applying behavioral principles and methods. Coverage usually includes maximizing parental attention and praise in response to appropriate child behavior, withholding attention (and praise) when behavior is inappropriate, developing reward and incentive systems (e.g., charts, points, tokens) to encourage desired behavior, and using time-out and mild punishment (e.g., losing a point or privilege) for noncompliance. Parents are also taught how to issue commands aligned with the child's ability to respond (e.g., issuing one directive at a time). Like BPT, teacher-focused CMT is aimed at helping teachers to establish and maintain contingencies at school that will reinforce self-control, attention to schoolwork, and appropriate social behavior with teachers and peers. Similar to BPT, coverage usually includes such behavioral interventions as developing reward and incentive systems (e.g., charts, points, tokens) to encourage desired behavior, issuing more appropriate instructions or commands, and organizing the classroom to help the child attend (e.g., seating the child near the front, removing distractions).

Summary and Recommendations

The evidence for the treatment of ADHD and associated symptoms supports two psychological interventions: relaxation training and multitargeted cognitive and behavioral treatment. Relaxation training has not been examined with children meeting diagnostic criteria for ADHD, and neither intervention has been examined in a controlled trial with children older than 13 years. In contrast, pharmacological interventions, and psychostimulants in particular, have shown consistently positive effects for children with ADHD (see Chapter 8C). Indeed, stimulant medication has repeatedly demonstrated superiority to psychological treatment (e.g., "Multimodal Treatment Study of Children with ADHD"[105] and Abikoff et al[106]), although controversy still exists regarding whether a combination of medication and multimodal psychological treatment may be superior to medication alone (e.g., Pelham et al[107]), especially in children with comorbid anxiety and behavior problems[108] or in children from more highly educated families.[109] In view of the available evidence, medications are currently the treatment of choice for ADHD. Cognitive and behavioral

interventions for the child, parent, and teacher may provide a helpful complement but are not recommended as the sole treatment for children with ADHD.

PSYCHOLOGICAL MANAGEMENT OF CONDUCT PROBLEMS

Child conduct problems include rule breaking (ranging from breaking household or school rules to breaking laws), oppositional behavior (e.g., refusing to comply with requests from adults), and physical aggression. The two most common diagnoses falling in this category are oppositional defiant disorder, characterized by habitual arguing with or defying adults and having difficulty controlling one's temper, and conduct disorder, characterized by severe delinquent or aggressive behavior. Estimates of the prevalence range from 2.21% to 5.5% for oppositional defiant disorder[97,110] and from 1.47% to 2.7% for conduct disorder.[52,110] For a more thorough review of the prevalence and characteristics of these behavior disorders, see Chapter 17.

Our review included treatment studies with children meeting criteria for oppositional defiant disorder, conduct disorder, or other disruptive behavior disorders (e.g., intermittent explosive disorder) and children with conduct problems that did not meet full criteria for a diagnosis. The psychological treatment literature has a long history of examining interventions for pediatric conduct problems and disorders, beginning in 1963 and totaling 100 randomized clinical trials (testing 155 treatment conditions) by the end of 2005. In 63 (63%) of these studies, investigators used a no-treatment or wait-list control group); of the remainder, 21 (21%) used an attention control condition and 16 (16%) used standard case management such as incarceration or probation. Several psychological interventions have yielded positive effects across two or more controlled trials (Table 8D-4), including relaxation training, reinforcement and response-cost programs, child-focused CBT, BPT, behavioral family therapy, teacher consultation and CMT, and multisystemic therapy. Other interventions have not shown consistently positive effects (e.g., client-centered therapy, insight-oriented therapy) or have not yet been examined in multiple controlled trials (e.g., multidimensional treatment foster care).

Relaxation Training

Relaxation training has been tested as a treatment for conduct problems in three studies, in both individual and group format, with children aged 9 to 18 years. As in the relaxation training studies for ADHD, relaxation training for conduct problems has not been

TABLE 8D-4 ■ Evidence-Based Psychological Treatments for Conduct Problems and Disorders in Children

Type of Intervention	No. Studies	Publication Dates	Ages	Gend	Race/Ethnicity	Symptom Severity
Child Focused						
Relaxation training	3	1981-2005	9-18	Both	Unknown	Elevated symptoms
Reinforcement and response-cost	5	1974-1995	7-17	Both	White, African American	Elevated symptoms
Cognitive-behavioral therapy	31	1977-2004	4-19	Both	White, African American, Hispanic/Latino, Asian, Native American	Elevated symptoms, diagnosed disorder
Parent Focused						
Behavioral parent training	23	1977-2005	2-12	Both	White, African American, Hispanic/Latino, Asian	Elevated symptoms, diagnosed disorder
Family Focused						
Behavioral family therapy	11	1973-2003	3-16	Both	White, African American, Hispanic/Latino, Asian, Native Australian	Elevated symptoms, diagnosed disorder
Teacher Targeted						
Teacher consultation/ CMT	2	1977-1981	7-12	Male	White, African American	Elevated symptoms
Multiple Systems Targeted						
Child and parent cognitive-behavioral therapy	8	1987-2004	4-14	Both	White, African American	Elevated symptoms, diagnosed disorder
Child or parent/ family cognitive-behavioral therapy and teacher consultation	5	1976-2003	4-17	Both	White, African American	Elevated symptoms, diagnosed disorder
Multisystemic therapy	3	1991-1997	10-17	Both	White, African American, Hispanic/Latino	Elevated symptoms

CMT, classroom management training.

tested with children who have a diagnosable oppositional defiant or conduct disorder or comorbid problems. The samples are also poorly described (e.g., no information is provided about the racial makeup of the samples). Thus, although relaxation training may be a worthwhile recommendation for children who show somewhat more anger or aggression than others do, it is unclear whether it would provide significant benefit for those with diagnosable conduct problems.

Reinforcement and Response-Cost Programs

The efficacy of implementing reinforcement and response-cost contingencies directly with children demonstrating disruptive behavior problems has been tested in five studies. In this format, therapists working directly with the children use behavioral procedures and contracts to reinforce prosocial, compliant behav-

ior with praise, attention, or points toward privileges; in contrast, inappropriate behavior is discouraged through selective ignoring or response costs, wherein children are fined by losing points or privileges. Such interventions have demonstrated positive effects across a wide range of ages, across diverse racial and ethnic groups, and with children who showed elevated levels conduct problems and those whose behavior met diagnostic criteria for oppositional defiant disorder or conduct disorder. No such studies have included children with comorbid conditions. These treatments have demonstrated beneficial effects with children in group settings such as schools,[111] residential treatment facilities,[112] and day treatment[113] (but this last study yielded somewhat less positive outcomes than the others). In all of these studies, mental health professionals were employed as therapists, but most of the investigators did not report providing extensive additional training, supervision, or manuals to guide intervention (it is not clear whether these efforts were not needed or because the investigators simply did not describe these efforts in publication).

Cognitive-Behavioral Therapy

Child-focused CBT has been tested in 31 controlled studies; it is thus the most widely investigated intervention for child conduct problems. It has demonstrated positive effects across a wide range of ages, across diverse racial and ethnic groups, and with children who show elevated levels of conduct and those whose behavior meet diagnostic criteria for oppositional defiant disorder and conduct disorder.[114-116] Several trials have revealed positive treatment effects even when participants have comorbid conditions in addition to their conduct problems.[114,116-119] It has been successfully administered in both individual and group formats. However, there is some evidence that administering treatment in a group format may, under some circumstances, actually increase pediatric conduct problems.[120] Dishion and associates[121] proposed that this results from a phenomenon they labeled *deviancy training,* in which the group format inadvertently encourages children to form relationships with other deviant peers in the group and to gain social reinforcement from those peers for their deviant behaviors (but see Weiss et al[122] for a critique of the deviancy training hypothesis).

In addition to showing beneficial effects when tested in research settings, CBT has also been used effectively in correctional settings,[123] residential treatment facilities,[112] inpatient psychiatric units,[114,116,117] and schools.[118,124-130] In the majority of successful trials, investigators employed mental health professionals. Some have successfully trained paraprofessionals, such as teachers[126] and nurses,[116] to implement the procedures, but others[131,132] were not successful when employing paraprofessional therapists.

CBT targets the emotional, behavioral and cognitive skills deficits most germane to conduct problems. Manuals include *Problem Solving Skills Training,*[133] *Anger Coping,*[134] and *Anger Control Training with Stress Inoculation.*[135] As applied to children with conduct problems, CBT includes the following:

- Affective education and monitoring (described previously).
- Relaxation training (described previously).
- Cognitive restructuring (the child learns to self-instruct or make self-statements to decrease his or her anger, such as "I can handle this" or "I can stay calm and in control," to challenge anger-provoking interpretations of events and to consider neutral alternative interpretations of events).
- Attention training (the child learns to direct his or her attention away from provocation).

- Problem-solving skills (describe previously).
- Social skills and conflict resolution (the child learns more effective, prosocial, assertive ways of communicating).
- Reinforcement and self-reinforcement (i.e., the child is rewarded and learns to reward himself or herself for appropriate, prosocial problem solving).

Behavioral Parent Training

After child-focused CBT, BPT is the most extensively tested form of treatment for child conduct problems and disorders. It has been tested in 23 studies with children aged 2 to 12 years. It has produced positive effects with diverse racial and ethnic groups, although it has been tested primarily with white families. It has been successful with children who show elevated levels of conduct problems, as well as those who meet diagnostic criteria for oppositional defiant disorder and conduct disorder,[136,137] and with children who have comorbid ADHD[136-138] and internalizing problems.[138] It has been administered successfully in both individual and group formats. It has also been administered successfully in video format, without a therapist present, in two studies,[139,140] but a third trial of video-administered parent training yielded little benefit.[141] In addition to BPT's showing beneficial effects when tested in research settings, one study demonstrated its effectiveness in a community-based mental health clinic,[142] but another community-based trial revealed little benefit.[143] With the exception of the video-administered parent training programs,[139,140] all successful trials of BPT for conduct problems involved mental health professionals, and the majority of investigators provided these therapists with a manual to guide intervention.

BPT programs for child conduct problems and disorders include several versions with manuals. The most widely studied programs are Webster-Stratton's *The Incredible Years,*[144] Patterson and colleagues Oregon model parent training,[145-149] Kazdin's *Parent Management Training,*[133,150] and Forehand and McMahon's parent training.[151] As applied to conduct problems, BPT typically includes the following:

- Psychoeducation about the treatment rationale (i.e., social learning theory).
- Supervision and monitoring (the parent learns how to provide the developmentally appropriate level of monitoring and supervision of the child's behavior).
- Appropriate command training (the parent learns how to appropriately issue requests or directives clearly, one at a time, in a calm but firm tone of voice, with time to comply).

- Positive reinforcement (the parent learns to regularly acknowledge and reward the child's appropriate behavior with strategic attention, labeled praise, and small prizes).
- Selective ignoring (the parent learns to ignore mildly negative behaviors).
- Time-out and response cost (the parent learns to use immediate time-out and appropriate mild punishment, such as work chores or loss of privileges, to decrease the child's inappropriate or rule-breaking behavior).
- Negotiation and problem solving (parents of older children and adolescents learn to negotiate developmentally appropriate rules with their child).

Teacher Consultation and Classroom Management Training

Teacher training and consultation in behavioral classroom management, as in ADHD, has been examined in two studies of children experiencing conduct problems. These interventions have been shown to be effective only with boys aged 7 to 12 and have not been tested with children meeting diagnostic criteria or experiencing comorbid conditions. It has also been examined as an added component to child CBT and BPT in five studies, and it has added some benefit to those interventions alone.[152,153] According to the available evidence, teacher consultation and CMT, although probably helpful in managing a classroom in general, and perhaps a worthwhile addition to child- and parent-focused interventions, is not the sole treatment of choice for a child with significant conduct problems.

Behavioral Family Therapy

Behavioral approaches combining contact with both parents and children have been tested in separate child-focused CBT and BPT (8 studies) and in behavioral family therapy with the child and parents in session together (11 studies). These interventions are effective across a wide range of ages and diverse racial and ethnic groups. They have been found to be effective with children with conduct problems and diagnoses of oppositional defiant disorder and conduct disorder. They have also been successful in studies allowing comorbid diagnoses, including ADHD, depression, and adjustment disorders.[136,154-156] These approaches have been administered successfully in both individual and group formats (bur see previous discussion regarding some concerns about child groups for conduct problems). In addition to showing beneficial effects when tested in research settings, they have also been used effectively in a psychiatric inpatient hospital[157] and in a medical hospital setting.[155] However, efforts to test these approaches in community[158] and school[159] settings have yielded more modest effects. In several studies, investigators employed paraprofessionals to implement these techniques; however, only one group was successful.[160] In the majority of successful trials, investigators employed mental health professionals as therapists and provided manuals to guide intervention.

The most widely researched behavioral family therapy technique, parent-child interaction therapy by Eyberg and colleagues,[161,162] combines a relationship-building parent-child intervention with BPT. Parent-child interaction therapy emphasizes building a warm, loving relationship between the parent and child, as well as improving the parent's ability to appropriately discipline the child. Typically, the therapist engages in live coaching of parents, often through a "bug-in-the-ear" microphone, as the parents practice the techniques in session with their child. Initially, parents are taught how to interact and play with their children in ways that improve the parent-child relationship and increase their ability to provide positive social reinforcement to the child (e.g., allowing the child to lead the play; providing strategic attention, such as moving closer and touching the child; or providing labeled praise, such as "I like how you put those toys away," to reinforce appropriate behavior). In the second phase, parents are given more extensive BPT training as described previously. If necessary, parents are taught self-relaxation techniques to use during discipline.

Multisystemic Therapy

We found three separate controlled studies of multisystemic therapy targeting severe delinquent behavior in children older than 10 years, across a diverse range of racial and ethnic groups.[163-165] Investigators in these studies did not assess diagnoses, but they focused on children at imminent risk of being placed in a facility for their delinquent behaviors. All three studies involved intensive, community-based interventions administered by a trained mental health professional who is provided with extensive specialized training, intensive ongoing supervision, and a manual to guide intervention. Multisystemic therapy has also shown positive effects with substance-abusing and substance-dependent adolescents,[166] those in psychiatric crisis,[167,168] and those with a history of sexual offenses.[169]

Multisystemic therapy treats seriously delinquent adolescents by reaching out to multiple aspects of their environment, often including siblings, parents, extended family, neighbors and neighborhood groups, peers, schools, churches, and juvenile justice personnel.[170] Multisystemic therapy is somewhat distinct from the interventions previously described in that the techniques are a fairly eclectic blend of evidence-based interventions aimed at addressing the specific behavior patterns that the therapist and treatment team hypothesize to underlie the child's problem behavior. In addition, therapists have daily contact with the child and family in a variety of settings (e.g., school, home, church). Typically, parents are taught to be stronger advocates for their family, to establish house rules, to improve monitoring of their child's whereabouts and behavior, and to provide appropriate social and tangible reinforcement for desired behavior, as well as appropriate negative consequences (e.g., providing additional chores, grounding) for unwanted behavior. The child is encouraged to decrease association with antisocial peers and to work toward development of a strong social support system of prosocial peers and adults. Rather than specifying core treatment techniques, multisystemic therapy is guided primarily by nine core principles:

- Finding the fit between the child's problem behavior and his or her environment (i.e., what purpose the behavior serves and how it makes sense in their environment).
- Interventions are positive and strength focused (therapists focus on using existing family strengths to move toward improvement).
- Interventions are focused on increasing responsibility (i.e., techniques are designed to encourage more responsible behavior among all family members).
- Interventions are present focused, action oriented, and well defined.
- Interventions target sequences of behaviors within and between systems that maintain the problem behavior.
- Interventions are developmentally appropriate to the child.
- Interventions are designed to require continuous (i.e., daily or weekly) effort on the part of the child and family.
- Intervention effectiveness is continuously examined, and multisystemic therapists are accountable for producing change in the child and family.
- Interventions are designed to promote generalization and long-term maintenance.

Summary and Recommendations

The evidence concerning the treatment of conduct problems in children indicates that several interventions are efficacious. With the exception of multisystemic therapy, which incorporates a variety of theoretical approaches, these interventions are all behavioral or cognitive-behavioral. For very young children, BPT has the most research support across a range of ethnic groups and severity levels, and it has been successfully administered in video format. However, in the absence of specialty videos and with children who have severe behavior problems, we recommend referral to a mental health professional trained to provide BPT or parent-child interaction therapy.

For older children and adolescents, child-focused CBT has the most consistent evidence across a wide range of ethnicities and severity levels. The evidence is mixed as to whether this intervention can be successfully administered by non–mental health professionals, and so we recommend referral to a mental health provider trained in CBT. Furthermore, because of the evidence that some forms of group-administered CBT may actually lead to increases in conduct problems, referrals to CBT groups should be made with caution.

Finally, for adolescents engaging in severe delinquent behaviors, multisystemic therapy is an appropriate treatment option. Because of the intense nature of this intervention, it is not yet available in many communities. However, multisystemic therapy is increasingly being offered as a treatment option through state juvenile justice and mental health systems, and so its availability may increase in the future.

FINAL THOUGHTS AND RECOMMENDATIONS

We reviewed the psychological clinical trials literature for children and adolescents with depression, anxiety, ADHD, and conduct problems. The evidence for the treatment of childhood depression provides the greatest support for CBT and, for Hispanic adolescents, interpersonal therapy. For childhood anxiety and fears, CBT with reinforcement, relaxation, modeling, and exposure currently has the strongest evidence base. For ADHD, the evidence does not support psychological treatment as the sole intervention. However, cognitive and behavioral treatments targeting the child, parent, and teacher may provide useful supplements to pharmacological treatments. The evidence for the treatment of conduct problems in children indicates that several interventions are efficacious; these include BPT for young children, CBT for older children and adolescents, and multisystemic therapy for adolescents who engage in severe delinquent behavior. Finally, relaxation training, including deep muscle relaxation and imagery, may be a worthwhile intervention for children and adolescent experiencing a range of subclinical emotional and behavioral problems.

We have described several psychological interventions that show consistent efficacy in the clinical trials research. Other interventions either have not yet been studied adequately to justify specific recommendations (e.g., attachment-based family therapy for depression, parent-focused therapy for anxiety) or have failed to show consistent benefit (e.g., child-focused CBT for ADHD, insight-oriented therapy for conduct problems). Therefore, we recommend that health care providers refer children to professionals who are specifically trained in the type of psychological intervention that research has shown beneficial for the kinds of difficulties being experienced by the child. Because not all interventions are equally supported, to simply advise parents to seek "therapy" for their child does not ensure that they will receive the intervention most likely to provide benefit.

The existing psychological clinical trials literature provides few examples of psychological interventions for child emotional and behavioral problems delivered in primary care settings. Clearly, improved coordination between primary care and mental health services is needed for optimal care of children and families. Currently, several studies are under way to examine both the feasibility and effect of such practices as routine screening and monitoring of emotional and behavioral problems and provision of psychological interventions within primary care practices. An important goal for the future may be to have psychological interventions increasingly integrated into primary care settings, with pediatricians and mental health professionals sharing office space to ease referral and to promote a collaborative working relationship in order to better meet the needs of children and families.

REFERENCES

1. Burns BJ, Costello EJ, Angold A, et al: DataWatch: Children's mental health service use across services sectors. Health Affair 14:147-159, 1995.
2. Weisz JR, Hawley KM, Doss AJ: Empirically tested psychotherapies for youth internalizing and externalizing problems and disorders. Child Adolesc Psychiatr Clin North Am Special Evid Based Pract I Res Update 13:729-815, 2004.
3. Casey RJ, Berman JS: The outcome of psychotherapy with children. Psychol Bull 98:388-400, 1985.
4. Kazdin AE, Bass D, Ayers WA, et al: Empirical and clinical focus of child and adolescent psychotherapy research. J Consult Clin Psychol 58:729-740, 1990.
5. Weisz JR, Weiss B, Alicke MD, et al: Effectiveness of psychotherapy with children and adolescents: A meta-analysis for clinicians. J Consult Clin Psychol 55:542-549, 1987.
6. Weisz JR, Weiss B, Han SS, et al: Effects of psychotherapy with children and adolescents revisited: A meta-analysis of treatment outcome studies. Psychol Bull 117:450-468, 1995.
7. Chambless DL, Hollon SD: Defining empirically supported therapies. J Consult Clin Psychol 66:7-18, 1998.
8. Chambless DL, Ollendick TH: Empirically supported psychological interventions: Controversies and evidence. Annu Rev Psychol 52:685-716, 2001.
9. Chambless DL, Sanderson WC, Shoham V, et al: An update on empirically validated therapies. Clin Psychol 49, 1996.
10. Chambless DL, Baker MJ, Baucom DH, et al: Update on empirically validated therapies, II. Clin Psychol 51:3-16, 1998.
11. Lonigan CJ, Elbert JC, Johnson SB: Empirically supported psychosocial interventions for children: An overview. J Clin Child Psychol 27:138-145, 1998.
12. Kaslow NJ, Thompson MP: Applying the criteria for empirically supported treatments to studies of psychosocial interventions for child and adolescent depression. J Clin Child Psychol 27:146-155, 1998.
13. Ollendick TH, King NJ: Empirically supported treatments for children with phobic and anxiety disorders: Current status. J Clin Child Psychol 27:156-167, 1998.
14. Rogers SJ: Empirically supported comprehensive treatments for young children with autism. J Clin Child Psychol 27:168-179, 1998.
15. Brestan EV, Eyberg SM: Effective psychosocial treatments of conduct-disordered children and adolescents: 29 years, 82 studies, and 5,272 kids. J Clin Child Psychol 27:180-189, 1998.
16. Pelham WE, Jr., Wheeler T, Chronis A: Empirically supported psychosocial treatments for attention deficit hyperactivity disorder. J Clin Child Psychol 27:190-205, 1998.
17. Mellon MW, McGrath ML: Empirically supported treatments in pediatric psychology: Nocturnal enuresis. J Pediatr Psychol 25:193-214, 2000.
18. McGrath ML, Mellon MW, Murphy L: Empirically supported treatments in pediatric psychology: Constipation and encopresis. J Pediatr Psychol 25:225-254, 2000.
19. Mindell JA: Empirically supported treatments in pediatric psychology: Bedtime refusal and night wakings in young children. J Pediatr Psychol 24:465-481, 1999.
20. Kerwin ME: Empirically supported treatments in pediatric psychology: Severe feeding problems. J Pediatr Psychol 24:193-214, 1999.
21. Jelalian E, Saelens BE: Empirically supported treatments in pediatric psychology: Pediatric obesity. J Pediatr Psychol 24:223-248, 1999.
22. Saunders BE, Berliner L, Hanson RF: Child Physical and Sexual Abuse: Guidelines for Treatment [Revised April 26, 2004]. Charleston, SC: National Crime Victims Research and Treatment Center. (Available at: *http://academicdepartments.musc.edu/ncvc/resources_prof/OVC_guidelines04-26-04.pdf;* accessed 10/31/06.)

23. Bukstein OG, Bernet W, Arnold V, et al: Practice parameter for the assessment and treatment of children and adolescents with substance use disorders. J Am Acad Child Adolesc Psychiatry 44:609-621, 2005.

24. Substance Abuse and Mental Health Services Administration National Registry of Evidence-Based Programs and Practices (NREPP). (Available at: *http://modelprograms.samhsa.gov/template.cfm?page-default;* accessed 10/31/06.)

25. Volkmar FR, Lord C, Bailey A, et al: Autism and pervasive developmental disorders. J Child Psychol Psychiatry 45:135-170, 2004.

26. Koegel RL, Koegel LK, Brookman LI: Empirically supported pivotal response interventions for children with autism. *In* Kazdin AE, Weisz JR, eds: Evidence-Based Psychotherapies for Children and Adolescents. New York: Guilford, 2003, pp 341-357.

27. Lovaas OI, Smith T: Early and intensive behavioral intervention in autism. *In* Kazdin AE, Weisz JR, eds: Evidence-based psychotherapies for Children and Adolescents. New York: Guilford, 2003, pp 325-340.

28. Weisz JR, Hawley KM: Finding, evaluating, refining, and applying empirically supported treatments for children and adolescents. J Clin Child Psychol 27:206-216, 1998.

29. Bickman L: A common factors approach to improving mental health services. Ment Health Serv Res 7:1-4, 2005.

30. Cohen J: Statistical Power Analysis for the Behavioral Sciences, 2nd ed. Hillsdale, NJ: Erlbaum, 1988.

31. Weisz JR, Hawley KM, Jensen Doss A, et al: The Effectiveness of Psychosocial Interventions with Children and Adolescents: A Meta-analysis for Clinicians and Researchers. Cambridge, MA: Harvard University, Judge Baker Children's Center, 2005.

32. Compton SN, Burns BJ, Egger HL, et al: Review of the evidence base for treatment of childhood psychopathology: Internalizing disorders. J Consult Clin Psychol 70:1240-1266, 2002.

33. Farmer EMZ, Compton SN, Burns JB, et al: Review of the evidence base for treatment of childhood psychopathology: Externalizing disorders. J Consult Clin Psychol 70:1267-1302, 2002.

34. Weisz JR, Hawley KM: Developmental factors in the treatment on adolescents. J Consult Clin Psychol 70:21-43, 2002.

35. Miller AL, Glinski J: Youth suicidal behavior: Assessment and intervention. J Clin Psychol 56:1131-1152, 2000.

36. Kahn JS, Kehle TJ, Jenson WR, et al: Comparison of cognitive-behavioral, relaxation, and self-modeling interventions for depression among middle-school students. School Psychol Rev 19:196-211, 1990.

37. Reynolds WM, Coats KI: A comparison of cognitive-behavioral therapy and relaxation training for the treatment of depression in adolescents. J Consult Clin Psychol 54:653-660, 1986.

38. Liddle B, Spence SH: Cognitive-behaviour therapy with depressed primary school children: A cautionary note. Behav Psychother 18:85-102, 1990.

39. Stark KD, Reynolds WM, Kaslow NJ: A comparison of the relative efficacy of self-control therapy and a behavioral problem-solving therapy for depression in children. J Abnorm Child Psychol 15:91-113, 1987.

40. Ackerson J, Scogin F, McKendree-Smith N, et al: Cognitive bibiliotherapy for mild and moderate adolescent depressive symptomatology. J Consult Clin Psychol 66:685-690, 1998.

41. Clarke GN, Lewinsohn PM, Hops H: Student Workbook: Adolescent Coping With Depression Course. Portland, OR: Kaiser Permanente, 1990.

42. Clarke GN, Lewinsohn PM, Hops H: Leader's Manual for Adolescent Groups: Adolescent Coping With Depression Course. Portland, OR: Kaiser Permanente, 1990.

43. Stark K, Kendall PC: Treating Depressed Children: Therapist Manual for Taking Action. Ardmore, PA: Workbook Publishing, 1996.

44. Weisz JR, Moore PS, Southam-Gerow M, et al: Primary and Secondary Control Enhancement Training (PASCET). Unpublished treatment manual, University of California, Los Angeles, 1999.

45. Clarke GN, Rohde P, Lewinsohn PM, et al: Cognitive-behavioral treatment of adolescent depression: Efficacy of acute group treatment and booster sessions. J Am Acad Child Adolesc Psychiatry 38:272-279, 1999.

46. Lewinsohn PM, Clarke GN, Hops H, et al: Cognitive-behavioral treatment for depressed adolescents. Behav Ther 21:385-401, 1990.

47. Mufson L, Weissman MM, Moreau D, et al: Efficacy of interpersonal psychotherapy for depressed adolescents. Arch Gen Psychiatry 56:573-579, 1999.

48. Rosello J, Bernal G: The efficacy of cognitive-behavioral and interpersonal treatments for depression in Puerto Rican adolescents. J Consult Clin Psychol 67:734-745, 1999.

49. Rudolph KD, Hammen C, Burge D, et al: Toward an interpersonal life-stress model of depression: The developmental context of stress generation. Dev Psychopathol 12:215-234, 2000.

50. Mufson L, Dorta KP: Interpersonal psychotherapy for depressed adolescents. *In* Kazdin AE, Weisz JR, eds: Evidence-Based Psychotherapies for Children and Adolescents. New York: Guilford, 2003, pp 148-164.

51. Mufson L, Dorta KP, Moreau D, et al: Interpersonal Psychotherapy for Depressed Adolescents, 2nd ed. New York: Guilford, 2004.

52. Costello EJ, Mustillo S, Erkanli A, et al: Prevalence and development of psychiatric disorders in childhood and adolescence. Arch Gen Psychiatry 60:837-844, 2003.

53. Boyd CP, Kostanski M, Gullone E, et al: Prevalence of anxiety and depression in Australian adolescents: Comparisons with worldwide data. J Genet Psychol 161:479-492, 2000.

54. Chavira DA, Stein MB, Bailey K, et al: Child anxiety in primary care: Prevalent but untreated. Depress Anxiety 20:155-164, 2004.

55. Ost L-G, Svensson L, Hellstroem K, et al: One-session treatment of specific phobias in youths: A randomized

clinical trial. J Consult Clin Psychol 69:814-824, 2001.

56. Cornwall E, Spence SH, Schotte D: The effectiveness of emotive imagery in the treatment of darkness phobia in children. Behav Change 13:223-229, 1996.

57. Dewis LM, Kirkby KC, Martin F, et al: Computer-aided vicarious exposure versus live graded exposure for spider phobia in children. J Behav Ther Exp Psychiatry 32:17-27, 2001.

58. Chemtob CM, Nakashima J, Carlson JG: Brief treatment for elementary school children with disaster-related posttraumatic stress disorder: A field study. J Clin Psychol 58:99-112, 2002.

59. Milos ME, Reiss S: Effects of three play conditions on separation anxiety in young children. J Consult Clin Psychol 50:389-395, 1982.

60. Furman W, Rahe DF, Hartup WW: Rehabilitation of socially withdrawn preschool children through mixed-age and same-age socialization. Child Dev 50:915-922, 1979.

61. Rosenfarb I, Hayes SC: Social standard setting: The Achilles heel of informational accounts of therapeutic change. Behav Ther 15:515-528, 1984.

62. Mann J: Vicarious desensitization of test anxiety through observation of videotaped treatment. J Counsel Psychol 19:1-7, 1972.

63. Tosi DJ, Upshaw K, Lande A, et al: Group counseling with nonverbalizing elementary students: Differential effects of Premack and social reinforcement techniques. J Counsel Psychol 18:437-440, 1971.

64. White WCJ, Davis MT: Vicarious extinction of phobic behavior in early childhood. J Abnorm Child Psychol 2:25-32, 1974.

65. Jakibchuk Z, Smeriglio VL: The influence of symbolic modeling on the social behavior of preschool children with low levels of social responsiveness. Child Dev 47:838-841, 1976.

66. King NJ, Tonge BJ, Heyne D, et al: Cognitive-behavioral treatment of school-refusing children: A controlled evaluation. J Am Acad Child Adolesc Psychiatry 37:395-403, 1998.

67. King NJ, Tonge BJ, Mullen P, et al: Treating sexually abused children with posttraumatic stress symptoms: A randomized clinical trial. J Am Acad Child Adolesc Psychiatry 39:1347-1355, 2000.

68. Spence SH, Donovan C, Brechman-Toussaint M: The treatment of childhood social phobia: The effectiveness of a social skills training-based, cognitive-behavioral intervention, with and without parental involvement. J Child Psychol Psychiatry 41:713-726, 2000.

69. Silverman WK, Kurtines WM, Ginsburg GS, et al: Contingency management, self-control, and education support in the treatment of childhood phobic disorders: A randomized clinical trial. J Consult Clin Psychol 67:675-687, 1999.

70. Silverman WK, Kurtines WM, Ginsburg GS, et al: Treating anxiety disorders in children with group cognitive-behavioral therapy: A randomized clinical trial. J Consult Clin Psychol 67:995-1003, 1999.

71. Flannery-Schroeder EC, Kendall PC: Group and individual cognitive-behavioral treatments for youth with anxiety disorders: A randomized clinical trial. Cognit Ther Res 24:251-278, 2000.

72. Shortt AL, Barrett PM, Fox TL: Evaluating the FRIENDS Program: A cognitive-behavioral group treatment for anxious children and their parents. J Clin Child Psychol 30:525-535, 2001.

73. Dadds MR, Heard PM, Rapee RM: The role of family intervention in the treatment of child anxiety disorders: Some preliminary findings. Behav Change 9:171-177, 1992.

74. Barrett PM: Evaluation of cognitive-behavioral group treatments for childhood anxiety disorders. J Clin Child Psychol 27:459-468, 1998.

75. Muris P, Meesters C, van Melick M: Treatment of childhood anxiety disorders; A preliminary comparison between cognitive-behavioral group therapy and a psychological placebo intervention. J Behav Ther Exp Psychiatry 33:143-158, 2002.

76. Kendall PC: Treating anxiety disorders in children: Results of a randomized clinical trial. J Consult Clin Psychol 62:100-110, 1994.

77. Kendall PC, Flannery-Schroeder E, Panichelli-Mindel SM, et al: Therapy for youths with anxiety disorders: A second randomized clinical trial. J Consult Clin Psychol 65:366-380, 1997.

78. Deblinger E, Lippman J, Steer R: Sexually abused children suffering posttraumatic stress symptoms: Initial treatment outcome findings. Child Maltreat 1:310-321, 1996.

79. Pediatric OCD Treatment Study (POTS) Team: Cognitive-behavior therapy, sertraline, and their combination for children and adolescents with obsessive-compulsive disorder: The Pediatric OCD Treatment Study (POTS) randomized controlled trial. JAMA 292:1969-1976, 2004.

80. Barrett P, Farrell L, Dadds M, et al: Cognitive-behavioral family treatment of childhood obsessive-compulsive disorder: Long-term follow-up and predictors of outcome. J Am Acad Child Adolesc Psychiatry 44:1005-1014, 2005.

81. Barrett P, Healy-Farrell L, March JS: Cognitive-behavioral family treatment of childhood obsessive-compulsive disorder: A controlled trial. J Am Acad Child Adolesc Psychiatry 43:46-62, 2004.

82. Beidel DC, Turner SM, Morris TL: Behavioral treatment of childhood social phobia. J Consult Clin Psychol 68:1072-1080, 2000.

83. Ahrens J, Rexford L: Cognitive processing therapy for incarcerated adolescents with PTSD. J Aggression Maltreat Trauma 6:201-216, 2002.

84. Aydin G, Yerin O: The effect of a story-based cognitive behavior modification procedure on reducing children's test anxiety before and after cancellation of an important examination. Int J Adv Couns 17, 1994.

85. Keller MF, Carlson PM: The use of symbolic modeling to promote social skills in preschool children with low levels of social responsiveness. Child Dev 45:912-919, 1974.

86. Wehr SH, Kaufman ME: The effects of assertive training on performance in highly anxious adolescents. Adolescence 22:195-205, 1987.

87. Williams CE, Jones RT: Impact of self-instructions on response maintenance and children's fear of fire. J Clin Child Psychol 18:84-89, 1989.

88. Kanfer FH, Karoly P, Newman A: Reduction of children's fear of the dark by competence-related and situational threat-related verbal cues. J Consult Clin Psychol 43:251-258, 1975.

89. Kendall P: Coping Cat Workbook. Ardmore, PA: Workbook Publishing, 1990.

90. Kendall PC, Kane M, Howard B, et al: Cognitive-Behavioral Therapy for Anxious Children: Treatment Manual. Ardmore, PA: Workbook Publishing, 1990.

91. Barrett PM, Lowry-Webster H, Turner C: FRIENDS Program for Children: Group Leaders Manual. Brisbane: Australian Academic Press, 2000.

92. Barrett PM, Lowry-Webster H, Turner C: FRIENDS Program for Children: Parents' Supplement, Brisbane: Australian Academic Press, 2000.

93. Barrett PM, Lowry-Webster H, Turner C: FRIENDS Program for Children: Participants Workbook, Brisbane: Australian Academic Press, 2000.

94. Beidel DC, Roberson-Nay R, eds: Treating childhood social phobia: Social effectiveness therapy for children. *In* Hibbs ED, Jensen, Peter S, eds: Psychosocial Treatments for Child and Adolescent Disorders: Empirically Based Strategies for Clinical Practice. Washington, DC: American Psychological Association, 2005, pp 75-96.

95. Barrett PM: Group family anxiety management: a treatment manual. Unpublished manuscript, Griffith University, School of Applied Psychology, Queensland, Australia, 1995.

96. Nauta MH, Scholing A, Emmelkamp PM, et al: Cognitive-behavioral therapy for children with anxiety disorders in a clinical setting: No additional effect of a cognitive parent training. J Am Acad Child Adolesc Psychiatry 42:1270-1278, 2003.

97. Canino G, Shrout PE, Rubio-Stipec M, et al: The *DSM-IV* Rates of Child and Adolescent Disorders in Puerto Rico. Arch Gen Psychiatry 61:85-93, 2004.

98. Redfering DL, Bowman MJ: Effects of a meditative-relaxation exercise on non-attending behaviors of behaviorally disturbed children. J Clin Child Psychol 10:126-127, 1981.

99. Klein SA, Deffenbacher JL: Relaxation and exercise for hyperactive impulsive children. Percept Mot Skills 45:1159-1162, 1977.

100. Omizo MM, Michael WB: Biofeedback-induced relaxation training and impulsivity, attention to task, and locus of control among hyperactive boys. J Learn Disabil 15:414-416, 1982.

101. Rivera E, Omizo MM: The effects of relaxation and biofeedback on attention to task and impulsivity among male hyperactive children. Except Child 27:41-51, 1980.

102. O'Leary KD, Pelham WE, Rosenbaum A, et al: Behavioral treatment of hyperkinetic children. Clin Pediatr 15:510-514, 1976.

103. Fehlings DL, Roberts W, Humphries T, et al: Attention deficit hyperactivity disorder: Does cognitive behavioral therapy improve home behavior? J Dev Behav Pediatr 12:223-228, 1991.

104. Pfiffner LJ, McBurnett K: Social skills training with parent generalization: Treatment effects for children with attention deficit disorder. J Consult Clin Psychol 65:749-757, 1997.

105. The MTA Cooperative Group. A 14-month randomized clinical trial of treatment strategies for attention-deficit/hyperactivity disorder. Multimodal Treatment Study of Children with ADHD. Arch Gen Psychiatry 56:1073-1086, 1999.

106. Abikoff H, Hechtman L, Klein RG, et al: Symptomatic improvement in children with ADHD treated with long-term methylphenidate and multimodal psychosocial treatment. J Am Acad Child Adolesc Psychiatry 43:802-811, 2004.

107. Pelham WE Jr, Gnagy EM, Greiner AR, et al: Behavioral versus behavioral and pharmacological treatment in ADHD children attending a summer treatment program. J Abnorm Child Psychol 28:507-525, 2000.

108. Jensen PS, Hinshaw SP, Kraemer HC, et al: ADHD comorbidity findings from the MTA study: Comparing comorbid subgroups. J Am Acad Child Adolesc Psychiatry 40:147-158, 2001.

109. Rieppi R, Greenhill LL, Ford RE, et al: Socioeconomic status as a moderator of ADHD treatment outcomes. J Am Acad Child Adolesc Psychiatry 41:269-277, 2002.

110. Ford T, Goodman R, Meltzer H: The British Child and Adolescent Mental Health Survey 1999: The prevalence of *DSM-IV* disorders. J Am Acad Child Adolesc Psychiatry 42:1203-1211, 2003.

111. Moracco J, Kazandkian A: Effectiveness of behavior counseling and consulting with non-Western elementary school children. Elem School Guid Couns 11:244-251, 1977.

112. Snyder JJ, White MJ: The use of cognitive self-instruction in the treatment of behaviorally disturbed adolescents. Behav Ther 10:227-235, 1979.

113. Basile VC, Motta RW, Allison DB: Antecedent exercise as a treatment for disruptive behavior: Testing hypothesized mechanisms of action. Behav Interv 10:119-140, 1995.

114. Kazdin AE, Esveldt-Dawson K, French NH, et al: Problem-solving skills training and relationship therapy in the treatment of antisocial child behavior. J Consult Clin Psychol 55:76-85, 1987.

115. Schneider BH, Bryne BM: Individualizing social skills training for behavior-disordered children. J Consult Clin Psychol 55:444-445, 1987.

116. Kolko DJ, Watson S, Faust J: Fire safety/prevention skills training to reduce involvement with fire in young psychiatric inpatients: Preliminary findings. Behav Ther 22:269-284, 1991.

117. Snyder KV, Kymissis P, Kessler K: Anger management for adolescents: Efficacy of brief group therapy. J Am Acad Child Adolesc Psychiatry 38:1409-1416, 1999.

118. Rosal ML: Comparative group art therapy research to evaluate changes in locus of control in behavior disordered children. Arts Psychother 20:231-241, 1993.

119. Ison MS: Training in social skills: An alternative technique for handling disruptive child behavior. Psychol Rep 88:903-911, 2001.

120. Dishion TJ, Andrews DW: Preventing escalation in problem behaviors with high-risk young adolescents: Immediate and 1-year outcomes. J Consult Clin Psychol 63:538-548, 1995.

121. Dishion TJ, McCord J, Poulin Fo: When interventions harm: Peer groups and problem behavior. Am Psychol 54:755-764, 1999.

122. Weiss B, Caron A, Ball S, et al: Iatrogenic effects of group treatment for antisocial youths. J Consult Clin Psychol 73:1036-1044, 2005.

123. Larson KA, Gerber MM: Effects of social metacognitive training for enhancing overt behavior in learning disabled and low achieving delinquents. Exceptional Children 54:201-211, 1987.

124. Deffenbacher JL, Lynch RS, Oetting ER, et al: Anger reduction in early adolescents. J Counsel Psychol 43:149-157, 1996.

125. Arbuthnot J, Gordon DA: Behavioral and cognitive effects of a moral reasoning development intervention for high-risk behavior-disordered adolescents. J Consult Clin Psychol 54:208-216, 1986.

126. Camp BW, Blom GE, Herbert F, et al: "Think aloud": A program for developing self-control in young aggressive boys. J Abnorm Child Psychol 5:157-169, 1977.

127. Feindler EL, Marriott SA, Iwata M: Group anger control training for junior high school delinquents. Cognit Ther Res 8:299-311, 1984.

128. Larkin R, Thyer BA: Evaluating cognitive-behavioral group counseling to improve elementary school students' self-esteem, self-control and classroom behavior. Behav Interv 14:147-161, 1999.

129. Lochman JE, Coie JD, Underwood MK, et al: Effectiveness of a social relations intervention program for aggressive and nonaggressive, rejected children. J Consult Clin Psychol 61:1053-1058, 1993.

130. Manning BH: Application of cognitive behavior modification: First and third graders' self-management of classroom behaviors. Am Educ Res J 25:193-212, 1988.

131. Coleman M, Pfeiffer S, Oakland T: Aggression replacement training with behaviorally disordered adolescents. Behavioral Disorders 18:54-66, 1992.

132. Huey WC, Rank RC: Effects of counselor and peer-led group assertive training on black adolescent aggression. J Counsel Psychol 31:95-98, 1984.

133. Kazdin AE. Problem solving and parent management in treating aggressive and antisocial behavior. In Hibbs ED, Jensen PS, eds: Psychosocial Treatments for Child and Adolescent Disorders: Empirically Based Strategies for Clinical Practice, (pp 377-408). Washington, D.C.: APA, 1996.

134. Larson J, Lochman J: Helping Schoolchildren Cope with Anger: A Cognitive-Behavioral Intervention. New York: Guilford, 2002.

135. Feindler EL: Adolescent Anger Control: Cognitive-Behavioral Techniques. New York: Pergamon Press, 1986.

136. Webster-Stratton C, Hammond M: Treating children with early-onset conduct problems: A comparison of child and parent training interventions. J Consult Clin Psychol 65:93-109, 1997.

137. Connell S, Sanders MR, Markie-Dadds C: Self-directed behavioral family intervention for parents of oppositional children in rural and remote areas. Behav Modif 21:379-407, 1997.

138. Beauchaine TP, Webster-Stratton C, Reid M: Mediators, moderators, and predictors of 1-year outcomes among children treated for early-onset conduct problems: A latent growth curve analysis. J Consult Clin Psychol 73:371-388, 2005.

139. Webster-Stratton C: Enhancing the effectiveness of self-administered videotape parent training for families with conduct-problem children. J Abnorm Child Psychol 18:479-492, 1990.

140. Webster-Stratton C, Kolpacoff M, Hollinsworth T: Self-administered videotape therapy for families with conduct-problem children: Comparison with two cost-effective treatments and a control group. J Consult Clin Psychol 56:558-566, 1988.

141. Webster-Stratton C: Individually administered videotape parent training: "Who benefits?" Cognit Ther Res 16:31-52, 1992.

142. Spaccarelli S, Cotler S, Penman D: Problem-solving skills training as a supplement to behavioral parent training. Cognit Ther Res 16:1-17, 1992.

143. Cunningham CE, Bremner R, Boyle M: Large group community-based parenting programs for families of preschoolers at risk for disruptive behaviour disorders: Utilization, cost effectiveness, and outcome. J Child Psychol Psychiatry 36:1141-1159, 1995.

144. Webster-Stratton C: The Incredible Years Parents and Children Training Series. Seattle, WA: Incredible Years, 2005.

145. Forgatch MS, Patterson GR: Parents and Adolescents Living Together, Part 2: Family Problem Solving. Eugene, OR: Castalia, 1989.

146. Patterson GR, Reid JB, Jones RR, et al: A Social Learning Approach to Family Intervention, Volume I: Families with Aggressive Children. Eugene, OR: Castalia, 1975.

147. Patterson GR: Living with Children: New Methods for Parents and Teachers. Champaign, IL: Research Press, 1980.

148. Patterson GR: Families. Champaign, IL: Research Press, 1975.

149. Patterson GR, Forgatch MS: Parents & Adolescents Living Together, Part 1: The Basics. Eugene, OR: Castalia, 1987.

150. Kazdin AE: Parent Management Training: Treatment for Oppositional, Aggressive, and Antisocial Behavior in Children and Adolescents. New York: Oxford University Press, 2005.

151. Forehand R, McMahon RJ: Helping the Noncompliant Child: A Clinician's Guide to Parent Training. New York: Guilford, 1981.

152. Reid M, Webster-Stratton C, Hammond M: Follow-up of children who received the Incredible Years intervention for oppositional-defiant disorder: Maintenance and prediction of 2-year outcome. Behav Ther 34:471-491, 2003.
153. Webster-Stratton C, Reid M, Hammond M: Treating children with early-onset conduct problems: Intervention outcomes for parent, child, and teacher training. J Clin Child Adolesc Psychol 33:105-124, 2004.
154. Eyberg SM, Boggs SR, Algina J: Parent-child interaction therapy: A psychosocial model for the treatment of young children with conduct problem behavior and their families. Psychopharmacol Bull 31:83-91, 1995.
155. Barrett P, Turner C, Rombouts S, et al: Reciprocal skills training in the treatment of externalising behaviour disorders in childhood: A preliminary investigation. Behav Change 17:221-234, 2000.
156. Schuhmann EM, Foote RC, Eyberg SM, et al: Efficacy of parent-child interaction therapy: Interim report of a randomized trial with short-term maintenance. J Clin Child Psychol 27:34-45, 1998.
157. Kazdin AE, Esveldt-Dawson K, French NH, et al: Effects of parent management training and problem-solving skills training combined in the treatment of antisocial child behavior. J Am Acad Child Adolesc Psychiatry 26:416-424, 1987.
158. Davidson WS, Redner R, Blakely CH, et al: Diversion of juvenile offenders: An experimental comparison. J Consult Clin Psychol 55:68-75, 1987.
159. Tremblay RE, Vitaro F, Bertrand L, et al: Parent and child training to prevent early onset of delinquency: The Montreal longitudinal-experimental study. *In* McCord J, Tremblay RE, eds: Preventing Antisocial Behavior: Interventions from Birth through Adolescence. New York: Guilford, 1992, pp 117-138.
160. Emshoff JG, Blakely CH: The diversion of delinquent youth: Family focused intervention. Child Youth Serv Rev 5:343-356, 1983.
161. Eyberg SM, Durning P: Parent-Child Interaction Therapy: Procedures Manual. Unpublished manuscript, University of Florida, Department of Clinical and Health Psychology, 1994.
162. Hembree-Kigin TL, McNeil CB: Parent-Child Interaction Therapy. New York: Plenum Press, 1995.
163. Henggeler SW, Borduin CM, Melton GB, et al: Effects of multisystemic therapy on drug use and abuse in serious juvenile offenders: A progress report from two outcome studies. Fam Dynamics Addict Q 1:40-51, 1991.
164. Henggeler SW, Melton GB, Brondino MJ, et al: Multisystemic therapy with violent and chronic juvenile offenders and their families: The role of treatment fidelity in successful dissemination. J Consult Clin Psychol 65:821-833, 1997.
165. Scherer DG, Brondino MJ, Henggeler SW, et al: Multisystemic family preservation therapy: Preliminary findings from a study of rural and minority serious adolescent offenders. J Emotional Behav Disord 2:198-206, 1994.
166. Henggeler S, Pickrel S, Brondino M: Multisystemic treatment of substance-abusing and dependent delinquents: Outcomes, treatment, fidelity, and transportability. Ment Health Serv Res 1:171-184, 1999.
167. Schoenwald SK, Ward DM, Henggeler SW, et al: Multisystemic therapy versus hospitalization for crisis stabilization of youth: Placement outcomes 4 months postreferral. Ment Health Serv Res 2:3-12, 2000.
168. Huey SJ Jr, Henggeler SW, Rowland MD, et al: Multisystemic therapy effects on attempted suicide by youths presenting psychiatric emergencies. J Am Acad Child Adolesc Psychiatry 43:183-190, 2004.
169. Borduin CM, Henggeler SW, Blaske DM, et al: Multisystemic treatment of adolescent sexual offenders. Int J Offender Ther Comp Criminol 34:105-113, 1990.
170. Henggeler SW, Schoenwald SK, Borduin CM, et al: Multisystemic Treatment of Antisocial Behavior in Children and Adolescents. New York: Guilford, 1998.

8E.
Complementary and Alternative Medicine in Developmental-Behavioral Pediatrics

EUGENIA CHAN

This chapter includes (1) a summary of the current evidence regarding the use of complementary and alternative interventions for developmental and behavioral disorders, particularly attention-deficit/hyperactivity disorder (ADHD), autism spectrum disorders (ASDs), cerebral palsy, and Down syndrome; (2) the theoretical background for selected therapy types; (3) specific examples with a review of evidence regarding their effectiveness and adverse effects; and (4) an approach to working with families interested in complementary and alternative interventions.

EPIDEMIOLOGY OF COMPLEMENTARY AND ALTERNATIVE MEDICINE USE

The use of complementary and alternative medicine (CAM) in the United States has become increasingly prevalent among adults, from 34% in 1993 to 62% in 2002.[1,2] Among children, the prevalence of use ranges from 1.8% to 2.0% nationally[3,4] to approximately 10% to 21% among children in community or primary care settings.[5-8]

CAM use is even more common among children with special health care needs.[9] Prevalence of CAM use in children with developmental-behavioral disorders has been estimated at up to 70% of children with Down syndrome,[10] 50% of children with autism,[11] 56% of children with cerebral palsy,[12] and 64% of children with ADHD.[13] The most common CAM interventions used for these populations vary by condition, geography, availability, and parental demand and may change from year to year as new therapies become popular and others are discredited or forgotten. Table 8E-1 lists popular therapies from prevalence studies.

Investigators in the field of mainstream medicine initially assumed that patients who sought CAM therapies were somehow dissatisfied with conventional medicine or saw alternative therapies as more congruent with their own beliefs and values about health and wellness.[14] Over time, results of studies of adult use of CAM have suggested that dissatisfaction with standard treatments is not a primary motivator for choosing CAM treatments. For example, a report from the Centers for Disease Control and Prevention[2] revealed that fewer than one third of adults nationwide worried that conventional medicine would not help their symptoms. Rather, nearly 55% used CAM because they believed that a combination of CAM and conventional medical treatments would help more, and 50% thought it would be "interesting" to try CAM (hence the term *complementary* medicine). The expense associated with conventional therapies is also beginning to emerge as a reason for choosing CAM.[2,15]

Demographic characteristics associated with CAM use in adults include increased educational attainment, female gender, race or ethnicity, and urban residence.[2] For example, black adults are more likely to use mind-body therapies, including specific prayer for healing, than are white or Asian adults, whereas white adults are more likely to use manipulative and body-based therapies than are black or Asian adults. Among children, CAM users are more likely to be white and female and to live in urban areas, particularly the West Coast.[3]

Investigators have found that the best predictor of CAM use in a child is CAM use by at least one parent, typically the mother.[3,4,9,12] In children with developmental disorders, the most common reason for using CAM is not the oft-cited "desperation" in search of a cure[16] but the desire to maximize a child's personal potential, improve quality of life, enhance conventional therapies, and have more control over treatment.[9,12,17] Cultural factors may also affect families' use of CAM and, on occasion, may contribute to a delay in seeking traditional medical care, accepting a diagnosis, or agreeing to conventional treatments.[18] Thus, clinicians involved in the care of children with developmental and behavioral conditions inevitably encounter families who use CAM, and the physicians should be knowledgeable about these interventions in order to work with families effectively.

WHAT IS CAM?

Definitions

The National Center for Complementary and Alternative Medicine (NCCAM), a component of the National Institutes of Health, defines CAM as "a group of diverse medical and health care systems, practices, and products that are not presently considered to be part of conventional medicine"—that is, medicine as practiced by those holding medical (M.D.) or osteopathy (D.O.) doctoral degrees and by allied health professionals, such as physical therapists, psychologists, and registered nurses.[19] Implicit in this definition is the ever-changing relationship between what is considered CAM and what is considered conventional, standard, or mainstream medicine. Therapies that were once thought of as alternative or nonstandard have gradually gained "conventional" status as evidence of effectiveness, new approaches to treatment, and willingness of third-party payers to reimburse for such therapies have emerged. An example is the use of acupuncture for acute and chronic pain.

An important consideration is how these unconventional interventions are used by patients and families in relation to standard medicine. Most families use unconventional therapies as adjuncts to complement standard treatments (hence the term *complementary* medicine). Fewer families use unconventional therapies as true alternatives to standard interventions. The terms *holistic medicine* and *integrative medicine* have emerged to designate an approach to care that is person-centered and embraces the full spectrum of possible therapies (both conventional and unconventional) to enhance overall well-being, as well as to target specific symptoms or conditions.[20]

Evidence-Based Complementary and Alternative Medicine

NCCAM noted that "While some scientific evidence exists regarding some CAM therapies, for most there are key questions that are yet to be answered through well-designed scientific studies," including their safety and efficacy.[19] Indiscriminate use of unproven CAM therapies in children is especially of concern because of children's particular physiological, developmental, cognitive, and societal vulnerabilities. Critics of CAM have been skeptical of the attractive, often inflated claims of effectiveness for various therapies in children with a broad range of disorders, citing both the "nonscientific" mechanism of action for some CAM therapies (e.g., homeopathy) and the general lack of research demonstrating effectiveness for most CAM interventions. As the importance and visibility of these therapies in mainstream medicine has increased,

TABLE 8E-1 ■ Most Common Complementary and Alternative Medicine Interventions Used in ADHD, ASD, Cerebral Palsy, and Down Syndrome

Condition	Sample	CAM Interventions Used*	% of Users
ADHD	Survey of 114 families of children with attention and hyperactivity problems (56% meeting *DSM-IV* criteria for ADHD) evaluated at a specialty clinic[17]	Expressive (e.g., sensory integration,* art, music,* dance, occupational therapy)	21
		Vitamins*	21
		Dietary manipulation* (e.g., Feingold, sugar elimination)	14
		Special exercises (e.g., yoga, tai chi)	10
		Relaxation techniques (e.g., meditation)	8
		Dietary supplements*	7
		Prayer	7
		Biofeedback*	5
		Chiropractic*	5
		Herbal remedies*	5
		Massage*	5
	Survey of 290 families of children meeting *DSM-III-R* criteria for ADHD seen in a child development center in western Australia[13]	Feingold-like diet*	44
		Sugar restriction diet*	34
		Allergy-based diet manipulation*	17
		Multivitaminsupplementation*	13
		Naturopathic supplementation	9
		Colored lenses*	4
ASD	Chart review of 284 children with autistic spectrum disorders (diagnosed from *DSM-IV-TR* checklist, Autism Diagnostic Observation Schedule, and/or Childhood Autism Rating Scale) seen at a regional autism center[139]	"Unproven benign biological treatments that have no basis in theory (such as vitamins,* gastrointestinal medications, antifungal agents)	16.9
		"Unproven benign biological treatment with some basis in theory" (such as gluten-free/casein-free diet,* vitamin C, secretin*)	15.5
		"Unproven, potentially harmful biological treatments" (e.g., anti-infectives, chelation,* vitamin A megadoses, withholding immunization)	8.8
		"Nonbiological treatments" (e.g., auditory integration training,* facilitatedcommunication,* interactive metronome, craniosacral manipulation)	3.9
Cerebral palsy	Survey of 213 families of children with cerebral palsy, seen at a tertiary pediatric rehabilitation clinic[12]	Prayer (as a treatment method)	40
		Massage*	25
		Aquatherapy	25
		Hippotherapy*	18
		Chiropractic manipulation*	12
		Conductive education	10
		Craniosacral therapy	8
		Euromed/Adeli suit	6
		Hyperbaric oxygen*	6
		Special dietary therapy*	6
Down syndrome	Interviews with 30 families of children with Down syndrome[10,16]	Nutritional supplements designed for Down syndrome*	N/A (Listed in order of most to least common; percentages not presented)
		Massage*	
		Herbal therapies*	
		Dietary modifications* (limit dairy, limit wheat, limit fat, limit processed foods and sweets)	
		Other nutritional supplements	
		Therapeutic horseback riding*	
		Faith/prayer healing	
		Piracetam	
		Chiropractic*	
		Homeopathy*	
		Osteopathy	
		Neurologically based movement programs*	
		Aromatherapy	
		Cell therapy	
		Yoga	

*Discussed in this chapter.
ADHD, attention-deficit/hyperactivity disorder; ASD, autism spectrum disorder; CAM, complementary and alternative medicine; *DSM-III-R, Diagnostic and Statistical Manual of Mental Disorders, Third Edition, Revised; DSM-IV, Diagnostic and Statistical Manual of Mental Disorders, Fourth Edition; DSM-IV-TR, Diagnostic and Statistical Manual of Mental Disorders, Fourth Edition, Text Revision;* N/A, not available.

serious attention to investigating CAM's effectiveness has also increased, culminating in the establishment of NCCAM to coordinate, prioritize, and fund research in this area.

Certainly, many studies supporting the effectiveness of CAM interventions do not conform to current standards of rigorous scientific inquiry. Interpreting the evidence base for CAM, especially with regard to children, requires a critical understanding of the elements of a rigorously designed randomized clinical trial, including potential sources of bias and applicability to diverse patient populations.[21,22] Special attention should be paid to appropriate comparison, placebo, or sham intervention groups; potentially powerful placebo effects[23]; and the need for preintervention titration trials, such as in homeopathy, that

may exert effects on measured outcomes independent of the actual therapy.

THE FIVE DOMAINS OF COMPLEMENTARY AND ALTERNATIVE MEDICINE

NCCAM groups CAM practices into five broad domains: biologically based therapies, mind-body medicine, energy therapies, manipulative and body-based therapies, and alternative medical systems (Table 8E-2). Some CAM interventions, such as hippotherapy or facilitated communication, may not fit neatly into any of these domains, and others could be

TABLE 8E-2 ■ Domains of Complementary and Alternative Medicine

Domain	Description	Examples of Therapeutic Approaches	Examples of Specific Therapies
Biologically based therapies	Use substances found in nature	Dietary supplements, including herbs, vitamins, minerals, enzymes, hormones*	Dimethylglycine* Essential fatty acids* Megavitamins/megaminerals* Melatonin* Pyridoxine* Targeted nutritional intervention (e.g., "U" series)* Valerian* Zinc*
		Whole diet modifications*	Feingold (additive free) diet* Oligoantigenic diet* Sugar elimination diet* Gluten-free/casein-free diet*
		Unconventional uses of medications*	Secretin* Chelation therapy* Hyperbaric oxygen*
Mind-body interventions	Techniques designed to enhance the mind's ability to affect bodily function and symptoms	Yoga Spirituality/prayer Relaxation	Biofeedback* Hypnosis* Sensory integration* Auditory integration training* Facilitated communication* Visual therapies* Music therapy*
Energy therapies	Use energy fields such as magnetic fields or energy fields surrounding and penetrating the human body (biofields)	Reiki Magnets Qi gong Acupuncture*	Tongue acupuncture*
Manipulative and body-based therapies	Manipulation, movement, or removal of one or more body parts	Massage* Chiropractic* Osteopathy Surgery	Plastic surgery* Bodywork (e.g., Feldenkrais method) Reflexology* Patterning* Hippotherapy*
Alternative medical systems	Complete systems of theory and practice, evolved separately from conventional medicine	Homeopathy* Naturopathy Ayurvedic medicine Traditional Chinese medicine	—

*Discussed in text.

categorized under several domains. Therapies such as acupuncture, hypnosis, and chiropractic depend on the training and skill of the practitioner.[19]

To discuss the vast number of CAM therapies that could be used for children with developmental-behavioral conditions is beyond the scope of this chapter. Instead, each domain of CAM is described, as is the available evidence for selected common and/or controversial CAM interventions that have been scientifically studied in developmental-behavioral pediatrics, including (but not necessarily limited to) ADHD, ASDs, cerebral palsy, and Down syndrome.

Biologically Based Therapies

Biologically based therapies entail the use of substances found in nature, such as herbs, foods, and vitamins. These may be the most commonly used CAM interventions in the United States (with the exception of specific prayer for healing purposes)[2] and include food supplements, herbal products, and whole diet interventions, as well as unconventional (not merely off-label) uses of pharmaceuticals and other products. Table 8E-3 summarizes the rationale and available evidence base for selected examples of

TABLE 8E-3 ■ Selected Examples of Biologically Based Therapies Used to Treat Developmental and Behavioral Disorders		
Therapy and Description	**Rationale/Mechanism of Action**	**Available Evidence Base for Some Developmental-Behavioral Disorders**
Herbs and Dietary Supplements Zinc		
Part of cytosolic copper-zinc-superoxide dismutase enzyme	Important in metabolism of oxygen-derived free radicals; cofactor for many enzymes involved with neural metabolism; essential for fatty acid absorption and melatonin production	**DS:** 13 of 16 studies revealed reduced levels of zinc in individuals with DS[24]; 1 crossover RCT revealed no changes in serum immune markers but fewer episodes of cough[140] **ADHD:** reports of zinc deficiency in children with ADHD in comparison with controls[141]; reports that response to stimulants may depend on adequate zinc stores[142]; no RCTs
Dimethylglycine (DMG) Metabolized in liver to glycine, an excitatory neurotransmitter	May help reduce lactic acid buildup in the blood during times of stress, enhance oxygen use during times of hypoxia, and reduce seizure threshold	**ASD:** 2 DB/PC studies suggested no benefit[143,144]
Essential fatty acids (e.g., linoleic acid, γ-linolenic acid) or **Polyunsaturated fatty acids,** often given as fish oil (omega 3 fatty acid) or evening primrose oil (omega 6 fatty acid)	Precursor for second messengers such as prostaglandins, prostacyclins, leukotrienes; essential to composition of neuronal membranes	**ADHD:** No clear benefit from several DB/PC RCTs[35] **ASD:** Case reports only[44] **DCD:** one DB/PC RCT revealed improvement in reading, spelling, and behavior but not in motor skills[145]
Melatonin Neurohormone produced in pineal gland	Thought to regulate circadian rhythm and sleep patterns by causing phase-shift of the endogenous disorders and sleep circadian pacemaker, reduction in core body temperature, and/or direction action on brain's somnogenic structures; also enhances immune system function	Case series in children with a variety of developmental cycle disturbances suggested improved sleep quality and duration[146] Primary sleep disorders: evidence review revealed melatonin not effective except for sleep onset difficulties in adults[147] and possibly in children with developmental disabilities[148]
Pyridoxine (vitamin B$_6$)	Involved in synthesis of many neurotransmitters, including dopamine, serotonin, norepinephrine, epinephrine, immune function; magnesium added to reduce undesirable side effects	**ASD** (frequently in combination with magnesium): no efficacy in 2 small DB crossover clinical trials[149] **DS** (frequently in combination with 5-hydroxytryptamine): 2 DB RCTs yielded no clinical improvements over 3 years of supplementation[150,151]
Megavitamin/megamineral supplementation (may include single vitamin or mineral megadoses or combination high-dose vitamins and/or minerals)	To correct relative deficiencies and enhance ability to correct damage caused by oxygen-derived free radicals; thought to be associated with premature aging, malignancy, and cognitive and immune problems in DS	**DS:** combination high-dose vitamins and minerals yielded no improvement in IQ, physical appearance, or general health in 6 RCTs[24]

TABLE 8E-3 ■ Selected Examples of Biologically Based Therapies Used to Treat Developmental and Behavioral Disorders—cont'd

Therapy and Description	Rationale/Mechanism of Action	Available Evidence Base for Some Developmental-Behavioral Disorders
Targeted nutritional intervention with "U" series, Haps Caps, MSB Plus, NuTriVene-D Mixtures of enzymes, minerals, and vitamins, often includes thyroid hormone	Thought to enhance capacity to deal with oxidative stress, immune dysfunction, and DNA damage caused by oxygen-derived free radicals	**DS:** 4 small RCTs did not produce improvement in cognitive or psychomotor function[25]
Valerian Herbal sedative	Traditionally used for insomnia and anxiety; often used in Europe as a substitute for benzodiazepines[152]	**Sleep problems:** 1 DB/PC crossover RCT in 5 boys with IQ < 70 (with or without epilepsy or hyperactivity) suggested improvements in sleep latency, total sleep time, and sleep quality[153]
Whole-Diet Modifications		
Feingold, Kaiser-Permanente (KP), or additive-free diet Elimination of salicylates (including aspirin, almonds, apples, berries, citrus, cucumbers, grapes, raisins, peaches, plums, nectarines, tomatoes, tea), artificial colors, flavors, and preservatives; modifications involve varying the combinations and extent of restriction	Individuals may have behavioral sensitivity to artificial or natural salicylates, artificial food colorings and flavorings, and artificial preservatives	**ADHD:** Meta-analysis and several reviews concluded that Feingold/KP diet is unlikely to be of benefit except for some children with true sensitivities to specific food additives[35]
Oligoallergenic diet Severely restricted diet typically limited to 2 meats (turkey, lamb), 2 carbohydrate sources (e.g., rice and potato), 2 fruits (e.g., bananas, apples, pears), some vegetables, water, salt, and pepper	Provocative foods or food components may precipitate "allergic" responses that are manifested behaviorally	**ADHD:** Equivocal results in several DB/PC crossover RCTs[35]
Sugar restriction or sugar elimination diet Restriction or elimination of refined sugars from the diet	Refined sugars may exert an adverse effect on behavior; too much sugar leads to hyperactivity	**ADHD:** Meta-analysis revealed no evidence of efficacy[39]
Gluten-free/casein-free diet Restriction or elimination of refined sugars from the diet	"Leaky gut" and inability to completely break down certain proteins may allow systemic absorption of peptide fragments (gliadinomorphins and casomorphins), which act as endogenous opioids	**ASD:** Small single-blind RCT demonstrated improvements in behavior and cognition[45]; preliminary DB/PC crossover RCT revealed no differences on objective measures of behavior and language[46]
Other Biologically Based Therapies		
Secretin Gastrointestinal hormone affecting brain GABA levels	Based on relationship between gut hormones and central nervous system	**ASD:** No evidence of efficacy in systematic reviews[49,50]
Chelation therapy Detoxification with agents such as DMSA	Environmental exposure to lead and mercury in early life may trigger or cause developmental regression and/or behavior problems	No specific data for ADHD, ASD, DS, or CP DB/PC RCT of succimer chelation in lead-exposed children revealed no effect on behavior, cognitive, or motor outcomes[51]
Hyperbaric oxygen therapy 100% oxygen at controlled pressures	Increase in blood oxygen levels may help "wake up" dormant areas of brain surrounding damaged motor areas	**CP:** Insufficient evidence of efficacy in systematic review[55]

ADHD, attention-deficit/hyperactivity disorder; ASD, autism spectrum disorder; CP, cerebral palsy; DB/PC, double-blind/placebo-controlled; DMSA, 2,3-dimercaptosuccinic acid; DS, Down syndrome; GABA, γ-amino butyric acid; RCT, randomized clinical trial.

biologically based therapies frequently encountered in developmental-behavioral pediatrics.

DIETARY SUPPLEMENTS, VITAMINS, MINERALS, AND HERBAL PRODUCTS

Dietary supplements, as defined by Congress in the Dietary Supplement Health and Education Act (DSHEA) of 1994, are nontobacco products taken by mouth that contain a "dietary ingredient" intended to supplement the diet. Such dietary ingredients may include vitamins; minerals; herbs or other botanicals; amino acids; and substances such as enzymes, organ tissues, and metabolites. These may be ingested alone or in various (often idiosyncratic) combinations.

The general reasons for using dietary supplements are (1) to address presumed deficiencies or relative deficiencies in bodily levels of specific substances such as vitamins or minerals (e.g., zinc for Down syndrome or ADHD); (2) to enhance specific body functions (e.g., dimethylglycine to reduce blood lactic acid levels in ASD; essential fatty acids to improve neural transmission in ADHD, ASD, and developmental coordination disorder; melatonin to regulate circadian rhythms in children with sleep disorders; and pyridoxine to enhance immune and neurotransmitter function in ASD and Down syndrome); and (3) to enhance overall well-being. Clinicians may encounter families who use typical doses of single vitamins, minerals, or other supplements, megadoses of single vitamins or minerals, or combinations of dietary substances in varying doses. The use of high-dose vitamins and minerals and targeted nutritional intervention mixtures of enzymes, minerals, and vitamins has been especially common for persons with Down syndrome, despite negative findings in several clinical trials.[24,25] The use of herbal products is usually based on traditional uses of the herbs. For example, sedative herbs such as valerian are often used to treat sleep difficulties and restlessness.

There are important safety issues to consider in counseling patients who use dietary supplements.[26] First, the U.S. Food and Drug Administration (FDA) regulates dietary supplements as foods, rather than as drugs, which means that studies in humans to demonstrate safety and effectiveness are not required before the supplements are marketed. The FDA can take action against a manufacturer or distributor only if a supplement is found to be unsafe once it is on the market. Second, although manufacturers must meet FDA Good Manufacturing Practices for foods, these standards for preparation, packaging, and storage are less stringent than those for drugs, and the FDA does not require that supplement labels be accurate. Contamination with other herbs, pesticides, herbicides, heavy metals, other environmental pollutants, and so forth, may occur at any stage of growth, harvesting,

preparation, and storage. In addition, because the active chemical constituents are not standardized, the potency of some supplements may differ from capsule to capsule even within the same bottle or production lot.

WHOLE DIET MODIFICATION

The notion that eliminating certain foods or food components from the diet can improve behavior dates from the early 1900s.[27] Interventions that involve such "whole diet" modifications appeal to families' desire to promote their children's overall health and well-being. Dietary interventions require a great deal of motivation and often must involve the entire family in order to promote successful adherence over the long term. Most whole diet modifications are reasonably safe as long as there is careful planning for adequate nutrition, especially certain vitamins and minerals, protein, and fiber, within the confines of the diet. Consultation with a dietician may be necessary for more restrictive diets.

Among the most common whole diet modifications used to treat developmental-behavioral conditions are the Feingold or additive-free diet, the sugar elimination diet, the oligoantigenic diet, and the gluten-free/casein-free diet.

The Feingold, or Additive-Free, Diet

This diet is one of the best-studied methods but one of the most enduring controversies in the alternative treatment of hyperactivity. The original Feingold diet is based on allergist Benjamin F. Feingold's observation that aspirin-sensitive adults experienced improved behavioral symptoms when on a diet free of artificial and natural salicylates and of artificial food colorings and flavorings. Feingold hypothesized that there was a link between the parallel rise in the incidence of learning disabilities and hyperkinesis and the increasing use of artificial colors and flavors, especially in commercially prepared foods.[28]

In multiple literature reviews[29-31] and one meta-analysis,[32] investigators considered double-blind, placebo-controlled trials with adequate sample size and appropriate outcome measures and concluded that the Feingold diet is not effective as a treatment for hyperactivity. A new generation of studies (in children whose symptoms do not necessarily meet criteria for ADHD) focusing on behavioral effects of specific food additives and preservatives such as tartrazine and calcium propionate suggest that this area is still open for further investigation.[33,34]

The Oligoantigenic (Oligoallergenic), or "Few Foods," Diet

This protocol is an extreme extension of the Feingold diet. It is based on the premise that behavioral symptoms in children can result from hypersensitivity to any number of potentially provocative foods and food additives, and its objective is to restrict the diet to a few relatively hypoallergenic foods. Enzyme-potentiated desensitization with intradermal injections of provoking food antigens may also follow a trial of the oligoantigenic diet as part of the treatment plan. This diet has been studied in children with ADHD, with equivocal results,[35] but has been adopted by parents for many other developmental and behavioral conditions, including autism. The severe restrictions make this diet very difficult to maintain, especially for children who are already picky or have other feeding issues. The likelihood of nutritional deficiencies is high.

The Sugar Elimination Diet

This dietary intervention is widely used by parents and perpetuated by the pervasive idea that refined sugars cause hyperactivity. Two hypotheses underlying the sugar elimination diet are that some children experience a "functional reactive hypoglycemia" after ingesting sugar[36] and that hyperactivity results from an allergy to refined sugar.[37] Little evidence supports a correlation between amount of ingested sugar and hyperactivity.[38] In a meta-analysis of 23 within-subject design studies in which sugar challenge tests were used with hyperactive children, so-called "sugar-reactors," and otherwise normal children, Wolraich and associates concluded that sugar does not affect child behavior or cognitive performance.[39] There have not been more recent investigations of the relationship between sugar and behavior in children, but studies in rats suggest that sugar dependence leads to behavioral and neural adaptations involving the dopamine system, similar to those occurring during stimulant sensitization.[40-42] However, these effects result in increased extracellular dopamine, which is contrary to the current understanding of dopaminergic function in ADHD.

Nevertheless, parents persist in attributing hyperactivity to ingested sugar and frequently restrict sugar in their child's diet. This intervention can be pursued with little cost or risk of adverse effects, unless parents substitute large amounts of artificial sweeteners (whose long-term effects are as yet unknown) for the refined sugars.

The Gluten-Free/Casein-Free Diet

One of the most commonly used dietary treatments for autism, this protocol is based on the "opioid-excess" theory that autism results from a metabolic disorder in which a "leaky gut," unable to break down proteins such as gluten and casein, allows the systemic absorption of peptide fragments (gliadinomorphins and casomorphins) that then act as endogenous opioids in the central nervous system.[43] This theory remains speculative.[44] Results of one small single-blind study

of the gluten-free/casein-free diet in 20 children with autism and abnormal urinary peptides suggested improvements in behavior and cognition.[45] However, results of a preliminary double-blind, placebo-controlled crossover trial in 15 children with autism revealed no significant differences on the Childhood Autism Rating Scale, on the Ecological Communications Orientation Language Sampling Summary, or in frequencies of behavior such as child initiation and child response.[46] These contradictory results reflect the lack of evidence supporting or refuting the effectiveness of the gluten-free/casein-free diet.

Disadvantages of the gluten-free/casein-free diet include the potentially higher cost of gluten-free/casein-free foods, the responsibility of parents to be vigilant in reading food labels, and the nutritional implications of eliminating milk products rich in calcium, vitamin D, and protein from the diet. In addition, maintaining adequate nutrition with this dietary intervention may be especially difficult for children who have unusual or restricted food preferences.

SECRETIN

Secretin is an example of an unconventional, off-label use of an FDA-approved medication. In 1998, Horvath and colleagues reported a case series of three children with autism who appeared to have improved eye contact, alertness, and expressive language after undergoing diagnostic endoscopy with secretin infusion.[47] Secretin, a gastrointestinal hormone usually used to examine pancreatic secretion during endoscopic procedures, is thought to act as a neuropeptide or, more specifically, as a brain-gut stress regulatory hormone that affects levels of γ-amino butyric acid in the brain.[48] This case report not only led to unprecedented demand for intravenous secretin to treat children with autism but also spurred a flurry of scientific investigation in the relationship between gut hormones and the central nervous system.

Levy and Hyman, in their review of novel treatments for ASDs,[44] noted that off-label use of secretin is the most carefully studied intervention for autism. At least 15 well-designed, randomized, double-blind, controlled trials involving more than 700 children, all published in peer-reviewed journals, failed to substantiate the therapeutic effect of secretin.[49,50] Nevertheless, this intervention continues to generate interest among families of children with ASDs.

CHELATION THERAPY

Chelation therapy is based on the hypothesis that environmental exposures in early life trigger or cause the developmental regression often seen in children with autism. Postulated environmental exposures include lead and mercury (especially through thimerosal-containing vaccines). Detoxification through chelating agents such as 2,3-dimercaptosuccinic acid (DMSA) has been shown to be effective at removing lead from the blood stream and periphery but may not produce benefits for long-term behavioral, cognitive, or neuromotor outcomes.[51] In addition, certain chelating agents such as sodium ethylenediaminetetraacetic acid (Na$_2$ EDTA) are associated with nephrotoxicity and hypocalcemia that can lead to tetany, cardiac arrest, and death.[52] As yet, there are no published studies of chelation in children with autism,[44] and the Institute of Medicine found no evidence to support its use in these children.[53]

HYPERBARIC OXYGEN THERAPY

In hyperbaric oxygen therapy (HBOT), commonly used in patients with severe burns or wounds, 100% oxygen is used at controlled pressures (typically 1.5 to 1.75 atm, equivalent to 16.5 to 25 feet below sea level) to increase the amount of oxygen at the cellular level. Treatments usually last 1 hour and are given once or twice daily, 5 to 6 days per week; 40 treatments are typical during the first phase of treatment.

The underlying rationale for HBOT in children with cerebral palsy is the theory that damaged motor areas of the brain are surrounded by so-called "dormant" areas that receive relatively less blood flow and thus less oxygen. By increasing blood oxygen levels, HBOT purportedly "wakes up" the brain cells in the dormant areas and also constricts blood vessels, thus reducing brain swelling and promoting growth of new brain tissue.[54] Potential risks include ear discomfort or trauma, pneumothorax, myopia, oxygen-induced convulsions, and fire or explosion.

According to an evidence report,[55] one fair-quality observational study and one fair-quality randomized controlled trial demonstrated improved motor and social function in the patients receiving HBOT.[56-58] However, in the randomized clinical trial, children who did not receive HBOT showed similar improvements. Overall, the report concluded that "there is insufficient evidence to determine whether the use of HBOT improves functional outcomes in children with cerebral palsy."[55] In a review of CAM therapies for cerebral palsy, the authors also noted that it seems unlikely that a single therapy could benefit as heterogeneous a disorder as cerebral palsy.[59]

Mind-Body Interventions

The basis for mind-body therapies is that frequent stress leads to physiological wear and tear as a result of either chronic overexposure or underexposure to stress mediators from the autonomic nervous system; from the hypothalamic-pituitary-adrenal axis; and from the cardiovascular, metabolic, and immune systems.[60] The overall hypothesis is that mind-body interventions increase awareness of the internal body state and elicit the relaxation response, leading to reductions in autonomic reactivity to stress, increases in an individual's sense of control and self-efficacy, and thus improved health and well-being. Mind-body therapies that have become mainstream include cognitive-behavioral therapy and biofeedback through electromyography. Other therapies frequently used in children with developmental-behavioral conditions include electroencephalographic (EEG) biofeedback, hypnosis, sensory integration, auditory integration training, facilitated communication, visual therapies (behavioral optometry), and music therapy (Table 8E-4).

ELECTROENCEPHALOGRAPHIC BIOFEEDBACK

Biofeedback through electroencephalography has been used since the early 1970s in the treatment of developmental-behavioral and psychiatric disorders, including ADHD, mental retardation, depression, mood disorders, and bipolar disorder.[61] In general, biofeedback involves the use of visual and auditory stimuli to make physiological processes such as heart rate, blood pressure, and skin temperature explicitly known to the individual. Through regular training sessions (typically once or twice a week for 40 to 50 weeks), patients learn to modulate these processes and, in turn, presumably affect their symptoms.

EEG biofeedback for ADHD and learning disabilities is based on a series of observations that children with these conditions may have higher rates of EEG abnormalities than do controls, including increased θ waves (associated with drowsiness), decreased β waves (associated with attention and memory processes), and decreased fast sensorimotor rhythms (inversely associated with movement).[62,63] Results of studies on the efficacy of EEG biofeedback in ADHD suggest that children can be taught to change their EEG wave patterns.[64] Whether EEG biofeedback also results in clinically significant changes in cognitive and behavioral outcomes pertinent to ADHD and/or learning disabilities remains to be seen, inasmuch as major design flaws, including lack of randomization, lack of appropriate comparison groups, small sample sizes, and differential attrition, significantly limit the interpretability of the available data.[35,65]

Biofeedback requires a great deal of motivation, expense, and time, and may not be available in certain geographic areas. Some children may be allergic to the adhesive used for EEG lead placement, and it may not be appropriate for children with visual processing difficulties, atypical visual system features, or very low cognitive levels.

TABLE 8E-4 ■ Selected Examples of Mind-Body Therapies Used to Treat Developmental and Behavioral Disorders

Therapy and Description	Rationale/Mechanism of Action	Available Evidence Base for Some Developmental-Behavioral Disorders
Biofeedback Visual and auditory stimuli help patients learn to control physiological processes such as heart rate and blood pressure	Children with ADHD and/or LD may have higher rate of EEG abnormalities (increased θ waves, decreased β waves, and fast sensorimotor rhythms)	**ADHD:** Children could be taught to change EEG wave pattern,[64] but evidence of clinical efficacy was equivocal in controlled trials of EEG biofeedback[35]
Hypnosis Various techniques are used induce an altered state of intense awareness and concentration	Hypnosis may allow individuals to self-regulate physiological and psychological processes such as heart rate, muscle tension, and anxiety	**Nocturnal enuresis:** insufficient evidence to support use[72] **LD:** 1 controlled trial demonstrated no differences in academic performance or self-esteem in comparison with untreated controls[73] **ADHD:** case reports, uncontrolled pretreatment/post-treatment results suggest benefit[75] **CP:** case reports and preliminary studies[76]
Sensory integration Individualized therapy involving tactile, vestibular, and proprioceptive experiences	Sensory processing difficulties are more prevalent among children with developmental disorders and may be associated with altered sympathetic and parasympathetic function	**MR:** insufficient evidence to support use[84] **LD:** insufficient evidence to support use[85] **ASD:** 4 small studies with objective measures (none with comparison group) yielded equivocal results[86]
Auditory integration training (AIT) Exposure to electronically modified music	Abnormal sound sensitivity is common in children with autism and other disorders; AIT may retrain perception of auditory stimuli	**ASD:** 6 RCTs with equivocal results[87]
Facilitated communication Trained facilitator supports a nonverbal person's hand to assist in using communication devices such as a computer keyboard	"Manual prompting" may provide access to expressive language abilities in individuals with physical disabilities, intellectual disabilities, and autism	**ASD/MR:** no evidence of efficacy[91]
Visual therapies (behavioral optometry) Trains visual system with eye tracking, accommodation, or convergence exercises; prism or colored lenses or overlays	Dysfunctional processing of visual information may affect attention, orientation, movement, and visual-motor coordination; children with specific reading disorders often exhibit impaired eye movements; children with autism often have visual stereotypies	**ASD:** 1 DB/PC crossover trial of ambient prism lenses demonstrated decreased behavior problem scores on Aberrant Behavior Checklist[93] **LD/dyslexia:** systematic review revealed insufficient evidence of efficacy[95]
Music therapy Active (musical improvisation) or receptive (listening to music) therapy to help develop communication skills and social interaction	Music is a nonverbal or preverbal language that may enable nonverbal individuals to communicate without words	**ASD:** meta-analysis of 9 studies suggested efficacy of music intervention[99]

ADHD, attention-deficit/hyperactivity disorder; ASD, autism spectrum disorder; CP, cerebral palsy; DB/PC, double-blind/placebo-controlled; EEG, electroencephalogram; LD, learning disability; MR, mental retardation; RCT, randomized clinical trial.

HYPNOSIS

Hypnosis creates an altered state of consciousness in which the individual experiences intensely focused attention, awareness, and self-control.[66] Accompanying autonomic changes such as decreased heart rate, increased skin temperature, and decreased electrodermal activity have been documented in children and adults.[67] The goal of hypnosis is to facilitate the patient's ability to self-regulate physiological and psychological processes through a variety of techniques, such as blowing or breathing, imagery, and suggestion. It is often used in combination with biofeedback and other types of relaxation training. Because of maturing cognitive processes, hypnotic responsivity is probably higher in children 8 years of age or older than in younger children.[68]

Hypnosis has been used successfully in a variety of childhood conditions, including postoperative pain,[69] recurrent headache,[70] and asthma.[71] Few well-conducted randomized controlled trials have evaluated the effect of hypnosis in children with developmental-behavioral conditions. For example, although hypnosis is often used to treat nocturnal enuresis, a systematic review uncovered only three poor-quality randomized clinical trials (one without formal statistical testing) and concluded that there was insufficient evidence to demonstrate effectiveness.[72] One controlled trial in 33 children with learning disabilities demonstrated no differences in reading performance, Wide Range Achievement Test scores, or Self-Esteem Inventory scores between the children who underwent self-hypnosis group and the untreated controls.[73] Another unblinded randomized controlled trial in 50 children with a variety of behavioral or somatic complaints (including recurrent headache, sleep problems, attention or hyperactivity problems, and recurrent abdominal pain) revealed reductions in both parent-reported behavioral symptoms on the Child Behavior Checklist and child-reported stress levels and psychosomatic complaints for the children receiving autogenic relaxation training in comparison with wait-list controls.[74] In an uncontrolled study of 19 children and adolescents with ADHD, mean scores on the parent-report Attention Deficit Disorders Evaluation Scale were reduced after hypnotherapy in comparison with baseline.[75] Case reports and one small pretrial/post-trial study suggested that children with cerebral palsy can use self-relaxation techniques to reduce muscle tension and improve functional abilities.[76]

SENSORY INTEGRATION

According to sensory integration theory, there is a linkage between difficulties in receiving, modulating, and integrating sensory input and adaptive behavior in some children with learning and behavior problems.[77] Sensory integration therapists provide individualized opportunities to actively engage the child in tactile, vestibular, and proprioceptive experiences in a therapeutic context, and they hope thereby to promote adaptive responses and behaviors. Therapists continually observe the child's ability to process and use sensory information and adjust the activity accordingly in order to provide a challenging and therapeutic experience.[78] Typically developing children may have sensory processing disorders,[79] but they are more prevalent among children with ASD, ADHD, mental retardation, the Fragile X syndrome, regulatory disorders, and environmental deprivation.[78]

Some evidence supports the idea that children with sensory integration difficulties have neural dysfunction that is related to sensory processing. For example, several investigators have found altered markers of sympathetic and parasympathetic function in children with poor sensory modulation, including children with the fragile X syndrome and ADHD, as well as children without a developmental diagnosis.[80-82] This will be an important area of research for the future.

Evidence of the efficacy of treatments aimed at sensory integration disorders is equivocal. Despite more than 80 studies in the current literature, methodological problems, such as lack of standardization across subjects and across studies, widely varying outcome measures, and small and heterogeneous samples, limit the comparability and interpretability of most studies.[83-86] From a practical standpoint, sensory integration therapy requires considerable time, motivation, and financial resources, as well as availability of properly trained therapists.

AUDITORY INTEGRATION TRAINING

Auditory integration training is a technique for improving abnormal sound sensitivity in individuals with autism, hyperactivity, and other behavior and learning disorders. Two half-hour daily sessions of exposure to electronically modified music over 10 days help "retrain" the ear's perception of auditory stimuli. Of six randomized controlled trials with varying outcome measures and methodological quality, three yielded some improvement and three yielded no benefit of auditory integration training over control conditions (e.g., listening to nonmodified music).[87] The American Academy of Pediatrics does not support the use of auditory integration training.[88]

FACILITATED COMMUNICATION

Facilitated communication, not to be confused with augmentative communication, is intended to assist a nonverbal person's use of a communication device, such as a computer keyboard, by supporting the individual's hand as he or she selects letters to spell out words. Proponents suggest that through facilitated communication, individuals with severe expressive language difficulties such as autism or mental retardation can demonstrate higher-than-expected literacy and communication skills.[89] The technique has been especially controversial because of some cases of alleged sexual abuse reported through the use of facilitated communication.[90] Controlled studies in individuals with ASD, mental retardation, and other developmental disabilities have been unable to demonstrate replicability or validity,[91] and the American Academy of Pediatrics does not recommend its use for children with disabilities.[88]

VISUAL THERAPIES (BEHAVIORAL OPTOMETRY)

Behavioral optometry has been used in a variety of developmental-behavioral conditions, including reading and other learning disabilities, ADHD, and autism. Individuals with specific reading disorder frequently exhibit impaired eye movements, such as incomplete saccades, poor tracking, poor convergence, and poor binocular control[92]; children with autism often rely on peripheral vision or have stereotypical behaviors involving the visual system.[93] Proponents of behavioral optometry hypothesize that dysfunctional processing of visual information affects attention, orientation, movement, and visual-motor coordination. Correcting or compensating for visual system defects is thought to alter the brain's processing of visual stimuli and thus improve academic and behavioral outcomes.[94] Some techniques include visual training with eye tracking, accommodation, and convergence exercises; "training" glasses with bifocals, prisms, or colored (Irlen) lenses; occlusion therapy; colored overlays or filters; and laterality or perceptual-motor training. These therapies may help improve convergence insufficiency and visual field deficits after brain damage, but evidence of their efficacy in learning disabilities or dyslexia is equivocal.[95] In one double-blind, placebo-controlled crossover trial in children with autism, investigators reported decreased average behavior problem scores on the Aberrant Behavior Checklist after 2 months of wearing ambient prism lenses, in comparison with placebo (clear) lenses.[93] The American Academy of Pediatrics, along with the American Academy of Ophthalmology and the American Association for Pediatric Ophthalmology and Strabismus, concluded that there is no known visual cause or effective visual treatment for learning disabilities.[94]

MUSIC THERAPY

Music may be useful in enhancing relaxation in stressful situations such as painful procedures. Specific music therapy, on the other hand, is designed to help individuals develop communication skills and social interaction through musical experiences such as listening, improvisation, and reflection on emotional responses or associations to music.[96] Music therapy may be active (musical improvisation) or receptive (listening to music). The underlying rationale for use of music therapy in individuals with communication disorders and autism is based on tonal (e.g., pitch, timbre, movement) and temporal (e.g., tempo, rhythm, timing) descriptions of sound dialogues between mothers and infants[97] and the belief that music therapy provides a nonverbal or preverbal language for communication.[96] Most music therapy for autism is individually based and focused on communication and behavioral goals.[98] A meta-analysis of nine studies in which music therapy was compared with no music therapy in children and adolescents with autism revealed overall benefits with music therapy.[99]

Energy Therapies

Energy therapies use manipulation of biofields and energy fields, which purportedly surround and penetrate the human body, to promote healing. The existence of such fields has not yet been scientifically proved.[19] Examples of biofield therapies include qi gong, acupuncture, Reiki, and therapeutic touch. Other energy therapies may involve the unconventional use of electromagnetic fields such as pulsed fields, magnetic fields, or alternating-current or direct-current fields. Only acupuncture has been studied scientifically (Table 8E-5).

ACUPUNCTURE

Acupuncture encompasses a group of healing procedures with its theoretical roots in East Asia. Two key concepts are the balance between yin (qualities of negative energy) and yang (qualities of positive energy) and *qi*, the vital energy surrounding and

---

TABLE 8E-5 ■ Selected Examples of Energy Therapies Used to Treat Developmental and Behavioral Disorders

Therapy and Description	Rationale/Mechanism of Action	Available Evidence Base for Some Developmental-Behavioral Disorders
Acupuncture Needles inserted into meridian points along the body restore flow of *qi*	Disruption of *qi* (vital energy) or imbalances in yin (negative energy) and yang (positive energy) leads to disease	**CP:** decreased muscle spasm, improved sleep, mood, and bowel function in uncontrolled studies[103,104] **Nocturnal enuresis:** insufficient evidence to support use[72]
Tongue acupuncture Needles inserted into meridian points along tongue	Repeated stimulation of tongue acupressure points augments neural pathways connected tomotor/somatosensory cortex	**CP:** RCT with sham tongue acupuncture control suggests improved gross motor function[105]

CP, cerebral palsy; RCT, randomized clinical trial.

flowing through the body.[100] Disease is thought to be caused by disruption of *qi* and/or by imbalances between yin and yang. In order to restore harmony to the body, fine needles are inserted into well-defined meridian points along the body, each with its own therapeutic action. Associated techniques include moxibustion, which involves burning the herb *Artemisia vulgaris* near the acupuncture point, hand pressure (acupressure), stimulation of needles with electrical current (electroacupuncture), concomitant use of traditional Chinese herbal medicine, and specialized acupuncture for tongue, ears, scalp, and hands. In most conditions, multiple acupuncture treatment sessions are necessary over an extended period of time in order to be effective. Although the existence of energy meridians has not been demonstrated, scientific research suggests that acupuncture may activate endogenous opioids and modulate pain transmission and pain response.[101]

There is growing evidence of acupuncture's efficacy in a variety of disorders in adults, including temporomandibular joint disorders; emesis related to cancer chemotherapy, surgery, and pregnancy; and osteoarthritis of the knee.[100] However, many randomized controlled trials have insufficient sample sizes, heterogeneous study samples, imprecise outcomes, high dropout rates, inadequate follow-up, difficulty with blind conditions for both acupuncturists and patients, and large placebo effects.[100] Although sham acupuncture (needle insertion at nonmeridian points in the body) is frequently used as a control treatment, it may not be a truly inert condition. A placebo acupuncture needle, which retracts back into the handle without entering the skin, may be a useful alternative.[102]

Acupuncture has been used in a variety of developmental disorders, but few well-designed controlled trials have been published in English. Results of uncontrolled studies suggest benefits in children with cerebral palsy, such as decreased painful muscle spasms,[103] more restful sleep, improved mood, and improved bowel function.[104] One small controlled trial of tongue acupuncture demonstrated improvements in gross motor function in 33 children with cerebral palsy,[105] and a pretreatment/post-treatment study reported amelioration in drooling in 10 children with neurological disabilities[106] A systematic review of acupuncture in nocturnal enuresis revealed that the three available randomized controlled trials were too methodologically poor to provide sufficient evidence of efficacy.[72] Studies of acupuncture in ADHD are currently ongoing.

The most common adverse effects of acupuncture in nine prospective studies were needle pain (1% to 45%), tiredness (2% to 41%), and bleeding (0.03% to 38%). More serious but rare adverse effects included pneumothorax, retention of broken needle remnants, transmission of infectious disease, syncope, and severe nausea.[107] Skilled acupuncturists should be able to insert needles painlessly, even in children. The National Commission for the Certification of Acupuncturists has developed standards for training and certification, and many states have guidelines for licensing acupuncturists.

Manipulative and Body-Based Methods

Manipulative and body-based methods involve the manipulation or movement of one or more parts of the body, such as in chiropractic and osteopathic manipulation, bodywork, and massage. From an integrative medicine framework, cosmetic surgery would also belong to this category of interventions (Table 8E-6).

SURGERY

Plastic surgery has been used for individuals with Down syndrome on the premises that altering the characteristic facial features would improve the individual's social acceptability and that decreasing the size of the tongue would improve oromotor functions such as speech, chewing, and swallowing and decrease drooling.[108] Studies of speech outcome[109-111] and observer perceptions of physical attractiveness and social acceptability before and after surgery have yielded mixed results.[112,113] In general, there is little enthusiasm for plastic surgery among parents of children with Down syndrome.[114]

CHIROPRACTIC

Chiropractic focuses on the relationship between bodily structures (primarily the spine) and function and the effects of this relationship on health. The hypothesis is that subluxation of the spinal segments causes nerve irritability, which in turn leads to agitation, decreased concentration, and abnormal behavior. There are sporadic case reports of chiropractic as a treatment for children with developmental disorders, including Down syndrome, ADHD, and ASD, but controlled studies are lacking. One randomized controlled trial of 46 children with nocturnal enuresis reported a lower mean frequency of wet nights after 10 weeks of chiropractic than with sham adjustment[115]; however, the chiropractic group had less severe enuresis at baseline, which suggests that randomization was inadequate.[72]

MASSAGE

Massage manipulates muscle and connective tissue to stimulate blood flow, enhance function, and promote relaxation and well-being. It is popularly used in children, both healthy and ill, and in adults. A few

TABLE 8E-6 ■ Selected Examples of Manipulative and Body-Based Therapies Used to Treat Developmental and Behavioral Disorders

Therapy and Description	Rationale/Mechanism of Action	Available Evidence Base for Some Developmental-Behavioral Disorders
Plastic surgery Surgery to alter external appearance	Surgical alteration of facial features and tongue size may improve an individual's social acceptability and oromotor functions	**DS:** No effect on speech intelligibility[109-111]
Chiropractic Manipulation of spinal segments	Subluxation of spinal segments may lead to nerve irritability and thus impaired concentration and behavior	**ADHD, DS, ASD:** case reports **Nocturnal enuresis:** 1 small RCT suggested benefits in comparison with sham adjustment[115]
Massage Kinesthetic and tactile stimulation of the body	Stimulation of blood flow may improve muscle and connective tissue function and promote relaxation	**ASD:** 2 small RCTs with raters unaware of experimental condition demonstrated improved social behavior and attention[117,118] **ADHD:** in 2 small controlled trials, investigators reported improved mood and decreased classroom hyperactivity[119,120]
Reflexology Pressure massage directed at reflex zones on the feet	Thought to facilitate homeostasis across body systems as represented by zones on the feet	**Encopresis:** pretreatment/post-treatment study (N = 50) with parent report of fewer soiling episodes per week[121]
Patterning Program of passive repetition of steps along normal motor development pathway	Believed to improve neurological organization in children with brain injury	**MR:** 4 studies with equivocal results[59]
Hippotherapy Therapeutic horseback riding	Riding a horse may improve muscle tone, head and trunk control, pelvic mobility, and equilibrium	**CP:** In 2 controlled studies, investigators reported improved gross motor function scores and muscle symmetry[125,126]

ADHD, attention-deficit/hyperactivity disorder; ASD, autism spectrum disorder; CP, cerebral palsy; DS, Down syndrome; GABA, γ-amino butyric acid; MR, mental retardation; RCT, randomized clinical trial.

preliminary studies of massage in children with developmental-behavioral disorders have yielded promising results. One exploratory study suggested that massage provided by primary caregivers of children with disabilities may help reduce anxiety and improve sleep, bowel function, and body movements.[116] In two small randomized controlled trials in which raters were unaware of experimental condition, investigators documented improvements in stereotypic behavior, social relatedness, and attention in preschool children with autism who received massage, in comparison with those who received either a reading control intervention[117] or a one-on-one play intervention.[118] In two small clinical trials of massage, investigators reported decreased classroom hyperactivity and improved mood among adolescent boys with ADHD.[119,120]

Reflexology is a specialized pressure massage directed at reflex zones on the feet. These reflex zones correspond to different parts of the body, and pressure on the zones is thought to facilitate balance among body systems. Most studies in reflexology have focused on adults. One study in 50 children with chronic consti-

pation and encopresis found that children and their parents reported fewer soiling episodes per week, in comparison to baseline, after 6 weeks of reflexology.[121]

PATTERNING

Patterning is based on the principle of "neurological organization," which suggests that failure to successfully master each step in a sequence of neurological development will adversely affect mastery of subsequent stages. As applied to children with actual or presumed brain injury, such as those with cerebral palsy, Down syndrome, autism, and learning disabilities, patterning is a program of passive repetition of steps in normal motor development, designed to improve a child's neurological organization. The treatment regimen is quite demanding, time-consuming, and inflexible and can cause a great deal of family distress.[122] Few well-designed studies support patterning as a treatment for children with disabilities, and the American Academy of Pediatrics Committee on Children with Disabilities discourages its use.[122,123]

HIPPOTHERAPY

Therapeutic horseback riding, also known as equine-assisted therapy or hippotherapy, was initially developed as a treatment for children with polio. This therapy is thought to improve muscle tone, head and trunk control, pelvic mobility, and equilibrium in children with cerebral palsy and other developmental disabilities.[124] Potential risks include trauma from falls and allergy to riding gear; other drawbacks include the time and expense involved. Although controlled studies are few, their results did suggest improved gross motor function[125] and symmetry of muscle activity.[126]

Alternative Medical Systems

Alternative medical systems are entire systems of theory and practice that have evolved separately from conventional biomedicine, both in Western cultures (e.g., homeopathy, naturopathy) and in non-Western cultures (e.g., Ayurvedic medicine, traditional Chinese medicine). Except for homeopathy, the efficacy of alternative medical systems in treating developmental-behavioral conditions has not been studied (Table 8E-7).

HOMEOPATHY

Homeopathy uses highly individualized remedies selected to address specific symptoms or symptom profiles, such as irritability, learning difficulties, impulsivity, social isolation, and restlessness, within the context of the whole child. Remedies generally seek to stimulate the body's natural defense mechanisms. Selecting a homeopathic remedy depends on two principles: (1) "like cures like" (a substance that causes symptoms in a healthy individual will cure the same symptoms in an affected individual) and (2) increasing dilutions increase the potency of a remedy because the bioenergy of molecules is maximized in extreme dilutions. Because dilutions range from 1 : 10 to 1 per billions, most homeopathic remedies are likely to be reasonably safe (although many contain alcohol). In addition, unlike dietary supplements, homeopathic remedies are subject to quality and production standards set by the Homeopathic Pharmacopoeia of the United States, which was enacted by Congress as part of the Food, Drug, and Cosmetics Act of 1939.[127]

Scientific support of homeopathy is limited by poor quality of methodology and overreporting of positive trials. A meta-analysis of 110 randomized, double-blind, placebo-controlled homeopathy trials, mostly among adults, and 110 matched conventional medicine trials concluded that, among the larger trials of higher quality, there was weak evidence for effect of homeopathy (odds ratio, 0.88; 95% confidence interval, 0.65 to 1.19) and strong evidence for effect of conventional medicine (odds ratio, 0.58; 95% confidence interval, 0.39 to 0.85), across a variety of disorders.[128] There have been multiple case reports but only four clinical trials of homeopathy for children with ADHD.[129-132] In three studies, investigators reported improvements in parent ratings of behavior, but the studies were limited by small sample sizes, incomplete naiveté to condition, and other methodological flaws.[129-131] The most recent study, which employed more rigorous double-blind, placebo-controlled, crossover trial methods, demonstrated improved parent Conners' Global Index ratings for children who received homeopathy in comparison with those receiving placebo.[132]

TABLE 8E-7 ■ **Example of an Alternative Medical System Used to Treat Developmental and Behavioral Disorders**

Therapy and Description	Rationale/Mechanism of Action	Available Evidence Base for Some Developmental-Behavioral Disorders
Homeopathy Individualized, often highly dilute remedies designed to address specific symptom profiles: for example, *Veratrum album* (restless, bossy, touch everything in sight, precocious); *Tarentula hispanica* (mischievous, cunning, impatient, hurried, destructive, agile); *Cina* (irritable, prefer not to be touched, may pinch or hit); *Calcarea phosphorica* (frustrated, dissatisfied, cranky, hard to please)	Remedies thought to stimulate the body's natural defense mechanisms; substances that cause symptoms in a healthy individual will cure the same symptoms in an affected individual; potency increases with increasing dilution	In 4 clinical trials (in 1, homeopathy was compared with methylphenidate) of varying quality, investigators reported improved parent ratings of behavior[129-132]

WORKING WITH FAMILIES INTERESTED IN COMPLEMENTARY AND ALTERNATIVE MEDICINE

Results of studies suggest that despite frequent use of CAM for developmental-behavioral conditions, as few as 11% of parents discuss such use with their child's health care providers,[17] and physicians are thus often unaware of concurrent CAM use.[133] In a survey of adults who used both conventional and CAM therapies, Eisenberg and colleagues found that the most common reasons for nondisclosure of CAM use were "It wasn't important for your doctor to know" and "Your doctor never asked."[134] Other reasons for nondisclosure included a sense of privacy ("None of your doctor's business") and fear of physician disapproval, discouragement, or abandonment. Parents often express a desire to discuss CAM use with their child's pediatrician[135] but have been disappointed by the physician's inexperience with or lack of knowledge about CAM therapies.[10,136] Because there is a real possibility for harm to result from indiscriminate or uninformed use of CAM, as either alternative or adjunctive therapy, it is essential for developmental-behavioral pediatricians and allied professionals to incorporate discussions about CAM therapies into their routine care of children with developmental-behavioral disorders.

The American Academy of Pediatrics recommends that clinicians provide families with information on a range of treatment options, including CAM.[133] This requires the clinician to seek education in CAM interventions, evidence of efficacy, side effects, and potential interactions and other risks (Table 8E-8). In initial discussions with families, clinicians should investigate what CAM therapies families have used and are currently using, the perceived efficacy of these therapies, and other therapies families may be interested in using in the future. Frank discussions to clarify the

---

TABLE 8E-8 ■ CAM Resources on the Web

General Information on CAM Therapies

National Center for Complementary and Alternative Medicine, NIH	*www.nccam.nih.gov* Are you considering using Complementary and Alternative Medicine? (*http://nccam.nih.gov/health/decisions/index.htm*) 10 Things to Know About Evaluating Medical Resources on the Web (*http://nccam.nih.gov/health/webresources/*) Selecting a Complementary and Alternative Medicine (CAM) Practitioner (*http://nccam.nih.gov/health/practitioner/index.htm*) Consumer Financial Issues in Complementary and Alternative Medicine (*http://nccam.nih.gov/health/financial/index.htm*) What's in the Bottle? An Introduction to Dietary Supplements (*http://nccam.nih.gov/health/bottle/*)	Premier national resource for health information, research, and alerts on CAM; CAM consumer guides
Office of Dietary Supplements, NIH	*www.ods.od.nih.gov*	Coordinates and conducts research on dietary supplements; compiles and disseminates research results

Evidence and Alerts for Safety, Interactions, and Effectiveness

CAM on PubMed	*www.nlm.nih.gov/nccam/camonpubmed.html*	Database of citations and abstracts of peer-reviewed scientific studies on CAM, developed by NCCAM and the National Library of Medicine
International Bibliographic Information on Dietary Supplements (IBIDS) Database, Office of Dietary Supplements, NIH	*www.ods.od.nih.gov/databases/ibids.html*	Database of citations and abstracts of scientific literature on dietary supplements, developed by the Office of Dietary Supplements, NIH
Center for Food Safety & Applied Nutrition, FDA	*www.cfsan.fda.gov*	Includes food and drug fact sheets and safety standards

TABLE 8E-8 ■ CAM Resources on the Web—cont'd

MedWatch, FDA	*www.fda.gov/medwatch/report/consumer/consumer.htm*	To report serious adverse events or illnesses related to FDA-regulated products such as drugs, medical devices, medical foods, and dietary supplements
Federal Trade Commission, Diet, Health, and Fitness Consumer Information	*www.ftc.gov/bcp/menu-health.htm*	Fraudulent claims and consumer alerts for specific therapies
Quackwatch and Autism Watch	*www.quackwatch.org* *www.autism-watch.org*	Addresses health-related frauds, myths, fads, and fallacies, including questionable claims, misleading advertising on the Internet, and illegal marketing; consumer protection and strategies

Continuing Education for Health Professionals

Complementary and Alternative Medicine Online Continuing Education Series	*http://nccam.nih.gov/videolectures*	Six video lectures (Overview of CAM, Herbs and Other Dietary Supplements, Mind-Body Medicine, Acupuncture, Manipulative and Body-Based Therapies, CAM and Aging) for health care providers and the public, with question and answer transcript and online test for CME and CUE credits
Northwest Area Health Education Center Online Professional Curriculum on Herbs and Supplements	*http://northwestahec.wfubmc.edu/learn/herbs/index.asp*	Online (email and Web-based) Continuing Education activity on herbs and dietary supplements; provides evidence-based, self-instructional modules on over 100 herbs and dietary supplements; teaches how to report any adverse effects; provides links to other resources
Wake Forest University Baptist Medical Center Program for Holistic and Integrative Medicine	*http://www1.wfubmc.edu/phim*	News articles, presentations, meeting schedules
Evidence-based Complementary and Alternative Medicine (Oxford Journal)	*http://ecam.oxfordjournals.org/*	International, peer-reviewed journal that seeks to encourage rigorous research in CAM; includes lecture series, reviews, education sections

CAM, complementary and alternative medicine; CME, continuing medical education; CUE, continuing university education; FDA, U.S. Food and Drug Administration; NCCAM, National Center for Complementary and Alternative Medicine; NIH, National Institutes of Health.

caregiver's treatment goals (e.g., prevention, cure, symptom management, simplifying therapy, minimizing medication side effects, promoting health) and expectations (e.g., target symptoms, degree of improvement, time frame for effects to occur, potential time lost by not using conventional treatments) can help reduce frustration for both families and clinicians.[137,138] Establishing a line of communication, with agreements on both sides to share information and in decision making, is essential for a successful therapeutic alliance that incorporates CAM use. Clinicians can also help parents become educated consumers and critical appraisers of CAM advertising by directing them to credible sources of information, particularly the NCCAM Web site, which has several useful consumer guides to CAM.

Finally, clinicians can also work closely with families to conduct systematic evaluations of a specific therapy by using an "N of 1" trial technique. In such a trial, the child serves as his or her own control in a series of crossovers from "on" (active therapy) and "off" (routine care or placebo, if available) conditions. With the use of objective measures and raters unaware of condition, this can be a powerful tool for demonstrating effectiveness of a CAM intervention and is the practicing clinician's best alternative to a large, well-designed, randomized controlled trial.

CONCLUSION

Health and other allied professionals who care for children with developmental-behavioral conditions inevitably encounter families who are interested in using complementary and alternative therapies to treat their child. Having an understanding of the variety of CAM modalities and specific therapies commonly used in this group of children, as well as a standard approach for incorporating CAM into clinical practice, allows clinicians to develop effective therapeutic alliances with families.

REFERENCES

1. Eisenberg DM, Kessler RC, Foster C, et al: Unconventional medicine in the United States. Prevalence, costs, and patterns of use. N Engl J Med 328:246-252, 1993.
2. Barnes PM, Powell-Griner E, McFann K, et al: Complementary and alternative medicine use among adults: United States, 2002. Adv Data (343):1-19, 2004.
3. Davis MP, Darden PM: Use of complementary and alternative medicine by children in the United States. Arch Pediatr Adolesc Med 157:393-396, 2003.
4. Yussman SM, Ryan SA, Auinger P, et al: Visits to complementary and alternative medicine providers by children and adolescents in the United States. Ambul Pediatr 4:429-435, 2004.
5. Ottolini MC, Hamburger EK, Loprieato JO, et al: Complementary and alternative medicine use among children in the Washington, DC area. Ambul Pediatr 1:122-125, 2001.
6. Sawni-Sikand A, Schubiner H, Thomas RL: Use of complementary/alternative therapies among children in primary care pediatrics. Ambul Pediatr 2:99-103, 2002.
7. Simpson N, Pearce A, Finlay F, et al: The use of complementary medicine in paediatric outpatient clinics. Ambul Child Health 3:351-356, 1998.
8. Spigelblatt L, Laine-Ammara G, Pless IB, et al: The use of alternative medicine by children. Pediatrics 94(6, Pt 1):811-814, 1994.
9. Sanders H, Davis MF, Duncan B, et al: Use of complementary and alternative medical therapies among children with special health care needs in southern Arizona. Pediatrics 111:584-587, 2003.
10. Prussing E, Sobo EJ, Walker E, et al: Communicating with pediatricians about complementary/alternative medicine: Perspectives from parents of children with Down syndrome. Ambul Pediatr 4:488-494, 2004.
11. Nickel R: Controversial therapies for young children with developmental disabilities. Infants Young Child 8:29-40, 1996.
12. Hurvitz EA, Leonard C, Ayyangar R, et al: Complementary and alternative medicine use in families of children with cerebral palsy. Dev Med Child Neurol 45:364-370, 2003.
13. Stubberfield T, Parry T: Utilization of alternative therapies in attention-deficit hyperactivity disorder. J Paediatr Child Health 35:450-453, 1999.
14. Astin JA: Why patients use alternative medicine: Results of a national study. JAMA 279:1548-1553, 1998.
15. Pagan JA, Pauly MV: Access to conventional medical care and the use of complementary and alternative medicine. Health Aff (Millwood) 24:255-262, 2005.
16. Prussing E, Sobo EJ, Walker E, et al: Between "desperation" and disability rights: A narrative analysis of complementary/alternative medicine use by parents for children with Down syndrome. Soc Sci Med 60:587-598, 2005.
17. Chan E, Rappaport LA, Kemper KJ: Complementary and alternative therapies in childhood attention and hyperactivity problems. J Dev Behav Pediatr 24:4-8, 2003.
18. Mandell DS, Novak M: The role of culture in families' treatment decisions for children with autism spectrum disorders. Ment Retard Dev Disabil Res Rev 11:110-115, 2005.
19. National Center for Complementary and Alternative Medicine, National Institutes of Health: What Is Complementary and Alternative Medicine (CAM)? (Available at: *http://nccam.nih.gov/health/whatiscam/*; accessed 11/1/06.)
20. Boon H, Verhoef M, O'Hara D, et al: From parallel practice to integrative health care: A conceptual framework. BMC Health Serv Res 4:15, 2004.
21. Guyatt GH, Sackett DL, Cook DJ: Users' guides to the medical literature. II. How to use an article about therapy or prevention. A. Are the results of the study valid? Evidence-Based Medicine Working Group. JAMA 270:2598-2601, 1993.
22. Guyatt GH, Sackett DL, Cook DJ: Users' guides to the medical literature. II. How to use an article about therapy or prevention. B. What were the results and will they help me in caring for my patients? Evidence-Based Medicine Working Group. JAMA 271:59-63, 1994.
23. Sandler A: Placebo effects in developmental disabilities: Implications for research and practice. Ment Retard Dev Disabil Res Rev 11:164-170, 2005.
24. Ani C, Grantham-McGregor S, Muller D: Nutritional supplementation in Down syndrome: Theoretical considerations and current status. Dev Med Child Neurol 42:207-213, 2000.

25. Salman M: Systematic review of the effect of therapeutic dietary supplements and drugs on cognitive function in subjects with Down syndrome. Eur J Paediatr Neurol 6:213-219, 2002.

26. National Center for Complementary and Alternative Medicine, National Institutes of Health: What's in the Bottle? An Introduction to Dietary Supplements. (Available at: *http://nccam.nih.gov/health/bottle/index.htm#q2;* accessed 11/1/06.)

27. Shannon W: Neuropathologic manifestations in infants and children as a result of anaphylactic reaction to foods contained in their diet. Am J Dis Child 24:89-94, 1922.

28. Feingold BE: Why Your Child is Hyperactive. New York: Random House, 1975.

29. Williams JI, Cram DM: Diet in the management of hyperkinesis: A review of the tests of Feingold's hypotheses. Can Psychiatr Assoc J 23:241-248, 1978.

30. Mattes JA: The Feingold diet: A current reappraisal. J Learn Disabil 16:319-323, 1983.

31. Wender EH: The food additive-free diet in the treatment of behavior disorders: A review. J Dev Behav Pediatr 7:35-42, 1986.

32. Kavale KA, Forness SR: Hyperactivity and diet treatment: A meta-analysis of the Feingold hypothesis. J Learn Disabil 16:324-330, 1983.

33. Bateman B, Warner JO, Hutchinson E, et al: The effects of a double blind, placebo controlled, artificial food colourings and benzoate preservative challenge on hyperactivity in a general population sample of preschool children. Arch Dis Child 89:506-511, 2004.

34. Dengate S, Ruben A: Controlled trial of cumulative behavioural effects of a common bread preservative. J Paediatr Child Health 38:373-376, 2002.

35. Rojas NL, Chan E: Old and new controversies in the alternative treatment of attention-deficit hyperactivity disorder. Ment Retard Dev Disabil Res Rev 11:116-130, 2005.

36. Langseth L, Dowd J: Glucose tolerance and hyperkinesis. Food Cosmet Toxicol 16:129-133, 1978.

37. Speer F: The allergic tension-fatigue syndrome. Pediatr Clin North Am 25:1029-1037, 1954.

38. Wolraich ML, Stumbo PJ, Milich R, et al: Dietary characteristics of hyperactive and control boys. J Am Diet Assoc 86:500-504, 1986.

39. Wolraich ML, Wilson DB, White JW: The effect of sugar on behavior or cognition in children. A meta-analysis. JAMA 274:1617-1621, 1995.

40. Avena NM, Hoebel BG: A diet promoting sugar dependency causes behavioral cross-sensitization to a low dose of amphetamine. Neuroscience 122:17-20, 2003.

41. Avena NM, Hoebel BG: Amphetamine-sensitized rats show sugar-induced hyperactivity (cross-sensitization) and sugar hyperphagia. Pharmacol Biochem Behav 74:635-639, 2003.

42. Avena NM, Rada P, Moise N, et al: Sucrose sham feeding on a binge schedule releases accumbens dopamine repeatedly and eliminates the acetylcholine satiety response. Neuroscience 139:813-820, 2006.

43. Shattock P, Whiteley P: Biochemical aspects in autism spectrum disorders: Updating the opioid-excess theory and presenting new opportunities for biomedical intervention. Expert Opin Ther Targets 6:175-183, 2002.

44. Levy SE, Hyman SL: Novel treatments for autistic spectrum disorders. Ment Retard Dev Disabil Res Rev 11:131-142, 2005.

45. Knivsberg AM, Reichelt KL, Hoien T, et al: A randomised, controlled study of dietary intervention in autistic syndromes. Nutr Neurosci 5:251-261, 2002.

46. Elder JH, Shankar M, Shuster J, et al: The gluten-free, casein-free diet in autism: Results of a preliminary double blind clinical trial. J Autism Dev Disord 36:413-420, 2006.

47. Horvath K, Stefanatos G, Sokolski KN, et al: Improved social and language skills after secretin administration in patients with autistic spectrum disorders. J Assoc Acad Minor Phys 9:9-15, 1998.

48. Kern JK, Espinoza E, Trivedi MH: The effectiveness of secretin in the management of autism. Expert Opin Pharmacother 5:379-387, 2004.

49. Sturmey P: Secretin is an ineffective treatment for pervasive developmental disabilities: A review of 15 double-blind randomized controlled trials. Res Dev Disabil 26:87-97, 2005.

50. Williams KW, Wray JJ, Wheeler DM: Intravenous secretin for autism spectrum disorder. Cochrane Database Syst Rev (3):CD003495, 2005.

51. Dietrich KN, Ware JH, Salganik M, et al: Effect of chelation therapy on the neuropsychological and behavioral development of lead-exposed children after school entry. Pediatrics 114:19-26, 2004.

52. Deaths associated with hypocalcemia from chelation therapy—Texas, Pennsylvania, and Oregon, 2003-2005. MMWR Morb Mortal Wkly Rep 55:204-207, 2006.

53. Institute of Medicine: Immunization Safety Review: Vaccines and Autism. Washington, DC: National Academies Press, 2004.

54. Chico Hyperbaric Center: Cerebral Palsy and HBO Therapy. (Available at: *http://www.hbotoday.com/treatment/cp;* accessed 11/1/06.)

55. McDonagh MS, Carson S, Ash JS, et al: Hyperbaric Oxygen Therapy for Brain Injury, Cerebral Palsy, and Stroke. Evidence Report/Technology Assessment No. 85 (Prepared by the Oregon Health & Science University Evidence-based Practice Center under Contract No. 290-97-0018). AHRQ Publication No. 04-E003. Rockville, MD: Agency for Healthcare Research and Quality, 2003.

56. Montgomery D, Goldberg J, Amar M, et al: Effects of hyperbaric oxygen therapy on children with spastic diplegic cerebral palsy: A pilot project. Undersea Hyperb Med 26:235-242, 1999.

57. Collet JP, Vanasse M, Marois P, et al: Hyperbaric oxygen for children with cerebral palsy: A randomised multicentre trial. HBO-CP Research Group. Lancet 357:582-586, 2001.

58. Hardy P, Collet JP, Goldberg J, et al: Neuropsychological effects of hyperbaric oxygen therapy in cerebral palsy. Dev Med Child Neurol 44:436-446, 2002.

59. Liptak GS: Complementary and alternative therapies for cerebral palsy. Ment Retard Dev Disabil Res Rev 11:156-163, 2005.

60. McEwen BS: Protective and damaging effects of stress mediators. N Engl J Med 338:171-179, 1998.

61. Nash JK: Treatment of attention deficit hyperactivity disorder with neurotherapy. Clin Electroencephalogr 31:30-37, 2000.

62. Lubar JF, Bianchini KJ, Calhoun WH, et al: Spectral analysis of EEG differences between children with and without learning disabilities. J Learn Disabil 18:403-408, 1985.

63. Mann CA, Lubar JF, Zimmerman AW, et al: Quantitative analysis of EEG in boys with attention-deficit-hyperactivity disorder: Controlled study with clinical implications. Pediatr Neurol 8:30-36, 1992.

64. Ramirez P, Desantis D, Opler L: EEG biofeedback treatment of ADD: A viable alternative to traditional medical intervention? Ann N Y Acad Sci 931:342-358, 2001.

65. Heywood C, Beale I: EEG biofeedback vs. placebo treatment for attention-deficit/hyperactivity disorder: A pilot study. J Atten Disord 7:43-55, 2003.

66. Sugarman LI: Hypnosis in a primary care practice: developing skills for the "new morbidities." J Dev Behav Pediatr 17:300-305, 1996.

67. Lee LH, Olness KN: Effects of self-induced mental imagery on autonomic reactivity in children. J Dev Behav Pediatr 17:323-327, 1996.

68. Vandenberg B: Hypnotic responsivity from a developmental perspective: Insights from young children. Int J Clin Exp Hypn 50:229-247, 2002.

69. Lambert SA: The effects of hypnosis/guided imagery on the postoperative course of children. J Dev Behav Pediatr 17:307-310, 1996.

70. Holden EW, Deichmann MM, Levy JD: Empirically supported treatments in pediatric psychology: Recurrent pediatric headache. J Pediatr Psychol 24:91-109, 1999.

71. Hackman RM, Stern JS, Gershwin ME: Hypnosis and asthma: A critical review. J Asthma 37:1-15, 2000.

72. Glazener CM, Evans JH, Cheuk DK: Complementary and miscellaneous interventions for nocturnal enuresis in children. Cochrane Database Syst Rev (2): CD005230, 2005.

73. Johnson LS, Johnson DL, Olson MR, et al: The uses of hypnotherapy with learning disabled children. J Clin Psychol 37:291-299, 1981.

74. Goldbeck L, Schmid K: Effectiveness of autogenic relaxation training on children and adolescents with behavioral and emotional problems. J Am Acad Child Adolesc Psychiatry 42:1046-1054, 2003.

75. Warner D, Barabasz A, Barabasz M: The efficacy of Barabasz's alert hypnosis and neurotherapy on attentiveness, impulsivity and hyperactivity in children with ADHD. Child Study J 30:43-49, 2000.

76. Mauersberger K, Artz K, Duncan B, et al: Can children with spastic cerebral palsy use self-hypnosis to reduce muscle tone? A preliminary study. Integr Med 2:93-96, 2000.

77. Ayres A: Sensory Integration and Learning Disorders. Los Angeles, CA: Western Psychological Services, 1972.

78. Schaaf RC, Miller LJ: Occupational therapy using a sensory integrative approach for children with developmental disabilities. Ment Retard Dev Disabil Res Rev 11:143-148, 2005.

79. Ahn RR, Miller LJ, Milberger S, et al: Prevalence of parents' perceptions of sensory processing disorders among kindergarten children. Am J Occup Ther 58:287-293, 2004.

80. Miller LJ, McIntosh DN, McGrath J, et al: Electrodermal responses to sensory stimuli in individuals with fragile X syndrome: A preliminary report. Am J Med Genet. 83:268-279, 1999.

81. Schaaf RC, Miller LJ, Seawell D, et al: Children with disturbances in sensory processing: A pilot study examining the role of the parasympathetic nervous system. Am J Occup Ther 57:442-449, 2003.

82. Mangeot SD, Miller LJ, McIntosh DN, et al: Sensory modulation dysfunction in children with attention-deficit-hyperactivity disorder. Dev Med Child Neurol 43:399-406, 2001.

83. Vargas S, Camilli G: A meta-analysis of research on sensory integration treatment. Am J Occup Ther 53:189-198, 1999.

84. Arendt RE, MacLean WE Jr, Baumeister AA: Critique of sensory integration therapy and its application in mental retardation. Am J Ment Retard 92:401-429, 1988.

85. Hoehn TP, Baumeister AA: A critique of the application of sensory integration therapy to children with learning disabilities. J Learn Disabil 27:338-350, 1994.

86. Dawson G, Watling R: Interventions to facilitate auditory, visual, and motor integration in autism: A review of the evidence. J Autism Dev Disord 30:415-421, 2000.

87. Sinha Y, Silove N, Wheeler D, et al: Auditory integration training and other sound therapies for autism spectrum disorders. Cochrane Database Syst Rev (1): CD003681, 2004.

88. Committee on Children with Disabilities: Auditory Integration Training and Facilitated Communication for Autism. Pediatrics 102:431-433, 1998.

89. Biklen D, Morton M, Gold D, et al: Facilitated communication: Implications for individuals with autism. Top Lang Disord 12:1-28, 1992.

90. Hostler S, Allaire J, Christoph R: Childhood sexual abuse reported by facilitated communication. Pediatrics 91:1190-1192, 1993.

91. Jacobson J, Mulick J, Schwartz A: A history of facilitated communication: Science, pseudoscience, and antiscience. Am Psychol 50:750-765, 1995.

92. Robinson R, Boyle P, Garvey P: Ocular interventions, excluding correction of significant refractive error, for specific reading disorder (Protocol). Cochrane Database Syst Rev (4):CD005140, 2004.

93. Kaplan M, Edelson SM, Seip JA: Behavioral changes in autistic individuals as a result of wearing ambient

transitional prism lenses. Child Psychiatry Hum Dev 29:65-76, 1998.

94. Committee on Children with Disabilities: Learning disabilities, dyslexia, and vision: A subject review. Pediatrics 102:1217-1219, 1998.

95. Rawstron JA, Burley CD, Elder MJ: A systematic review of the applicability and efficacy of eye exercises. J Pediatr Ophthalmol Strabismus 42:82-88, 2005.

96. Gold C, Wigram T: Music therapy for autistic spectrum disorder. Cochrane Database Syst Rev (3):CD004381, 2003.

97. Trevarthen C: Musicality and the intrinsic motive pulse: Evidence from human psychobiology and infant communication. Musicae Scientiae (Special Issue 1999-2000):155-215, 1999.

98. Kaplan RS, Steele AL: An analysis of music therapy program goals and outcomes for clients with diagnoses on the autism spectrum. J Music Ther 42:2-19, 2005.

99. Whipple J: Music in intervention for children and adolescents with autism: A meta-analysis. J Music Ther 41:90-106, 2004.

100. Kaptchuk TJ: Acupuncture: Theory, efficacy, and practice. Ann Intern Med. 136:374-383, 2002.

101. He LF: Involvement of endogenous opioid peptides in acupuncture analgesia. Pain 31:99-121, 1987.

102. Streitberger K, Kleinhenz J: Introducing a placebo needle into acupuncture research. Lancet 352:364-365, 1998.

103. Sanner C, Sundequist U: Acupuncture for the relief of painful muscle spasms in dystonic cerebral palsy. Dev Med Child Neurol 23:544-545, 1981.

104. Duncan B, Barton L, Edmonds D, et al: Parental perceptions of the therapeutic effect from osteopathic manipulation or acupuncture in children with spastic cerebral palsy. Clin Pediatr (Phila) 43:349-353, 2004.

105. Sun JG, Ko CH, Wong V, et al: Randomised control trial of tongue acupuncture versus sham acupuncture in improving functional outcome in cerebral palsy. J Neurol Neurosurg Psychiatry 75:1054-1057, 2004.

106. Wong V, Sun JG, Wong W: Traditional Chinese medicine (tongue acupuncture) in children with drooling problems. Pediatr Neurol 25:47-54, 2001.

107. Ernst E, White AR: Prospective studies of the safety of acupuncture: A systematic review. Am J Med 110:481-485, 2001.

108. Roizen NJ: Complementary and alternative therapies for Down syndrome. Ment Retard Dev Disabil Res Rev 11:149-155, 2005.

109. Klaiman P, Witzel MA, Margar-Bacal F, et al: Changes in aesthetic appearance and intelligibility of speech after partial glossectomy in patients with Down syndrome. Plast Reconstr Surg 82:403-408, 1988.

110. Margar-Bacal F, Witzel MA, Munro IR: Speech intelligibility after partial glossectomy in children with Down's syndrome. Plast Reconstr Surg 79:44-49, 1987.

111. Parsons CL, Iacono TA, Rozner L: Effect of tongue reduction on articulation in children with Down syndrome. Am J Ment Defic 91:328-332, 1987.

112. Strauss RP, Mintzker Y, Feuerstein R, et al: Social perceptions of the effects of Down syndrome facial surgery: A school-based study of ratings by normal adolescents. Plast Reconstr Surg 81:841-851, 1988.

113. Arndt EM, Lefebvre A, Travis F, et al: Fact and fantasy: Psychosocial consequences of facial surgery in 24 Down syndrome children. Br J Plast Surg 39:498-504, 1986.

114. Goeke J, Kassow D, May D, et al: Parental opinions about facial plastic surgery for individuals with Down syndrome. Ment Retard 41:29-34, 2003.

115. Reed WR, Beavers S, Reddy SK, et al: Chiropractic management of primary nocturnal enuresis. J Manipulative Physiol Ther 17:596-600, 1994.

116. Cullen LA, Barlow JH: A training and support programme for caregivers of children with disabilities: An exploratory study. Patient Educ Couns 55:203-209, 2004.

117. Escalona A, Field T, Singer-Strunck R, et al: Brief report: Improvements in the behavior of children with autism following massage therapy. J Autism Dev Disord 31:513-516, 2001.

118. Field T, Lasko D, Mundy P, et al: Brief report: Autistic children's attentiveness and responsivity improve after touch therapy. J Autism Dev Disord 27:333-338, 1997.

119. Field TM, Quintino O, Hernandez-Reif M, et al: Adolescents with attention deficit hyperactivity disorder benefit from massage therapy. Adolescence 33:103-108, 1998.

120. Khilnani S, Field T, Hernandez-Reif M, et al: Massage therapy improves mood and behavior of students with attention-deficit/hyperactivity disorder. Adolescence 38:623-638, 2003.

121. Bishop E, McKinnon E, Weir E, et al: Reflexology in the management of encopresis and chronic constipation. Paediatr Nurs 15:20-21, 2003.

122. Committee on Children with Disabilities: The treatment of neurologically impaired children using patterning. Pediatrics 104:1149-1151, 1999.

123. Michaud LJ, Committee on Children with Disabilities: Prescribing therapy services for children with motor disabilities. Pediatrics 113:1836-1838, 2004.

124. Sterba JA, Rogers BT, France AP, et al: Horseback riding in children with cerebral palsy: Effect on gross motor function. Dev Med Child Neurol 44:301-308, 2002.

125. Cherng R, Liao H, Leung H, et al: The effectiveness of therapeutic horseback riding in children with spastic CP. Adapt Phys Activ Q 21:103-121, 2004.

126. Benda W, McGibbon NH, Grant KL: Improvements in muscle symmetry in children with cerebral palsy after equine-assisted therapy (hippotherapy). Jl Altern Complementary Med 9:817-825, 2003.

127. Homeopathic Pharmacopoeia Convention of the United States: The Homeopathic Pharmacopoeia of the United States. (Available at: *http://www.hpus.com/*; accessed 11/1/06.)

128. Shang A, Huwiler-Muntener K, Nartey L, et al: Are the clinical effects of homoeopathy placebo effects?

Comparative study of placebo-controlled trials of homoeopathy and allopathy. Lancet 366:726-732, 2005.

129. Lamont J: Homeopathic treatment of attention deficit disorder. Br Homeopath J 86:196-200, 1997.

130. Strauss L: The efficacy of a homeopathic preparation in the management of attention deficit hyperactivity disorder. Biol Ther 18:197-201, 2000.

131. Frei H, Thurneysen A: Treatment for hyperactive children: Homeopathy and methylphenidate compared in a family setting. Br Homeopath J 90:183-188, 2001.

132. Frei H, Everts R, von Ammon K, et al: Homeopathic treatment of children with attention deficit hyperactivity disorder: A randomised, double blind, placebo controlled crossover trial. Eur J Pediatr 164:758-767, 2005.

133. Committee on Children with Disabilities: Counseling families who choose complementary and alternative medicine for their child with chronic illness or disability. Pediatrics 107:598-601, 2001.

134. Eisenberg DM, Kessler RC, Van Rompay MI, et al: Perceptions about complementary therapies relative to conventional therapies among adults who use both: Results from a national survey. Ann Intern Med 135:344-351, 2001.

135. Sibinga EMS, Ottolini MC, Duggan AK, et al: Parent-pediatrician communication about complementary and alternative medicine use for children. Clin Pediatr 43:367-373, 2004.

136. Kemper KJ, O'Connor KG: Pediatricians' recommendations for complementary and alternative medical (CAM) therapies. Ambul Pediatr 4:482-487, 2004.

137. Chan E: The role of complementary and alternative medicine in attention-deficit hyperactivity disorder. J Dev Behav Pediatr 23(1 Suppl):S37-S45, 2002.

138. Kemper KJ: Integrative medicine: Talking with families about complementary, alternative, and mainstream medical therapies in acute care settings. Emerg Office Pediatr 13:45-49, 2000.

139. Levy SE, Mandell DS, Merhar S, et al: Use of complementary and alternative medicine among children recently diagnosed with autistic spectrum disorder. J Dev Behav Pediatr 24:418-423, 2003.

140. Lockitch G, Puterman M, Godolphin W, et al: Infection and immunity in Down syndrome: A trial of long-term low oral doses of zinc. J Pediatr 114:781-787, 1989.

141. Bekaroglu M, Aslan Y, Gedik Y, et al: Relationships between serum free fatty acids and zinc, and attention

deficit hyperactivity disorder: A research note. J Child Psychol Psychiatry 37:225-227, 1996.

142. Arnold LE, Votolato NA, Kleykamp D, et al: Does hair zinc predict amphetamine improvement of ADD/hyperactivity? Int J Neurosci 50:103-107, 1990.

143. Kern JK, Miller VS, Cauller PL, et al: Effectiveness of *N,N*-dimethylglycine in autism and pervasive developmental disorder. J Child Neurol 16:169-173, 2001.

144. Bolman WM, Richmond JA: A double-blind, placebo-controlled, crossover pilot trial of low dose dimethylglycine in patients with autistic disorder. J Autism Dev Disord 29:191-194, 1999.

145. Richardson AJ, Montgomery P: The Oxford-Durham study: A randomized, controlled trial of dietary supplementation with fatty acids in children with developmental coordination disorder. Pediatrics 115:1360-1366, 2005.

146. Jan JE, O'Donnell ME: Use of melatonin in the treatment of paediatric sleep disorders. J Pineal Res 21:193-199, 1996.

147. Buscemi N, Vandermeer B, Pandya R, et al: Melatonin for Treatment of Sleep Disorders. Evidence Report/Technology Assessment No. 108 (Prepared by the University of Alberta Evidence-based Practice Center, under Contract No. 290-02-0023.) AHRQ Publication No. 05-E002-2. Rockville, MD: Agency for Healthcare Research and Quality, 2004.

148. Willey C, Phillips B: Is melatonin likely to help children with neurodevelopmental disability and chronic severe sleep problems? Arch Dis Child 87:260, 2002.

149. Nye C, Brice A: Combined vitamin B_6–magnesium treatment in autism spectrum disorder. Cochrane Database Syst Rev (4):CD003497, 2005.

150. Pueschel SM, Reed RB, Cronk CE, et al: 5-Hydroxytryptophan and pyridoxine. Their effects in young children with Down's syndrome. Am J Dis Child 134:838-844, 1980.

151. Coleman M, Sobel S, Bhagavan HN, et al: A double blind study of vitamin B_6 in Down's syndrome infants. Part 1—Clinical and biochemical results. J Ment Defic Res 29(Pt 3):233-240, 1985.

152. Hrastinger A, Dietz B, Bauer R, et al: Is there clinical evidence supporting the use of botanical dietary supplements in children? J Pediatr 146:311-317, 2005.

153. Francis AJ, Dempster RJ: Effect of valerian, *Valeriana edulis*, on sleep difficulties in children with intellectual deficits: Randomised trial. Phytomedicine 9:273-279, 2002.

Adaptation to General Health Problems and Their Treatment

OLLE JANE Z. SAHLER

This chapter reviews (1) how children learn to distinguish being sick from being healthy, what causes one to feel sick, and how to get better; (2) how sick children's understanding of health and illness states is similar to and yet different from that of healthy children; (3) how children adapt to or cope with stress; (4) how chronic illness stresses the child and family unit; (5) children's competency in medical decision making; (6) the importance of proactively transitioning chronically ill young adults to adult care; and (7) children's understanding of death. The crucial role of the cognitive developmental sequence in determining what pediatric patients understand and why they respond as they do to the need for adherence to treatment regimens is evident in virtually every aspect of any medical encounter. Time and repetition remain key elements in fostering understanding of illness and promoting healthy behaviors.

CHILDREN'S UNDERSTANDING OF HEALTH AND ILLNESS

In 1986, the First International Conference on Health Promotion defined child health as "the extent to which individual children or groups of children are able or enabled to: a) develop and realize their potential; b) satisfy their needs; and c) develop the capacities that allow them to interact successfully with their biological, physical, and social environments."[1] In 1997, the World Health Organization defined health as a state of complete physical, social, and mental well-being.[2]

Children are likely to give a fundamentally different answer to the question "What is health?" by defining what it is not: disease or disability. Much as a young child is more likely to learn the word *dead* before learning the word *alive* (because, to the anthropomorphic child, everything is alive), the young child is more likely to learn the word *sick* or *sickness* (as dif-ferent from the way a person feels every day) before learning the words *healthy* or *health*.

What is the child's conceptualization of illness? A number of investigators surveying children with a variety of illness types and in a variety of cultures[3-9] have consistently found that the child's understanding of illness is a stepwise process that evolves in a systematic and predictable sequence. A useful, although by no means the only, framework for understanding this evolution is Piaget's theory of cognitive development.[10,11] According to this paradigm, both biological and cognitive maturation and the accumulation of experiences facilitate a progression to sequentially more sophisticated stages of understanding. Salient characteristics of each stage include the progressive ability to engage in logical (operational) thought, to separate internal realities (wishes, desires, thoughts) from the external world, and to distinguish other people's points of view from one's own.

Children with almost any type of chronic illness have a more sophisticated understanding of disease, especially their own, than do healthy children, and their knowledge base can expand quickly with increasing experience with the disease.[12-14] Similarly, children in the general population have a better understanding of "everyday"-type illnesses—which they or a family member or friend have experienced—than they do of less common or unusual illnesses.[15] However, even younger children (e.g., those in kindergarten through sixth grade) can benefit from appropriate, developmentally based instruction about relatively complicated conditions, such as acquired immunodeficiency syndrome (AIDS), without engendering fear of contracting or being harmed by the illness.[5,16,17] Thus, acquired knowledge plays a role in children's conceptual development that augments gains in understanding purely from the maturational process or experience.

Understanding of illness in children as young as 4 to 6 years includes such dimensions as *identity* (what the illness is, including labels and symptoms); *consequences* (the short- and long-term effects); *time frame* (how long the illness usually lasts or how long it will take to get better); *cause* (factors contributing to the onset of the illness); and *cure* (actions needed to become well again). Young children's understanding of these dimensions of illness is similar to, although less mature and informed than, that of adults and appears to be an important influence on health-related beliefs and behavior.

Although preschool-aged children have limited understanding of their role in illness causation, most understand that they have a role to play in the remediation of illness, probably because they have already been asked to do so (e.g., take medication, drink lots of fluids, stay in bed). Thus, if clinicians desire to involve children in health decisions, they should provide appropriate, structured choices regarding the various treatment options available to encourage a patient's willing participation.[15]

Symptoms are the outward manifestation of disease and serve as the cues that enable children to identify and recognize illness. Studies of how children understand illness have typically been based on the conceptual complexity, factual content, and accuracy of their responses about causation and transmission.[4,5,18] Brewster[12] outlined a three-stage sequence of conceptual development in children's understanding of illness causation: (1) illness is caused by human action, (2) illness is caused by germs, and (3) illness is caused by physical weakness or susceptibility. Perrin and Gerrity[3] reinterpreted these findings as follows: (1) illness is the consequence of transgression against rules, (2) illness is caused by the mere presence of germs in the environment, and (3) illness may have many causes, including the body's particular response (host factor) to a variety of external agents that either cause or cure disease.

Piagetian Framework of Illness Conceptualization

Piaget[19] demonstrated that children exhibit a system of logic that is fundamentally different from that of adults, as they try to understand and explain basic concepts such as space, time, number, and causality. As the child's understanding of the world increases, the system of logic follows a developmental sequence that appears to be independent of specific cultural differences, although it is influenced by age, particularly developmental age, and by experience. In a landmark 1980 study, Bibace and Walsh[11] investigated the relationship between children's assimilation of their illness experience and Piaget's stages of cognitive development, especially causal reasoning. In particu-

lar, they investigated the degree of differentiation between self and others as a major determinant of differences in children's conceptions of health and illness.

PRELOGICAL CONCEPTUALIZATIONS

According to Piaget,[20] children between the ages of about 2 and 6 years are egocentric and unable to separate themselves from their environment. They are also anthropomorphic and bound by magical thinking. These characteristics typically result in explanations of causality that are undifferentiated, logically circular, and superstitious and that reflect the immediate spatial or temporal cues that dominate their experience. Juxtaposition in time or space is interpreted as having a cause-and-effect relationship (syncretism). They are unable to understand processes and mechanisms because they focus solely on one aspect of a situation or an object without attending to the whole. (For example, if a child of this age looks at two pencils of equal length that are aligned so that one pencil is placed below and an inch to the right of the upper pencil, the child will designate the lower pencil as longer if he or she focuses on the right side and will designate the upper pencil as longer if he or she focuses on the left side.) Children of this age also have little understanding of being sick, except as this is told to them ("Your face feels warm; you should go to bed" or, conversely, "You don't have a fever; go out and play"). Whereas getting sick may be seen as the consequence of a misbehavior ("If you had worn your boots as I told you to, you wouldn't have gotten sick"), getting well is seen as the result of following certain rules ("You'll get better if you stay in bed and drink lots of orange juice").[21] This just-world view (good behavior is rewarded and bad behavior is punished, or people get what they deserve) occurs when fairness judgments predominate over physical causality and is referred to as *immanent justice*. In the youngest children, the outcome of an act is more important than intent (breaking three dishes while helping to clear the dinner table is worse than breaking one dish when climbing up to a cupboard to get some forbidden candy stored there).

Two types of explanation about illness are characteristic of prelogical thinking: phenomenism and contagion. *Phenomenism* is considered the most developmentally immature explanation of illness causality. In this conceptualization, the child is unable to explain how spatially or temporally remote phenomena, which they ascribe as the causes of illnesses, actually have that effect. Example: "How do people get colds?" "From the sun." "How does the sun give you a cold?" "It just does, that's all."[11] *Contagion* theory explains the cause of illness as people or objects that are proximate, but not touching, the person. The link explaining how the illness is transmitted is magical. Example: "How do people get colds?" ". . . when someone else gets near you." "How?" "I don't know—by magic, I think."[11]

Raman and Gelman,[22] investigating children's understanding of transmission of genetic disorders and contagious illnesses, found that children as young as early school age were able to distinguish genetic disorders from contagious illnesses in the presence of kinship cues (e.g., "Someone else in the family has this condition."). In contrast, in the presence of contagion cues (e.g., "Someone coughed in your face."), preschoolers selectively applied contagious links primarily to contagious illnesses. When they were presented with descriptions of novel illnesses, children were most likely to infer that permanent illnesses were probably transmitted by birth parents rather than by contagion. Thus, even at the late preoperational stage, children appear to recognize that not all disorders are transmitted exclusively by germ contagion.

CONCRETE OPERATIONAL CONCEPTUALIZATIONS

Children aged about 7 to early adolescence are able to distinguish between self and others.[19] Unlike younger children, who have a univariate view of the world, older children are able to understand phenomena from multiple points of view and can understand relationships between events or objects (the pencils from the previous example are understood to be of equal length, just placed differently in space). By manipulating objects, the older child is also able to understand reversibility. However, hypothesis formation is not yet possible. In terms of understanding health and illness, the older child is likely to see external agents causing illness; getting well is a passive experience in which body systems play little or no role.

Two explanations are particularly salient: contamination and internalization. *Contamination* explanations are characterized by beginning to understand the cause of an illness and how this cause might act. Example: "How do people get [colds]?" "You're outside without a hat and you start sneezing. Your head would get cold—the cold would touch it—and then it would go all over your body."[11] *Internalization* refers to understanding that the cause of illness (person, object) might be outside the body, but it causes an illness that is inside the body by being incorporated within it. Typically, the child has little understanding of organs and organ systems. Example: "How do people get colds?" "In winter, they breathe in too much air into their nose, and it blocks up the nose." "How does this cause colds?" "The bacteria get in by breathing. Then the lungs get too soft [child exhales],

and it goes to the nose." "How does it get better?" "Hot fresh air, it gets in the nose and pushes the cold air back."[11]

FORMAL OPERATIONAL CONCEPTUALIZATIONS

Adolescence is marked by the transition to formal operational thinking: the ability to clearly differentiate self from others, the capability for logical thought, and freedom from the need to respond to or be circumscribed by immediate stimuli or real (concrete) objects (i.e., the ability to hypothesize). Adolescents are also able to fill in gaps of knowledge by reasoning from generalizations gleaned from their understanding of the concrete world. The most important feature of this stage is the ability to understand that the source of an illness may be located within the body (host response), even though an external agent interacting with the body may be the ultimate cause of the illness. Thus, they are capable of understanding the general principles of infection, health maintenance, and treatment. Adolescents also can define illness as an internal feeling of not being well, even in the absence of external signs or symptoms.

Formal operational explanations tend to be physiological or psychophysiological. *Physiological* explanations place the source or nature of an illness within specific body parts or functions. Example: "What is a cold?" "It's when you get all stuffed up inside, your sinuses get filled up with mucus . . . ." "How do people get colds?" "They come from viruses. . . . Other people get the virus and it gets into your bloodstream."[11] *Psychophysiological* explanations are among the most sophisticated responses. Building on the physiological model, the child recognizes that thoughts or feelings can affect how the body functions. Example: "What is a heart attack?" "It's when your heart stops working right. Sometimes it's pumping too slow or too fast." "How do people get a heart attack?" ". . . You worry too much. The tension can affect your heart."[11]

SICK CHILDREN'S UNDERSTANDING OF ILLNESS

Children process information about their own illnesses according to a predictable sequence of cognitive maturation[12] that is similar to their understanding of illness in general. They understand first human causation (especially doing something "wrong"), followed by the germ theory, the differentiation of causes depending on the type of condition, and finally an interactional model, in which physical or psychological susceptibility and external factors act together to cause illness. Although this sequence is no different from that in healthy children, having an illness can influence the rapidity with which children pass through the various stages of understanding. Crisp and colleagues[14] found that experience with a chronic illness (present for 3 or more months, involving repeated hospitalizations, or interfering with normal childhood activity) increases children's understanding at various ages; this increase may be especially prominent at the transition points between Piaget's stages of cognitive functioning. However, this greater sophistication does not necessarily generalize beyond the child's specific condition. For example, children with cancer do not necessarily know more than their healthy peers about the common cold.[14] Krishnan and associates[23] actually raised the question about whether children with a chronic disease are resistant to learning about new medical information that has no bearing on their own illness.

What Is Being "Sick"?

An important issue is the child's perception of what is considered illness in the context of self and what is not. Note, for example, the following exchange with an 8-year-old boy with Legg-Perthes disease, published by Brewster:[12] "How does someone get sick?" "Because they touch something. I mean because they eat junk." "How did you get sick?" "I didn't." "Why did you come?" "My leg got hurt." "How?" "I was born with a leg like this." "How did it happen?" "I don't know." For this boy, having Legg-Perthes disease fits into the same category of personal physical characteristics as having brown eyes or curly hair: "I have it, it's a fact of my life." In contrast, being "sick" is a state other than baseline, and the most common sicknesses are viral infections, especially gastroenteritis or colds. When children of this age think about illnesses, they are most likely to consider those conditions that they, their family, and their friends have experienced that preclude them from their usual participation in activities of daily living (e.g., school, playing).

This perception of Legg-Perthes disease or such chronic disorders as cystic fibrosis or inflammatory bowel disease as "not sick" protects the child from feeling different or having to play the sick role continuously. In fact, "forgetting" that he or she has a chronic disease and incorporating the condition into the child's perception of self can serve as a useful adaptive mechanism. Being sick then becomes a state of having another, different condition that acutely changes or limits the child's activity or behavior. Maladaptation arises when the child denies an underlying condition that requires special, specific treatments (e.g., enzyme therapy, prophylactic antibiotic therapy, immunosuppression), even when he or she is feeling well. This is especially true when children must alter typical, everyday behaviors (e.g., stop playing) to receive treatment (chest physical therapy), in order to avoid some potential negative outcome (inspissated mucus plugging) in the future.

Did I Cause My Illness?

Despite an advanced understanding of their own disease, children may experience egocentric or magical thinking, especially about causation. In fact, adults may also experience such egocentrism ("I know that my child's cancer is caused by bad white blood cells, but I wonder if I did something to cause it"). Brewster[12] found that such magical thinking was especially likely to occur at times of great stress, when temporary regression to earlier developmental stages is common. This regression results in a state of "cognitive dissonance." For example, children (and adults) may maintain a notion of personal culpability (sense of guilt) despite "knowing better" and understanding logical explanations for illness causation.

In the mid-20th century, Gardner[24] hypothesized that guilt (acknowledgment of "something bad I did") served to protect parents of children with severe physical illnesses against the feelings of helplessness that might otherwise overwhelm them were they to believe that their child's condition was merely the result of random chance. In this context, Gardner urged health care personnel to be wary of assuaging guilt feelings of parents—and older children, especially adolescents—too quickly, if such feelings serve a useful purpose in the search for meaning. Eliminating a defense is hazardous without some reasonable expectation that a more constructive concept will take its place. In the final analysis, the clinician's hearing and understanding what the patient or parent is saying and why are more important than the patient's or parent's hearing and understanding what the clinician is saying.

The Evolution of the Concept of Being Sick

Table 9-1 provides insight into the evolution of sick children's thinking about health—and death—as their illness progresses. This particular schema is most useful when there is an abrupt onset of "disease," so that the moment of diagnosis is a discrete event coinciding with a perceived state of illness. This is different for children with cystic fibrosis, for example, when the "diagnosis" typically occurs as the result of a laboratory study performed in the context of ongoing concern about the child's growth or general state of health, rather than in response to an acute event that is easily recognized as signaling being "sick." In this

TABLE 9-1 ■ Stages in Sick Children's Acquisition of Information about Their Illness			
Stage	Medical Status	Child's Information	Child's Self-Concept
First	Diagnosis	"It" is a serious illness (may not know disease name)	I was well but am now sick.
Second	Remission (child meets/talks to other ill children)	Names of drugs, how given, and side effects	I am sick but will get better.
Third	First relapse	Purposes of procedures/treatments; relationship between procedures and particular symptoms	I am always sick but will get better.
Fourth	Several relapses and remissions	Disease perceived as an endless series of relapses and remissions	I am always sick and will never get better.
Fifth	Child learns of the death of an ill peer	Disease perceived as a series of relapses and remissions ending in death	I am dying.

Adapted from Bluebond-Langer M: The Private Worlds of Dying Children. Princeton, NJ: Princeton University Press, 1978.

instance, the moment of diagnosis is less clear and the transition from "maybe" being sick to "really" being sick is more problematic. For children who experience a gradually progressive, almost imperceptible decline over long intervals, the series of discrete steps exemplified by cancer relapse and remission is not as obvious. Over time, however, the general principles of increasing experience, interaction with others in similar circumstances, and the growing understanding that certain skills or functions are being either lost or never fully developing, serve as the basis for these patients' advanced knowledge about their illness.

Unlike children with cancer or other progressively deteriorating conditions, children with non–life-threatening handicapping conditions typically do not progress to the fifth stage (see Table 9-1). Instead, they habituate to the fourth stage. Instead of seeing themselves as "sick," they are more likely to see themselves as "different." In fact, children with such conditions as spina bifida, seizure disorder, hemophilia, or cerebral palsy reject the notion of sickness unless they have an illness (e.g., a cold, gastroenteritis) that any member of the general population would consider a sign of being sick.

Hidden Disabilities

Children with such "hidden" disabilities as diabetes, sickle cell anemia, dyslexia or other learning disability, or a psychiatric disorder such as anxiety face unique challenges. In the optimal scenario, such children develop a self-perception that positively integrates their experience of disability and enables them to cope with their limitations and adjust to the expectations of society.[25] Unfortunately, this is a cognitive process that frequently does not become manifest until late adolescence or young adulthood, if ever. In the meantime, dependence on peers and diminished

acceptance by the peer group, which can be particularly cruel to anyone who is perceived as different, can result in years of social isolation that is either imposed by the group or self-imposed.

Disclosure to Friends

The desire to not tell friends or classmates about an illness or condition is common, especially among preteenagers and young adolescents who are most concerned with social acceptance. Children with an acute onset of disease, such as cancer, frequently have little choice regarding disclosure, because disfigurement (e.g., alopecia, loss of a limb, steroid-induced obesity) is obvious and can lead to merciless taunting if no explanation is offered. News of a diagnosis of cancer tends to spread quickly and the community often reacts with compassion, tempered by misperceptions of what causes cancer and concerns about its transmissibility. Social reintegration after hospitalization may be promoted through, for example, meetings with school personnel and classmates to explain the disease, the side effects of medication, the potential need for frequent hospitalizations, and the fact that cancer is not a contagious disease.

For the child or teenager with a chronic underlying condition such as sickle cell anemia, social reintegration after hospitalization for a pain crisis, for example, is typically less formal and frequently, at the child's insistence on secrecy, not done at all. Interestingly, the rise of human immunodeficiency virus (HIV) infection and AIDS has had a beneficial effect on the disclosure of sickle cell disease. Because both are blood diseases, children with sickle cell disease who were once reluctant to disclose their condition now prefer to do so, so that classmates will not assume that they have HIV infection or AIDS. In effect, they make their decision on the basis of what they perceive as the "lesser of two evils."

For other children, whether to disclose their illness can become an inescapable issue when asked to participate in sleepovers and class trips. Such interventions as insulin injections, chest physiotherapy, or colostomy bags may be impossible to hide. Most children are surprised when their friends and classmates are, aside from curious, also supportive.

The Role of Health Education

Health care personnel often assume that providing information to a child will lead to greater understanding and, as a result, better adherence to treatments. Yet this outcome is rarely realized, for several reasons: (1) children have their own conceptualization of what is happening to them; (2) their ability to assimilate information may be limited by their general level of cognitive functioning; and (3) other factors, particularly emotional factors, may further impede understanding.[12]

Although many educational interventions have been implemented in attempts to increase adherence to treatment regimens, only modest improvements have been found in certain clinical outcomes. A meta-analysis of educational programs for children with asthma revealed small to moderate gains in lung function, activity level, school attendance, and self-efficacy and decreases in emergency room visits.[26] Such modest findings are fairly typical for educational interventions, especially among children with chronic but nondisabling conditions. Current approaches must be modified in order to realize significant benefits.

In contrast, children and adolescents diagnosed with potentially life-threatening illnesses such as cancer are interested in knowing about their disease and treatment.[1] Knowledge appears to reduce anxiety and depression and to increase self-esteem. For teenagers, increased knowledge leads to more trusting relationships with staff and enhanced coping with painful procedures. The process of information sharing is not a one-time event but rather extends over a series of sessions that address the child's status and any anticipated changes in treatment.

Differences between children's views of cancer and asthma probably reflect the acuity, novelty, and perceived seriousness of the cancer diagnosis, as opposed to the low-level chronicity and the mistaken perception that asthma is not a life-threatening condition. Motivation is a key element in learning. Helping child and adolescent patients understand the long-term seriousness of a particular condition is hampered by their limited ability to understand consequences that are not immediately observable. Concrete information (e.g., viewing radiographs, seeing pulmonary function test results) and repeated experience may be helpful in hastening the process of understanding.

Before information is given, it is crucial to discover the child's conceptions about the medical situation and how such understanding may comfort the child. For example, an 8-year-old girl was watching the birth of her sibling. As the head emerged, she called out, "Her brains are coming out!" The obstetrician became extremely upset at what he perceived the girl to be saying and later vowed that he would never again have a sibling present at a delivery. However, on later investigation, the girl's exclamation was a purely observational comment. The whitish-gray vernix covering the molded head reminded her of pictures of the brain that she had seen in a magazine. She was not upset but instead excited and even delighted that she could relate the delivery to something in her experience. A more appropriate response from the obstetrician would have been "Yes, you're right. The baby's head is coming out, and the brains are inside the head."

This vignette emphasizes the importance of accurate communication between health care providers and children, in order to avoid the pitfalls of literal interpretation. In this instance, the child used imagery that was familiar to her to matter-of-factly describe an event. However, her comment was misinterpreted and inadvertently put the physician into a state of distress. How often do physicians do this to patients when they say that an injection is like a bee sting (and, therefore, something to be dreaded and avoided) or that an injection will not hurt (and, as a consequence, lose all credibility)? Clearly, a more appropriate preparation might be "This is going to hurt. You can cry or sing as loud as you want. If you sing, can I sing, too?"

CHILDREN'S ADAPTATION TO STRESS

Coping, or adaptation to stress, entails managing emotions, thinking constructively, regulating and directing behavior, controlling autonomic arousal, and acting on both social and physical environments to alter or decrease stressors.[27] Both mental and physical health are strongly influenced by exposure to and ability to cope with stress.

Eisenberg and colleagues[28] defined three aspects of coping, or self regulation: regulation of emotion (emotion-focused coping or emotional regulation); regulation of the situation (problem-focused coping); and regulation of emotionally driven behavior (behavior regulation). Compas and colleagues[27] add that the child's or adolescent's developmental level both contributes to and constrains the repertoire of mechanisms available for coping. Thus, infants have the capacity to self-soothe (e.g., sucking), a primitive, automatic, reflexive behavior. Conscious, volitional self-regulation does not appear until the development of the concept of intentionality, representational language, metacognition, and the capacity for delay. These are characteristics that first begin to emerge during the late preoperational or early concrete operational stages and are unlikely to be seen until early school age.

Rudolph and colleagues,[29] when considering a child's reaction to a stressor, identified three particular portions of that reaction: the *coping response* (the intentional physical or emotional action in response to a stress); the *coping goal* (the objective or intent of the coping response, which is usually to reduce the aversive effects of the stressor); and the *coping outcome* (the specific consequences of the person's deliberate, volitional attempts to reduce the stress). Attempts at coping may become maladaptive when the consequences of the coping response meet the initial coping goal but create a more severe stressor in its place. For example, a child might develop a headache in anticipation of a math test. The headache is severe enough that the child stays home from school. Absence results in not having to take the math test (realization of primary goal) but also causes the student to miss a key lesson in social studies, which then causes him or her to fall behind in that subject. Unless the student makes up the work quickly and does extra studying (added stress), it is likely that another headache will occur at the time of the social studies test. Over time, the headache becomes recurrent because of sequential isolated stress and then, eventually, progresses to chronic, persistent pain because of anxiety about poor academic performance in many areas (overwhelming stress).

Coping responses can be characterized according to a number of different types. *Behavioral versus cognitive coping* distinguishes between external modes of coping (e.g., overt, observable actions such as seeking information or support; holding someone's hand) and internal modes of coping (e.g., constructive self-talk such as "I can do this"; diversionary thinking). Another type distinguishes between *problem-focused coping* (eliminating or altering a distressing situation; constructive problem solving) and *emotion-focused coping* (regulating one's emotional reaction to a situation: positive reframing, acceptance). *Primary versus secondary coping* highlights the differences between altering the situation and maximizing the person's fit to the current situation in ways that are similar to problem-versus emotion-focused coping. *Approach versus avoidance* might be described as information seeking versus information avoiding or attention versus distraction. For example, during venipuncture,

some children want to see the needle, watch the needle being inserted, and calculate how long it will take for the tube to be filled with blood; other children want to look away and do not want to be told when the needle will be inserted, preferring to carry on a loud, unrelated conversation with a parent. Finally, another way to look at coping style is what Field and associates[30] described as sensitizers versus repressors. Sensitizers exhibit higher levels of anxiety before procedures, whereas repressors tend to be more fearful and disruptive during procedures and rate themselves as more distressed after procedures. Sparse research focuses on the efficacy of different coping approaches or whether it is more desirable for a child to have a few successful coping strategies[31] or many coping strategies in order to be prepared for a novel stressor.[32]

In summary, children's coping is a complex phenomenon. We should view coping not in terms of single, mutually exclusive categories of responses but rather as a multifaceted process. Crouch[33] developed a multidimensional model, COPE, that classifies coping along four separate, non-orthogonal dimensions: (1) control—primary versus secondary; (2) orientation (toward or away from the stressor)—attention versus distraction; (3) process (specific categories of coping thoughts and behaviors)—information seeking, support seeking, emotional regulation, and direct action; and (4) environmental match—the degree of match or mismatch between the child's coping goals or responses and the parent's or other caregiver's method of facilitating coping. This classification is a reminder that giving the child some level of control over how he or she will handle the stressor is crucial for successful coping. Furthermore, we can promote constructive coping by helping the child at his or her level of understanding and incrementally molding the response to become increasingly adaptive.

CHILDREN'S UNDERSTANDING OF DEATH

Until the mid-1970s, it was unusual for children to be given information about their illness. In particular, little was said about potentially fatal illness. Pioneering work by Spinetta,[34,35] among others, led to the discovery that children who were uninformed about their illness, its treatment, and the prognosis often felt lonely and isolated and were subject to frightening fantasies about their condition. These findings have led to greater openness, more developmentally appropriate explanations, and frequent invitations to the child to ask questions and express wishes and worries. Greater awareness of how children understand their illness and the unnecessary stress imposed by silence has led to better understanding of how children conceptualize death in general and how terminally ill children conceptualize their own death specifically.

Development of the Concept of Death

The acquisition of four basic cognitive concepts frames the stages of understanding death: *irreversibility* (death is permanent), *inevitability* or *universality* (all living things eventually must die), *finality* or *nonfunctionality* (dead people no longer have experiences or feelings), and *causality* (why a death occurs).[36]

A Piagetian framework helps explain observable behaviors that reflect cognitive understanding of death, like that of health and illness (Table 9-2). This, like all stage-based frameworks, represents only a guide to common behavior in the general population of children. The time at which children display these behaviors is clearly influenced by personal experience, such as the death of a family member, friend, or pet and by their specific education about death.

Children at the *sensorimotor stage* have limited language skills that are typically "instrumental," used to make known simple wants and needs (e.g., "ba-ba" for bottle, or "go car" to signal going for a ride). Their emotions are expressed primarily through behaviors such as laughing, tugging at someone or something, or crying. Children of this age are uncomfortable with separation from familiar people or surroundings, as evidenced by separation anxiety and stranger anxiety. They react to pain by crying, because they do not understand that they might have some control over the intensity of their experience of pain, despite

TABLE 9-2 ■ Development of the Concept of Death in Healthy Children			
Age Range (Years)	Piagetian Developmental Stage	Specific Age Period (Years)	Concept of Death
0-2	Sensorimotor Preverbal Reflex activity → purposeful activity Rudimentary thought	Infancy	Expresses discomfort with separation; fears pain
2-6	Preoperational Prelogical	3	Uses the word *dead* but only to indicate "not alive"
	Development of representational or symbolic language Initial reasoning	4	Limited understanding of finality; may express no personal emotion but may associate death with sorrow of others
	Juxtaposition of events in time perceived as cause and effect (syncretism)	5	Avoids dead things; imagines death as a personified being (ghost, bogeyman); believes he or she will always live
	Magical thinking, egocentrism	6	Associates death with "old age"; may be violent and emotional about death, including representations (magazine pictures), or display intense curiosity about dead things
7-12	Concrete operational Logical Problem-solving restricted to physically present, real objects that can be manipulated	7	Great interest in details (graveyards, coffins, possible causes); seeks answers through observation of decomposition and other death-related processes; suspects he or she, too, may die
	Development of logical functions (e.g., conservation of mass)	8	Less morbid, more expansive; interest in what happens after death; accepts that he or she, too, will die
		9-10	Understands biological (e.g. absence of pulse) essentials of death; understands concrete explanations of the dying process
12+	Formal operational Abstract Comprehension of abstract or symbolic content Development of advanced logical functions (hypothesis formation)	Adolescence	Meaning of death appreciated, but reality of personal death not accepted

Adapted from Sahler OJZ, Friedman SB: The dying child. Pediatr Rev 3:159-165, 1981.

past successful experiences with such approaches as distraction.

Children at the *preoperational stage* of development are what Piaget termed *prelogical*. Their increasing verbal skills allow researchers to discover that their reasoning is characterized by magical thinking (e.g., "My wish caused something to happen"), egocentrism (e.g., "What I wish or desire will happen; the world is limited to what I know, say, or do"), and a belief that two events that happen in close temporal relationship are also related by cause and effect (syncretism). Children this age believe in animism (every object, including trees, toys, and rocks, is a living, sentient being). However, what about the worm crushed on the sidewalk after a rain storm? Or the baby bird that has fallen from the nest to its death? Most children will pick up the worm or bird and carry it to a parent, wondering why the worm is not squirming or the bird is not flapping its wings. Typically, the parent will say, "Poor worm [or bird] is dead." The child comes to realize that there is a state in which an animal or bird does not do the things that they expect it to do and that state is "dead." Thus, at about age 3, children learn the word *dead* before they learn the word *alive*.

By about age 4, the child realizes that this designation is usually accompanied by tears ("Aunt Mary died last night," says a crying mother). Because the child has no understanding of the finality or irreversibility of death, however, sadness is momentary; the child is quickly off doing other things and may ask later, "When will Aunt Mary come to visit us again? I really like her."

Around the age of 5, children begin to personify death and, when asked to depict death, are likely to draw a picture of a ghost or skeleton, especially one that comes in the night and spirits people away. This is also about the time that children remember dreams and ask for night lights because of fear of the dark. This association should remind adults never to describe death as "going to sleep."

Around age 6, children enter the transitional stage to concrete operational thought. Their interest in death assumes a morbid quality that includes great interest in the technical aspects of dying and decomposition. Because children may still not understand the finality of death, they may wish to bury pets with supplies of food or toys for them to use in "pet heaven." Children between the ages of 6 and 8 years also may dig up animals after burial to determine what occurs following death and to better understand parents' descriptions of the death process through their own observations.

By the second or third grade, children may hear about the death of similar-aged or even younger schoolmates or relatives. They begin to understand that they, too, may die. This is a marked change from their earlier belief that "only old people die."

By the age of 9 to 10 years, most children can offer a reasonably logical, biological explanation of death. Through health and science classes, they are aware of the absence of a pulse, respirations, and movement in people or animals that are dead. They appear dispassionate on the subject of death, reflecting, perhaps, reaction formation (i.e., substituting nonchalance for anxiety) or, especially in boys, the need to be stoic and macho.

Adolescents entering the stage of formal operations can clearly conceptualize both the finality and the inevitability of death. However, they also have a sense of personal invulnerability that makes it difficult for them to conceive of their own personal death. Death-denying or death-defying behaviors (e.g., drinking and driving, playing around with firearms) are common. Their view of themselves as an integral part of a world in which there is truth and justice further contributes to their sense of invincibility: "If I'm this important, certainly I can't die." This thinking contributes to injuries: drunken driving and other risk-taking behaviors are the most common causes of death among 15- to 24-year-olds.

Terminally Ill Children's Perceptions of Their Own Death

Like adults, children vary in their readiness to talk about the end of their life. Although young children do not understand time, the future, or the finality of death, they are likely to ask questions about it, using language and imagery that reflect their understanding of death and the afterlife. Some terminally ill children wonder about impending death ("When I'm an angel, will I still be able to go to the zoo with you?" "When I'm in heaven, will I see Grandma?" "Will it hurt to die?"). Many wish to stop searching for a cure ("I'm so tired of being sick, but my mom will be disappointed if I stop treatment." "Do you really think I'll ever get better?" "I would rather go home and be with my friends than stay here. I know what that means."). Virtually all children desire honest discussion ("I'm not getting better, am I?"). Answers to such questions are challenging for child health care providers and we worry about getting it right. A more useful response is one that can uncover the issues uppermost in the child's mind and lead to a meaningful discussion: "Tell me what you're thinking about."

Clarifying the terminally ill child's concerns can be emotionally difficult for the caregiver who understands the finality of death and the pain of loss. Adults may believe that discussion will provoke, rather than allay, children's fear and anxiety. However, speaking directly with a dying child is the most effective way to explore the range of issues that preoccupy such children. Some children are most concerned with the

iding their own death. Questions such
Barbie with me?" "Will Dr. X and my
) the funeral?" or "What will heaven
eeking reassurance about the continu-
.. .. familiar and comfortable. Comments
such as "Don't cry a lot, Daddy" reflect the child's
concern for the welfare of others. Questions such as
"Will you keep my pictures in the album?" are efforts
to gain assurance that their lives have been meaningful and that they will be remembered.

End-of-Life Care

Many children have difficulty expressing their preference for forgoing further care. They are particularly
concerned about disappointing their parents by not
continuing to "fight." Interestingly, parents often
admit their own and their child's exhaustion. Helping
parents express to the child that he or she has endured
a very long and hard battle, is understandably physically and emotionally exhausted and that the child
has their permission to stop treatment can
be a turning point in setting appropriate goals for
end-of-life care. Without permission to let go, children will try to keep fighting if they perceive that this
is their parents' wish. The peace that accompanies
acceptance and mutual agreement makes the dying
process more comfortable and less terrifying for the
entire family.

Some children are most concerned about the effect
of their death on others. In particular, they worry
about their parents and how they will deal with the
loss. The majority of children, when asked, will state
a preference to die at home, surrounded by their toys,
pets, and friends and family, rather than in the hospital. Most families try to accommodate their child's
wish. However, clinicians should maintain the option
of hospitalization (or hospice, if available) if the
burden of care or family anxiety makes dying at home
too challenging. A few children state a preference to
die in the hospital. Typically, they worry that going
home will be too difficult for their parents, especially
their mother, and hope hospital personnel will provide
critical family support.

CHRONIC ILLNESS AS A PARADIGM OF STRESS

Diagnosis of a significant chronic health condition in
child of any age has a profound effect on the entire
family. Level of adaptation is directly related to the
success of the various coping mechanisms available to
each individual. Parental adjustment to chronic and
life-threatening illness in children remains an impor-

tant focus of psychosocial investigation because
parental adjustment influences not only parent but
also child-patient and sibling adaptation within the
dynamic family system.[37-39]

Parental Adjustment to a Child's Chronic Illness

One of the most studied groups of parents of children
with chronic illness has been parents of children with
cancer. Since the 1970s, cancer has evolved from an
almost universally rapidly fatal disease into a chronic
illness with a long-term survival (>5 years) of about
80% for all types. Certain characteristics of this condition make it particularly worthy of study as a serious
and, importantly, unpredictable illness: (1) it is one
of the few acute-onset, chronic illnesses of childhood
(an apparently healthy child can become significantly
ill within a matter of hours, requiring immediate
initiation of treatment); (2) treatment is long (2 or
more years for acute lymphoblastic leukemia, the
most common type), painful (lumbar punctures and
bone marrow aspirations may be performed a dozen
or more times a year), disfiguring (from chemotherapy or surgery), and socially isolating (repeated,
sometimes prolonged hospitalizations); (3) long-term
survival is not a cure (relapse remains a possibility for
years after completing treatment); and (4) treatment
itself carries a major risk of inducing a second malignancy, even decades later.

In studies of parental adjustment to childhood
cancer, investigators have documented increased
levels of emotional distress, typically heightened
anxiety and depression.[40-45] However, mothers and
fathers appear to differ in their responses. For example,
Barrera and colleagues[40] found higher levels of distress among mothers of children with cancer than
among mothers of children with acute illnesses, and
Noll and associates[46] similarly reported greater distress in mothers of children with cancer than in
mothers of classmates without a chronic illness but
found no differences for fathers. Additional studies
have confirmed that mothers of children with cancer
experience higher levels of distress than do fathers.[44,47]
Most longitudinal studies suggest that any increased
levels of distress in parents of children with cancer
attenuate to normal levels over 6 to 12 months,[48-51]
although some have revealed no significant decreases
up to 18 months after diagnosis.[44,52]

Studies of the effects of being persistently exposed
to a major stressor, such as cancer in their children,
suggest that mothers are especially at risk for post-
traumatic stress symptoms (PTSS), with an incidence
as high as 40%.[38,53-59] Overall, it appears that mothers
of children with cancer represent a group prone to

high levels of emotional distress and that the period after their child's diagnosis and the initiation of treatment may be particularly traumatic.[51,60]

Dolgin and colleagues[61] reported on a multisite, longitudinal study, monitoring more than 200 English-speaking and newly immigrated Spanish-speaking mothers for 6 months, beginning about 8 weeks after diagnosis of cancer in their children. These mothers received no intervention except "usual psychosocial care" (mental health, financial, and education assessments typically provided at the cancer center where their children were treated). As a group, the mothers displayed moderately elevated levels of negative affectivity (anxiety, depression) and PTSS during the period immediately after diagnosis. These levels were higher than those reported for general populations of adults without a child with cancer and also higher than those reported for mothers of long-term survivors.[38] Distress declined steadily, in line with previous studies documenting moderate initial levels of distress that diminish over the year after diagnosis.[49-52,62]

Dolgin and colleagues[61] were able to identify specific trajectories of maternal adjustment over time, with three distinct patterns emerging from the sample as a whole: mothers whose initial distress levels were comparatively low and remained so over time (stable-low); mothers who exhibited moderate levels of initial distress that remained so over time (stable-moderate); and mothers who had very high initial distress levels that declined over time (early-high). Trajectory analyses may help target those most likely to benefit from intervention efforts.

PREDICTORS OF PARENTAL ADJUSTMENT

Studies of predictors of parental adjustment to childhood cancer often focus on such variables as social support and parental coping style.[47,48,63] In Dolgin and colleagues'[61] report, maternal personality traits (i.e., neuroticism) and problem-solving ability (to be discussed) were significant predictors of initial distress levels, as well as the rate of improvement over time. Mothers with higher levels of neuroticism and poorer problem-solving skills had initially increased negative affectivity and PTSS.

Culture and language also emerged as significant predictors, specifically in relation to PTSS. Mothers whose primary language was Spanish reported higher levels of initial PTSS. This suggests that populations subject to cumulative stressors, such as immigration and acculturation, are more vulnerable. Perhaps this serves as a reminder that having a child with cancer is not the only stressor, or in some cases, even the primary stressor that parents may be experiencing. These findings underscore the potentially critical contribution of sociocultural characteristics to parental adjustment.

The model presented by Dolgin et al[61] suggests that quantifiable personality characteristics (neuroticism, extroversion, agreeability, problem-solving ability) in combination with readily available sociodemographic data (marital status, ethnicity, and education level) can be meaningful predictors of how a mother will adjust. Developing robust screening tools that incorporate identified predictors can assist in targeting intervention services and allocating clinical resources. Between one third and one half of the total sample reported on by Dolgin and colleagues had a stable-low distress adjustment trajectory, which suggests that delayed distress, or late-onset adjustment difficulties, are unlikely to occur in parents who are doing well initially, if their children continue to do well (the children of the mothers in this study were all clinically stable). Targeting individuals with a stable-moderate or early-high distress trajectory for intervention would be clinically most sensible, as well as resource efficient.

Interventions designed to improve parental adaptation to childhood cancer are increasingly available. Kazak and associates[64] developed a promising four-session intervention integrating cognitive-behavioral and family therapy approaches to reduce PTSS in childhood cancer survivors and their parents. The report by Dolgin and colleagues[61] demonstrated the benefits of an eight-session cognitive-behavioral intervention based on the five steps of problem-solving therapy ("Identify the problem"; "Determine your options"; "Evaluate your options, and pick the one most likely to succeed *in your hands*"; "Act"; and "See whether it worked").[65]

Little work has been done thus far investigating parents'—as well as children's—response to multiple relapses and remissions and the effects on family dynamics and adaptation. Such investigations are clearly needed in order to better inform the cost-benefit analysis of repeated therapeutic interventions of escalating invasiveness and morbidity.

The Stress of Procedural Pain

For many children with chronic conditions, including those with cancer, the disease itself is only occasionally painful. The most difficult and stressful aspect of such an illness is pain associated with procedures such as repeated venipuncture, lumbar puncture, or bone marrow aspiration.

HOW CHILDREN PERCEIVE THE INTENT OF PROCEDURES

A child's conceptualization of the value, function, and consequences of the procedure has implications for the coping process.[29] A child who appreciates the secondary gain of expressing feelings of pain may view it as an opportunity to garner sympathy or a reward, whereas a child who views a medical procedure as unnecessary may recount all the dangers and side effects; a child who understands the benefits may focus on the positive aspects of the procedure and its potential results (perhaps indicating that no further [painful] treatment is required).

Children's understanding of the *intent* of medical procedures and the role of medical personnel parallels their changing concept of illness and reflects their general understanding of intentionality and social roles. In the very earliest stage, the child perceives medical treatment or procedures as punishment for some undesired behavior. This is much the same as the child's perception that illness is a punishment. In the next stage, children perceive painful procedures as something done to help them, but they are unable to infer the good intent of the care providers. Thus, they typically believe that the providers will know that the procedure is painful only if the child cries, which typically elicits a response like "I'm sorry. I don't mean to hurt you." In the final stage, children are able to understand that the intent is to help them and that providers are aware of the pain they are causing ("because they were kids once") and that providers would not inflict the pain if they could avoid it. Children also develop the perception, frequently carried into adulthood, that others who have not suffered as they have cannot fully understand their distress ("Sometimes I feel nobody understands what's really happening to me, I think because I've had it and other people don't, so they don't know").[12]

THE EXPERIENCE OF PROCEDURAL PAIN

Fordyce[66] distinguished four basic facets of a pain episode: nociception (physiological signal that alerts the central nervous system to an aversive stimulus), pain (the sensory perception of the stimulus), suffering (the affective reaction to the stimulus, such as fear or distress), and pain behavior (the person's actions in response to the stimulus).

The experience of pain is unique to each individual. What may be merely a minor inconvenience to one child may be debilitating to another. Until improvements were made in nonverbal and indirect techniques to assess pain, clinicians believed that children had a lower sensitivity to pain perception than did adults, commonly attributed to immaturity of the nervous system or high levels of resilience. These assumptions frequently led to underestimates of perceived pain and undertreatment.[67] In fact, current evidence suggests that neonates experience more pain sensitivity than do older age groups.[68] Furthermore, although critically ill neonates may demonstrate little visible response to pain, they mount impressive hormonal, metabolic, and cardiovascular responses to invasive procedures.[69]

In early investigation of the possible neurophysiological repercussions of early exposure to painful stressors, Barr and colleagues[70] hypothesized that repeated exposure may redirect the growth of neural pathways and result in a "nociceptive neural architecture that renders the individual pain vulnerable or pain resilient." Specifically, an increase in dendritic branching may accompany the experience of pain, producing a permanently lowered pain threshold. Anand and Scalzo,[71] reporting on the effects of repeated pain experiences in animal models, demonstrated that the plasticity of the neonatal brain responds by altering pain sensitivity and anxiety levels. These alterations result in an increased occurrence of, for example, stress disorders in adults. Among children, pain, fear, and separation anxiety all are likely to contribute to the child's perception of invasive medical procedures as bodily threats and even punishments.

Inadequately managed procedural pain associated with common childhood experiences (e.g., immunization, venipuncture, laceration repair) can have long-term, negative effects on future pain tolerance and pain responses.[72] These findings have contributed to increased attention to pain management in all clinical settings, including the emergency department[72,73] and the inpatient hospital setting,[74] with the use of both pharmacological and nonpharmacological approaches.[29,31,32,75-77]

Most children do not habituate to repeated painful procedures.[78] Although sedation may remove the memory of the event, the pain itself is nonetheless experienced. Furthermore, it distorts thinking and may interfere with the child's understanding during the procedure. Of even more concern is that sedation has been associated with airway obstruction, hypoxia, and apnea, especially when used with other central nervous system depressants (e.g., opiates). Such side effects as simple pooling of secretions can be life-threatening in children who have impaired pulmonary functioning, such as those with cerebral palsy who undergo painful Botox injections.[79]

Recollection of Pain

Despite advances in pediatric pain management, misconceptions persist. Some providers believe that children do not remember pain or do not experience pain as intensely as do adults. In fact, children as young as age 2 years can recall a painful procedure (e.g., voiding cystourethrogram) up to 6 months later. As expected, older children provide more complete and accurate reports than do younger children. The specific behaviors recalled by children are influenced by various factors: crying during a procedure is inversely correlated with the ability to report correct information; procedure-related talk is positively associated with correct information; and distraction is negatively associated with the accuracy of recall.[80]

Children as young as 5 years can provide detailed information about their pain, using a variety of descriptors. They can reliably discriminate among the sensory (quality, duration), affective (tension, fear), and evaluative (intensity) components of pain.[81] By school age, children can recall painful experiences, understand the nature of pain causality, and associate pain with certain feelings, such as fear, anxiety, and embarrassment.[82] However, children also have conceptual deficiencies in understanding. For example, few school-aged children can identify how pain is transmitted (e.g., "It's a signal sent by a nerve")[82] or identify a beneficial function (e.g., a warning about being burned by a hot stove).[83] Children at this age are, however, well aware of the secondary gain derived from having pain (e.g., missing school, avoidance of responsibilities). Children and teenagers functioning at the formal operational level show advanced understanding of the physiological, biological, and psychosocial aspects of pain.[84]

COPING WITH PROCEDURAL PAIN

Several child-specific variables moderate or affect the strength of coping responses to procedural pain, including age or developmental level, gender, prior experience,[29] and temperament.

Age/Developmental Level

Younger children are more likely to use loud verbalizations (crying, screaming) and whole body contortions (squirming); older children are likely to exhibit verbal expressions of pain and greater muscular rigidity. Increasing age is also associated with increasing information seeking, higher levels of direct problem solving, lower levels of problem-focused avoidance, more cognitive self-distraction, and less rumination about escape strategies.[29]

Gender

Girls are likely to report more pain and anxiety when coping with medical procedures.[85] Girls are also more likely to cry, cling, and seek emotional support, whereas boys are more likely to be uncooperative. These differences are probably the result of typical socialization processes that encourage boys to adopt stoic attitudes about pain and encourage girls to be more passive and affective in their expression of pain. This responsiveness to social expectations tends to increase these gender differences as children mature into adolescents.[29]

Prior Experience

Repeated pain may have significant negative effects on brain development. Whether children beyond early infancy are able to habituate to painful procedures is unclear. In some instances, experience may facilitate the purposeful development of adaptive skills such as information-seeking strategies[86] to reduce current anxiety. In other instances, especially among younger children, responses to feared stressors are more likely to be automatic and conditioned. Thus, unpleasant or painful memories of experiences may increase the negative emotions associated with procedures and interfere with coping.[87]

In general, the *quality* of past experiences may be a more accurate predictor of coping response than is the *quantity*. For example, negative experiences appear to be predictive of parental, staff, and observer ratings of children's increased anxiety and distress during medical examinations.[88] However, it is also possible that there is some expectation, perhaps unconscious, on the part of parents or staff about how the child will react, and this can become a self-fulfilling prophecy.

Temperament

Temperament may also play a role in how a child copes with painful procedures. Psychologically, temperament is classically defined as an inborn dispositional difference in behavioral style and self-regulation or variability in individual behavioral responses to external stimuli.[89] Physiologically, temperament is conceptualized in terms of individual differences in reactivity to stress and focuses on, for example, cardiovascular and neuroendocrine responsiveness (heart rate, blood pressure, vagal tone, cortisol levels).[90] Children with temperaments characterized by higher levels of behavioral or physiological reactivity, lower levels of adaptability, and lower thresholds for behavioral or physiological responsiveness to stimuli demonstrate higher levels of distress when confronted with medical stressors and seem to prefer coping responses that decrease their perception of the stressor (avoidance, distraction). From a physiological viewpoint, such coping responses may downregulate a child's reaction to the stressor. Children with less reactive and more adaptable temperaments, who demonstrate lower levels of distress, may be able to take better advantage of coping responses that involve direct confrontation with the stressor (information seeking, observation).[29]

PREPARATION OF THE CHILD FOR PAINFUL PROCEDURES

Reviews of how best to prepare children for painful procedures focus primarily on two approaches: the use of pharmacological therapies[91,92] and the use of nonpharmacological, complementary, or alternative therapies.[93] In fact, as advocated by Kazak and associates,[94] a combination of the two approaches is most likely to achieve maximal benefit for the majority of children. The primary goal should be adequate pain control with the minimum amount of sedation while helping the child develop a sense of mastery from self-regulation through distraction (e.g., music, puppets), education about the procedure, or mind-body (e.g., self-hypnosis) techniques. Studies have repeatedly demonstrated cognitive-behavioral therapies, in particular, to be effective in pain management.[95] (See Chapter 21 for more details on pain.)

The most important principle in developing a procedural pain management plan is that children of different personality types require different approaches to coping with stress. The child who adapts well to preparation and anticipatory guidance may benefit from knowing about an upcoming procedure in advance (hours or even days), whereas the child who becomes anxious and cannot easily adapt to anticipated events may best be "surprised." During the procedure, children may choose to watch or to be distracted. After the procedure, children may want to be comforted, or they may want to just get on to the next activity.

There is no "correct" way for an individual child to respond; similarly, there is no absolute preparation that is helpful to every child. Parents are good judges of their child's coping style. Discussion of options and what other children have found useful may be helpful to parents and contribute to the development of more effective coping strategies tailored to the child's temperament.

THE ROLE OF PARENTS DURING PROCEDURES

Nonpharmacological strategies, such as distraction, are useful as pain-controlling maneuvers, because children are particularly responsive to imaginative play. Imaginative play delivered by a parent or other familiar figure to provide comforting physical contact and distraction is even more powerful.[96]

Parental assistance appears to be crucial for addressing the three stages of coping with procedure-associated pain: anticipation of the procedure (i.e., whether it is appraised as a harm/loss, a threat, a challenge to be overcome, or an activity that is ultimately valuable in fighting disease); the actual procedure (encounter); and the aftermath (recovery) period. The anticipation stage may be associated with apprehension and psychological distress; coping responses during this stage may be directed toward managing anxiety or fear. The encounter stage is characterized not only by psychological distress but also by physiological sensations of pain. The recovery phase may include coping with feelings of having been assaulted and may also require coping that reduces pain or regulates reactions to pain. Not surprisingly, children may cope in different ways during different stages of

medical stressors. For example, children are more likely to engage in verbal coping (humor) during the nonpainful stages, and audible, deep breathing is more frequent during the painful stages.[29]

Data on the effect of parental presence during stressful medical procedures are mixed.[97] Much depends on the parents' tolerance for pain in their child, which is based on their understanding the reason for the procedure and the intent of the person doing the procedure. Parental support may facilitate children's adaptive coping responses. Alternatively, certain parental behaviors, such as empathic comments, apologies to the child, criticism, undue reassurance, and affording the child control over when the procedure begins, actually increase the child's distress.[97] This variability in research findings on parental presence may also relate to parental characteristics. For example, children with anxious mothers exhibit greater anxiety in their mother's presence, whereas children with mothers who are not anxious show more distress in their mother's absence.[29]

THE COMPETENCY OF MINORS TO MAKE MEDICAL DECISIONS

Most pediatric providers would agree that a 4-year-old with acute leukemia can decide the arm for intravenous insertion, but not whether an intravenous line is needed. Most providers would also allow a 10-year-old the same option. What about the 14-year-old? Or the 17-year-old? Does it make any difference whether this is a new diagnosis, the second relapse, or the second relapse after stem cell transplantation? Does it make any difference whether the patient and family agree or disagree, or whether the physician agrees or disagrees?

Being considered competent to make a decision implies being able to understand the risks, benefits, and alternatives when choices are available and to express a choice between the alternatives; to demonstrate logical and rational reasoning; to make a "reasonable" choice; and to make a choice without coercion. Children in Piaget's preoperational stage are unable to reason beyond their own personal experiences and are limited in their understanding of cause-and-effect relationships. During the concrete operational stage, children begin to think logically, but only about things that are physically present or that they have experienced. However, in the formal operational stage, children show an intellectual capacity to reason, generalize beyond personal experience, deal with abstract ideas, and hypothesize or predict potential consequences of actions. Apart from inexperience, most individuals 14 years of age and older have the same capacities for processing information

25. Olney MF, Kim A: Beyond adjustment: Integration of cognitive disability into identity. Disabil Soc 16:563-583, 2001.

26. Richardson CR: Educational interventions improve outcomes for children with asthma. J Fam Pract 52:764-766, 2003.

27. Compas BE, Connor-Smith JK, Saltzman H, et al: Coping with stress during childhood and adolescence: Problems, progress, and potential in theory and research. Psychol Bull 127:87-127, 2001.

28. Eisenberg N, Fabes RA, Guthrie I: The roles of regulation and development. *In* Sandler JN, Wolchik SA, eds: Handbook of Children's Coping with Common Stressors: Linking Theory, Research, and Intervention. New York: Plenum Press, 1997, pp 41-70.

29. Rudolph KD, Denning MD, Weisz JR: Determinants and consequences of children's coping in the medical setting: Conceptualization, review, and critique. Psychol Bull 118:328-357, 1995.

30. Field T, Alpert B, Vega-Lahr N, et al: Hospitalization stress in children: Sensitizer and repressor coping styles. Health Psychol 7:433-445, 1988.

31. Siegel LJ: Hospitalization and medical care of children. *In* Walker E, Roberts M, eds: Handbook of Clinical Child Psychology. New York: Wiley, 1983, pp 1089-1108.

32. Worchel FF, Copeland DR, Barker DG: Control-related coping strategies in pediatric oncology patients. J Pediatr Psychol 12:25-38, 1987.

33. Crouch MD: Children with Cancer: A Study of Coping in the Medical Setting. Los Angeles: University of California, 1999 (Dissertation).

34. Spinetta JJ: The dying child's awareness of death: A review. Psychol Bull 81:256-260, 1974.

35. Spinetta JJ: Adjustment in children with cancer. Pediatr Psychol 2:49-51, 1977.

36. Schonfeld DJ: Talking with children about death. J Pediatr Health Care 7:269-274, 1993.

37. Dolgin M, Phipps S: Reciprocal influences in family adjustment to childhood cancer. *In* Baider L, Cooper C, Kaplan de-Nour A, eds: Cancer and the Family. Oxford, UK: Wiley, 1996, pp 73-92,

38. Kazak AE, Alderfer M, Rourke MT, et al: Posttraumatic stress disorder (PTSD) and posttraumatic stress symptoms (PTSS) in families of adolescent childhood cancer survivors. J Pediatr Psychol 29:211-219, 2004.

39. Sahler OJ, Roghmann KJ, Mulhern RK, et al: Sibling adaptation to childhood cancer collaborative study: The association of sibling adaptation with maternal well-being, physical health, and resource use. J Dev Behav Pediatr 18:233-243, 1997.

40. Barrera M, D'Agostino NM, Gibson J, et al: Predictors and mediators of psychological adjustment in mothers of children newly diagnosed with cancer. Psychooncology 13:630-641, 2004.

41. Landolt MA, Vollrath M, Ribi K, et al: Incidence and associations of parental and child posttraumatic stress symptoms in pediatric patients. J Child Psychol Psychiatry 44:1199-1207, 2003.

42. Lansky SB, Cairns NU: The Family of the Child with Cancer. New York: American Cancer Society, 1979.

43. Overholser JC, Fritz GK: The impact of childhood cancer on the family. J Psychosoc Oncol 8:71-85, 1990.

44. Sloper P: Predictors of distress in parents of children with cancer: A prospective study. J Pediatr Psychol 25:79-91, 2000.

45. Steele RG, Dreyer ML, Phipps S: Patterns of maternal distress among children with cancer and their association with child emotional and somatic distress. J Pediatr Psychol 29:507-517, 2004.

46. Noll RB, Gartstein MA, Hawkins A, et al: Comparing parental distress for families with children who have cancer and matched comparison families without children with cancer. Fam Syst Med 13:11-28, 1995.

47. Frank NC, Brown RT, Blount RL, et al: Predictors of affective responses of mothers and fathers of children with cancer. Psycho-oncology 10:293-304, 2001.

48. Hoekstra-Weebers JEHM, Jaspers JPC, Kamps WA, et al: Psychologic adaptation and social support of parents of pediatric cancer patients: A prospective longitudinal study. J Pediatr Psychol 26:225-235, 2001.

49. Steele RG, Long A, Reddy KA, et al: Changes in maternal distress and child-rearing strategies across treatment for pediatric cancer. J Pediatr Psychol 28:447-452, 2003.

50. Kupst MJ, Schulman JL: Long-term coping with pediatric leukemia: A six-year follow-up study. J Pediatr Psychol 13:7-22, 1988.

51. Sawyer M, Antoniou G, Toogood I, et al: Childhood cancer: A 4-year prospective study of the psychological adjustment of children and parents. J Pediatr Hematol Oncol 22:214-220, 2000.

52. Manne S, Miller D, Meyers P, et al: Depressive symptoms among parents of newly diagnosed children with cancer: A 6-month follow-up study. Child Health Care 25:191-209, 1996.

53. Brown RT, Madan-Swain A, Lambert R: Posttraumatic stress symptoms in adolescent survivors of childhood cancer and their mothers. J Trauma Stress 16:309-318, 2003.

54. Hall M, Baum A: Intrusive thoughts as determinants of distress in parents of children with cancer. J Appl Soc Psychol 25:1215-1230, 1995.

55. Kazak AE, Boeving CA, Alderfer MA, et al: Posttraumatic stress symptoms during treatment in parents of children with cancer. J Clin Oncol 23:7405-7410, 2005.

56. Nelson AE, Miles MS, Reed SB, et al: Depressive symptomatology in parents of children with chronic oncologic or hematologic disease. J Psychosoc Oncol 12:61-75, 1994.

57. Pelcovitz D, Goldenberg B, Kaplan S, et al: Posttraumatic stress disorder in mothers of pediatric cancer survivors. Psychosomatics 37:116-126, 1996.

58. Stuber ML, Christakis DA, Houskamp B, et al: Posttrauma symptoms in childhood leukemia survivors and their parents. Psychosomatics 37:254-261, 1996.

59. Stuber ML, Gonzales S, Meeske K, et al: Posttraumatic stress after childhood cancer II: A family model. Psychooncology 3:313-319, 1994.

60. Wallander JL, Varni JW: Effects of pediatric chronic physical disorders on child and family adjustment. J Child Psychol Psychiatry 39:29-46, 1998.

61. Dolgin MJ, Phipps S, Fairclough DL, et al: Trajectories of adjustments in mothers of children with newly diagnosed cancer: A natural history investigation. J Pediatr Psychol (in press).

62. Dahlquist LM, Czyzewski DI, Jones CL: Parents of children with cancer: A longitudinal study. J Pediatr Psychol 21:541-554, 1996.

63. Manne S, DuHamel K, Redd WH: Association of psychological vulnerability factors to post-traumatic stress symptomatology in mothers of pediatric cancer survivors. Psychooncology 9:372-384, 2000.

64. Kazak AE, Alderfer MA, Streisand R, et al: Treatment of posttraumatic stress symptoms in adolescent survivors of childhood cancer and their families: A randomized clinical trial. J Fam Psychol 18:493-504, 2004.

65. Sahler OJ, Fairclough DL, Phipps S, et al: Using problem-solving skills training to reduce negative affectivity in mothers of children with newly diagnosed cancer: Report of a multisite randomized trial. J Consult Clin Psychol 73:272-283, 2005.

66. Fordyce WE: Pain and suffering: A reappraisal. Am Psychol 43:276-283, 1988.

67. Thompson KL, Varni JW: A developmental cognitive-biobehavioral approach to pediatric pain assessment. Pain 25:283-296, 1986.

68. Anand KJS: Clinical importance of pain and stress in preterm neonates. Biol Neonate 73:1-9, 1998.

69. Johnston CC, Stevens BJ, Yang F, et al: Differential response to pain by very premature neonates. Pain 61:471-479, 1995.

70. Barr RG, Boyce WT, Zeltzer LK: The stress-illness association in children: A perspective from the biobehavioral interface. In Haggerty RJ, Sherrod LR, Garmezy N, et al, eds: Stress, Risk, and Resilience in Children and Adolescents: Processes, Mechanisms, and Interventions. Cambridge, UK: Cambridge University Press, 1994, pp 182-224.

71. Anand KJ, Scalzo FM: Can adverse neonatal experiences alter brain development and subsequent behavior? Biol Neonate 77:69-82, 2000.

72. Young KD: Pediatric procedural pain. Ann Emerg Med 45:160-171, 2005.

73. Bauman BH, McManus JG Jr: Pediatric pain management in the emergency department. Emerg Med Clin North Am 23:393-414, 2005.

74. Greco C, Berde C: Pain management for the hospitalized pediatric patient. Pediatr Clin North Am 52:995-1027, 2005.

75. Hain RD, Miser A, Devins M, et al: Strong opioids in pediatric palliative medicine. Paediatr Drugs 7:1-9, 2005.

76. Chitkara DK, Rawat DJ, Talley NJ: The epidemiology of childhood recurrent abdominal pain in Western countries: A systematic review. Am J Gastroenterol 100:1868-1875, 2005.

77. Mercadante S: Cancer pain management in children. Palliat Med 18:654-662, 2004.

78. Kuttner L: Management of young children's acute pain and anxiety during invasive medical procedures. Pediatrician 16:39-44, 1989.

79. http://www.centerwatch.com/patientdrugs/dru246.html [database online]. 2004.

80. Salmon K, Price M, Pereira JK: Factors associated with young children's long-term recall of an invasive medical procedure: A preliminary investigation. J Dev Behav Pediatr 23:347-352, 2002.

81. McGrath P: Psychological aspects of pain perception. In Schecter N, Berde C, Yaster M, eds: Pain in Infants, Children and Adolescents. Baltimore: Williams & Wilkins, 1993, pp 39-63.

82. Ross DM, Ross SA: Childhood pain: The school-aged child's viewpoint. Pain 20:179-191, 1984.

83. Savedra M, Tesler M, Ward J, et al: Descriptions of the pain experience: A study of school-age children. Issues Compr Pediatr Nurs 5:373-380, 1981.

84. Gaffney A: Cognitive developmental aspects of pain in school-age children. In Schecter N, Berde C, Yaster M, eds: Pain in Infants, Children and Adolescents. Baltimore: Williams & Wilkins, 1993, pp 75-83.

85. Weisz JR, McCabe M, Denning MD: Primary and secondary control among children undergoing medical procedures: Adjustment as a function of coping style. J Consult Clin Psychol 62:324-332, 1994.

86. Smith KE, Ackerson JP, Blotchy AD, et al: Preferred coping styles of pediatric cancer patients during invasive medical procedures. J Psychosoc Oncol 8:59-70, 1991.

87. Siegel L, Smith KE: Children's strategies for coping with pain. Pediatrician 16:110-118, 1989.

88. Lumley MA, Melamed BG, Abeles LA: Predicting children's presurgical anxiety and subsequent behavior change. J Pediatr Psychol 18:481-497, 1993.

89. Thomas A, Chess S: Temperament and Development. New York: Brunner/Mazel, 1977.

90. Boyce WT, Barr RG, Zeltzer LK: Temperament and the psychobiology of childhood stress. Pediatrics 90:483-486, 1992.

91. Evans D, Turnham L, Barbour K, et al: Intravenous ketamine sedation for painful oncology procedures. Paediatr Anaesth 15:131-138, 2005.

92. Krauss B, Green SM: Procedural sedation and analgesia in children. Lancet 367:766-780, 2006.

93. Kuppenheimer WG, Brown RT: Painful procedures in pediatric cancer: A comparison of interventions. Clin Psychol Rev 22:753-786, 2002.

94. Kazak AE, Penati B, Brophy P, et al: Pharmacologic and psychological interventions for procedural pain. Pediatrics 102:59-66, 1998.

95. Powers SW: Empirically supported treatments in pediatric psychology: Procedure-related pain. J Pediatr Psychol 24:131-145, 1999.

96. Gerik SM: Pain management in children: Developmental considerations and mind-body therapies. South Med J 98:295-302, 2005.

97. Blount R, Davis N, Powers S, et al: The influence of environmental factors and coping style on children's coping and distress. Clin Psychol Rev 11:93-116, 1991.

98. Doig C, Burgess E: Withholding life-sustaining treatment: Are adolescents competent to make these decisions? CMAJ 162:1585-1588, 2000.

99. Rozovsky LE: Children, Adolescents, and Consent. The Canadian Law of Consent to Treatment. Toronto: Butterworths, 1997, pp 61-75.

100. Gaylin W: The competence of children: No longer all or none. Hastings Cent Rep 12:33-38, 1982.

101. American Academy of Pediatrics, Committee on Bioethics: Guidelines on foregoing life-sustaining medical treatment. Pediatrics 93:532-536, 1994.

102. Sigman G, Silber TJ, English A, et al: Confidential health care for adolescents: Position paper of the Society for Adolescent Medicine. J Adolesc Health 21:408-415, 1997.

103. Schidlow DV: Transition in cystic fibrosis: Much ado about nothing? A pediatrician's view. Pediatr Pulmonol 33:325-326, 2002.

104. Hagood JS, Lenker CV, Thrasher S: A course on the transition to adult care of patients with childhood-onset chronic illness. Acad Med 80:352-355, 2005.

Developmental-Behavioral Aspects of Chronic Conditions

10A.
Effects of Adverse Natal Factors and Prematurity

EDWARD GOLDSON
SANDRA L. GARDNER

At the beginning of the 21st century, many infants with very low birth weight (VLBW) (weight, <1500 g) are surviving the neonatal intensive care experience and are being discharged home to their families. Their posthospital care has become increasingly important for the primary care pediatrician as well as for the developmental pediatrician and clinical researcher.[1,2] The pediatrician's skills must meet these infants' complex medical needs, as well as meet the associated developmental and psychological challenges that many of these children and their families present.

In 2002, there were 4,019,280 children born in the United States, a birth rate of 13.9 per 1000. Of these infants, 12% were born prematurely: that is, before 37 weeks' gestation. This is an increase from 9.4% of such births in 1981 to 10.6% in 1990. These preterm births occurred primarily among non-Hispanic white women. Similarly, there has been an increase in the percentage of children born with birth weights lower than 2500 g. Such infants represented 6.7% of the births in 1984 and 7.8% of the births in 2002. Also, there was steady increase in the number of infants with VLBW from the 1980s through the 1990s (1.15% in 1980 to 1.45% in 1999 and 2002). Moreover, 95% of children with birth weights between 1250 and 1499 g currently survive.[3] Thus, as noted by the March of Dimes, approximately one per eight infants is born prematurely and is at risk for later problems. Such children present a significant public health issue that must be addressed.

In the past, pediatricians were concerned primarily with the survival of infants with VLBW and with the medical and developmental sequelae of their prenatal, perinatal, and postnatal experiences. Although these remain critical issues for the neonatologist and primary care physician, the affective and cognitive consequences of VLBW are now emerging as significant public health issues, as children who were born with VLBW confront the challenges of education and school performance. In this chapter, we provide a brief historical overview of the advances in neonatal intensive care, examine the short-term and long-term developmental and behavioral outcomes of premature infants, and provide recommendations for the follow-up care and assessment of this high-risk population of children.[4]

HISTORICAL OVERVIEW

Although the development of centers for the care of premature infants began in the 1950s, these centers had very little effect on the outcome of infants with VLBW; the reported mortality rate continued to be about 75% for the next 10 years.[5] Of the infants who did survive, some did relatively well.[6,7] However, it was not until the major advances in basic scientific knowledge and technology of the 1960s led to more rigorous neonatal intensive care that survival increased. In 1960, Alexander Schaffer coined the term *neonatology* to identify the newly emerging pediatric subspecialty that was to devote itself to the care of the sick and premature infants and those with low birth weight.

Two major factors proved critical for the later advances made in the care of these infants. The first was an increase in the understanding of fetal and neonatal physiology, which led to advances in technology. Recognition of the significance of maintaining normal body temperature, providing adequate nutrition, and preventing infection led to the development of the early neonatal intensive care nursery.[8] The understanding of the effect of oxygen and its use in the treatment of respiratory distress was also a significant achievement.[9] Although an incomplete understanding of the properties of oxygen and its toxicity resulted in retrolental fibroplasia (now called *retinopathy of prematurity*), the introduction of oxygen resulted in the survival of many small infants who, in the past, would have died. Another example was the appreciation of the role of bilirubin in the etiology of kernicterus and athetoid cerebral palsy. Recognition of the association between blood group incompatibilities and hemolytic anemia of the newborn led to the development of $Rh_O(D)$ immune globulin (RhoGAM) and a marked diminution in the incidence of severe hyperbilirubinemia and kernicterus. A further example was recognition of the need for prompt feeding of the newborn.[10,11] Consequently, nurseries stopped waiting the customary 24 hours before feeding the infant, thus avoiding hypoglycemia and other metabolic disturbances of delayed feeding.

The technology that developed as a result of this expanded knowledge of physiology played a major role in the survival of the small infant. Although small babies had been ventilated in the 1950s and 1960s, the development of continuous positive airway pressure, which evolved in response to an understanding of lung and chest wall mechanics, had a great impact on the survival of the small infant.[12] Continuous positive airway pressure stabilizes the alveoli, prevents atelectasis, and facilitates respiration. This technique also led to the development of more efficient and effective ventilators. The design of sophisticated monitoring systems, including the capability for monitoring blood gases noninvasively,[13-16] allowed for better control of oxygenation with the aim of decreasing the incidence of the complications of oxygen therapy. The discovery of phototherapy for the treatment of hyperbilirubinemia led to a decrease in the incidence of kernicterus. The development of hyperalimentation[17] and its application to premature infants facilitated care for infants with significant bowel disturbances and those too small or too sick to feed on their own. Natural and synthetic surfactant are now being administered to infants with VLBW at birth to prevent the major pulmonary complications of surfactant deficiency.[18-22] Most recently, with the discovery of the vasodilator properties of nitric oxide, there is more hope for the survival of infants with VLBW with such problems as persistent pulmonary hypertension.[23]

In summary, the care of very small infants since the early 1980s has progressed from minimal support to intensive intervention, as a consequence of the expansion of knowledge of neonatal physiology and significant technological advances. Infants surviving today are smaller and sicker than those who survived 30 years ago. Their survival has stimulated a wide range of investigations in which researchers monitor mortality and morbidity,[24,25] evaluate long-term outcome, determine the quality of their lives,[26] and debate the ethics of applying technological advances to prolong survival of severely premature infants.[27] Such debate is crucial as resources become increasingly limited. At the same time, survival of these infants has stimulated a wide range of questions about such issues as mother-infant attachment,[28,29] the temperament of premature infants,[30,31] and the effect of the premature and potentially disabled or chronically ill infant on the family.

FOLLOW-UP STUDIES OF INFANTS WITH VERY LOW BIRTH WEIGHT

Over the years, researchers have gathered considerable information on the outcome of infants with VLBW and those with extremely low birth weight (ELBW) (i.e., birth weight <1000 g). Data from perinatal programs document the effectiveness of neonatal intensive care.[32] In early studies, all premature infants were grouped together, and an increase in survival was demonstrated after the introduction of intensive care. However, it soon became apparent that this group of babies was not homogeneous; for example, there are significant differences between an infant weighing 2000 g at birth and one weighing 1250 g and between an infant who is of appropriate size for gestational age and one who is small for gestational age.[33] Moreover, investigators performed many of these studies over relatively short time periods and tended to focus on gross abnormalities and to ignore more subtle, long-term issues. As a result, the understanding of the outcome of these babies was limited and superficial. Furthermore, the failure to consider more subtle but important adverse outcomes contributed to an unrealistically positive impression of the effectiveness of intensive interventions.

To better understand findings from longitudinal studies, clinicians should consider factors that confound the interpretation of data from a variety of settings. Follow-up studies on the outcomes of prematurity vary in several ways: (1) reporting and defining of handicapping conditions (e.g.. mild, moderate, severe)[34]; (2) inclusion of appropriate controls (e.g., full-term neonates and classmates)[35]; (3) use of retrospective versus prospective study designs; (4)

addressing sources of bias (e.g., evaluators' unawareness of experimental condition; parental compliance with follow-up; selection of study subjects)[36,37]; (5) use of birth weight or gestational age to measure morbidity; (6) use of a single center, multicenter, and population-based paradigm[35,38]; (7) definition of outcome measures (e.g., what/how/when to measure[34,35] and the "disability paradox" in quality of life studies)[39]; and (8) and study length (e.g., subject attrition; ages at follow-up).[40-43]

Place of birth (i.e., type of facility), characteristics of the neonatal intensive care unit (NICU) (e.g., approaches to management, the general environment, and use of technology), and parental factors influence both short- and long-term outcomes. Research findings from as long ago as the 1970s have documented better outcomes for infants with ELBW or VLBW born in Level III perinatal centers than for those born in Levels I and II centers.[44,45] Use of developmental care in the NICU has been shown to alter brain function and structure,[46] to have physiological benefits (e.g., less intraventricular hemorrhage, chronic lung disease/bronchopulmonary dysplasia, retinopathy of prematurity, ventilator and oxygen use), and to have developmental benefits (e.g., improvements in behavior organization, self-regulation, interactive capability and quality with parents, ability of mother to read and respond to infant's cues, and cognitive function/IQ; fewer behavior problems and attention difficulties).[46,47] Advances in neonatal intensive care with the development of new technologies (e.g., high-frequency ventilation, inhaled nitric oxide) and use of drugs influence outcomes of premature infants.[48-50] For example, use of one course of antenatal steroids and surfactant replacement lowers rates of morbidity and mortality, whereas multiple courses of antenatal steroids and use of postnatal steroids results in long-term central nervous system deficits. Indeed, the short-term benefits (e.g., earlier weaning from the ventilator) of postnatal steroid use are offset by their long-term consequences (e.g., effect on the developing brain).[51] Well-documented variations in outcome morbidity (e.g., chronic lung disease/bronchopulmonary dysplasia, retinopathy of prematurity, infection, intraventricular hemorrhage) among NICUs have a myriad of causes, including different centers' approaches to infants at the "limits of viability" and the use of and expertise with technologies, nutritional management, pain relief, and infection control.[49,50,52-54] International comparisons are made difficult by the greater sociodemographic diversity of the United States population in comparison with those of many European countries (e.g., socioeconomic, educational, and marital status; ethnic or cultural differences; access to community resources or supports).[52,55]

Finally, parental factors have an important effect on the outcomes of the preterm infant. Parent-infant interaction is influenced by preterm birth and, in turn, influences the outcome of the preterm infant. Characteristics such as maternal responsiveness, the physical appearance of the infant, parental expectations for the child, and child-rearing abilities have been shown to influence both caretaking ability and children's subsequent cognitive and academic achievement.[55-60] These confounders and variations make comparisons between different studies often difficult, if not impossible.

In the late 1970s and early 1980s, investigators began to examine different populations of infants more closely and to consider the effect of factors other than birth weight and gestational age more rigorously, including perinatal and postnatal complications (e.g., intracranial hemorrhage, bronchopulmonary dysplasia), socioeconomic status, access to care, and place of birth.

Early Studies

Douglas[6] reported on 163 infants with birth weights of 2000 g or less born in the United Kingdom during a single week in 1946. Some of the babies were born at home and some in the hospital. Of those cared for in a hospital, 18 received oxygen, and 11 were in incubators. None of the infants weighing less than 1000 g, whether born at home or in the hospital, survived; only 32% of the infants weighing 1001 to 1500 g lived. Of the infants weighing 1500 to 2000 g who did survive, none had handicaps. Of the infants weighing less than 1500 who survived, 17% had significant physical, neurological, mental, or behavioral problems. In 1958, Dann and associates[7] described the outcomes for 73 of 116 infants born in the New York City area between 1940 and 1952 with birth weights of 1000 g or less or whose weight dropped below 1000 g during their hospitalization. The infants were kept in incubators, and most received oxygen and meticulous but nonintrusive medical support. The children were evaluated between 1950 and 1957. All 73 studied, who were among the 116 survivors, were found to have generally good physical health with few neurological defects. Most had achieved normal height, but often not until after 4 years of age. However, the IQs of 84%, while in the average range, were below those of their full-term siblings. Sixteen percent had IQs below 80. After considering variables such as birth weight, gender, race, and socioeconomic status, Dann and associates found that the infants with the highest IQs were from families with higher socioeconomic status.

Both of these studies are unique in that they preceded, by approximately two decades, the establishment of modern neonatal intensive care. As a result, they provide a historical perspective and also demonstrate that even without neonatal intensive care, some infants with low birth weight did survive and did well. With the introduction of new methods of care, survival increased and outcomes improved, although other issues have emerged.[61-63] In the next section of this chapter, we review later follow-up studies on the infants with VLBW and those with ELBW.

Studies from 1979 to the Early 1980s

Studies published after 1979[1,64-70] documented the results of the emergence of the modern age of neonatology and the progress in the evolution of care for the infant with VLBW. With technological advances and recognition of the importance of continuous and comprehensive assessment of outcomes, findings extend beyond morbidity, mortality, and medical issues to include such issues as the psychosocial, neurodevelopmental, educational, and behavioral sequelae of premature birth for children and their families.

INFANTS WITH BIRTH WEIGHTS OF 1000 TO 1500 GRAMS

In 1982, Orgill et al.[71] published 6- and 12-month follow-up findings on 123 survivors of a cohort of 148 infants born between January 1979 and July 1980, with birth weights of 1500 g or less. Twenty-one infants had birth weights of 1000 g or lower. At 18 months, 84 (57%) were alive. Of this group of infants, 16 (19%) were handicapped (i.e., had a developmental level 2 standard deviations below the norm, cerebral palsy, visual deficits, or sensorineural deafness.) There were no reports of bronchopulmonary dysplasia, but one child had retinopathy of prematurity. The authors acknowledged their very short-term follow-up, the small number of subjects, and the inability to generalize to other populations.

In 1981, Rothberg and colleagues[65] reported on the 2-year outcome of 28 infants with birth weights lower than 1250 g who were born between May 1, 1973, and July 31, 1976 and had been mechanically ventilated. It is noteworthy that these authors addressed not only survival and early morbidity but also the effect of various complications of prematurity, aspects that had not been examined in earlier studies. These 28 infants were the survivors of a population of 144 infants, of whom 22% were inborn and 78% were outborn then transported to the authors' neonatal intensive care unit. Thus, it can be seen from this small sample, despite the numerous advances in neonatal intensive care in the 1970s, the mortality and morbidity for these small infants remained high.

It was suggested that if the best results were to be obtained, these infants should be delivered in perinatal centers; if they are not, such infants with VLBW should be expeditiously transferred to a tertiary care nursery.

INFANTS WITH BIRTH WEIGHTS OF 800 TO 1000 GRAMS

In 1979, Yu and Hollingsworth[72] reported on 55 infants with birth weights of 1000 g or less who were born in 1977 and 1978. The overall survival rate was 60%; 44% of infants weighing 501 to 750 g and 67% of infants weighing 751 to 1000 g survived. The authors reported no major abnormalities and suggested that the prognosis for these very small infants was good. However, these investigators based this suggestion on only a 1-year follow-up period, during which time no formal neurodevelopmental assessments were performed. The investigators also did not identify whether there were complications of prematurity, and they did not compare their results with those of earlier studies. Nevertheless, this work set the stage for researchers in the 1980s, who maintained that the chances of the very small infant surviving were improving, as were the developmental outcomes.

Saigal and associates,[69] in a study of children born between 1973 and 1978, found that among the 294 infants weighing between 501 and 1000 g, there was a 31.9% survival rate. The investigators monitored 37 discharged infants in this weight group for a minimum of 2 years and found that 9 (24.3%) had some functional handicap. Of the 35 patients they evaluated, 21 (60%) had some dysfunction, whereas they determined 14 (40%) to be normal. Among the 21 with some dysfunction, 9 had neurological impairments, including hydrocephalus and cerebral palsy. Factors associated with poor outcome included ventilatory support and intracranial hemorrhage. As with the previous study, these authors suggested improvement in the outcome for this population, although they acknowledged the underestimation of minor disabilities in younger infants.

Ruiz and colleagues[66] reported the 1-year outcome for 38 infants born between 1976 and 1978 with birth weights lower than 1000 g. These infants were selected from a cohort of 134 infants, 47 (35%) of whom survived. The investigators concluded the ventilated infants seemed to fare worse than the nonventilated infants. Multiple disabilities were common, with overlap between neuromuscular and developmental problems. Of the 38 infants studied, 20 (53%) had no problems, 17 (45%) had multiple disabilities, and 3 (8%) had severe neurological or developmental impairment.

Driscoll and associates[67] reported on a prospective study of 54 infants born in 1977 and 1978 who survived with birth weights lower than 1000 g, half of whom were born in a center with a NICU. None of the infants with birth weights lower than 700 g survived. On the basis of their results, the authors concluded that there had been improvement in the survival of these small infants but that there was a high complication rate, including intellectual impairment in 30% of the group. Unfortunately, they did not separate the outcome of children with bronchopulmonary dysplasia and/or intracranial hemorrhage from that of children without these complications, and thus the characterization of the population studied is incomplete.

Kitchen and associates[73] reported on 351 infants born in one region in Australia with birth weights of 500 to 999 g who were monitored for 2 years. Eighty-nine (25.4%) survived, and investigators evaluated 83. Overall, 22.5% had severe functional handicaps, 29.2% had moderate-to-mild handicaps, and 48.3% had no handicap; 13.5% had cerebral palsy, 3.4% had bilateral blindness, and 3.4% had severe sensorineural hearing loss. Those born in tertiary care centers did better than those who were born elsewhere, as reflected in a significantly lower incidence of functional handicaps and higher scores on the Mental Developmental Index of the Bayley Scales of Infant Development. The authors concluded that to optimize outcome, infants with VLBW should be delivered in the setting most capable of responding to their unique needs. This view is similar to that of Rothberg and colleagues[65] and Lubchenco and coworkers.[74]

Kitchen and associates[75] also reported on 54 children with birth weights of 500 to 999 g born during 1977 to 1980 and seen at 2 years of corrected age. Fifty of these children were also seen at age $5^1/_2$ years. There was a 39.6% survival rate with a mean birth weight of 864 g. At age 2 years, on the Bayley Scales of Infant Development, the study children had a mean Mental Developmental Index score of 91.1 (standard deviation, 16.5) and a mean Psychomotor Developmental Index score of 87.7 (standard deviation, 17.0), both of which are below the population mean. Of the 50 children evaluated at $5^1/_2$ years of corrected age, 30 (60%) had no impairment, 5 (10%) had severe sensorineural hearing loss or intellectual deficits, 5 (10%) had mild-to-moderate impairment, and 10 (20%) had minor neurological abnormalities. Three children had spastic diplegia. The authors also noted a small number of patients with sensorineural deficits and blindness. The mean score on the full Wechsler Preschool and Primary Scales of Intelligence was 101.8. This study suggested that outcome may improve from ages 2 to $5^1/_2$ years among VLBW survivors.

Nevertheless, even at the later time, 40% of survivors had some difficulty.

In another population, Kitchen and associates[76] reported on the 5-year outcome for the same weight group (500 to 999 g) born during 1979 and 1980. The survival rate in this group was 25.4%; investigators evaluated 83 of 89. Of the 83, 60 (72%) had no functional impairment, 16 (19%) had severe impairment, 4 (5%) had moderate impairment, and 3 (4%) had mild involvement. In this regional study, the patients who were not born at the tertiary care center did worse than those born at the center. Eight children had cerebral palsy, six were blind, and four had sensorineural or mixed deafness. Once again, the authors found that the outcome at 5 years was better than at 2 years. However, they did not comment on whether these children had been in any kind of therapy or early intervention program.

INFANTS WITH BIRTH WEIGHTS LOWER THAN 800 GRAMS

Britton and colleagues[26] questioned whether intensive care was justified for infants weighing less than 801 g at birth. They examined a population of 158 infants weighing less than 801 g born between 1974 and 1977 who were transported to the intensive care unit. The infants with birth weights higher than 750 g did somewhat better than those with lower birth weights.

Hirata and associates[77] obtained similar findings in 22 infants with birth weights 501 to 750 g, 36.7%. Of these 22 infants, 18 were monitored from ages 20 months to 7 years. The investigators found that 11% had neurological sequelae, 22% were functional and of borderline or below-average intelligence, and 67% were normal. Thus, the results of these studies suggested that the outcome for children with birth weights higher than 750 g was better than previously expected and that aggressive therapy improved the outcome, although many survivors had significant neurodevelopmental problems.

The reports on the survival and follow-up study of children born in the 1970s were largely optimistic. There was a definite increase in the survival of small infants receiving intensive care, including those with birth weights lower than 800 g. Moreover, the infants who did survive, including those of extremely low birth weight, seemed to do fairly well, at least over the short term. Thus, clinicians believed that they should provide every possible support for these infants. However, a nagging concern began to emerge: that although many of these infants survived and did fairly well, they would have problems as they grew up. Furthermore, the appreciation that premature infants were not a homogeneous group and that multiple factors affected outcomes influenced the follow-up study of premature infants in the 1980s and 1990s.

Studies in the Late 1980s

In 1989, Hack and Fanaroff[1] reported on the outcome of infants with birth weights lower than 750 g born between 1982 and 1988. Ninety-eight infants were born between July 1982 and June 1985 (period 1), and 120 infants were born between July 1985 and June 1988 (period 2). There was some increase in survival from period 1 to period 2 among infants with gestational ages between 25 and 27 weeks (52% vs. 71%), but the overall rates of neonatal morbidity in the two groups were similar. The neurodevelopmental outcomes were also similar. Period 1 children had Bayley motor and mental scores of 90 ± 17 and 88 ± 14, respectively, at 20 months of corrected age. The period 2 children were seen at 8 months of corrected age and had motor and mental scores of 77 ± 25 and 81 ± 30. There was more aggressive intervention with the period 2 children who had many complications, including bronchopulmonary dysplasia, septicemia, retinopathy of prematurity, intraventricular hemorrhage, and deficits in neurodevelopmental function.

O'Callaghan and coworkers[78] reported on the 2-year outcome of 63 children with ELBW born between 1988 and 1990 and cared for in a neonatal intensive care unit. Findings provide some insight into how more recent cohorts of children with ELBW may be functioning at 2 years of age. Investigators compared the children to full-term matched controls by using a cognitive function measure, a neurosensory motor developmental assessment, and a medical assessment. Furthermore, they studied these children as a whole group and as a subset, a low-risk group, which included children with no intracranial hemorrhage, periventricular leukomalacia, or chronic lung disease (i.e., bronchopulmonary dysplasia). The interesting findings very much mirrored those of earlier studies. The total ELBW group differed significantly from the control group (children born at term) with regard to cognitive and personal-social functioning, although they scored in the average range. The low-risk ELBW group did not differ from the control group. There were more striking differences with review of the neurosensory motor findings. Both the total ELBW group and the low-risk ELBW group had poorer total scores than did the control group, as well as poorer gross and fine motor subscale scores.

In the past, there was interest primarily in the IQs of children born very early. Most investigators assessed early neurodevelopmental functioning and found that, as a group, the infants with VLBW did not do as well as the older and heavier premature infants or

a matched control group of infants born at term. However, investigators are now able to assess more subtle aspects of central nervous system function that have an effect on cognitive functioning.

Herrgaard and colleagues[79] undertook a 5-year neurodevelopmental assessment of 60 children born before 32 weeks of gestation. These children were matched with 60 full-term controls. Assessment tools used included a standardized neurological examination, a neuropsychological assessment, an audiological examination, and an ophthalmological examination. Included in the preterm group were children thought to be handicapped (children with cerebral palsy, mental retardation [IQ < 70], bilateral hearing loss, visual impairment, and epilepsy) and those not disabled. With regard to IQ, there were significant differences between the entire preterm group and the control group, as well as significant differences between the handicapped and nonhandicapped preterm groups. The control group had the highest IQs, the nonhandicapped preterm group had lower IQs, and the handicapped group had the lowest IQs. The neurodevelopmental profile was composed of eight functional entities: gross motor, fine motor, visual-motor, attention, language, visual-spatial, sensorimotor, and memory skills. The investigators noted several interesting findings. First, all of the children born preterm had difficulty with gross, fine, and visual-motor skills. They also had difficulty with language, sensorimotor, visual-spatial, and memory skills. Second, the nonhandicapped children with minor neurodevelopmental difficulties had a similar spectrum of problems, although their IQs were in the average range, with some even in the exceptional range.

These findings are similar to those of Sostek[80] in her study of children born before 33 weeks of gestational age and with a mean birth weight of 1358 g, in comparison with children born at term. None of the premature children had lung disease, intracranial hemorrhage, or other medical problems. Although these children had normal IQs, they were compromised with regard to perceptual-motor integration and recognition, perceptual performance tasks, quantitative tasks, memory, and visual-motor skill and were found to be more distractible and to have poorer attention and less readiness for kindergarten than were full-term controls. These findings emphasize the importance of assessing neurodevelopmental profiles, rather than relying on global measures of intelligence.

Teplin and associates[81] assessed the neurodevelopmental, health, and growth status at 6 years of age in 28 children with birth weights lower than 1001 g. In comparison with 26 control children born at term, the children with ELBW had significantly more mild or moderate-to-severe neurological problems (61% vs. 23%) including cerebral palsy; abnormalities of muscle tone; and immaturities of balance, speech, and articulation. In cognitive function, the controls scored significantly higher than the children with ELBW. However, more than half of the children with ELBW with normal IQs had mildly abnormal neurological findings, whereas the controls with normal IQs had normal neurological findings. When they determined the overall functional status, the investigators found that 46% of children with ELBW were normal, 36% were mildly disabled, and 18% were moderately to severely disabled; in comparison, 75% of the controls were normal, only 4% were significantly disabled, and the remainder had some mild degree of abnormality. In contrast to other reports, attentional disturbances were not a problem for the preterm groups described in these two studies.[82,83]

Halsey and colleagues[84] conducted another provocative and important study on children with VLBW when they were in preschool. They studied 60 white, middle-class children with VLBW and compared them with a matched peer group. They used a general developmental scale and a scale of visual-motor integration. They found that the VLBW group's mean scores were significantly lower than those of the controls, although they were still within one standard deviation of the mean. Of the children with VLBW, 23% were clearly disabled, 51% obtained borderline scores, and 26% were average. The control group had cognitive scores 15 to 18 points higher than those of the VLBW group and were 2.5 times more likely to have normal development. The authors were reluctant to make any predictions on the basis of these data but expressed concern that this pattern of performance placed the children with VLBW at higher risk for later difficulties. A subsequent study, to be discussed later,[90] confirmed that these data are indeed predictive of later difficulties. Thus, follow-up studies suggest that premature infants with VLBW, despite relatively intact cognitive skills as evidenced by normal IQs, appear to have neuropsychological and neuromotor disturbances that can adversely affect their school performance, self-esteem, and behavior.

The studies of the 1980s, in which children were monitored to only the preschool years, reinforced the concerns of the 1970s. Although investigators did note an increase in survival and found that many children did well, they also noted that these children were functioning at lower levels than their peers and with a variety of neurodevelopmental problems that earlier studies had not identified. These problems included deficiencies in their perceptual skills, social skills, and level of maturity.

We have thus far reviewed reports on infants with VLBW evaluated after only 2 to 6 years. However,

among the most important indicators of successful outcome are the child's social-emotional adaptation and how well the child does in school. Studies have acknowledged that many infants with VLBW have significant difficulties that persist throughout their lives. Although such children may have IQs in the average range, they do not perform as well as controls on measures of fine and gross motor and visual-motor tasks and display so-called "minor disabilities" that become more apparent in school. An important question, then, is what effect these difficulties have on school performance and peer relationships. Eilers and associates[85] studied a group of children with birth weights of 1250 g or lower who were born between July 1974 and July 1978. There were 43 survivors, 33 of whom were studied at 5 to 8 years of age. Of the 33 children, 16 were functioning at an age-appropriate level, 3 had major handicaps, and 14 were in regular classes but needed remedial help. The authors noted that 51.5% of this group required special education support, in comparison with 21.4% of the general school population.

Vohr and Garcia Coll[86] reported on a 7-year longitudinal study of children with birth weights lower than 1500 g who were born in 1975. Of their original population, 62 (51.2%) survived, and 42 (67%) were monitored. The investigators evaluated patterns of neurological and developmental functioning at 1 year of age and compared them with normal functioning children at age 7. Using a classification of "normal," "suspect," and "abnormal," they found that the patterns at 1 year were significantly related to those at 7 years and that 54% of the total sample required special education or resource help at 7 years. Furthermore, those who had abnormal findings at 1 year were most likely to have difficulties at 7 years. This was less clear for the groups with suspect and normal functioning. Based on their identification at age 1 year, 27% of the children with normal patterns, 50% of the children with suspect patterns, and 87% of the children with abnormal patterns required special educational services by age 7. The investigators also noted that 45% of the children with normal patterns, 75% of those with suspect patterns, and 100% of those with abnormal patterns had visual-motor disturbances.

Another study[87] revealed that even among a relatively normal group of children with birth weights of 1500 g or lower, there was an increased incidence of visual-motor problems. Klein and coworkers[83] found that a group of children with VLBW scored lower at 9 years of age on tests measuring general intelligence, visual or spatial skills, and academic achievement than did full-term controls. Klein and coworkers found that a subset of children with VLBW but normal IQs showed significant deficits in mathematics skills. Crowe and associates[88] reported on 90 children born between 24 and 36 weeks of gestation who participated in a longitudinal follow-up program; children with such major neurological impairments as cerebral palsy were excluded from study. Crowe and associates found that motor development at $4^1/_2$ years of corrected age was relatively intact, but children with birth weights of about 1000 g displayed significantly poorer motor skills. Moreover, such children with symptomatic intracranial hemorrhage also had significantly poorer motor performance.

Saigal and associates[82] conducted a longitudinal, regionally based study over many years and reported on the cognitive and school abilities at 8 years of a cohort of relatively socioeconomically advantaged infants with birth weights of 501 to 1000 g who were born between 1977 and 1981. The investigators compared the children's intellectual, motor, visual-motor, and adaptive capabilities and their teachers' perceptions to those of a matched group of children born at term. They found that the majority of children with ELBW had IQs in the normal range but significantly lower than those of the controls. This was true even when handicapped children were excluded from the analysis. Moreover, the ELBW group was significantly disadvantaged on every measure. Furthermore, the teachers rated the ELBW group as performing below grade level. Interestingly, neurologically normal children also performed below the normal range on tests of visual-motor and motor abilities.

Hack and coworkers[89] reported on the 8-year neurocognitive abilities of a group of 249 infants with VLBW born between 1977 and 1979, in comparison with 363 randomly selected normal children born at the same time. The investigators administered a neurological examination and tests of intelligence, language, speech, reading, mathematics, spelling, visual and fine motor abilities, and behavior. Twenty-four (10%) of the children with VLBW had a major neurological abnormality. None of the controls had such a finding. With the exception of speech and total behavior scores, the VLBW group scored significantly more poorly than did the controls on all tests. Even neurologically intact children with VLBW but normal IQs had significantly poorer scores than did the controls in expressive language, memory, visual-motor function, fine motor function, and measures of hyperactivity. When the investigators controlled for social risk as a significant determinant of poor outcome, VLBW still had an adverse affect on functioning, with the exception of verbal IQ. The investigators concluded that prematurity may contribute only minimally to the negative effect of a poor psychosocial environment in this area. In contrast, biological factors may have a greater effect on the deficits of more advantaged children, in comparison with their peers.

In a more recent study, Hille and associates[90] assessed the school performance at 9 years of age of children with VLBW born in the Netherlands. They were able to gather data on 84% ($N = 813$) of the survivors from an almost complete birth cohort at 9 years of age. Nineteen percent were in special education programs, half of whom had been placed since 5 years of age for identified problems. Of the children with VLBW in mainstream classes, 32% were in a grade below their age level, and another 38% required special assistance. Of the children who were retained, 60% required special assistance, in comparison with 28% of children in an age-appropriate grade. The authors identified a number of factors at 5 years of age that were predictive of school difficulties at 9 years. These included developmental delays, speech and language delay, behavioral problems, and low socioeconomic status, which confirmed the findings of Hack and coworkers[89] and Halsey and colleagues.[84]

A final issue to consider with this group of children is the possible effect of VLBW on behavior. We noted previously that many of these children have significant problems with hyperactivity and attention. Weisglas-Kuperus and colleagues[91] addressed the issue of behavior problems in this group of children. In a study of 73 children with VLBW who were compared with 192 full-term children at $3^1/_2$ years of age, the authors found a significant degree of behavioral disturbance in the VLBW group. Problems included depression and internalizing difficulties.

Studies in the 1990s

Follow-up studies proliferated throughout the 1990s. These studies focused not only on the improved survival of the infant with VLBW as a result of further technological advances but also, of even more importance, on developmental, cognitive, academic, and social outcomes. Investigators noted the improved survival rates among infants with VLBW, as well as among infants with ELBW, during this period, in comparison with the 1970s and 1980s. As a group, the studies addressed cognition (IQ), academic performance, behavioral issues and social competence, health, language development, and visual and fine motor capacities. These follow-up studies were of longer term than previous studies, extending up to 11 to 13 years of age. As in the 1980s, the investigators divided the infants into groups of those with birth weight lower than 750 g, 750 to 1000 g, 1001 to 1499 g, and 1500 to 2500 g and used as controls children with birth weights higher than 2500 g, who were also matched for gender and socioeconomic status.

The prenatal and perinatal factors with the greatest effect on outcome included birth weight, gestational age, whether the infant was born in or outside of a special care center, and the nature and degree of the complications of premature birth. These complications included chronic lung disease and the need for oxygen, the presence of intraventricular hemorrhage and its complications, and the presence of seizures. Of note, many of these children had significant infections and gastroenterological problems, including necrotizing enterocolitis and undernutrition. In addition, many of these children had recurrent ear infections, which often necessitated myringotomy and tubes retinopathy of prematurity. The lighter and more immature the infant, the more prevalent were complications and so the higher was the risk for a more adverse outcome. Thus, the smallest infants who survived, those with birth weight lower than 750 g, had the worst outcomes. As a group, they had an increased incidence of cerebral palsy, mental retardation, autism, attention-deficit/hyperactivity disorder, and learning disability and had lower IQs than their peers. In addition, these children were less socially adept than their heavier or full-term peers. This same pattern appeared with other premature infants of greater birth weights.

Ross and associates[92] measured the academic and social competence at 7 to 8 years of age of boys and girls with birth weights lower than 1501 g. They found that, as group, these children had lower scores than their full-term peers on measures of social competence and cognitive functioning and had a greater incidence of conduct disorders. Differences were greatest for children from the lower socioeconomic groups and for boys.

Investigators in Canada have been effective in capturing regional cohorts. Saigal and associates[82] examined the 8-year outcome of somewhat socioeconomically advantaged children with birth weights of 501 to 1000 g and compared them with a matched group of children born at term. They found that the majority of children with ELBW had IQs in the normal range but lower than those of the full-term controls. Moreover, 8% to 12% of the children with ELBW scored in the "abnormal range," in comparison with only 1% to 2% of the controls. Even the children with ELBW who were neurologically "normal" were performing below grade level, according to their teachers' ratings, and had difficulties with visual-motor tasks. In a later study, Saigal and associates[93] evaluated children with birth weights lower than 1500 g and compared them to full-term children at ages 8 to 9 years. Very few of the children with ELBW had no functional limitations, and significant numbers of these children had cognitive problems

and difficulties with mobility and the processing of sensory information.

In the United States, the studies of Hack and coworkers are of particular interest because their follow-up program has continued for many years, entails evaluation of infants admitted to a single tertiary care unit, and has had excellent subject retention. Hack and coworkers[89] compared children with birth weights lower than 1500 g to full-term children at ages 8 to 9 years. They found that 10% of the infants with VLBW had major neurological deficits and an additional 21% had IQ scores lower than 85. Although the neurologically intact infants with VLBW had IQs similar to those of full-term controls, they had significantly poorer scores on tests of expressive language, memory, and visual–fine motor skills and had a higher incidence of hyperactivity. These differences persisted even after the investigators controlled for social risks.

In another study, Hack and coworkers[94] evaluated a small group of children with birth weights lower than 1000 g and found that those with birth weights lower than 750 g did much worse in school than did premature children with higher birth weights. In turn, the latter performed more poorly than did matched full-term controls. Interestingly, abnormal head ultrasonograms and prolonged oxygen dependence were associated with mental retardation and cerebral palsy. In a similar study, Halsey and colleagues[95] monitored 210 children with birth weights lower than 800 g into the school years and found that although many of these children scored in the cognitively normal range, their scores were significantly lower than those of matched full-term children. In addition, 20% of this group had disabilities, including cerebral palsy, mental retardation, autism, and learning problems, and half of the children with ELBW required special educational services. Similar patterns were reported by Taylor and associates[96] and LaPine and coworkers.[97]

Kilbride and Daily[98] performed an 8-year follow-up study on 114 children with birth weights of 500 to 750 g. Of this group, 30% were considered normal at 3 years and 89% were in regular classes without educational assistance. Fifty percent had suspect IQ scores (69 to 83) and motor quotients at age 3 years. Of importance, 20% of these children were in special education classes and 33% were held back a grade and were receiving learning support. Forty-six percent were functioning in an age-appropriate class, although only 15% were not receiving additional services. (Twenty percent were abnormal at 3 years.) Seventy-five percent of there children with combined cognitive-motor concerns were in special remedial classes. This study revealed that performance at 3 years of adjusted age was predictive of functioning at 8 years.

This pattern of outcome is described by a number of other reports from different centers.[82,90,92-126]

These studies from the 1990s documented an increase in survival of children with VLBW and ELBW in comparison with earlier decades, but they also documented significant morbidity. Even among children who seem "normal," there are ongoing major academic and behavioral challenges necessitating educational interventions and supports.

More recent studies, published between 1999 and 2005, focused primarily on infants with VLBW or ELBW.[127-167] Although most earlier studies were conducted in the United States, Canada, and Australia, later studies documented outcomes from Germany, as well as other European countries. In the Bavarian Longitudinal Study,[127] investigators reviewed the outcomes from multiple centers in Germany, assessing at 6 years of age children born with gestational ages of less than 32 weeks and comparing them with matched, full-term controls. The investigators found that the children born before term scored significantly lower on cognitive, language, and prereading skills than did the controls and were more likely to have deficits in simultaneous processing. Preterm birth had a greater effect on outcome than did socioeconomic status.

Investigators in the Epidemiological Project for ICU Research and Evaluation (EPICure) study[129,130] evaluated children with gestational ages of less than 25 weeks when they were 30 months old and then at 6 years of age. The investigators found that severe disability at 30 months was predictive of outcome at 6 years. At the 6-year pediatric visit, 46% of the 78% of surviving children who had participated at 30 months had cognitive and neurological impairments. Twenty-one percent had moderate to severe cognitive impairments in comparison to test norms, 41% had moderate to severe impairments in comparison with their classmates, 22% had severe developmental disability, 24% had moderate disability, 34% had mild disability, and 12% had disabling cerebral palsy and cognitive deficits. Thirty-eight percent whose impairments were classified as "other disability" at 30 months of age had severe disability at 6 years. Twenty-four percent who had been classified as having no disability at 30 months had significant disability at 6 years of age. Vohr[132] reported the same pattern of outcome for a large multicenter cohort of children with birth weights of 501 to 1000 g. Significant numbers of these children had neurodevelopmental disorders, cerebral palsy, and Bayley scores lower than 70, in addition to hearing and vision impairments.

Follow-up studies from this period in which investigators evaluated very premature children and children with VLBW at 7 to 12 years of age reveal significant, previously undetected deficits in social functioning, academic performance, and atten-

tion.[133,134] The increasing survival of more immature and lighter babies is evident in comparisons of outcomes with earlier time periods. However, the consequences of this survival are increasing numbers of children with significant neurodevelopmental problems and the emergence during the school-age years of previously undetected social, academic, and behavioral difficulties.

IMPLICATIONS FOR CLINICAL ASSESSMENT, MONITORING, AND CHILD HEALTH SUPERVISION

Findings from longitudinal follow-up studies raise the question of whether a more aggressive and proactive approach to detection of potential learning problems during the preschool years would be worthwhile in preventing or ameliorating later difficulties. The earlier identification of such problems may improve the overall outcome for the child and family. Helpful implications from follow-up studies include the observations that any child requiring neonatal intensive care is at risk for later difficulties (medical, developmental, behavioral, and psychological) and that the smaller and more immature (in weight and gestational age) the infant, the greater is the risk for complications and adverse outcomes.

Study findings suggest that all children born prematurely should be evaluated and monitored by a multidisciplinary team of clinicians to identify strengths and weaknesses, suggest intervention strategies, assess the efficacy of the interventions, and monitor the child's progress into the early school years. These evaluations and early interventions should inform educational and psychological strategies whose objectives are to optimize outcome in this high-risk population of children.[168]

With regard to child health supervision services, children "born too soon and too small" require care and monitoring beyond that indicated for most children born at term. At the time of discharge from the nursery, the clinician should clearly identify the infant's needs and establish a plan for medical and developmental follow-up. Infants with conditions such as bronchopulmonary dysplasia, intracranial hemorrhage and possible hydrocephalus, or other serious complications of prematurity require close follow-up by a primary care provider and appropriate subspecialists and may benefit from referral for occupational, physical, and speech therapy. Assessment should include tests of hearing and vision. Children with previously identified problems should be assessed at least every 6 months through the first 2 years and then yearly until school entry. Evaluation before school entry is crucial for facilitating appropriate school placement. Assessments should include intelligence testing, as well as evaluations of language, social maturity, and behavioral status and functioning.

Premature infants in apparently good health also require careful monitoring. We suggest that such children be evaluated between the ages of 3 and 4 months, 6 and 8 months, and 12 and 14 months and at 18 months and 2 years of age. Measurements of height, weight, and head circumference should be obtained at every health supervision visit, as should an assessment of general health and well-being.[169] Evaluation during the first 2 years of life should include developmental and language assessments, as well as evaluations by an occupational and physical therapist. We also recommend evaluation between the ages of 3 and 5 years to help determine school readiness and during the school-age years to monitor educational progress.

CONCLUSIONS

The introduction of neonatal intensive care has had a dramatic effect on the prognosis of premature infants. Ongoing research will undoubtedly contribute to new approaches to management and further changes in outcome. We draw the following conclusions from our review of longitudinal studies to date:

- Important clinical advances since the early 1970s have resulted in increasing numbers of infants with VLBW who survive the neonatal period. Whether the absolute number of children surviving with some disability is also increasing is controversial. Stewart[62] maintained that the number of surviving children with disabilities is not increasing, whereas Paneth and colleagues,[25] Pharoah and coworkers,[170] and Bhushan and associates[171] reported the opposite. We believe that the current data suggest that the incidence of cerebral palsy and major disability has not increased since the first reports of the 1960s but that the absolute numbers of children with some disabilities has increased.

- The 2-year outcome for these children is related to birth weight, gestational age, and neonatal morbidity. The smaller the infant, the greater is the risk for prenatal and postnatal complications and the higher is the incidence of such early morbid conditions as respiratory distress syndrome and intracranial hemorrhage and such subsequent, long-term morbid conditions as bronchopulmonary dysplasia, chronic lung disease, and cerebral palsy. Infants with bronchopulmonary dysplasia, intraventricular hemorrhage and periventricular leukomalacia, and severe

retinopathy of prematurity and significant sensorineural hearing loss are at greater risk for significant, long-term, neurodevelopmental impairments. Being born outside a perinatal center, low maternal education, and low socioeconomic status are among the other factors contributing to poor outcome.

- Our review of 2- and 5-year developmental outcomes demonstrates the effects of clinical advances since the early 1970s. However, 20% to 60% of survivors still have some difficulties; approximately 10% to 20% have significant neurodevelopmental disability. Moreover, even those who initially appear well subsequently experience more difficulties in school than does the general population. Even neurologically intact infants with VLBW may have significant, pervasive multisystem problems that are not evident until school age. For example, a normal neonatal head ultrasonogram is not necessarily correlated with or predictive of long-term outcome.

- In studies of school performance at 6 to 8 years of age, investigators have reported a significant incidence of learning and behavioral disorders among children born with ELBW and VLBW, including those without significant disabling conditions. This high-risk population of children requires monitoring for such "sleeper effects" of prematurity.

REFERENCES

1. Hack M, Fanaroff AA: Outcomes of extemely low-birth-weight infants between 1982 and 1988. N Engl J Med 321:1642-1647, 1989.
2. Allen MC, Donohue PK, Dusman AB: The limit of viability—Neonatal outcome of infants born at 22 to 25 weeks' gestation. N Engl J Med 329:1597-1601, 1993.
3. Arias E, MacDorman M, Stubino D, et al: Annual summary of vital statistics—2002. Pediatrics 112:1215-1230, 2003.
4. MacDorman M, Minino A, Strobino D, et al: Annual summary of vital statistics—2001. Pediatrics 110:1037-1052, 2002.
5. Hess JH: Experiences gained in a thirty-year study of prematurely born infants. Pediatrics 11:425-434, 1953.
6. Douglas JWB: Premature children at primary school. BMJ 1:1008-1013, 1960.
7. Dann M, Levine SZ, New EV: The development of prematurely born children with birth weights or minimal postnatal weights of 1,000 grams or less. Pediatrics 22:1037-1052, 1958.
8. Gordon HH: Perspectives on neonatology. *In* Avery GB, ed: Neonatology. Philadelphia: JB Lippincott, 1975.
9. Silverman WA: Retrolental Fibroplasia: A Modern Parable, New York: Grune & Stratton, 1980.
10. Davies PA, Russel H: Later progress of 100 infants weighing 1000 to 2000 grams at birth fed immediately

with breast milk. Dev Med Child Neurol 10:725-735, 1968.

11. Rawlings G, Reynolds EOR, Stewart AL, et al: Changing prognosis for infants of very low birth weight. Lancet 1:516-519, 1971.

12. Gregory GA, Kitterman JA, Phibbs RH, et al: Treatment of idiopathic respiratory-distress syndrome with continuous positive airway pressure. N Engl J Med 284:1333-1340, 1971.

13. Huch R, Huch A, Albani M, et al: Transcutaneous PO_2 monitoring in routine management of infants and children with cardiorespiratory problems. Pediatrics 57:681-690, 1976.

14. Conway M, Durbin GM, Ingram D, et al: Continuous monitoring of arterial oxygen tension using a catheter-tip polarographic electrode in infants. Pediatrics 57:244-250, 1976.

15. Aoyagi T, Kishi M, Yamaguchi K, et al: Improvement of the earpiece oximeter. *In* Abstracts of the Japanese Society of Medical Electronics and Biological Engineering, Tokyo, 1974, pp 90-91.

16. Poets CF, Southall DP: Noninvasive monitoring of oxygenation in infants and children: Practical considerations and areas of concern. Pediatrics 93:737-746, 1994.

17. Heird WC: Nutritional support of the pediatric patient. *In* Winters RW, Green HL, eds: Nutritional Support of the Seriously Ill Patient. New York: Academic Press, 1983, pp 157-179.

18. Gitlin JD, Soll RF, Parad RB, et al: Randomized controlled trial of exogenous surfactant for the treatment of hyaline membrane disease. Pediatrics 79:31-37, 1987.

19. Robertson CMT: Surfactant replacement therapy for severe neonatal respiratory distress syndrome: An international randomized clinical trial. Pediatrics 82:683-691, 1988.

20. Dunn MS, Shennan AT, Hoskins EM, et al: Two-year follow-up of infants enrolled in a randomized trial of surfactant replacement therapy for prevention of neonatal respiratory distress syndrome. Pediatrics 82:543-547, 1988.

21. Vaucher YE, Merritt TA, Hallman M, et al: Neurodevelopmental and respiratory outcome in early childhood after human surfactant treatment. Am J Dis Child 142:927-930, 1988.

22. Survanta Multidose Study Group: Two-year follow-up of infants treated for neonatal respiratory distress syndrome with bovine surfactant. J Pediatr 124:962-967, 1991.

23. Abman SH, Kinsella JP: Nitric oxide in the pathophysiology and treatment of neonatal pulmonary hypertension. Neonat Respir Dis 4:1-11, 1994.

24. Kiely J, Paneth N, Stein Z, et al: Cerebral palsy and newborn care. II. Mortality and neurological impairment in low-birth weight infants. Dev Med Child Neurol 5:650-666, 1981.

25. Paneth N, Kiely L, Stein Z, et al: Cerebral palsy and newborn care. III. Estimated prevalence rates of cerebral palsy under differing rates of mortality and impairment of low-birth weight infants. Dev Med Child Neurol 23:801-817, 1981.

26. Britton SB, Fitzhardinge PM, Ash by S: Is intensive care justified for infants weighing less than 801 gm at birth? J Pediatr 99:937-943, 1981.

27. Shelp EE: Born to Die? Deciding the Fate of Critically Ill Newborns. New York: Free Press, 1986.

28. Klaus MH, Kennell JH: Parent-Infant Bonding, 2nd ed. St. Louis: CV Mosby, 1982.

29. Plunkett JW, Meisels SJ, Stiefel GS, et al: Patterns of attachment among preterm infants of varying biological risk. J Am Acad Child Psychiatry 25:794-800, 1986.

30. Washington J, Minde K, Goldberg S: Temperament in preterm infants: Style and stability. J Am Acad Child Psychiatry 25:493-502, 1986.

31. Oberklaid F, Prior M, Sanson A: Temperament of preterm versus full-term infants. Dev Behav Pediatr 7:159-162, 1986.

32. Cohen RS, Stevenson DK, Malachowski N, et al: Favorable results of neonatal intensive care for very low-birth-weight infants. Pediatrics 69:621-625, 1982.

33. Lubchenco LO, Searls DT, Brazie IV: Neonatal mortality rate: Relationship to birth weight and gestational age. J Pediatr 1972; 81:814-822, 1972.

34. Vohr B, O'Shea M, Wright L: Longitudinal multicenter follow-up of high-risk infants: Why, who, when and what to assess. Semin Perinatol 27:333-342, 2003.

35. Johnson A: Disability and perinatal care. Pediatrics 95:272-274, 1995.

36. Castro L, Yolton K, Haberman B, et al: Bias in reported neurodevelopmental outcomes among extremely low birth weight survivors. Pediatrics 114:404-410, 2004.

37. Evans D, Levene M: Evidence of selection bias in preterm survival studies: A systematic review. Arch Dis Child Fetal Neonatal Ed 84:F79-F84, 2001.

38. Vohr BR, Wright LL, Dusick AM, et al: Center differences and outcomes of extremely low birth weight infants. Pediatrics 113:781-789, 2004.

39. Albrecht G, Devlieger P: The disability paradox: High quality of life against all odds. Soc Sci Med 48:977-988, 1999.

40. Escobar G, Littenberg B, Petitti D: Outcome among surviving very low birth weight infants: A metaanalysis. Arch Dis Child 66:204-211, 1991.

41. Gross S, Slagle T, D'Eugenio D, et al: Impact of a matched term control group on interpretation of developmental performance in preterm infants. Pediatrics 90:681-687, 1992.

42. Harrison H: The principles of family-centered neonatal care. Pediatrics 92:643-650, 1993.

43. Vohr B, Msall M: Neuropsychological and functional outcomes of very low birth weight infants. Semin Perinatol 21:202-220, 1997.

44. Hernandez J, Hall D, Goldson E, et al: Impact of infants born at the threshold of viability on the

neonatal mortality risk rate in Colorado. J Perinatology 1:21-26, 2000.

45. Johansson S, Montgomery S, Ekbom A, et al: Preterm delivery, level of care, and infant death in Sweden: A population-based study. Pediatrics 113:1230-1235, 2004.

46. Als H, Duffy F, McNulty G, et al: Early experience alters brain function and structure. Pediatrics 113:846-857, 2004.

47. Gardner S, Goldson E: The neonate and the environment: Impact on development. In Merenstein G, Gardner S, eds: Handbook of Neonatal Intensive Care, 6th ed. St.Louis: Mosby, 2006

48. Bennett F, Scott D: Long-term perspective on premature infant outcome and contemporary intervention issues. Semin Perinatol 21:190-201, 1997.

49. Fanaroff A, Hack M, Walsh M: The NICHD Research Network: Changes in practice and outcomes during the first 15 years. Semin Perinatol 27:281-287, 2003.

50. Perlman J: Cognitive and behavioral deficits in premature graduates of intensive care. Clin Perinatol 29:779-797, 2002.

51. Finer N, Craft A, Vaucher Y, et al: Postnatal steroids: Short term gain, long term pain? J Pediatrics 137:9-13, 2000.

52. Vohr B, Msall M: Neuropsychological and functional outcomes of very low birth weight infants. Semin Perinatol 21:202-220, 1997.

53. Clark R, Thomas P, Peabody J: Extrauterine growth restriction remains a serious problem in prematurely born neonates. Pediatrics 111:986-990, 2003.

54. Clark R, Wagner C, Merritt R, et al: Nutrition in the neonatal intensive care unit: How do we reduce the incidence of extrauterine growth restriction? J Perinatol 23:337-344, 2003.

55. Leonard C, Piecuch R: School age outcome in low birth weight preterm infants. Semin Perinatol 21:240-253, 1997.

56. Badr L, Abdallah B: Physical attractiveness of premature infants affects outcome at discharge from the NICU. Infant Behav Dev 24:129-133, 2001.

57. Poehlmann J, Fiese B: Parent-infant interaction as a mediator of the relation between neonatal risk status and 12-month cognitive development. Infant Behav Dev 24:171-188, 2001.

58. Raval V, Goldberg S, Atkinson L, et al: Maternal attachment, maternal responsiveness and infant attachment. Infant Behav Dev 24:281-304, 2001.

59. Schraeder B, Heverly M, O'Brien C, Goodman R: Academic achievement and educational resource use of very low birth weight (VLBW) survivors. Pediatr Nurs 23:21-25, 1997.

60. Ziva Y, Cassidy J: Maternal responsiveness and infant irritability: The contribution of Crockenberg and Smith's "Antecedents of mother-infant interaction and infant irritability in the first 3 months of life." Infant Behav Dev 25:16-20, 2002.

61. Koops BL, Harmon RJ: Studies on long-term outcome in newborns with birth weights under 1500. Adv Behav Pediatr 1:1-28, 1980.

62. Stewart AL: Follow-up studies. In Robertson NRC, edr: Textbook of Neonatology, Edinburgh: Churchill Livingstone, 1986.

63. Goldson E: Follow-up of low birth weight infants: A contemporary review. In Wolraich M, Routh DL, eds: Advances in Developmental and Behavioral Pediatrics, vol 9. London: Jessica Kingsley Publishers, 1992, pp 159-179.

64. Peacock WG, Hirata T: Outcome in low-birth-weight infants (750 to 1,500 grams): A report on 164 cases managed at Children's Hospital, San Francisco, California. Am J Obstet Gynecol 140:165-172, 1981.

65. Rothberg A, Maisels J, Bagnato S, et al: Outcome for survivors of mechanical ventilation weighing less than 1,250 grams at birth. J Pediatr 98:106-111, 1981.

66. Ruiz M, LeFever J, Hakanson D, et al: Early development of infants of birth weight less than 1,000 grams with reference to mechanical ventilation in newborn period. Pediatrics 68:330-335, 1981.

67. Driscoll J, Driscoll Y, Steir M, et al: Mortality and morbidity in infants less than 1,001 grams birth weight. Pediatrics 69:21-26, 1982.

68. Knobloch H, Malone A, Ellison P, et al: Considerations in evaluating changes in outcome for infants weighing less than 1,501 grams. Pediatrics 69:285-295, 1982.

69. Saigal S, Rosenbaum P, Stoskopf B, et al: Follow-up of infants 501-1,500 grams birth weight delivered to residents of a geographically defined region with perinatal intensive care facilities. J Pediatr 100:606-613, 1982.

70. Klein N, Hack M, Breslau N: Children who were very low birth weight: Development and academic achievement at nine years of age. Dev Behav Pediatr 10:32-37, 1989.

71. Orgill AA, Astbury I, Bajuk B, et al: Early neurodevelopmental outcome of very low birthweight infants. Aust Paediatr J 18:193-196, 1982.

72. Yu VYH, Hollingsworth E: Improving prognosis for infants weighing 1000 g or less at birth. Arch Dis Child 55:422-426, 1979.

73. Kitchen W, Ford G, Orgill A, et al: Outcome of infants with birth weight 500 to 999 gm: A regional study of 1979 and 1980 births. J Pediatr 104:921-927, 1984.

74. Lubchenco LO, Butterfield LI, Delaney-Black V, et al: Outcome of very-low-birth-weight infants: Does antepartum versus neonatal referral have a better impact on mortality, morbidity, or long-term outcome? Am J Obstet Gynecol 160:539-545, 1989.

75. Kitchen WH, Ford GW, Rickards AL, et al: Children of birthweight < 1000 g: Changing outcome between ages 2 and 5 years. J Pediatr 110:283-288, 1987.

76. Kitchen W, Ford G, Orgill A, et al: Outcome in infants of birth weight 500 to 999 g: A continuing regional study of 5-year-old survivors. J Pediatr 111:761-766, 1987.

77. Hirata T, Epcar IT, Walsh A, et al: Survival and outcome of infants 501-750 grams: A six-year experience. J Pediatr 102:741-748, 1983.

78. O'Callaghan MI, Burns Y, Gray P, et al: Extremely low birth weight and control infants at 2 years corrected age: A comparison of intellectual abilities, motor performance, growth and health. Early Hum Dev 40:115-125, 1995.

79. Herrgaard E, Luoma L,Tuppurainen K, et al: Neurodevelopmental profile at five years of children born at ≈ 32 weeks gestation. Dev Med Child Neurol 135:1083-1086, 1993.

80. Sostek AM: Prematurity as well as intraventricular hemorrhage influence developmental outcome at 5 years. *In* Friedman SL, Sigman MD, eds: The Psychological Development of Low Birthweight Children. Norwood, NJ: Ablex, 1992, pp 259-274.

81. Teplin SW, Burchinal M, Johnson-Martin N, et al: Neurodevelopmental, health, and growth status at 6 age years of children with birth weights less than 1001 grams. J Pediatr 118:768-777, 1991.

82. Saigal S, Szatmari P, Rosenbaum P, et al: Cognitive abilities and school performance of extremely low birth weight children and matched term control children at age 8 years: A regional study. J Pediatr 118:751-760, 1991.

83. Klein NK, Hack M, Breslau N: Children who were very low birth weight: Development and academic achievement at nine years of age. Dev Behav Pediatr 10:32-37, 1989.

84. Halsey CL, Collin MF, Anderson CL: Extremely low birth weight children and their peers: A comparison of preschool performance. Pediatrics 91:807-811, 1993.

85. Eilers BL, Desai NS, Wilson MA, et al: Classroom performance and social factors of children with birth weights of 1250 grams or less: Follow-up at 5 to 8 years of age. Pediatrics 77:203-208, 1986.

86. Vohr BR, Garcia Coll CT: Neurodevelopmental and school performance of very low birth weight infants: A seven-year longitudinal study. Pediatrics 76:345-350, 1985.

87. Klein N, Hack M, Gallagher I, et al: Preschool performance of children with normal intelligence who were very low-birth-weight infants. Pediatrics 75:531-537, 1985.

88. Crowe TK, Deitz IC, Bennett FC, et al: Preschool motor skills of children born prematurely and not diagnosed as having cerebral palsy. Dev Behav Pediatr 9:189-193, 1988.

89. Hack M, Breslau N, Aram D, et al: The effect of very low birth weight and social risk on neurocognitive abilities at school age. J Dev Behav 13:412-420, 1992.

90. Hille ETM, Den Ouden A, Bauer L, et al: School performance at nine years of age in very premature and very low birth weight infants: Perinatal risk factors and predictors at five years of age. J Pediatr 125:426-434, 1994.

91. Weisglas-Kuperus N, Koot HM, Baerts W, et al: Behaviour problems of very low-birthweight children. Dev Med Child Neurol 35:406-416, 1993.

92. Ross G, Lipper E, Auld PAM: Social competence and behavior problems in premature children at school age. Pediatrics 86:391-397, 1990.

93. Saigal S, Rosenbaum P, Stoskopf B, et al: Comprehensive assessment of the health status of extremely low birth weight children at eight years of age: Comparison with a reference group. J Pediatr 125:411-417, 1994.

94. Hack M, Taylor H, Klein N, et al: School-age outcomes in children with birth weights under 750 grams. N Engl J Med 331:753-759, 1994.

95. Halsey C, Collin M, Anderson C: Extremely low-birth-weight children and their peers: A comparison of school-age outcomes. Arch Pediatr Adolesc Med 150:790-794, 1996.

96. Taylor HG, Hack M, Klein N, et al: Achievement in children with birth weight less than 750 grams with normal cognitive abilities: Evidence for specific learning disabilities. J Pediatr Psychology 20:703-719, 1995.

97. LaPine T, Jackson JC, Bennett F: Outcome of infants weighing less than 800 grams at birth: 15 years' experience. Pediatrics 96:479-483, 1995.

98. Kilbride H, Daily D: Eight year educational outcomes of 801 gram and below birth weight infants: Relationship to assessment at 3 years of age. Pediatr Res 39:269A, 1996.

99. McCormick M, Gortmaker S, Sobol A: Very low birth weight children: Behavior problems and school difficulty in a national sample. J Pediatr 117:687-693, 1990.

100. The Infant Health and Development Program: Enhancing the outcomes of low-birth-weight, premature infants: A multisite, randomized trial. JAMA 263:3035-3042, 1990.

101. Brooks-Gunn J, McCarton C, Casey P, et al: Early intervention in low-birth-weight premature infants: Results through age 5 years from the Infant Health and Development Program. JAMA 272:1257-1262, 1994.

102. McCarton C, Brookes-Gunn J, Wallace I, et al: Results at age 8 years of early intervention for low-birth-weight premature infants. JAMA 277:126-132, 1997.

103. Hoy E, Sykes D, Bill J, et al: The effects of being born of very-low-birthweight. Ir J Psychol 12:182, 1991.

104. Oberklaid F, Sewell J, Sanson A, et al: Temperament and behavior of preterm infants: A six-year follow-up. Pediatrics 87:854-861, 1991.

105. Johnson A, Townshend P, Yudkin P, et al: Functional abilities at age 4 years of children born before 29 weeks of gestation. BMJ 306:1715-1718, 1993.

106. Whyte H, Fitzhardinge P, Shennan A, et al: Extreme immaturity: Outcome of 568 pregnancies of 23-26 weeks' gestation. Obstetr Gynecol 82:1-7, 1993.

107. Allen M, Donohue P, Dusman A: The limit of viability—Neonatal outcome of infants born at 22 to 25 weeks' gestation. N Engl J Med 329:1597-1601, 1993.

108. Collin M, Halsey C, Anderson C: Emerging developmental sequelae in the "normal" extremely low birth weight infant. Pediatrics 88:115-120, 1991.

109. Pharoah P, Stevenson C, Cooke R, et al: Clinical and subclinical deficits at 8 years in a geographically

defined cohort of low birthweight infants. Arch Dis Child 70:264-270, 1994.

110. Breslau N, Brown G, DelDotto J, et al: Psychiatric sequelae of low birth weight at 6 years of age. J Abnorm Child Psychol 24:385-400, 1996.

111. Hack M, Friedman H, Fanaroff A: Outcomes of extremely low birth weight infants. Pediatrics 98:931-937, 1996.

112. O'Callahan M, Burns Y, Gray P, et al: School performance of ELBW children: A controlled study. Dev Med Child Neurol 38:917-926, 1996.

113. Botting N, Powls A, Cooke R, et al: Attention deficit hyperactivity disorders and other psychiatric outcomes in very low birthweight children at 12 years. J Child Psychol Psychiatry 38:931-941, 1997.

114. Fazzi E, Orcesi S, Telesca C, et al: Neurodevelopmental outcome in very low birth weight infants at 24 months and 5 to 7 years of age: Changing diagnosis. Pediatr Neurol 17:240-248, 1997.

115. O'Shea T, Klinepeter K, Goldstein D, et al: Survival and developmental disability in infants with birth weights of 501-800 grams, born between 1979 and 1994. Pediatrics 100:982-986, 1997.

116. Powls A, Botting N, Cooke R, et al: Visual impairment in very low birthweight children. Arch Dis Child 76: F82-F82, 1997.

117. Schraeder B, Heverly M, O'Brien C, et al: Academic achievement and educational resource use of very low birth weight (VLBW) survivors. Pediatr Nurs 23:21-25, 1997.

118. Sykes D, Hoy E, Bill J, et al: Behavioral adjustment in school of very low birthweight children. J Child Psychol Psychiatry 38:315-325, 1997.

119. Victorian Infant Collaborative Study Group: Improved outcome into the 1990s for infants weighing 500-999 grams at birth. Arch Dis Child Fetal Neonatal Ed 77: F91-F94, 1997.

120. Whitaker A, Van Rossem R, Feldman J, et al: Psychiatric outcomes in low-birth-weight children at age 6 years: Relation to neonatal cranial ultrasound abnormalities. Arch Gen Psychiatry 54:847-856, 1997.

121. Whitfield M, Grunau R, Holst L: Extremely premature (<800 g) schoolchildren: Multiple areas of hidden disability. Arch Dis Child 77:F85-F90, 1997.

122. Goyen T, Lui K, Woods R: Visual-motor, visual-perceptual, and fine motor outcomes in very-low-birthweight children at 5 years. Dev Med Child Neurol 40:76-81, 1998.

123. Horwood L, Mogridge N, Darlow B: Cognitive, educational, and behavioral outcomes at 7 to 8 years in a national very low birthweight cohort. Arch Dis Child Fetal Neonatal Ed 79:F12-F20, 1998.

124. Resnick M, Gomatam S, Carter R, et al: Educational disabilities of neonatal intensive care graduates. Pediatrics 102:308-314, 1998.

125. Ehrenkranz R, Younes N, Lemons J, et al: Longitudinal growth of hospitalized very low birth weight infants. Pediatrics 104:280-289, 1999.

126. Stewart A, Rifkin L, Kirkbride V, et al: Brain structure and neurocognitive and behavioral function in adolescents who were born very preterm, Lancet 353:1653-1657, 1999.

127. Wolke D, Meyer R: Cognitive status, language attainment and prereading skills of 6 year old very preterm children and their peers: The Bavarian Longitudinal Study. Dev Med Child Neurol 41:94-109, 1999.

128. Hack M, Fanaroff A: Outcomes of children of low birth weight and gestational age in the 1990's. Early Hum Dev 53:193-218, 1999.

129. Costeloe K, Hennessey E, Gibson A, et al: The EPICure study: Outcomes to discharge from hospital for infants born at the threshold of viability. Pediatrics 106:659-671, 2000.

130. Wood N, Marlow N, Costeloe K: Neurologic and developmental disability after extremely preterm birth. EPICure Study Group. N Eng J Med 343:378-384, 2000.

131. Marlow N, Wolke D, Bracewell M, et al: Neurologic and developmental disability at six years of age after extremely preterm birth. N Engl J Med 352:9-19, 2005.

132. Vohr, B, Wright L, Dusick M, et al: Neurodevelopmental and functional outcomes of Child Health and Human Development Neonatal Research Network, 1993-1994. Pediatrics 105:1216-1226, 2000.

133. Barlow J, Lewandowski L: Ten-Year Longitudinal Study of Preterm Infants: Outcome and Predictors. Presented at the annual meeting of the American Psychological Association, Washington, DC, August 8, 2000.

134. Buck G, Msall M, Schisterman E, et al: Extreme prematurity and school outcomes, Paediatr Perinat Epidemiol 14:324-331, 2000.

135. Hack M, Wilson-Costello D, Friedman H, et al: Neurodevelopmental and predictors of outcomes of children with birth weights of less than 1000 grams: 1992-1995. Arch Pediatr Adolesc Med 154:725-731, 2000.

136. Hack M, Taylor H, Klein N, et al: Functional limitations and special health care needs of 10-to-14 year old children weighing less than 750 grams at birth. Pediatrics 106:554-560, 2000.

137. Palta M, Sadek-Badawi M, Evans M, et al: Functional assessment of a multicenter very low-birth-weight cohort at 5 years. Arch Pediatr Adolesc Med 154:23-30, 2000.

138. Taylor HG, Klein N, Minich N, et al: Middle-school-age outcomes in children with very low birthweight. Child Dev 71:1495-1511, 2000.

139. Saigal S, Hoult L, Streiner D, et al: School difficulties at adolescence in a regional cohort of children who were extremely low birth weight. Pediatrics 105:325-331, 2000.

140. Tideman E, Ley D, Bjerre I, et al: Longitudinal follow-up of children born preterm: Somatic and mental health, self-esteem and quality of life at age 19. Early Hum Dev 61:97-110, 2001.

141. Vanhaesebrouck P, Allegaert K, Bottu J, et al: The EPIBEL study: Outcomes to discharge from the hospital for extremely preterm infants in Belgium. Pediatrics 114:663-675, 2004.

142. Allegaert K, de Coen K, Devlieger H, et al: Threshold retinopathy at threshold of viability: The EpiBel study, Br J Opthalmol 88:239-242, 2004.

143. Larroque B, Breart G, Dehan M, et al: Survival of very preterm infants: EPIPAGE, a population based cohort study. Arch Dis Child Fetal Neonatal Ed 89:F139-F144, 2004.

144. Larroque B, Marret S, Ancel P, et al: White matter damage and intraventricular hemorrhage in very preterm infants: The EPIPAGE study. J Pediatr 143:477-483, 2003.

145. Elgen I, Sommerfelt K, Markestad T: Population based, controlled study of behavioral problems and psychiatric disorders in low birthweight children at 11 years of age. Arch Dis Child Fetal Neonatal Ed 87:F128-F132, 2002.

146. Hack M, Flannery D, Schuluchter M, et al: Outcomes in young adulthood for VLBW infants. N Engl J Med 346:149-157, 2002.

147. Bhutta A, Cleves M, Casey P, et al: Cognitive and behavioral outcomes of school-aged children who were born preterm: A meta-analysis. JAMA 288:728-737, 2002.

148. Ment L, Vohr B, Allan W, et al: Change in cognitive function over time in very low-birth-weight infants. JAMA 289:705-711, 2003.

149. Aylward G: Cognitive function in preterm infants: No simple answers. JAMA 289:752-753, 2003.

150. Sweet M, Hodgman J, Pena I, et al: Two-year outcome of infants weighing 600 grams or less at birth and born 1994-1998. Obstet Gynecol 101:18-23, 2003.

151. Rijken M, Stoelhorst G, Martens S, et al: Mortality and neurologic, mental, and psychomotor development at 2 years in infants born less than 27 weeks' gestation: The Leiden Follow-up Project on Prematurity. Pediatrics 112:351-358, 2003.

152. Saigal S, den Ouden L, Wolke D, et al: School-age outcomes in children who were extremely low birth weight from four international population-based cohorts. Pediatrics 112:943-950, 2003.

153. Short E, Klein N, Lewis B, et al: Cognitive and academic consequences of bronchopulmonary dysplasia and very low birth weight: 8-year-old outcomes. Pediatrics 112:e359, 2003.

154. Sullivan M, McGrath M: Perinatal morbidity, mild motor delay, and later school outcomes. Dev Med Child Neurol 45:104-112, 2003.

155. Vohr B, Allan W, Westerveld M, et al: School-age outcomes of very low birth weight infants in the indomethacin intraventricular hemorrhage prevention trial. Pediatrics 111: e340-e346, 2003.

156. Wood N, Marlow N, Costeloe K: Neurologic and developmental disability after extremely preterm birth. N Engl J Med 343:378-384, 2000.

157. Anderson P, Doyle L, and the Victorian Infant Collaborative Study Group: Executive functioning in school-aged children who were born very preterm or with extremely low birth weight in the 1990's. Pediatrics 114:50-57, 2004.

158. DeVries L, Van Haastert I, Rademaker K, et al: Ultrasound abnormalities preceding cerebral palsy in high-risk preterm infants. J Pediatr 144:815-820, 2004.

159. Fearon P, O'Connell P, Frangou S, et al: Brain volumes in adult survivors of very low birth weight: A sibling-controlled study. Pediatrics 114:367-371, 2004.

160. Klassan K, Shoo L, Raina P, et al: Health status and health-related quality of life in a population-based sample of NICU graduates. Pediatrics 113:594-600, 2004.

161. Gardner F, Johnson A, Yudkin P, et al: Behavioral and emotional adjustment of teenagers in mainstream school who were born before 29 weeks' gestation. Pediatrics 114:676-688, 2004.

162. Gray R, Indurkhya A, McCormick M: Prevalence, stability and predictors of clinically significant behavior problems in low birth weight children at 3, 5, and 8 years of age. Pediatrics 114:736-743, 2004.

163. Hoekstra R, Ferrara TB, Couser R, et al: Survival and long-term neurodevelopmental outcome of extremely premature infants born at 23-26 weeks' gestational age at a tertiary center. Pediatrics 113: e1-e6, 2004.

164. Kilbride H, Thorstad K, Daily D: Preschool outcome of less than 801 gram preterm infants compared with full-term siblings. Pediatrics 113:742-747, 2004.

165. Hack M, Taylor H, Drotar D, et al: Chronic conditions, functional limitations, and special health care needs of school-aged children born with extremely low-birth-weight in the 1990s. JAMA 294:318-325, 2005.

166. Hintz S, Kendrick D, Vohr B, et al: Changes in neurodevelopmental outcomes at 18-22 months' corrected age among infants of less than 25 weeks' gestational age born in 1993-1999. Pediatrics 115:1645-1651, 2005.

167. Wilson-Costello D, Friedman H, Minich N, et al: Improved survival rates with increased neurodevelopmental disability for extremely low birth weight infants in the 1990s. Pediatrics 115:997-1003, 2005.

168. Glascoe F: Detecting developmental, behavioral and school problems. *In* Wolraich M, ed: Disorders of Development and Learning, 3rd ed. Philadelphia: BC Decker, 2003, pp 61-79.

169. Vohr B, Wright L, Hack M, et al, eds: Follow-up care of high-risk infants. Pediatrics 114(5, Suppl):1377-1397, 2004.

170. Pharoah POD, Cooke T, Cooke RW, et al: Birthweight specific trends in cerebral palsy. Arch Dis Child 65:602-606, 1990.

171. Bhushan V, Paneth N, Kiely JL: Impact of improved survival of very low birth weight infants on recent secular trends in the prevalence of cerebral palsy. Pediatrics 91:1094-1111, 1993.

10B.
Genetics in Developmental-Behavioral Pediatrics

PAUL WANG

For 21st-century practitioners of developmental-behavioral pediatrics (DBP), it is almost axiomatic that genetic disorders and differences can be associated with characteristic profiles of behavior and development. However, many patients' families and other clients of DBP practitioners may not understand, for example, that genetic disorders can be associated not simply with mental retardation but also with specific profiles of strengths and weaknesses within the larger context of mental retardation. Some people may still hold the concept that young children are tabula rasa (blank slates), although it is clear that these children—like all children—have genetic proclivities that help to shape their personalities and cognitive profiles. (Real-life parents, in contrast, have probably always known the tabula rasa idea to be foolish.)

The evidence is clear that both genetics and environment play important roles in shaping the developmental trajectories that children follow, as well as the mature profiles of skills and behavior in which those trajectories result. Indeed, the resolution of the "nature versus nurture" debate is moving away from both the genetic and the behaviorist extremes toward a middle ground that highlights the interaction of biological and environmental forces.

This chapter provides an overview of the genetic differences that can affect child development and behavior. Research since the 1990s has demonstrated that not only the so-called disorders but also single-gene differences can have important implications for development and behavior. The small but growing body of evidence on the interaction of genetic differences with environmental factors is also reviewed. Finally, the value of genetic diagnosis and the clinical approach to these diagnoses are discussed. Thus, this chapter is an attempt to provide both theoretical and practical contexts in which to evaluate new findings on the importance of genetics and environment to behavior and development.

MECHANISMS OF GENETIC DISORDERS AND DIFFERENCES

The human genome and its replication are phenomenally complex. In view of this complexity, it is not surprising that a large variety of abnormal genetic mechanisms, from meiotic nondisjunction to simple base pair substitution, can perturb the typical course of child development. As a correlate, disorders of development and behavior have been prominent in the history of genetic research; several well-known DBP conditions serve as prototypes of pathological genetic processes. (Genetic concepts that are discussed in this chapter but are not specifically referenced are described more fully by Nussbaum et al.[1]) A summary of these genetic disease mechanisms and their developmental-behavioral exemplars are provided in Table 10B-1.

Chromosomal Aneuploidy

Down syndrome, formerly known as "mongolism," which most commonly results from trisomy 21, is the best-known example of chromosomal aneuploidy. Early theories of its etiology drew from the mistaken biological and racist theories of the time (that ontogeny recapitulated phylogeny and that "Mongols" represented an evolutionarily primitive stage of development); awareness of the trisomy etiology of Down syndrome is now common in the general populace. Trisomy 13 and trisomy 18 are other examples of autosomal aneuploidies that are sometimes compatible with fetal and neonatal survival, but they carry devastating implications for behavior, development, and all aspects of health.[2] Turner syndrome (45,XO), Klinefelter syndrome (47,XYY), and other less common disorders associated with sex chromosome aneuploidy are associated with phenotypes that are medically less severe than the autosomal aneuploidies but that have important developmental and behavioral implications.[2] Chromosomal aneuploidy typically results from meiotic nondisjunction, which is progressively more likely to occur as maternal age increases. Although all chromosomes can be affected by meiotic nondisjunction, it is believed that aneuploidy of chromosomes other than 21 (the smallest chromosome) almost invariably leads to fetal demise. Chromosomal aneuploidy is easily detected by conventional karyotype testing.

Other Chromosomal Anomalies

Some sporadic cases of developmental disabilities and organ malformation are associated with visible deletions of a chromosome. The loss of such substantial amounts of chromosomal material implies that these conditions are associated with the deletion of many genes, ranging in number possibly into the hundreds, depending on the specifics of the deletion. Conversely, some disorders of development and behavior may result from duplication of a portion of a chromosome,

TABLE 10B-1 ■ Mechanisms of Genetic Difference and Common Examples

Mechanism of Genetic Difference	Diagnostic Approach	Examples of Disorders
Aneuploidy	Karyotype	Down syndrome (usually trisomy 21) Sex chromosome aneuploidies, such as XO (Turner) syndrome, XXY (Klinefelter) syndrome, and XYY syndrome
Chromosomal deletions and duplications (large)	Karyotype; may be associated with translocations, ring chromosomes, and other chromosomal anomalies	Wilms tumor, aniridia, genitourinary anomalies, mental retardation (WAGR syndrome): 11p$^-$
Telomeric rearrangements (deletions or duplications)	FISH testing; occasionally visible on karyotype	Cri-du-chat syndrome (telomere at chromosome 5p)
Microdeletions; contiguous gene deletion syndromes	FISH testing	DiGeorge/velocardiofacial syndrome (del 22q11.2) Williams syndrome (del 7q11.23)
Single gene disorders; may result from substitutions or deletions of one or more DNA base pairs or from trinucleotide repeats	Specific tests of DNA or metabolic products; for some conditions, the diagnosis is established clinically in most instances	Lesch-Nyhan syndrome (testing of enzyme activity is diagnostic; DNA tests also available) Fragile X syndrome (DNA testing for trinucleotide repeat length) Tuberous sclerosis (diagnosis is typically clinical; DNA testing is available) Neurofibromatosis type 1 (diagnosis is typically clinical; DNA testing is available)
Mitochondrial gene disorders	Various tests, including clinical, tissue pathology, and DNA analysis	Syndrome of mitochondrial myopathy, encephalopathy, lactic acidosis, and strokelike episodes (MELAS)
Allelic differences and multigene disorders	Testing generally available for research purposes only	Reading disorder Autistic spectrum disorders ADHD
Epigenomic regulation	Testing for epigenomic factors is generally available for research purposes only	Imprinting: Angelman, Prader-Willi, and Turner syndromes Lyonization: fragile X syndrome, Rett syndrome, and other X-linked disorders

ADHD, attention-deficit/hyperactivity disorder; FISH, fluorescence in situ hybridization.

resulting in "overdosage" of the genes on the duplicated segment of chromosome. Chromosomal anomalies such as ring chromosomes, derivative chromosomes (in which portions of multiple chromosomes re-form into a single atypical chromosome), and balanced and unbalanced translocations can be associated with developmental and behavioral disorders when chromosomal material (i.e., multiple genes) is lost in formation of the new chromosomes or when the "breakpoint" of the original chromosome or chromosomes occurs in a gene that becomes dysfunctional as a result of the break. All these types of chromosomal anomalies can be detected on a conventional karyotype.

Telomeric Abnormalities

The telomeres and the subtelomeres, which are the ends of each chromosome and the regions immediately adjacent, are unique chromosomal regions that contain long stretches of DNA but do not contain genes. The understanding of telomeric function and telomeric molecular biology is still developing, but it is already appreciated that chromosomal rearrangements in the subtelomeres can be associated with cancer and with perturbations to the processes of cell senescence.

Rearrangements in the subtelomeric regions appear to be responsible for 5% to 10% of cases of moderate and severe mental retardation.[3] Most cases of subtelomeric rearrangement are associated with novel or unnamed syndromes of disability. Subtelomeric rearrangements can include both deletions and duplications of chromosomal material and are very difficult to detect with conventional karyotyping. However, these subtelomeric rearrangements can be identified with specialized diagnostic methods. It is believed that individuals with subtelomeric rearrangements typically have evidence of dysmorphology and/or congenital malformations, in addition to their neurodevelopmental symptoms. As the understanding of telomeric function and dysfunction expand, their role in development and behavior will also become better understood.

Contiguous Gene Deletion Syndromes

Williams syndrome[4] and velocardiofacial/DiGeorge syndrome[5] are two well-known examples of contiguous gene deletion syndromes. In these genetic disorders, a submicroscopic portion of a chromosome is deleted, at 7q11.23 and 22q11.2, respectively, resulting in the deletion of all of the genes that are physically contiguous on that portion of the chromosome. In a majority of cases, these deletions occur spontaneously, but similar deletions occur in unrelated persons because of a common peculiarity of the chromosome in these regions. In Williams syndrome, for example, the deleted region is bounded on both ends by repetitive chromosomal segments that are duplicates of each other. As a consequence, these homologous regions can mispair during meiosis, which results in the deletion of the intervening region of chromosome. The same mechanism is believed to operate in velocardiofacial/DiGeorge syndrome. The risk of recurrence in affected families appears to be greater than the incidence in the general population, perhaps because these families have a particularly high degree of homology between the bounding segments.

Persons affected by contiguous gene deletion syndromes are haploid for the genes that are deleted; that is, they are missing one copy of the deleted genes. However, because humans have two copies of each autosomal chromosome, the affected persons still have one copy of these genes on the unaffected member of the chromosomal pair. Contiguous gene deletion syndromes thus highlight the concept of *haploinsufficiency.* Whereas normal development and physiological function may be possible with only one copy of some genes, two copies may be necessary for other genes. When only one copy of a gene from the latter category exists, the affected person is said to be *haploinsufficient.* In contiguous gene deletion syndromes, it is the haploinsufficiency of certain genes that contributes to the atypical phenotype. Research is active on Williams, velocardiofacial/DiGeorge, and other contiguous gene deletion syndromes to determine which of the deleted genes are haploinsufficient and thereby contribute to the phenotypes associated with these syndromes.

As is true for almost all genetic disorders, contiguous gene deletion syndromes can produce large variability in the phenotype of individual patients. Researchers initially hypothesized that this variability was related to variability in the number of genes that were deleted in each patient; that is, all patients with a specific syndrome would have a core group of genes deleted, but some patients would have a larger chromosomal deletion, with differences in phenotype accounted for by the exact number and identity of the additional genes deleted. In fact, it is now understood that the large majority of patients with a specific syndrome have exactly the same gene deletions. For example, about 95% of patients with Williams syndrome have a common deletion involving at least 23 genes at chromosome 7q11.23,[6] and about 70% of patients with velocardiofacial/DiGeorge syndrome have a common deletion involving about 15 genes at chromosome 22q11.2.[5] Variability in these syndromes arises from the specific alleles that the patient carries for the other copy of the deleted genes, from "background genetic effects" (i.e., the effects of the remainder of the person's genome), and from other biological and experiential factors.[7]

The variability in phenotype for patients with a common genetic disorder sometimes led historically to a proliferation of diagnoses despite unitary etiologies. For example, the "conotruncal anomaly face syndrome," DiGeorge syndrome, velocardiofacial syndrome, and some cases of "Opitz G/BBB" syndrome were thought to be distinct diagnoses, but all are now known to result from a contiguous gene deletion at chromosome 22q11.2.[8]

In contiguous gene deletion syndromes, the deleted chromosomal segment is typically too small to be detected by conventional microscopic karyotyping. Instead, the deletion must be probed for and found absent, through the fluorescent in situ hybridization (FISH) test. As previously stated, these disorders most commonly occur spontaneously (de novo), but vertical transmission can occur.

Single-Gene Disorders

The effects of single-gene abnormalities on development and behavior can be as powerful clinically as the effects of chromosomal disorders, whether the single-gene abnormality results from gene deletion, base pair mutation, or other genetic mechanisms. For example, Lesch-Nyhan syndrome results from a mutation in the gene *HGPRT* and is associated with a phenotype of severe mental retardation and self-injurious behavior. The study of Lesch-Nyhan syndrome led to the first known usage of the term *behavioral phenotype,* referring to the concept that genetic differences can be associated with specific phenotypes of behavior.[9] This statement was one of the earliest and most powerful medical refutations of the concept of tabula rasa that had been championed by behavioral psychology in the first half of the 20th century.

The etiology of the fragile X syndrome, another single-gene disorder, was elucidated more recently. The clinical syndrome was described in 1943, but the specific underlying genetic mechanism, an extended repeat of three base pairs ("triplet repeat") on the X chromosome, was not discovered until 1991. The triplet repeat mechanism of genetic disease had never been described in any condition before then, but it is now known to underlie not only the fragile X syndrome but also Huntington disease, myotonic dystrophy, several spinocerebellar ataxia syndromes, and other disorders.[10]

It is now appreciated that the fragile X syndrome is the most common single-gene etiology for mental retardation and the most common heritable cause of mental retardation. Down syndrome is the most common genetic etiology but is rarely transmitted vertically, whereas the fragile X syndrome is less common overall but typically results when a mother has a slightly expanded triplet repeat, known as a "premutation," that expands into a "full mutation" in gamete formation. The phenomenon of triplet repeat expansion manifests itself clinically in the greater phenotypic severity of patients with a full mutation in comparison with patients with a shorter premutation. Research continues on the molecular implications and clinical correlates of the premutation in the fragile X syndrome, as well as on the full range of clinical manifestations associated with the full mutation.[11]

Single-gene disorders can be diagnosed only through directed testing, triggered by clinical suspicion, and cannot be detected through nonspecific tests such as karyotyping. The specific tests for a single-gene disorders range from metabolic testing of urine or serum to gene sequencing and to other molecular diagnostic assessment, such as the test commonly used to determine triplet repeat length in the fragile X syndrome. For neurofibromatosis type 1 and tuberous sclerosis, as well as for many other single-gene disorders, diagnoses are typically made clinically, with DNA testing reserved for confirmatory testing, prenatal diagnosis, or other uncommon situations. In most cases other than the fragile X syndrome, the diagnostic testing for single-gene disorders is directed by a genetic or metabolic specialist.

Mitochondrial Genes

In addition to the nuclear genomes of both the sperm and the egg, all human embryos receive a genetic endowment from the mitochondria of the ovum. (Mitochondria from the sperm do not survive in the zygote, and thus no mitochondria from the father are passed on to the child.[12]) The mitochondria contain a genome that is much smaller than the genome that is in the nucleus of cells. The mitochondrial genome contains only about 37 genes, and all of these genes appear to be important for mitochondrial function. (There are other genes in the nuclear genome that also are important for mitochondrial function.) In this age of assisted reproductive technologies, it is useful to note that children who are conceived from donor eggs are genetically related to the egg donor through both the nuclear genome and the mitochondrial genome of the donor egg.

Despite the small number of genes in the mitochondrial genome, mutations in these genes appear to be very likely to affect brain development or function, perhaps because the high energy demand of the brain makes it particularly dependent on mitochondrial function. Examples of disorders resulting from mutations in mitochondrial DNA include the syndromes of mitochondrial myopathy, encephalopathy, lactic acidosis, and strokelike episodes (MELAS) and of myoclonic epilepsy associated with ragged-red fibers (MERFF). Some clinical syndromes, such as MELAS, may be attributable to mutations in one of several different genes. These disorders are typically diagnosed when clinical suspicion leads to pediatric neurological evaluation, followed by specific testing that sometimes requires muscle or other tissue biopsies.[13] For some of these mitochondrial disorders, DNA testing also is available for confirmatory or prenatal testing.

Multiple-Gene Disorders and Allelic Differences

In contrast to the chromosomal disorders and single-gene disorders such as Lesch-Nyhan and the fragile X syndromes, which typically result in complete inactivation or overdose of one or more genes and have severe effects on development and behavior, many genes exert their influences on development and behavior through more subtle, additive effects. Reading disabilities[14,15] and autistic disorder[16] are examples of this. The complex behavioral phenomena of these disorders are believed to result from the effects of multiple genes. Mutations or allelic differences in only one of the implicated genes may have only minor effects or no effect at all. However, if several of these genes are abnormal or are present in the form of a "pathological" allele, then full-fledged dyslexia or autism may result. If the abnormalities are present in only one or a few of these genes, then they may manifest only as a shy temperament or a tendency toward perseveration. Abnormalities that are limited to another few genes might manifest as a restricted range of interest. When a critical number of the implicated genes are abnormal or are present in the pathological allele, then the full clinical picture of autism may emerge.

Allelic gene differences are known to influence the susceptibility of an individual to a phenotypic disorder. One of the best known examples of this, from outside the field of DBP, is the susceptibility to breast cancer that is associated with mutations in the gene *BRCA1*.[17] These mutations do not directly cause breast cancer, but they raise the risk of breast cancer substantially, because the mutations affect the ability of the BRCA1 protein to regulate the cell cycle. Other genes are believed to influence development and behavior through their effects on complicated pathophysiological processes that involve other genetic and biological factors, as well as environmental factors. Some examples of susceptibility genes and their interaction with environmental factors are described later in this chapter.

Chapter 16 reviews some of the genes that have been linked to attention-deficit/hyperactivity disorder (ADHD).[18] It is not yet understood how certain alleles of these genes act to increase the likelihood that a person will have ADHD, but it is clear that these genetic differences alone do not completely prevent or cause ADHD by themselves, Instead, they presumably exert their influence through some interaction with other genes and/or with environmental factors. Background genetic effects are likely to have a strong influence on the phenotypic expression of "susceptibility genes," just as they do on contiguous gene deletion syndromes and other genetic mechanisms affecting development and behavior.

The Epigenome

Discussions of genetic effects on phenotype typically focus on the genome—that is, on the specific genes on the chromosomes and in the mitochondrial DNA—and on the sequence of noncoding base pairs that are found between genes. There is a growing appreciation, however, that the "epigenome" also exerts important effects on the phenotype. The epigenome is defined as the entire array of gene expression states imposed by chromatin and nonhistone regulators on the genome. The two examples of epigenomic regulation that are most familiar to developmental-behavioral pediatricians are gene inactivation by *methylation* and X chromosome inactivation through the normal process known as *lyonization.*

Genomic imprinting, in which a cell can "tell" whether a specific gene is from the maternally inherited chromosome or the paternally inherited one, is commonly implemented through a process of methylation, in which a methyl group becomes bonded to the DNA in the promoter region of certain genes. One example of the significance of imprinting is found in the social skills of girls with Turner syndrome. Such girls who inherit their single X chromosome from their father exhibit social skills that are relatively superior in comparison to those of such girls who inherit their X chromosome from their mother.[18a]

Another example of imprinting is found in Angelman and Prader-Willi syndromes, which result from deletions at chromosome 15q11-q13 on the maternally derived chromosome (Angelman) or the paternally derived chromosome (Prader-Willi). Alternatively, either of these disorders may result from uniparental disomy, the condition in which both copies of a particular chromosome are derived from the same parent, rather than one from the mother and one from the father.

In the fragile X syndrome, the inactivation of the mutated *FMRP1* gene is associated with methylation of the *FMRP1* gene. There are reports of rare cases in which there is a "full mutation" of the *FMRP1* gene, but the gene is still at least partially expressed because it has somehow escaped methylation. Individuals in which this occurs exhibit less severe phenotypic effects than in most cases of full mutation, in which gene methylation results in complete absence of gene expression.[11]

Lyonization is an early embryonic process by which one of the two X chromosomes in females is inactivated in each cell of the embryo, which results in the formation of the Barr body. For female patients who are carriers of an X-linked disorder, the random process of lyonization sometimes results in the inactivation of the normal allele of a disease gene in an unusually high (or low) percentage of cells. In the fragile X syndrome, the severity of the clinical phenotype in female carriers of the full mutation is correlated with the lyonization ratio for the abnormal versus the normal X chromosome.[11] Analogous findings have been reported for female carriers of the gene for Rett syndrome.[19]

The effects of epigenomic phenomena are thus evident in multiple disorders relevant to DBP, including Prader-Willi and Angelman syndromes and X-linked disorders such as Rett syndrome, Turner syndrome, and the fragile X syndrome. The possible effects of environmental factors on the epigenome are discussed in greater detail as follows.

Genomics and Proteomics

Although the sequencing of the entire human genome was a major research achievement, that accomplishment highlighted the fact that knowing the order of the billions of base pairs in the genome is only an intermediate milestone in understanding human molecular biology. The task that researchers now face is known as *genomics research:* elucidating the function and interactions of the more than 25,000 genes that every human being carries.[20] The role of regulatory genes, the poorly understood significance of gene introns and of the "junk DNA" that is found between genes, the extent to which alternative splicing occurs to create different transcripts from a single gene, and other mysteries all remain to be explored as part of genomics research. A potentially even more complex challenge is the understanding of proteomics: how the myriad protein translation products of the genes interact with each other in the physiological processes that ultimately manifest themselves in the typical or atypical growth, development, and behavior of children and adults.[20] Beyond genomics and proteomics lies the even larger challenge of understanding how environmental factors interact with these biological processes.

PHENOTYPES

Genotypic abnormalities and differences can be associated with a wide range of phenotypic manifestations. Well-known genetic disorders such as Down syndrome illustrate the breadth of potential phenotypic manifestations, from facial abnormalities and congenital organ malformations to neuropsychological profiles and neurodegenerative conditions.

Medical Phenotypes

Genetic disorders and differences appear to be associated with a very wide variety of medical phenotypic manifestations. The most obvious are the congenital malformations that characterize many chromosomal disorders. In these conditions, malformations may affect any organ system and often affect multiple organ systems in a single individual. Some of these malformations may be considered major, in that they are incompatible with life or necessitate surgical intervention to establish a normal range of function, whereas other malformations may be considered minor or cosmetic.

When the best medical care is accessible, advances in medical, surgical, and chronic care have led to enormous improvements in the life expectancy and the quality of life of many individuals with chromosomal and other genetic disorders that are associated with major medical morbidity. For example, as recently as the 1960s, the congenital malformations that affect most newborns with Down syndrome, especially cyanotic cardiac defects, implied a very short life expectancy. Advances in cardiac diagnosis and surgical intervention now enable almost all such infants to survive and often to thrive with full physiological repairs of their malformations. Whereas it used to be common and acceptable to allow such neonates to die without heroic medical intervention, it is now considered unethical in many parts of the industrialized world to withhold medical intervention unless there are at least two major congenital malformations. Thus, it can be fairly asserted that in affluent communities, the effect of medical phenotypes on

and across the lifespan has changed dramatically. Advances in educational and related therapeutic services also have had a dramatic effect on the development and quality of life of older children and adults with Down syndrome.[21]

Research on medical phenotypes continues to have real clinical significance nonetheless. As a direct result of the improvements in and greater availability of treatment for congenital malformations, and consequent increases in life expectancy, one area in which research is most active is the late-adult phenotype associated with genetic disorders. In Down syndrome, for example, the early onset of Alzheimer-like dementia was not recognized until sufficiently large numbers of individuals with Down syndrome began to survive into the middle-adult years.

The fragile X syndrome provides a vivid example of how new aspects of the medical phenotype are still being brought to light for a disorder that was recognized before 1950. (In this case, the new recognition is not simply the result of increased survival, but of persistent inquiry and keen clinical acumen, combined with advances in genetic diagnostics.) A new syndrome of tremor and ataxia has been identified in adults with premutations of the *FMRP1* gene, and female carriers of the premutation appear to have an increased incidence of premature ovarian failure.[11] In many other genetic disorders, increasing survival into the adult years has called attention to the need for careful medical surveillance and systematic study of possible late manifestations of the medical phenotype.

Pharmacogenomics

Although the topic of pharmacogenomics—genetically based differences in drug pharmacology—usually is not included in DBP reviews of medical phenotype, it is a topic of enormous clinical relevance, for which the knowledge base is likely to grow very quickly.[22] Researchers have begun to identify specific genes that affect both pharmacokinetics (the effects of the body on the drug: namely, absorption, distribution, metabolism, and elimination) and pharmacodynamics (the effects of the drug on the body). In the case of drug metabolism, the genetic basis for individual differences in the rate of metabolism of certain drugs has been found. Patients who are "poor metabolizers," "extensive metabolizers," and "ultra-rapid metabolizers" of various antidepressants and antipsychotics are now known to have different genotypes for the cytochrome P-450 2D6 enzyme (CYP2D6). The poor metabolizers carry alleles for this gene that code for a relatively low-activity version of the enzyme, whereas the ultra-rapid metabolizers carry a higher activity allele and have extra copies of these genes.

Behavioral Phenotypes

Lesch-Nyhan syndrome is the vivid exemplar for which the term *behavioral phenotype* was first coined; the behavioral phenotypes associated with other genetic disorders and differences are, in general, less striking.[23-25] These phenotypes span the range from other dramatic but circumscribed behaviors to temperamental characteristics, profiles of cognitive ability, and trajectories of cognitive development. Other examples of phenotypes that comprise circumscribed behaviors include the hand-wringing associated with Rett syndrome and the spasmodic "self-hug" that has been described in Smith-Magenis syndrome.[26] On the border between circumscribed behaviors and more generalized behavioral and temperamental phenotypes are the hyperphagia associated with Prader-Willi syndrome and the extreme difficulty with sleep seen in many individuals with Smith-Magenis syndrome (which may be related to an abnormal circadian rhythm for melatonin secretion[27]). Temperamental or personality phenotypes have been described for several genetic disorders, including Williams, Prader-Willi, Angelman, and velocardiofacial syndromes.[4,28,29] Well-recognized (if not fully understood) developmental trajectories include the degenerative patterns of Rett syndrome and of Down syndrome (in adulthood), the onset of hyperphagia in Prader-Willi after early hypotonia and motor delays improve, and the apparent acceleration of language development often seen in toddlers and preschoolers with Williams syndrome (although this may be analogous to the language burst that many typically developing children seem to show around ages 2 and 3).[30] Some genetic conditions also appear to be associated with an increased risk of psychiatric disorders. Examples include the possible increased incidence of internalizing disorders in adults with Williams syndrome[4] and the complex relationships between the fragile X syndrome and autism[11] and between velocardiofacial disorder and both mood and psychotic disorders.[30a] Table 10B-2 depicts the different facets of behavioral phenotypes that are relevant to DBP.

Cognitive profiles are probably the most extensively investigated type of behavioral phenotype in children and adults with genetic disorders. Down syndrome, Williams syndrome, velocardiofacial/DiGeorge syndrome (del 22q11.2), the fragile X syndrome, neurofibromatosis type 1, Turner syndrome, and Duchenne muscular dystrophy are among the disorders that have been the subject of extensive psychoeducational and cognitive investigation. Progress in the understanding of their cognitive behavioral phenotypes often follows a similar pattern: early publications report on the typical IQ, academic achievement, and functional profiles, whereas in later studies,

TABLE 10B-2 ■ Facets of Genetically Based Phenotypes

Phenotypic Facet	Example
Circumscribed behavior	Self-injury in Lesch-Nyhan syndrome Spasmodic "self-hug" in Smith-Magenis syndrome Hand-wringing in Rett syndrome Hyperphagia in Prader-Willi syndrome
Cognitive/neuropsychological	Phonological/verbal memory impairment in Down syndrome Spatial memory and visual-motor impairments in Williams syndrome "Nonverbal learning disability" profile in Turner syndrome
Developmental-behavioral trajectories over time	Emergence of hyperphagia and resolution of severe hypotonia in preschool-aged children with Prader-Willi syndrome "Early onset" senile dementia in Down syndrome
Temperament and personality	Sociability in Williams syndrome
Psychiatric diatheses	Fragile X disorder and autistic symptoms Williams syndrome and internalizing disorders Velocardiofacial/DiGeorge syndrome and mood and psychotic symptoms
Biobehavioral	Sleep disorders and melatonin dysregulation in Smith-Magenis syndrome Pharmacogenomic effects; e.g., differences in hepatic metabolism

investigators attempt to elucidate the fundamental neuropsychological or cognitive profiles that lie at their heart. In many cases, there also are neuroanatomical and other biomedical studies (including structural and functional neuroimaging, as well as postmortem neuropathological characterization) in which researchers examine the biological basis for the behavioral phenotypes, such as the discovery that the sleep difficulties in Smith-Magenis syndrome are associated with abnormal melatonin physiology. There seems to be little reason to doubt that progress in understanding brain-behavior relationships will eventually erase, or at least blur, the distinction between medical and behavioral phenotypes.

The psychiatric literature contains an analogous line of investigation that uniquely employs the term *endophenotype,* which refers to traits that are believed to be at the core of the complex processes that ultimately manifest as psychiatric disease or risk for psychiatric disease.[31] Most commonly, the endophenotypic traits are neuropsychological or neurophysiological in nature. For example, verbal short-term memory, eye blink conditioning, and saccadic eye movements all have been studied as endophenotypes for various psychiatric diagnoses, and the genetics of these traits are studied as possible clues to the genetics of psychiatric disease. Implicit in the research on endophenotypes is the recognition that psychiatric disorders are extremely complex phenomena that probably result from developmental pathology or deviance in multiple underlying processes.

A number of caveats need to be considered carefully in interpreting the research on behavioral phenotypes.[32] These caveats pertain both to the description of the phenotypes and to the "immutability" that is often incorrectly ascribed to them because of their genetic basis.

1. The description of behavioral phenotypes must be methodically rigorous.[33] Research on Williams syndrome and on neurofibromatosis provides two examples of the importance of carefully selected control groups for research in which investigators seek to describe behavioral phenotypes. In the case of Williams syndrome, early research in which subjects with Williams syndrome were compared with subjects with Down syndrome, matched for age and IQ, was often misinterpreted as showing that language skills in Williams syndrome were higher than expected for IQ. This interpretation failed to account for the fact that language skills in Down syndrome are often below the level expected for a given level of general intelligence. Furthermore, interpretations that language skills in Williams syndrome were fully preserved despite general cognitive impairments neglected to account for ceiling effects on many of the tasks that were administered and for the associated fact that typically developing 7- or 8-year-old children have already mastered most of the grammar of their native languages. Later research in which subjects with Williams syndrome were compared with age-matched and developmentally matched healthy children showed that, in fact, language skills in Williams are not fully preserved, although they do tend to be among the strengths in the Williams syndrome cognitive profile.[34]

   Research on neurofibromatosis illustrated the perils of ascertainment bias and the difficulty of identifying subtle differences in cognitive phenotype. In early studies, researchers often reported data from children with neurofibromatosis who were recruited through learning disorder clinics. As a consequence, these subjects typically showed cognitive profiles characteristic of the type of learning disorder that the research clinics commonly evaluated.[35] It was not until patients with neurofibromatosis were compared with their own siblings as controls that the subtle cognitive profile associated with the disorder was identified.

2. Developmental considerations must be taken into account. Basic psychological research conducted on subjects with genetic disorders highlights the importance of studying trajectories of development and of studying behavioral phenotypes at different ages. In the case of Williams syndrome, although older children and adults with the disorder show stronger language skills but weaker arithmetic skills than do individuals with Down syndrome, studies of toddlers with Williams and Down syndrome show that they have relatively similar early vocabulary and numerical skills.[4] For clinical purposes, these data illustrate that behavioral phenotypes identified in one age group with a disorder should not be assumed to apply to other age groups. For theoretical purposes, these findings are a reminder that genotype cannot directly specify the behavioral phenotype of a mature individual; it can only contribute to specifying the starting point and the trajectory for an individual's developmental course.

3. Individual variability must be taken into account. The behavioral phenotype that typifies a disorder is not likely to characterize all individuals with that disorder equally well. As discussed previously, background genetic effects and allelic gene differences are sources of variability among individuals with the same genetic disorder. Environmental effects also provide a source of variability in phenotype among individuals with a shared genotypic disorder. Together, these factors help account for atypical individuals, such as the woman with Down syndrome who speaks three languages with good grammatical skills[36] and the girl with Williams syndrome who is a prize-winning painter, in contrast to the classic behavioral phenotype of both syndromes.

4. Historical variability must be taken into account. A final caveat is that behavioral phenotypes, and clinicians' understanding of them, can change over time. These changes can be attributed to both environmental factors and medical advances. Among individuals with Down syndrome, for example, it has been estimated that typical IQ scores have risen 10 to 20 points since the 1950s.[21] One large reason, of course, is the categorical shift from a standard practice of institutional care to the current standard of home care for children with Down syndrome. With the richer, more nurturing environment provided by their parents and through the educational system

of today with its better resources, children and adults with Down syndrome commonly reach levels of academic achievement that used to be thought impossible for them. Advances in medical care, such as cardiac diagnostics and cardiac surgery, are probably contributors to this change as well.

Advances in medical diagnostics also account for changes in typical levels of cognitive ability in individuals with other disorders. Disorders in higher functioning individuals who do not have major medical stigmata are now diagnosed by FISH or other techniques, whereas they would not have been diagnosed previously. Thus, for disorders such as Williams, the fragile X, and Smith-Magenis syndromes, the availability of modern diagnostics has shifted the range of individuals who receive diagnoses, resulting in a shift of our understanding of the typical behavioral phenotype, whereas in Down syndrome, the phenotype itself has shifted as a result of improvements in the environment that these children typically encounter during the course of their development.

INTERACTION OF GENETICS AND ENVIRONMENT

One of the most dangerous fallacies in the understanding of the phenotypes associated with genetic disorders is that they cannot be modified by environmental factors. In fact, it is inappropriate to state that behavioral phenotypes are genetically determined. Environmental factors (i.e., educational and other interventions, home environment, life experiences of all sorts) are of potentially critical importance, regardless of genetic endowment. This fact is established most clearly by studies of monozygotic twins, who fail to show 100% concordance for any neurodevelopmental outcome that has been studied, despite the fact that they have identical genotypes (Fig. 10B-1).[37] Whether the outcome examined is a cognitive trait such as IQ, a disability such as dyslexia, or psychiatric disorders such as autism, ADHD, or depression, identical twins are not uniformly alike. (The same finding holds true for other medical outcomes such as cancer, inflammatory bowel disease, height, and weight.) Indeed, prominent scholars have noted that the study of genetic effects has yielded some of the strongest evidence for the importance of environmental factors.[37]

Behavioral genetic analyses often generate an estimate of a parameter known as *heritability* and symbolized as h^2. In statistical terms, this parameter is the proportion of variance in the outcome variable that is attributable to genetics. For example, in some behav-

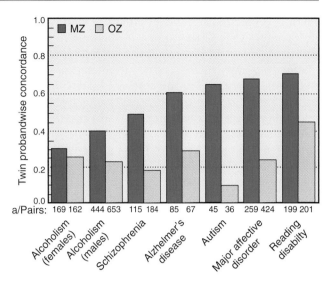

FIGURE 10B-1 **Monozygotic (MZ) and dizygotic (DZ) twin concordances for behavioral disorders.** (From Plomin R, Owen MJ, McGuffin P: The genetic basis of complex human behaviors. Science 264:1733-1739, 1994.)

ioral genetic studies of intelligence, investigators estimated h^2 to range from 0.4 to 0.8. Unfortunately, estimates of heritability are often misinterpreted; in the same example, they would be misinterpreted to mean that intelligence is 60% genetic. Such interpretations are specious: What could "60% genetic" possibly mean? Heritability (h^2) is only a mathematical construct; it does not mean that 60 IQ points of 100 come from the genes, or that 60 of 100 cases of mental retardation result from genetic etiologies, or that any given case of mental retardation is 60% attributable to genetic differences and 40% to other factors. Furthermore, estimates of the heritability of any trait are strictly valid only within the context in which they were studied. Fine-grained analyses suggest that the heritability of IQ score is dependent on the socioeconomic status of the population in which it is studied.[38] Specifically, IQ score is highly "heritable" among affluent families but much less so among impoverished families. Thus, the interpretation of statistical estimates of heritability must account for the nongenetic factors that might have influenced the trait under study and for the possibility that there were other unrecognized, nongenetic factors at play.

The increase in functional and cognitive abilities among individuals with Down syndrome that resulted from deinstitutionalization is one of the best illustrations of how environmental factors can dramatically affect the behavioral phenotype associated with a genetic disorder. The effects of early intervention in general are further evidence of the capacity of environmental manipulation to alter genetically influenced phenotypes. Although chromosomal disorders such as Down syndrome obviously exert strong effects on phenotype, the significant effects of environmental variables suggest that other, less extensive genetic difference may be better viewed as risk factors for phenotypic impairments, rather than as causative of a specific phenotypic outcome. In particular, the fragile X syndrome may be a risk factor for autism, and Smith-Magenis syndrome may be a risk factor for sleep disorders, with ultimate phenotypic outcome dependent on other genetic effects and environmental variables. Many allelic differences are indeed thought of as susceptibility factors for specific neurodevelopmental outcomes. Genes that increase the risk for reading disorder,[14,15] autistic spectrum disorders,[16] and ADHD[39] have been identified, each gene incrementally increasing the risk for its corresponding disorder, but none of the genes is sufficient cause by itself to result in the full developmental phenotype.

The best understood examples of the interaction of genetic and environmental factors to influence neurobehavioral outcome is found in the psychiatric literature. Studies of allelic differences in the monoamine oxidase A gene show that the allele that codes for a high-activity form of the enzyme is associated with a lower risk of conduct disorder and other antisocial

behaviors. However, the difference in risk is much stronger for children who have been maltreated, and in the absence of child maltreatment, the risk is essentially identical to that in individuals with the low-activity allele (Fig. 10B-2).[40] Similarly, various alleles of the gene for a serotonin transporter are associated with differences in risk for depression. In this case, however, the genetic difference interacts with environmental stressors in such a way that individuals who encounter multiple stressful life events have very different risks for depression, but individuals who encounter fewer significant life stresses show little effect of the serotonin transporter gene on risk for depression.[41] A third example is found in research on the relationship between birth weight (as a marker of prenatal adversity) and the alleles of the gene for catechol-O-methyltransferase (COMT), a gene involved in the metabolism of many neurotransmitters. This research revealed that the risk for antisocial behavior among children with a diagnosis of ADHD is much higher when low birth weight occurs in the context of one particular allele of COMT than when either low birth weight or that allele occurs in the absence of the other.[42]

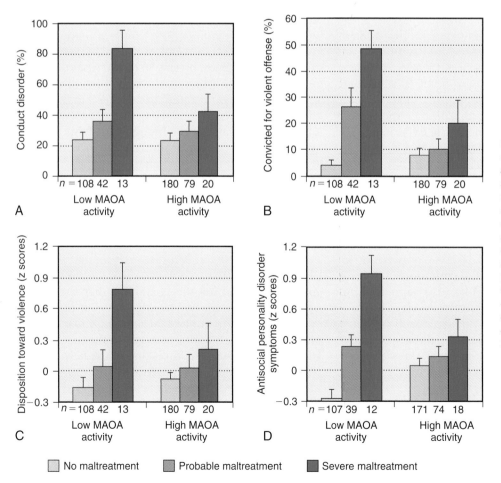

FIGURE 10B-2 Interaction of monoamine oxidase A genotype and child maltreatment. The association between childhood maltreatment and subsequent antisocial behavior as a function of monoamine oxidase A gene activity. This activity is the gene expression level associated with allelic variants of the functional promoter polymorphism. (From Caspi A, McClay J, Moffitt TE, et al: Role of genotype in the cycle of violence in maltreated children. Science 297:851-854, 2002.)

The interaction of genetic differences in the mono-amine oxidase A, serotonin, and COMT genes with environmental factors presumably takes place in the neurotransmitter pathways of the central nervous system, although the specific mechanisms of these interactions are currently unknown. Another mechanism by which environmental and genetic factors can interact is through the environmental modification of the epigenome. That the environment can affect neurobiology has been known at least since the study of rats after they were raised in enriched versus deprived environments,[43] but it was not until 2005 that it was found that the environment can affect gene expression. Specifically, it was found that the methylation state of many genes in identical twins differs increasingly as they age and differs more if the twins live apart than if they live together.[44] These findings show that environmental factors not only interact with genetic factors to influence behavioral outcome but also may actually act upon the genes themselves.

GENETIC DIAGNOSIS

Despite the many caveats that apply to genotype-phenotype correlations, there are many benefits to establishing a patient's precise genetic diagnosis. Genetic disorders and differences can have clinically significant and extensive effects on development and behavior, and the anticipation of possible phenotypic consequences of a genetic diagnosis allows patients, families, physicians, and other professionals to put into action the therapies and interventions that can shape the developmental and behavioral outcomes for those patients.

To begin with, the current and potential medical needs of patients with genetic disorders are more likely to be understood when the patient's precise diagnosis is established.[45] Recommendations for the screening, treatment, and ongoing medical surveillance of patients with many genetic conditions are now the subject of evidence-based practice guidelines issued by the American Academy of Pediatrics.[3] The optimization of patients' medical condition, including their ophthalmological and auditory function, is appropriately regarded as a foundation for developmental and behavioral care. Even in conditions such as Rett syndrome or other neurodegenerative diagnoses, an understanding of diagnosis and prognosis is necessary to ensure that appropriate supports are in place for child and family when they are needed. Similarly, for conditions in which development continues to move forward, prognostic information is useful for predicting which therapeutic and educational supports will optimize developmental-behavioral outcome.

The potentially most valuable benefits of establishing a genetic diagnosis are psychological and social in nature. Many parents harbor unstated but profound concerns that their actions were responsible for their children's disabilities, as well as potentially disabling uncertainties about their child's prognosis. Establishing a precise genetic etiology appears to alleviate many of these concerns and uncertainties.[46] One particularly supportive resource that families can draw upon after receiving a genetic diagnosis for their children is that of diagnosis-driven family support groups. As for families of children with other chronic health conditions, these groups serve as warehouses of information and psychosocial support. Other, more experienced families who are faced with similar challenges can provide practical information on medical care, school district politics, extracurricular activities, transition to adulthood, and many other topics about which even the best clinicians have limited knowledge, and these families can also provide a forum through which to share and thereby relieve some of the stresses and burdens of their unique parenthood experiences.

Approach to Diagnostic Evaluation

Until every newborn receives exhaustive testing for all possible genetic disorders and differences, the diagnosis of these conditions will remain driven largely by clinical suspicion; that is, genetic conditions can be diagnosed only if they are suspected and if appropriate diagnostic tests are then requested. Although the most common genetic cause of mental retardation, Down syndrome, is in most cases easily recognized and is diagnosable by routine karyotype, specific testing is required for diagnosis of most of the other recognizable patterns of human malformation. For conditions that involve gene deletion, diagnosis is typically by FISH testing, through use of a molecular probe that is specific for the suspected condition. Thus, the diagnosis is not made unless a specific clinical suspicion engenders specific testing. Other conditions that result from defined molecular genetic abnormalities can be diagnosed with directed testing of other sorts, but these tests also must be specifically requested on the basis of a specific suspicion. Only a few commonly occurring disorders besides Down syndrome (notably, the sex chromosome aneuploidies) are diagnosable by routine karyotype.

Rapid advances in molecular biological technology may soon make suspicion-driven diagnosis obsolete. So-called microarray methods are able to assess the expression of hundreds or thousands of genes simultaneously, with very small samples of blood or other tissue.[3] It may soon be possible for the developmental-behavioral pediatrician to send a single blood specimen for genetic testing, with a note on the clinical context for testing, and for the laboratory to screen rapidly and inexpensively for any of thousands of genetic disorders or differences that are known to be associated with that clinical history.

The decision on when to request genetic testing is one whose answer is evolving as well. Classically, the only children who underwent genetic testing were those with multiple congenital anomalies or with dysmorphology, because they were the only ones in whom testing was likely to yield informative results. As diagnostic methods advanced, and as the spectrum of diagnosable genetic differences widened, the population of patients who might benefit from genetic testing grew very quickly as well. Many authorities now recommend that all children with significant developmental delays of unknown etiology should be considered for testing that includes a karyotype, subtelomeric probes, and DNA testing for the fragile X syndrome, because abnormal findings on any of these tests can be associated with seemingly nonspecific developmental impairment.[3] For children with autistic spectrum disorders, additional testing might be recommended, as discussed in Chapter 15. Of course, a neurodegenerative history or the presence of certain other neurological signs and symptoms is an indication for testing for various metabolic and storage diseases that manifest in these types of presentation and are discussed in Chapter 10C. Here again, advances in diagnostic methods that allow simple and inexpensive testing for many conditions simultaneously may soon make an encyclopedic knowledge of genetic disorders obsolete at the diagnostic stage of care. One algorithm for the approach to diagnostic testing is illustrated in Figure 10B-3.

For conditions and genetic disorders whose phenotypes are less pervasive than for the chromosomal and similar disorders, diagnosis will probably remain driven by specific clinical questions, at least for the near future. As an example, if and when pharmacogenomic research is able to determine who will respond best to which drugs, it will be the physician's responsibility to request the appropriate genetic testing to guide prescribing practice.

Some patients and families are unmotivated to undergo or even resistant to diagnostic testing. In these cases, the possibility of diagnostic testing should be revisited at a later time because of possible implications for reproductive decisions by the patient or by other family members and because the benefits associated with establishing a diagnosis are likely to increase as research advances.

Treatment Implications

With relatively few exceptions, genotypic diagnosis does not currently lead to specifically effective recommendations for developmental and behavioral intervention. Research remains focused on phenotypic description, which despite its challenges, remains a much simpler task than the identification of diagnosis-specific treatments and behavioral interventions.

Special education and neuropsychology are two disciplines that have led in the development of diagnosis-specific treatment strategies. For example, children with Down syndrome typically show particular impairment in auditory-based phonetic and phonological skills, which results in significant compromise in the development of their spoken language abilities.[47,48] When the communicative abilities of these individuals are below the level of their general cognitive abilities, behavioral consequences may result. Many experts therefore recommend the extensive use of sign language for young children with Down syndrome, taking advantage of their better preserved capacities for learning a nonverbal, nonauditory language. Although some are concerned that the use of sign language will delay or impair the development of spoken language skills, the studies that exist suggest that this concern is generally unwarranted and that the early introduction of sign language is associated with lasting benefits to the communicative and social skills of children with Down syndrome.[49]

Other examples of therapeutic interventions that are diagnostically specific include the use of "verbal mediation" techniques for children with Williams syndrome and the use of intensive oral drills for teaching arithmetic to children with velocardiofacial/DiGeorge syndrome. In the case of Williams syndrome, this educational/therapeutic approach is driven by the neuropsychological profile that is associated with the syndrome, in which verbal and auditory skills are strengths that can be used to support other functions that are not as strong.[4] In the case of velocardiofacial/DiGeorge syndrome, the suggestion to use a specific educational approach is driven largely by repeated anecdotal reports from parents. In both cases, the suggested therapeutic approaches remain open to rigorous validation, but they appear to be promising with regard to the potential for diagnostically driven intervention.

As discussed in the section on phenotypic variability, care providers and parents must remember that every child is unique and that the therapeutic suggestions intended to benefit most children with a specific diagnosis may not be valid for a specific child. For the purpose of educational programming and related therapeutic intervention, a thorough psychoeducational and/or neuropsychological evaluation of the individual child is the most helpful diagnostic assessment that can be made. Knowledge of the typical phenotype associated with the genetic diagnosis is

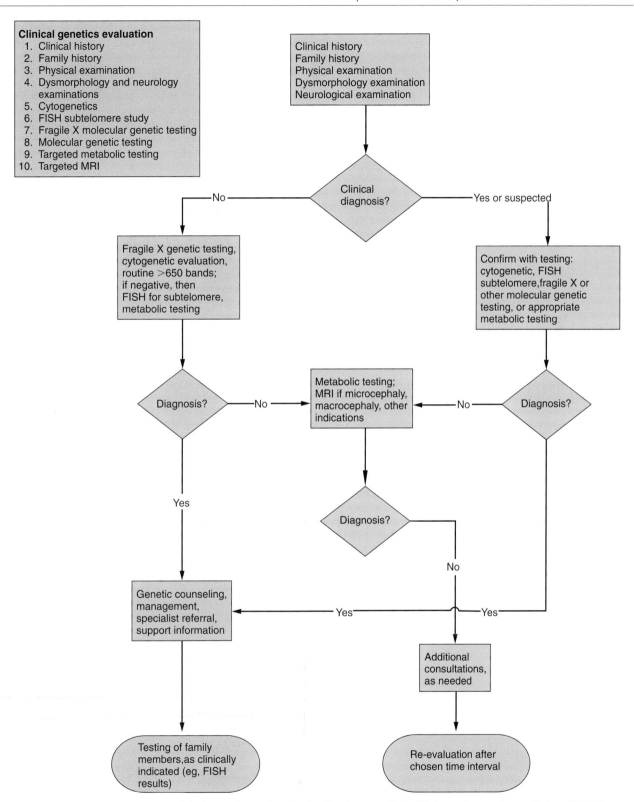

Clinical genetics evaluation
1. Clinical history
2. Family history
3. Physical examination
4. Dysmorphology and neurology examinations
5. Cytogenetics
6. FISH subtelomere study
7. Fragile X molecular genetic testing
8. Molecular genetic testing
9. Targeted metabolic testing
10. Targeted MRI

FIGURE 10B-3 Approach to the clinical genetics evaluation for developmental disabilities and mental retardation. FISH, fluorescent in situ hybridization; MRI, magnetic resonance imaging. (From Moeschler JB, Shevell M, American Academy of Pediatrics Committee on Genetics: Clinical genetic evaluation of the child with mental retardation or developmental delays. Pediatrics 117:2304-2316, 2006.)

best used to guide the psychological assessment and to supplement its results.

Gene therapy for neurodevelopmental disorders remains entirely hypothetical. Because a genetic diagnosis must be made before any specific genetic therapy can be instituted, and because genetic disorders affecting development and behavior are rarely diagnosed before the brain has completed all of its prenatal and much of its postnatal development, it is not clear what effect genetic therapies could have. Many genetic disorders affect brain function, as well as brain development, but it seems naive to believe that postnatal therapies could reverse developmental abnormalities that have already been completed. In the event that a genetic disorder is diagnosed in the course of prenatal genetic testing, the opportunity to intervene in the processes of brain development may be present, but there is currently no paradigm for prenatal genetic therapy.

COMPENDIUM OF DEVELOPMENTAL-BEHAVIORAL PHENOTYPES

The study of behavioral phenotypes has increased at a seemingly exponential rate since the late 20th century. Textbook descriptions of behavioral phenotypes quickly become dated and, in any case, cannot be comprehensive when journal reviews of single disorders are several pages in length. Fortunately, medical periodicals are increasingly available through the Internet, and dedicated Internet databases also provide comprehensive and frequently updated reviews. Authoritative Internet databases on genetic disorders (Online Mendelian Inheritance in Man [OMIM][50] and GeneReviews[51]) are sponsored by the federal government of the United States, and they provide reliable information on both medical and behavioral phenotypes.

The following listings focus on key aspects of the behavioral phenotypes of some of the most common and best studied genetic disorders (listed alphabetically by their commonly used names). The list does not include descriptions of genes implicated in the etiology of multiple-gene disorders such as dyslexia and also does not include information on the medical phenotypes of the disorders listed. That information also is available in general pediatric references, in the public Internet databases mentioned previously, and in guidelines for medical care published by the American Academy of Pediatrics and other groups.

In general, this listing focuses on phenotypic features that are believed to be of specific interest for the disorders discussed, rather than on developmental and behavioral characteristics that are found commonly in many disorders. Examples of such characteristics include broadly decreased IQ scores, language delay commensurate with overall IQ, and the diagnosis of ADHD. "Executive function deficits" also have been described in a large number of genetic conditions, and it is not clear to what extent these deficits are specific to any particular disorder or whether they reflect impairments in general cognitive functions.

Down Syndrome[52]

ETIOLOGY

Causes are trisomy 21, partial trisomy 21, unbalanced translocations involving chromosome 21, and related mosaic genotypes.

DEVELOPMENTAL-BEHAVIORAL PHENOTYPE[48]

General cognitive abilities in adulthood range from normal-level intelligence (in individuals with mosaic trisomy) to moderate and severe mental retardation; IQ scores are most commonly in the range of mild-moderate retardation. Most prominent in the neuropsychological profile is the impairment of verbal memory skills and other verbal processing abilities. Linguistic skills are almost always poorer than general cognitive skills, with grammar most severely affected. Receptive vocabulary can continue to increase through young adulthood. Visual-spatial short-term memory span often exceeds verbal short-term memory span; this situation is exceptionally rare in typically developing children and adults. Many affected infants seem to show a deceleration in developmental rate around a year of age, although this may be related to the increasing rate of language-related development that is expected at this age. Most patients show the onset of an Alzheimer-like dementia sometime during the fourth decade of life. Affect is often relatively flat, and depression is often present.

IMPLICATIONS

It is important to support the development of communication skills, in order to facilitate other aspects of development and to avert behavioral complications. As discussed previously, sign language may be acquired more easily than spoken language and does not decrease the level of skill in spoken language that is ultimately achieved. Depression can be difficult to recognize when communication skills are poor.

RESEARCH DIRECTIONS

Down syndrome is often featured as a comparison group in research on other genetic disorders, because of its relatively high prevalence. It has been the subject of studies of the effect of pharmacological treatment on cognitive abilities (piracetam, donepezil) and is likely to be the subject of similar future studies.

Fragile X Syndrome[11,53]

ETIOLOGY

The cause is a triplet repeat expansion in an untranslated segment at the 5′ end of the gene for FMR1 protein. "Premutation carriers" have an intermediate expansion of the triplet repeat, and their offspring are at risk of repeat expansion. Expansion results in hypermethylation of the gene and failure to produce FMR1 protein.

DEVELOPMENTAL-BEHAVIORAL PHENOTYPE

In boys and men with the full mutation and hypermethylation of the FMR1 gene, no protein product is found after early fetal development, and IQ is typically in the range of moderate or severe mental retardation. IQ is correlated with levels of FMR1 protein. Protein levels are a function of gene methylation and, in girls and women, X activation ratios (percentage of cells in which the normal X chromosome is the active X chromosome). IQ often declines in the adolescent years, not because cognitive abilities regress, but because development of more abstract reasoning does not occur. Various impairments in executive functions believed to reflect the operation of the prefrontal lobes have been reported.

Symptoms such as auditory and tactile hypersensitivity, gaze aversion, stereotypic behaviors such as hand-flapping, and perseveration lead to a suspicion of autistic disorders in many affected persons, but this diagnosis should not be assumed in the fragile X syndrome. In some patients, these symptoms are accompanied by social disinterest meriting the autism diagnosis, but in others the presence of social anxiety also results in the "satisfaction" of diagnostic criteria for autism but presents a subtly different picture. Other psychiatric symptoms and diagnoses are common among girls and women with the full mutation, particularly anxiety disorders. Premutation carriers also may show a related phenotype and have a heightened risk of affective disorders as well.

IMPLICATIONS AND RESEARCH DIRECTIONS

As reviewed previously, the phenotypes of the fragile X syndrome and of carriers of the premutation remain under active investigation. New data show that the premutation carriers may show significant behavioral symptoms at some point in their lives, and so psychiatric and medical support are appropriate. For boys with the full mutation, extensive early intervention and special educational services are indicated. Many small studies of pharmacological treatment for various symptoms have been published, but therapy remains largely empirical.

Muscular Dystrophy (Duchenne and Becker)

ETIOLOGY

These diseases are caused by a mutation in the gene for dystrophin. In Duchenne muscular dystrophy, the protein product is absent; in Becker muscular dystrophy, the protein product is present but functionally abnormal.

DEVELOPMENTAL-BEHAVIORAL PHENOTYPE

In the older medical literature, authors consistently reported Wechsler Full-Scale IQ scores typically in the 80s, with Verbal IQ score often lower than Performance IQ score, but more recent research results are less consistent.[54] Neuropsychological assessment commonly reveals deficits in verbal short-term memory. Preliminary evidence suggests that this is not the case in Becker muscular dystrophy. Research on behavioral and other psychological consequences of Duchenne muscular dystrophy is relatively early.[55]

IMPLICATIONS AND RESEARCH DIRECTIONS

The precise developmental and behavioral implications of Duchenne muscular dystrophy remain to be defined. The physical disability associated with this condition is expected to be associated with the potential for major psychological sequelae.

Neurofibromatosis Type I[56]

ETIOLOGY

This disease is caused by a mutation in the gene for neurofibromin; many distinct mutations have been described, and diagnosis is clinical.

DEVELOPMENTAL-BEHAVIORAL PHENOTYPE[57]

As reviewed previously, the behavioral phenotype of neurofibromatosis type 1 is subtle and was not well understood until patients with neurofibromatosis type 1 were carefully compared with sibling controls. Brain lesions that are apparent on magnetic resonance imaging or other neuroimaging procedures have not been clearly related to the developmental-behavioral phenotype. Various developmental psychiatric diagnoses are found with increased prevalence in neurofibromatosis type 1,[58] as are impairments in social skills.[59]

IMPLICATIONS

This disorder illustrates the importance of comprehensive and thorough individualized psychoeducational testing, to develop the most appropriate individualized educational plan for every affected child. Although syndrome-specific patterns of impairment exist, these patterns are variable.

Prader-Willi Syndrome

ETIOLOGY

This disorder arises from the absence of paternally derived chromosome 15q11-q13, through deletion or uniparental (maternal) disomy

DEVELOPMENTAL-BEHAVIORAL PHENOTYPE

The hyperphagia and obsessive food-seeking behavior are well known. These do not emerge in infancy, which instead is characterized by extreme hypotonia and associated feeding difficulties. The hyperphagia emerges in the late preschool years, as can other obsessive behaviors. Obesity is common as a result of uncontrolled eating. Cognitive abilities are classically described in the range of mild to moderate retardation, but molecular diagnostics have revealed many individuals in the borderline or normal range of intelligence to have the 15q deletion. Patients with uniparental disomy (as opposed to deletion) may be more likely to show autistic-type symptoms[60] and psychotic symptoms.[61]

IMPLICATIONS AND RESEARCH DIRECTIONS

The specific genes causing Prader-Willi syndrome have not been identified, nor is the pathophysiology of the hyperphagia understood. Elucidation of these etiological questions will provide important clues for the management of Prader-Willi syndrome. The usefulness of growth hormone supplementation is uncertian. The molecular diagnosis of individuals with this disorder (and with Smith-Magenis syndrome, described later) who have IQ scores in the normal range is an example of the evolution in our understanding of behavioral phenotypes. Research on Prader-Willi syndrome is yielding data on the role and importance of genetic imprinting in humans.

Rett Syndrome

ETIOLOGY

This disorder is known to be caused by a mutation in the gene *MECP2*. Mutations in *CDKL5* have also been found to cause Rett disorder.

DEVELOPMENTAL-BEHAVIORAL PHENOTYPE

Rett syndrome illustrates how developmental-behavioral phenotypes can in some cases be characterized by a specific developmental trajectory (here, a degenerative process after up to 2 years of typical development) and by motoric stereotypies (hand-wringing). This condition is discussed more extensively in Chapter 15.

Sex Chromosome Aneuploidies (Besides Turner syndrome)

ETIOLOGY

Aneuploidy of the X and/or the Y chromosome. Klinefelter syndrome results from a 47,XXY genotype.

DEVELOPMENTAL-BEHAVIORAL PHENOTYPE[24]

Increasing numbers of either the X or the Y chromosome are associated with lowered IQ scores. The X polysomy disorders are not as well studied as Turner syndrome, but language impairments are common, and reading achievement may be poorer than arithmetic achievement in both affected boys and girls. Risk of psychiatric diagnoses is raised, with affective disorders possibly most likely.

In boys and men with polysomy of the Y chromosome, relatively few controlled studies have been conducted. IQ is lower than in sibling controls, and it appears that learning disorders have an increased incidence. Limited controlled data show no significant incidence of incarceration, but the risk for behavioral problems, including inattention, impulsivity, and aggression, is increased. Testosterone levels have not been shown to be correlated with levels of aggression on psychological testing.

IMPLICATIONS

Androgen replacement in X polysomy appears to be associated with improvement of psychological status, possibly from both direct and indirect effects.

Smith-Magenis Syndrome

ETIOLOGY

This disorder results from a contiguous gene deletion at 17p11.2, typically about 5 megabases in size.

DEVELOPMENTAL-BEHAVIORAL PHENOTYPE[62,63]

IQ scores are believed to be most commonly in the range of moderate mental retardation, but there appears to be wide variation; some affected patients have IQs in the normal range and receive little or no special educational support. Self-injurious behaviors and sleep difficulties are the best-known features of this condition. No specific understanding of the self-injurious behavior has been achieved, but some cases appear to be associated with anxiety. The sleep difficulties are associated with abnormal rhythms for the secretion of melatonin.[27]

IMPLICATIONS

Prompt evaluation, including functional analysis, should be performed if self-injurious behaviors are noted. This may be helpful in many cases to prevent escalation of these behaviors. Melatonin administration may improve sleep patterns.

Tuberous Sclerosis

ETIOLOGY

This disorder is caused by a mutation in the gene for either TSC1 (hamartin) or TSC2 (tuberin); diagnosis is clinical.

DEVELOPMENTAL-BEHAVIORAL PHENOTYPE[64,65]

Many developmental and behavioral issues have been associated with tuberous sclerosis, but research has focused primarily on its relationship with autism. One study of patients with tuberous sclerosis suggests that the risk of autistic disorder, and of low IQ, is much greater for patients with a mutation in TSC2 than for those with a mutation in TSC1.

IMPLICATIONS AND RESEARCH DIRECTIONS

There may be other putatively unitary conditions that, like tuberous sclerosis, can actually arise from more than one etiology. The discovery of these distinct causes may lead to the recognition that one or some causes carry a greater risk of certain developmental-behavioral outcomes than do other causes, which highlights the benefits of genotypic diagnosis for the future.

Turner Syndrome[66]

ETIOLOGY

This disorder is characterized by a 45,X karyotype or mosaic.

DEVELOPMENTAL-BEHAVIORAL PHENOTYPE[18a]

General cognitive abilities are slightly lower than average, but the majority of affected patients have IQs in the normal range. Many patients have a nonverbal learning disability profile, with deficiencies in math achievement but often with unusually strong reading skills. This can be accompanied by a discrepancy between Wechsler Verbal IQ scores (higher) and Performance IQ scores, and this is most likely before adolescence. As described previously, socials skills may be stronger in those whose X chromosome is paternally derived, whereas autism may be more common in those with a maternally derived X chromosome. In early development, motor delays are common. ADHD symptoms are common in childhood, at least in a subset of patients.

IMPLICATIONS

Early physical therapy is indicated for many affected patients. Surveillance for arithmetic disabilities and initiation of appropriate supports should be accomplished as soon as indicated. Estrogen replacement therapy may affect development and behavior both directly through effects on brain development and indirectly through psychosocial benefits associated with normalized sexual maturation.

RESEARCH DIRECTIONS

Active research on arithmetic abilities is likely to yield guidelines on the best educational methods and supports for this population.

Velocardiofacial/DiGeorge Syndrome

ETIOLOGY

This disorder arises from a contiguous gene deletion at 22q11.2, encompassing about 3 megabases in most patients. It is also known as Shprintzen syndrome and conotruncal anomaly face syndrome, and the gene deletion accounts for some cases of Opitz G/BBB syndrome.

DEVELOPMENTAL-BEHAVIORAL PHENOTYPE[30a,67,68]

General cognitive abilities in adults range from normal to mild retardation, with many in borderline range. A profile of nonverbal learning disabilities is common, with reading achievement superior to arithmetic achievement. Neuropsychological assessment reveals weakness in visual-spatial memory. In early childhood, severe language delays are common, not only in relation to velopharyngeal insufficiency and phonetic difficulties but also in acquisition of grammar and vocabulary. Psychiatric problems are common and often severe, starting in childhood for many patients. The diagnostic formulation of these psychiatric problems is disputed; some experts argue that they represent a primary psychotic diathesis, and others interpret them as bipolarity.[69] When these problems are absent, the possibility of high-functioning, undiagnosed cases in the community is very high, because dysmorphology is subtle and severity of medical phenotype is quite variable.

IMPLICATIONS

Sign language very helpful for affected children. Otolaryngological management also is key. In the school years, a rote approach to arithmetic may be most effective (e.g., the Kumon approach to tutoring). Possible psychiatric symptoms should be evaluated immediately, with treatment as indicated.

RESEARCH DIRECTIONS

Risk factors for psychiatric problems and possibility of prophylactic treatments, including pharmacological prophylaxis, should be identified. A specific allele of the gene for COMT, one copy of which is deleted in this condition, may be associated with higher risk for developmental, behavioral, and psychiatric complications.[70]

Williams Syndrome[71]

ETIOLOGY

This disorder arises from a contiguous gene deletion at 7q11.23, encompassing about 2 megabases.

DEVELOPMENTAL-BEHAVIORAL PHENOTYPE[4,72,73]

Attention has focused primarily on language skills in this condition, but it is now appreciated that language skills are generally at the level expected for the overall cognitive level (this may be unusual among syndromes associated with mental retardation). IQ scores generally range from the upper reaches of moderate mental retardation into the borderline range, with outliers at either end of this distribution. Auditory and verbal skills are clearly superior to visual-spatial skills, and academic achievement shows a similar discrepancy between reading and spelling versus arithmetic. Despite this profile in later life, infants and toddlers show major delays in language development. Behavioral symptoms include auditory and tactile hypersensitivity, feeding difficulties often associated with extreme selectivity, and severe colic in infancy. Interest and skills in music are often surprisingly high, and this is probably related to the same fundamental cognitive skills that support language processing.

More recently, investigators have focused on the temperamental characteristics of high emotionality and sociability. The latter may be the true hallmark of the syndrome. The desire for social interaction and for the approval of others is a key motivator. For many individuals with disabilities, the opportunity for social interaction is lost at the end of schooling, and this loss is associated with depressive symptoms in many cases. Other psychiatric concerns include specific phobias and generalized anxiety in some patients, as well as ADHD. Musical therapy to support developmental activities and to address psychiatric symptoms appears to be well received by many.[74]

IMPLICATIONS

Extensive early intervention services are required, despite the relative strength in communication skills later in life. Attention to possible psychiatric symptoms is important, starting at least with the transition to adulthood.

RESEARCH DIRECTIONS

This is another syndrome that is the subject of intensive cognitive research; investigators have examined the fundamental cognitive skills and impairments that support language-related and other higher order cognitive skills. Research also focuses on the temperamental characteristics of the syndrome and its biological basis.

CONCLUSION

Genetic factors play a central role in shaping human development and behavior. In most cases, the effects of these genetic factors are mediated by other genetic factors and by environmental factors as well. Indeed, some genetic differences may produce phenotypic effects only in specific "at-risk" environments. As a corollary, substantial individual variability is found in the developmental-behavioral manifestations of genetic syndromes and other genetic differences.

Despite this caveat, genetic diagnoses often yield valuable insights for patient management and for prognostication. Genetic testing may soon be relevant not only for the diagnosis of the classic genetic syndromes but also for understanding the basis of multiple-gene disorders, such as dyslexia and autism in an individual patient, and for individualized pharmacotherapy. The literature on the developmental-behavioral facets of genetics is already quite large, and clinicians and researchers will have to rely increasingly on electronic resources to help them manage this corpus of knowledge.

REFERENCES

1. Nussbaum RL, McInnes RR, Willard HF: Thompson & Thompson Genetics in Medicine, Revised Reprint, 6th ed. Philadelphia: Elsevier, 2004.
2. Jones KL: Smith's Recognizable Patterns of Human Malformation. Philadelphia: WB Saunders, 1997.
3. Moeschler JB, Shevell M, American Academy of Pediatrics Committee on Genetics: Clinical genetic evaluation of the child with mental retardation or developmental delays. Pediatrics 117:2304-2316, 2006.
4. Morris CA, Lenhoff HM, Wang PP, eds: Williams-Beuren Syndrome: Research, Evaluation, and Treatment. Baltimore: Johns Hopkins University Press, 2006.
5. Emanuel BS, McDonald-McGinn D, Saitta SC, et al: The 22q11.2 deletion syndrome. Adv Pediatr 48:39-73, 2001.
6. Osborne LR: The molecular basis of a multisystem disorder. *In* Morris CA, Lenhoff HM, Wang PP, eds: Williams-Beuren Syndrome: Research and Clinical

Perspectives, Baltimore: Johns Hopkins University Press, 2006, pp 18-58.

7. Bucan M, Abel T: The mouse: Genetics meets behaviour. Nat Rev Genet 3:114-123, 2002.

8. McDonald-McGinn DM, Tonnesen MK, et al: Phenotype of the 22q11.2 deletion in individuals identified through an affected relative: Cast a wide FISHing net. Genet Med 3:23-29, 2001.

9. Nyhan W: Behavioral phenotypes in organic genetic disease. Pediatr Res 6:1-9, 1972.

10. Cunniff C: Molecular mechanisms in neurologic disorders. Semin Pediatr Neurol 8:128-134, 2001.

11. Hagerman RJ: Lessons from fragile X regarding neurobiology, autism, and neurodegeneration. J Dev Behav Pediatr 27:63-74, 2006.

12. Sutovsky P, Schatten G: Paternal contributions to the mammalian zygote: Fertilization after sperm-egg fusion. Int Rev Cytol 195:1-65, 2000.

13. DiMauro S, Andreu-Antoni L, De Vivo DC: Mitochondrial disorders. J Child Neurol 17(Suppl 3):3S35-3S45, 2002.

14. Fisher SE, Francks C: Genes, cognition and dyslexia: Learning to read the genome. Trends Cogn Sci Regul Ed 10:250-257, 2006.

15. Fisher SE, DeFries JC: Developmental dyslexia: Genetic dissection of a complex cognitive trait. Nat Rev Neurosci 10:767-780, 2002.

16. Coon H: Current perspectives on the genetic analysis of autism. Am J Med Genet C Semin Med Genet 142:24-32, 2006.

17. Deng CX: *BRCA1:* Cell cycle checkpoint, genetic instability, DNA damage response and cancer evolution. Nucleic Acids Res 34:1416-1426, 2006.

18. Thapar A, O'Donovan M, Owen MJ: The genetics of attention deficit hyperactivity disorder. Hum Mol Genet 14(Spec No. 2):R275-R282, 2005.

18a. Ross J, Roeltge D, Zinn A: Cognition and the sex chromosomes: Studies in Turner syndrome. Horm Res 65:47-56, 2006.

19. Hoffbuhr K, Devaney JM, Lafleur B, et al: *MeCP2* mutations in children with and without the phenotype of Rett syndrome. Neurology 56:1486-1495, 2001.

20. Childs B: Genomics, proteomics, and genetics in medicine. Adv Pediatr 50:39-58, 2003.

21. Epstein CJ: Foreword. *In* Lott IT, McCoy EE, eds: Down Syndrome: Advances in Medical Care. New York: Wiley-Liss, 1992, pp ix-x.

22. Sadee W, Dai Z: Pharmacogenetics/genomics and personalized medicine. Hum Mol Genet 14(Spec No. 2): R207-R214, 2005.

23. Dykens E: Introduction to the special issue on behavioral phenotypes. Am J Ment Retard 106:1-3, 2001.

24. O'Brien G, Yule W, eds: Behavioural Phenotypes. London: MacKeith, 1995.

25. Cassidy SB, Morris CA: Behavioral phenotypes in genetic syndromes: Genetic clues to human behavior. Adv Pediatr 49:59-86, 2002.

26. Finucane BM, Konar D, Haas-Givler B, et al: The spasmodic upper-body squeeze: A characteristic behavior in Smith-Magenis syndrome. Dev Med Child Neurol 36:70-83, 1994.

27. De Leersnyder H, De Blois MC, Claustrat B, et al: Inversion of the circadian rhythm of melatonin in the Smith-Magenis syndrome. J Pediatr 139:111-116, 2001.

28. Cassidy SB, Dykens E, Williams CA: Prader-Willi and Angelman syndromes: Sister imprinted disorders. Am J Med Genet 97:136-146, 2000.

29. Prinzie P, Swillen A, Vogels A, et al: Personality profiles of youngsters with velo-cardio-facial syndrome. Genet Couns 13:265-280, 2002.

30. Bates EA: Explaining and interpreting deficits in language development across clinical groups: Where do we go from here? Brain Lang 88:248-253, 2004.

30a. Murphy KC: Annotation: Velo-cardio-facial syndrome. J Child Psychol Psychiatry 46:563-571, 2005.

31. Gottesman II, Gould TD. The endophenotype concept in psychiatry: Etymology and strategic intentions. Am J Psychiatry 160:636-645, 2003.

32. Finegan J: Study of behavioral phenotypes: Provocations from the new genetics. Am J Med Genet 81:148-155, 1998.

33. Hodapp RM, Dykens EM: Measuring behavior in genetic disorders of mental retardation. Ment Retard Dev Disabil Res Rev 11:340-346, 2005.

34. Vicari S, Bates E, Caselli MC, et al: Neuropsychological profile of Italians with Williams syndrome: An example of a dissociation between language and cognition? J Int Neuropsychol Soc 10:862-876, 2004.

35. Cutting LE, Koth CW, Denckla MB: How children with neurofibromatosis type 1 differ from typical learning disabled clinic attenders: Nonverbal learning disabilities revisited. Dev Neuropsychol 17:29-47, 2000.

36. Vallar G, Papagno C: Preserved vocabulary acquisition ion Down's syndrome: The role of phonological short-term memory. Cortex 29:467-483, 1993.

37. Plomin R, Owen MJ, McGuffin P: The genetic basis of complex human behaviors. Science 264:1733-1739, 1994.

38. Turkheimer E, Haley A, Waldron M, et al: Socioeconomic status modifies heritability of IQ in young children. Psychol Sci 14:623-628, 2003.

39. Thapar A, O'Donovan M, Owen MJ: The genetics of attention deficit hyperactivity disorder. Hum Mol Genet 14(Spec No. 2):R275-R282, 2005.

40. Caspi A, McClay J, Moffitt TE, et al: Role of genotype in the cycle of violence in maltreated children. Science 297:851-854, 2002.

41. Caspi A, Sugden K, Moffitt TE, et al: Influence of life stress on depression: Moderation by a polymorphism in the 5-HTT gene. Science 301:386-389, 2003.

42. Thapar A, Langley K, Fowler T, et al: Catechol *O*-methyltransferase gene variant and birth weight predict early-onset antisocial behavior in children with attention-deficit/hyperactivity disorder. Arch Gen Psychiatry 62:1275-1278, 2005.

43. Volkmar FR, Greenough WT: Rearing complexity affects branching of dendrites in the visual cortex of the rat. Science 176:1445-1447, 1972.

44. Fraga MF, Ballestar E, Paz MF, et al: Epigenetic differences arise during the lifetime of monozygotic twins. Proc Natl Acad Sci U S A 2005. 102: 10604-10609.

45. Dykens EM, Hodapp RM: Research in mental retardation: Toward an etiologic approach. J Child Psychol Psychiatry 42:49-71, 2001.

46. Lenhard W, Breitenbach E, Ebert H, Schindelhauer-Deutscher HJ, Henn W. Psychological benefit of diagnostic certainty for mothers of children with disabilities: lessons from Down syndrome. Amer J Med Genet A 133:170-5, 2005.

47. Wang PP. A neuropsychological profile of Down syndrome: cognitive skills and brain morphology, Ment Retard Devel Disabil Res Rev 2:102-108, 1996.

48. Chapman RS, Hesketh LJ. Behavioral phenotype of individuals with Down syndrome. Ment Retard Dev Disabil Res Rev 6:84-95, 2000.

49. Clibbens J. Signing and Lexical Development in Children with Down Syndrome. Down Syndr Res Prac 7:101-105, 2001.

50. OMIM™—Online Mendelian Inheritance in Man™. (Available at: http://www.ncbi.nlm.nih.gov/omim/; accessed 11/14/06.)

51. GeneReviews. Available at: http://www.genetests.org/; accessed 11/14/06.)

52. American Academy of Pediatrics Committee on Genetics: Health supervision for children with Down syndrome. American Academy of Pediatrics. Pediatrics 107:442-449, 2001.

53. Health supervision for children with fragile X syndrome. American Academy of Pediatrics Committee on Genetics. Pediatrics 98:297-300, 1996.

54. Wicksell RK, Kihlgren M, Melin L, et al: Specific cognitive deficits are common in children with Duchenne muscular dystrophy. Dev Med Child Neurol 46:154-159, 2004.

55. Nereo NE, Hinton VJ: Three wishes and psychological functioning in boys with Duchenne muscular dystrophy. J Dev Behav Pediatr 24:96-103, 2003.

56. Health supervision for children with neurofibromatosis. American Academy of Pediatrics Committee on Genetics. Pediatrics 96:368-372, 1995.

57. Kayl AE, Moore BD 3rd: Behavioral phenotype of neurofibromatosis, type 1. Ment Retard Dev Disabil Res Rev 6:117-124, 2000.

58. Johnson H, Wiggs L, Stores G, et al: Psychological disturbance and sleep disorders in children with neurofibromatosis type 1. Dev Med Child Neurol 47:237-242, 2005.

59. Barton B, North K: Social skills of children with neurofibromatosis type 1. Dev Med Child Neurol 46:553-563, 2004.

60. Milner KM, Craig EE, Thompson RJ, et al: Prader-Willi syndrome: Intellectual abilities and behavioural features by genetic subtype. J Child Psychol Psychiatry 46:1089-1096, 2005.

61. Vogels A, De Hert M, Descheemaeker MJ, et al: Psychotic disorders in Prader-Willi syndrome. Am J Med Genet A 127:238-243, 2004.

62. Shelley BP, Robertson MM: The neuropsychiatry and multisystem features of the Smith-Magenis syndrome: A review. J Neuropsychiatry Clin Neurosci 17:91-97, 2005.

63. Gropman AL, Duncan WC, Smith ACM: Neurologic and developmental features of the Smith-Magenis syndrome (del 17p11.2). Pediatr Neurol 34:337-350, 2006.

64. Prather P, de Vries PJ: Behavioral and cognitive aspects of tuberous sclerosis complex. J Child Neurol 19:666-674, 2004.

65. Asato MR, Hardan AY: Neuropsychiatric problems in tuberous sclerosis complex. J Child Neurol 19:241-249, 2004.

66. Frias JL, Davenport ML, Committee on Genetics and Section on Endocrinology: Health supervision for children with Turner syndrome. Pediatrics 111:692-702, 2003.

67. Wang PP, Solot C, Moss EM, et al: Developmental presentation of 22q11.2 deletion (DiGeorge/velocardiofacial syndrome). J Dev Behav Pediatr 19:342-345, 1998.

68. Shprintzen RJ, Higgins AM, Antshel K, et al: Velo-cardio-facial syndrome. Curr Opin Pediatr 17:725-730, 2005.

69. Jolin EM, Weller EB, Weller RA: Velocardiofacial syndrome: Is there a neuropsychiatric phenotype? Curr Psychiatry Rep 8:96-101, 2006.

70. Shashi V, Keshavan MS, Howard TD, et al: Cognitive correlates of a functional COMT polymorphism in children with 22q11.2 deletion syndrome. Clin Genet 69:234-238, 2006.

71. Committee on Genetics: American Association of Pediatrics: Health care supervision for children with Williams syndrome. Pediatrics 107:1192-1204, 2001.

72. Mervis CB, Klein-Tasman BP: Williams syndrome: Cognition, personality, and adaptive behavior. Ment Retard Dev Disabil Res Rev 6:148-158, 2000.

73. Karmiloff-Smith A, Brown JH, Grice S, et al: Dethroning the myth: Cognitive dissociations and innate modularity in Williams syndrome. Dev Neuropsychol 23:227-242, 2003.

74. Dykens EM, Rosner BA, Ly T, et al: Music and anxiety in Williams syndrome: A harmonious or discordant relationship? Am J Ment Retard 110:346-358, 2005.

10C.
Metabolic Disorders

MARSHALL SUMMAR

This chapter addresses the role of metabolic disease in human development. Although it does not provide an exhaustive overview of all metabolic diseases, it does categorize the types of disease that result in aberrant development, some of their root causes, and strategies for both diagnosis and treatment. The brain represents one of the most metabolically active organs in the human body and has tremendous needs for both energy and the production of biomolecules on a constant basis. Mild variations in metabolic processing affect the brain at a much earlier stage and more severely than they affect other more robust organs, such as the liver, kidneys, or heart. Therefore, most metabolic diseases result in aberrant development. Developmental delay is often the first sign of an underlying inborn error of metabolism.

When the role of metabolic disease in development is explored, a standard approach can be quite useful. Although these disorders are individually rare, they pose a significant burden of disease as a group. It is essential to consider them in a patient without an obvious cause of either developmental delay or neurological dysfunction. The importance of diagnosing them lies in the availability of treatment options for several diseases or the ability to perform presymptomatic diagnostic testing on other family members.

Many practitioners are reluctant to approach the diagnosis of these conditions, because the definitive diagnosis typically requires rather esoteric testing. However, both categorizing and responding to these patients can be accomplished with laboratories that are typically nearby.[1] As with most conditions, clues from the history, examination, family, and course of disease are immensely valuable. This approach is presented in a useful manner.

TYPES OF INBORN ERRORS OF METABOLISM THAT AFFECT DEVELOPMENT

Disorders in Energy Metabolism

These diseases are related to the ability to generate adenosine triphosphate or other energy substrates that are vital for normal cellular function. Among the best known of this group are the mitochondrial diseases. The majority of proteins involved in mitochondrial energy metabolism are encoded by nuclear rather than the small mitochondrial genome.[2] These diseases typically result in poor energy production and overproduction of lactic acid.[3,4] A second type of energy problem involves glucose metabolism.[5] Conditions such as glycogen storage defects and gluconeogenic defects result in decreased supplies of energy substrate to the brain.[6,7] The disorders of fatty acid oxidation can also result in a limited glucose supply with similar effects.[8,9] This can rapidly result in depletion of both adenosine triphosphate and energy.

Disorders of Biomolecule Conversion

This group consists of defects in systems that convert one molecule to another. Examples include phenylketonuria, homocystinuria, hyperglycinemia, tyrosinemia, and the organic acidemias. In these diseases, failure of molecule conversion results in an oversupply of the one or more precursor metabolites and an undersupply of the products. Phenylketonuria is an excellent example of this concept. Absence of phenylalanine hydroxylase results in the accumulation of phenylalanine, which at high levels is toxic to neurons.[10-12] The inability to convert phenylalanine to tyrosine results in the conversion of tyrosine to an essential amino acid. Galactosemia is another example in which galactose cannot be isomerized to glucose.[13] The unconverted galactose results in neurotoxicity and hepatotoxicity, and the potential energy from the glucose is lost.

Disorders of Biomolecule Clearance

These diseases are somewhat similar to the disorders of molecule conversion but occur in systems specifically designed to clear molecules that are toxic in large quantities. The urea cycle is an excellent example.[14,15] With turnover and dietary intake, the body must clear waste nitrogen on a regular basis. This nitrogen appears in the blood stream as ammonia, levels of which can elevate rapidly if the urea cycle cannot convert it to the readily excreted molecule urea. Another example is the breakdown of the simplest amino acid, glycine. Failure of the glycine cleavage complex results in its accumulation in the central nervous system, where glycine's neurotransmitter properties interfere with function at many levels.[16] In the purine metabolic pathway, defects in clearance result in toxic buildups in Lesch-Nyhan syndrome.[17,18] Disorders of biomolecule clearance also include the lysosomal storage disorders, which remove relatively inert molecules such as mucopolysaccharides and oligosaccharides.[19] These molecules accumulate over time, and their occupation of cellular space leads to their toxicity.

Disorders of Cellular Function

Defects in basic cellular function constitute this group of disorders. The defects in aspartate transport (citrin deficiency, or citrullinemia type II) result in poor metabolism of both glucose and ammonia.[20,21] These disorders affect cerebral development and also result in long-term toxicity. The peroxisomal disorders, such as Zellweger syndrome, represent whole organelle failure, which results in damage to the brain and other organs.[22,23] These disorders are characterized by their effects on a wide range of cellular metabolic functions.

TIMING OF DEVELOPMENTAL DELAY AND METABOLIC CONSIDERATIONS

A first step in categorizing the effects of metabolites on the brain is temporal. The timing of the disruption in development offers substantial clues to the nature of the disease.

Acute

Some metabolites cause rapid damage only during an acute crisis episode. Examples of this damage are the rapid cerebral edema caused by ammonia in urea cycle defects and the acute hypoglycemia resulting from fatty acid oxidation defects such as medium-chain acyl–coenzyme A dehydrogenase deficiency.[8,14] Patients are often normal until the insult and then remain stable afterwards unless another crisis occurs. Long-term damage results from neuronal injury during the acute episode and can often produce strokelike residual problems.

Progressive

Patients with progressive disorders start out with normal development, but then their developmental trajectory is lost and they lose acquired skills. Examples of this scenario include the neurotoxic metabolites of phenylalanine and homocysteine, long-term exposure to mildly elevated ammonia levels, and the lysosomal storage disorders. The clinical course for these patients reflects the ongoing neurotoxicity and cell death from the toxins. Disorders in chronic energy metabolism (such as mitochondrial metabolism) also manifest in this manner.[24]

Prenatal Onset

We also find patients whose developmental problems precede birth, such as those with hyperglycinemia or peroxisomal disorders.[16,22] The metabolites in these disorders accumulate beyond the ability of the placenta's biofilter capacity or result in intracellular toxicity. These disorders continue to cause neurological deterioration after birth and are usually refractory to treatment.

Combined

Some disorders combine these features. Patients with urea cycle disorders develop acute hyperammonemia with damage to the brain but also have long-term neurotoxic effects from the chronic elevations of ammonia and other cycle intermediates such as arginine.[25,26] Patients with disorders resulting in lactic acidosis (such as pyruvate dehydrogenase) can have acute episodes of lactic acidosis but also suffer from chronic loss of neuronal tissue.[5]

A key point is that a downward progression of development and the loss of milestones is very suggestive of an ongoing toxic metabolic process, as is a change in development after an unexplained medical crisis.

CLUES IN THE HISTORY THAT SUGGEST A METABOLIC DISEASE IN THE DEVLOPMENTALLY DELAYED PATIENT

A careful history of a developmentally delayed patient may suggest the need for a workup concerning a metabolic disease and can often suggest which direction to pursue.

Timing and Progression

As noted in the previous section, the timing of the developmental delay can often provide clues to the type of problem. A developmental course with steady deterioration of function is suggestive of a chronic neurotoxic metabolite, whereas a sudden onset of delay is produced by a different set of disorders. As a rule, fixed developmental delays without progression are less likely to represent metabolic disease than are progressive disorders.

Family History

Although all of the metabolic diseases discussed result from genetic defects, there is often no family history of problems, because most genetic defects are autosomal recessive. Several exceptions should be remembered. Patients with disorders on the X chromosome typically have a family history of affected male relatives over several generations. Examples include the urea cycle disorder ornithine transcarbamylase and the purine metabolic disorder Lesch-Nyhan syndrome. With both of these disorders, there is a substantial number of female relatives partially or even fully affected as a result of nonrandom X chromosome inactivation.[27] The disorders of mitochondrial dysfunction resulting from mutations in mitochondrial DNA manifest with a family history of maternal lineage, because mitochondria are passed on only through the ovum and not through the sperm. Finally, the family should be asked about any type of consanguinity that may exist. This circumstance dramatically increases the risk of rare autosomal recessive metabolic diseases.

Common Illnesses

The course of diseases accompanied by common illnesses such as colds and ear infections should be obtained. Patients with partial defects in metabolic systems typically become symptomatic with other illnesses.[26] Prolonged lethargy, slow recovery from common viral illnesses, and increased frequency of infections are all suggestive of an underlying metabolic disease. The onset of seizures with a mild illness is also highly suggestive of metabolic disease.

Seizures

The development of seizures in a patient with developmental delay is often suggestive of the presence of a toxic metabolite, which is the cause of both.[28] Prolonged seizures can be particularly related.

Neonatal History

The neonatal period is one of the most stressful metabolic periods for everyone. Lethargy, excessive sleeping, poor feeding, abnormal behaviors, seizures, and temperature irregularities are all indicators that a toxic metabolite may have been present. Most of these patients undergo a workup for sepsis that reveals no pathogen. By the time the sepsis workup is complete, the metabolic disease may have stabilized and become dormant.

Specific Findings in the History That Suggest Metabolic Disease

1. Hiccups: For reasons not entirely clear, patients with defects in glycine metabolism have a history of persistent hiccups.[29] A history of the gestation usually reveals consistent hiccups during the third trimester. It is, however, normal for there to be some hiccups during the third trimester.
2. Night terrors: These are also found in patients with elevations in glycine in the cerebrospinal fluid (personal observation in three patients).
3. Autistic behavior: In patients with autistic-type behaviors (poor communication abilities), developmental delay, microcephaly, and either hiccups

or night terrors, hyperglycinemia should be considered.

4. Protein avoidance: Patients with urea cycle defects become "autoselective vegetarians" because they subconsciously condition themselves to avoid the nitrogen in the protein that results in hyperammonemia and neurological dysfunction.[26]
5. Slow hair growth: In patients with certain urea cycle defects or chronic metabolic dysfunction (such as organic acidemias), the growth of hair is very slow.[30] In argininosuccinic lyase deficiency (a urea cycle defect), the hair becomes brittle (trichorrhexis nodosa) and is always short.[31]
6. Pale blond hair: In patients with untreated phenylketonuria, the phenylalanine cannot be converted to tyrosine, which is a pigment precursor. Such patients have a fair complexion and pale blond hair.[10] This appearance is similar to that of albinism.
7. Bacterial infections: In galactosemia, there is a particular predilection for bacterial infections of all types but specifically gram-negative sepsis (such as that caused by *Escherichia coli*).[32-34]
8. Peculiar odors: The most reliable of the smells is that produced by maple syrup urine disease; parents of affected infants report a pancake syrup smell to the diaper.[35] Isovaleric acidemia produces a strong odor of sweaty socks.
9. Cataracts: The storage disorders and galactosemia can manifest with cataracts.[13,19]
10. Unusual rashes: In disorders of amino acid metabolism, the deficiencies often result in generalized skin rashes and breakdown.[36-38] These problems are particularly prominent in lysinuric protein intolerance (lysine transport defect), in which lysine is almost absent.
11. Facial feature change: In the storage disorders, the facial bone structure can change as the bones and tissues thicken with accumulated material.[39,40] Examination of old photographs of the patient can be particularly useful.
12. Neonatal microcephaly: The presence of microcephaly at birth is suggestive of a metabolic process present before birth. Hyperglycinemia manifests with this finding.[41]
13. Frequent feeding: Patients with fatty acid oxidation or glycogen storage defects may present with a history of food-seeking behavior or frequent feeding. This is possibly in response to the hypoglycemia they develop when they cannot access their secondary energy stores.
14. Strokes or thrombosis: Patients with homocystinuria have altered coagulation and may present with neonatal stroke (or later onset) and/or thromboembolism later in life.[42-44]

15. Self-mutilation: Patients with Lesch-Nyhan syndrome and elevations of uric acid have altered pain sensation, and many chew through their lips and deeply damage their hands. Many of these patients have a history of gouty tophi (nodules of uric acid crystals).[18]

CLUES IN THE PHYSICAL EXAMINATION THAT ARE SUGGESTIVE OF A METABOLIC DISEASE IN THE DEVELOPMENTALLY DELAYED PATIENT

Many metabolic diseases do not produce specific physical findings, but there are a few manifestations that may help in pursuing the workup.

General Examination

Poor growth and an appearance of chronic illness are suggestive of an underlying process in developmentally delayed patients. Disrupted cellular metabolism from toxins or absence of vital substrate results in poor growth of both brain tissue and is also reflected in short stature and an emaciated appearance.

Head, Ears, Eyes, Nose, and Throat (HEENT)

Both microcephaly and macrocephaly are features of metabolic diseases. In the amino acid metabolism defects and in diseases with sudden onset of metabolic crisis, microcephaly most commonly results from loss of neuronal tissue. In disorders of glutaric acid metabolism, macrocephally is present and is often associated with abnormal ventricles visible on imaging.[45] A large fontanelle is present in patients with the peroxisomal disorder such as Zellweger syndrome.[23] The presence of clouding of the cornea is suggestive of a storage disorder, and cataracts often result from deposits of metabolites (this is fairly common in galactosemia).[19] In patients with homocystinuria, displacement of the lens results from breakage of the fibrils holding the lens in place.[46] Examination under slit-lamp conditions by an ophthalmologist is often of particular use because the retina can also be examined for the cherry-red spots that occur in several storage disorders. Chewing of the lip is observed in patients with decreased pain sensation, as in Lesch-Nyhan syndrome.

Hair

The hair is useful in medical assessment of metabolic disorders. Hair growth requires protein manufacture and collagen crosslinking. In disorders of amino acid metabolism, the growth may be slowed as a result of deficiencies.[30,38] In the urea cycle disorders (particularly argininosuccinic lyase deficiency), the patients cannot make arginine and develop a characteristic finding of trichorrhexis nodosa. Microscopic examination reveals a bamboo appearance of the hair with numerous fragile points in the hair, which makes it breakable.[31] Hair that has a very coarse or kinky texture is indicative of a defect in copper metabolism, which affects collagen crosslinking.[47] Microscopic examination reveals twists in the hair known as pili torti. This most closely resembles the twists seen in a cocktail stirring stick. Hair without pigment or very little pigment is suggestive of phenylketonuria or a defect in metabolism of tyrosine, which makes pigment.

Abdomen

The presence of chronic hepatomegaly is suggestive of a stored product. Glycogen storage disorders can manifest with this finding, and when accompanied by splenomegaly, it is suggestive of a storage disorder.

Skin

The presence of generalized rashes can indicate a lack of a key metabolic building block such as an amino acid (lysinuric protein intolerance, for instance) or buildup of an unprocessed metabolite, such as fatty acids in some of the fatty acid oxidation defects.[48,49]

Neurological

Few specific findings in the neurological examination point toward a specific metabolic disease. The presence of hypotonia or poor muscle development in excess of the overall neurological state is suggestive of a mitochondrial myopathy, but it is difficult to distinguish from generalized hypotonia.

LABORATORY TESTS FOR THE WORKUP OF METABOLIC DISEASE IN DEVELOPMENTAL DELAY

The laboratory information in the diagnosis of metabolic diseases is not necessarily obtained through the use of rare and obscure tests. A layered approach is often appropriate and helps direct the workup.

Common Laboratory Measurements

RED AND WHITE BLOOD CELL COUNTS

The production of red and white blood cells in the bone marrow can be affected by a number of abnormal metabolites. The organic acidemias suppress bone marrow function, which results in pancytopenia. The production of abnormal white blood cells (such as Gaucher cells) and overall decreases in marrow production can reflect occupation of the marrow spaces in the storage (mucopolysaccharide and oligosaccharide) disorders. Disorders in cellular function, such as those involving peroxisomes, can also lower overall cell counts. Finally, in chronic metabolic disease, anemia can result from the overall stress to the individual.

ELECTROLYTES AND BICARBONATE

Measurements of electrolytes and bicarbonate are useful in determining the amount of unexplained acid that is circulating in the blood stream. Calculating the anion gap (anion gap = sodium – chloride – bicarbonate) can reveal an increase in a biological acid. Both the organic acids and increases in lactic acid produce increases in the anion gap. As the gap approaches 15 or more, an investigation for one of these compounds should be considered.

GLUCOSE

In the defects of energy metabolism, the circulating levels of glucose (particularly during a crisis) can reveal an underlying problem. In the fatty acid oxidation disorders (most notably those involving medium-chain fatty acids), a low glucose level is a common finding and can cause many of the associated symptoms. In the organic acidemias, as well as in pyruvate carboxylase deficiency, gluconeogenesis is suppressed by the acids. In defects involving the storage of glucose (glycogen), hypoglycemia is a common finding and is related to much of the toxicity.

BLOOD UREA NITROGEN

The measurement of urea is often used to determine fluid status and kidney function in patients. A low or very low blood urea nitrogen concentration may reflect a defect in the urea cycle and necessitates further workup.

pH

Like the anion gap, the blood pH can be used to measure the presence of unexplained acids in the system. Patients with severe metabolic derangements present with acidosis. An elevation in the blood pH can reflect a respiratory alkalosis, which in cerebral edema results from elevations in ammonia.

URINE KETONES

Ketones in the urine reflect the use of fatty acids in energy metabolism. In organic acidemias, glycogen storage diseases, and other mitochondrial diseases in which normal energy metabolism is disrupted, an elevation should be expected. In patients with severe developmental delays, this can also occur as a result of poor nutritional status. In patients with low blood glucose levels, the absence of ketones is suggestive of a defect in fatty acid oxidation, which necessitates further workup.

URINE REDUCING SUBSTANCE

The presence of reducing substances in the urine suggests that reducing sugars are being spilled in the urine. Galactose or fructose would be the most common abnormal metabolites in this group. Care should be taken because most penicillin-related antibiotics produce a positive reaction as well.

Readily Available but Not Commonly Drawn Laboratory Measurements

LACTATE

Blood lactate levels are elevated in diseases affecting energy metabolism. Lactate is an intermediate product produced in the breakdown of glucose. Its elevation reflects either overuse of the system or a direct block (such as block by pyruvate dehydrogenase or pyruvate carboxylase). Disorders in mitochondrial energy metabolism or fatty acid oxidation defects also produce elevations in lactate. Levels must be carefully drawn from a free-flowing blood source (no tourniquet) and processed rapidly to prevent a false reading of elevation. Hypoxia, rapid exertion (such as in a seizure or heavy exercise), or cardiac disease can also result in significant elevations in lactate. Besides being a measure of metabolic abnormality, lactate is also toxic to neurons at elevated concentrations. Whenever possible, a pyruvate level should be obtained at the same time, because this can distinguish between primary and secondary defects in glucose breakdown.

AMMONIA

Elevations of ammonia above 100 µmol/L in children and above 50 µmol/L in adults are considered abnormal and may necessitate further workup.[15] When combined with a low urea level, an elevated ammonia level is suggestive of a urea cycle defect. Organic acids also interfere with urea cycle function and can manifest with elevated ammonia levels. Disorders such as viral hepatitis and certain chemicals that severely disrupt liver function can also cause hyperammonemia. The drug valproic acid, which is used in treatment of a number of developmental disorders, can also cause interference with the urea cycle and elevate ammonia level.

Radiological Tests

Although few radiographic findings are specific for metabolic diseases, some findings are more frequent than others. Partial or total agenesis of the corpus callosum, in addition to overall maldevelopment of the brain, is noted in patients with hyperglycinemia.[50] Enlargement of the ventricles with macrocephaly occurs in patients with glutaric aciduria. Disorders of energy metabolism with lactic acidosis affect the basal ganglia early in the course of disease and are often described as having a Swiss cheese appearance on magnetic resonance imaging. This is often described as Leigh encephalopathy by radiologists. Generalized loss of neuronal tissue observed on magnetic resonance imaging is also suggestive of an underlying metabolic toxin or process. Enlargement of the liver or spleen visible on abdominal imaging is suggestive of a storage disorder. Cardiomegaly or hypertrophy is also suggestive of either a metabolic myopathy or a storage disorder such as Pompe disease.

Assessments Specific for Metabolic Disease

These tests are conducted in specialized laboratories that require careful quality control. The tests are usually offered at major university hospitals and a select number of reference laboratories. Interpretation of the results is often difficult and requires the assistance of a specialist in biochemical genetics. Tests employing paper chromatography are less reliable and should be avoided. At the time of publication, a number of companies are offering "comprehensive" metabolic profiles to consumers, who are typically families with a child with a developmental disability. The same companies typically find a number of metabolic abnormalities that often lead to recommendations for a product or service that they also provide. Use of these companies should be discouraged because it can often delay a correct diagnosis or lead to treatments for the patient that may be harmful. The Society for the Study of Inborn Errors of Metabolism lists Clinical Laboratory Improvement Amendments (CLIA)–certified laboratories on its Web site (http://www.ssiem.org), as well as clinics specializing in metabolic diseases. Another good rule is that in the absence of overwhelming levels of a metabolite, a repeat sample is needed for confirmation. It is often best to conduct these tests when the patient is ill from the suspected underlying defect, because a higher diagnostic yield is obtained. However, acute illness from any cause can result in elevations or depressions

of many of the tested elements and should always be considered. Finally, the use of parenteral nutrition can affect the levels of metabolites in these tests. As much information as possible about these issues should be provided to the testing laboratory, so that a proper interpretation can be made in context of the patient's condition. Another helpful piece of information to include on the test request is the name and telephone number of a contact individual for discussion of abnormal results and suggestions for additional testing.

PLASMA AMINO ACIDS

The plasma amino acid test measures the concentration of free amino acids in a separated plasma sample. Urine amino acids are difficult to interpret and may demonstrate numerous false elevations; therefore, this test is best used in a workup for a specific disorder. Plasma levels should not typically be measured immediately after a meal or feeding (a 2-hour gap is best but not always practical). This test will detect amino acid processing defects such as phenylketonuria, tyrosinemia, hyperglycinemia, branched-chain amino acidopathies (such as maple syrup urine disease), homocystinuria, methionine defects, and lysine transport defects. It also detects problems with urea cycle function through measurement of arginine and other cycle intermediates. Disorders that affect the health of the liver manifest with elevations of the hepatic processed amino acids phenylalanine, tyrosine, methionine, homocysteine, leucine, isoleucine, and valine. Amino acid measurements can verify elevations in lactic acid, inasmuch as its precursor pyruvate can also convert to alanine.

URINE ORGANIC ACIDS

Urine organic acid analysis detects a wide range of compounds. It is an excellent diagnostic test for the organic acidemias involving propionic, methylmalonic, and isovaleric acids. It also detects glutaric acid, which is a progressive neurotoxic defect in biomolecule conversion. The fatty acid oxidation defects also result in abnormal compounds in the urine. The presence of succinylacetone is a hallmark of tyrosinemia; similarly, the presence of isoleucine metabolites is a hallmark of maple syrup urine disease. Lactic acid and ketones are also detectable on organic acid analysis but are not always well correlated with plasma levels.

BLOOD ACYL-CARNITINE PROFILE

This test is available from only a few national reference laboratories (Duke University Medical Center, Baylor Clinic, and Mayo Clinic) but is extremely useful. It can performed on a blood spot sample, which increases its utility further. It detects defects in fatty acid oxidation, because these compounds readily bind to carnitine and are exported from the mitochondria. A number of other compounds, such as the organic acid defects and the urea cycle intermediate argininosuccinate, also bind to carnitine and are readily detectible.

PLASMA LONG-CHAIN FATTY ACIDS

Qualitative and quantitative analysis of plasma long-chain fatty acids is performed at the Kennedy Krieger Institute at Johns Hopkins University.[22] This profile is needed to assess function of peroxisomes and is very useful for diagnosing the adrenal-leukodystrophies and Zellweger syndrome.

TRANSFERRIN ELECTROPHORESIS

This test is used to detect defects in the attachment of carbohydrates to proteins after translation. This relatively new group of disorders can manifest with very vague problems in development and cognition and is worth consideration in the workup.

MITOCHONDRIAL MUTATION

Although DNA is not typically used as a screening test for metabolic disease, the difficulty in testing mitochondrial function from muscle makes it an acceptable substitute. Laboratories performing this test should screen for defects that cause the syndromes of myoclonus, epilepsy, and ragged red fibers (MERRF) and of mitochondrial myopathy, encephalopathy, lactic acidosis, and strokelike episodes (MELAS) and other common mutation disorders. New technologies in which the entire mitochondrion is screened would be preferable. The user should remember that the majority of enzymes used in energy metabolism in the mitochondria are encoded in the genomic DNA and are not detected in this highly specific screen.

URINE MUCOPOLYSACCHARIDE/ OLIGOSACCHARIDE SCREEN

Screening the urine for mucopolysaccharides and oligosaccharides is very useful for detecting lysosomal storage disorders.

Disease-Specific Tests

These tests are typically difficult to perform, are expensive, and require carefully processed testing material (often biopsy material). It is recommended that they be performed by a biochemical geneticist or in consultation with another highly experienced individual.

Neonatal Screening Testing

As more and more states move to the expanded neonatal screening, a powerful tool has become available to the diagnostician. The tandem mass spectrometry employed in neonatal screening detects organic acids and most of the compounds involved in fatty acid oxidation that bind to carnitine. It also detects phenylketonuria and tyrosinemia through their secondary metabolites. This test can be used in the clinical setting as a cost-effective screening tool, with an understanding of what it does not detect. It does not detect storage disorders, mitochondrial defects, glycogen storage defects, most urea cycle defects, amino acid transport defects, long-chain fatty acids, glycoprotein defects, and many other disorders. It otherwise is an excellent part of a general workup if it was not performed on the patient in the neonatal period. If the neonatal information is available, it can be very useful to the clinician during workup of the developmentally delayed patient. A careful check of which metabolites are reported by the specific state should be made because the test detects more compounds than many state programs report.

APPROACH TO DIAGNOSING METABOLIC DISEASE IN A PATIENT WITH DEVELOPMENTAL PATHOLOGY

As outlined in the previous sections, a thorough history and physical examination constitute an excellent starting point when metabolic disease is suspected. These often provide an indication of what to look for; however, there are often no strong clues in a normal-appearing patient with developmental delay. An often-asked question is what constitutes a reasonable workup for such a patient. While a workup for chromosomal and syndromic problems is under way, a reasonable approach of a few screening laboratory studies should be considered. A plasma amino acid profile, a urine organic acid profile, an acylcarnitine profile, and possibly transferrin electrophoresis will detect a very high percentage of the more common metabolic diseases that result in developmental delay. If the patient shows evidence of progression of neurological disease, then the addition of urine mucopolysaccharide and oligosaccharide testing, along with plasma long-chain fatty acid analysis, is probably warranted. If the suspicion for metabolic disease is low, then tandem mass spectrometry of a blood sample (as used in neonatal screening) could be considered. For the developmental specialist, this should be a sufficient approach. A more detailed or exhaustive investigation should be performed by a metabolic specialist to control both costs and properly direct the search.

SUMMARY

Although this chapter does not cover each metabolic disease in depth, it does provide an approach to both the pathological processes and the workup of these diseases. There are numerous excellent textbooks on metabolic disease. The most widely used is *Scriver's The Metabolic and Molecular Basis of Inherited Disease*,[51] which is available in an online searchable form in many medical libraries. By thinking about how the process is affecting the brain and development, the clinician can compose a sensible and appropriate workup of the patient.

REFERENCES

1. Saudubray JM, Nassogne MC, de Lonlay P, et al: Clinical approach to inherited metabolic disorders in neonates: An overview. Semin Neonatol 7:3-15, 2002.
2. Wallace DC: The mitochondrial genome in human adaptive radiation and disease: On the road to therapeutics and performance enhancement. Gene 354:169-180, 2005.
3. Wallace DC: Mitochondrial defects in cardiomyopathy and neuromuscular disease. Am Heart J 139(2, Pt 3):S70-S85, 2000.
4. Wallace DC: Mitochondrial diseases in man and mouse. Science 283:1482-1488, 1999.
5. Kerr DS: Lactic acidosis and mitochondrial disorders. Clin Biochem 24:331-336, 1991.
6. Chen YT, Bali D, Sullivan J: Prenatal diagnosis in glycogen storage diseases. Prenat Diagn 22:357-359, 2002.
7. Talente GM, Coleman RA, Alter C, et al: Glycogen storage disease in adults. Ann Intern Med 120:218-226, 1994.
8. Bennett MJ, Rinaldo P, Strauss AW: Inborn errors of mitochondrial fatty acid oxidation. Crit Rev Clin Lab Sci 37:1-44, 2000.
9. Rinaldo P, Matern D, Bennett MJ: Fatty acid oxidation disorders. Annu Rev Physiol 64:477-502, 2002.
10. Scriver CR, Eisensmith RC, Woo SL, et al: The hyperphenylalaninemias of man and mouse. Annu Rev Genet 28:141-165, 1994.
11. Scriver CR, Clow CL: Phenylketonuria: epitome of human biochemical genetics (first of two parts). N Engl J Med 303:1336-1342, 1980.
12. Scriver CR, Clow CL: Phenylketonuria and other phenylalanine hydroxylation mutants in man. Annu Rev Genet 14:179-202, 1980.
13. Hansen RG: Hereditary galactosemia. JAMA 208:2077-2082, 1969.
14. Summar M: Current strategies for the management of neonatal urea cycle disorders. J Pediatr 138(1 Suppl):S30-S39, 2001.
15. Summar M, Tuchman M: Proceedings of a consensus conference for the management of patients with urea cycle disorders. J Pediatr 138(1 Suppl):S6-S10, 2001.
16. Kure S, Tada K, Narisawa K: Nonketotic hyperglycinemia: Biochemical, molecular, and neurological aspects. Jpn J Hum Genet 42:13-22, 1997.
17. Jinnah HA, Visser JE, Harris JC, et al: Delineation of the motor disorder of Lesch-Nyhan disease. Brain 129(Pt 5):1201-1217, 2006.
18. Nyhan WL: Inherited hyperuricemic disorders. Contrib Nephrol 147:22-34, 2005.
19. Vellodi A: Lysosomal storage disorders. Br J Haematol 128:413-431, 2005.
20. Saheki T, Kobayashi K, Iijima M, et al: Adult-onset type II citrullinemia and idiopathic neonatal hepatitis caused by citrin deficiency: Involvement of the aspartate glutamate carrier for urea synthesis and maintenance of the urea cycle. Mol Genet Metab 81(Suppl 1):S20-S26, 2004.
21. Saheki T, Kobayashi K, Iijima M, et al: Pathogenesis and pathophysiology of citrin (a mitochondrial aspartate glutamate carrier) deficiency. Metab Brain Dis 17:335-346, 2002.
22. Moser HW, Bergin A, Cornblath D: Peroxisomal disorders. Biochem Cell Biol 69:463-474, 1991.
23. Moser HW, Moser AB, Chen WW, et al: Adrenoleukodystrophy and Zellweger syndrome. Prog Clin Biol Res 321:511-535, 1990.
24. Gropman AL: Diagnosis and treatment of childhood mitochondrial diseases. Curr Neurol Neurosci Rep 1:185-194, 2001.
25. Brusilow SW: Urea cycle disorders: Clinical paradigm of hyperammonemic encephalopathy. Prog Liver Dis 13:293-309, 1995.
26. Summar ML, Barr F, Dawling S, et al: Unmasked adult-onset urea cycle disorders in the critical care setting. Crit Care Clin 21(4 Suppl):S1-S8, 2005.
27. Maestri NE, Lord C, Glynn M, et al: The phenotype of ostensibly healthy women who are carriers for ornithine transcarbamylase deficiency. Medicine (Baltimore) 77:389-397, 1998.
28. Pearl PL, Bennett HD, Khademian Z: Seizures and metabolic disease. Curr Neurol Neurosci Rep 5:127-133, 2005.
29. Wallace AH, Manikkam N, Maxwell F: Seizures and a hiccup in the diagnosis. J Paediatr Child Health 40:707-708, 2004.
30. Wiest LG, Lutz P, Jung EG, et al: [Morphological and biochemical investigations of hairs in inborn errors of amino acid metabolism (author's transl)]. Arch Dermatol Res 256(1):53-65, 1976.
31. Hartlage PL, Coryell ME, Hall WK, et al: Argininosuccinic aciduria: Perinatal diagnosis and early dietary management. J Pediatr 85:86-88, 1974.
32. Henderson H, Leisegang F, Brown R, et al: The clinical and molecular spectrum of galactosemia in patients from the Cape Town region of South Africa. BMC Pediatr 2:7, 2002.
33. Kelly S: Septicemia in galactosemia. JAMA 216:330, 1971.

34. Levy HL, Sepe SJ, Shih VE, et al: Sepsis due to *Escherichia coli* in neonates with galactosemia. N Engl J Med 297:823-825, 1977.

35. Rizzo WB, Roth KS: On "being led by the nose." Rapid detection of inborn errors of metabolism. Arch Pediatr Adolesc Med 148:869-872, 1994.

36. Bos JD: Atopiform dermatitis. Br J Dermatol 147:426-429, 2002.

37. Fisch RO, Tsai MY, Gentry WC Jr: Studies of phenylketonurics with dermatitis. J Am Acad Dermatol 4:284-290, 1981.

38. Irons M, Levy HL: Metabolic syndromes with dermatologic manifestations. Clin Rev Allergy 4:101-124, 1986.

39. Klock JC, Starr CM: The different faces of disease. FACE diagnosis of disease. Adv Exp Med Biol 376:13-25, 1995.

40. Ries M, Moore DF, Robinson CJ, et al: Quantitative dysmorphology assessment in Fabry disease. Genet Med 8:96-101, 2006.

41. Tada K, Kure S, Takayanagi M, et al: Non-ketotic hyperglycinemia: A life-threatening disorder in the neonate. Early Hum Dev 29(1-3):75-81, 1992.

42. Brattstrom L, Lindgren A: Hyperhomocysteinemia as a risk factor for stroke. Neurol Res 14(2 Suppl):81-84, 1992.

43. Gaustadnes M, Rudiger N, Rasmussen K, et al: Intermediate and severe hyperhomocysteinemia with thrombosis: A study of genetic determinants. Thromb Haemost 83:554-558, 2000.

44. Kelly PJ, Furie KL, Kistler JP, et al: Stroke in young patients with hyperhomocysteinemia due to cystathionine beta-synthase deficiency. Neurology 60:275-279, 2003.

45. Hoffmann GF, Zschocke J: Glutaric aciduria type I: From clinical, biochemical and molecular diversity to successful therapy. J Inherit Metab Dis 22:381-391, 1999.

46. White HH, Rowland LP, Araki S, et al: Homocystinuria. Arch Neurol 13:455-470, 1965.

47. Moore CM, Howell RR: Ectodermal manifestations in Menkes disease. Clin Genet 28:532-540, 1985.

48. Nagata M, Suzuki M, Kawamura G, et al: Immunological abnormalities in a patient with lysinuric protein intolerance. Eur J Pediatr 146:427-428, 1987.

49. Rajantie J, Perheentupa J: Lysinuric protein intolerance. Lancet 2:978, 1980.

50. Hoover-Fong JE, Shah S, Van Hove JL, et al: Natural history of nonketotic hyperglycinemia in 65 patients. Neurology 63:1847-1853, 2004.

51. Scriver CR, Beaudet AL, Sly WS, et al, eds: The Metabolic and Molecular Basis of Inherited Disease, 7th ed. New York: McGraw-Hill, 1995.

10D.
Developmental and Behavioral Outcomes of Infectious Diseases

MARSHA D. RAPPLEY
MARIA J. PATTERSON

Infectious diseases can adversely affect the growth and development of children far beyond the damage that a specific organism might cause. The developmental-behavioral pediatrician might be consulted on a broad scope of services, including organizing efforts to change high-risk sexual behaviors in high schools,[1] assisting parents in disclosing developmentally appropriate information about catastrophic illness,[2] and working with foster care personnel in placing chronically ill children.[3] All of these services depend on the basic skills of the developmental-behavioral pediatrician. However, certain infections require a greater awareness and surveillance because they profoundly affect a child's entire life, such as human immunodeficiency virus (HIV) and congenital syphilis, in which effects can develop years after the initial infection, or cytomegalovirus infections, in which a child can have later effects in the absence of symptoms with the initial infection.

Infections, particularly those of the central nervous system, are often associated with long-term sequelae that affect cognition, learning, and behavior. Although these issues are not foremost in the minds of parents and physicians when the child is acutely ill, subsequent assessments at critical points in development are essential. These include cognitive development in the early years of language acquisition, at preschool entry, and at school entry, and learning activities of the early elementary years through adolescence. In addition, assessment of the child's attachment to parents, social support network, and development of interpersonal relationships is important. Children may be perceived as vulnerable, even after recovery from life-threatening infection.

Infections that highlight this broad effect on the growth and development of a child and family are described. Two case studies illustrate the complex interplay of illness, family, health, and social systems.

INFECTIONS OF THE NEONATE AND INFANT

Infection acquired in utero and in the first months of life can result in especially severe sequelae. Hearing and vision are the sensory modalities most often affected in such infants.

Cytomegalovirus

Cytomegalovirus affects approximately 1% of all newborns in the United States, which represents 30,000 to 40,000 infants per year; only 5% to 10% of these infants are symptomatic (Table 10D-1). The mortality rate among symptomatic infants is 12%, and most who survive have sequelae. Of less severely affected infants, 20% will have hearing loss, difficulties with speech perception, slowed auditory processing, and microphthalmia. Even infants who are asymptomatic may be found later to have hearing loss and/or learning disabilities.[4]

Rubella

Rubella also affects both hearing and vision in the neonate. Although the incidence of rubella was reduced by 99% with initiation of the second measles-mumps-rubella vaccine in 1969, resurgence occurred in the early 1990s as a result of inadequate immunization. Children and young women who have poor access to health care, those born in other countries, and communities with sizable groups opposed to immunization continue to be at risk for disease.[5,6] All organ systems can affected by congenital rubella, which creates a grim prognosis for a number of the children affected. Cataracts and hearing loss are frequent; microphthalmia is possible.

Toxoplasmosis

The incidence of neonatal infection with *Toxoplasma gondii* ranges from 1 to 8 per 1000 live births and is higher in warmer climates. Most congenital cases occur with a primary infection of the mother during pregnancy; it is rare with chronic infection. When primary infection occurs in the last trimester, the predilection of the parasite for the placenta is so strong that it is considered an obligatory infection.[7] About half of infected children are asymptomatic as neonates, but 85% have ocular involvement and possibly hearing loss at a later age, including glaucoma, cataracts, chorioretinitis, and deafness. Isolated ocular toxoplasmosis may also occur, with retinal infiltrates developing in the early adult years.[4]

Group B Streptococcal Infection

Progress has been made in reducing the incidence of group B streptococcal (GBS) infection. However, it continues to be the dominant pathogen both for perinatal infection of the mother and for neonatal meningitis. Early-onset GBS infection usually occurs within the first 24 hours of life and may occur at up to age 6 days. Infection with early-onset GBS has declined 70% since 1970, in association with preventive measures for mother and infant, to approximately 0.5 cases per 1000 live births. Late-onset GBS infection occurs at 3 to 4 weeks of age and may occur any time from 7 days to 3 months of age. Late-onset GBS infection has not declined in incidence over time and is more likely to include meningitis. The case:fatality ratio for both early- and late-onset GBS infection is now 4%; severe neurological sequelae occur in 20% to 30% of cases. Milder but significant consequences, including bilateral deafness and cortical blindness, occur in another 15% to 25%.[8]

Syphilis

Syphilis is transmitted to the fetus at high rates for the first 4 years that a woman is infected. Primary and secondary syphilis occur at a rate of 2.7 per 100,000, 4.7 among men, and 0.8 among women.[9] Of 7980 cases reported in 2004, 84% were men; men having sex with men are at the highest risk. Also in 2004, for the first time since 1991, the incidence of new cases among women did not decline but stayed the same. The disparity in incidence of syphilis between African Americans and others in the United States is growing, and rates overall are at greatest increase in the southern states.[9] Because antigens are formed 4 to 8 weeks after infection is acquired, serological testing during the incubation or early primary stage of syphilis can yield false-negative results. It is recommended that if a woman with a child younger than 1 year of age receives a diagnosis of early-stage syphilis, the infant should be evaluated and treated for syphilis. It was previously thought that infection of the fetus could not occur before the fifth month of gestation. However, evidence of infection is found as early as 9 weeks. Lesions characteristic of syphilis, perivascular lymphocytic infiltration, occur in all organs.[7] Early sequelae of congenital syphilis are often not present at birth and develop over weeks to months. Almost every organ system is involved, and the mortality rate is 40%. Deafness, glaucoma, chorioretinitis, and blindness may result, as well (see Table 10D-1).

TABLE 10D-1 ■ Infections, Sequelae, and Major Symptoms

Infectious Agent	Transmission	IUGR	Vision	Hearing	Neurocognitive	Other	Special Risk/Comments
						Symptoms	
Candida albicans	Prenatal Perinatal Postnatal	No	Yes	No	No	Multiorgan and system	Immunocompromise
Chlamydia trachomatis	STD Perinatal	No	Yes	No	No	Trachoma, pneumonia, genital tract infection, lymphogranuloma venereum	Most common reportable sexually transmitted disease
Cytomegalovirus (CMV)	Secretions Prenatal Perinatal Postnatal Breast milk Transfusion	Yes	Yes	Yes	Microcephaly, seizures, motor impairment	Often asymptomatic at birth; or jaundice, purpura, hepatosplenomegaly, microcephaly, intracerebral calcifications; prolonged fever, mild hepatitis in adolescent and adult	Immunocompromise
Enterovirus	Fecal-oral Respiratory Perinatal	No	Yes	No	Seizures, motor impairment	Nonspecific fever, upper and lower respiratory tract infection, exanthema, aseptic meningitis, encephalitis, paralysis, vomiting, diarrhea, abdominal pain, hepatitis, myopericarditis	Highest incidence in young children, tropical climate, summer and early fall in temperate climate
Group A *Streptococcus*	Respiratory Food-borne illness Skin Perinatal	No	No	No	PANDAS (see text)	Pharyngotonsillitis, otitis media, sinusitis, cervical adenitis, scarlet fever, skin infection, rheumatic fever, erysipelas, cellulitis, vaginitis, bacteremia, pneumonia, endocarditis, pericarditis, septic arthritis, necrotizing fasciitis, toxic shock syndrome, osteomyelitis, myositis, puerperal sepsis, neonatal omphalitis	Highest incidence among school-aged children and adolescents; incidence of invasive form highest in infants and elderly persons
Group B *Streptococcus*	Perinatal Gastrointestinal, genitourinary secretions	No	Yes	Yes	Hydrocephaly, brain atrophy, seizures, hypothalamic dysfunction, quadriplegia, hemiplegia	In pregnancy: bacteremia, endometritis, chorioamnionitis, urinary tract infection In neonates: respiratory distress, apnea, shock, pneumonia, meningitis, osteomyelitis, septic arthritis, adenitis, cellulitis	Immunocompromise
Haemophilus influenzae	Respiratory Secretions Perinatal	No	No	Yes	Meningitis, encephalitis Learning disorders	Upper and lower respiratory tract infections, fever and bacteremia, epiglottitis, septic arthritis, cellulitis, otitis media, pericarditis, endocarditis, endophthalmitis, osteomyelitis, peritonitis, chorioamnionitis	Unimmunized and younger than 4 years; immunocompromise; sickle cell disease

TABLE 10D-1 ■ Infections, Sequelae, and Major Symptoms—cont'd

Infectious Agent	Transmission	IUGR	Vision	Hearing	Neurocognitive	Other	Special Risk/Comments
Human immunodeficiency virus (HIV/AIDS)	STD Percutaneous Mucus membranes Prenatal Perinatal Postnatal Breast milk	Yes	No	No	Microcephaly, hyperreflexia, clonus	Lymphadenopathy, hepatomegaly, splenomegaly, opportunistic infections, diarrhea, parotitis, cardiomyopathy, hepatitis, nephropathy, pneumonia, neoplasm	Mother-to-child transmission accounts for most infections in preadolescent children
Herpes simplex virus (HSV)	Prenatal Perinatal Postnatal Breast milk	No	Yes	No	Microcephaly, brain atrophy	Neonatal: disseminated disease, CNS disease, seizures, skin and mucus membrane ulcers	Mother has primary HSV; prematurity of infant
Listeria monocytogenes	Food-borne illness Prenatal Perinatal	No	No	No	Meningitis, brainstem encephalitis, brain abscess	Maternal: fever, malaise, headache, vomiting, diarrhea, back pain, amnionitis, abortion, preterm delivery and fetal death Neonate: early and late onset (similar to Guillain-Barré syndrome), granulomatosus infantisepticum, meningitis, endocarditis	Immunocompromise, old age, pregnancy, neonatal period
Borrelia burgdorferi (Lyme disease)	Tick bite	No	No	No	Cranial nerve palsies, lymphocytic meningitis, peripheral neuropathy	Early localized: erythema migrans; early localized and disseminated: fever, malaise, headache, neck stiffness, myalgia arthralgia, conjunctivitis, fatigue; carditis; late: pauciarticular arthritis of large joints	Untreated children: 50% arthritis, 10% CNS, <5% cardiac; late disease uncommon if treated in early stage
Neisseria gonorrhoeae gonorrhea	STD Perinatal	No	Yes	No	Meningitis	Vaginitis, disseminated, arthritis; urethritis in prepubertal boys uncommon; pharyngitis, anorectal infection, endocervicitis, salpingitis, epididymitis, pelvic inflammatory disease, perihepatitis, ectopic pregnancy, infertility, arthritis-dermatitis, tenosynovitis, endocarditis	Reported incidence highest among girls 15 to 19 years old

Symptoms

Organism	Transmission				Clinical Manifestations	Comments
Neisseria meningitidis	Respiratory	No	Yes	Yes	Abrupt onset with fever, chills, malaise, prostration, rash; Waterhouse-Friderichsen syndrome: purpura, disseminated intravascular coagulation, shock, coma, death; pneumonia, conjunctivitis, arthritis, myocarditis, pericarditis, endophthalmitis, digit or limb amputation	Peak attack at ages < 1 year, between ages 2 and 5 years, and 15-18 years; complement deficiency and asplenia
Taenia solium	Food-borne illness	No	Yes	Seizures, obstructive hydrocephalus, gait disturbance, back pain, transverse myelitis	Nausea, diarrhea, abdominal pain, subcutaneous cysts	Poor sanitation; in most U.S. cases, patients are from Latin America and Asia
Rubivirus (rubella)	Secretions Prenatal Breast milk	Yes	Yes	Yes	Congenital: cardiac, pneumonitis, bone radiolucencies, hepatosplenomegaly, thrombocytopenia, dermal erythropoiesis Many postnatal infections are subclinical	—
Streptococcus pneumoniae	Respiratory	No	Yes	Yes	Otitis media, invasive bacterial infections, upper and lower respiratory tract infections, conjunctivitis, periorbital cellulites, endocarditis, osteomyelitis, pericarditis, peritonitis, pyogenic arthritis, soft tissue infection	Highest rates in infants, young children, elderly persons, African Americans, native Americans; immunocompromised patients; patients with asplenia, cochlear implants
Treponema pallidum (syphilis)	STD Secretions Prenatal Perinatal	No	Yes	No	Stillbirth, hydrops fetalis, preterm birth Neonates: hepatosplenomegaly, snuffles, lymphadenopathy, skin lesions, osteochondritis, pseudoparalysis, edema, hemolytic anemia, thrombocytopenia Late (after age 2 years): CNS, bones, joints, teeth, eyes affected; primary stage: chancre; secondary stage: rash, lymphadenopathy, condylomata lata, fever, malaise, splenomegaly, pharyngitis, headache, arthralgia; latent: after infection but asymptomatic; tertiary: gumma formation of skin, bone, viscera, aorta	Rise in 1980s and early 1990s, subsequent decline; highest rates in large urban centers, in southern United States

TABLE 10D-1 ■ Infections, Sequelae, and Major Symptoms—cont'd

Infectious Agent	Transmission	Symptoms					Special Risk/Comments
		IUGR	Vision	Hearing	Neurocognitive	Other	
Toxoplasma gondii	Food-borne illness Water Soil Transfusion Perinatal	Yes	Yes	Yes	Microcephaly, hydrocephaly, cerebral calcifications, encephalitis, hypotonia, seizures	Congenital: rash, lymphadenopathy, hepatosplenomegaly, jaundice, thrombocytopenia Acquired after birth: milder illness, fever, malaise, pharyngitis, myalgia, lymphadenopathy, myocarditis, pericarditis, pneumonitis	Immunocompromise
Varicella zoster virus	Respiratory Secretions Prenatal Perinatal Postnatal	No	Yes	No	Acute cerebellar ataxia, encephalitis,	Rash, fever, superinfection of skin, pneumonia, thrombocytopenia, glomerulonephritis, arthritis, hepatitis; later activation of zoster Fetus and infant: fetal death, limb hypoplasia, cutaneous scarring	Immunocompromise, Highest risk for neonate is maternal varicella 5 days before to 2 days after birth
West Nile virus	Mosquito bite Transfusion Prenatal Breast milk (probable)	No	Yes	Possible	<1% neuroinvasive: aseptic meningitis, encephalitis, flaccid paralysis, movement disorders, seizures, Guillain-Barrè syndro me	Most often asymptomatic; self-limited febrile illness; persistent fatigue, malaise, weakness	Older age, male gender Transplant recipients

Data from American Academy of Pediatrics[4] and Remington et al.[7]

"Transfusion" includes transplantation.

CNS, central nervous system; IUGR, intrauterine growth restriction; PANDAS, pediatric autoimmune neuropsychiatric disorders associated with streptococcal infections; STD, sexually transmitted disease.

Other Neonatal Infections

Other neonatal infections include herpes simplex virus, which causes retinopathy; varicella zoster virus, which causes cataracts; and candidal infection in immunosuppressed infants, which leads to endophthalmitis and chorioretinitis. *Neisseria gonorrhoeae* is a major sexually transmitted pathogen, but neonatal infection with *N. gonorrhoeae* occurs in less than 1% of the overall U.S. population, probably because of prenatal care and early treatment of pregnant women. Gonococcal ophthalmitis appears at 1 to 4 days of age. Infection with *Chlamydia trachomatis,* the most common cause of preventable blindness in the world, is commonly concurrent with *N. gonorrhoeae* infection and also causes neonatal ophthalmitis. Approximately 20% to 30% of pregnant women in the United States have cervical chlamydial infection, most often asymptomatic. Administration of silver nitrate, erythromycin, or tetracycline ophthalmic solution is recommended for neonatal ophthalmic prophylaxis. If left untreated, 30% to 50% of infants born to these mothers will develop neonatal conjunctivitis, which may lead to corneal ulceration, scarring, and blindness.[4]

Many of these same infections result in impairment of learning, behavior and cognition for both neonates and older children. Cytomegalovirus, rubivirus (which causes rubella), and group B streptococcal (GBS) infection are associated with profound to moderate retardation in severely infected children; significant learning problems and language delays are seen in those with less severe infection. Rubivirus infection is associated with autistic spectrum disorders, as well. Toxoplasmosis, syphilis, and *Listeria monocytogenes* infection are more often associated with cognitive impairment. Congenital syphilis may manifest in adolescence with the classic deterioration of neurological function, cognition, and behavioral regulation. This is described as juvenile paresis and includes adolescent onset of behavioral change, focal seizures, and cognitive impairment. Juvenile tabes, blindness, and deafness may also result.[4]

Monitoring and Treatment of Children Who Had Neonatal or Infant Infections

All children with a history of in utero infection, meningitis, or childhood infection associated with sensorineural hearing loss require assessment at birth and regular intervals, in addition to careful surveillance at well-child visits with parent questionnaires (see Chapter 7B).

For infants, assessment of hearing is indicated at birth for all infants, at 6 months of age, and at any sign of delayed acquisition of language. This guideline requires close assessment of language development and behavioral response to sound, cooing, babbling, and development of consonant and vowel sounds as expected for age (see Chapters 7D). Evaluations of auditory brainstem response and evoked otoacoustical emissions are appropriate tests for infants. However, although they assess the integrity of the auditory pathway, they are not true tests of hearing. For this reason, results from these examinations may be normal in newborns even when hearing may subsequently be found to be impaired. Therefore, close monitoring of hearing is required until a child is mature enough for behavioral audiography. Children as young as 9 to 12 months may be tested by an audiologist with conditioned oriented responses or visual oriented audiometry. Toddlers may be tested with play audiometry and older children with conventional audiometry. Any abnormal finding or delay in language acquisition should prompt referral to pediatric otolaryngologists, audiologists, and speech and language pathologists for specific diagnosis, counseling, and treatment.[10]

All children with a history of in utero infection, meningitis, or childhood infection associated with visual impairment should have a comprehensive pediatric medical eye examination at birth, at the time of diagnosis, or at the age of 6 months. An assessment of visual acuity should occur by age 3 years, and children who cannot perform such an assessment or who are at risk for structural damage should be referred for ophthalmological evaluation. The periodicity of subsequent assessments can then be determined.[11] For newborns of mothers with West Nile virus infection, a specific recommendation is made for hearing evaluation at birth and at 6 months and for ophthalmological evaluation at birth.[12]

Interventions for impairment of hearing and vision are primarily educational and are indicated for hearing and visual impairment of any etiology. They include accommodation in education, patient and family education, and establishing connections to important social service and community agencies (see Chapter 10F).

Monitoring over time for learning, behavior, and language delays is important for the child who experiences less severe infection and no apparent delays immediately after the infection. Neuropsychological evaluation before a child or teenager returns to the school environment is important for provision of appropriate educational services. Specific areas to address are cognitive status, academic achievement, language development, visuospatial and constructional functioning, sensory and motor development, memory and learning, behavioral development, and problem solving.[13]

INFECTIONS OF CHILDREN AND ADOLESCENTS

Meningitis and encephalitis continue to be serious infections of childhood and adolescence. *Neisseria meningitidis* and *Streptococcus pneumoniae* are currently the leading causes of meningitis in young children.[4] *Enterovirus* organisms continue to be a common cause of viral meningitis. *Haemophilus influenzae* bacterial meningitis is less prevalent since effective immunization was implemented in 1988. While most children who survive *S. pneumoniae, N. meningitidis,* and *H. influenzae* infections and enteroviral meningitis are healthy and attend school, they are more likely than their siblings to demonstrate inattention, hyperactivity, and impulsiveness and to have diagnoses of ADHD.[14] Hearing impairment and speech and language delay may also result from meningitis.[15-17] Encephalitis caused by West Nile virus is severe in fewer than 1% of children affected, but it may involve optic neuritis, uveitis, and chorioretinitis. Hearing loss is possible as well. Of 388 cases reported from 26 states in the first 9 months of 2006, 158 included meningitis, encephalitis, and myelitis.[18]

Group A Streptococcal Infection

Group A streptococcal infection is a common infection causing pharyngitis in children and adolescents. The pediatric autoimmune neuropsychiatric disorders associated with streptococcal infections (PANDAS) are similar symptomatically and possibly in etiology to Sydenham chorea, obsessive-compulsive disorder, tic disorder, and Tourette syndrome.[19] Five clinical characteristics identify PANDAS (Table 10D-2). Onset of symptoms is abrupt, with relapse and remission in association with group A β-hemolytic streptococcal infection. The most prominent symptoms are ticlike movements and obsessive thoughts and compulsions. Although this disorder is the subject of much research because of the link among these behaviors, infection, and immune response, this disorder is not likely to explain most of the new onset of obsessive-compulsive disorder or tic disorders of childhood. Patients whose symptoms meet criteria may be considered for treatment with penicillin as symptoms recur, but this is not yet a firm recommendation; further research with randomized, placebo-controlled design might provide stronger evidence for the efficacy of this treatment.[20] Immunotherapy, such as plasma exchange or intravenous immune globulin, is not recommended outside of research studies.

TABLE 10D-2 ■ Clinical Features of Pediatric Autoimmune Neuropsychiatric Disorders Associated with Streptococcal Infections (PANDAS)[19]

The presence of a tic disorder
Prepubertal onset, usually between 3 and 12 years of age
Earlier onset than usual for tic disorder and obsessive-compulsive disorder
Abrupt symptom onset and/or episodic course of symptom severity
Tic disorder and obsessive-compulsive disorder more gradual or waxing and waning in onset and relapse
Temporal association between symptom exacerbations and streptococcal infections
Presence of neurological abnormalities during periods of symptom exacerbation
Additional symptoms commonly seen during exacerbation:
　Emotional lability
　Problems with attention
　Separation anxiety
　Motor hyperactivity
　Enuresis
　Deterioration of handwriting
　Choreiform movements of hands and fingers

OTHER, LESS COMMON INFECTIONS ASSOCIATED WITH BEHAVIORAL SYMPTOMS

Neurocysticercosis

Neurocysticercosis is increasingly identified in the United States, both domestically acquired and among immigrants and travelers abroad. It is the most common parasitic infection of the central nervous system and is endemic in areas of Africa, Asia, and Latin America. Ong and associates[21] described neurocysticercosis in 2% of more than 1000 patients presenting to emergency departments with seizures, with prevalence exceeding 10% in the southwest. The larval form of *Taenia solium* infests pork and is transferred to humans through consumption of eggs. This most often occurs by ingestion of undercooked pork or exposure to food contaminated by human fertilizer or unwashed hands. Focal seizures are the most common symptom in children, but psychosis and dementia may be presenting symptoms. Diagnosis is confirmed by imaging studies. Treatment depends on the presenting symptoms; antihelmintics may cause more morbidity than improvement, and supportive therapy may be indicated.[22,23]

Lyme Disease

Lyme disease is caused by the transmission of *Borrelia burgdorferi* through the bite of the deer tick. More than 90% of cases come from the northeastern, mid-Atlantic, and northern Midwestern states and from northern California. The incidence is highest among children 5 to 9 years old. The neurological symptoms are most often associated with chronic infection and occur in 15% of patients. These include neuropathy of cranial nerves such as Bell's palsy, meningitis, and radiculopathy. Chronic Lyme disease may also be associated with difficulty with memory and concentration, fatigue, irritability, and depression.[22] In a study in which 20 children with cognitive problems after Lyme disease were compared with matched healthy controls, cognitive and psychiatric problems were identified, after the investigators controlled for anxiety, depression, and fatigue.[24] Diagnosis requires serological confirmation. The acute disease is treated with doxycycline (not often used in children), ceftriaxone, or amoxicillin for 2 to 4 weeks. Infection of the central nervous system is treated with intravenous ceftriaxone; however, patients with the chronic condition do not clearly benefit from antibiotic therapy. A vaccine was introduced in 1998, but controversy regarding its risks and benefits resulted in its being withdrawn by the manufacturer in 1999.[4]

HUMAN IMMUNODEFICIENCY VIRUS

Current estimates are that 11,000 children in the United States are infected with HIV. The global picture is much grimmer; 2.3 million children live with HIV infection, and many die before the age of 3 from diarrhea, malnutrition, respiratory infection, and tuberculosis.[25] In the United States, however, infection is no longer uniformly fatal and now most often results in chronic illness. Cognitive, emotional, and social development require careful attention in the long-term management of children with HIV infection and for those who develop the life-threatening symptoms of immunodeficiency, the acquired immunodeficiency syndrome (AIDS).[26]

More than half of persons infected with HIV develop neurological disease. The pathophysiological process of the central nervous system damage is related to the ability of HIV to cross the blood-brain barrier early after infection. Damage is not limited to infected cells; it is widely distributed, occurring in all types of cells within a given area. Clusters of HIV-infected microglial cells lead to spongiform lesions. The toxicity is associated with release of proteins and products of infected cells. In patients with access to antiretroviral therapy, peripheral neuropathy and cognitive dysfunction continue to occur. However, antiretroviral therapy may produce reversal of dementia in children.[27]

Transmission of HIV to newborns occurs in utero, during the time of delivery, and postnatally through breastfeeding. Infants affected earlier during gestation typically have the most severe disease. Studies in industrialized countries indicate that most cases of vertical transmission occur during the intrapartum period. The strongest predictor of HIV infection in an infant is the viral load carried by the mother. Because primary infections are associated with high viral loads, the infant exposed during primary infection, whether in utero, during birth, or through breastfeeding, will have the greatest risk. Thus, antiretroviral therapy has been successful in reducing the rate of vertical transmission by decreasing the viral load of the mother.[27]

An understanding of the epidemiological characteristics of HIV infection and AIDS is important for the developmental-behavioral pediatrician, as awareness of who continues to be at greatest risk is essential to prevention, identification, and timely intervention.

The incidence of AIDS peaked in 1992 and has declined in all U.S. populations, stabilizing in 1998 at approximately 40,000 new cases per year. Although the numbers of new cases of AIDS are declining in all sectors, women and minority populations are now disproportionately affected by AIDS. Among new cases reported from 2001 to 2004, the proportion of female patients increased to 27%; the proportion of affected children younger than 13 years old declined to 0.2%. Although initially the affected persons were largely white, this has shifted so that approximately 50% of new cases are among African Americans, 30% are in white persons, and 20% are in Hispanics. The highest transmission rate continues with male-to-male sexual contact at 47%. However, heterosexual transmission is increasing, now representing 34% of new cases. Other routes of transmission are injection drug use (17%), both sexual contact and injection drug use (4%), and perinatal transmission (0.6%).[28]

The Centers for Disease Control and Prevention estimated that approximately 300,000 persons in the United States are unaware that they are infected with HIV. The onset of symptoms occurs, on average, 8 to 11 years after infection; thus, a large group of people, unaware that they are infected, are also unaware that they may transmit HIV to others, including their newborns. Approximately 7000 seropositive women become pregnant each year in the United States. The rate of transmission of HIV from infected mothers to their infants is now less than 2%. Unfortunately, lapses occur in the delivery of effective treatment and prevention. In 2004, 7% of infants in whom HIV or AIDS was diagnosed had mothers who were not known to have HIV infection before delivery. It is interesting to note that between 2001 and 2004 approximately 6% of mothers of HIV exposed infants did not have a prenatal care visit.[29]

The possibility of an infant unexpectedly found to have HIV infection is further complicated by reports of mothers whose HIV test results were negative during pregnancy and went on to deliver HIV-positive infants.[30] The actual number of reported perinatal cases of AIDS is now very low: 48 cases in 2004, in comparison with 945 cases in 1992.[29] This remarkable change resulted from increased identification of HIV infection in pregnant women; the effectiveness of the antiretroviral therapy given prenatally, perinatally, and postnatally; avoidance of breastfeeding; and cesarean delivery as needed.[28] However, more than 11,000 children continue to live with this chronic and serious condition, and it is still possible for children to be born with HIV infection and for the infection to remain asymptomatic and undetected for many years.

Studies of cognitive function of children with HIV infection and those with AIDS are difficult to aggregate because of the rapid changes in the ability to deliver effective treatment since the 1990s, the longer life span associated with treatment, limited control groups, and the variety of methods employed. Together, however, they suggest that children with serious complications of HIV infection are most at risk for poor cognitive function and that decline in language and cognitive function may be a very early predictor of disease progression (Table 10D-3). These studies also demonstrate that many children with HIV infection are performing within the expected range for age but must be carefully monitored for decline.[31-36]

Children infected with HIV or who have AIDS should undergo baseline neurological and ophthalmological examination. Clinicians should specifically investigate the possibility of developmental delay, loss of milestones, microcephaly or deceleration of head growth, abnormal muscle tone and reflexes, focal findings, and speech and language delays. If delays are noted and the child is otherwise stable, these should be reevaluated in 3 months. The ophthalmological examination should be repeated yearly. Developmental assessment with reliable and validated instruments appropriate for the infant and preschool-aged child (see Chapter 7C) should occur at regular intervals to allow early detection of deterioration and promote intervention. Neuropsychological evaluation for the school-aged child is informative before school entry, upon reentry to school after illness, and at any indication of learning difficulty. Interventions require teams of professionals representing health, education, and social service, with the underlying premise that HIV infection and AIDS are chronic conditions,

managed with family education and support. The following case illustrates the compelling circumstances presented by HIV infection and AIDS, including tremendous loss of family and support networks for both mother and child.

Case Study: Janae

Janae was born to Theresa, aged 20 years, before prenatal antiretroviral therapy was known to be effective, and HIV infection was diagnosed at birth as a result of her mother's prenatal care. Janae's family included her mother and a 3-year-old brother who did not have HIV infection. Her father died of AIDS before her birth. Theresa had a fragile relationship with Janae's paternal uncle, who also had AIDS but overall was a supportive father figure for the family. Theresa's sister was very supportive but also had AIDS and no children of her own. Theresa's other sister and parents were largely estranged from Theresa and her family because of Theresa's previous issues with substance abuse. Theresa was not actively abusing any substances, nor did she have any other sexually transmitted diseases during this pregnancy or thereafter.

Janae failed to thrive as an infant. She had repeated oral and pharyngeal candidal infections, which complicated eating. She was slow to develop language and had delayed motor skills, but social interaction was positive. Janae and Theresa had a loving relationship, and her mother was diligent in keeping medical and social service appointments for the child. She did not follow through on medical care for herself, despite urging of the child's health providers, and seemed depressed. Theresa became symptomatic of AIDS when Janae was approximately 3 years old. Janae was placed in preprimary education after much deliberation by the education team, because of concern for exposure to other children. She had limited expressive language, good receptive language, and poor fine and gross motor skills. Evaluation with McCarthy Scales of Children's Abilities demonstrated a mean profile approximately one standard deviation below the norm. Her weight, height, and head circumference were at less than the third percentile for age. Janae made steady progress in language development and age-appropriate play with other children. She entered kindergarten at 6 years of age as a special education student, receiving services in speech and language, physical therapy, and occupational therapy. School staff appointed a primary contact person in the school who provided counseling for Janae's mother with regard to child development and parenting. Janae learned to read picture books by the end of second grade, at the age of 8 years. At this time, fatigue and lassitude became characteristic, and the

TABLE 10D-3 ■ Studies of Cognitive Function Associated with HIV Infection

Investigators	Study Question	Children Studied	Measures	Results
Smith et al[31]	Effect of HIV status on cognitive ability	539 exposed to HIV, aged 3 to 7 years 33 infected/serious complication 84 infected/no serious complication 422 not infected	McCarthy Scales of Children's Abilities Administered every 6 months between 3 and 7 years of age	Serious complication of AIDS associated with 1 SD below mean, in comparison to others Rates of development of cognitive skills from age 3 to 7 years were similar for all three groups
Jeremy et al[32]	Effect of treatment for HIV infection on neuropsychological function	489 infected with HIV, aged 4 months to 17 years Assigned to three treatment groups	Bayley Infant Development Scale Wechsler Preschool and Primary Scale of Intelligence Conners Parent Rating Scale Measures administered at varying intervals per study protocols	The 13% of children with serious complication of AIDS had IQ, short-term memory, and vocabulary scores 1 SD below norm Behavior rating scale scores significantly higher in conduct disorder, learning disorder, psychosomatic complaints, impulsivity, and hyperactivity than norm, but not associated with increased viral load Combination protease inhibitor/ antiretroviral therapy dramatically reduced viremia but had little effect on cognitive function
Mellins et al[33]	Influence of HIV status, prenatal drug exposure, and environmental factors	307 exposed to HIV, aged 3 to 8 years 96 infected 211 not infected	Conners Parent Rating Scale Administered every 6 months between 3 and 8 years of age	Neither HIV status nor prenatal drug exposure was related to hyperactivity, impulsivity, or conduct problems
Chase et al.[34]	Factors associated with abnormal cognitive development in infants exposed to HIV	595 exposed to HIV, aged newborn to 30 months 114 infected 481 not infected	Bayley Scales of Infant Development Psychomotor Developmental Index Administered at 4, 9, 12, 15, 18, 24, 30 months of age	HIV infection, prematurity, and maternal education <9th grade were predictive of abnormal development Prenatal drug exposure and primary language other than English were not predictive of abnormal development
Pearson et al[35]	Usefulness of neuropsychological testing, motor dysfunction, and cortical atrophy in predicting disease progression	490 infected with HIV, aged 3 months to 18 years Not previously treated with antiretroviral therapy	Bayley Scales of Infant Development McCarthy Scales of Children's Abilities Wechsler Adult Intelligence Scale and Wechsler Intelligence Scale for Children Administered serially, according to age	Poor performance on global neuropsychological measures and poor motor function were predictive of progression of disease, over and above the ability of laboratory data to predict progression MRI and CT of cortical atrophy were not predictive of progression
Coplan et al[36]	Compare language development in HIV-exposed infants and young children	78 exposed to HIV, aged 6 weeks to 5 years 9 infected 69 not infected Studied before wide availability of antiretroviral therapy	Early language Milestone Scale administered every 3 months Periodic assessment with Neurologic Examination for Children	Language deterioration signaled deterioration of global cognitive ability Language deterioration common in the presence of normal neurological and laboratory findings

AIDS, acquired immunodeficiency syndrome; CT, computed tomography; HIV, human immunodeficiency virus; MRI, magnetic resonance imaging; SD, standard deviation.

cross-disciplinary team had difficulty ascertaining whether the child's symptoms were caused by progression of disease, depression of the child related to mother's depression and increasing debilitation, or both.

These symptoms preceded decline of the laboratory indices by a few months, which indicated progression of the disease. Janae was admitted to the hospital in end stages of opportunistic infection at age 9 years. Janae's brother, now 12 years old, was placed with a relative. Theresa was symptomatic at this time and often would go from the child's bedside to the hospital emergency department for episodic care after the child fell asleep. Both her significant other and her sister had died of AIDS. Theresa's greatest fear was that she would die before Janae, and indeed she died approximately 3 months before Janae; both died of opportunistic infection. At the time of Theresa's death, the estranged grandparents came forward and accepted both children.

This case illustrates the disintegration of family support that occurs for the child and parent with HIV infection that progresses to AIDS. It is consistent with the findings of Pelton and Forehand,[37] who examined the reactions of 100 noninfected African American children, ages 6 to 11 years, with an HIV-infected mother; their control group consisted of 149 noninfected children and noninfected mothers. They described both internalizing and externalizing problems of children before the death of their mothers and internalizing problems 2 years after the death. Rotheram-Borus and colleagues[38] described 6-year follow-up of 414 adolescents living with 272 parents with HIV infection. More than 1 year before the death of a parent, the adolescents had elevated levels of isolation, fearfulness, and irritability; many depressive symptoms and somatic complaints; and contact with the juvenile justice system. Depressive symptoms persisted for 1 year after the death. Both of these studies indicate the need for close assessment of children well before and after the death of a parent with AIDS.

This case also illustrates the problems of finding care for children who lose a parent to AIDS. It is estimated that in 1998, 50,000 to 60,000 children younger than 21 years were orphaned by AIDS.[39] Worldwide, the United Nations estimates that number at more than 8.2 million; 90% of these children live in Africa.

The experience of Harlem Hospital is that developmental, behavioral, and long-term problems of orphaned infected children include mental health disorders and aggression, as they survive longer and grow older.[40] Foster and adoptive parents must be ready to accept a child who is likely to survive into young adult years. The American Academy of Pediatrics has specific recommendations for HIV testing of children in foster care and adoptive homes and recommends permanency planning with a mother before her death, to include the medical, mental health, and social service disciplines important to the health and psychological well-being of these children.[3]

The phenomenon of HIV and the medical and social problems that it causes have a developmental trajectory of their own. Because of effective treatment, young men and women infected prenatally are now of childbearing age, sexually active, and giving birth. To date, case reports indicate that older teenagers' compliance with preventive measures is suboptimal, but aggressive management of parents and newborns can result in seronegative newborns.[41] The issue of prevention of HIV infection in infants of these survivors of HIV is paramount and daunting. In addition, the effect of HIV infection across generations is demonstrated in the study of parents with HIV infection, their daughters, and their grandchildren. Rotheram-Borus and colleagues demonstrated significant and persistently lower levels of cognitive development for grandchildren in comparison to norms for similar socioeconomic status, but they also demonstrated positive effects of a family-based, skill-focused intervention on behavioral symptoms, cognitive outcomes, and enriching home environments in families with HIV infection.[42] These studies illustrate the importance of the developmental perspective in addressing the HIV epidemic.

In anticipation of recommendations to come from the Centers for Disease Control and Prevention, Bayer and Fairchild[43] called strongly for eliminating the obstacles to successful screening for HIV infection among pregnant women. Harwell and Obaro[25] recommended that strategies be implemented for the identification and treatment of all HIV-infected infants through comprehensive programs of antenatal testing and close follow-up. They noted that a family-centered model begins with a healthy pregnancy and recognizes the survival advantage of a child with a healthy parent.

THE VULNERABLE CHILD SYNDROME

In 1964, Green and Solnit[44] described the vulnerable child syndrome, in an article subsequently reviewed in 1998,[45] as highly relevant to pediatrics and the well-being of children and families. The following case study illustrates the complicated and far-reaching effect of a serious infection on a child and family and the intervention of the developmental-behavioral pediatrician.

Case Study: Michael

Michael, aged 3 years, and his mother were referred to a developmental-behavioral pediatrician by a pediatric infectious disease specialist and the primary care pediatrician. Michael was born at 32 weeks' gestation and developed meningitis caused by *L. monocytogenes* in the neonatal intensive care unit. He underwent 3 weeks of intravenous therapy with ampicillin and gentamicin. He recovered without apparent sequelae and was discharged home from the neonatal intensive care unit. From ages 1 month to 3 years, Michael underwent four courses of intravenous antibiotics for 3 to 6 weeks each, in treatment of recurrent infection of the eyes that was thought to be related to the initial meningitis. Each treatment decision was based primarily on history; physical examination and laboratory studies consistently yielded normal results. The child grew along the fifth percentile, had normal hearing, and normal developmental milestones except mild delay in expressive language according to assessments at 6- to 12-month intervals. He was shy but easily engaged and most often playful and vigorous.

Physicians, social workers, and nursing staff discussed a differential that included Munchausen syndrome by proxy. Staff could not find evidence that the child was purposefully infected but believed that the mother overinterpreted normal conditions as serious and that the medical team responded to her anxiety with treatment of the child. A referral was made to Child Protective Services, and the referral to the developmental-behavioral pediatrician was initiated to help in this determination.

The child visited the developmental-behavioral pediatrician 3 weeks after completion of the fourth round of intravenous antibiotics. The child lived with his mother, father, and older sister, aged 5 years, who had asthma. His father worked, and all appointments were kept by his mother. His sister did well in kindergarten and first grade. His maternal grandmother was supportive of the family and often provided child care. His family history was not remarkable. His physical examination findings were normal. The vital signs, including temperature, were normal. However, his mother reported that the child indeed had a fever and, once again, eye drainage.

The infectious disease specialist was invited to the first visit and examined the child with the developmental-behavioral pediatrician. Together they addressed each physical sign the mother described and informed her that these were variations of normal and did not indicate infection. The mother then agreed to weekly scheduled visits with the developmental-behavioral pediatrician. This pediatrician began steering the interview away from possible signs of infection to discussions of normal developmental issues of early childhood. The mother chose the issue that was to be monitored over the next few visits, such as progress with the child's accepting a variety of foods.

Visits occurred weekly to monthly for 12 months. Calls to the office decreased from three to four per week to once per month. The mother began counseling with a therapist and attended approximately eight sessions, the maximum covered by her insurance. The father did not participate because of his work hours. Approximately 6 months of visits with the developmental-behavioral pediatrician were devoted to mother's anxiety about letting Michael go to school. The virtual absence of the father in the care of the children was noted. The child was eventually placed in a preprimary classroom for speech and language services. His level of delay was not significant enough to warrant this placement; however, because of the circumstances, the school staff agreed that this was in the best interest of the child.

After 1 year, Michael remained free of diagnosis or treatment of serious infection. He continued to grow well and entered kindergarten without need of special services. At this time, Michael's sister, aged 7 years, suffered exacerbation of her asthma, previously well controlled. She was admitted from the emergency department to the pediatric intensive care unit with status asthmaticus and discharged home from the intensive care unit in good condition after 3 days. The pattern of repeatedly seeking care for unsubstantiated symptoms developed with Michael's sister. The mother again saw a therapist. The developmental-behavioral pediatrician was not consulted, and it was possible that the mother declined this referral. A case was opened with child protective services on behalf of the sister.

Over the next few years, the mother became a family advocate for mothers of premature infants and began providing child care for children who required tracheotomy care and oxygen at home. Follow-up with Michael at age 10 years revealed a healthy, robust boy with growth parameters at the 25th percentile who did well in school and was gregarious and endearing. His sister's asthma continued to be poorly managed, and she frequently missed school and was under assessment for depression.

This case illustrates what Green and Solnit[44] and Shonkoff[45] described as the therapeutic nature of the office visit and the importance of relationship and doctor patient communication. It makes clear the critical role of cross-disciplinary collaboration, including education. Unfortunately, this case also illustrates the elusive nature of vulnerability and the complex interplay among illness, psychological state, and family dynamics.

REFERENCES

1. Brener N, Kann L, Lowry R, et al: Trends in HIV-related risk behaviors among high school students—United States, 1991-2005. Morb Mortal Wkly Rep 55:851-854, 2006.

2. Corona R, Beckett MK, Cowgill BO, et al: Do children know their parent's HIV status? Parental reports of child awareness in a nationally representative sample. Ambul Pediatr 6:138-144, 2006.

3. Identification and care of HIV-exposed and HIV-infected infants, children, and adolescents in foster care. American Academy of Pediatrics. Committee on Pediatric AIDS. Pediatrics 106:149-153, 2000.

4. Pickering LK, ed: Red Book: 2006 Report of the Committee on Infectious Diseases, 27th ed. Elk Grove, IL: American Academy of Pediatrics, 2006.

5. Parker AA, Staggs W, Dayan GH, et al: Implications of a 2005 measles outbreak in Indiana for sustained elimination of measles in the United States. N Engl J Med 355:447-455, 2006.

6. Mulholland EK: Measles in the United States, 2006. N Engl J Med 355:440-443, 2006.

7. Remington JS, LKlein JO, Wilson CB, et al: Infectious Diseases of the Fetus and Newborn Infant, 6th ed. Philadelphia: Elsevier, 2006.

8. Schrag S, Gorwitz R, Fultz-Butts K, et al: Prevention of perinatal group B streptococcal disease. Revised guidelines from CDC. MMWR Recomm Rep 51(RR-11):1-22, 2002.

9. Centers for Disease Control and Provention (CDC): Primary and secondary syphilis—United States, 2003-2004. MMWR Morb Mortal Wkly Rep 55:269-273, 2006.

10. Cunningham M, Cox EO: Hearing assessment in infants and children: Recommendations beyond neonatal screening. Pediatrics 111:436-440, 2003.

11. American Academy of Ophthalmology Pediatric Ophthalmology Panel: Pediatric Eye Evaluations Preferred Practice Pattern. San Francisco: American Academy of Ophthalmology, October 22, 2002.

12. Centers for Disease Control and Prevention (CDC): Interim guidelines for the evaluation of infants born to mothers infected with West Nile virus during pregnancy. MMWR Morb Mortal Wkly Rep 53:154-157, 2004.

13. Obrecht RE, Patrick PD: Neuropsychological sequelae of adolescent infectious diseases. Adolesc Med 13:663-681, 2002.

14. Berg S, Trollfors B, Hugosson S, et al: Long-term follow-up of children with bacterial meningitis with emphasis on behavioural characteristics. Eur J Pediatr 161:330-336, 2002.

15. Bent JP 3rd, Beck RA: Bacterial meningitis in the pediatric population: Paradigm shifts and ramifications for otolaryngology–head and neck surgery. Int J Pediatr Otorhinolaryngol 30:41-49, 1994.

16. Wellman MB, Sommer DD, McKenna J: Sensorineural hearing loss in postmeningitic children. Otol Neurotol 24:907-912, 2003.

17. Oostenbrink R, Maas M, Moons KG, et al: Sequelae after bacterial meningitis in childhood. Scand J Infect Dis 34:379-382, 2002.

18. Centers for Disease Control and Prevention: West Nile Virus Activity—United States, January 1–August 15, 2006. Morb Mortal Wkly Rep 55:879-880, 2006.

19. Snider LA, Swedo SE: PANDAS: Current status and directions for research. Mol Psychiatry 9:900-907, 2004.

20. Snider LA, Lougee L, Slattery M, et al: Antibiotic prophylaxis with azithromycin or penicillin for childhood-onset neuropsychiatric disorders. Biol Psychiatry 57:788-792, 2005.

21. Ong S, Talan DA, Moran GJ, et al: Neurocysticercosis in radiographically imaged seizure patients in U.S. emergency departments. Emerg Infect Dis 8:608-613, 2002.

22. Schneider RK, Robinson MJ, Levenson JL: Psychiatric presentations of non-HIV infectious diseases. Neurocysticercosis, Lyme disease, and pediatric autoimmune neuropsychiatric disorder associated with streptococcal infection. Psychiatr Clin North Am 25:1-16, 2002.

23. Singhi P, Singhi S: Neurocysticercosis in children. J Child Neurol 19:482-492, 2004.

24. Tager FA, Fallon BA, Keilp J, et al: A controlled study of cognitive deficits in children with chronic Lyme disease. J Neuropsychiatry Clin Neurosci 13:500-507, 2001.

25. Harwell JI, Obaro SK: Antiretroviral therapy for children. Substantial benefit but limited access. JAMA 296:330-331, 2006.

26. Mok J, Cooper S: The needs of children whose mothers have HIV infection. Arch Dis Child 77:483-487, 1997.

27. Mandell GL, Bennett JE, Dolin R: Principles and Practice of Infectious Disease, 6th ed. Oxford, UK: Churchill Livingstone, 2005.

28. Centers for Disease Control and Prevention (CDC): Epidemiology of HIV/AIDS—United States, 1981-2005. MMWR Morb Mortal Wkly Rep 55:589-592, 2006.

29. Centers for Disease Control and Prevention (CDC): Reduction in perinatal transmission of HIV infection—United States, 1985-2005. MMWR Morb Mortal Wkly Rep 55:592-597, 2006.

30. Warren B, Glaros R, Hackel S, et al: Residual Perinatal HIV Transmission in 25 Births Occurring in New York State. Presented at the National HIV Prevention Conference, Atlanta, GA, June 12-15, 2005.

31. Smith R, Malee K, Leighty R, et al: Effects of perinatal HIV infection and associated risk factors on cognitive development among young children. Pediatrics 117:851-862, 2006.

32. Jeremy RJ, Kim S, Nozyce M, et al: Neuropsychological functioning and viral load in stable antiretroviral therapy-experienced HIV-infected children. Pediatrics 115:380-387, 2005.

33. Mellins CA, Smith R, O'Driscoll PO, et al: High rates of behavioral problems in perinatally HIV-infected children are not linked to HIV disease. Pediatrics 111:384-393, 2003.

34. Chase C, Ware J, Hittelman J, et al: Early cognitive and motor development among infants born to women infected with human immunodeficiency virus. Women

and Infants Transmission Study Group. Pediatrics 106(2):E25, 2000.

35. Pearson DA, McGrath NM, Nozyce M, et al: Predicting HIV disease progression in children using measures of neuropsychological and neurological functioning. Pediatric AIDS Clinical Trials 152 Study Team. Pediatrics 106(6):E76, 2000.

36. Coplan J, Contello KA, Cunningham CK, et al: Early language development in children exposed to or infected with human immunodeficiency virus. Pediatrics 102(1):e8, 1998.

37. Pelton S, Forehand R: Orphans of the AIDS epidemic: An examination of clinical levels of problems of children. J Am Acad Child Adolesc Psychiatry 44:585-591, 2005.

38. Rotheram-Borus MJ, Weiss R, Alber S, et al: Adolescent adjustment before and after HIV-related parental death. J Consult Clin Psychol 73:221-228, 2005.

39. Lee LM, Fleming PL: Estimated number of children left motherless by AIDS in the United States, 1978-1998. J Acquir Immune Defic Syndr 43(2):231-236, 2003.

40. Nicholas SW, Abrams EJ: Boarder babies with AIDS in Harlem: Lessons in applied public health. Am J Public Health 92:163-165, 2002.

41. Levine AB, Aaron E, Foster J: Pregnancy in perinatally HIV-infected adolescents. J Adolesc Health 38:765-768, 2006.

42. Rotheram-Borus MJ, Lester P, Song J, et al: Intergenerational benefits of family-based HIV interventions. J Consult Clin Psychol 74:622-627, 2006.

43. Bayer R, Fairchild AL: Changing the paradigm for HIV testing—The end of exceptionalism. N Engl J Med 355:647-649, 2006.

44. Green M, Solnit AA: Reactions to the threatened loss of a child: A vulnerable baby syndrome. Pediatrics 34:58-66, 1964.

45. Shonkoff JP: Reactions to the threatened loss of a child: A vulnerable child syndrome, by Morris Green, MD, and Albert A. Solnit, MD: Reactions to the threatened loss of a child: A vulnerable child syndrome, Pediatrics, 1964;34:58-66. Pediatrics 102(1 S1):239-241, 1998.

10E.
Central Nervous System Disorders

DEAN P. SARCO
DOUGLAS L. VANDERBILT
JAMES J. RIVIELLO, JR.

The spectrum of central nervous system (CNS) disorders in childhood leads to wide variability in developmental outcomes. Fundamental factors that influence developmental outcomes include the timing in development of the CNS insult, the severity and type of disorder, and the location of the CNS lesion. In this chapter, we consider the basic aspects of common CNS disorders encountered by the developmental-behavioral pediatrician and the relevant developmental considerations for each. We begin with a brief review of the neurological examination, because this provides the clues that may alert the developmental-behavioral pediatrician to a potential underlying neurological disorder.

THE NEUROLOGICAL EVALUATION

The pediatric neurological examination complements a detailed history and general examination. It also allows for an assessment of CNS function and the stage of development. A delay, plateau, or regression in the acquisition of normal developmental milestones is a concern. Likewise, lack of the proper temporal acquisition and loss of certain developmental reflexes may signify underlying neurological dysfunction, as may an abnormal neurological examination finding. We review the relevant aspects of the pediatric neurological evaluation, which may yield clues about an underlying neurological disorder. A specific diagnosis, when possible, is often crucial in understanding the developmental outcome in a child.

The Clinical History

A complete and accurate history yields clues about the presenting problem, if not the specific diagnosis. A detailed understanding of the prenatal, perinatal, and developmental histories must be ascertained, as must the family history. Defining the chronology and nature of the problem, notably whether the onset of the disorder is acute or chronic and whether the course is static or progressive, is imperative. Progressive disability may reflect a potential underlying metabolic or neurodegenerative disorder, whereas static disability may reflect a past and stable neurological insult, as in neonatal hypoxic-ischemic encephalopathy. Understanding the neurological disorder, whether acute or chronic, progressive or static, aids in understanding the impact on a child's developmental outcome.

The General Examination

The general examination should include the measurement and plotting of standard growth parameters, including head circumference. The rate of brain growth is reflected in the head circumference, and any deviation from the normal trajectory, or greater than two standard deviations, is cause for concern.

A head circumference smaller than two standard deviations defines *microcephaly*. A head circumference greater than two standard deviations defines macrocephaly. Either of these may be congenital or acquired in etiology, and both warrant evaluation by a neurologist. Head circumference abnormalities may aid in diagnosing a specific developmental disorder, which may indicate the developmental and neurological prognosis.

Several aspects of the routine pediatric examination are of particular importance in the neurological assessment. The size and tenseness of the anterior fontanelle must be assessed in infants. A bulging and tense fontanelle may indicate increased intracranial pressure, whereas a small fontanelle may be present with microcephaly. In addition, hair texture and color may be suggestive of certain neurological disorders; for example, sparse, wiry hair is characteristic in trichopoliodystrophy (Menkes disease), and premature graying, in ataxia-telangiectasia.

The presence of dysmorphic features in combination with neurological findings may be suggestive of an underlying genetic or metabolic disorder. Examples include hypotonia in association with Down or Prader-Willi syndrome, or mental retardation in association with the fragile X syndrome. Ataxia and seizures are characteristic in Angelman syndrome, and cranial nerve and tone abnormalities in storage disorders such as Gaucher or Niemann-Pick disease.

Skin should be examined for lesions that are associated with certain neurocutaneous disorders. These commonly include the hyperpigmented café-au-lait patches of neurofibromatosis, the hypopigmented ash-leaf spots of tuberous sclerosis, or a port-wine stain over the upper face that is suggestive of Sturge-Weber disease. Any concerns necessitate further investigation.

The Neurological Examination

An extensive neurological examination is not required for all children presenting for developmental assessment; however, understanding and performing a brief examination will aid in assessing neurological function and maturity. A brief screening examination may be performed in several minutes, and proficiency is achieved by practicing it in the same sequence each time. A more complete discussion of the finer points of the neurological examination is available in the literature dedicated to this subject.[1] The examination is divided into the following parts: mental status, cranial nerve, motor, sensory, and coordination testing.

The focus of the neurological examination varies, depending on the presenting symptoms. In addition, dysfunction at different levels of the nervous system may manifest with similar symptoms and examination findings, which by themselves may be nonspecific, as in hypotonia. However, certain manifestations have common specificities as follows:

1. Alteration of awareness is suggestive of either diffuse bilateral cortical or brainstem involvement.
2. Cranial nerve abnormalities, particularly ipsilateral (same side) in association with contralateral (opposite side) motor or sensory findings, are suggestive of brainstem involvement.
3. Incoordination, ataxia, or tremor is suggestive of cerebellar dysfunction.
4. Bilateral lower extremity weakness, hyperreflexia, a sensory level deficit, or bowel or bladder dysfunction, or a combination of these, is suggestive of spinal cord dysfunction.
5. Paresthesias, dysesthesias, or autonomic dysfunction is suggestive of peripheral nerve involvement.

The location of abnormality in the nervous system may be broadly divided into the CNS (brain, brainstem, and spinal cord) or peripheral nervous system (anterior horn cell, peripheral nerve, neuromuscular junction, and muscle). Examination findings suggestive of CNS involvement, or upper motor neuron signs, include brisk deep tendon reflexes, hypertonia, absence of muscle fasciculations, and extensor plantar response. Examination findings suggestive of peripheral nervous involvement, or lower motor neuron signs, include depressed or nonexistent deep tendon reflexes, hypotonia, and muscle fasciculations.

Mental Status Assessment

Assessment of mental status begins by describing the level of alertness and the interactions that a child has with his or her environment. The mental status examination evaluates speech and language, attention, memory, concentration, fund of knowledge, abstract thinking, and visual-spatial skills. If aphasia, apraxia, neglect, or visual-spatial impairment is present, its character may suggest a localization or lateralization of cortical impairment.

Cranial Nerve Examination

Impairment of cranial nerve function often reflects dysfunction either within the brainstem, such as a stroke or mass lesion, or along the course of the nerve, as in Bell's palsy. Table 10E-1 outlines the examination of the cranial nerves and their function.

Motor Examination

The motor examination involves assessment of the appearance, bulk, tone, and strength of individual

TABLE 10E-1 ■ Cranial Nerve Examination

Cranial Nerve Function	Functional Testing
I: Olfactory Nerve	
Olfaction	Examine by testing various non-noxious odors
II: Optic Nerve	
Vision	Examine by testing visual acuity, visual fields, and fundi
III, IV, and VI: Oculomotor, Trochlear, and Abducens Nerves	
Oculomotor function	Examine pupil size and light reflex, eye position in primary gaze, and extraocular movements
V: Trigeminal Nerve	
Motor function to masseter muscle	Examine by jaw opening and closing
Sensory function in face	Examine facial sensation, sensory limb of corneal reflex
VII: Facial Nerve	
Motor movements of face	Examine facial movements, motor limb of corneal reflex
VIII: Vestibulocochlear Nerve	
Hearing and vestibular function	Examine by testing hearing, balance
IX and X: Glossopharyngeal and Vagus Nerves	
Motor and sensory innervation of pharynx, larynx, and palate	Examine gag reflex, palatal rise
XI: Spinal Accessory Nerve	
Sternocleidomastoid and trapezius muscles	Examine neck movements, shoulder elevation
XII: Hypoglossal Nerve	
Tongue movements	Examine tongue position, strength, and movements

muscles. The presence of atrophy or hypertrophy, or abnormal movements such as fasciculations, are indicative of underlying primary or secondary disorders of muscle. Muscle tone, the resistance to passive movement at rest, may be increased (hypertonia) or decreased (hypotonia). Different types of increased tone are suggestive of their localization within the nervous system. The most common hypertonia found in children, spasticity, reflects a lesion of the descending motor tracts from motor cortex.

Strength in infants and young children may be assessed primarily through observation and may be formally tested in older cooperative children. The presence of Gower's sign (using the hands to assist in rising from the floor with pelvic weakness), or pronator drift with outstretched arms, indicates weakness. Lower extremity or trunk weakness may also be detected by having the child walk. Heel or toe gait may be impaired with lower extremity weakness. The biceps, triceps, brachioradialis, patellar, and Achilles deep tendon reflexes may also be tested for strength and asymmetry. An extensor plantar response (Babinski's sign) indicates upper motor neuron disease in the proper context.

The pattern of weakness helps the clinician localize a lesion within the CNS or the peripheral nervous system. Weakness in the arm extensor and leg flexors may be present with upper motor neuron lesions. Proximal and trunk weakness is suggestive of a muscular disorder, such as muscular dystrophy or myopathy. Distal weakness is suggestive of a peripheral neuropathy. Cortical lesions involving primarily the face and arm may result from a middle cerebral artery distribution injury, whereas lower extremity weakness corresponds more to an anterior cerebral artery distribution.

The onset and disappearance of neonatal reflexes have been well defined.[2] Asymmetry discovered when these maneuvers are performed may be indicative of lower motor neuron dysfunction, as in weakness from a brachial plexus injury. Reflexes may be depressed or absent entirely with lower motor neuron lesions.

At the least, examination of muscle bulk, assessment of muscle tone in the extremities, testing for pronator drift, symmetry of deep tendon reflexes, and heel and toe gait should be observed.

Sensory Examination

The sensory examination is limited in a young child because it depends on patient cooperation and feedback. Light touch, pain, temperature, vibratory sensation, proprioception, and cortical sensations may be assessed. At the least, presence of and asymmetry in reactions to light, touch, and temperature (cold tuning fork) in an extremity may be assessed in most children. The presence of Romberg's sign (unable to sustain upright posture while standing with eyes closed) is indicative of proprioceptive dysfunction.

Coordination

Coordination refers to fluid and accurate motor movements. Abnormality in cerebellar and/or extrapyramidal system function may result in decreased muscle tone, incoordination, abnormal posture or gait (ataxia), or tremor. The patient should be observed at rest and while performing volitional movements. Common maneuvers for testing coordination include finger-to-nose movements, rapid alternating finger movements, hand pronation/supination, foot tapping, and heel-to-shin maneuvers.

EPILEPSY

Epilepsy occurs in approximately 0.5% to 1% of the population.[3] The onset of epilepsy has a higher incidence during the first year of life, which then decreases into childhood and adolescence. In addition, children with developmental disorders such as mental retardation and cerebral palsy have a higher incidence of epilepsy than do normal children.[4] Although the many children with the traditional "benign" childhood epilepsy syndromes have a favorable developmental outcome, this is not the case for many other children with epilepsy. Certain "catastrophic" epilepsy syndromes may profoundly affect development, and accumulating data are evidence of cognitive and behavioral impairments in some children with "benign" childhood epilepsies.

From infancy through childhood, basic developmental skills are acquired and refined. Younger onset of epilepsy has more potential for interference in development. How an epileptic disorder results in cognitive and behavioral impairment is poorly understood. The effects of recurrent seizures, the underlying etiology of the epilepsy, and the potential side effects of therapies may contribute to developmental disability, although their contribution does not adequately explain the degree of impairment seen in many children. The extent and significance of ongoing abnormal electrical activity and metabolic changes in epilepsy, and their effects on development, necessitate further investigation.

Definition

Seizures may have clinical signs or symptoms, or may be clinically silent. Seizures without clinical symptoms are also termed *electrographic seizures,* as they are detected only with electroencephalographic (EEG) recording. The clinical symptoms of a seizure are variable and dependent on the regions of cortex involved. Seizures by nature are sudden and involuntary. Stressors such as fevers, illness, or sleep deprivation may precipitate them. Clinical manifestations may include loss or alteration of consciousness, involuntary movements, or abnormal sensations. These may involve a specific area of cortex (partial, or focal) or spread throughout both hemispheres (generalized). A postictal state is typical, consisting of brief lethargy and occasionally transient neurological deficits.

The term *epilepsy* refers to recurrent, unprovoked seizures resulting from abnormal cerebral electrical activity. There are many causes of epilepsy. Single or recurrent seizures with an acute provocation are not considered epilepsy. Such seizures do not occur spontaneously and are not associated with altered developmental outcomes.

Classification and Clinical Characteristics

Although no scheme is perfect, categorizing seizures and epilepsy syndromes is helpful in guiding further evaluation and treatment and in generating a prognosis. Seizures may be broadly classified into either partial or generalized events (Table 10E-2; see also

---

TABLE 10E-2 ■ Classification of Seizures

Partial (Focal, Local) Seizures

Simple Partial Seizures (Consciousness Not Impaired)

With motor signs
With somatosensory or special sensory symptoms
  Somatosensory
  Visual
  Auditory
  Olfactory
  Gustatory
  Vertiginous
With autonomic symptoms and signs
With psychic symptoms (impaired higher cortical function)
  Speech disturbance (dysphasia)
  Memory disturbance (e.g., dèjà vu)
  Cognitive disturbance (e.g., dissociative states)
  Affective disturbance (e.g., fear, anger)
  Illusions
  Structured hallucinations

Complex Partial Seizures (Consciousness Impaired)

Simple partial onset followed by impairment of consciousness
Impairment of consciousness at onset

Partial Seizures (Simple or Complex) Evolving to Secondarily Generalized Seizures

Generalized Seizures (Bilateral, Symmetrical, without Focal Onset)

Absence seizures
  With impairment of consciousness only
  With clonic components
  With tonic components
  With atonic components
  With automatisms
  With autonomic components
Atypical absence seizures (more dramatic tone changes, less abrupt onset/end)
Myoclonic seizures
Clonic seizures
Tonic seizures
Tonic-clonic seizures ("grand-mal" seizures)
Atonic seizures

Unclassified Seizures

Data from Commission on Classification and Terminology of the International league Against Epilepsy. Proposal for revised clinical and electroencephalographic classification of epileptic seizures. Epilepsia 1981;22:489-501.

Table 10E-1). It is also useful to define certain epilepsy syndromes, because they can be divided by their effects on developmental outcome.

Partial seizures begin in a focal region of cortex and may remain focal or become secondarily generalized. They are categorized as simple partial seizures or complex partial seizures, depending on whether consciousness is impaired.

Simple partial seizures themselves do not impair memory or cognitive function; thus, patients can respond during the seizure and recall the event afterwards. Patients may recall motor symptoms, such as stiffening or jerking, or sensory changes, such as tingling in an extremity. Special sensory symptoms, such as unusual smells, tastes, or abdominal sensations, may also occur. Autonomic involvement includes changes in heart rate, changes in respiratory rate, and flushing. Other symptoms may include "out-of-body" experiences or depersonalization, emotional changes such as fear or anger, or memory disturbances such as déjà vu (the incorrect sensation that the same situation has occurred before).

During a complex partial seizure, consciousness is impaired but not completely lost. Memory for the event is often absent or impaired. Normal behavior ceases, frequently with staring and unresponsiveness. Automatisms frequently seen include lip-smacking, grunting, or chewing movements.

Partial seizures may also become secondarily generalized. Patients may recall the onset of a seizure, although they have no recollection of events once the seizure has generalized. Rapid secondary generalization may be difficult to distinguish clinically from primary generalization; thus, EEG monitoring is helpful in making the distinction.

A generalized seizure involves the entire cortex at onset. The mechanism is unclear, although it may involve rapid secondary generalization from other focal areas. These frequently appear as generalized convulsions, such as those seen with "grand mal" or generalized tonic-clonic seizures. In childhood epilepsy, a common nonconvulsive generalized seizure type is absence, or "petit mal," seizures, which may occur in young school-aged children. A generalized, nonconvulsive seizure may be difficult to differentiate by clinical appearance from a complex partial seizure, although they can be readily differentiated by EEG recording.

Other seizures types can also occur. Myoclonic seizures manifest as a rapid, involuntary jerks, which may occur individually or in clusters. These may be associated with specific epilepsy syndromes or neurological disorders. Clonic seizures involve repetitive and rhythmic muscle contractions. Tonic seizures involve sustained muscle contractions and stiffening. Atonic seizures involve loss of muscle tone, ranging

in severity from brief head drops to dangerous generalized drop attacks. Clonic, tonic, and atonic seizures may occur in combination in certain epilepsy syndromes, such as Lennox-Gastaut syndrome.

Epileptic seizures may also be classified into various epilepsy syndromes. The determination of a specific epilepsy syndrome is based on the seizure type and characteristics, the findings on the neurological examination, and supportive data from studies such as EEG monitoring.

These syndromes may be grouped by their effect on developmental outcome into the descriptively named "benign" and "malignant" epilepsies of childhood. The benign epilepsies of childhood are characterized by infrequent or mild seizures, a good developmental outcome, and no significant psychosocial effects (Table 10E-3). In contrast, the malignant epilepsies are characterized by frequent and often intractable seizures and associated with significant cognitive and developmental impairment. Affected patients' response to medications is often poor (Table 10E-4). This distinction is not absolute, but it is useful in many cases.

TABLE 10E-3 ■ Benign Epilepsies of Childhood

Generalized

Benign familial neonatal convulsions
Benign idiopathic neonatal convulsions
Benign myoclonic epilepsy of infancy
Childhood absence epilepsy
Juvenile absence epilepsy
Juvenile myoclonic epilepsy

Partial

Benign childhood epilepsy with centrotemporal spikes
Childhood epilepsy with occipital paroxysms
Early-onset benign childhood occipital epilepsy
  (Panayiotopoulos type)
Late-onset childhood occipital epilepsy (Gastaut type)

TABLE 10E-4 ■ Malignant Epilepsies of Childhood

Neonatal

Early myoclonic encephalopathy

Infancy

Early infantile epileptic encephalopathy (Ohtahara syndrome)
Severe myoclonic epilepsy of infancy (Dravet syndrome)
Infantile spasms (West syndrome)

Childhood

Lennox-Gastaut syndrome
Myoclonic-astatic epilepsy (Doose syndrome)
Landau-Kleffner syndrome
Electrical status epilepticus of sleep

Of the benign epilepsies of childhood, benign rolandic epilepsy with centrotemporal spikes (BRECTS) is most frequent, accounting for approximately 15% of cases of pediatric epilepsy.[5] The episodes are typically nocturnal, partial seizures in children with motor and sensory involvement of one side of the face, sometimes accompanied by guttural sounds or other unusual vocalizations. The incidence peaks at 3 to 10 years of age, disappearing by adolescence. Seizures may occur during the daytime and may also secondarily generalize. The EEG recording reveals characteristic epileptiform abnormalities in the centotemporal regions, exacerbated in sleep. There is a good response to anticonvulsant medications.

Data have indicated that the course of BRECTS may not be entirely benign in some children. A subset of patients may experience mild neuropsychological deficits and behavioral problems. Significant language impairment, attentional difficulties, behavioral problems, and visual-spatial impairment have been described in comparison to normal children.[6,7] Children with benign childhood epilepsy with occipital paroxysms have been found to score lower in visual transformation tasks than do normal children, and to have impaired attention and memory.[8]

Continuous spike-waves in slow-wave sleep constitutes a unique syndrome in which very frequent generalized spike-wave discharges are associated with significant cognitive dysfunction but few or no clinical seizures.[9]

Landau-Kleffner syndrome is another epilepsy syndrome associated with primarily cognitive dysfunction. Receptive language regression occurs in a previously normal child, followed by expressive language regression. Seizures and behavioral problems are present in most affected children, and the EEG recording shows very frequent epileptiform activity, present primarily in sleep and described as electrical status epilepticus of slow-wave sleep. Language impairment may persist in some children despite treatment.

A more frequently seen severe epilepsy syndrome is the Lennox-Gastaut syndrome, characterized by a mixture of seizure types, including tonic, atonic, and myoclonic. EEG recordings reveal a typical slow spike-and-wave pattern, with persistent seizures. Mental retardation is, unfortunately, present in most affected children.

Etiology

There are numerous causes of seizures, and the prognosis is dependent primarily on the underlying cause and other associated neurological abnormalities. In approximately 25% to 45% of cases in children, a specific cause is found.[10] Causes considered in children include birth trauma, cerebral malformations, cerebrovascular disorders, metabolic disorders, neurocutaneous disorders, CNS infections, brain tumors, traumatic brain injury (TBI), neurodegenerative disorders, and genetically inherited predisposition to epilepsy. Each of these has its own implications in terms of the course of epilepsy and developmental outcome.

The siblings of individuals affected with epilepsy have a 2.5 fold increased risk of epilepsy.[11] The incidence of trauma as the cause of epilepsy ranges from 4% to 10%, and such trauma is more prevalent in children older than 5 years.[10] CNS infections are associated with a three-fold increased risk of epilepsy overall.[12] Certain causes, such as a structural malformations, tumor, or stroke, may produce more severe seizures.

The causes of seizures are often divided into the following categories: idiopathic, cryptogenic, and symptomatic. *Idiopathic* epilepsies are those without an identifiable etiology and normal evaluation findings. In general, patients with these forms have a better prognosis, and these forms may include many genetic causes. *Cryptogenic* epilepsy refers to a suspected symptomatic cause from neurological abnormalities, although no specific diagnosis has been identified. *Symptomatic* epilepsy is associated with a known underlying cause. Cryptogenic and symptomatic epilepsies are associated with poorer developmental outcomes overall. A well-described example of this scenario is infantile spasms. This is an age-related seizure type also referred to as West syndrome, which describes the triad of infantile spasms, developmental delay, and the characteristic chaotic and disorganized EEG pattern described as "hypsarrhythmia." The majority of children with infantile spasms who develop further seizure types have either cryptogenic or symptomatic causes. In one series of children who developed cryptogenic infantile spasms that then resolved, 12 of 18 had normal intelligence by age 5 years, and 5 had specific cognitive deficits. Three had a mild learning disability.[13]

Diagnosis of Seizures

Epilepsy is a clinical diagnosis that is based on the description of the event, either by the history or actual observation. The evaluation of suspected seizures should include a thorough history and examination. Metabolic causes should be evaluated, including measurements of glucose and electrolytes with calcium and magnesium (see Chapter 10C for more detail). Hepatic and renal function should be assessed. Toxicology screening should be considered, and the cerebrospinal fluid (CSF) should be examined if infection is a possibility. An EEG study should be obtained in order to help clarify the diagnosis and potentially identify an epilepsy syndrome. In general, imaging should be obtained if the history is suggestive of seizures, if there is an abnormality on neurological examination, or if the EEG findings are abnormal. The purpose is to find an underlying structural cause of seizures. Computed tomography (CT) is useful for rapid evaluation if hemorrhage or hydrocephalus is suspected. Magnetic resonance imaging (MRI) provides significantly higher resolution than does CT in visualizing the brainstem and posterior fossa, as well as in describing cerebral structures.

With a sufficient history, convulsive seizures may be easy to distinguish from nonconvulsive events; however, other possibilities need to be considered and evaluated. The differential diagnosis often includes syncope, breath-holding spells, or normal movements. Other movement disorders that must be distinguished include dystonia, tics, stereotypies, and chorea. Sleep events, such as nonepileptic myoclonus, night terrors, or somnambulism may also be considered. Also, nonepileptic seizures, or pseudoseizures, may be suggested by a poor response to medications, normal findings on repeated studies, and psychosocial issues. Nonconvulsive seizures, as may be seen in complex partial or absence seizures, may be more difficult to diagnose by history. If the history is suggestive of seizures, or unclear, then an EEG study is warranted. Electrographic seizure activity correlated with an event is diagnostic of an epileptic seizure. Epileptiform abnormalities in between seizures are evidence of an underlying seizure disorder; however, they not diagnostic. A normal EEG result does not support a diagnosis of seizures, but it does not exclude the possibility.

Unusual behaviors or changes in behaviors can be difficult to differentiate from epileptic events, particularly in children with an underlying disability such as mental retardation or autism. If events are frequent, then prolonged EEG monitoring may be particularly useful in order to capture the events and obtain a clinical and electrographic correlation. This may occur in the outpatient setting through ambulatory EEG recording or in the inpatient setting through video-EEG recording. The latter has the added benefit of video recording to correlate specific events with the EEG recording; however, it is more disruptive, requiring hospitalization for at least 24 hours in most cases.

Another potential option is a trial of anticonvulsant therapy. However, abnormal movements such as dystonia or myoclonus that are not epileptic seizures may respond to treatment with anticonvulsants. Anticonvulsants such as valproate and topiramate are also used in the treatment of affective disorders and may improve symptoms; thus, it is often useful to clarify

a diagnosis of epilepsy before the initiation of treatment.

Treatment

Anticonvulsant medications are usually not initiated after a first seizure. When a decision to treat is made, the choice of anticonvulsant medication is dependent on multiple factors, including seizure type and epilepsy syndrome, etiology, pharmacokinetics, and the efficacy and tolerability profile. This is particularly important in children with developmental disabilities, who may be more sensitive to certain adverse effects and who may experience more functional impairment than a neurologically normal child. Understanding medication side effects and simplifying anticonvulsant regimens are crucial for avoiding excessive sedation, cognitive dulling, or behavioral problems. Overall, the newer anticonvulsants have fewer cognitive and behavioral adverse effects than do older medications. Table 10E-5 lists the more common antiepileptic drugs.

Febrile seizures, which do not adversely affect development, are the most frequently encountered seizures in childhood. The National Collaborative Perinatal Project found no significant motor or cognitive effects of febrile seizures, although other researchers have suggested that there may be intelligence deficits with repeated simple and complex febrile seizures.[14,15] Anticonvulsant prophylaxis is rarely recommended.[16]

With anticonvulsant treatment, further cognitive impairment may occur in an already challenged child. Phenobarbital, the benzodiazepines, and phenytoin may be associated with excessive sedation and cognitive dulling. Data regarding the newer anticonvulsants are limited; however, topiramate has been associated with cognitive dulling and word-finding difficulty. These effects are reversible with discontinuation of the agent and may be reduced with slower titration.[17]

TABLE 10E-5 ■ Commonly Used Anticonvulsant Medications	
Older	**Newer**
Carbamazepine	Felbamate
Clonazepam	Gabapentin
Diazepam	Lamotrigine
Ethosuximide	Levetiracetam
Lorazepam	Oxcarbazepine
Phenobarbital	Pregabalin
Phenytoin	Tiagabine
Valproate	Topiramate
	Zonisamide

Behavioral problems, which may already be present in some children with developmental disabilities, may be exacerbated by certain anticonvulsants, including phenobarbital, the benzodiazepines, gabapentin, and levetiracetam. Valproate has been linked to reduced aggression, although further studies are required.[18] Table 10E-6 lists additional risk factors for behavioral problems in children with epilepsy.

Depressive symptoms have been reported with phenobarbital.[19] In contrast, valproate and other newer anticonvulsants have been used as mood stabilizers and may benefit patients with comorbid affective disorders.

The effect of anticonvulsant medications on comorbid conditions should also be considered. There may be a small but increased risk of seizures in association with some antidepressant medications, including bupropion, clomipramine, and maprotiline.[20,21] No well-designed study thus far has shown that stimulant treatment of attention-deficit/hyperactivity disorder (ADHD) is associated with an increased risk of seizures, and several studies have supported its safety in children with epilepsy.[22] One study in children with epilepsy and ADHD revealed that long-acting methylphenidate improved ADHD symptoms, with no increase in seizure frequency.[23]

In children with medically refractory seizures, consideration should be given to other therapies, including the ketogenic diet, vagus nerve stimulation, and epilepsy surgery. Epilepsy surgery may have a significant developmental effect on young children with catastrophic epilepsy with developmental failure. There appears to be a less vigorous effect on development in older children with focal epilepsy.[24]

Developmental and Behavioral Implications

Certain developmental disabilities, such as ADHD, autism, depression, and anxiety, are present more frequently in children with epilepsy than in nonepileptic children.[25] In addition, many authors have noted that children with developmental disabilities are more likely to develop multiple seizure types and to develop medically refractory epilepsy than are nonepileptic children.[26]

An increased incidence of attentional difficulties and hyperactivity is reported in children with epilepsy.[27] The reported prevalence of epilepsy in children with ADHD has been highly variable. In an attempt to define more precisely the prevalence of epilepsy in this population, Dunn and colleagues studied a series of 175 children with epilepsy and reported an ADHD incidence of 38%, in comparison with a 5% to 10% incidence in the general population.[28]

Cerebral palsy and mental retardation have a significant association with epilepsy. Approximately 15% to 35% of cases of childhood epilepsy are associated with cerebral palsy or mental retardation.[29,30] In addition, epilepsy has an earlier onset in children with mental retardation and/or cerebral palsy.[31] Neurological evaluation should be conducted in such children when possible seizures are suspected.

Children with autistic spectrum disorders also have an increased incidence of epilepsy, estimated at 8% to 28%. This risk is increased if comorbid cerebral palsy or mental retardation is present.[32-34] Valproate appears to have some efficacy in improving autistic behaviors in children with epilepsy; however, further studies are required in this population.[35]

TABLE 10E-6 ■ Risk Factors for Academic and Behavioral Problems in Pediatric Epilepsy
Neurological Dysfunction
EEG abnormalities, especially in slow-wave activity
Neurological Dysfunction
EEG abnormalities, especially in slow-wave activity
Structural abnormalities on CT or MRI
Mental retardation
Severe epileptic syndromes
Seizure Variables
Early age at onset
Long seizure duration
High seizure frequency
Multiple seizure types
Prior unrecognized seizures
Neuropsychological Dysfunction
Mental retardation
Language
Attention
Psychomotor speed
Memory and learning
Problem solving
Side Effects of Medication
Poor Child and Family Response to the Epilepsy Conditions
Family stress
Low family adaptive resources
Negative perceptions or attitudes
Maladaptive coping behaviors
External locus of control
Child's satisfaction with family relationships

From Fastenau P, Dunn D, Austin J: Pediatric epilepsy: Risk factors for academic and behavioral problems in pediatric epilepsy in childhood. *In* Rizzo M, Eslinger P, eds: Principles and Practice of Behavioral Neurology and Neuropsychology. Philadelphia: Elsevier, 2004, p 968.
CT, computed tomography; EEG, electroencephalographic; MRI, magnetic resonance imaging.

Children with epilepsy also appear to have a higher prevalence of behavioral, cognitive, and developmental difficulties in comparison with children who have other types of chronic illness. Autistic features, temper tantrums, aggression, inattentiveness, hyperactivity, and impulsivity are more frequent.[19] Symptoms of anxiety occur in 16% to 23% of children with epilepsy, and symptoms of depression in 26%.[36,37] The origin of such difficulties is probably multifactorial, including the underlying cause, the effect of chronic seizures, medication side effects, and the potential effect of interictal epileptiform discharges. In addition, the fear associated with unpredictable seizures, parental stress, associated cognitive and academic problems, social stigma, and misinformation about the disorder all contribute to the psychosocial difficulties that children with epilepsy experience.[38,39]

HYDROCEPHALUS

Significance

Hydrocephalus is the most common cause of increased intracranial pressure in children. Rates of morbidity and mortality decrease significantly with appropriate treatment, especially if carried out early. Hydrocephalus has been noted to affect several domains of development, including memory, mathematical skills, visual-spatial skills, and general cognition.[40-42]

Definition and Etiology

In hydrocephalus, excess CSF accumulates in the ventricular system of the brain. This often signifies increased intracranial pressure within the skull, which results in the associated signs and symptoms. The normal production of CSF occurs primarily within the choroid plexus, structures found within the ventricular system. This fluid flows out from the lateral ventricles, through the third and fourth ventricles, and out the foramina of Magendie and Luschka. From there it bathes the spinal cord and outer surfaces of the brain, to be resorbed at the arachnoid villi and granulations on the internal surface of the skull. When this flow is altered and the CSF volume within the skull increases, it displaces either blood or brain, which eventually results in either infarction or herniation.

Hydrocephalus in children, which may be congenital or acquired, has been divided into communicating and noncommunicating types. In communicating hydrocephalus, the ventricular system is patent; the disorder is caused by either overproduction of CSF or impaired resorption of CSF at the villi and granulations. In noncommunicating hydrocephalus, there is a blockage within ventricular system proximal to the foramina of and Magendie, resulting in a buildup of pressure proximal to the obstruction or stenosis. In hydrocephalus ex vacuo, a type of communicating hydrocephalus, there are excessive CSF spaces secondary to brain atrophy.

Overall, hydrocephalus has been estimated to affect 1 per 500 children.[43] The incidence in neonates varies from 0.4 to 0.8 per 1000 live births and stillbirths.[44] Aqueductal stenosis accounts for 80% of neonatal hydrocephalus and 60% of all cases.[45] X-linked hydrocephalus accounts for approximately 5% of total cases.[44] Table 10E-7 lists potential causes of childhood hydrocephalus.

Communicating hydrocephalus comprises approximately 30% of cases of childhood hydrocephalus.[46] Benign external hydrocephalus is associated with enlarged bifrontal subarachnoid spaces, normal or mildly enlarged ventricles, and mild gross motor delay. This type of hydrocephalus usually resolves spontaneously within the second year of life. Gliosis, or scarring within the CNS may occur after an insult, such as infection or hemorrhage. Meningeal scarring results in impaired resorption of CSF at the arachnoid villi, which causes hydrocephalus. Various tumors involving the meninges, including lymphoma, may also obstruct CSF resorption. A choroid plexus

TABLE 10E-7 ■ Causes of Hydrocephalus
Communicating
Benign external hydrocephalus
Post-hemorrhagic
Post-meningitic
Meningeal tumors
Choroid plexus papilloma
Noncommunicating
Aqueductal stenosis
Post-infectious
Post-hemorrhagic
Genetic disorders (X-linked, autosomal recessive, other syndromes)
Chemical irritation
Chiari malformations
Dandy-Walker malformation
Foramen of Monroe stenosis
Skull base abnormalities
Mass lesions
Tumors
Cysts (arachnoid cysts, colloid cysts)
Abscess
Vascular malformations

papilloma is a rare tumor that may result in excessive CSF production, thereby causing hydrocephalus.

Noncommunicating hydrocephalus often results from stenosis of the cerebral aqueduct between the third and fourth ventricles. The small diameter of the cerebral aqueduct, estimated at 0.5 mm^2, makes it particularly susceptible to inflammation or compression.[47] Gliosis of the aqueduct may occur after intraventricular hemorrhage, meningitis, or ventriculitis. Genetic disorders may result in congenital stenosis. The most common of these are the X-linked hydrocephalus syndromes, associated with mental retardation. A gene mutation at Xq28, encoding for the L1 cell adhesion molecule, is responsible. Less common autosomal recessive forms of congenital hydrocephalus also exist. Various genetic syndromes such as Walker-Warburg or Hunter syndromes may also be associated with hydrocephalus.

Structural malformations may also obstruct CSF flow, which results in noncommunicating hydrocephalus. Chiari malformations result in posterior fossa abnormalities, including downward displacement of the cerebellar tonsils, the vermis, and possibly the lower medulla. Dandy-Walker malformation is associated with posterior fossa abnormalities, including enlargement of the fourth ventricle and dysplasia of the cerebellar vermis, among other cerebral malformations. Hydrocephalus typically develops during the first year of life.

Mass lesions often compress the cerebral aqueduct to obstruct CSF flow; they may also locally obstruct flow at any location to cause hydrocephalus. Supratentorial tumors, such as astrocytomas, or infratentorial tumors, such as medulloblastoma, may result in such compression. Arachnoid cysts may obstruct flow. A colloid cyst of the third ventricle may cause intermittent obstruction with an acute or prolonged course. Vascular malformations include vein of Galen or other arteriovenous malformations, which may cause chronic symptoms.

Clinical Characteristics

The clinical features of hydrocephalus are variable, depending on the rate of progression. Acute hydrocephalus may manifest dramatically, as in the case of certain tumors that obstruct ventricular CSF flow. Chronic hydrocephalus, in contrast, may manifest with a history of worsening chronic headaches in the absence of other neurological signs or symptoms.

Congenital hydrocephalus may manifest at birth with failure of labor to adequately progress. Cephalopelvic disproportion may be noted. In neonates, the fontanels may appear tense or bulging, and the sutures may be splayed. The head may appear enlarged, and scalp veins may be dilated. An infant may display the "setting sun" sign, consisting of impaired upward gaze and a downward gaze preference with lid retraction. Horizontal gaze impairment caused by abducens nerve palsies may be present. Lethargy, emesis, irritability, and seizures may also occur.

In older children and adolescents, acute onset of hydrocephalus may manifest with progressive lethargy, emesis, headache, abducens nerve palsies, and progressive worsening into coma. Pupillary dilation secondary to oculomotor nerve palsy may occur with acute and rapid hydrocephalus, resulting in herniation. Papilledema may be noted on funduscopic examination.

A more subacute or chronic presentation may be found by charting the trajectory of head circumference growth. An increase in head circumference faster than the expected growth velocity may also represent the first signs of developing hydrocephalus. Failure or delay of normal developmental reflexes may occur. Spasticity may be noted in the lower extremities over time as compression of lower extremity motor fibers occurs.

A more chronic course may manifest as a progressively worsening new-onset headache. Typical characteristics of headaches associated with increased intracranial pressure include worsening in the early morning, night-time awakening, worsening with coughing or the Valsalva maneuver, and a progressive course. Lethargy, emesis, and papilledema also develop as hydrocephalus worsens.

Diagnosis

The signs and symptoms of the hydrocephalus are also dependent on the underlying cause. For example, a progressively expanding mass lesion such as a tumor would probably also produce other signs and symptoms that suggest its location. A right frontal tumor, for example, may manifest with a progressive left-sided hemiparesis.

Evaluation should occur promptly when there is suspicion of hydrocephalus or increased intracranial pressure. If macrocephaly is noted, then imaging must be conducted to determine whether increased head size is caused by increased CSF, brain, or blood volume. Increased brain volume may be present in some metabolic disorders such as Alexander disease. Increased blood volume may occur with epidural or subdural hemorrhage.

In infants, head ultrasonography or CT is useful in emergency cases if a hemorrhage that may necessitate acute neurosurgical intervention is suspected. Ultrasonography is readily available in many hospitals and allows for monitoring after a diagnosis is made. MRI provides higher resolution and better visualization of the cerebral aqueduct and posterior fossa than does

CT or ultrasound. Magnetic resonance angiography with contrast material may be necessary to differentiate mass lesions such as tumors and arteriovenous malformations. MRI sequences can be used to assess cerebral aqueduct flow. Reconstruction of the skull on CT may be used to evaluate the cranial sutures if premature craniosynostosis is suspected, as in Crouzon syndrome. Nuclear medicine studies are also available to assess CSF clearance.

Treatment

Medical therapy for hydrocephalus with acetazolamide or furosemide serves as a temporizing measure and is not curative. Once a diagnosis is made, neurosurgical consultation is required in most cases in order to correct CSF flow. Milder degrees of hydrocephalus may be monitored by neuroimaging studies, serial head circumference measurements, and developmental assessments. Severe hydrocephalus necessitates diversion of CSF flow from the ventricular system to an extraventricular site; such diversion includes ventriculoperitoneal, ventriculoatrial, ventriculopleural, or lumboperitoneal shunting. Long-term complications of shunting include shunt infection and malfunction.

Developmental and Behavioral Implications

Recognizing and treating hydrocephalus rapidly is imperative. Untreated, hydrocephalus is associated with a mortality rate of 50%; 50% to 60% of survivors have mental retardation.[48,49]

Treated hydrocephalus is associated with normal IQ in approximately two thirds of patients.[46] Deficits in intelligence, language, visual-spatial skills, memory, and fine motor skills may be present.[50]

Children with very low birth weight or grade IV intraventricular hemorrhage and subsequent hydrocephalus are at high risk for neurodevelopmental difficulties. The prognosis appears to depend to a greater degree on the extent and timing of parenchymal injury caused by hemorrhage rather than on the degree of ventricular dilatation.[51] Benign external hydrocephalus is associated with delays in gross motor or language skills, which resolve in most patients by age 2 years.[52]

STROKE

Significance

Childhood stroke continues to gain recognition as a cause of significant childhood morbidity and mortal-

ity, including cerebral palsy. Poor understanding of the various risk factors and proper management may result in delays in diagnosis.

Definition

Stroke occurs when there is insufficient blood flow to a region of brain, caused by either hemorrhage or ischemia and resulting in injury. Hemorrhagic stroke results from rupture of arterial supply, such as that caused by an aneurysm or trauma. Ischemic strokes in children may occur in sickle cell disease, congenital heart disease, or moya-moya disease. Most strokes are arterial in etiology; however, venous infarctions may occur, as in the case of venous sinus thrombosis.

Strokes are defined by location (i.e., epidural, subdural, subarachnoid, intraparenchymal, or intraventricular) and by their mechanism (i.e., thrombotic or embolic). Thrombotic infarction occurs when clot forms within the blood vessels at the site of occlusion, as in sickle cell disease. Embolic infarction refers to a clot that has traveled from a distant location, as may occur with congenital cardiac disease. A transient ischemic attack is defined as the presence of transient symptoms of a stroke followed by the reestablishment of blood flow. A transient ischemic attack should be considered a harbinger of stroke, and prompt evaluation is imperative.

Etiology

In the United States, the annual incidence of stroke has been estimated at 2.3 per 100,000 children, with an incidence of 1.2 for ischemic and 1.1 for hemorrhagic strokes.[53] Approximately 60% of childhood strokes are idiopathic, which reflects our limited understanding of the disease pathophysiology.[54] In infants, the incidence is even higher; prematurity is another increasingly frequent risk factor for stroke. The incidence of perinatal arterial ischemic stroke has been estimated at 20 per 100,000 live births.[55] Table 10E-8 lists the causes of stroke in children. This list continues to expand as a better understanding of childhood stroke evolves, such as the identification of new prothrombotic factors.

Clinical Characteristics

The clinical manifestations of stroke depend on the location of injury within the CNS. Any new neurological deficit necessitates prompt evaluation. Symptoms are typically maximal at onset, with slow improvement afterwards over weeks to months. Stroke may occur in a vascular distribution, and examination findings may be referable to one

TABLE 10E-8 ■ Causes of Ischemic and Hemorrhagic Pediatric Stroke

Cardiac Abnormalities and Events

Arrhythmia
Bacterial endocarditis
Cardiac catheterization
Cardiomyopathy
Cyanotic congenital defects
Masses (i.e., atrial myxoma, rhabdomyoma)
Rheumatic heart disease
Valve disease

Cerebrovascular Malformations

Arteriovenous malformations
Fibromuscular dysplasia
Hereditary hemorrhagic telangiectasia
Sturge-Weber syndrome

Coagulopathies/Hemoglobinopathies

Antiphospholipid antibodies/lupus anticoagulant
Congenital coagulation defects
Disseminated intravascular coagulation
Drug-induced (e.g., medications, cocaine, amphetamines)
Malignancy
Polycythemia
Sickle cell anemia/disease
Thrombocytopenic purpura

Trauma

Arterial dissection
Chiropractic manipulation
Intraoral trauma
Neck trauma

Vasculitis

Hemolytic-uremic syndrome
Kawasaki disease
Meningitis
Primary central nervous system vasculitis
Systemic inflammatory disorders (i.e., systemic lupus erythematosus)
Takayasu arteritis
Varicella infection

Vasculopathies

Amino and organic acidopathies
Complicated migraine
Mitochondrial disorders
Moya-moya disease

Adapted from Fenichel GM: Hemiplegia. *In* Fenichel GM, ed: Clinical Pediatric Neurology: A Signs and Symptoms Approach, 5th ed. Philadelphia: Elsevier, 2005, pp. 256.

location, as with focal ischemic or hemorrhagic infarction, but multifocal or nonspecific involvement may also be present. Stroke from multiple emboli may cause multifocal neurological symptoms but are often limited to a vascular distribution. Venous infarctions may manifest as headache and nonspecific neurological complaints.

Acute sensory or motor deficits, including numbness or weakness, particularly on one side of the body, are suggestive of stroke in the contralateral hemisphere. Acute aphasia with difficulty speaking or understanding should raise concern about a dominant hemisphere stroke involving branches of the middle cerebral artery territory. Visual impairment may occur in one eye if the ipsilateral ophthalmic artery is occluded. A visual field deficit may be present in both eyes if arterial supply to the optic radiations or the occipital lobe is compromised. An acute difficulty in gait, balance, or coordination may result from a cerebellar infarction. New-onset seizures may occur after cortical injury. A severe headache may occur with venous infarction, as in the case of superior sagittal sinus thrombosis. Large strokes involving either both hemispheres or the brainstem may produce lethargy or coma.

Diagnosis

Prompt evaluation is important in order to identify the etiology of the stroke and to guide further treatment. In documenting the history, the clinician should inquire about any recent trauma; medications, including oral contraceptives; substance abuse, including cocaine and amphetamines; underlying predisposing medical conditions; family history of coagulopathy or early stroke; and associated systemic symptoms that may be indicative of an underlying systemic condition, such as vasculitis. Evaluation of hypertension, cardiac abnormalities, bruits, funduscopic examination, and a careful neurological examination are essential.

Imaging to evaluate for infarction, hemorrhage, arteriovenous malformations, or other mass lesions affecting blood supply must be done expediently. Neuroimaging should include emergency CT if a significant hemorrhage that may necessitate neurosurgical intervention is suspected. In other cases, however, MRI is the preferred study, with magnetic resonance angiography for visualization of the vasculature. MRI also has the capability of providing diffusion-weighted images for visualization of areas of infarction and perfusion-weighted images to identify areas at risk from hypoperfusion. In neonates, ultrasonography may insert grossly show areas of hemorrhage until more definitive imaging is obtained. The head and neck may be visualized if vertebral or carotid pathological processes are suspected, as in the case of neck trauma and vertebral dissection. Cerebral angiography may be considered if vasculitis is a possibility.

If an embolic etiology is suspected, cardiac evaluation, including echocardiography and electrocardiography, is warranted. Laboratory assessment should include a basic metabolic evaluation, as well as serum and urine toxicology screening. A complete hypercoagulable evaluation should include measurement of antiphospholipid antibodies, apolipoproteins, cholesterol, erythrocytes, factor VIII C, factor IX, factor XII, homocysteine, lactate, lupus anticoagulant, plasminogen, protein S, protein C, and triglycerides; assessments for antithrombin III deficiency, sedimentation rate, factor V Leiden mutation (activated protein C resistance), and prothrombin G20210A mutation; and a complete blood cell count.

Treatment

The treatment of the acute cerebral injury caused by pediatric stroke is primarily supportive. With large strokes, intracranial pressure and vital signs need to be closely monitored and treated. Significant edema or hemorrhage necessitate surgical intervention. Seizures may occur and should be treated accordingly. In the case of hemorrhage, prophylactic anticonvulsant therapy should be considered.

If a cause is found, treatment of the predisposing condition is warranted. Data regarding the efficacy of various treatments, dosages, and duration of therapy are insufficient. Accumulating evidence regarding heparin, warfarin, and aspirin in children supports the safety and tolerability of these agents. Their use is similar to that in adulthood stroke, although optimal strategies are still under investigation.

Developmental and Behavioral Implications

Neuropsychological deficits secondary to stroke include cognitive delay; language impairment; and disturbances in visual memory, perceptual organization, and processing speed.[56] One study showed no difference in IQ between children with sinovenous stroke and those with arterial ischemic stroke; both were in the normal range.[57] Comorbid seizures herald poorer outcomes, including lower intelligence, social impairment, nonspecific behavioral problems, and limitations in the child's activities of daily living.[58-60] Different locations of stroke lead to different developmental outcomes. For example, approximately 60% of children with subcortical stroke have motor deficits.[56]

Overall, most neonates who have had a cerebral infarction have good neurodevelopmental outcomes, with significant recovery of motor functions, and one third ultimately have normal long-term development.[61,62] Prenatal or perinatal unilateral brain damage from stroke, especially in the parietal region, results in a disturbance in facial recognition ability that is independent of the side of the lesion.[63] Perinatal arterial ischemic stroke in neonates lead rates of cerebral palsy, epilepsy, language de behavioral problems.[64]

TRAUMATIC BRAIN INJURY

Significance

TBI is the most common cause of neurological morbidity in children in the United States, resulting in a significant effect on society.[65] Most frequent are insignificant head injuries without loss of consciousness in young children. More severe injuries may significantly impair developmental progress.

Definition

TBI may result from either closed or open head injuries. Closed head injury refers to a nonpenetrating skull injury and accounts for the majority of pediatric head trauma. This type of blunt trauma may result in vascular and/or brain parenchymal injury. Arterial and/or venous hemorrhage may result in epidural or subdural hematoma. Parenchymal injury may occur as a result of either diffuse axonal injury or cerebral contusion, explained further in this section. The secondary effects of such injury further impair developmental outcome.

Open head injuries—that is, those penetrating the skull—often result in a broader range of injury. Hemorrhage and infection are more likely to occur as a result of disruption of the integrity of the blood-brain barrier. Parenchymal injury may result from diffuse axonal shear injury, cerebral contusion, or direct parenchymal injury caused by the skull itself or a foreign object.

The Glasgow Coma Scale was designed to provide an efficient and standardized assessment of level of consciousness after TBI. Scoring is dependent on eye opening, motor responsiveness, and verbal responsiveness (Table 10E-9). A higher score denotes increased level of consciousness; 15 denotes normal. 12 to 14 denote mild TBI, 9 to 11 denote moderate TBI, and less than 8 denotes severe injury. The lowest attainable score is 3, indicating complete unresponsiveness and severe coma. Glasgow Coma Scale scoring overall is well correlated with mortality.[66] The correlation with other prognoses is less clear.

This scale has been adapted for children as the Pediatric Coma Scale, the Pediatric Glasgow Coma Scale, and the Modified Glasgow Coma Scale for more accurate and reliable assessment of verbal function in younger children. Pediatric Coma Scale scores have been shown to be correlated broadly with neurological outcome.[67]

TABLE 10E-9 ■ Glasgow Coma Scale	
Response	Score
Eye Opening	
Spontaneously	4
To speech	3
To pain	2
None	1
Motor Response	
Obeys	6
Localizes	5
Withdraws	4
Abnormal flexion	3
Abnormal extension	2
None	1
Verbal Response	
Oriented	5
Confused conversation	4
Inappropriate words	3
Incomprehensible sounds	2
None	1

Etiology and Pathophysiology

In children, TBI commonly results from falls, motor vehicle accidents, abuse, and physical activities, including sports. In the newborn population, perinatal injury accounts for most depressed skull fractures. Severe falls resulting in a depressed skull fracture is a common mode of open skull injury in older children. In older children and adolescents, sports activities account for approximately 300,000 concussions per year.[68] An important cause of closed head injury is "nonaccidental" trauma, or shaking injury. This occurs most frequently during the first year of life and accounts for a significant number of cases of inflicted trauma and associated morbidity and mortality. The incidence has been estimated between near 30 per 100,000 person-years.[69] The mortality rate is estimated at 13% to 36%.[70]

Closed head trauma results from the acceleration-deceleration forces applied to the brain. A shearing force is often created when adjacent tissue moves in opposite directions, depending on the location and magnitude of the force applied. This may result in injury to brain parenchyma and blood vessels. An acceleration force may cause a compression injury at the site of impact (coup injury), as well as injury on the opposite side of the skull (contrecoup injury). The inferior frontal and temporal lobes are particularly susceptible to this type of injury.

Diffuse axonal injury occurs from stretching or shearing of axonal connections to and from the cortex. This mode of injury may occur in the cerebrum, cerebellum, or brainstem. Injury may range from mild cognitive difficulty to severe or even fatal injury if brainstem connections are sufficiently involved. Evidence of injury may be found on examination and on imaging. Cerebral contusion, or bruising of the brain, may also be present when a large area of parenchyma is injured, with resultant hemorrhage and edema.

Open or penetrating head injury from either a depressed skull fracture or a foreign body may cause cerebral lacerations, in addition to arterial and venous injury. Hemorrhage may occur, as in closed head injury, although epidural hematoma is more likely because of the susceptibility of the middle meningeal artery to laceration with skull fracture. The risk of infection rises because of tearing of the meninges, which sets the stage for abscesses or meningoencephalitis, which in turn may further cause injury and potentially worsen prognosis.

In addition to the primary injury incurred from closed or open TBI, secondary damage may result from cerebral swelling, arterial or venous hemorrhage, ischemic injury, increased intracranial pressure, and excitotoxic and free radical-induced cell injury and death. This secondary injury accounts for many of the long-term developmental complications seen in more severe cases of TBI.

Such injury can be prevented through appropriate safety measures, including proper use of seat belts, car seats, helmets, protective sports gear, and proper storage of weapons.

Clinical Characteristics

Initial evaluation includes rapid assessment and assignment of a Glasgow Coma Scale or Pediatric Coma Scale score. A brief but focused neurological examination should occur, as should assessment and treatment of other significant injuries concurrently.

Neonatal assessment should include examination of the anterior fontanel. Depressed consciousness, poor suck or feeding, bradycardia, apnea, or other cardiorespiratory abnormalities may be suggestive of increased intracranial pressure in a newborn with a depressed skull fracture. Seizures may also occur with severe injury.

Infants may present with depressed consciousness, irritability, and seizures after TBI. Retinal hemorrhages found on funduscopic examination in an infant are evidence of nonaccidental trauma. When abuse is suspected, evidence of other and prior injury must be sought, the safety of the child must be ensured, and the appropriate protection agencies must be contacted.

Children and adolescents with TBI commonly present with depressed consciousness. Loss of consciousness may or may not occur, although generally occurs with more severe injury. A child may show impairment immediately after injury or may begin to decline several minutes to hours afterwards; thus, observation after injury is essential. Confusion, agitation, mood changes, and disorientation may also be present after acute injury. Progressive decline of consciousness, confusion, and development of other signs, including nausea and vomiting, are suggestive of increased intracranial pressure or herniation, necessitating emergency evaluation and treatment.

Focal neurological deficits may be present with open skull injury, and they are correlated with the area of involvement, as well as the extent of injury. Amnesia is often associated with TBI. This includes amnesia for the event itself, with a brief retrograde amnesia immediately before, and variable anterograde amnesia after.

As defined by the American Academy of Neurology, a concussion is a trauma-induced alteration in mental status, which may or may not involve loss of consciousness.[71] Concussions are characterized by confusion and amnesia for the event. Neuroimaging may show evidence of injury, which may not necessarily be well correlated with cognitive outcome.

Clinically, coup or contrecoup injuries may result in cerebral contusion, or bruising, with radiographic evidence of petechial hemorrhage and edema. The inferior brain surfaces adjacent to the skull are most susceptible; thus, severe injury may be detected in the inferior frontal or temporal lobes. The resultant vascular injury often accounts for most of the injury afterwards.

Diagnosis

The history and examination often yield clues to the mechanism and severity of head injury. Neuroimaging is most readily available through CT, which demonstrates skull fractures and hemorrhages, as well as parenchymal injury. Further assessment with MRI yields higher resolution of the brain parenchyma and may demonstrate more subtle areas of hemorrhage and edema, as may occur with mild diffuse axonal injury. In a symptomatic child, serial neurological examinations are warranted, as is repeat imaging if neurological deterioration is suspected.

Other studies are not routinely indicated in the evaluation of TBI. There are emerging data that serum markers of neuronal injury may indicate and be correlated with the extent of injury in TBI. Most notable are S100B protein and neuronal specific enolase, levels of which have been shown to have a good correlation with Glasgow Coma Scale score and may aid in indicating outcome.[72] The effect of TBI on the neurochemical systems and behavior are poorly understood and being explored.

Treatment

Acute management of TBI is primarily supportive dependent on the severity and location of injury. Acute interventions attempt to minimize the extent of injury to the brain, primarily from secondary complications such as cerebral edema and hemorrhage. Secondary complications of more severe injury may include seizures, stroke, hemorrhage, and increased intracranial pressure. Subacute complications include pneumocephalus after basilar skull fractures, persistent CSF leakage, posthemorrhagic hydrocephalus, and skull deformities.

In the long term, assessment and monitoring of neurological deficits and developmental progress is vital. Close monitoring enables the clinician to determine appropriate rehabilitation to maximize developmental and psychosocial outcomes.

Developmental and Behavioral Implications

Many developmental and behavioral domains can be affected by TBI and depend on time since injury and on location and severity of injury. Although a developing brain has more plasticity, and may thus have better outcome, than the adult brain, extensive injury may limit a child's ability to acquire given functions, which may have a significant effect on academic performance, behavior, and psychosocial outcome. Table 10E-10 lists the major domains affected by significant TBI.

With an acute concussion or closed head injury, the patient may exhibit confusion, disorientation, agitation, and mood changes in the period immediately after injury. Amnesia is also often present, as described previously. This typically improves so that only a brief period of amnesia, consisting of the moments preceding injury, as well as the injury itself, may remain. Over time, the delirium may resolve, or the patient may develop a postconcussion disorder. The prevalence of these immediate symptoms has been estimated between 80% and 100% in the first month after injury.[73] Persistence past 1 year occurs in a minority of patients with mild TBI; however, most patients have resolution of symptoms by 3 months.[73]

Postconcussion disorder may include many symptoms, such as fatigue, headaches, and sleep difficulty. Behavioral changes may include anxiety, aggression, depression, and emotional lability.[74] Cognitive effects such as slow information processing, inattentiveness, impaired concentration, and poor judgment are commonly reported.[74,75] It has been suggested the prolonged persistence of symptoms may be driven by underlying psychological factors rather than organic neurological impairment. Brief psychological

TABLE 10E-10 ■ Consequences of Significant Traumatic Brain Injury in Childhood	
Domain	**Deficit**
Language	Reduced expressive skills Impaired pragmatics
Motor skills	Gross motor problems Poor balance Fine and visuomotor incoordination
Memory	Reduced learning Poor storage skills Retrieval problems
Attention	Fluctuating attention Impulsivity
Executive function	Poor planning and organization Impaired reasoning Reduced monitoring
Education	Poor reading comprehension Poor mathematics Slow, untidy writing
Behavior/social skills	Social difficulties Reduced self-esteem Irritability Low frustration tolerance

From Anderson V: Pediatric head injury: Consequences of significant TBI in childhood. *In* Rizzo M, Eslinger P, eds: Principles and Practice of Behavioral Neurology and Neuropsychology. Philadelphia: Elsevier, 2004, p 872.

treatment may help reduce the severity and duration of symptoms.[76]

In children experiencing more severe TBI and diffuse injury, behavioral and cognitive problems have persisted for years after injury. Risk factors for persistent behavioral problems included socioeconomic disadvantage and adverse family outcomes, in addition to underlying neurological injury.[77] In general, a more severe injury increases the probability of longer-lasting cognitive and behavioral effects. Common deficits with more severe or diffuse TBI include slowed information processing speed, impaired attention and concentration, impaired learning, personality changes, and memory difficulty.[78] Effects on verbal learning and memory may outlast other symptoms. Frontal lobe injury may result in poor planning, poor organization, poor judgment, poor abstraction, and impulsiveness.[79] In one study, behavioral, emotional, memory, and attention problems were reported by one third of subjects with severe injury, 25% with moderate injury, and 10% to 18% with mild injury.[80] Personality changes were most prevalent in subjects with severe TBI, and social deprivation was significantly correlated with a poorer outcome. In a series of children with severe head injury before preschool age, 30% were found to have below-average IQ scores when retested as adults.[81]

The affective and cognitive dysfunction present after TBI results in part from the susceptibility of the frontal and temporal lobes to injury, in view of their placement in the base of the skull. Injury to the frontal and temporal lobes, notably the hippocampus and limbic system, may result in personality changes, disinhibition, affective disorders, memory impairment, and executive dysfunction.[82,83] Subtle slowing of reaction times and overall motor slowing have also been reported, independent of other cognitive deficits.[84]

Neurological and behavioral disorders have been described to emerge long after TBI. These include significant increases in rates of depression, seizures, and behavioral problems.[85] The risk of each of these is greatly increased with a second TBI. The incidence of depression after TBI has been found to range between 10% and 77%.[86] Psychosis and mania occurs in rare cases. Phobias, academic difficulties, rage attacks, and episodic depression occurred in a pediatric series with minor trauma, including head injury.[87] Negative social outcomes among children with moderate to severe TBI result from deficits in executive functions, pragmatic language, and social problem solving.[88]

Post-traumatic seizures after TBI have been well described. *Immediate seizures* occur within 1 hour of injury, and *early seizures* occur within the first week after injury. Many studies have found early seizures associated with a 15% to 50% increased risk of late post-traumatic seizures.[89] The risk of late-onset seizures has been associated with acute hematoma, depressed skull fracture, and early seizures.[90] Late-onset seizures appear to have a prevalence lower than the 5% reported for adults with TBI.[89] Tics have also been observed less frequently after TBI, without any clear association on neuroimaging.[91]

Penetrating brain injury is associated with higher rates of CNS and other systemic complications and comorbid conditions than are closed head injury cases.[92] A case series of 780 pediatric patients with gunshot injuries revealed that younger age was associated with poorer neurological outcome.[93]

Secondary attention-deficit disorder has been reported in approximately 16% of children in the first 6 months after injury, 15% between 6 and 12 months after injury, and 21% in the second year after injury.[94,95]

Infants who survive TBI as a result of shaken-infant syndrome have a very poor long-term prognosis, correlated with injury severity. In one case series, sequelae included motor deficits (60%), visual deficits (48%), epilepsy (20%), speech and language abnormalities (64%), and behavioral problems (52%).[70] The severity and outcome with inflicted head injury are worse than in any other type of childhood head injury overall.[96]

TBI causes significant family concern and hardship, leaving families vulnerable to further disruption from family conflict.[97,98] Family reactions to their child's TBI can include stages such as shock, expectancy, reality, mourning, and finally adjustment.[99]

Neurological function should be monitored carefully after TBI. Neuropsychological testing is useful for quantifying and monitoring cognitive deficits over time. Behavioral changes such as post-traumatic stress disorder may occur and should be monitored with the use of appropriate behavioral rating scales. In difficult cases, appropriate pharmacotherapy to aid in behavioral management may be necessary. Communication with a child's teacher or school may be helpful in managing such changes. Several TBI-specific assessments have been created, including the Rivermead Post-Concussion Symptoms Questionnaire and the Galveston Orientation and Amnesia Test.[100,101] These tools appear to be useful adjuncts to neuropsychiatric testing.

Assessment and close surveillance of development after injury is important for providing appropriate services and aiding families in coping with the emotional trauma of TBI. Evaluation by physical, occupational, and/or speech therapists should be considered, depending on the extent of injury. Repeat neuroimaging after the acute period may be helpful in defining the extent of chronic injury. Long-term MRI changes, particularly loss of hippocampal volume, have been shown to be of greater prognostic significance than initial severity of injury.[102] Such hippocampal atrophy is correlated with impaired memory and executive functions. White matter injury has been shown to be correlated with slower visual and reaction times.[103]

TUMORS OF THE CENTRAL NERVOUS SYSTEM

Significance

In children, brain tumors are the second most common cause of cancer death, and their overall incidence is estimated between 1 and 5 per 100,000.[104,105] In addition to the effects of the tumor itself, the lasting effects of treatment, including surgery, chemotherapy, and radiation, may adversely affect the development of a child.

Definition and Etiology

Tumors arising from CNS tissue are termed *primary,* as opposed to *metastatic* tumors. Primary tumors in young children are predominantly supratentorial in location. After 4 years of age, they generally occur in the posterior and middle fossa. In adults, the most frequent location again becomes supratentorial within the cerebral hemispheres. The reasons for the shift in locations according to age are not known.

In most children, there are no clear factors predisposing to CNS tumors, even in family history. Most tumors in patients younger than 2 years of age are congenital, differing in etiology and behavior from tumors in older children. Certain genetic syndromes, such as neurofibromatosis, tuberous sclerosis, or ataxia-telangiectasia, may be associated with an increased risk of specific tumor types. The genetics of certain tumors are better understood, as in the case of retinoblastoma; however, an understanding of the pathophysiological processes of most CNS tumors remains poor. Active research is under way to identify genetic loci associated with tumor predisposition and to understand the role of oncogenes in carcinogenesis.

Brain tumors in childhood may be classified according to their location. Table 10E-11 lists the most common tumor types in children and their location. Classifying by type, gliomas are the most frequent pediatric brain tumor, constituting approximately 70% of cases. Of gliomas, astrocytoma accounts for 30%, medulloblastoma for 20%, and ependymoma for 10%.[106]

Clinical Characteristics

Brain tumors cause a variety of neurological symptoms, depending on their location. More diffuse neurological symptoms may predominate if increased intracranial pressure is present, whereas focal neurological abnormalities may occur with localized tumors that impair specific functions.

Infants may present with more subtle signs, including irritability, listlessness, vomiting, failure to thrive, and progressive macrocephaly.[107] In one large series of children with tumors in the first year of life, Raimondi and Tomita[108] found that hydrocephalus was present in 82% and that progressive enlargement of head circumference was the most common reason for referral. In older children, increased intracranial pressure may cause headache, lethargy, and nausea and/or vomiting. Focal lesions may result in vision or hearing problems, behavioral and cognitive problems, motor problems, and incoordination. In a review of 200 patients, Ferris and colleagues[109] found headache to be the most common symptom in childhood brain tumors (56%), followed by vomiting, behavioral problems, unsteadiness, and visual problems. The most common abnormalities found on neurological examination included cranial nerve abnormalities (49%), cerebellar signs (48%), and papilledema (38%).[109] Seizures may arise from either focal cerebral abnormality or increased intracranial pressure.

TABLE 10E-11 ■ Brain Tumors in Children

Supratentorial Tumors

Angioma
Astrocytoma
Central neurocytoma
Dysembryoplastic neuroepithelial tumor
Ependymoma
Meningioma
Metastatic tumors
Oligodendroglioma
Primitive neuroectodermal tumors (PNETs)

Ventricular Tumors

Choroid plexus papilloma
Colloid cyst
Giant cell astrocytoma
Meningioma

Midline Tumors (involving thalamus, hypothalamus, optic pathways, pineal region)

Astrocytoma
Choroid plexus papilloma
Craniopharyngioma
Ependymoma
Germ cell tumors
Glioma
Pineal parenchymal tumors

Posterior Fossa Tumors

Astrocytoma
Brainstem tumors
Ependymoma
Hemangioblastoma
Medulloblastoma

With progressive expansion of a focal mass eventually comes increased intracranial pressure, resulting either from obstruction of CSF flow or, in the rare case of choroid plexus papillomas, from overproduction of CSF. With severe increased intracranial pressure from a large mass effect or compromised CSF flow, the Cushing triad of hypertension, irregular respiratory rate, and bradycardia may be seen. Herniation, most often of the cerebellar tonsils, may then occur, to be followed by brainstem dysfunction and death.

Diagnosis

The diagnosis of a tumor begins with a careful history and neurological examination, including funduscopic examination. Headaches associated with increased intracranial pressure tend to be of new onset and progressive, often worse in the morning and worsened by cough or Valsalva maneuver. If tumor is suspected, then neuroimaging via MRI or CT is required for diagnosis. Imaging of the spine may also reveal involvement of the spinal cord with certain tumors.

After an abnormality has been found, further imaging may be necessary to further identify the type of mass found, because different tumors have their own imaging characteristics. MRI enhancement with gadolinium improves delineation of a tumor and aids in correct identification.

Ancillary studies include lumbar puncture for measurement of intracranial pressure, as well as for cell count and differential, protein, and glucose, and cytological assessment, which may aid in identifying an abnormality. Because of the risk of herniation with a lumbar puncture, neuroimaging should be obtained first if a mass lesion is suspected. EEG monitoring is warranted if seizures are present or suspected. In some cases, positron emission tomography and magnetic resonance spectroscopy may be useful in diagnosis.

Treatment

Available treatment options include surgery, radiation, and chemotherapy. If there is significant edema or increased intracranial pressure, steroids may be administered to improve symptoms and facilitate surgery. Surgical biopsy may be diagnostic, and resection, if possible, aims at maximizing tumor removal while avoiding significant neurological deficits. Modern advances have improved the safety of resective surgery.

Radiation therapy is useful as an adjunct to surgical resection or as the primary means of treatment for some inoperable malignancies. Improvements in radiotherapy techniques have minimized toxicity to brain tissue adjacent to targeted areas with the goal of improved cognitive outcome.[106]

Chemotherapy is frequently adjunctive to surgical therapy or is the primary treatment for nonresectable tumors. Many chemotherapeutic agents themselves have neurotoxic potential adverse effects. Various chemotherapeutic regimens exist for different malignant tumors.

Developmental and Behavioral Implications

Greater cognitive declines in children with CNS tumors can be attributed to rapid tumor growth rate; location in the supratentorial and hypothalamic regions; younger age at onset; and treatment effects of surgery, radiation, and chemotherapy.[110] These factors also affect memory, visual-spatial processing, and attention, which creates learning disabilities.[110] Significant behavioral problems are seen in half of children with CNS tumors and include depression, oppositional behavior, anxiety, and hyperactivity.[110]

The extent of developmental and functional impairment caused by a tumor depends on its size, location, and rate of growth. Treatment itself is associated with substantial development and neurological morbidity. One study revealed impairments on measures of motor output, verbal memory, and visual-spatial organization in children after tumor resection; this finding reflects a moderate degree of neuropsychological morbidity before stereotactic radiation therapy.[111] Thus, the tumor and surgery itself appear to be associated with neurocognitive impairment, even before radiation treatment. Inattentiveness and slow reaction times have also been described in children after tumor resection without radiation treatment.[112]

Younger age is associated with worse developmental outcomes and IQ decline.[113] Children younger than 7 years appear to fare worse in terms of academic achievement and overall cognitive function.[114] Those younger than 2 years have an even poorer prognosis with regard to mortality, morbidity, and quality of life.[115] Survivors treated with surgery and chemotherapy generally have better intellectual functioning than do patients treated with surgery and radiation, with or without chemotherapy.[115]

Radiotherapy has well-described long-term cognitive effects. The mechanism of injury appears to be radiation-induced vascular injury. This results in small-vessel thrombosis and infarction, causing white matter injury. During acute radiation treatment, this may result in edema and injury to small blood vessels, which in turn result in fatigue and encephalopathy.

Long-term complications include cognitive difficulties, impaired growth, and increased risk of later malignancies. Cognitive decline may occur as long as a decade after irradiation.[116] With irradiated posterior fossa tumors, Full-Scale IQ score continues to decline more than 4 years after the diagnosis, although the rate of decline slows over time.[117] In patients undergoing local or whole brain irradiation, the incidence of Full-Scale IQ decline reported ranges from 10% to 80%.[118] Impairments in verbal fluency, short-term memory, visual-spatial skills, and fine motor skills; learning disabilities; dementia; and mental retardation have been described in children after irradiation.[108,118,119] Newer techniques to limit radiation exposure may improve cognitive outcome without worsening disease control.

Children treated with chemotherapy alone are also at risk for cognitive decline; however, the effects do not appear to be as severe as with radiation therapy.[116] In particular, frequent, high-dose administration of methotrexate is linked to a higher incidence of cognitive dysfunction.[116] Regardless of the treatment rendered, children with brain tumors require close monitoring of developmental progress and neurological function.

Associated long-term effects of treatment include impaired growth, precocious puberty, hypothyroidism, poor nutrition, increased risk of stroke, increased risk of secondary tumors, sleep abnormalities, and significant emotional difficulties.[120] Survivors of CNS tumors reportedly were more likely than controls to have educational problems and fewer close friends.[121] Brain tumor survivors and their parents have been reported to experience symptoms of post-traumatic stress disorder.[122] Ongoing counseling and education have been advocated in order to maximize quality of life and social-emotional functioning in children with brain tumors.[123]

NEUROCUTANEOUS DISORDERS

Significance

The most common neurocutaneous disorders are neurofibromatosis and tuberous sclerosis. These disorders consist of CNS abnormalities and unique associated skin findings. They are also associated with various systemic findings and often include a predisposition to neoplasms. Their effect on development varies in severity, depending on the disorder and its phenotype.

The basis of these disorders is a common embryological formation. Both the skin and the CNS are derived from neural crest cells. Specific genetic abnormalities are associated with some of these disorders.

Neurofibromatosis

Neurofibromatosis (NF), also referred to as von Recklinghausen disease, is inherited in an autosomal dominant manner. Neurofibromatosis may be divided into types 1 (NF-1) and 2 (NF-2). NF-1 affects primarily the CNS, whereas NF-2 affects the peripheral nervous system.

NF-1 is the most common neurocutaneous disorder, with an incidence of 2 to 3 per 10,000 live births.[124] The genetic abnormality occurs on chromosome 17q, and a variety of different mutations have been described. The abnormal gene product has been termed *neurofibromin*. The phenotype for NF-1 is somewhat variable, although two of the following seven findings must be present for diagnosis: (1) six or more café-au-lait spots larger than 5 mm in prepubertal individuals, or larger than 15 mm in postpubertal individuals; (2) two or more neurofibromas, or one plexiform neurofibroma; (3) axillary or inguinal freckling; (4) greater than two iris hamartomas (Lisch nodules); (5) optic glioma; (6) osseous lesion (sphenoidal dysplasia, long bone thinning); and (7) an affected first-degree relative. Café-au-lait spots, peripheral neurofibromas, and Lisch nodules are the most common manifestations.

NF-2 is less prevalent than NF-1, and at least one of the following is required for diagnosis: (1) bilateral cranial nerve VIII tumors (vestibular schwannomas); (2) an affected first-degree relative with NF-2 and either unilateral cranial nerve VIII mass, or two of the following: neurofibroma, meningioma, glioma, schwannoma, or juvenile posterior subscapular lenticular opacity.

The diagnosis is made on clinical grounds according to criteria just mentioned. Affected individuals require ophthalmologic examinations for development of Lisch nodules and brain MRI imaging if optic glioma is suspected. There is an increased risk of various tumors, including peripheral system tumors, optic pathway gliomas, meningiomas, and gliomas.[125] There is also an increased incidence of non-neural tumors.

Several cognitive deficits have been described in children with NF-1, including nonverbal and verbal learning disabilities in approximately 30% to 65%, as well as deficits in IQ, executive function, attention, and motor skills.[126] Dysfunction in visual perception and in visual-spatial skills, executive skills (planning and abstract concept formation), and attention (sustained and switching) has also been described.[127] Rates of mental retardation are 8 to 10% higher than in the general population.[128] Brain MRI imaging may reveal multifocal areas of increased signal, which may be associated with slightly lower IQ in this subset of patients with neurofibromatosis.[129]

Tuberous Sclerosis

Tuberous sclerosis complex is an autosomal dominant disorder with variable phenotypic expression. Mutations in the genes *TSC1* on chromosome 9q34 and *TSC2* on chromosome 16p13.3 are responsible for the disorder. There is no clear difference in phenotype based on whether *TSC1* or *TSC2* is affected.

The most common clinical manifestations of tuberous sclerosis include seizures, mental retardation, renal abnormalities, and hypopigmented ash-leaf spots. Table 10E-12 lists the proposed clinical criteria for diagnosis. Brain MRI reveals characteristic cortical tubers, or hamartomas. Other systemic manifestations include retinal hamartomas, cardiac rhabdomyomas, renal angiomyolipomas, and other tumors of bone and lung. Infantile spasms are

---

TABLE 10E-12 ■ Diagnostic Criteria for Tuberous Sclerosis Complex

Major Features

Facial angiofibromas or forehead plaque
Nontraumatic ungual or periungual fibroma
Hypomelatonic macules (three or more)
Shagreen patch (connective-tissue nevus)
Multiple retinal nodular hamartomas
Cortical tubers
Subependymal nodule
Subependymal giant-cell astrocytoma
Cardiac rhabdomyoma, single or multiple
Lymphangiomyomatosis
Renal angiomyolipoma

Minor Features

Multiple, randomly distributed pits in dental enamel
Hamartomatous rectal polyps
Bone cysts
Cerebral white matter radial migration lines
Gingival fibromas
Nonrenal hamartoma
Retinal achromic patch
"Confetti" skin lesions
Multiple renal cysts

Definite Tuberous Sclerosis Complex

Either two major features or one major feature plus two minor features

Probable Tuberous Sclerosis Complex

One major plus one minor feature

Possible Tuberous Sclerosis Complex

Either one major feature or two or more minor features

From Roach ES, DiMario FJ, Kandt RS, et al: Tuberous Sclerosis Consensus Conference: Recommendations for diagnostic evaluation. National Tuberous Sclerosis Association. J Child Neurol 14:401-407, 1999.

---

a common seizure type in infancy, and at least mild developmental delay is often present. As the child ages, intractable epilepsy and mental retardation may occur.

The incidence of mental retardation is variable. Approximately half of individuals diagnosed with tuberous sclerosis complex have global intellectual impairment.[130] Even those with normal cognitive function have an increased risk of behavioral, learning, and other psychiatric disorders. An autistic phenotype also has been described. A series of 21 children revealed that 24% met *Diagnostic and Statistical Manual of Mental Disorders,* 4th edition (*DSM-IV*), criteria for autism, and another 19% met criteria for pervasive developmental disorder not otherwise specified.[131] Frequent seizures and the side effects of anticonvulsant medications may compound underlying difficulties.

Other Neurocutaneous Syndromes

Sturge-Weber syndrome is characterized by a facial port-wine stain in the distribution of cranial nerve V. Associated abnormalities include glaucoma and leptomeningeal angioma. Epilepsy, which may be severe, occurs in approximately 75% of patients.[132] Mental retardation, hemiparesis, and hemiatrophy also occur. Of the affected children with seizures in the first year of life, approximately 80% have developmental delay. Other children exhibit learning disabilities, attention disorders, and behavioral disturbances.[133]

Ataxia-telangiectasia has classic dermatological findings, as well as CNS manifestations and autoimmune dysfunction. Choreoathetosis or ataxia develops during the first year of life, followed by abnormal eye movements. Telangiectasias develop over the bulbar conjunctivae, ears, face, and flexor surfaces. There is an increased risk of sinopulmonary infections and malignancies. There is normal development initially, followed by regression. Approximately one third of affected children have mental retardation.[134]

Incontinentia pigmenti is a rare X-linked disorder with characteristic skin lesions. Blister-like lesions appear in infancy, progressing to vesiculobullous lesions in a linear pattern on the trunk or extremities. These then evolve into hyperpigmented macules, which may be linear or occur in whorls. Seizures may occur, and mental retardation is reported in 15% of sporadic cases and 3% of familial cases.[135]

Linear sebaceous nevus manifests with multiple epidermal nevi, which enlarge with age. Severe epilepsy often occurs, and mental retardation is present in approximately 50% to 60% of affected patients.[136]

Xeroderma pigmentosum consists of a group of disorders with photosensitivity and progressive neurological deterioration. Defects in DNA repair result in the predisposition to skin cancer. Microcephaly and cognitive deterioration occur.

Any child with potential neurocutaneous lesions should undergo further neurological evaluation to aid in diagnosis, so that proper management, prognostic information, and genetic counseling may be provided.

CONCLUSION

The presence of underlying neurological dysfunction may have significant developmental and behavioral implications on the infant and child, as well as on the family. The neurological examination is a useful screening tool in identifying neurological disorders. Within this high-risk population, developmental, neuropsychological, academic, behavioral, and psychiatric assessments are necessary to prevent and ameliorate adverse outcomes.

REFERENCES

1. Riviello JJ: Neurological examination. *In* Maria BL, ed: Current Management in Child Neurology. Hamilton, Ontario: BC Decker, 1999, pp 24-29.
2. Volpe JJ: Neurological examination: Normal and abnormal features. *In* Volpe JJ, ed: Neurology of the Newborn. Philadelphia: WB Saunders, 2001, pp 103-133.
3. Hauser WA, Annegers JF, Kurland LT: Prevalence of epilepsy in Rochester, Minnesota: 1940-1980. Epilepsia 32:429-445, 1991.
4. Annegers JF: The epidemiology of epilepsy. *In* Wyllie E, ed: The Treatment of Epilepsy: Principles and Practice. Philadelphia: Lippincott Williams & Wilkins, 2001, pp 131-138.
5. Astradsson A, Olafsson E, Ludvigsson P, et al: Rolandic epilepsy: An incidence study in Iceland. Epilepsia 39:884-886, 1998.
6. Croona C, Kihlgren M, Lundberg S, et al: Neuropsychological findings in children with benign childhood epilepsy with centrotemporal spikes. Dev Med Child Neurol 41:813-818, 1999.
7. Weglage J, Demsky A, Pietsch M, et al: Neuropsychological, intellectual, and behavioral findings in patients with centrotemporal spikes with and without seizures. Dev Med Child Neurol 39:646-651, 1997.
8. Gulgonen S, Demirbilek V, Korkmaz B, et al: Neuropsychological functions in idiopathic occipital lobe epilepsy. Epilepsia 41:405-411, 2000.
9. Camfield P, Camfield C: Epileptic syndromes in childhood: Clinical features, outcomes, and treatment. Epilepsia 43(Suppl 3):27-32, 2002.
10. Cowan LD: The epidemiology of the epilepsies in children. Ment Retard Dev Disabil Res Rev 8:171-181, 2002.
11. Annegers JF, Rocca WA, Hauser WA: Causes of epilepsy: Contributions of the Rochester epidemiology project. Mayo Clin Proc 71:570-575, 1996.
12. Annegers JF, Hauser WA, Beghi E, et al: The risk of unprovoked seizures after encephalitis and meningitis. Neurology 38:1407-1410, 1988.
13. Gaily E, Appelqvist K, Kantola-Sorsa E, et al: Cognitive deficits after cryptogenic infantile spasms with benign seizure evolution. Dev Med Child Neurol 41:660-664, 1999.
14. Nelson KB, Ellenberg JH: Prognosis in children with febrile seizures. Pediatrics 61:720-727, 1978.
15. Smith JA, Wallace SJ: Febrile convulsions: Intellectual progress in relation to anticonvulsant therapy and to recurrence of fits. Arch Dis Child 57:104-107, 1982.
16. Practice parameter: Long-term treatment of the child with simple febrile seizures. American Academy of Pediatrics. Committee on Quality Improvement, Subcommittee on Febrile Seizures. Pediatrics 103:1307-1309, 1999.

17. Aldenkamp AP, Baker G, Mulder OG, et al: A multicenter, randomized clinical study to evaluate the effect on cognitive function of topiramate compared with valproate as add-on therapy to carbamazepine in patients with partial-onset seizures. Epilepsia 41:1167-1178, 2000.

18. Lindenmayer JP, Kotsaftis A: Use of sodium valproate in violent and aggressive behaviors: A critical review. J Clin Psychiatry 61:123-128, 2000.

19. Brent DA, Crumrine PK, Varma RR, et al: Phenobarbital treatment and major depressive disorder in children with epilepsy. Pediatrics 80:909-917, 1987.

20. Montgomery SA: Antidepressants and seizures: Emphasis on newer agents and clinical implications. Int J Clin Pract 59:1435-1440, 2005.

21. Harden CL, Goldstein MA: Mood disorders in patients with epilepsy: Epidemiology and management. CNS Drugs 16:291-302, 2002.

22. Hemmer SA, Pasternak JF, Zecker SG, et al: Stimulant therapy and seizure risk in children with ADHD. Pediatr Neurol 24:99-102, 2001.

23. Gonzalez-Heydrich J, Whitney J, Hsin O, et al: Tolerability of OROS-MPH for Treatment of ADHD Plus Epilepsy. Meeting poster presentation. Presented at the International Epilepsy Congress, Paris, 2005.

24. Shields WD: Effects of epilepsy surgery on psychiatric and behavioral comorbidities in children and adolescents. Epilepsy Behav 5(Suppl 3):S18-S24, 2004.

25. Pellock JM: Understanding co-morbidities affecting children with epilepsy. Neurology 62:S17-S23, 2004.

26. Shinnar S, Pellock JM: Update on the epidemiology and prognosis of pediatric epilepsy. J Child Neurol 17(Suppl 1):S4-S17, 2002.

27. Schubert R: Attention deficit disorder and epilepsy. Pediatr Neurol 32:1-10, 2005.

28. Dunn DW, Austin JK, Harezlak J, et al: ADHD and epilepsy in childhood. Dev Med Child Neurol 45:50-54, 2003.

29. Singhi P, Jagirdar S, Khandelwal N, et al: Epilepsy in children with cerebral palsy. J Child Neurol 18:174-179, 2003.

30. Berg AT, Shinnar S: The contributions of epidemiology to the understanding of childhood seizures and epilepsy. J Child Neurol 9(Suppl 2):19-26, 1994.

31. Bouma PA, Bovenkerk AC, Westendorp RG, et al: The course of benign partial epilepsy of childhood with centrotemporal spikes: A meta-analysis. Neurology 48:430-437, 1997.

32. Wong V: Epilepsy in children with autistic spectrum disorder. J Child Neurol 8:316-322, 1993.

33. Olsson I, Steffenburg S, Gillberg C: Epilepsy in autism and autisticlike conditions. A population-based study. Arch Neurol 45:666-668, 1988.

34. Tuchman RF, Rapin I, Shinnar S: Autistic and dysphasic children. II: Epilepsy. Pediatrics 88:1219-1225, 1991.

35. Hollander E, Dolgoff-Kaspar R, Cartwright C, et al: An open trial of divalproex sodium in autism spectrum disorders. J Clin Psychiatry 62:530-534, 2001.

36. Williams J, Steel C, Sharp GB, et al: Anxiety in children with epilepsy. Epilepsy Behav 4:729-732, 2003.

37. Ettinger AB, Weisbrot DM, Nolan EE, et al: Symptoms of depression and anxiety in pediatric epilepsy patients. Epilepsia 39:595-599, 1998.

38. Solomon GE, Pfeffer C: Neurobehavioral abnormalities in epilepsy. In Frank Y, ed: Pediatric Behavioral Neurology. Boca Raton, FL: CRC Press, 1996, pp 269-287.

39. Aldenkamp AP, Mulder OG: Psychosocial consequences of epilepsy. In Goreczny A, Hersen M, eds: Handbook of Pediatric and Adolescent Health Psychology. Boston: Allyn & Bacon, 1999, pp 105-144.

40. Barnes MA, Pengelly S, Dennis M, et al: Mathematics skills in good readers with hydrocephalus. J Int Neuropsychol Soc 8:72-82, 2002.

41. Scott MA, Fletcher JM, Brookshire BL, et al: Memory functions in children with early hydrocephalus. Neuropsychology 12:578-589, 1998.

42. Soare PL, Raimondi AJ: Intellectual and perceptual-motor characteristics of treated myelomeningocele children. Am J Dis Child 131:199-204, 1977.

43. National Institute of Neurological Diseases and Stroke: Hydrocephalus Fact Sheet. Bethesda, MD: National Institutes of Health. 2006.

44. Schrander-Stumpel C, Fryns JP: Congenital hydrocephalus: Nosology and guidelines for clinical approach and genetic counselling. Eur J Pediatr 157:355-362, 1998.

45. Laurence KM: The pathology of hydrocephalus. Ann R Coll Surg Engl 24:388-401, 1959.

46. Sarnat HB: Neuroembryology, genetic programming, and malformations of the nervous system. In Menkes JH, Sarnat HB, Maria BL, eds: Child Neurology. Philadelphia: Lippincott Williams & Wilkins, 2006, pp 259-366.

47. Emery JL, Staschak MC: The size and form of the cerebral aqueduct in children. Brain 95:591-598, 1972.

48. Laurence KM, Tew BJ: Follow-up of 65 survivors from the 425 cases of spina bifida born in South Wales between 1956 and 1962. Dev Med Child Neurol 9(Suppl 13):1-4, 1967.

49. Laurence KM: Neurological and intellectual sequelae of hydrocephalus. Arch Neurol 20:73-81, 1969.

50. Prigatano GP, Zeiner HK, Pollay M, et al: Neuropsychological functioning in children with shunted uncomplicated hydrocephalus. Childs Brain 10:112-120, 1983.

51. Futagi Y, Suzuki Y, Toribe Y, et al: Neurodevelopmental outcome in children with posthemorrhagic hydrocephalus. Pediatr Neurol 33:26-32, 2005.

52. Alvarez LA, Maytal J, Shinnar S: Idiopathic external hydrocephalus: Natural history and relationship to benign familial macrocephaly. Pediatrics 77:901-907, 1986.

53. Fullerton HJ, Wu YW, Zhao S, et al: Risk of stroke in children: Ethnic and gender disparities. Neurology 61:189-194, 2003.

54. Strater R, Becker S, von Eckardstein A, et al: Prospective assessment of risk factors for recurrent stroke during childhood—A 5-year follow-up study. Lancet 360:1540-1545, 2002.

55. Lee J, Croen LA, Backstrand KH, et al: Maternal and infant characteristics associated with perinatal arterial stroke in the infant. JAMA 293:723-729, 2005.

56. Hartel C, Schilling S, Sperner J, et al: The clinical outcomes of neonatal and childhood stroke: Review of the literature and implications for future research. Eur J Neurol 11:431-438, 2004.

57. Hetherington R, Tuff L, Anderson P, et al: Short-term intellectual outcome after arterial ischemic stroke and sinovenous thrombosis in childhood and infancy. J Child Neurol 20:553-559, 2005.

58. Ganesan V, Hogan A, Shack N, et al: Outcome after ischaemic stroke in childhood. Dev Med Child Neurol 42:455-461, 2000.

59. Hurvitz EA, Beale L, Ried S, et al: Functional outcome of paediatric stroke survivors. Pediatr Rehabil 3:43-51, 1999.

60. Laucht M, Esser G, Baving L, et al: Behavioral sequelae of perinatal insults and early family adversity at 8 years of age. J Am Acad Child Adolesc Psychiatry 39:1229-1237, 2000.

61. Miller V: Neonatal cerebral infarction. Semin Pediatr Neurol 7:278-288, 2000.

62. Sreenan C, Bhargava R, Robertson CM: Cerebral infarction in the term newborn: Clinical presentation and long-term outcome. J Pediatr 137:351-355, 2000.

63. Ballantyne AO, Trauner DA: Facial recognition in children after perinatal stroke. Neuropsychiatry Neuropsychol Behav Neurol 12:82-87, 1999.

64. Lee J, Croen LA, Lindan C, et al: Predictors of outcome in perinatal arterial stroke: A population-based study. Ann Neurol 58:303-308, 2005.

65. Kraus JF, Rock A, Hemyari P: Brain injuries among infants, children, adolescents, and young adults. Am J Dis Child 144:684-691, 1990.

66. Kuhls DA, Malone DL, McCarter RJ, et al: Predictors of mortality in adult trauma patients: The physiologic trauma score is equivalent to the Trauma and Injury Severity Score. J Am Coll Surg 194:695-704, 2002.

67. Simpson DA, Cockington RA, Hanieh A, et al: Head injuries in infants and young children: The value of the Paediatric Coma Scale. Review of literature and report on a study. Childs Nerv Syst 7:183-190, 1991.

68. Sports-related recurrent brain injuries—United States. MMWR Morb Mortal Wkly Rep 46:224-227, 1997.

69. Keenan HT, Runyan DK, Marshall SW, et al: A population-based study of inflicted traumatic brain injury in young children. JAMA 290:621-626, 2003.

70. Barlow KM, Thomson E, Johnson D, et al: Late neurologic and cognitive sequelae of inflicted traumatic brain injury in infancy. Pediatrics 116:e174-e185, 2005.

71. Practice parameter: The management of concussion in sports (summary statement). Report of the Quality Standards Subcommittee. Neurology 48:581-585, 1997.

72. Sawauchi S, Taya K, Murakami S, et al: [Serum S-100B protein and neuron-specific enolase after traumatic brain injury]. No Shinkei Geka 33:1073-1080, 2005.

73. Bohnen N, Jolles J, Twijnstra A: Neuropsychological deficits in patients with persistent symptoms six months after mild head injury. Neurosurgery 30:692-695, 1992 [discussion, Neurosurgery 30:695-696, 1992].

74. Ryan LM, Warden DL: Post concussion syndrome. Int Rev Psychiatry 15:310-316, 2003.

75. Levin HS, Mattis S, Ruff RM, et al: Neurobehavioral outcome following minor head injury: A three-center study. J Neurosurg 66:234-243, 1987.

76. Miller LJ, Mittenberg W: Brief cognitive behavioral interventions in mild traumatic brain injury. Appl Neuropsychol 5:172-183, 1998.

77. Schwartz L, Taylor HG, Drotar D, et al: Long-term behavior problems following pediatric traumatic brain injury: prevalence, predictors, and correlates. J Pediatr Psychol 28:251-263, 2003.

78. Scheid R, Walther K, Guthke T, et al: Cognitive sequelae of diffuse axonal injury. Arch Neurol 63:418-424, 2006.

79. Fortin S, Godbout L, Braun CM: Cognitive structure of executive deficits in frontally lesioned head trauma patients performing activities of daily living. Cortex 39:273-291, 2003.

80. Hawley CA, Ward AB, Magnay AR, et al: Outcomes following childhood head injury: A population study. J Neurol Neurosurg Psychiatry 75:737-742, 2004.

81. Koskiniemi M, Kyykka T, Nybo T, et al: Long-term outcome after severe brain injury in preschoolers is worse than expected. Arch Pediatr Adolesc Med 149:249-254, 1995.

82. Jorge RE, Robinson RG, Starkstein SE, et al: Depression and anxiety following traumatic brain injury. J Neuropsychiatry Clin Neurosci 5:369-374, 1993.

83. Bergeson AG, Lundin R, Parkinson RB, et al: Clinical rating of cortical atrophy and cognitive correlates following traumatic brain injury. Clin Neuropsychol 18:509-520, 2004.

84. Gray C, Cantagallo A, Della Sala S, et al: Bradykinesia and bradyphrenia revisited: Patterns of subclinical deficit in motor speed and cognitive functioning in head-injured patients with good recovery. Brain Inj 12:429-441, 1998.

85. Gualtieri T, Cox DR: The delayed neurobehavioural sequelae of traumatic brain injury. Brain Inj 5:219-232, 1991.

86. Alderfer BS, Arciniegas DB, Silver JM: Treatment of depression following traumatic brain injury. J Head Trauma Rehabil 20:544-562, 2005.

87. Basson MD, Guinn JE, McElligott J, et al: Behavioral disturbances in children after trauma. J Trauma 31:1363-1368, 1991.

88. Yeates KO, Swift E, Taylor HG, et al: Short- and long-term social outcomes following pediatric traumatic brain injury. J Int Neuropsychol Soc 10:412-426, 2004.

89. Arzimanoglou A, Guerrini R, Aicardi J: Aicardi's Epilepsy in Children, 3rd ed. Philadelphia: Lippincott Williams & Wilkins, 2004, p 516.

90. Jennett B, Miller JD, Braakman R: Epilepsy after nonmissile depressed skull fracture. J Neurosurg 41:208-216, 1974.

91. Krauss JK, Jankovic J: Tics secondary to craniocerebral trauma. Mov Disord 12:776-782, 1997.

92. Black KL, Hanks RA, Wood DL, et al: Blunt versus penetrating violent traumatic brain injury: Frequency and factors associated with secondary conditions and complications. J Head Trauma Rehabil 17:489-496, 2002.

93. Levy ML, Masri LS, Levy KM, et al: Penetrating craniocerebral injury resultant from gunshot wounds: Gang-related injury in children and adolescents. Neurosurgery 33:1018-1024, 1993 [discussion, Neurosurgery 33:1024-1015, 1993].

94. Max JE, Schachar RJ, Levin HS, et al: Predictors of attention-deficit/hyperactivity disorder within 6 months after pediatric traumatic brain injury. J Am Acad Child Adolesc Psychiatry 44:1032-1040, 2005.

95. Max JE, Schachar RJ, Levin HS, et al: Predictors of secondary attention-deficit/hyperactivity disorder in children and adolescents 6 to 24 months after traumatic brain injury. J Am Acad Child Adolesc Psychiatry 44:1041-1049, 2005.

96. Goldstein B, Kelly MM, Bruton D, et al: Inflicted versus accidental head injury in critically injured children. Crit Care Med 21:1328-1332, 1993.

97. Inzaghi MG, De Tanti A, Sozzi M: The effects of traumatic brain injury on patients and their families. A follow-up study. Eura Medicophys 41:265-273, 2005.

98. Wade SL, Taylor HG, Drotar D, et al: Parent-adolescent interactions after traumatic brain injury: Their relationship to family adaptation and adolescent adjustment. J Head Trauma Rehabil 18:164-176, 2003.

99. Ponsford J, Willmott C, Rothwell A, et al: Factors influencing outcome following mild traumatic brain injury in adults. J Int Neuropsychol Soc 6:568-579, 2000.

100. Crawford S, Wenden FJ, Wade DT: The Rivermead head injury follow up questionnaire: A study of a new rating scale and other measures to evaluate outcome after head injury. J Neurol Neurosurg Psychiatry 60:510-514, 1996.

101. Levin HS, O'Donnell VM, Grossman RG: The Galveston Orientation and Amnesia Test. A practical scale to assess cognition after head injury. J Nerv Ment Dis 167:675-684, 1979.

102. Himanen L, Portin R, Isoniemi H, et al: Cognitive functions in relation to MRI findings 30 years after traumatic brain injury. Brain Inj 19:93-100, 2005.

103. Mathias JL, Bigler ED, Jones NR, et al: Neuropsychological and information processing performance and its relationship to white matter changes following moderate and severe traumatic brain injury: A preliminary study. Appl Neuropsychol 11:134-152, 2004.

104. Berg BO: Principles of Child Neurology. New York: McGraw-Hill, Health Professions Division, 1996, p 1799.

105. Aicardi J: Diseases of the Nervous System in Childhood, 2nd ed. London: Mac Keith Press, 1999, p 491.

106. Maria BL, Menkes JH: Tumors of the central nervous system. In Menkes JH, Sarnat HB, Maria BL, ed: Child Neurology. Philadelphia: Lippincott Williams & Wilkins, 2006, pp 739-802.

107. Albright AL: Brain tumors in neonates, infants, and toddlers. Contemp Neurosurg 7:1-6, 1985.

108. Raimondi AJ, Tomita T: Brain tumors during the first year of life. Childs Brain 10:193-207, 1983.

109. Ferris R, Kennedy C, Nathwani A: Meeting Presenting Features of Brain Tumours. Presented at the International Symposium on Pediatric Neuro-oncology, Boston, 2004.

110. Duffner PK, Jackson LA, Cohen ME: Neurobehavioral abnormalities resulting from brain tumors and their therapy. In Frank Y, ed: Pediatric Behavioral Neurology. Boca Raton, FL: CRC Press, 1996, pp 302-303.

111. Carpentieri SC, Waber DP, Pomeroy SL, et al: Neuropsychological functioning after surgery in children treated for brain tumor. Neurosurgery 52:1348-1356, 2003 [discussion, Neurosurgery 52:1356-1347, 2003].

112. Merchant TE, Kiehna EN, Miles MA, et al: Acute effects of irradiation on cognition: Changes in attention on a computerized continuous performance test during radiotherapy in pediatric patients with localized primary brain tumors. Int J Radiat Oncol Biol Phys 53:1271-1278, 2002.

113. Duffner PK, Cohen ME, Parker MS: Prospective intellectual testing in children with brain tumors. Ann Neurol 23:575-579, 1988.

114. Radcliffe J, Packer RJ, Atkins TE, et al: Three- and four-year cognitive outcome in children with noncortical brain tumors treated with whole-brain radiotherapy. Ann Neurol 32:551-554, 1992.

115. Cohen BH, Packer RJ, Siegel KR, et al: Brain tumors in children under 2 years: Treatment, survival and long-term prognosis. Pediatr Neurosurg 19:171-179, 1993.

116. Duffner PK: Long-term effects of radiation therapy on cognitive and endocrine function in children with leukemia and brain tumors. Neurologist 10:293-310, 2004.

117. Kieffer-Renaux V, Viguier D, Raquin MA, et al: Therapeutic schedules influence the pattern of intellectual decline after irradiation of posterior fossa tumors. Pediatr Blood Cancer 45:814-819, 2005.

118. Duffner PK, Cohen ME: The long-term effects of central nervous system therapy on children with brain tumors. Neurol Clin 9:479-495, 1991.

119. Kieffer-Renaux V, Bulteau C, Grill J, et al: Patterns of neuropsychological deficits in children with medulloblastoma according to craniospatial irradiation doses. Dev Med Child Neurol 42:741-745, 2000.

120. Anderson NE: Late complications in childhood central nervous system tumour survivors. Curr Opin Neurol 16:677-683, 2003.

121. Barrera M, Shaw AK, Speechley KN, et al: Educational and social late effects of childhood cancer and related clinical, personal, and familial characteristics. Cancer 104:1751-1760, 2005.

122. Barakat LP, Kazak AE, Meadows AT, et al: Families surviving childhood cancer: A comparison of posttraumatic stress symptoms with families of healthy children. J Pediatr Psychol 22:843-859, 1997.

123. Sands SA, Milner JS, Goldberg J, et al: Quality of life and behavioral follow-up study of pediatric survivors of craniopharyngioma. J Neurosurg 103:302-311, 2005.

124. Rosser T, Packer RJ: Neurofibromas in children with neurofibromatosis 1. J Child Neurol 17:585-591, 2002 [discussion, 602-604, 646-651, 2002].

125. Hughes RC: Neurological complications of neurofibromatosis. In Hughes RAC, Huson SM, eds: The Neurofibromatoses: A Pathogenetic and Clinical Overview. London: Chapman & Hall, 1994, pp 204-232.

126. Rosser TL, Packer RJ: Neurocognitive dysfunction in children with neurofibromatosis type 1. Curr Neurol Neurosci Rep 3:129-136, 2003.

127. Descheemaeker MJ, Ghesquiere P, Symons H, et al: Behavioural, academic and neuropsychological profile of normally gifted neurofibromatosis type 1 children. J Intellect Disabil Res 49:33-46, 2005.

128. Riccardi VM, Eichner JE: Psychosocial aspects. In Riccardi VM, Eichner JE, eds: Neurofibromatosis: Phenotype, Natural History and Pathogenesis. Baltimore: Johns Hopkins University Press, 1986, pp 150-168.

129. North K, Joy P, Yuille D, et al: Specific learning disability in children with neurofibromatosis type 1: Significance of MRI abnormalities. Neurology 44:878-883, 1994.

130. Prather P, de Vries PJ: Behavioral and cognitive aspects of tuberous sclerosis complex. J Child Neurol 19:666-674, 2004.

131. Hunt A, Shepherd C: A prevalence study of autism in tuberous sclerosis. J Autism Dev Disord 23:323-339, 1993.

132. Sujansky E, Conradi S: Sturge-Weber syndrome: Age of onset of seizures and glaucoma and the prognosis for affected children. J Child Neurol 10:49-58, 1995.

133. Thomas-Sohl KA, Vaslow DF, Maria BL: Sturge-Weber syndrome: A review. Pediatr Neurol 30:303-310, 2004.

134. Fenichel GM: Hemiplegia. In Fenichel GM, ed: Clinical Pediatric Neurology. Philadelphia: Elsevier, 2005, pp 239-254.

135. Landy SJ, Donnai D: Incontinentia pigmenti (Bloch-Sulzberger syndrome). J Med Genet 30:53-59, 1993.

136. Lovejoy FH Jr, Boyle WE Jr: Linear nevus sebaceous syndrome: Report of two cases and a review of the literature. Pediatrics 52:382-387, 1973.

10F.
Sensory Deficits

DESMOND P. KELLY

THE SENSORY SYSTEMS

Human experience is dependent on sensory input through multiple modalities. The senses enable humans to learn about their world, to detect changes in their environment, and to adjust their behavior accordingly. Sensory input is also crucial for brain development. This is most clearly demonstrated in the phenomenon of "experience-expectant synaptogenesis," in which a sensory experience, such as visual input, is necessary for neuronal organization.[1] In this example, the visual cortex "expects, "and is genetically programmed, to usze visual stimulation, and any interruption in this sensory input has deleterious effects on brain architecture and function.

The "input" loop of the central nervous system includes the five major sensory modalities: auditory (detection of sound, or pressure waves in the air); visual (detection of light by the retina); olfactory (detection of molecules in the air by receptors high in the nasal cavity); gustatory (detection of selected organic compounds and ions by the tongue); and tactile (detection of changes in pressure, temperature, and other sensations by skin receptors). In addition, the proprioceptive system provides sensory input from the bones and joints, and the vestibular system provides the brain with input regarding the body's movement through space. Each of the sensory systems contains specialized sensory neurons that transmit nerve impulses to the central nervous system. In the brain, these signals are processed and integrated with previously acquired and stored information to yield a perception that may trigger a change in behavior. Deficits in sensation can occur at the peripheral receptor level, along the neural pathways connecting receptors to the central nervous system, or at the cortical level. In this chapter, we describe how insults to the nervous system that impede sensory function in one system may affect other senses and overall neurodevelopmental functioning.

Although all sensory modalities are active at birth, development is particularly rapid in the first 3 months, with increasingly sophisticated ability to perceive environmental stimuli. During the sensorimotor stage of development, behavioral responses to novel sensations are relatively unmodulated. Maturation of the nervous system enables more efficient processing of sensory input with regulation and modulation of responses on the basis of other potentially mitigating factors (e.g., the need to attend to auditory input from a teacher in preference to the visual input from the window into the playground).

Brain plasticity enables compensatory changes in certain conditions of sensory deficit.[2] However, the timing of the onset of the sensory deficit or its duration can have a significant effect on outcome and function. *Sensitive periods* are unique periods in brain development when specific structures or functions become especially susceptible to particular experiences in ways that alter their structure or function. Sensitive periods for vision and for hearing and language development have been clearly demonstrated. For example, exposure to a specific language in the first 6 months of life alters an infant's phonetic perceptions. This ability to distinguish sounds used in nonnative languages begins to decline by 10 to 12 months.[3] Thus, the early detection of any sensory deficit is crucial in order for intervention to optimize development and functional outcome.

HEARING IMPAIRMENT

Deficits in hearing have their most negative effect on language development and in turn can profoundly disrupt social communication and learning.[4] The manifestations of hearing impairment can be subtle during the first year or two of life, which raises the risk of missed diagnoses and neglected opportunities for intervention during a critical period of language development. Fortunately, the adoption of universal screening of hearing in newborns in the United States has significantly lowered the average age at identification of hearing loss in this country, but in many parts of the developing world, hearing impairment in children is still diagnosed too late.[5] Comprehensive programs incorporating early amplification, interventions to aid communication, support for parents and families, and surgical interventions such as cochlear implants have revolutionized management of this sensory deficit. The potential for a successful developmental outcome, even in a child with profound hearing loss, has improved significantly, but health professionals who have contact with hearing-impaired children must be knowledgeable about the multiple factors that can influence this success.

Terminology

Hearing impairment can be classified by degree, type, cause, and age at onset.[6] Hearing is measured in terms of loudness at varying frequencies of sound waves. Figure 10F-1 illustrates the frequency (pitch) and loudness (intensity) of common sounds. Speech sounds range from about 500 hertz (Hz) (vowel sounds and certain consonant sounds such as /m/ and /b/ are of lower frequency) to 4000 Hz (consonant sounds such as /s/ and /f/).[5] The degree of hearing loss is usually categorized by the average threshold for hearing (measured in decibels) across the speech frequencies. Table 10F-1 illustrates the categories and functional effects of hearing loss of varying degrees. Any hearing loss for sounds softer than 15 dB can influence speech perception in young children. People with hearing loss for sounds softer than 70 dB are sometimes referred to as "hard of hearing," and hearing loss for sounds in the 70- to 90-dB range is referred to as "partial hearing." "Deafness" denotes a profound degree of hearing loss, with a hearing threshold greater than 90dB.

The type of hearing loss is categorized by the anatomical level at which hearing is interrupted. *Conductive hearing loss* follows an interruption of the mechanical elements required for the transduction of sound waves in air into hydraulic waves in the inner ear. These elements include the pinna, the external ear canal, the tympanic membrane, and the middle ear ossicles connecting to the oval window. Accumulation of fluid in the middle ear secondary to otitis media is the most common cause of conductive hearing loss. Conductive hearing loss is usually limited to sounds softer than 50 dB, inasmuch as sounds louder than this are conducted directly via the

TABLE 10F-1 ■ Hearing Loss		
Classification	Hearing Level (dB)*	Functional Effect
Normal	0-15	None
Minimal	16-25	In children, hearing loss >15 dB can affect language development
Mild	26-30	Difficulty with soft spoken speech at distance >3 feet from source
Moderate	31-50	Conversational speech may be heard at 3 to 5 feet
Moderate to Severe	51-70	Ability to hear only very loud speech <3 feet from source; vowels but not consonants may be distinguished
Severe	71-90	Awareness of loud voices 1 foot from ear
Profound	>90	Awareness of vibrations; inability to distinguish any elements of spoken language

*Loudness at which sound is first heard.

Frequency (Hz) →	125	250	500	1000	2000	4000	8000
Hearing level (dB) ↓							
0				Leaf rustling			
10	Faucet dripping					Bird chirping	
20		"z" "v"		"p" "h" / "g"	Whisper / "k"	"f" "s" "th"	
30			Conversational speech	"ch" / "sh"			
40	"j"	"m" "d" / "b" / "h" / "n" "g" / "e" "f" / "u"	"j" / "a" / "o" / "r"				
50							
60			Baby crying		Vacuum		
70		Dog barking					
80				Piano			
90					Telephone		
100							Motorcycle
110		Lawnmower			Saw		Helicopter
120	Jack-hammer			Rock band		Jet engine	
>120			Firecracker		Gunfire		

FIGURE 10F-1. Range of familiar sounds.

temporal bone to the cochlea. *Sensorineural hearing loss* refers to involvement of the cochlea, or the neural connections to the auditory cortex via cranial nerve VIII and central pathways. The impairment typically is greater for higher frequency sounds, which are usually of lower intensity. Not infrequently, there is a combination of these types of loss, termed a *mixed hearing loss*. *Auditory neuropathy* is a neural conduction disorder that has been recognized more frequently and that has a variable prognosis.[7,8] This can occur without concomitant sensory (outer hair cell) dysfunction and involves dysfunction of the nerve conduction to the cortex. In rare cases, hearing impairment can occur centrally at the *cortical* level with difficulty related to auditory perception or discrimination.

Congenital hearing loss is present at birth. This can be *hereditary* (as an isolated disorder or part of a syndrome) or *acquired* (such as loss secondary to congenital infection). Hearing loss of postnatal onset is usually acquired, although some forms of hereditary deafness have delayed onset and can be associated with progressive loss. *Prelingual deafness* refers to hearing impairment with onset before acquisition of expressive language (2 to 3 years). *Unilateral hearing loss* can remain undetected, and is associated with behavioral difficulties and academic problems.

Epidemiology

Estimates of the prevalence of hearing loss vary, depending on populations studied; rates of congenital severe to profound bilateral sensorineural hearing loss have been reported to be 1 to 2 per 1000 live births.[6] An additional 2 to 3 persons per 1000 subsequently acquire severe loss. If cases of mild through moderately severe loss are included, this number increases further by 2 per 1000, and inclusion of unilateral hearing loss raises the incidence to 10 per 1000.[9] Populations at high risk, such as infants treated in intensive care units, have higher reported rates of 2 to 4 per 100. Since the 1960s, the incidence of acquired sensorineural hearing loss among children in developed countries has dropped as a result of medical advances in primary prevention, such as immunizations against viral infections (measles, mumps, and rubella) and bacterial causes of meningitis. In turn, there has been a relative increase in the proportion of inherited forms of hearing loss.[9] These patterns have not been seen in less developed countries, where the prevalence of consanguinity is high and both genetic and acquired forms of hearing loss are more common.

Etiology

Sensorineural hearing loss has genetic causes in 30% to 50% of cases. Prenatal insults account for 10% of cases; perinatal causes, 5% to 15%; and childhood infections, head injuries, or exposure to ototoxic medications, the remaining 20% to 30%.[10]

PRENATAL CAUSES

Deafness can be *inherited* as an autosomal dominant, autosomal recessive, or X-linked condition and can be an isolated trait or constitute one component of a recognizable syndrome. Molecular genetic testing has enabled identification of more than 60 loci for genes associated with nonsyndromic hearing impairment.[11] Autosomal recessive patterns of inheritance account for 70% to 80% of cases. Mutations in the gap junction proteins β2 and β6 (GJβ2 and GJβ6) are known to cause hearing impairment; a mutation of GJβ2, which encodes the connexin protein 26 (key to potassium homeostasis in the cochlea), has been reported as responsible for up to 50% of the hearing loss in certain populations.[12] More than 90 mutations have been described, of which the 35delG is the most common. The hearing loss is usually moderate to severe and bilateral, but it can be mild, asymmetrical, and progressive.

More than 500 syndromic forms of deafness have been identified.[11] Table 10F-2 lists the associated clinical findings in some of the more common syndromes of hearing loss. In addition, many mitochondrial genes for syndromic and nonsyndromic hearing impairment have been identified.

Prenatal *acquired* causes of hearing impairment include the congenital infections toxoplasmosis, rubella, cytomegalovirus, and herpes simplex. These infections can be asymptomatic apart from the hearing loss or can involve multiple organ systems. The hearing loss can be progressive. Prenatal exposures to toxins such as alcohol, trimethadione, and mercury have also been linked to hearing loss.[13]

PERINATAL CAUSES

Extremely premature infants are at increased risk of hearing loss as a result of various factors, including hypoxia, acidosis, hypoglycemia, hyperbilirubinemia, high levels of ambient noise, and ototoxic drugs such

TABLE 10F-2 ■ Common Hearing Loss Syndromes	
Syndrome	Associated Clinical Features
Autosomal Dominant	
Waardenburg	White forelock; heterochromia iridis Lateral displacement of inner canthus of each eye
Alport	Nephritis
Branchio-oto-renal	Branchial arch anomalies; renal anomalies; mixed hearing loss; temporal bone abnormalities may be present
Stickler	Flat facies; myopia; spondyloepiphyseal dysplasia; hypotonia
Treacher-Collins	Malar hypoplasia; downward-slanting palpebral fissures; malformation of external ear (conductive hearing loss)
Autosomal Recessive	
Usher	Retinitis pigmentosa; vestibular function absent in type 1 with profound hearing loss, normal in type 2 with moderate hearing loss, and variable in type 3 with progressive hearing loss
Pendred	Enlarged vestibular aqueduct Goiter; thyroid function can be normal
Jervell and Lange-Nielsen	Cardiac conduction problems (prolonged QT interval)

as aminoglycosides. It is likely that these influences are additive.[13] Kernicterus is now a much less common condition, but there is still uncertainty as to which levels of bilirubin are harmful in premature infants with associated stresses such as infection and acidosis. Neonatal infections, including meningitis, confer a relatively high risk for hearing loss.

POSTNATAL CAUSES

Bacterial meningitis is linked to sensorineural hearing loss in up to 10% of cases.[14] The introduction of immunizations has decreased the incidence of some forms of meningitis, but children who suffer this infection require close audiological follow-up because the hearing loss can be progressive. Viral infections such as mumps can cause hearing impairment, although this is a rare complication. Prolonged exposure to loud noise, either environmental or recreational, can damage cochlear hair cells and result in a predominantly high-frequency loss. The surge in popularity of personal audio devices, often with earphones worn within the external ear canal, has significantly raised this risk.

Causes of *conductive hearing loss* include congenital conditions such as anomalies of the pinna or external canal, as well as congenital cholesteatoma. Acquired causes of conductive loss include otitis media, ossicular discontinuity (resulting from infection, trauma, or cholesteatoma), tympanosclerosis, tumors (histiocytosis), otosclerosis, fibrous dysplasia, and osteopetrosis.[10] Conditions such as Down syndrome and cleft palate are associated with a higher risk of conductive hearing loss.

Developmental and Behavioral Effects

By as early as 26 weeks' gestation, the fetus responds behaviorally to sounds, and the newborn infant shows a preference for the mother's voice over that of other female voices. By 2 to 3 months of age, infants are able to detect and discriminate most speech sounds and recognize prosodic elements of their native language. Thus, much language development related to auditory input occurs from the earliest stages of brain development.

There are many determinants of developmental outcome in children with hearing impairment, in addition to the more obvious factors such as age at onset and degree of hearing loss. These include the origin of the hearing impairment, quality of early communication, and diversity of social experience.[15] Research findings have emphasized the critical role of early diagnosis and intervention.[16]

LANGUAGE DEVELOPMENT

Speech and language are the domains of development at greatest risk in children with hearing impairment. Children who have had the opportunity to acquire language before losing their hearing are more likely to be able to communicate orally than are those with deafness of prelingual onset. Children whose hearing loss is identified early (especially before 6 months of age) have been shown to have significantly higher language developmental quotients than do those whose loss is identified at a later age.[16] Before adoption of universal neonatal hearing screening, when the average age at diagnosis of hearing loss was 30 months, deaf children born into families with other deaf members were reported to demonstrate more advanced language skills. This probably reflected the positive effects of earlier adaptations and efforts to promote communication.[17]

MOTOR DEVELOPMENT

Although motor milestones are generally reached within the expected age ranges, some studies suggest that children with hearing loss walk at a slightly older age than do children with normal hearing.[18] There are group differences in balance, probably secondary to vestibular dysfunction.[19] Children with deafness appear to have more difficulty mastering complex motor sequences (repetitive, alternating, and sequential movements) that require mobilization of multiple muscle groups, even in the absence of other neurological disorders. Subtle differences have also been demonstrated in visual-motor skills (such as performance on video game tasks).[18] It is postulated that the hearing sensory deficit has some effect on mastery of these more complex motor actions.

COGNITIVE DEVELOPMENT

Measurement of intelligence in children with deafness is challenging and prone to inaccuracy because of the heavy emphasis on reading and language abilities in the majority of standardized intelligence tests. Although early studies suggested that deaf individuals had below-average intelligence, more recent investigations indicate that, in general, the performance of deaf children on nonverbal measures of intelligence is in the average range.[17,20] The range of intelligence varies among children with profound deafness just as it does among those with normal hearing. Debate continues as to the role of standard language in facilitating abstract thought. Deaf children, although often being described as concrete and rigid in their thinking, are reported to have creative abilities equal to those of hearing children.[17]

The cause of the hearing loss influences cognitive abilities and academic achievement.[20] Deaf students as a group are reported to have significantly lower levels of academic achievement; deaf high school graduates are reported have average reading levels at a fourth to fifth grade level, with math skills somewhat stronger, at an average seventh grade level. These data relate to children whose hearing loss, on average, was identified at an older age than is currently the case. The influence of early detection and intervention on subsequent academic achievement remains to be determined.

SOCIAL AND EMOTIONAL DEVELOPMENT

Children who are deaf have been described as socially immature with a tendency to be egocentric and aggressive in expressing their complaints.[21] An increased frequency of impulsivity has also been described, although this might also reflect acquired patterns of social interaction and response (such as sometimes having to touch people to get their attention) rather than specific deficits in inhibition. One population-based study indicated that nearly half of a group of children who had been fitted with hearing aids were reported by their parents to have a significant behavior problem. Of these children, 56% had mood problems, 25% had conduct problems, and 19% had both. Teachers reported behavior problems in fewer children (20%) than did parents.[22] It is not clear how early intervention and improved language abilities would influence the development of these problems.

Although the overall prevalence of attention deficits does not appear to be increased in children who have hearing impairments, certain subgroups, such as those with acquired deafness, do appear to be at higher risk.[23] Studies of outcomes in children with profound deafness who have received cochlear implants, in comparison with those who have not, are suggestive of improved abilities on visual perception and understanding tasks, which raises questions about the role of auditory input in spatial integration and sustained attention.[24]

Visual impairment, neuromotor difficulties, seizure disorders, and/or learning disabilities are present in up to 30% of children with deafness, especially those with acquired causes such as congenital infections or extreme prematurity, which reflects more diffuse damage to the central nervous system.

Identification

The key to an optimal outcome for the child with a hearing impairment is early identification and intervention. In its Year 2000 Position Statement, the Joint Committee on Infant Hearing[7] endorsed early detection of, and intervention for, hearing loss in infants through integrated interdisciplinary state and national systems of universal neonatal hearing screening. More than 40 states have already adopted legislation mandating universal screening of newborns for hearing loss, and 5 have achieved universal screening without legislation. It is also recommended that all infants who have risk indicators for delayed-onset or progressive hearing loss should undergo regular assessment of hearing every 6 months until age 3 years. Table 10F-3 lists risk factors indicating need for follow-up hearing evaluations.

Reliance on behavioral symptoms to identify hearing loss is not recommended, although such symptoms might lead parents to raise concerns. The obvious manifestations of hearing loss include failure of an infant to startle in response to loud noises or to turn in the direction of a sound. Toddlers might not respond to environmental sounds or might appear to ignore requests or instructions. They might also position themselves closer to sound sources. Most often, however, hearing impairment is subtle and can quite easily elude detection. Infants with even a profound hearing loss begin to vocalize before 6 months of age; delays in further language development become apparent only later. Children with severe to profound hearing loss fail to develop "canonical babbling" (use of discrete syllables such as /ba/, /da/, and /na/) by 11 months.[25] Delayed development of speech is a universal symptom of hearing impairment, and even milder degrees of hearing impairment can cause difficulties with language development. For

TABLE 10F-3 ■ Risk Factors for Delayed Onset of Hearing Loss
History
Parental or caregiver concern regarding hearing, speech, language, and/or developmental delay
Family history of permanent childhood hearing loss
Neonatal Indicators
In utero infections: cytomegalovirus infection, rubella, syphilis, herpes, or toxoplasmosis
Hyperbilirubinemia at a serum level necessitating exchange transfusion
Persistent pulmonary hypertension
Use of extracorporeal membrane oxygenation
Postnatal Indicators
Syndrome associated with sensorineural and/or conductive hearing loss or eustachian tube dysfunction
Syndromes associated with progressive hearing loss such as neurofibromatosis, osteopetrosis, and Usher syndrome
Neurodegenerative disorders such as Hunter syndrome
Sensory motor neuropathies such as Friedreich ataxia and Charcot-Marie-Tooth syndrome
Postnatal infections associated with sensorineural hearing loss, including bacterial meningitis
Head trauma
Recurrent or persistent otitis media with effusion for at least 3 months

From Joint Committee on Infant Hearing: Year 2000 Position Statement: Principles and Guidelines for Early Hearing Detection and Intervention Programs. Pediatrics 106:798-817, 2000.

example, children who are unable to discriminate phonemes, especially the softer, higher frequency sounds such as consonants, may develop speech and language dysfunction. Behavioral problems and/or impaired social interactions secondary to hearing problems sometimes are ascribed incorrectly to disorders such as autism, oppositional defiant disorder, or mental retardation.

Clinicians must be alert to parental concerns regarding a child's hearing, delays in language development, and significant articulation deficits. Parents' responses to developmental screening questionnaires reveal concerns regarding delays in communication and language development.[26,27] Other instruments that more directly assess language include the Early Language Milestone Scale and the Clinical Linguistic and Auditory Milestone Scale.[28,29] In children with otitis media and persistent middle ear effusion, the level of hearing loss should be documented and monitored closely.

Methods of Hearing Assessment

Perfunctory assessments of hearing in a clinic setting can be misleading. Response to a bell, hand clap, or other loud sound does not rule out milder levels of hearing loss and does not differentiate thresholds of hearing at various frequencies. If there is *any* question of hearing impairment, the child should be referred for formal audiological evaluation.

OBJECTIVE AUDIOMETRY

Auditory evoked potentials are electrophysiological responses with which to assess auditory function and neurological integrity. Auditory brainstem evoked response (ABR) testing is the most clinically useful in newborns, infants, and difficult-to-test children. It is accurate and reliable and can also detect unilateral loss. A click is introduced by an inserted earphone or a headphone at the external canal, and the transmission of the low energy evoked potential through the brainstem pathways to the auditory cortex is recorded by means of scalp electrodes. Although clicks have a broad frequency range and provide little information about hearing in the lower frequency range, tone bursts can be used to provide more frequency specificity if necessary.[5] ABR testing does not measure how the sound is being interpreted and processed, and it should be used in conjunction with behavioral audiometry whenever possible. Automated ABR tests (in which responses are interpreted by computer and reported as "pass" or "fail") are used frequently in neonatal hearing screening programs.

Otoacoustic emissions offer a clinical technique for measuring the integrity and sensitivity of the cochlea, as well as indirectly reflecting middle ear status. Otoacoustic emissions are a form of acoustic energy produced by active movements of the outer hair cells of the cochlea in response to sound. Otoacoustic emission testing entails the introduction of a click via a probe in the ear canal with measurement of the emissions from the inner ear by a microphone. In *transient-evoked* otoacoustic emissions testing, a brief click stimulus is applied to elicit the hair cell response. *Distortion-product* otoacoustic emissions are recorded from hair cells when two tones of different frequency are presented to the external auditory canal simultaneously. The latter entails the use of specific frequency stimuli to measure specific regions of the cochlea. Otoacoustic emissions testing is relatively simple and highly sensitive but is less specific than ABR testing and can be affected by outer ear canal obstruction and middle ear effusion. In neonatal screening, if otoacoustic emissions testing indicates hearing loss, follow-up with ABR is recommended. Another helpful application of otoacoustic emissions is in the identification of infants and children with auditory neuropathy, in which cochlear function is normal (normal otoacoustic emissions) but the more rostral regions of the auditory pathways are dysfunctional (as measured by ABR).[5]

Immittance audiometry is another objective measure whereby the physical volume of the external auditory canal and the compliance of the middle ear system can be assessed. In tympanometry, acoustic energy passed through the middle ear system (admittance) or reflected back (impedance) is measured. Mobility of the tympanic membrane and middle ear pressure can be gauged. This technique is very helpful in the assessment of middle ear effusions. There are three measurable patterns of middle ear compliance: normal (peaked, or type A), noncompliant (flat, or type B), and retraction (negative pressure, or type C). The presence of the acoustic reflex (contraction of the stapedius muscle in response to sounds of greater than 70 dB) confirms the presence of hearing but is not sensitive to lesser degrees of hearing loss. When there is a normal measure on tympanometry but the acoustic reflex is absent, sensory hearing loss is a prime consideration, and additional testing is required. An excessively large external auditory canal volume with a flat tympanogram indicates a perforation of the tympanic membrane.[5]

OPERANT CONDITIONING

Hearing tests that elicit behavioral responses allow for more frequency specific testing and confirmation that sound is being perceived by the child.

Behavioral observation audiometry can be used in very young infants (birth to age 6 months) to establish estimated levels of hearing. This technique entails observation of an infant's behavioral response to sound stimulation under controlled conditions. These responses include the aural-palpebral reflex, startle and arousal responses, and rudimentary head turning. There are several limitations, including the need for a high-intensity stimulus and the potential for examiner bias, which can contribute to false-negative and false-positive responses.[5]

Visual reinforcement audiometry can be used for children by 6 months of age and is particularly helpful in children aged 1 to 4 years. In this technique, the systematic reinforcement of behavioral responses is used. In the typical application, the child is seated on the parent's lap in the sound booth with animated lighted toys placed in such a way that when the child turns in response to sound from the speaker, the toy at that speaker is lit to reinforce the response. After conditioning, the sound is presented before the toy lights up, and thus the child's response to the varying auditory stimuli can be measured. The learning curve is short, and accurate frequency-specific thresholds for various stimuli (tones, speech, and noise) can be obtained. This method does rely on the experience, skill, and patience of the audiologist.

Play audiometry can be used in children aged 2 years and older as attention spans increase. The child responds to sound by performing tasks such as dropping or stacking blocks or placing rings on pegs.

Pure tone and speech audiometry provides more accurate measurement of response to pure tones or speech. Older children are asked to respond to signals generated by a calibrated audiometer. Pure tone assessment can measure air conduction (by speaker or headphone) and bone conduction (by bone vibrator). Use of speakers has the limitation of reflecting hearing only in the "better-hearing ear." Once children accept the use of headphones, more accurate assessments can be made in each ear. In addition to pure tone testing, speech reception threshold and speech recognition scores are a standard component of a basic auditory test battery. Speech reception thresholds are the lowest (softest) level in dB at which a patient can repeat approximately 50% of a list of spondaic (two-syllable) words. If young children do not respond verbally, they can be asked to point to pictures, objects, or body parts. For very young children, this measure might be limited to assessment of "speech detection," in which behavioral responses such as eye widening and head turning are recorded. Speech recognition is the ability of a child to repeat a list of phonetically balanced words correctly. These words are presented to the child at a level 30 dB above the speech reception thresholds. The results of hearing tests are described graphically on an audiogram, which displays auditory threshold in decibels as a function of frequency that ranges from 250 to 8000 Hz.[5]

Medical Evaluation

When hearing loss has been identified, further medical assessment is necessary.[10,30,31] A thorough history can establish risk factors and potential causes. In children with sensorineural hearing loss, it is essential to rule out any associated treatable conductive component that could be adding to the hearing deficit. A detailed general physical examination should include pneumatic otoscopy and tests of vestibular function. Comprehensive evaluation is important to look for associated disabilities. For example, unexplained fainting spells in a deaf child might signal a cardiac conduction defect (long QT interval) characteristic of Jervell and Lange-Nielsen syndrome. Other associated findings are listed in Table 10F-2. Ophthalmological evaluation is also essential for confirming or ruling out conditions such as retinitis pigmentosa with progressive loss of vision, which occurs in children with Usher syndrome. Chorioretinitis accompanies some of the congenital infections, and this finding might help establish an etiological diagnosis. Routine evaluation for refractive errors is important for ensuring optimal vision for children who are more reliant on visual input for communication and learning.

Although there are numerous special tests that could be ordered to rule out all possible underlying or associated causes, most of these have a low yield, and the clinical significance of the findings can be challenging to interpret. According to current recommendations, imaging of the temporal bone and genetic testing should be a part of the workup for every child with sensorineural hearing loss.[10] High-resolution computed tomographic scan of the temporal bone is strongly recommended. In some clinical studies, up to 20% of children with sensorineural hearing loss have demonstrated abnormalities on this scan. The most common of these is enlarged vestibular aqueduct (associated with progressive hearing loss) and abnormalities of the cochlea and semicircular canals. These children can also have intermittent vertigo. Magnetic resonance imaging does not have as high a yield, but it can also identify anatomical abnormalities or neoplasms, and a computed tomographic brain scan might also reveal calcifications indicating congenital infection.

Genetic testing should include DNA testing for genes such as connexin 26 and 30 and for mitochondrial mutations such as A1555G (increased susceptibility to aminoglycoside toxicity) and PDS (pendrin, present in Pendred syndrome).[10]

Other special investigations should be dictated by the specific clinical characteristics of each case and might include tests of renal function or metabolic function, immunological testing, or electrocardiography. If congenital or acquired infection is suspected, consultation with a pediatric infectious disease specialist is helpful in ordering and interpreting immunological tests (cytomegalovirus, toxoplasmosis, rubella, herpes, and syphilis). Certain forms of hearing loss can be progressive, and the level of hearing loss should be reevaluated routinely on an annual basis.

Treatment

Comprehensive management should include attention to medical conditions, interventions to promote language development, educational interventions, use of assistive devices, and support and advocacy.[32,33] This is best accomplished by a team of professionals working in partnership with families, including a pediatrician or primary care physician, otolaryngologist, audiologist, speech-language pathologist, and an educator of children who are deaf or hard of hearing.

The primary care physician working with the parents and other health professionals provides the medical home to facilitate and coordinate many of these interventions. Audiologists confirm the existence and degree of hearing loss through comprehensive audiological assessment and evaluate candidacy for amplification and assistive technology, as well as recommendations and follow-up for amplification devices. Otolaryngologists are able to assess middle ear function and to evaluate for any surgically correctable causes of hearing loss such as cholesteatoma, ossicular abnormalities, or other anomalies of the conductive system. They can also provide consultation with regard to candidacy for cochlear implantation. In children with sensorineural hearing loss, any associated conductive losses secondary to persistent middle ear effusions should be treated more aggressively than might be the case in children with normal hearing.

SOUND AMPLIFICATION

When a significant hearing loss has been discovered, the child should be fitted with a hearing aid as soon as possible. Hearing aids can be fitted in infants on the basis of estimates of hearing thresholds from ABR measurements. Once a child is old enough to participate in behavioral hearing tests, these results can be incorporated into more precise calibration of hearing aids. The goal of amplification is to make speech and other environmental sounds audible while avoiding high-intensity sound levels that are aversive or could damage residual hearing. A variety of forms of amplification are available. The original body-worn receivers have generally been replaced by behind-the-ear or ear-level hearing aids that fit behind the pinna with amplified sound transmitted to the ear canal via the custom-fit ear mold. Technological advances have resulted in devices that amplify sounds differentially in the frequency spectra most affected in that individual. These devices can also be used with telephones and with direct input from frequency modulation auditory trainers in which the primary speaker (usually the classroom teacher) wears a lapel-type microphone that transmits the speaker's voice directly to the hearing aid. Bone conduction devices are used for children with certain types of conductive hearing loss, such as atresia of the external auditory canal.

COCHLEAR IMPLANTS

Although hearing aids are effective for children with moderate to severe hearing loss, cochlear implants are revolutionizing the management of children with profound hearing loss.[24] A cochlear implant is an electronic device, of which part is surgically implanted into the cochlea and the remaining part is worn externally. It functions as a sensory aid converting mechanical sound energy into a coded electric stimulus that bypasses damaged or missing cochlear hair cells and directly stimulates remaining auditory neural elements. Cochlear implants have two major components. An external speech processor consists of a microphone, usually worn behind the ear, that transmits sounds to a speech-processing computer that in turn converts the sound into an electric code. An external coil then transmits the signal across the skin to the internal receiver system implanted within the temporal bone and connected to multichannel electrodes placed within the cochlea. The electrodes are located at different sites to utilize the tonotopic organization of the spiral ganglion cells within the cochlea. Clinical trials have indicated positive outcomes with significant improvement in appreciation of sound in everyday situations, speech recognition and understanding, and expressive language abilities.[34] The implantation procedure appears to be well tolerated, and a follow-up survey of patients who received cochlear implants 10 to 13 years earlier (when devices were less sophisticated and the mean age at surgery was 9 years) indicated that 88% would choose again to undergo the procedure.[24] More recent studies have demonstrated positive functional outcomes and lack of significant surgical complications even in children who receive their implants before 12 months of age.[35] Implantation before 2 years of age has been found to provide the most advantage with regard to speech perception and language development; studies have suggested that a majority of children with profound deafness who receive implants between 12 and 24 months of age enter school with near-normal language skills.[3]

Children who use any form of amplification device, and especially those who have cochlear implants, need auditory training to help them understand the meaning of the newly amplified sounds.

OTHER ASSISTIVE DEVICES

A number of assistive devices are available including telecommunication devices for the deaf (TDD), closed captioning of television, and adapted warning devices, such as flickering lights to indicate a ringing alarm or telephone. Advances in information technology have, of course, enormously increased opportunities for communication for individuals with hearing impairment. The Internet and email, as well as voice-to-text technology, have broken down barriers at many levels. The pervasive use of "instant messaging" on computers linked to the Internet, email communications on personal digital assistants, and "text messaging" on cellular mobile phones are prime examples of these gains as they have become preferred methods of communication among children and young adults, regardless of hearing status.

EARLY INTERVENTION

Early intervention to promote language development remains the most critical management challenge for children with hearing impairment. The child with profound hearing loss, his or her parents, and other caregivers should receive professional assistance in establishing a functional system of communication as soon as possible. There are many differing opinions regarding the most appropriate communication and instructional techniques. Options include sign language (manual communication), lip reading and use of speech (oral communication), and a combination (total communication).[36] Children with profound hearing loss who have not received cochlear implants usually experience great difficulty learning to read lips and speak fluently and are best served by early exposure to visual and manual forms of communication such as sign language. However, children with milder degrees of loss and those who have received cochlear implants are better able to communicate with most of the people who are not hearing impaired by development of their oral language skills.

The advent of universal neonatal hearing screening has provided a unique opportunity to study the effects of early intervention on child development, particularly in relation to hearing impairment. Studies involving children in the Colorado Home Intervention Program have definitively established that early intervention services for families with infants with hearing loss identified in the first few months of life result in significantly better language, speech, and social-emotional development. Earlier diagnosis allows the families to obtain information and receive counseling and support over a longer period of time.[16] Children in whom impairment is diagnosed and who receive services before 6 months of age did significantly better than those with later diagnoses, in whom intervention kept language delays from increasing but did not enable them to catch up with regard to delays that were already present at the time of diagnosis.

Educational interventions should be tailored to the individual needs of each child. These services are mandated through the Individuals with Disabilities Education Act. Options for children whose hearing loss has not been fully corrected range from use of interpreters in a regular school and classroom to special programs in a regular school or enrollment in a school for the deaf. Children with hearing impairment must have the opportunity for full participation in academic and social activities. The optimal school setting to achieve this goal depends on individual characteristics of the child and the educational system in that geographical region. The clinician should be familiar with local educational resources, including the institutions of higher learning for the deaf, such as Gallaudet University and the National Technical Institute for the Deaf.

Parents of the child with newly diagnosed hearing loss are dealing with significant grief and, at the same time, are faced with enormous amounts of information and the need to make decisions regarding treatment approaches. Counseling can be helpful in assisting the parents work through their feelings and adapt to their new roles.[37] The primary care clinician or developmental-behavioral pediatrician is a vital source of information and support for the families of children with severe hearing impairment within the medical home. Parents might receive conflicting advice regarding both medical and educational interventions deemed necessary for the child. They face numerous stresses, including adjustment to the diagnosis and the need to learn new forms of communication and access the most appropriate therapies and interventions for their child.

Summary

The outlook for children with hearing impairment has improved quite dramatically since the 1960s. Increased knowledge related to the genetic basis of hearing loss has greatly decreased the ranks of those with hearing impairment of "undetermined etiology" and enabled more accurate diagnosis and genetic counseling. Likewise, efforts at primary prevention such as immunizations against the infectious agents responsible for meningitis have decreased the incidence of some forms of acquired deafness. The very positive outcomes for early identification and intervention for children with hearing loss have become a model for the evidence base supporting early intervention for many forms of developmental dysfunction. Cochlear implants have also radically changed the scenario regarding treatment options. New technology has broadened the opportunities for communication for individuals with hearing impairment. All of these options increase the responsibility of the physician to be alert to early signs of hearing problems and to ensure that children with this sensory deficit have access to all the advances in management that will enable them to be successful.

VISUAL IMPAIRMENT

Loss of vision profoundly effects development and lifestyle. It has been estimated that up to 80% of the information from the outside world is incorporated through visual pathways.[38] Although impairments in vision are usually more obvious in the early months of life than are hearing deficits, children with vision problems more frequently have other neurodevelopmental challenges, and visual impairment can also be missed in children with multiple handicaps.

Terminology

Legal blindness is the term used when central visual acuity is 20/200 or less in the better eye with corrective lenses or there is a restriction in the visual field of 20 degrees or less in the better eye. However, *blindness* rarely means a complete loss of vision; the legal definition is used more often to determine eligibility for benefits and services from government or educational agencies. Up to 75% of legally blind individuals have some residual visual function, and many of them can read large print.[39] Students are classified as *educationally visually impaired* if their central acuity is 20/70 or worse. They usually require at least some modification of educational materials in the classroom. *Partially sighted* individuals are those with visual acuity of between 20/70 and 20/200 in the better eye, corrected. The World Health Organization has developed a graded system of visual impairment that is summarized in Table 10F-4. Other systems assign a percentage of impairment to the whole visual system that is based on loss of vision in one or both eyes.[40]

For children with extremely limited vision (below about 20/400), functional designations can be used: for example, *hand motion* or *object perception* (ability to detect presence and motion of nearby objects), *light projection* (ability to determine the direction of a light source), *light perception* (ability to notice whether there is light present), and *no light perception* (total blindness). Children with some residual vision can be referred to as having *low vision*. *Functional vision* refers to qualities of vision that are important in determining how efficiently residual vision is used. For example, two children may have identical distance visual acuities (e.g., 20/400), but, because of other aspects of functional vision, one child may be able to read large print, whereas for the other, use of Braille for reading may be more efficient.

Nystagmus can be congenital or acquired. Congenital nystagmus is either sensory or motor. *Sensory nystagmus* develops as a result of afferent pathway disease (globes, optic nerves, optic chiasm or tracts) before 4 to 6 months of age and usually varies according to the level of vision loss. If visual impairment occurs 6 months, a child will not develop sensory nystagmus. *Motor nystagmus* occurs secondary to an anomaly of the central oculomotor control system and is usually present within weeks of birth.[41] *Spasmus nutans* is an acquired form of nystagmus that includes head nodding and torticollis. It develops between 6 and 12 months of age and usually resolves by 4 years with normal vision.

Cortical visual impairment (previously called *cortical* or *central blindness*) refers to vision loss secondary to disorders of the optic radiations, striate, and peristriate cortex of the occipital lobe. *Delayed visual maturation* is a term used retrospectively for children who initially appear to have cortical visual impairment but later achieve normal or nearly normal vision. Proposed causes for this condition include immaturity of visual association areas, delayed striate cortex development, or overall delayed myelination.[40] These children have a higher incidence of other developmental-behavioral disorders. *Amblyopia* refers to unilateral decrease in visual acuity in the absence of physical disorder of that eye. This is usually secondary to sensory deprivation, as result of anisometropia (eyes with unequal refractive power), which leads to ocular misalignment and neglect of visual input from one eye.

Epidemiology

The prevalence of blindness and severe visual impairment among children is estimated to be 2 to 10 per 10,000.[42,43] If lesser degrees of visual impairment are included, this number is significantly higher. One population-based study indicated that 12.5% of the children in that population had significant visual disorders, including strabismus, anisometropia or ametropia (with myopia, hypermetropia, or astigmatism), and organic defects.[44] The concept of visual impairment in children has evolved, with an overall decrease in the number of children with an isolated visual problem and an increase in the number of those with visual impairment and an associated neurological disability. In one survey, 43% of children with visual impairment were found to have more global developmental or learning disabilities. Additional medical problems were present in 79%.[45]

Etiology

In developed countries, approximately half of all congenital and late-onset blindness is of genetic origin, including many types of cataracts, albinism, and a variety of retinal dystrophies.[42] Other congenital causes include intrauterine infections (rubella, cytomegalovirus, and toxoplasmosis) and malformations

Category	Terminology	Vision
1	Visually impaired	<20/30-20/200
2	Severely impaired	20/200-20/400
3	Blind	20/400-20/2400
4	Blind	20/400-Light Perception
5	Blind	No Light Perception

TABLE 10F-4 ■ World Health Organization Classification of Visual Impairment

of the eye (coloboma, microphthalmia, anophthalmia), the optic nerve (optic nerve hypoplasia, optic atrophy), and the brain. Sometimes such malformations are associated with chromosomal abnormalities (e.g., trisomy 13, trisomy 21) or other syndromes (the syndrome of coloboma, heart disease, atresia choanae, retarded growth and development, genital hypoplasia, and ear anomalies [CHARGE]). The most common perinatal causes of visual impairment include hypoxic-ischemic damage to cortical visual pathways and retinopathy of prematurity, a vasoproliferative disorder that currently affects primarily extremely premature infants. With technological advances enabling the survival of increasingly premature infants, the prevalence of visual impairment secondary to retinopathy of prematurity increased during the 1980s and 1990s, accounting for approximately 400 to 500 significantly visually impaired infants each year in the United States during the early 1990s.[46] Research on its pathogenesis is revealing complex interactions between genetic predisposition, immature retinal vascular endothelium, oxygen exposure, and the effects of locally produced vascular endothelial growth factors.[47] A significant proportion of children with visual impairment secondary to retinopathy of prematurity have other neurodevelopmental disabilities.[48] Close ophthalmological monitoring of premature infants at high risk and prompt laser treatment of "threshold" retinopathy of prematurity can prevent retinal detachment in a significant proportion, although the risk of later ophthalmological sequelae of this disorder (e.g., strabismus, myopia, glaucoma, late-onset retinal detachment) persists.[49]

Cortical visual impairment is associated with damage to the optic radiations and occipital cortex. Causes include perinatal and postnatal hypoxia, periventricular and intraventricular hemorrhage, cerebral malformations, head trauma, metabolic and neurodegenerative conditions, meningitis, and hydrocephalus or ventricular shunt failure.[40] Major causes of acquired or later onset visual impairment include tumors such as retinoblastoma (often diagnosed in the preschool years), genetic conditions such as retinitis pigmentosa (also a finding in Usher syndrome), accidental head and eye trauma, and child abuse (particularly shaking-related injuries of the brain). Common causes of amblyopia include unilateral visual deprivation (e.g., cataract), prolonged strabismus (ocular misalignment), and anisometropia (a significant difference between the two eyes in the refractive error).

Developmental and Behavioral Impact

The heterogeneity of the population of children with visual impairment precludes precise prognostication regarding outcome for any individual child. Many of these children have other neurological deficits, and the causes of vision loss, and anatomical location of the impairment, have significant bearing on the developmental effects. Visual disorders such as cortical visual impairment and nystagmus are associated with specific developmental challenges.

Factors influencing development in children with visual impairment are similar to those related to children with hearing impairment and include specific causes of the visual impairment, the severity of the visual impairment, the age at onset (e.g., congenital vs. acquired after several years of age), the presence of additional disabilities and/or chronic illness, individual temperamental characteristics, and the psychosocial environment in which the child is raised. In general, with the provision of appropriate opportunities for development and learning, young blind children can progress through many of the same developmental phases as their sighted peers. However, some important qualitative differences and variations in sequence of developmental patterns of blind and sighted children are often apparent. Patterns of development are correlated with the amount of residual functional vision. Children with visual acuity worse than 20/800 appear to be at significantly greater risk for slower developmental progress than are children with visual acuities in the range of 20/500 to 20/800.[50]

MOTOR DEVELOPMENT

In the absence of specific neuromotor disabilities, such as cerebral palsy, most young children who are visually impaired can achieve postural milestones, such as sitting and standing, at about the same age as infants with sight. In contrast, skills involving movement through space, such as crawling and walking, are often delayed. The young child who is visually impaired must first learn through repeated experience that the sounds he or she hears represent objects that can be touched or held if he or she moves toward that sound. Mild hypotonia and the element of insecurity—having to move through "unknown" space—may also initially impede motivation to move.[51] Even after walking is achieved, many severely visually impaired children without other disabilities have continuing motor difficulties related to low muscle tone and decreased balance. They tend to have poor posture with stooping of the head and/or trunk, and a broad-based, toe-out gait. Early intervention and ongoing feedback about posture from parents, physical therapists, and teachers can minimize these motor patterns. Improved stability of the head and trunk can be beneficial with regard to oculomotor control and functional vision in children with visual impairment in association with severe motor disabilities such as quadriplegic cerebral palsy.[52]

COGNITIVE DEVELOPMENT

Children who are visually impaired may lag in acquisition of concepts and knowledge about their environment, such as understanding object permanence. They tend to be more concrete and less abstract in their description of objects. There is wide variability among samples of visually impaired children.[53] In the absence of associated learning problems and when given appropriate learning opportunities, children with severe visual impairment can eventually master the same general concepts as do their sighted peers. *Tactile defensiveness* (an excessive sensitivity and resistance to touching certain textures) is sometimes a problem, posing the threat of further sensory deprivation. This can also affect feeding practices, as many blind children go through a prolonged phase of tolerating only soft foods, rejecting many harder textured foods that require chewing.

LANGUAGE DEVELOPMENT

Language is a critical interface between child with the severe visual impairment and his or her environment. Early acquisition of vocabulary occurs at a rate similar to that of children with sight, but qualitative differences often emerge during the second year. Blind children's vocabulary consists of more words describing objects and people than actions. Some blind children succeed in rote-learning words, but experiential limitations may render these words with little if any true meaning for the child (so-called verbalism).[54] Similarly, there may also be a prolonged phase of echolalia, the child repeating what he or she has heard. There is also confusion about pronouns (e.g., "I" vs. "you") at younger ages. Caregivers and others working with visually impaired children can facilitate stronger cognitive connections between words and their meanings by providing meaningful experiences that match the child's words.

SOCIAL AND EMOTIONAL DEVELOPMENT

Stages of emotional attachment for children who are visually impaired generally follow the same timetable as those for sighted peers. There is stronger reliance on other sensory input; for example, recognition of a parent's voice and demonstration of anxiety when the child is held by a stranger are strong indicators of a visually impaired infant's attachment. Nevertheless, babies with visual handicaps may be at increased risk for attachment disorders. Parents might be misled by the fact that infants who are visually impaired do not smile as easily as sighted babies. This, in addition to their lack of eye contact, delayed reaching out, and tendency to be passive may give the impression of a lack of emotional connection or of cognitive slowness, which adds to the emotional vulnerability of the parents. In turn, parents' feelings of guilt, stress, and inadequacy may lead to lowered expectations for their infant's development. For some parents who lack adequate social supports or information, this combination of miscues between parents and child can lead to inadvertent parental emotional withdrawal or have the opposite effect of intrusion and overprotectiveness.[55]

Preschool children who are blind tend to be more passive in their play and less likely to initiate social interactions during play than are their sighted peers.[56] This isolation is often compounded if the child with visual impairment is the only one in his or her school to have such special needs. In addition to the importance of learning how to interact with his or her sighted peers in a "sighted world," the visually impaired child's self-esteem can be enhanced by opportunities to meet other children with similar disabilities.

Adolescence provides further challenges, and the normal social and emotional tasks, especially the need for growing independence, can be significantly complicated by visual impairment that impedes function. Creativity and advocacy are required of parents and others to encourage increasing individuation, peer affiliation, and the beginnings of preparation for a career and more independent living as an adult.[57]

There is limited information regarding the impact of *nystagmus* on visual and social function. One questionnaire survey of children with nystagmus (predominantly of idiopathic origin) and their parents indicated quite significant impairment of visual function (only slightly better than for individuals with macular degeneration). One third of the children indicated that they worried a great deal about their eyesight, and 26% reported being bullied frequently.[41]

Identification

In contrast to most children with hearing impairments whose disabilities elude detection until well after their first birthday, many children with significant visual impairment are brought to the clinician's attention during the first year of life. By the time the infant is 3 to 6 months old, parents are usually quick to notice their infant's poor visual attention to, or tracking of, objects or people and may readily detect such important ophthalmological signs as nystagmus, "lazy eye" (strabismus), and excessive tearing in the absence of crying. The presence of sensory nystagmus in a visually impaired child is an obvious sign reflecting visual impairment of very early onset.[52] Other signs and symptoms that may be clues to a possible visual impairment include lack of accurate reaching for objects by 6 months, haziness of the cornea, persisting photophobia, persistent conjunctival erythema, persisting head tilt, asymmetry of pupillary size, and abnormalities of pupillary shape (e.g., "keyhole" defect indicating a coloboma of the iris).

A variety of behavioral manifestations of children with severe visual impairments may also be apparent to parents and clinicians. Common behaviors include stereotyped movements, such as rocking, hand-flapping, exaggerated finger play, rhythmic head or body swaying, and prolongation of echolalic speech patterns. A long-term follow-up study of severely impaired children showed that many of these stereotypical behaviors had been spontaneously abandoned by the time of adulthood.[58] Light-gazing and brief, sideways-glancing at objects and people seem to be more characteristic of children with cortical, rather than ocular, visual impairment.[58] Forceful eye rubbing (with the thumb or fist), the oculodigital reflex, is suggestive of retinal disease. The force to the eye causes mechanical stimulation of the retina with triggering of ganglion cell action potentials, which creates flashes of light, or phosphenes.[40] This is not usually dangerous or self-injurious, as opposed to eye-poking, which can cause damage to the eye.[59]

Approximately 50% to 60% of children with severe visual impairment have additional neurodevelopmental and behavioral disabilities, including cerebral palsy, mental retardation, autism, hearing impairment, and epilepsy.[42,60,61] In children with visual impairment who have multiple disabilities, the visual problems may be less obvious than the other neurological problems, and thus their detection is delayed or missed altogether. The clinician needs to maintain a high index of suspicion and systematically check visual function in children who have other disabilities. Likewise, it is important to consider the possibility of additional disabilities in a child with obvious visual impairment.

Assessment of Vision

Although ophthalmologists are best able to do the necessary detailed assessment of a child's eyes and visual function, the American Academy of Pediatrics and the U.S. Preventive Services Task Force reaffirmed recommendations regarding the role of the pediatrician in the early detection and prompt treatment of ocular disorders in children.[62,63] Newborns should be examined for ocular structural abnormalities such as cataract, corneal opacities, and ptosis. At well-child visits, there should be ongoing monitoring for retinal abnormalities, glaucoma, retinoblastoma, strabismus, and neurological disorders. Visual function should be assessed from birth, with measurement of visual acuity beginning at the earliest age possible, usually 3 years.[62] Despite these recommendations,

there is still much room for improvement of vision and eye screening programs in primary care settings.[62-64]

Soliciting parents' descriptions of and concerns about a child's visual behavior is a crucial part of the assessment. Physical examination techniques further define the existence and nature of any visual problem. In the neonatal period, ocular history; external inspection of the eyes and lids; ocular motility assessment; and checking for symmetrical red reflexes, pupillary shape, and response to light are important. Standard assessment should include determination of whether each eye can fixate on an object, maintain fixation, and then follow the object into various gaze fixations. An inability to successfully perform these maneuvers indicates significant visual impairment. Most newborns with normal vision are capable of limited visual tracking of slow-moving, high-contrast targets about 8 to 12 inches from their faces during alert periods. By the time an infant is 2 to 4 months of age, parental reports of social smiling and nearly automatic visual tracking of people and bright objects should be elicited, as well as observations of eye alignment. Examination should include elicitation of a social smile, visual tracking of the examiner's face and/or a bright toy across the infant's visual field, observations of pupillary light reactions, checking for red reflexes, and at least brief glimpses of the fundi. By 6 to 8 months, visual function can be further documented through observations of an infant's reaching for and attempted grasping of nearby small objects (1-mm cake sprinkle, 6-mm candy bead, 1-cm Cheerio, 1-inch red cube, and so forth), as well as obvious reactions to more distant people or large objects. Visually searching for a silently dropped bright object is also notable after about 5 to 6 months. Screening for visual acuity, alignment of the eyes (using the cover-uncover test), and ocular diseases at 4 to 6 months is crucial for timely detection of conditions such as strabismus and cataracts, which, if left untreated, can eventually lead to amblyopic visual loss.[65] Photoscreening, although innovative and potentially useful in detecting strabismus, media opacities, and significant refractive errors in children's eyes, still has associated methodological problems as a vision screening technique. The American Academy of Pediatrics recommended that this method be studied more extensively before its routine use by pediatricians is recommended.[66]

A number of tests are available to the pediatrician for measuring visual acuity in older children.[38] Tests involving cards with symbols or pictures, such as the Allen cards, are suitable for children aged 2 to 4 years. Children older than 4 years can be tested with wall charts containing the Snellen letters or numbers, the tumbling E test, and the HOTV test. Many pediatric practices use vision-testing machines, but administration of these tests can be difficult for children 4 years or younger. Criteria for referral for children aged 3 to 5 years include describing fewer than four of six stimuli correctly from 20 feet away (less than 20/40) or a two-line difference between eyes, even within the passing range (e.g., 20/25 and 20/40/). Children aged 6 years and older should be referred if distance acuity is less than 20/30 or if there is a two-line difference within this passing range (20/20 and 20/30).[38] External examination of the eye should include the lids, conjunctiva, sclera, cornea, and iris. Tearing or discharge can be a sign of infection, allergy, or glaucoma, or it might be caused by nasolacrimal duct obstruction. Cloudy or asymmetrically enlarged corneas are indicative of glaucoma and the need for prompt ophthalmological evaluation. Unilateral ptosis could cause amblyopia, and bilateral ptosis would raise suspicion for myasthenia gravis. Strabismus can develop at any age, and ocular alignment should be checked carefully. The corneal reflex test (with a penlight held 2 feet in front of the face and the child fixating on the light) and the cross-cover test (child looks at an object 10 feet away, and one eye is covered with an occluder while the clinician observes for movement of the other eye) are useful in differentiating true strabismus from pseudostrabismus. Pseudostrabismus is most commonly a result of prominent epicanthal lid folds covering the medial portion of the sclera. Slowly or poorly reactive pupils may reflect significant retinal or optic nerve dysfunction. Asymmetrical pupil size could be caused by sympathetic disorder (Horner syndrome) or parasympathetic abnormality (third nerve palsy). All children with ocular abnormalities or who perform poorly on vision screening should be referred to a pediatric ophthalmologist or eye care specialist appropriately trained to treat pediatric patients.[62]

It is important for each primary care clinician to have a close working relationship with an ophthalmologist who is comfortable in examining infants and children and is knowledgeable about their eye problems. However, many ophthalmologists have little or no training in children's development and should not necessarily be expected to know how to guide or support parents of severely visually impaired children with regard to interventions to promote optimal development.

A child with severe visual impairment, just like one with any other type of developmental disability, needs to have an initial interdisciplinary evaluation as the foundation of an intervention plan, as specified by the Individuals with Disabilities Education Act. Knowledge of the ophthalmologist's diagnosis and visual acuity data is crucial for such an evaluation but may be insufficient to adequately describe important qualitative aspects of the child's day-to-day visual functioning, such as the extent to which sounds are distracting, whether the child's medications affect visual function, and how the ambient lighting and contrast of the toys or written materials affect the child's performance. The presence on the assessment team of a person with expertise and experience in working with children with severe visual impairments helps ensure that cognitive and other types of testing are done in a way that takes advantage of the child's best use of any residual vision and does not unfairly bias the results on the basis of the visual impairment.

Treatment

In addition to standard general medical care, children with visual impairment may have additional specialized medical issues, depending on the nature of the child's neuro-ophthalmological status (e.g., monitoring growth and endocrinological parameters in children with optic nerve hypoplasia; addressing the frequent problems with sleep and feeding that many young children who are blind encounter).[67]

After the initial ophthalmological and developmental evaluations, intervention strategies can be planned, with professionals and parents collaborating on goals, priorities, and the optimal use of community and educational resources. Early intervention service systems vary from state to state; therefore, clinicians need to be aware of how and to whom to make referrals and how they can participate in the planning and monitoring process. In most states, a state-level agency or consultant to the department of public instruction is designated to assist local school systems with planning appropriate services and specialized materials for their students with visual impairments. At the local level, larger and/or urban school districts may have their own teachers for students who are blind or visually impaired. In smaller and/or more rural areas, these specialized teachers may be more itinerant, providing consultation to many schools throughout the region. Orientation and mobility instructors are trained professionals who teach individuals who are blind or visually impaired to travel safely and efficiently (e.g., proper use of a cane).

As the child passes from preschool to school age, families, eye-care specialists, and child educators must usually face a series of educational decisions.[55,68] What will be the most appropriate classroom setting (residential school vs. self-contained class vs. resource class vs. "inclusion" in the regular classroom)? Will the child most likely have sufficient visual function to proceed with learning to read print, or will Braille be a more efficient system? What visual and/or technological aids are most helpful and most acceptable to the child (large print, closed-circuit television, hand-held magnifier, stand-magnifier, magic marker rather than pencil, and so forth)? Some students benefit from technology that allows blind students to convert print media to Braille; Braille-to-speech output; and/or computer software that facilitates Internet browsing, word-processing, and most other computer functions that sighted peers are accessing. Depending on the child's eye condition, possibly changing visual function, and academic abilities, initial educational decisions may need to be reassessed periodically to determine whether new approaches are indicated.

Deaf-Blindness (Combined Hearing and Visual Impairments)

In the United States, an estimated 10,000 children who were deaf-blind, from birth to 21 years of age, received special education services in schools during 1994, and about 85% had additional disabilities, most commonly mental retardation, speech impairments, and orthopedic handicaps.[69] The usual external stimuli that serve as motivators for mobility, communication, and learning about the environment are beyond access or are distorted for these children, which limits their initial awareness to the confines of their "random reach."[70] Traditional tests of vision, hearing, and cognitive abilities are frequently inappropriate in the evaluation of such children, and medical and educational specialists who are trained and experienced with this population need to be involved early on in the diagnostic and intervention-planning phases of care. When a child has a combination of impairments of both the auditory and visual channels, uniquely adaptive interventions need to address the important areas of communication, socialization, concept formation, and mobility.[71] The use of mechanical or electrical vibrotactile devices has been shown to be a feasible type of assistive technology for children who are deaf-blind.[72] For the child who loses the second sensory function adventitiously (the child with Usher syndrome who is deaf from birth but only gradually loses vision from retinitis pigmentosa as adolescence approaches), helping the child and family cope emotionally with this loss is crucial. The clinician also needs to guard against an unfounded bias in assuming that the child with deaf-blindness must be "profoundly retarded" and/or "unable to learn."

Summary

The diagnosis of visual impairment can be missed in infants and in children with multiple disabilities. Children with visual impairment frequently have other neurodevelopmental and behavioral conditions. Early diagnosis and implementation of a coordinated treatment approach are crucial for optimal outcome. (*The author acknowledges the significant contribution of Stuart W. Teplin MD to the Visual Impairment section.*)

OTHER SENSORY DEVIATIONS

Olfactory Impairments

Olfaction, or smell, occurs when chemicals stimulate olfactory receptors high in the nasal cavity. There are many different classes of odor stimuli that affect different receptor proteins on the membranes of the cilia of olfactory neurons. Odor can reach these receptors from the nostrils during inhalation and from the back of the nasopharynx during chewing and swallowing (which probably explains the close links between taste and smell). Shortly after birth, infants can detect a wide variety of odors, as evidenced by the research on feeding that indicates the ability of an infant to quickly identify his or her mother by odor alone.

Anosmia refers to a complete absence of olfactory functioning. *Hyposmia* refers to diminished functioning that may be specific to a particular odorous compound (also referred to as *specific anosmia*). *Dysosmia* or *paraosmia* refers to distortions in smell.[73] Dysfunction in smell can result from nasal obstruction, allergic or chronic rhinitis, and nasal polyps. Head trauma is a less frequent cause of olfactory loss in children than in adults. Traumatic injury can include shearing of the olfactory nerves, hemorrhage into the olfactory bulb, and fractures of the cribriform plate, but their exact effect on chemosensation is unclear.

Genetic disorders can affect smell with Kallmann syndrome being the most common (anosmia, and hypogonadotropic hypogonadism).[74] Adults with Down syndrome have decreased ability to smellm but this is not evident in children with Down syndrome. Medicationsm including opiates and antibiotics such as doxycycline, and anesthetics, including tetracaine, can inhibit smell. Certain metals (cadmium and zinc), tobacco products, and industrial chemicals can also have an effect.

Gustatory Impairments

Taste, or gustation, is mediated by receptors that respond to chemical stimulation on the dorsum of the tongue and in parts of the larynx, pharynx and epiglottis. Studies of premature infants have indicated that the sense of taste is developed before birth and that newborns show distinct responses to sweet, sour, and bitter tastes, with an early preference for sweet taste. Loss of taste, *ageusia* or *hypogeusia*, can accompany genetic disorders such as familial dysautonomia; surgical procedures (tonsillectomy with damage to the lingual branch of the glossopharyngeal nerve); and endocrine, metabolic, and nutritional disorders.[73]

Insensitivity to Pain

There is a wide range of normal levels of sensitivity to pain among children. A higher prevalence of *relative insensitivity to pain* has been reported in children with certain developmental disorders such as autism. However, investigators using objective measures of behavioral response to a painful stimulus (venipuncture) in children with autism found typical responses to pain but low concordance with parental reports of the child's reaction.[75] Variations in pain threshold have been reported in other populations, with mixed reports of increased thresholds in children with eating disorders and increased sensitivity to pain in children born prematurely.[76]

There is a distinct group of genetic disorders characterized by *congenital insensitivity to pain.* Affected individuals also manifest dysfunction of the autonomic nervous system, and these conditions are known as the *hereditary sensory and autonomic neuropathies* (HSANs).[77] The best known of these conditions is *familial dysautonomia,* or *Riley-Day syndrome* (HSAN type III). Onset is at birth, and the autonomic dysfunction can overshadow the sensory neuropathy. Early signs of the condition include feeding difficulties caused by poor oral coordination and hypotonia, with increased risk of aspiration. Pain and temperature perception is decreased but not absent in skin and bones, but visceral pain is intact. Autonomic disturbances include absence of tears with emotional crying. The "dysautonomic crises" that are characteristic of the condition include protracted episodes of nausea and vomiting triggered by emotional or physical stress. Vasomotor manifestations include erythematous skin blotching and hyperhidrosis. There is also relative insensitivity to hypoxemia. The disorder is seen only in individuals both of whose parents are of Ashkenazi Jewish extraction. Definitive diagnosis can be made by DNA molecular diagnostics. Diazepam is effective in treating the dysautonomic vomiting crisis and clonidine works synergistically and aids in management of associated diastolic hypertension.[77]

Congenital insensitivity to pain with anhidrosis (HSAN type IV) is the second most common hereditary sensory and autonomic neuropathy. The cardinal feature is absence of or markedly decreased sweating (probably secondary to impaired thoracolumbar sympathetic outflow). Anhidrosis is associated with episodic fevers and extreme hyperpyrexia and contributes to thickened skin with lichenification of palms, dystrophic nails, and areas of hypotrichosis on the scalp.

There is profound insensitivity to pain, with self-mutilation, autoamputation, and corr___ ring. Fractures are slow to heal, and repeated trau__ can lead to Charcot joints and osteomyelitis. Hypotonia is frequent, along with neurodevelopmental and behavioral problems, including learning disorders, emotional lability, and hyperactivity. Treatment is focused on controlling hyperthermia and prevention of self-mutilation and orthopedic problems. Some children require smoothing of teeth or extraction to prevent unintended damage to tongue and lips.[77] The other HSANs involve varying degrees and distribution of sensory loss and autonomic dysfunction. Sensory involvement includes pain, temperature, tactile, and vibration sense deficits, which can be stable or progressive.

SENSORY INTEGRATION

Some children who do not have specific sensory deficits nevertheless appear to experience sensory dysfunction as a result of difficulty modulating and integrating sensory input. Some find tactile or auditory stimulation aversive, even at levels that cause no negative perception among their peers. Others find particular textures or smells of food to be noxious. In contrast, another group of children appear to have *diminished* responsiveness to sensory input and crave levels of stimulation that most people would consider aversive. These symptoms occur with increased frequency in children with identified developmental-behavioral disorders such as attention-deficit/hyperactivity disorder and autism spectrum disorders.[78]

The theory of sensory integration was first introduced by A. Jean Ayres in the 1970s to explain the perceptual, sensory, and motor difficulties that she had observed in children with learning disabilities. Ayres postulated that some children with learning disorders had difficulty with the process of reception, modulation, and integration of sensation from their bodies and thus had difficulty using their bodies effectively within the environment.[79] The dysfunction was thought to involve impairment of the vestibular, proprioceptive, and tactile systems. Sensory integrative therapy is the approach developed by Ayres that is said to restore effective neurological processing by enhancing each of these systems.[80] The sensory integrative approach is used most frequently by occupational therapists.[81] Although the theory was developed to treat children with learning disabilities, it is now more frequently applied to children with autistic spectrum disorders, attention-deficit/hyperactivity disorder, and genetic disorders such as the fragile X syndrome.

The construct of sensory integration and the application of sensory integrative therapy remains the source of considerable controversy. Although the numbers of children receiving this form of therapy continue to increase, there remains a lack of well-established scientific evidence to support its efficacy. The field of sensory integration has been inhibited by the lack of controlled clinical trials, and many of the claims of efficacy are based on nonblinded trials and anecdotal reports. Some efforts are under way to address this challenge.[81]

Terminology

Ayres first defined *sensory integration* as "the neurological process that organizes sensation from one's own body and from the environment and makes it possible to use the body effectively within the environment."[79] She postulated that integration of sensory input was necessary for high-level cognitive functioning; that is, the more primitive subcortical pathways ("inner senses") such as the vestibular, proprioceptive, and tactile systems must develop before the optimal formation and function of advanced cortical systems, including vision and hearing ("outer senses"), that mediate more complex cognitive skills. This approach was based on the old theory that development of human function mirrors the evolutionary development of the species ("ontogeny recapitulates phylogeny").[80]

Vestibular dysfunction is postulated to manifest as poor posture and dyspraxia; *proprioceptive dysfunction* is associated with stereotyped movements; and *tactile dysfunction* is evidenced by oversensitivity or undersensitivity to sensory stimuli. The basic principles of sensory integration theory are that (1) sensory integration matures along a predictable developmental sequence; (2) the central nervous system is plastic; (3) sensory integration therapy attempts to revisit and restructure the development of sensory integration where the normal development has been disrupted; (4) adaptive responses are linked to sensory input; and (5) children have an innate drive to integrate information.[82]

Updates to the theory have been proposed since its original description. Schaaf and Miller[81] noted that new scientific findings and knowledge confirm that the nervous system is more complex than Ayres believed when the theory was first developed. They proposed a classification system related to patterns of dysfunction in three areas[81]: sensory modulation, sensory discrimination, and sensory-based motor disorders. *Sensory modulation* is the pattern that has been studied most extensively, and is described as the process of perceiving sensory information and generating responses that are appropriately graded to, or congruent with the situation. Children with sensory modulation disorder are reported to have difficulty regulating responses, being either overresponsive or underresponsive to normal levels of stimuli with unusual behavioral patterns of sensation seeking or sensation avoiding (such as tactile defensiveness).

Epidemiology

The prevalence of sensory modulation disorder has been estimated at up to 10% of the general population and 30% of children with developmental disabilities.[83] Studies of children with attention-deficit disorder have indicated that these children as a group display greater abnormalities in sensory modulation than do their typical peers; some authors describe more than two thirds of children with ADHD as having sensory modulation dysfunction.[78] Conversely, 40% of a sample of children with poor sensory modulation also had symptoms of attentional deficits.[84] Ahn and colleagues used the Short Sensory Profile to establish the prevalence of sensory processing disorders among incoming kindergarteners in a public school system. Approximately 5% in this population met criteria for the condition.[84]

Etiology

Any attempt to assign etiology to a condition that itself lacks clear definition is liable for inaccuracy. Many of the causes of other developmental disorders have been described as possible etiological factors, including genetic inheritance, prenatal exposure to toxins, prematurity, perinatal complications, and postnatal insults such as environmental toxins.[85] What could be postulated is that there are individual variations in the ability to modulate and regulate sensory input that are likely to be genetically determined and that might be susceptible to other disruptive influences.

Developmental and Behavioral Impact

The behavioral symptoms that have been proposed as manifestations of sensory integration dysfunction are broad and overlap with many of the characteristics of developmental-behavioral disorders discussed elsewhere in this book. Proponents of sensory integration theory describe symptoms related to sensory difficulties that manifest as either "oversensitivity" or "undersensitivity" in distinct domains as follows.[85]

TOUCH

"Oversensitive" children avoid being touched by objects or people. This is also referred to as *tactile defensiveness*. Clinical manifestations have been grouped as (1) avoidance of touch, in the form of certain textures, contact with other children (including avoidance of play involving contact), and a tendency to pull away from anticipated touch; (2) aversive responses to non-noxious touch, such as struggling when picked up or hugged or aversion to baths, haircuts, having nails cut, dental care, and similar activities; and (3) atypical affective response to non-noxious tactile stimuli, such as responding with aggression to light touch or being physically close to people. Children who are "undersensitive" to touch may appear relatively unaware of pain and temperature and have been described as enjoying playing in mud, rubbing against walls and furniture, and bumping into people.

MOVEMENT

"Oversensitive" children are said to manifest gravitational insecurity, becoming anxious when tipped off balance. They may avoid running, climbing, sliding, or swinging and have motion sickness in cars or elevators. "Undersensitive" children are described as craving fast movements such as swinging, rocking, and spinning and assuming unusual positions when sitting or lying.

BODY POSITION

The "oversensitive" child may be tense, stiff, and uncoordinated, whereas the "undersensitive" may slump, be clumsy, bump into objects, stamp feet, and move fingers repetitively.

VISUAL AND AUDITORY STIMULI

With regard to visual stimuli, "oversensitivity" might lead to covering eyes in response to heightened visual input, avoidance of eye contact, or "hypervigilance," whereas "undersensitivity" is said to contribute to missing visual cues. "Auditory oversensitivity" might manifest as aversive responses to fire alarms, vacuum cleaners, and blenders; auditory "undersensitivity" may manifest as ignoring when spoken to, speaking loudly, and preferring louder volume for the radio or television. Variations in sensitivity are also seen in response to stimuli such as smell, tastes, textures, and temperatures of foods.

ASSOCIATED SYMPTOMS

Associated behavioral problems have been described, including unusually high or low activity levels; problems with muscle tone and coordination; motor planning (praxis); lack of hand preference by age of 4 or 5; difficulties with transitions; problems with self-regulation; and various academic, social, and emotional problems. The overlap of these symptoms with those of other developmental and behavioral disorders is obvious.

Identification

Ayres developed an integrated battery of tests in 1989 for children 4 through 8 years with mild to moderate learning, behavioral, or developmental irregularities. The Sensory Integration and Praxis Tests consist of 17 tests that were designed to measure broad groups of function including[79] tactile and vestibular-proprioceptive sensory processing (e.g., kinesthesia; graphesthesia, postrotatory nystagmus, balance); form and space perception and visuomotor coordination (e.g., figure-ground perception; motor accuracy, constructional praxis); and praxis (design copying; postural, sequencing, and oral praxis). A number of other measures have subsequently been developed, including the Sensory Profile, the Infant/Toddler Sensory Profile, and the Adult Sensory Profile, parent or self-completed questionnaires that describe responses to sensations during daily life activities.[81] Studies of autonomic function in children with poor sensory modulation in which measures of electrodermal activity were used have demonstrated sympathetic markers of dysfunction with increased amplitudes of electrodermal response, more frequent responses, and less habituation to repeated stimulation.[86]

Treatment

In sensory integration therapy, sensory motor activities that provide tactile, vestibular, and proprioceptive sensations are used. Activities such as swinging, rolling, jumping on a trampoline, riding on scooter boards, or completing obstacle courses are intended to stimulate the vestibular system. Brushing the body, providing joint compression, and applying pressure to the body between pads or pillows and with the use of ball pits purportedly address the tactile and proprioceptive systems. The therapist usually monitors the child's responses during these activities and modifies the sensory and motor demands, recording observable changes in ability to participate in the activities, regulate arousal level, and ability to participate in daily living activities. Therapists then make recommendations to parents, teachers, and others regarding the child's behavior from a sensory perspective and provide suggestions for adaptations to the environment. A related clinical practice is the application of a "sensory diet" in which individual activity plans are designed to meet the presumed sensory needs of the patient (such as wearing weighted vests, conducting oral-motor exercises, and modifying the environment).

Discussion

Many children with symptoms of sensory integration dysfunction appear to demonstrate a short-term positive response to sensory integration therapy with diminished levels of disruptive or dysfunctional behavior. Long-accepted practices such as swaddling and rocking infants to soothe them, or relaxing in rocking chairs and hammocks, could also be described as sensory therapy. The time and individual attention provided by the therapist and the sense of empowerment by parents who are given lists of structured activities to perform with their child are indisputably productive. However, the scientific evidence that this technique actually accomplishes the effects that have been postulated is still lacking. It is well recognized that the placebo effect accounts for more than 30% of improvement in symptoms, regardless of the modality of therapeutic intervention or the condition being treated.

There is no shortage of published reports on sensory integration therapy. Results of many studies suggest that the intervention works, but many studies have also concluded that it does not work.[87] Unfortunately, *none* of the investigators has adhered to rigorous criteria for randomized controlled trials. There is also no reliable evidence to support a basic tenet of sensory integration theory: that integration of sensory input is necessary for high-level cognitive functioning.

There are concerns regarding the widespread application of sensory integration theory and interventions without the support of scientific evidence. A particular concern is the use of this diagnosis to explain the origin of ill-defined developmental problems without more diligent pursuit of potential underlying medical diagnoses. For example, for a child with poor posture who is clumsy, tends to bump into objects, fatigues easily, prefers to have the volume of radio and television loud, and is underachieving at school, a diagnosis of sensory integration disorder might be used to explain these symptoms; however, they might represent a mitochondrial disorder with encephalomyopathy and mild hearing impairment. Numerous similar examples could be cited. Likewise, clinicians must understand that sensory integration therapy approaches should not be used to the exclusion of other therapeutic interventions that have scientifically proven efficacy.

If families do decide to pursue this therapeutic approach for their children, they should develop a plan for objectively evaluating its efficacy. This should include selection of target behaviors to be addressed and methods for measuring changes in these behaviors. The type of intervention to address these behaviors must be defined, as must the duration of the therapy. Target behaviors should be measured at baseline and after the treatment phase.

Current efforts to more rigorously study the construct of sensory integration and the efficacy of intervention are to be lauded and encouraged. It is hoped that clinicians will in the future have scientific evidence on which to base their advice to patients and families regarding decisions about sensory integration therapy.

REFERENCES

1. Greenough WT, Black JE: Induction of brain structure by experience: Substrates for cognitive development. Dev Behav Neurosci 24:155-200, 1992.
2. Schlumberger E, Narbona J, Manrique M: Non-verbal development of children with deafness with and without cochlear implants. Dev Med Child Neurol 46:599-606, 2004.
3. Svirsky MA, Teoh, S, Neuburger H: Development of language and speech perception in congenitally profoundly deaf children as a function of age of cochlear implantation. Audiol Neurotol 9:224-233, 2004.
4. Task Force on Newborn and Infant Hearing, American Academy of Pediatrics: Newborn and infant hearing loss: Detection and intervention. Pediatrics 103:527-530, 1999.
5. Jacobson J, Jacobson C: Evaluation of hearing loss in infants and young children. Pediatr Ann 33:812-821, 2004.
6. Davidson J, Hyde ML, Alberti PW: Epidemiologic patterns in childhood hearing loss. Int J Pediatr Otorhinolaryngol 17:239, 1989.
7. Joint Committee on Infant Hearing: Year 2000 Position Statement: Principles and Guidelines for Early Hearing Detection and Intervention Programs. Pediatrics 106:798-817, 2000.
8. Berlin CI: Role of infant hearing screening in health care. Semin Hear 17:115-123, 1996.
9. Smith RJ, Bale JF, White KR: Sensorineural hearing loss in children. Lancet 365:2085-2086, 2005.
10. Kenna MA: Medical management of childhood hearing loss. Pediatr Ann 33:822-832, 2004.
11. Greinwald JH, Hartnick CJ: The evaluation of children with hearing loss. Arch Otolaryngol Head Neck Surg 128:84-87, 2002.
12. Frei K, Ramsebner R, Lucas T, et al: GJβ2 mutations in hearing impairment: Identification of a broad clinical spectrum for improved genetic counseling. Laryngoscope 115:461-465, 2005.
13. Roizen NR: Etiology of hearing loss in children: Nongenetic causes. Pediatr Clin North Am 46:49-61, 1999.
14. Dodge P, Davis H, Feigin R, et al: Prospective evaluation of hearing loss as a sequela of acute bacterial meningitis. N Engl J Med 311:869-874, 1984.
15. Meadow KP: Deafness and Child Development. Berkeley: University of California Press, 1980.
16. Yoshinaga-Itano C: From screening to early identification and intervention: Discovering predictors to successful outcomes for children with significant hearing loss. J Deaf Stud Deaf Educ 8:11-30, 2003.
17. Marschak M: Psychological Development of Deaf Children. New York: Oxford University Press, 1993.
18. Schlumberger E, Narbona J, Manrique M: Non-verbal development of children with deafness, with and

without cochlear implants. Dev Med Child Neurol 46:599-606, 2004.

19. Butterfield SA, Ersing WF: Influence of age, sex, etiology and hearing loss on balance performance by deaf children. Percept Mot Skills 62:653-659, 1986.

20. Vernon M: Fifty years of research on the intelligence of deaf and hard-of-hearing children: A review of the literature and discussion of implications. J Deaf Stud Deaf Educ 10:225-231, 2005.

21. Ita C, Friedman H: The psychological development of children who are hard of hearing: A critical review. Volta Rev 101:165-181, 1999.

22. Wake M, Hughes EK, Poulakis Z, et al: Outcomes of children with mild-profound hearing loss at 7 to 8 years: A population study. Ear Hear 25:1-8, 2004.

23. Kelly DP, Kelly BJ, Jones ML, et al: Attention deficits in children and adolescents with hearing loss: A survey. Am J Dis Child 147:737-741, 1993.

24. Haensel J, Engelke JC, Ottenjam W, et al: Long-term results of cochlear implantation in children. Otolaryngol Head Neck Surg 132:456-458, 2005.

25. Eilers RE, Oller DK: Infant vocalizations and the early diagnosis of severe hearing impairment. J Pediatr 124:199-203, 1994.

26. Glascoe FP: Parents' Evaluations of Developmental Status. Nashville, TN: Elsworth & Vandermeer, 2005.

27. Bricker D, Squires J: Ages & Stages Questionnaire: A Parent-Completed, Child-Monitoring System, 2nd ed. Baltimore: Paul H. Brooks, 1999.

28. Coplan J: The Early Language Milestone Scale. Tulsa, OK: Modern Education Corp., 1987.

29. Capute AJ, Shapiro BK, Wachtel RC, et al: The Clinical Linguistic and Auditory Milestone Scale (CLAMS): Identification of cognitive deficits in motor-delayed children. Am J Dis Child 140:694, 1986.

30. Brookhouser PE: Sensorineural hearing loss. Pediatr Clin North Am 43:1195-1216, 1996.

31. Pickett BP, Ahlstrom K: Clinical evaluation of the hearing impaired infant. Otolaryngol Clin North Am 32:1019-1033, 1999.

32. Rapin I: Hearing Disorders. Pediatr Rev 14:43, 1993.

33. Brookhouser PE, Beauchaine MA, Osberger MJ: Management of the child with sensorineural hearing loss. Pediatr Clin North Am 46:121-141, 1999.

34. Slattery WH, Fayad JN: Cochlear implants in children with sensorineural inner ear hearing loss. Pediatr Ann 28:359-363, 1999.

35. Waltzman SB, Roland JT: Cochlear implantation in children younger than 12 months. Pediatrics 116(4): e487-e493, 2005.

36. Reamy CE, Brackett D: Communication methodologies: Options for families. Otolaryngol Clin North Am 32:1103-1115, 1999.

37. Luterman D: Counseling families with a hearing-impaired child. Otolaryngol Clin North Am 32:1037, 1999.

38. Kniestedt C, Stamper RL: Visual acuity and its measurement. Ophthalmol Clin North Am 16:155-170, 2003.

39. Buncic JR: The blind child. Pediatr Clin North Am 34:1403-1414, 1987.

40. Thompson L Kaufman LM: The visually impaired child. Pediatr Clin North Am 50:225-238, 2003.

41. Pilling RF, Thompson JR, Gottlob I: Social and visual function in nystagmus. Br J Ophthalmol 89:1278-1281, 2005.

42. Baird G, Moore AT: Epidemiology. *In* Fielder AR, Best AB, Bax MCO, eds: The Management of Visual Impairment in Childhood. London: MacKeith Press, 1993.

43. Gilbert CE, Anderton L, Dandona L, et al: Prevalence of visual impairment in children: A review of available data. Ophthalmol Epidemiol 6:73-82, 1999.

44. Donnelly UM, Stewart NM, Holinger M: Prevalence and outcome of childhood visual disorders. Ophthalmol Epidemiol 12:243-250, 2005.

45. Flanagan NM, Jackson AJ, Hill AE: Visual impairment in childhood: Insights from a community survey. Child Care Health Dev 29:493-499, 2003.

46. Phelps D: Retinopathy of prematurity. Pediatr Rev 16:50-56, 1995.

47. Reynolds JD: The management of retinopathy of prematurity. Paediatr Drugs 3:263-272, 2001.

48. Msall ME, Phelps DL, DiGaudio KM, et al: Severity of neonatal retinopathy of prematurity is predictive of neurodevelopmental functional outcome at age 5.5 years. Pediatrics 106:998-1005, 2000.

49. Clemett R, Darlow B: Results of screening low-birth-weight infants for retinopathy of prematurity. Curr Opin Ophthalmol 10:155-163, 1999.

50. Hatton DD, Bailey DB, Burchinal MR, et al: Developmental growth curves of preschool children with vision impairments. Child Dev 68:788-806, 1997.

51. Warren DH: Blindness in children—An individual differences approach. Part I. a. Motor and locomotor interaction with the physical world. Cambridge, UK: Cambridge University Press, 1994, pp 30-55.

52. Jan JE, Groenveld M: Visual behaviors and adaptations associated with cortical and ocular impairment in children. J Vis Impair Blind 87:101-105, 1993.

53. Warren DH: Blindness in children—An individual differences approach. Part II. b. Executive functions: memory attention, and cognitive strategies. Cambridge, UK: Cambridge University Press, 1994, pp 152-153.

54. Andersen ES, Dunlea A, Kekelis LS: Blind children's language: Resolving some differences. J Child Lang 11:645-664, 1984.

55. Teplin SW: Developmental issues in the care of blind infants and children. Pediatr Rounds Growth Nutr Dev 3(2):1-6, 1994.

56. Rettig M: The play of young children with visual impairments: Characteristics and interventions. J Vis Impair Blind 88:410-420, 1994.

57. Uttermohlen TL: On "passing" through adolescence. J Vis Impair Blind 1997; 91:309-314.

58. Hoyt CS: Visual function in the brain-damaged child. Eye 17:369-384, 2003.

59. Freeman R, Goetz E, Richards D, et al: Defiers of negative prediction: A 14-year follow-up study of legally blind children. J Vis Impair Blind 85:365-370, 1991.

60. Jan JE, McCormick AQ, Scott EP, et al: Eye pressing by visually impaired children. Dev Med Child Neurol 25:755-762, 1983.

61. Hatton DD: Model registry of early childhood visual impairment: First-year results. J Vis Impair Blind 95:418-433, 2001.

62. Committee on Practice and Ambulatory Medicine, Section on Ophthalmology, American Association of Certified Orthoptists; American Association for Pediatric Ophthalmology and Strabismus; American Academy of Ophthalmology: Eye examination in infants, children, and young adults by pediatricians. Pediatrics 111:902-907, 2003.

63. U.S. Preventive Services Task Force: Screening for visual impairment in children younger than five years: Recommendation statement. Am Fam Physician 71:333-336, 2005.

64. Simon JW, Kaw P: Vision screening performed by the pediatrician. Pediatr Ann 30:446-452, 2001.

65. Magramm I: Amblyopia: Etiology, detection, and treatment. Pediatr Rev 13:7-14, 1992.

66. Committee on Practice and Ambulatory Medicine and Section on Ophthalmology: American Academy of Pediatrics: Use of photoscreening for children's vision screening. Pediatrics 109:524-525, 2002.

67. Kelly DP, Teplin SW: Disorders of sensation: Hearing and visual impairment. *In* Wolraich ML, ed: Disorders of Development and Learning, 3rd ed. Philadelphia: BC Decker, 2002, pp 329-343.

68. Teplin SW: Developmental issues in blind infants and children. *In* Silverman WA, Flynn JT, eds: Retinopathy of Prematurity. Oxford, UK: Blackwell, 1985, p 286.

69. Demographic update: The number of deaf-blind children in the United States. J Vis Impair Blind News Serv 89(3):13, 1995.

70. McInnes JM, Treffry JA: Deaf-Blind Infants and Children—A Developmental Guide. Toronto: University of Toronto Press, 1982.

71. Miles B, Riggio M, eds: Remarkable Conversations—A Guide to Developing Meaningful Communication with Children and Young Adults Who Are Deafblind. Watertown, MA: Perkins School for the Blind, 1999.

72. Franklin B: Tactile sensory aids for children who are deaf-blind. Traces (Teaching Research Assistance to Children and Youth Experiencing Sensory Impairments) 1(3):2-3, Summer 1991.

73. Menella JA: Taste and smell. *In* Swaiman KF, Ashwal S, eds: Pediatric Neurology: Principles ad Practice. St. Louis: CV Mosby, 1999, pp 104-113.

74. MacColl G, Quinton R: Kallman's syndrome: bridging the gaps. J Pediatr Endocrinol Metab 18(6):541-543, 2005. Kallman syndrome

75. Nader R, Oberlander TF, Chambers CT, et al: Expression of pain in children with autism. Clin J Pain 20(2):88-97, 2004.

76. Buskila D, Neumann L, Zmora E, et al: Pain sensitivity in prematurely born adolescents. Arch Pediatr Adolesc Med 157:1079-1082, 2003.

77. Axelrod FB, Hilz MJ: Inherited autonomic neuropathies. Semin Neurol 23:381-390, 2003.

78. Mangeot SD, Miller LJ, McIntosh DN, et al: Sensory modulation dysfunction in children with attention-deficit–hyperactivity disorder. Dev Med Child Neurol 43:399-406, 2001.

79. Ayres AJ: Sensory Integration and Learning Disorders. Los Angeles: Western Psychological Services, 1972, p 11.

80. Smith T, Mruzek DW, Mozingo D: Sensory integrative therapy. *In* Jacobson JW, Foxx RM, Mulick JA, eds: Controversial Therapies for Developmental Disabilities. Mahwah, NJ: Erlbaum, 2005, pp 331-350.

81. Schaaf RC, Miller LJ: Occupational therapy using a sensory integrative approach for children with developmental disabilities. Ment Retard Dev Disabil Res Rev 11:143-148, 2005.

82. Bundy AC, Lane SJ, Fisher AG, et al: Sensory Integration Theory and Practice. Philadelphia: FA Davis, 2002.

83. Baranek GT, Foster LG, Berkson G: Sensory defensiveness in persons with developmental disabilities. Occup Ther J Res 17:173-185, 1997.

84. Ahn RR, Miller LJ, Milberger S, et al: Prevalence of parents' perceptions of sensory processing disorders among kindergarten children. Am J Occup Ther 58:287-293, 2004.

85. Kranowitz CS: The Out-of-Sync Child. New York: Berkley Publishing, 1998.

86. McIntosh DN, Miller LJ, Shyu V, et al: Sensory-modulation disruption, electrodermal responses, and functional behaviors. Dev Med Child Neurol 41:608-615, 1999.

87. Miller LJ: Empirical evidence related to therapies for sensory processing impairments. NASP Communiqué 31(5):34-37, 2003.

Cognitive and Adaptive Disabilities

WILLIAM O. WALKER, JR. ■ CHRIS PLAUCHÉ JOHNSON

PURPOSE

The initial diagnosis of mental retardation brings uncertainty to the family of the affected child; they do not know what this diagnosis will mean for their child now or in the future. At the same time, the physician is also uncertain, as he or she may not have a clear explanation of either the cause of these specific delays or the types of interventions and support services that are appropriate and necessary for a child, teenager, young adult, or adult with this diagnosis. Individuals with mental retardation now live much longer lives and often do so in community, rather than institutional, settings.

The direct and indirect economic costs associated with mental retardation in the United States are significant: $51.2 billion (2003 dollars) for persons born in 2000.[1] The proportion of school-aged children classified as having "mental retardation" and receiving services in federally funded educational programs in the United States has stabilized since the early 1990s between 1.26% and 1.28%.[2] The Centers for Disease Control and Prevention currently estimate that mental retardation is diagnosed in 12 per 1000 U.S. school-aged children; the result in annual special education costs is $3.3 billion.

The goal of this chapter is to provide information about how clinicians establish this diagnosis by using well-accepted definitions, appropriate testing instruments, and an evidence-based etiological evaluation method, in conjunction with developing effective support systems across the entire lifespan.

TERMINOLOGY DEBATE

The terminology used to describe mental retardation has changed since the 19th century, reflecting an increased sensitivity to the rights of and opportunities for persons with mental retardation, an increased effort to mainstream individuals with mental retarda-

tion into society to improve their quality of life, and a decreased tolerance for stigmatizing and limiting "labels" that focus on the disability rather than on the individual. The terms *imbecility* and *idiocy* were used in the late 19th century to describe different levels of intellectual functioning on the basis of decreasing language and speech abilities. Less affected individuals were referred to as being "feeble-minded." At that time, the outcome for individuals with mental retardation was believed to be predetermined; their ability to participate in everyday activities and within typical environments was limited. In the mid-20th century, terms such as *trainable* and *educable* were used to characterize persons with mental retardation, often to suggest what type of educational experience was most appropriate. Newer educational interventions that emphasize mainstreaming have reversed this focus on limiting participation and minimizing progress. What has remained, however, is the need to distinguish between a label, the specific difficulties faced by an individual with that label, and the social judgments associated with that label.[3] Effective differentiation between the label and the individual and advocacy for the integration of these children and their families into every aspect of society is an essential responsibility of developmental-behavioral pediatricians and every other member of the multidisciplinary teams providing their care.

There are numerous negative connotations associated with the term *mental retardation*. There is no agreement on a more preferred term at either the international or national level. Other terms that have been proposed include *intellectual disability/disabilities, developmental disabilities, mentally challenged,* and *cognitive adaptive disability or delay.* In the United Kingdom, the term *learning disability* is used, whereas *intellectual disability* is preferred in Japan and is increasingly the label of choice among the international community.[4]

As it prepared to revise its 1992 definition for mental retardation, the American Association on

TABLE 11-1 ■ Current Definitions of Mental Retardation

Feature	AAMR, 2002	DSM-IV-TR
Intellectual functioning	Significant limitations in intellectual functioning	Significantly subaverage IQ of approximately 70 or below on an individually administered standardized test of intelligence
Adaptive functioning	Significant limitations in adaptive behaviors as expressed in conceptual, social, and practical adaptive skills	Concurrent impairments in two of the following areas: communication, self-care, home living, social skills, community skills, self-direction, functional academic skills, work, leisure, health, and safety
Age at onset	Before 18 years	Before 18 years

AAMR, American Association on Mental Retardation[5]; DSM-IV-TR, Diagnostic and Statistical Manual of Mental Disorders, 4th ed, text revision (American Psychiatric Association[6]).

Mental Retardation (AAMR) asked for comments and recommendations for an alternative term that would better describe these individuals. One strongly considered proposal was *cognitive adaptive disability.* Interestingly, this evolving discussion of a "best" or "better" term eventually led to a change in the name of the President's Committee on Mental Retardation to the President's Committee on Intellectual Disability. There are very strong arguments that any other term selected to describe this group of individuals will quickly assume similar negative connotations. It is also important to realize that what is "acceptable" to professionals may not be so readily accepted by affected individuals and their families. There have also been concerns that changing the term used to describe these individuals might adversely affect their eligibility for services specifically defined in statute for "persons with mental retardation" (supplemental Social Security payments) and for unique legal protections provided by this diagnosis (death penalty exclusions). The debate over the correct terminology for this condition continues. In January 2007, the American Association on Mental Retardation (AAMR) officially changed the organization's name to the American Association on Intellectual and Developmental Disabilities (AAIDD). Although they recognize that the condition "mental retardation" they have defined for over 100 years still exists, the AAMR/AAIDD leadership feels that this change is "an idea whose time has come."

DEFINITION AND CRITERIA

The AAIDD and predecessor organizations have updated their definition 10 times since Alfred F. Tredgold proposed this definition in 1908:

A state of mental defect from birth, or from an early age, due to incomplete cerebral development, in consequence of which the person affected is unable to perform his duties as a member of society in the position of life to which he is born.[5]

There are two generally well-accepted organizational definitions of mental retardation: the AAMR's and the American Psychiatric Association's as described in the *Diagnostic and Statistical Manual of Mental Disorders,* fourth edition, text revision *(DSM-IV-TR)* (Table 11-1).[5,6] The two schemes have common elements: the use of standardized measures of intelligence and adaptive abilities to define levels of significant subaverage intellectual and adaptive functioning and evidence of the disability's presence before 18 years of age. In current definitions, mental retardation is no longer described as a state of "global incompetence." Instead, they refer to an overall pattern of limitations and describe how individuals typically, not ideally, function in various contexts of their everyday life.

There are differences between the AAMR and *DSM-IV-TR* definitions and their classification of "significant subaverage intellectual functioning." Until 1973, the AAMR criterion for significant subaverage intellectual functioning was one, rather than two, standard deviations below the mean. AAMR now defines the upper limit of mental retardation as a range of standardized IQ scores (70 to 75), whereas the *DSM-IV-TR* definition maintains the upper limit of normal at the traditional level IQ score of 70. The current AAMR cutoff scores are approximately two standard deviations below the mean score on standardized measures of intelligence. However, use of a range, rather than a specific score to define mental retardation actually doubles the number of persons who could be described as having "mental retardation:" from 2.27% of the general population with scores less than 70 to 4.85% with scores less than 75.

In discussions with families, it is very important to remember that *cognition, intelligence,* and *IQ* are not synonymous terms; confusion and disagreement often occur when they are used interchangeably. *Intelligence* is a combination of the ability to learn and to pose and solve problems.[7] Various schemas for intelligence have been proposed with complementary and overlapping features.

The requirement to consider adaptive abilities was first included in the 1959 AAMR definition. Adaptive behavior encompasses the application of conceptual, social, and practical skills to daily life. Significant limitations in adaptive behavior affect a person's daily life and his or her ability to respond to a particular situation or environment. Adaptive areas typically evaluated include communication, self-care, home living, social skills, community use, self-direction, health and safety, functional academics, leisure, and work. There are well-accepted standardized measures used to quantify adaptive behaviors, such as the Vineland Adaptive Behavior Scales. These measures are standardized with regard to the general population, which includes persons with and without disabilities.

Levels of Mental Retardation

Efforts to classify mental retardation by level of severity have a long and rather colorful history. Specific terms to describe different levels of impairment have evolved over time to help differentiate individuals and their outcome with the understanding that a variety of comorbid medical, psychiatric, and behavioral disorders also affect outcome. The outcome of individuals with mental retardation is affected by the severity of both their adaptive and intellectual disabilities. Identifying a specific cause, rather than an "idiopathic" cause, may also affect any ability to predict outcome.

In the traditional classification schema, continued in the *DSM-IV-TR* system, the number of standard deviations below the mean is its basis (Table 11-2). There are both advantages and disadvantages to this schema. It is often preferable for research purposes because of its ability to better define a "homogeneous" population. However, the fact that a numerical "score" from a standardized measure of intelligence may vary by as much as 5 points higher or lower (95% confidence interval) still limits the effectiveness of a specific score as a method of differentiation across severity levels. In other schemas, particularly for epidemio-

logical analyses, an IQ cutoff score of 50 is used to differentiate between "mild" and "severe" mental retardation.[8] The reason for this division was to define and describe individuals who would benefit from a formal/academic education program (mild) from those who would benefit more from a life skills education program (severe). Likewise, the same differentiation could be applied to individuals who would be able to live independently (mild) from those more likely to need a guardian and additional supervision (severe).

Levels of Support

The 1992 edition of AAMR's definition of mental retardation introduced a significant change in the organizational and descriptive approach to individuals with mental retardation: the concept of "levels of support." AAMR further developed this concept and proposed the current definition in 2002: "Supports are resources and strategies that aim to promote the development, education, interests and personal well being of a person and that enhance individual functioning."[5]

The supports approach purpose is to evaluate the specific needs of the individual and then suggest strategies, services, and supports that will optimize individual functioning across the various dimensions of intellectual functioning. These resources and strategies can be the result of a person's own efforts or help from other individuals (natural sources), or it can be the result of additional technology, agencies, or service providers (service-based sources). The goal of these interventions is to improve personal functioning, promote self-determination and societal inclusion, and improve the personal well-being and functional abilities and outcomes of a person with mental retardation. In many ways, this method parallels the evolving attention to not only the cognitive and adaptive limitations but also the specific abilities of an individual.[5] In an effort to provide a comprehensive assessment, an evaluation is recommended in at least nine key areas: human development, teaching and education, home living, community living, employment, health and safety, behavior, social function, and pro-

TABLE 11-2 ■ Levels of Mental Retardation			
Level	% of Total Mentally Retarded Population	IQ Range	Standard Deviations Below Mean
Mild	85%	From 50-55 to approximately 70	2-3
Moderate	10%	From 35-49 to 50-55	3-4
Severe	3.5%	From 20-25 to 35-40	4-5
Profound	1.5%	<20-25	>5

From the American Psychiatric Association: *Diagnostic and Statistical Manual of Mental Disorders*, 4th ed, text revision. Washington, DC: American Psychiatric Association, 2000.

TABLE 11-3 ■ Dimensions of Mental Retardation

Intellectual abilities	Communication, functional academics, vocational skills
Adaptive behavior	Self-care, home living, integrated vocational opportunities
Social roles, participation, interactions*	Community living, friendships, self-esteem, social skills, leisure activities
Health concerns (physical, mental, etiological)	Etiology and conditions related to biological processes; comorbid disorders
Context considerations	Environments, cultures

From American Association on Mental Retardation. *In* Luckasson RA, Schalock RL, Spitalnik DM, et al, eds: Mental Retardation: Definition, Classification, and Systems of Support, 10th ed. Washington, DC: American Association on Mental Retardation, 2002, pp 99-121.
*New dimension as of 2002.

TABLE 11-4 ■ Support Intensity Levels

Intermittent	Will require support only on an "as needed" basis
	Episodic or short-term support (least affected individuals)
Limited	Will require support on a constant but not permanent basis
	Consistent, time-limited support
Extensive	Will require constant, lifelong support
	Regular involvement in an aspect of the person's environment
	This support may not apply to all environments
Pervasive	Will require constant, lifelong support in all environments
	Potentially life-sustaining support
	(Most seriously affected individuals)

From American Association on Mental Retardation. *In* Luckasson RA, Schalock RL, Spitalnik DM, et al, eds: Mental Retardation: Definition, Classification, and Systems of Support, 10th ed. Washington, DC: American Association on Mental Retardation, 2002, pp 145-168.
*New dimension as of 2002.

tection and advocacy. Within these areas, such supports as teaching, befriending, financial planning, employee assistance, behavioral support, in-home living assistance, community access and use, and health assistance may be required. The level of support method recognizes that an individual's needs and circumstances change over time and are influenced by an individual's environment. Supports are dynamic.

As a support schema is developed, two additional characteristics must be considered: support dimensions and support intensity. Five dimensions of intellectual ability in which an individual may require additional support have been identified (Table 11-3). Each individual has different needs and therefore requires different supports in each of these dimensions. The intensity, frequency, and acuity of what an individual requires in support are also not uniform across these various dimensions (Table 11-4).

The most recent evolution in this method is the AAIDD's development of the Supports Intensity Scales.[9] This instrument provides a direct assessment of the support needed on an individual basis that is not inferred from a "score" derived from other instruments whose norms are based on the general population and not specifically on individuals with disabilities.[10]

Prevalence

The statistical prevalence of mental retardation is approximately 2% to 3%, although the actual prevalence may be closer to 1%. The estimate varies according to the particular study, specific ascertainment methods, the age of the cohort being studied (lower prevalence among subjects aged <5 years and >18 years—i.e., non–school-aged cohorts), and the level of impairment. Multiple studies and surveys have demonstrated that specific populations are overrepresented; the label "mental retardation" is more likely

to be applied to individuals of lower socioeconomic status, ethnic groups, and cultural minority groups; those in institutions; and those with related conditions (cerebral palsy, spina bifida, autism).[11-13] The prevalence of severe mental retardation (IQ < 50) has remained stable at approximately 0.4% to 0.5%; it is much more likely to be associated with organic disorders and causes. Because of the more variable upper diagnostic limits, the prevalence of mild mental retardation (IQ of 50 to ≤70-75) is more difficult to ascertain. Nevertheless, the vast majority (approximately 85%) of persons with mental retardation have IQ scores in the "mild" range.

ETIOLOGY

Risk Factors in Mental Retardation

A distinction must be made between "causes of" and "risk factors for" mental retardation. There are well-established medical and genetic disorders consistently associated with mental retardation (e.g., trisomy 21, congenital hypothyroidism, untreated phenylketonuria) that represent an established cause. A carefully documented history may reveal biological events with significant potential to impair future cognitive functioning (prematurity, hypoxic-ischemic encephalopathy) that represent a biological risk. Likewise, significant environmental deprivation (of nutritional or social stimulation) may place an individual at increased risk for mental retardation.

Studies of intelligence with standardized IQ measures have produced evidence for a significant genetic influence, although experience and environment also influence this innate ability: 50% of the IQ test score variation can be attributed to genetic variation.[14] Heritability estimates for general intelligence appear to be approximately 0.45 to 0.75; longitudinal studies have shown this factor to increase steadily from infancy through adulthood.[15] Different genes may play a role, each with a varying degree of effect (quantitative trait loci).[15] Children with birth defects are 27 times more likely to have mental retardation by 7 years of age than are children without a diagnosed birth defect, regardless of the type of defect.[16]

Different risk factors for mild and severe levels of mental retardation are known. Sameroff and associates[17] found that the presence of multiple risk factors at age 4 were an important predictor of children's IQ at age 13. The cumulative effect of multiple risk factors can have an adverse effect on academic success from 1st through 12th grade, overcoming any bolstering effect of intelligence and positive mental health.[18] Low maternal education level continues to be the strongest predictor of mild mental retardation. Women with less than 12 years of schooling are more likely to have a child with a mental retardation placement in school than are mothers with some degree of post-secondary education.[19] Women with only high-school diplomas still have an increased, albeit lower, risk. Numerous studies have demonstrated an increased risk for isolated severe mental retardation in boys and men (1.4:1) and in nonwhite populations (2:1).[20] Therefore, both nature and nurture play important roles in cognitive development. Genetics appears to provide the cognitive potential that is then shaped and developed by environmental and self-selected experiences that further modify a person's behavior.

Etiological Diagnosis of Mental Retardation

Efforts to identify specific causes of mental retardation are driven by the hope that defining a cause will improve the ability to prevent mental retardation from that cause. However, an etiological diagnosis is made in less than one half of individuals with mental retardation.[21] A major challenge in defining an etiology for mental retardation remains in characterizing the contribution and interaction of various socioeconomic factors and other factors in association with prenatal, perinatal, and postnatal events. The number of cases attributed to specific diagnostic categories varies according to the degree of mental retardation, patient selection criteria (including age of the patient), study protocols, technological advances over time, and definitions of diagnoses.[22] Because of these issues, classification systems based only on timing or etiology, although more frequently used, may be incomplete. Moog[23] proposed a "dynamic classification system" that distinguishes among genetic, unknown, and acquired causes with additional consideration to the degree of diagnostic certainty.

"Diagnostic uncertainty" has a significant effect on families and their ability to cope with the stresses associated with a child having mental retardation. In one comparison of levels of anxiety, feelings of guilt, and emotional burdens of mothers of children with Down syndrome and mothers of children with an undefined reason for their mental retardation, the latter group was found to be at a significant psychoemotional disadvantage.[24] Therefore, defining an etiology goes beyond identifying recurrence risk and intervention planning; the process and its outcome may provide a significant emotional support to that family by addressing issues of guilt and in establishing connections with other similarly affected families through support groups.

MOST COMMON IDENTIFIABLE ETIOLOGIES

The three most common identifiable causes of mental retardation are fetal alcohol syndrome (FAS), the fragile X syndrome, and Down syndrome. In individual children with FAS, IQ measures range from 20 to 120, with a mean of 65.[25] In comparison, IQ scores of affected male patients with the fragile X syndrome range from 25 to 65, and those of children with Down syndrome range from 40 to 60.[26,27]

Fetal Alcohol Syndrome

FAS is the most common preventable, nongenetic cause of mental retardation.[28] Mental retardation is the abnormality most often associated with the diagnosis of FAS. Estimates of birth prevalence vary among countries. The critical period for alcohol exposure appears to be in the initial 3 to 6 weeks of brain development. The term *fetal alcohol spectrum disorders* has been suggested to describe the range of impairments in this disorder.[29] Other terms such as *fetal alcohol effects, prenatal alcohol effects,* and *alcohol-related neurodevelopmental disabilities or birth defects* have been proposed.[29] There is no reliable biological marker for FAS. Therefore, the diagnosis is based on clinical criteria that include evidence of prenatal and postnatal growth deficiency, characteristic facial features, and central nervous system anomalies and/or dysfunction.[30] Although a history of maternal alcohol use during the pregnancy should be present, exposure is frequently underreported. The differences in growth and facial features vary with the patient's age and ethnicity.[25] Multiple efforts have been made at establishing a paradigm or tool to evaluate and diagnose these affected children, including the Institute of Medicine's criteria for FAS/fetal alcohol effects published in 1996[28] and the four-digit system proposed by Astley and Clarren.[31]

In comparison with other individuals with an identifiable cause of mental retardation, FAS-affected children are at an increased risk for behavioral and psychiatric disorders. Children with FAS exhibit early deficits in measures of attention, learning, executive functioning, and visual-spatial processing. Their social abilities often plateau at the 6-year-old level. Individuals with FAS/fetal alcohol effects demonstrate significant problems with adaptive behavior, which continue into adulthood. One of the strongest correlates with this adverse outcome was the lack of an early diagnosis.[32] Young adults with FAS and normal IQs (>70) demonstrate deficits in the areas of attention, verbal learning, and executive function that are more severe than suggested by IQ alone. FAS-affected children with normal IQ scores may still have significant neurobehavioral and adaptive deficits. Some of these behavioral issues may be complicated by the association between several forms of hearing loss and FAS: delays in auditory maturation, sensorineural hearing loss, and intermittent hearing loss secondary to chronic serous otitis media.

Fragile X Syndrome

The fragile X syndrome (also see Chapter 10B for more information) is the most common inherited form of mental retardation and has been identified in every racial and ethnic group studied. It is the leading cause of inherited mental retardation, affecting approximately 50,000 persons in the United States alone (prevalence, 1 per 4000 boys and men, 1 per 6000 girls and women). X-linked factors are believed to be responsible for 10% to 12% of mental retardation in boys and men.[33] Fragile X represents the most common (15% to 25%) of the numerous loci identified on the X chromosome that are associated with mental retardation. The fragile X syndrome is the result of an expansion of an unstable cytosine-guanine-guanine (CGG) repeat within the *FMR1* gene at Xq27.3. The reason for this expansion is unknown. Four allele patterns have been defined: normal (6 to 50 repeats), intermediate/"gray" (45 to 50), permutation (55 to 200) and full mutation (>200). Once the expansion reaches 200 repeats, the entire *FMR1* gene region is methylated (silenced) and FMR1 protein is not produced. It is the absence of FMR1 protein that leads to the characteristic cognitive and clinical features of the syndrome.[34]

The cognitive profile in the fragile X syndrome is similar in both affected male and female patients, with observed weaknesses in the areas of short-term memory for complex sequential information, visual-spatial skills, planning, and verbal fluency. Many of these areas are often subsumed under the term *executive functioning*.[35] In the fragile X syndrome, the social deficits that make up part of the full mutation phenotype range from autistic features to social anxiety and pragmatic language deficits. As many as 25% to 35% of individuals with full mutations meet diagnostic criteria for autism.[36]

The physical characteristics are much more obvious in affected boys and men, evolving over time so that they become more apparent during adolescence and adulthood. The two most frequently described findings are large ears and macro-orchidism. Other physical findings include a long, narrow face; a high arched palate; loose connective tissue (hyperextensible fingers, flat feet); and mitral valve prolapse.

Boys and men with the full mutation usually exhibit moderate to severe intellectual impairment, characteristic language disorders (cluttering; stronger receptive than expressive skills), and social and behavioral difficulties, including problems with at-tention, impulsivity, anxiety, social avoidance, and arousal. There does not appear to be any relationship between the number of CGG repeats and IQ score in boys and men with the full mutation. Boys and men with the fragile X syndrome exhibit a decline in cognitive, language, and adaptive skills measures during the school years. A specific cause of this decline is not known.[26]

Approximately 30% to 50% of girls and women with the full fragile X mutation have IQ scores in the mental retardation range. In addition, they often exhibit a characteristic behavioral phenotype of extreme shyness and decreased eye contact. The remaining female patients may present with borderline to normal intellectual functioning, learning disabilities related to executive functioning, and/or other psychosocial difficulties. There does appear to be a relationship between IQ score and chromosome X activation scores and between IQ score and FMR1 protein levels in affected women.[37]

The ability to identify children with the fragile X mutation through genetic testing is of particular benefit to physicians and families. DNA studies for the fragile X syndrome have been readily available since 1991 and should be strongly considered in every affected child, boy or girl, in whom the cause of mental retardation is unknown. Despite the availability of this technology, the average age at diagnosis in boys with the fragile X syndrome is 3 years; it is even later in girls.[38] In a survey of 274 families with a child with the fragile X syndrome, a number of variables affected making the diagnosis of the syndrome in a timely manner.[38] As is the case in other cause of developmental delay, there is often a lag between when the parent expresses concern and when the professional agrees that there is a problem. More than one half of the families expressing a concern about their child were told to "wait and see; he might improve" or that their child was developing normally. In families with affected children born after 1991, the average time between the parent's first concern and the ordering of the fragile X test was 18 months. More than 50% of the families had already had another child before the diagnosis of fragile X syndrome was made.[38] Although some authorities have argued for its implementation, the fragile X syndrome does not meet the traditional criteria for neonatal screening, because an identifiable intervention that could change the course of the disorder does not exist.

Down Syndrome

Down syndrome occurs in 1 per 800 live births and 1 per 1000 conceptions and is the most common genetic disorder causing mental retardation. It is usually readily identified at or near birth by characteristic physical features: hypotonia, hyperflexibility of joints, flat facial profile, slanted palpebral fissures, poor Moro reflex, excess skin on the back of the neck, abnormal ears, dysplasia of the midphalanx of the fifth finger, and a single palmar crease. Other frequently associated conditions include congenital heart disease (40%) and gastrointestinal abnormalities (5%).[39] There exist artistic representations of persons with Down syndrome from as early as 500 A.D. Because no combination of these features is specific to Down syndrome, the diagnosis is confirmed by routine chromosome analysis; three abnormalities are possible. The most common finding on chromosomal analysis is a true trisomy for chromosome 21 (in 95% of affected patients); unbalanced robertsonian translocations (3% to 4%), and mosaicism (1% to 2%) account for the other affected individuals. Triplication of a specific region of the long arm of chromosome 21 (21q22.2) is sufficient to produce the clinical phenotype.[40] Although there are many similarities in this group, individual variation must also be recognized. The range of outcome can be quite broad. Most affected patients have mild to moderate mental retardation. Mental retardation in children with Down syndrome is not an "across-the-board" phenomenon; thus, there are strengths, as well as deficits.

The profile of cognitive impairment in Down syndrome appears to differ from that of other forms of mental retardation. In much of the work involving children with Down syndrome, investigators have studied their language difficulties, especially in the areas of phonological, grammar, and syntactic skills. Expressive language skills are often more delayed than are cognitive and receptive language skills.[40,41] There is also strong evidence that these patients have specific difficulties in other areas of learning and memory, such as poor verbal working memory. Affected individuals show relative strengths in visual motor skills. Although children with Down syndrome continue to learn new skills, they appear to be subject to instability of acquisition and rapid forgetting. Their rate of learning is not only delayed but appears to follow a different path.[42] The measured IQ of individuals with Down syndrome typically declines through the first 10 years of life, reaching a plateau in adolescence that continues into adulthood.[43,44] These functional deficits may be explained by differences in the hippocampal and prefrontal cortex regions of their brains.

Although fetal brains of individuals with Down syndrome are normal, they do not develop the increasing dendritic complexity or number seen in unaffected individuals.[42] Delayed myelination of these structures is seen in 25% of children with Down syndrome. Anatomical studies have demonstrated neuropathological changes earlier than in the general population. Some of these changes are similar to those seen in association with Alzheimer disease. However, although 100% of individuals with Down syndrome eventually exhibit these changes, only 50% have clinical evidence of the associated dementia.[42] Individuals with Down syndrome have behavioral and psychiatric problems but often less frequently than children with other types of mental retardation.[40] From childhood and into adolescence, the most frequent problems are disruptive behavior disorders, including attention-deficit/hyperactivity disorder (ADHD) and oppositional defiant disorder. Approximately 5% to 10% also meet criteria for autism.[45] As adults, individuals with Down syndrome are more likely to have a major depressive disorder or demonstrate aggressive behaviors.[46]

TIMING OF CAUSE

There have been numerous efforts to categorize mental retardation on the basis of timing of the "cause:" prenatal, perinatal, and postnatal. A limitation of using this time-based approach exclusively is that it requires the assignment of a single causative factor and does not account for the role of multiple events that may contribute to mental retardation.

Prenatal

Most cases of mental retardation have prenatal causes: 70% of cases of severe mental retardation and 51% of cases of mild mental retardation.[47] Children with birth defects, regardless of the type of defect, are significantly more likely to be identified with mental retardation than are children without birth defects; the risk tends to be the highest among children with central nervous system and heart defects.[16] Environmental exposures during the prenatal period (e.g., to alcohol) and intrauterine infections (e.g., cytomegalovirus) also contribute to the overall incidence of mental retardation. Placental insufficiency for any variety of reasons may result in fetal malnutrition and subsequent intrauterine growth retardation; in the most significant cases of intrauterine growth retardation, affected infants demonstrate evidence of microcephaly at birth.

Perinatal

Individuals in this group are most often affected by the sequelae of low birth weight (<2500 g) and prematurity (<37 weeks of gestation). These complications represent about 4% of identifiable causes of severe mental retardation and 5% of identifiable cases of mild mental retardation. Perinatal infections, including herpes simplex virus and group B streptococcal infections, also often produce serious long-term cognitive effects.[9]

Postnatal/Acquired

Typically, some specific event or exposure can be identified in children in this group. These patients represent 5% of cases of severe mental retardation and 1% of cases of mild mental retardation. Examples include traumatic brain injury, infection/meningitis, central nervous system malignancy and significant environmental insults, psychosocial deprivation, and severe malnutrition.

Unknown

This group includes individuals in whom no obvious hereditary, perinatal, or postnatal event is identified by history. Their physical examination findings, in fact, are usually normal. This group may also be affected by environmental factors to a lesser degree than in cases attributed to a postnatal/acquired etiology.

NATURE OF INSULT

Classification efforts by insult alone may be equally incomplete, inasmuch as there are cases in which more than one insult is involved. Likewise, the timing of that insult affects the final outcome and its severity.

Genetic

The number of known genetic causes of mental retardation now exceeds 1000 and represents the largest proportion of known causes of mental retardation (also see Chapter 10B). This number is expected to increase as genetic techniques, such as subtelomeric fluorescent in situ hybridization (FISH) and comparative genomic hybridization, evolve and the ability to identify specific entities associated with cognitive impairment improves.[48,49] Genetic causes are currently believed to be responsible for 7% to 15% of all cases of mental retardation and for 30% to 40% of cases with known causes.[50,51] When a specific cause can be identified, genetic causes are typically identified in 30% of patients with severe mental retardation and in 4% to 8% of patients with mild mental retardation.[52]

Teratogenic

In utero exposures to teratogenic agents such as valproic acid and hydantoin and the effects of maternal cigarette smoking are associated with an increased risk for mental retardation.[52,53] The effects of intrauterine exposure to alcohol may manifest across a spectrum of clinical conditions: fetal alcohol syndrome, alcohol-related birth defects, and alcohol-related neurodevelopmental disorder.[54] Postnatal exposure to agents such as lead, methyl mercury, and polychlorinated biphenyls is also of concern.

Infectious

Although the effects of many infectious causes have been dramatically reduced with improved prenatal care and the introduction of several vaccinations (rubella, *Haemophilus influenzae*), this category still is important when specific causes of mental retardation are considered. Although the human immunodeficiency virus continues to be of concern, the effectiveness of methods to reduce maternal fetal transmission may have lessened its effect.[9]

Traumatic

Many cases of trauma-induced mental retardation are preventable. Closed head injuries associated with child battering, with lack of restraint in automobile accidents, and with not wearing a bicycle helmet are avoidable.

Psychosocial

In cases of mild mental retardation, low socioeconomic status, however it is measured, is strongly and inversely related to prevalence.[9,52] In theory, this is related to a lack of opportunity and/or stimulation in the home environment. The logical extension of that theory is that these cases are therefore preventable if identified early. It is this conclusion that formed the basis for the initial development of Head Start and other early intervention programs (EIPs).

Idiopathic

Reducing the number of cases of "idiopathic" mental retardation is the goal of combining newer technologies with a measured and appropriate diagnostic approach. The numerous variances within this group make it very difficult to predict the success of interventions and outcome.

CLINICAL MANAGEMENT

Importance of Assessing All Developmental Domains

The evaluation of a child with any type of delay in development should begin with a broadly based assessment in which all functional areas, not just the identified area of concern, are considered. This approach is consistent with the American Academy of Pediatrics' recommendation for pediatricians to survey and screen routinely and repeatedly for development.[55] Cognitive deficits may initially manifest as delays in language or social skills. Mental retardation may not be the only reason for this pattern of delay, but it must be considered and not immediately discarded as a "rare" problem in children. Relying on only clinical observation or informal checklists without specific cutoff scores or validation may cause the clinician to overlook affected children, delaying both identification and intervention.[55]

The level of cognitive involvement may be of primary importance in defining what is "normal" for a particular child in other developmental areas as patterns of developmental delay are described. For example, if a child has delays in both cognitive and social skills, the clinician must determine whether these deficits are similar in level or disparate, which would suggest other possible explanations or diagnoses, such as autism spectrum disorder. The incidence of pervasive developmental disorders in children with mental retardation is between 8% and 20%.[56] With the increasing efforts by numerous organizations to identify children with autism spectrum disorder at the earliest possible age, the confounding effect of cognitive delay may be inappropriately ignored or minimized.

LANGUAGE SKILLS

Because of the breadth of potential causes of language delay, some schedule and method of standardized screening by the primary care provider are priorities. Although the most common clinical manifestation in children with mental retardation is delay in both receptive and expressive language, mental retardation is not the only reason for such a delay. Other causes and presumed explanations (bilingualism, "late talkers in the family") should be carefully investigated and not presumed to be the actual reason. Neither the family or physician should presume that the child will simply "grow out of" these delays.

A child with a language delay should always receive a formal audiological evaluation as part of their assessment. No child is too young to be tested. Language development in a child with normal hearing is the best indicator of future intelligence. Language delay in association with atypical social and play skills should always raise the possibility of the autism spectrum disorders as a cause.

ADAPTIVE OR SELF-HELP SKILLS

Parents may become concerned when their child is unable to become independent in eating, dressing, and/or toileting skills or has a pattern of immature behaviors. A younger sibling surpassing the affected child or the inability of parents to find a daycare center or preschool willing to enroll the child may prompt parents to consult their pediatrician. Adaptive skills can be taught and learned; success can often be attributed to the efforts of parents and EIPs. Frequently, it is the stronger abilities in these areas that form the basis of parents' denial of any significant delay in their child's cognitive abilities and the use of qualifying statements such as "high functioning."

MOTOR SKILLS

Some disorders associated with mental retardation (Down syndrome and Prader-Willi syndrome) are also associated with neuromuscular abnormalities that result in motor delays (hypotonia in both). Although children with severe mental retardation may have delayed motor milestones, motor development is never a reliable predictor of cognitive development. Children with mild to moderate mental retardation usually master early gross motor milestones "on time." Subsequently, more complex gross motor skills and some fine motor skills may appear to be delayed as a result of the child's inability to comprehend verbal directions or to focus and concentrate on the specific desired task.

SOCIAL SKILLS

Children with undiagnosed mild mental retardation may exhibit poor attention skills during the early elementary school years. What the teacher may perceive as "ADHD" may instead be a set of social skills that are actually more consistent with the child's mental, rather than chronological, age. Evaluation of social skills should not be simply a checklist approach; qualitative as well as quantitative characteristics of social skills must be integrated into the assessment of the child's overall development.

Timing of Presentation

Is there a "best" or "typical" time to identify a child with mental retardation? Although the degree of severity affects the timing of diagnosis, there are other factors to consider. The parents' expectations of their child and the opportunities for the child to interact with other children also affect the presentation timing.

NATURE OF PARENTS' CONCERNS

In every case, it is extremely important for medical providers to listen to and address the concerns of a parent or care provider. It is extremely rare for parents' chief complaint to be "I think my child is mentally retarded." Instead they may report their own, or perhaps a teacher's, concern that the child is "immature." A child may initially present with behavioral problems, being described as "stubborn" or "oppositional." The child's inconsistent performance on structured, multiple-step tasks may be presented as proof that the child could do the work if he or she wanted to. Judgmental decisions by adults that the child is "just lazy" without an effort to assess the child's true abilities may further delay the diagnosis. Provider reassurances that the child "will grow out of it" or that he or she "looks fine to me" have repeatedly been shown to be significantly frustrating for parents seeking help for their child.[57]

THE EFFECT OF MENTAL RETARDATION SEVERITY ON MANIFESTATION

Despite their frequently identified delays in language skills, children with mild mental retardation may not be formally identified as such until they enter an academic setting in which their difficulties with processing increasingly complex and novel information become apparent. For some children, this may be their first experience with such activities and with specific performance expectations. Parents may not have a realistic expectation of what children can and should be doing at different ages. These increasing problems in more structured and academic settings may result in formal IQ and adaptive skills testing, which are essential prerequisites for establishing a formal diagnosis of mental retardation. This delay in diagnosis may occur in spite of the identification of earlier language or other associated delays. However, with careful surveillance of language, visual-problem solving, and adaptive skills, most children with milder levels of mental retardation can be identified as such by 3 to 4 years of age.

Moderate mental retardation in a child is often diagnosed between 3 and 4 years of age. The effect of their cognitive and social/adaptive differences is much more likely to bring them to the attention of parents and providers than are their language delays alone.

Severe mental retardation is often diagnosed by 1 year of age, especially when dysmorphic features are present. In addition, the effects of their associated medical conditions and the greater likelihood of global developmental delays, including motor delay, may explain their earlier identification.[58]

CLINICAL DIAGNOSIS

A number of misconceptions that have been identified over the years have delayed acknowledgment of "mental retardation" as an appropriate clinical possibility, by both parents and physicians: "cute children" cannot have mental retardation; "ambulatory children" cannot have mental retardation; children younger than a certain age are "too young to test."[59] When these and other barriers are finally overcome, the clinical diagnosis of mental retardation can be considered as a possible explanation for a child's pattern of developmental differences. A comprehen-

sive and appropriate assessment should then be initiated to confirm the diagnosis.

Establishing the Diagnosis of Mental Retardation with the AAMR Three-Step Assessment

STEP 1

Step 1 is to use established criteria and standardized tests to assess current levels of functioning in the cognitive and adaptive domains.

Cognitive tests of infant and early childhood cognitive abilities, except in the most severely affected cases, are poor predictors of later academic success, an ability that is currently best represented by an IQ score. The developmental abilities of typical children in this age range are rapidly changing.[60] IQ testing is possible during the preschool years; however, the label "mental retardation" is usually not applied until the child is of school age, because IQ tests are not well correlated with later measures of IQ until 3 to 5 years of age. At that point, formal IQ testing is more reliable, and results better reflect a child's long-term abilities (see Chapter 7C for more information). Several frequently used instruments are briefly described in this chapter. Lichtenberger[61] published a more detailed review of formal measures of preschool cognitive assessment. Whichever particular instrument is selected, it must match the purpose of the assessment: to establish eligibility for services, to assist in planning intervention strategies and programs, or to provide support benefits and/or legal protection. Interpretation of test results always requires careful consideration of several variables: Was this a typical performance for the child? Were all sociocultural biases considered during test development and administration? Did the child understand the test instructions/format? Were special modifications required because of other developmental disabilities (motor, sensory, communication deficits)?[61]

- Bayley Scales of Infant Development–III: Provides a core battery of five sclaes. Three scales administered with child interaction—cognitive, motor, language. Two Scales conducted with parent questionnaires—social-emotional, adaptive behavior. Used in very young children (aged 1 to 42 months).[62]
- Stanford-Binet Intelligence Scale (5th edition): Provides a full scale score, two domain scores (verbal and nonverbal IQ), and several factor indexes for individuals aged 2 to 85 years.[63]
- Kaufman Assessment Battery for Children II: Provides a global measure of ability (Mental Processing Composite IQ) for children as young as 3 years old.

Additional scales and indices are added across the age range of the instrument (3 years 0 months to 18 years 11 months).[64]

- Wechsler Preschool and Primary Scale of Intelligence III (WPPSI III): Provides Full Scale, Verbal, and Performance scores (FSIQ, VIQ, and PIQ). The latest edition (2002) adds a General Language Composite for measuring both expressive and receptive but not higher order language functioning. For older children (aged 4 years 0 months through 7 years 3 months), a Processing Speed Quotient has been added. The WPPSI III is an appropriate instrument for children aged 2 years 6 months to 7 years 3 months.[65]
- Wechsler Intelligence Scale for Children (WISC-IV): Provides Verbal, Performance, and Full Scale IQ scores for children aged 6 years to 12 years.[66]

Adaptive behavior scales focus on the skill level a person typically displays when performing tasks in his or her environment, whereas IQ tests focus on the maximal performance of an individual on tasks related to conceptual intelligence. Adaptive behavior scales measure aspects of conceptual, practical, and social intelligence, even though performance on tasks requiring social intelligence is often underrepresented on adaptive behavior scales. In addition to providing diagnoses, adaptive behavior scales are useful in identifying educational or training-related goals. Examples of commonly used measures of adaptive behavior include the following:

- Vineland Adaptive Behavior Scales II[67]
- Adaptive Behavior Assessment Scale II (ABAS—II)[68]
- Scales of Independent Behaviors—Revised[69]

STEP 2

Step 2 is to describe strengths and weaknesses across the five dimensions of mental retardation.

Describing strengths and weaknesses represented a dramatic shift for the AAIDD and other organizations working with individuals with mental retardation. These organizations began to address the effect of mental retardation on such individuals and on society, focusing on intervention and service planning rather than simply a "level of severity" classification system approach. These five dimensions are a key component of the 2002 AAMR comprehensive model of mental retardation (see Table 11-3). (See also the section "Levels of Support" earlier in this chapter.)

STEP 3

Step 3 is to determine needed supports and classify by intensity of service.

In a supports-based approach to the delivery of necessary services, the individual, rather than a spe-

cific program, is the focus. Supports enhance functioning and facilitate an individual's inclusion in his or her natural community. Characterizing a person's strengths and weaknesses is of no benefit unless some additional effort is made to define the necessary intensity level of those supports. It is important to recognize that the intensity of supports is independent of the location where the support needs to be delivered and may vary across the various areas of need. The judicious use of supports should improve a person's level of functioning. Specific levels of support intensity have been defined (see Table 11-4). (See also the section "Levels of Support" earlier in this chapter.)

Identifying strengths and weaknesses across the five dimensions was integrated with the concept of "levels and intensity of support" in the AAIDD's Supports Intensity Scales.[10] There is frequent confusion about how the Supports Intensity Scales differ from a standardized measure of adaptive skills. A key distinction between the two approaches is that adaptive behavior measurements address "skills" needed for an individual to successfully function in society (the level of mastery), whereas the Supports Intensity Scales address activities that a person engages in during the course of participating in everyday life and how much support he or she needs to complete those activities.[11]

Etiological Diagnostic Workup: "The Search"

OVERVIEW: WHY ASK "WHY?"

Any number of reasons can be given for asking why a particular child has mental retardation. The search for a reason may be initiated by the family or the physician; each may have a very different focus. Physicians may direct their efforts toward defining the expected natural history of a particular condition, determining the recurrence risk, initiating a prevention program, determining whether this might be a treatable condition, and/or to take advantage of new diagnostic tools as they are developed. Families may feel that finding an explanation or "label" means that the condition might be curable. Families may demand extensive evaluations to provide a sense of closure and to empower them to focus on intervention rather than explanation.

Lenhard and associates[24] described a number of psychological benefits for families attributed to diagnostic certainty. Families were frequently confronted in their physician's office with an approach that Lenhard and associates characterized as "diagnostic minimalism"—the argument of health care providers that the assignment of a diagnosis of mental retardation rarely led to more effective treatments. The reluctance of physicians and other professionals (i.e., school personnel) working with the child and family to make and discuss this diagnosis may eliminate essential pathways to facilitate the family's coping. It is also much easier for parents of children with a specific diagnosis to join and form associations and provide mutual support. Having a name for their child's condition may improve the family's access to systems of public support.

There is *no* standard workup for mental retardation or global developmental delay. There are numerous consensus guidelines regarding the appropriate degree and order of assessment in children diagnosed with mental retardation: two from genetics organizations, one from the American Academy of Neurology, and one from the American Academy of Pediatrics.[50,51,70,70a] A useful comparison of the similarities and differences among these statements was included in the article by Roberts and colleagues.[71]

COMPONENTS OF THE SEARCH

Each series of investigations should be tailored to the individual patient. The investigation should be directed by findings from the patient's history, the family history, and the physical examination. In a systematic analysis, van Karnebeek and associates[72] reported the results of several diagnostic investigations. Their recommendations included obtaining a clinical history and physical examination with emphasis on the neurological and dysmorphological examinations, obtaining standard cytological studies in all cases, ordering fragile X studies in all male patients, and requesting FISH subtelomeric studies based on established checklists. Metabolic studies were not recommended as a first-line investigation. Van Karnebeek and associates also concluded that neuroradiological studies had a high yield for identifying brain anomalies but a low yield for establishing an etiological diagnosis.[72]

CLINICAL EVALUATION

A thorough history and careful physical examination should initiate any diagnostic search. Information about the prenatal and birth history should be reviewed: How was the mother's health during the pregnancy? Were there any teratogenic exposures? Is there a history of pregnancy loss? Other illnesses or patterns of illness experienced by the child may be suggestive of an underlying diagnosis. A family history of similar problems or of consanguinity is contributory, and it is important to obtain a three-generation family pedigree. Environmental effects (deprivation, nutrition, lead) should be clarified. The child's pattern of development over time should be described: Has there been any loss or regression of skills? The physi-

cal examination should focus on the presence of dysmorphic features, neurological examination findings, and possible behavioral phenotypes. Characteristic physical findings may be suggestive of a particular syndrome associated with mental retardation. Focal neurological findings or a history of stereotypical movements may lead to other diagnostic studies. Many of the conditions associated with mental retardation have very specific behaviors: for example, the hand wringing by girls with Rett syndrome. If there are no obvious clues on the initial examination, the clinician should remember that many of these conditions evolve over time; serial examinations may reveal the necessary clue the next time.

HEARING AND VISION EVALUATIONS

Individuals with developmental delay and/or mental retardation are at increased risk for primary sensory impairments: vision abnormalities in 13% to 50% and audiological abnormalities in 18%.[51] Formal assessments of hearing and vision are an integral part of the evaluation of these children.

LANGUAGE

Delays in receptive and expressive language are often the presenting concern about children with mental retardation. Because language skill is the best predictor of future cognitive abilities, the physician's recognition of such delays is an important first step. Minimizing the degree of involvement, predicting that things "will be fine soon," or ignoring the concerns of the family only delays the evaluation process and potentially beneficial interventions.

GENETIC TESTING: INDICATIONS AND YIELD

Cytogenetically visible rearrangements are present in about 1% of newborns with a standard karyotype study (500 bands). The clinical significance of these rearrangements is not known. Chromosomal abnormalities are seen in approximately 25% of individuals with mental retardation: 40% of cases of severe mental retardation and 10% of cases of mild mental retardation. The presence of two or more minor dysmorphic features detected on physical examination also increases the likelihood that a chromosomal abnormality will be identified from 3.7% to 20% in affected individuals. The fragile X has been identified in 2% to 6% of male patients and in 2% to 4% of female patients with mental retardation. An increase in diagnostic yield from 2.6% to 7.6% is seen when decisions to obtain DNA fragile X studies are combined with physical examination findings.[21]

There is an increased percentage of genes in the telomeric regions of the chromosomes. Currently, these areas can best be examined with FISH. This technique identifies differences in 0.9% of normal controls, 1.1% of individuals with mild mental retardation, and 6.6% of individuals with moderate to severe mental retardation. At some point in the future, subtelomeric abnormalities may well become the primary cause of what had previously been described as "idiopathic mental retardation." A checklist has been developed to improve the diagnostic yield of this method: family history of mental retardation; prenatal onset of growth retardation; postnatal poor growth/overgrowth; two or more facial dysmorphic features; and one or more nonfacial dysmorphic features and/or congenital abnormalities. The most significant predictors of a subtelomeric deletion are intrauterine growth retardation and a family history of mental retardation.[73]

NEUROIMAGING: INDICATIONS AND YIELD

Any explanation to parents about mental retardation includes some attribution to effects on the central nervous system, although a specific area or cause may not be identified. Many parents assume that an imaging study of the brain will identify the "problem area." They are frequently confused when an imaging study is not recommended by their physician or when the result of a completed study is "normal."

There is an increased chance of an abnormal finding on head imaging study in the presence of an IQ of less than 50 in a child who has one of the following: microcephaly or macrocephaly, an abnormal cranial contour, midline and/or multiple dysmorphic features, an abnormal neurological examination finding, seizures, neurocutaneous findings, or a history of developmental milestone loss.[74,75] Both the American College of Medical Genetics and the American Academy of Neurology recognize these as indications for obtaining a head imaging study. The American Academy of Neurology also recommends a head imaging study in cases of mental retardation associated with intrapartum asphyxia.[50,51,58] The current yield from head imaging studies in children with mental retardation ranges from 33% in children without any other signs or symptoms to 63% to 73% in children with both mental retardation and cerebral palsy.[21,51]

METABOLIC TESTING: INDICATIONS AND YIELD

Relatively few metabolic conditions cause mental retardation in isolation; other neurological symptoms are commonly found (see Chapter 10C for more information). The presence of such symptoms in the child and in family members should be pursued. Many researchers assessing the yield of routine metabolic investigations in the child with mental retardation have concluded that there is little usefulness in such screening.[50,51,70] The presence of a positive family history or other specific signs and symptoms identi-

fied in the history and physical examination may increase the yield of metabolic screening from 1% to 5%.

Generally accepted indications for additional metabolic investigations in children with mental retardation include episodic vomiting or lethargy, poor growth, seizures, evidence of storage disease, unusual odors, the loss of or a plateau of developmental skills, the presence of a movement disorder (chorea, dystonia), a new sensory loss (especially with retinal abnormality), or an acquired cutaneous disorder. The yield of directed and focused metabolic testing that is based on symptoms and performed in a stepwise manner may approach 14%.[76]

Expanded neonatal screening, now available in 23 states in the United States, tests for 20 or more of the 29 conditions recommended by the American College of Medical Genetics.[77,78] The expansion in neonatal screening has allowed for the identification and treatment of inborn errors of metabolism in many children who might otherwise have died with the conditions undetected or become handicapped before any therapeutic interventions could be initiated. Although 15 states screen for fewer than 10 conditions, screening for congenital hypothyroidism and phenylketonuria is universal. Information from these screening programs should always be included in the evaluation of a child suspected to have mental retardation.

Differential Diagnosis

The differential diagnosis may best be organized around a number of "yes/no" questions. The specific order of these questions will vary, depending on the clinical information already available in each case. However, each should be considered in every case.

1. Is the delay in learning or communication isolated, rather than a global or uniform pattern of delay across all developmental domains? A symmetrical pattern of delay across all developmental domains would be more typical in a child with mental retardation, although gross motor skills may be least affected. An isolated delay in communication skills, without delays in problem solving or social relatedness, is suggestive of developmental language impairment. A delay in learning without significant language or social relatedness delays is suggestive of a specific learning disability.

2. Are there significant deficits (quantitative and qualitative) in social relatedness in comparison with the overall level of functioning? The combination of delays in language use, social relatedness, and stereotypical/restrictive behaviors is suggestive of autism spectrum disorder. Deficits in joint attention, pointing, and imaginative play are much more

common in autism spectrum disorder than in mental retardation alone. Preferences for routine and occasional stereotypical behaviors are not discriminating features between these two populations.

3. Are there associated conditions that limit the child's ability to perform during the testing situation? Sensory (hearing, vision) impairments or limitations in motor ability may adversely affect the ability of the child to best complete the testing. Nonverbal instruments may be required for a hearing-impaired child. "Motor free" assessments or response modifications may be required for a child with cerebral palsy.

4. Are there other factors that have not been considered that affect the child's ability to perform during the testing situation? Other medical conditions (seizures, nutritional status) and/or other psychosocial effects (language, culture, and environmental experiences) may adversely affect the child.

Breaking the News

The diagnosis and evaluation steps in this process usually have a beginning and an end. Whether the diagnosis occurs in infancy or later, management begins with breaking the news in a sensitive, compassionate, and culturally appropriate manner. When the clinician breaks the news, it is important to emphasize the child's strengths, as well as the deficits. It is also important to be realistic without taking away hope. Parents should be informed that the child will continue to progress but at a slower pace. In addition, the child's progress will be dependent on direct training rather than simply on the modeling of parents and siblings. If the child is less than 6 years of age at the time of diagnosis and does not have a syndrome known to be associated with mental retardation, it may be more appropriate to use the term *global developmental delay*. One problem in using the term *delay* lies in the fact that some parents may misconstrue the term as indicating that the condition is only temporary and that their child will some day catch up. This may indeed be the case when developmental quotients are marginal and/or unreliable because of the child's lack of cooperation during testing. For the most part, developmental quotients below 50 in a cooperative child almost always indicate long-term impairment. When the child enters elementary school and standardized testing is more reliable and predictive of long-term cognitive status, the diagnosis may be revised as mental retardation. In any case, it is important to help parents maintain a level of expectation that is consistent with the child's potential in order to enable the child to reach his or her maximum potential. When the child has a known syndrome that is causing the delays, the family should receive appropriate genetic counseling, be provided with up-to-date literature on the syndrome, and be linked to local (when available) and national syndrome-specific support groups, as well as more general support groups such as Family Voices or The Arc of the United States.[79] (See later section on "Parent-Centered Supports.")

When all of the history questions have been asked, when all of the medical and psychological tests are done, and when all of the other diagnostic possibilities have been considered, the physician and the family are left with one final (or initial) question: "What are we going to do?" That process and management evolves and grows to incorporate a broad range of support services for the child and the family.

MANAGEMENT

Historical Overview of the Management of Individuals with Mental Retardation and Associated Conditions

To review the care and management of children and adults with mental retardation since the 1950s, it is useful to consider separately those with mild mental retardation and those with severe mental retardation. Care for children with *mild* mental retardation, without dysmorphic features or a known syndromic cause, has not markedly changed over the years. Previously, most such children were not identified until school age. Most of these individuals usually lived at home with their families and attended regular school, at least in the early years. Because formal testing was not available in all communities, some cases might not have even been diagnosed as mental retardation. These children learned to read, some as high as the sixth grade level. As school became more and more challenging, many dropped out and entered the unskilled or semiskilled work force early. Because most were healthy and without comorbid disorders, they received medical care similar to that of their unaffected siblings. As adults, they may have had some functional limitations and lived with their parents for a longer time than usual. Many were successful at work if they had developed a good work ethic and if their duties were matched to their strengths. Eventually, many married, parented children, and lived independently unless they had impairing behaviors.

On the other hand, the care of individuals with *severe* mental retardation has markedly changed since the 1950s. These children were readily recognized by their dysmorphic features, although many current syndromes were not known by name, and/or by their severe cognitive and adaptive impairments. At that time, funding to support families raising children with severe disabilities was almost nonexistent. When families felt overwhelmed with their child's challenging behaviors or when the extra caregiving duties required, parents' only choice was to relinquish their child with severe mental retardation to an institution. Although the first institutions were built in the 1880s, enrollment in large facilities did not become a matter of routine until the mid-1900s.[80] Enrollment peaked in 1967, when these facilities served almost 200,000 individuals.[81]

In the 1960s and 1970s, the social revolution fostered mainstreaming of children with disabilities into integrated settings, encouraged freedom of choice, and promoted a better quality of life for persons with mental retardation. These trends were accelerated by shocking exposés on public television revealing the status of individuals who were living in institutions. Federal legislation began to support families raising their children with severe disabilities, including mental retardation, at home. In 1974, the Supplemental Security Income (SSI) program became the cornerstone of a national commitment to support children with disabilities. SSI is a federally funded income subsidy program designed to provide monthly cash benefits to low-income families of children with disabilities. In 1975, the Education of All Handicapped Children Act (Public Law 94-142) ensured that all children, regardless of the degree of their impairments, were entitled to a free and appropriate public education. In 1981, the Tax Equity and Fiscal Responsibility Act allowed states to disregard parental income in determining the eligibility of a children with disabilities for Medicaid services and other disability supports. Also known as the Katie Becket option or waiver, the Tax Equity and Fiscal Responsibility Act provided funds that enabled parents to hire providers in order to receive respite from caring for a child with severe disabilities at home rather than in a hospital, nursing home, or institutional setting. In 1990, the Americans with Disabilities Act mandated community inclusion and prohibited discrimination against people with disabilities. Among other issues, it addressed equal opportunities for work participation, community living, and removal of architectural barriers. Philosophically, it introduced "people first" language and promoted the dignity of persons with disabilities (including mental retardation) throughout all aspects of society. The outcomes of the Americans with Disabilities Act were greatest for adults with disabilities; additional legislation in 1990 dramatically affected children with mental retardation. The Individuals with Disabilities Education Act (IDEA) of 1990 replaced 1975's Public Law 94-142 and promoted inclusion of children with disabilities in regular classrooms and introduced the concept of

"least restrictive environment." It also promoted transition services for teenagers and ensured that children with disabilities received individualized educational and support services from the time of diagnosis of the disability through age 21 years. IDEA was amended and re-authorized in 1997 and again in 2004.

Since 1990, family and disability advocates have worked tirelessly to promote inclusion, increase funding for family support, and prevent out-of-home placements. New admissions to institutions, especially of children, have been curtailed, and many adults with mental retardation have moved out of large institutions into community-based group homes or to independent living settings. By 2000, only 15% (43,000) of individuals with severe disabilities lived in state-administrated institutions.[81] One of the many goals included in Healthy People 2010, a road map for public health initiatives over the next decade for the entire population, was to "reduce the number of persons with disabilities living in congregate care facilities...to 0 by 2010 for persons aged 21 years and under."[82] The American Academy of Pediatrics supported this Healthy People 2010 goal with the publication of "Helping Families Raise Children with Disabilities at Home."[83] In 2005, several states reported having already met this goal by using innovative strategies such as recruiting support families to help a birth or adoptive family with the day-to-day child-rearing activities, as well as providing some extended respite services.[80]

The concept of providing appropriate supports was not new; what was new was the belief that appropriate supports could improve the functional outcomes of individuals with mental retardation. The introduction by the AAIDD of the supports-based approach in 1992 affected education and adult habilitation programs by promoting a more natural, efficient, and ongoing basis for enhancing an individual's functional status.[84] Despite that document's emphasis on appropriate supports to improve the functional outcome of individuals with mental retardation, community living, and supported employment, fewer than 10% of the states had fully embraced these concepts by 2000.[85] However, a landmark Supreme Court decision (Olmstead v. L.C. Decision (527 U.S. 581, 138 F.3d 893, 1999) upheld the rights of individuals with mental retardation to live in community settings rather than in institutions. The decision emphasized community supports, independent individual assessment, and self-determination and choice as viable principles for persons with mental retardation, even those with severe mental retardation. It was a strong "voice" for a support-based approach. The Developmental Disabilities Assistance and Bill of Rights Act of 2000 (Public Law 106-402) further advanced the case for self-determination. Because of changing societal expectations, legislation, and judicial decisions, management strategies since the 1950s for persons with mental retardation have evolved from segregation (1960 to the 1980s) to deinstitutionalization (1990s) and to the current situation in which community membership—a concept that embraces true participation rather than simply living in community settings—is the norm.[5]

Management Priorities

The following sections describe various systems of care and supports that are crucial for children with mental retardation and their families: health; developmental, educational, and vocational services; and community/public supports. For persons with mental retardation, community membership depends on many available and appropriate supports throughout their lives. For children with mental retardation, supports begin with appropriate health care, EIPs, and schools. Of these, the educational system often has the potential to provide the greatest and most important effects. When transitions dismantle a parent's previously attained equilibrium with the grieving process, the parent too may need extra support, regardless of the degree of the child's mental retardation.

Children with mild idiopathic mental retardation may not require many of the interventions or management strategies to be described except for special education services. Even in that setting, most demonstrate steady progress, although at a slower rate, and should be integrated into the regular classroom to the greatest extent possible. Typically, the most important aspect of their management plan is the promotion of independence, adaptive skill development, decision-making skills, and good study and work habits. With these skills and other necessary supports, many of these children grow up, marry, have a family, are successfully employed, and become productive members of the community.

In children with severe mental retardation, supports addressing their comorbid health and/or psychiatric disorders may assume primary importance. For example, during infancy and early childhood, medical and surgical subspecialists may be of primary importance for a child with Down syndrome to manage the cardiac complications. As a child with severe mental retardation ages, behavior problems may prevent participation in inclusive school and community settings. Addressing these new challenges must then become the focus of intervention and management strategies. Success always requires coordination among medical, psychiatric, behavioral, and educational professionals.

Health Care

DEFINING HEALTH

Health is a state of physical, mental, and social well-being. For the majority of persons with mental retardation, physical and mental health concerns are similar to those of the general population. In the past, these concerns were addressed in a purely medical model. More recently, health care professionals, particularly those specializing in disabilities, have realized that societal attitudes, roles, and policies can have a major influence on the ways that individuals experience health disorders. Today, it is recognized that disability reflects a complex interaction among health conditions, functional impairments, and social roles; the interactions among these three areas are also influenced by personal and environmental factors.

ROUTINE SURVEILLANCE AND CARE

As with typically developing children, children with mental retardation benefit from ongoing health care within the context of a "medical home."[86,87] Health care should be family-centered, accessible, continuous, comprehensive, culturally sensitive, and developmentally appropriate. Unfortunately, the quality of health care for persons with mental retardation has often been significantly below established standards. Because many individuals with mental retardation now live longer, do so in communities rather than institutions, and are at an increased likelihood to live in poverty, these differences in health care have become more obvious. Transitions to adult systems of care have also been difficult for individuals with mental retardation and their families because of both availability and expertise.[88] These challenges prompted a working conference and led to the report *Closing the Gap: A National Blueprint to Improve the Health of Persons with Mental Retardation*.[11] This "blueprint," designed to be an agenda for action, outlined goals to improve health care delivery, including integrating quality health care into communities (as opposed to institutions), improving the current unwieldy system of health care financing, developing more extensive resources, and increasing public knowledge and health professional training regarding the unique and specialized needs of individuals with mental retardation through research and new partnerships. If this agenda can be implemented, the key factors identified during a plenary presentation to that conference will be addressed: access, affordability, availability, and acceptability.[11]

Parent-professional partnerships are especially important for children with chronic disorders such as mental retardation. In addition to the child's needs, the needs of the parents should always be given consideration in medical decision making. Except for the extra time and effort needed to communicate with schools and community agencies, the routine health maintenance of children with idiopathic mild mental retardation is very similar to that of typically developing children. The clinician should specifically address safety issues (because the child may not understand danger and environmental hazards), attainment of future developmental milestones, prevention of behavior problems, and early and ongoing promotion of independence through a program of anticipatory guidance.

Particular attention should be given to healthy lifestyles, good nutrition, and physical fitness. It appears that individuals with mental retardation have a much higher prevalence of obesity and cardiovascular disease than does the general population.[89,90] These disorders are associated with lower rates of physical exercise, especially after graduation from high school, when there are fewer opportunities for organized sporting events such as the Special Olympics. Primary care physicians should monitor growth curves and advise parents early on when an increase in weight in relation to height is first noticed.

Dental surveillance and preventive care is also a challenging but vital aspect of care that is often neglected. Oral health disorders are more common among children with mental retardation than among the general population: 25% to 56% have caries, and 60% to 90% have gingivitis.[91] This increased prevalence is associated with irregular brushing of teeth, the gingival hyperplasia seen with some anticonvulsant medications, and excessive dryness of the mouth caused by the anticholinergic side effects of certain medications. Dental treatment of children with severe mental retardation is more problematic because of the inability of such children to cooperate and their high levels of anxiety. Sometimes, restraints or general anesthesia is needed to facilitate restorative care.[92]

ROLE OF THE DEVELOPMENTAL-BEHAVIORAL PEDIATRICIAN

The developmental-behavioral pediatrician can assist the primary care provider in providing care to children with mental retardation within the context of the medical home. It can be difficult to predict outcomes in very young children with developmental delays. There are no standardized IQ tests for this age group, and developmental scores may not be correlated with long-term outcomes because of environmental factors, sickness, lack of cooperation, and deficient examiner skills, among other reasons. Prediction may be somewhat easier in children with known genetic syndromes for which long-term outcome studies exist. The

developmental-behavioral pediatrician can play an important role in educating and guiding the child's primary care provider with regard to appropriate anticipatory guidance for parents as they journey through various stages of their child's development. Ongoing care issues such as parent education and support, adoption of realistic goals that are based on standardized test results, assessment of new and challenging behaviors, health and fitness, adolescent sexuality, and transition to adulthood are all areas in which the developmental pediatrician is often the "expert" in assessing and coordinating local community and national resources, as well as public services available to families of children with mental retardation.

In addition to routine visits with their primary care provider, most children with mental retardation also benefit from periodic visits, at least annually, to a developmental-behavioral pediatrician. The developmental-behavioral pediatrician's role in the ongoing care of children with mental retardation varies, depending on whether the child has mild or severe mental retardation and whether there are comorbid physical, health, psychiatric, or behavioral issues. This role demarcation begins early in the child's life.

The developmental-behavioral pediatrician may be the first to diagnose mental retardation in a child without dysmorphic features (or at least with more subtle ones) and milder degrees of cognitive deficit. These children may present with speech delay during the preschool years or for an evaluation of learning difficulties during the early school years. The developmental-behavioral pediatrician may "discover" mental retardation during an evaluation for behavior problems that were not recognized as possible signs of mental retardation by the referring primary care provider. Other than determining the reason for the difficulties or behaviors, the developmental-behavioral pediatrician may not be involved in the child's routine management except in support of the primary care provider.

More severe mental retardation, especially in children with dysmorphic features and/or neurological deficits, may be diagnosed at birth or during infancy by a geneticist or neurologist. The developmental-behavioral pediatrician may be asked to evaluate a child with severe global developmental delay, especially in language and adaptive skills. However, this pediatrician may not become involved until later when the child's primary care provider has questions about the developmental or functional status of the child, requests information about supports for the family, or needs assistance with comorbid disorders (health, behavioral, educational) that are unique to the child's condition. Among the several medical subspecialists caring for a child with mental retardation, accessing and coordinating various systems of care is an area of expertise that is often unique to the developmental-behavioral pediatrician or neurodevelopmental disability physicians.

ADDITIONAL ETIOLOGICAL SEARCHES

One aspect of health care management is specific to individuals without an identifiable cause for their mental retardation: a repeated neurogenetic search. It is wise to consider this reevaluation every 5 years, because new and more precise techniques are constantly being developed. As with the original search, a search should be repeated while the patient's behavior and physical phenotypes are considered, especially when new symptoms appear with maturation. Although many new tests are developed each year, availability of a new test, in and of itself, is not an adequate reason to order it. Idiopathic mental retardation is static; if regression becomes evident in the absence of the emergence of a new comorbid disorder or secondary disability, the child must be evaluated for a central nervous system lesion, a metabolic or storage disease, or a known degenerative syndrome. Regression might also manifest as a side effect of a medication, particularly with polypharmaceutical treatment.

Management of Associated and Comorbid Disorders

CLASSIFICATION SYSTEMS

In 1980, the World Health Organization developed a model describing how an intrinsic *disease* could *impair* body functioning that could result in a *disability* and put the individual at a social disadvantage *(handicap)*.[93,94] This model was later revised to expand the idea that disease resulted in bodily impairments, limitations of activities, and restrictions in societal roles.[95] These philosophical constructs are best captured in the International Classification of Functioning, Disability and Health (ICF) (see Chapter 6 for more information).[95] On the other hand, the International Classification of Disease (ICD), also developed by the World Health Organization and most recently revised in 1993 as the 10th edition, provides a coding system for both physical and mental diseases.[96] Although similar to ICD standards, the guidelines and classification procedures for mental health disorders published in the *DSM-IV-TR*[6] are often preferred by clinicians in the United States (see Chapter 6 for more information). All three systems may play a role in the characterization and care of individuals with mental retardation, especially those with more severe forms of mental retardation. The ICF describes and quantifies the individual's impairments and disabilities within a functional context, whereas the ICD classifies physical health conditions; the *DSM-IV-TR* classifies mental health conditions (including levels of mental retardation).

EFFECT OF MENTAL RETARDATION SEVERITY ON COMORBIDITY

These system characterizations (ICF, ICD, *DSM-IV-TR*) may not be essential for anticipating interventions for those individuals with *mild* mental retardation. Most children with mild mental retardation do not experience significant impairments or societal limitations and have fewer physical comorbid conditions. They are much more likely to demonstrate difficulties in areas of behavior, psychosocial issues, educational expectations, and decision making. Because the prevalence of mild mental retardation far outranks that of severe mental retardation, the management of the "typical child with mental retardation" is very similar to that of any "typical child." The majority of children with mild mental retardation do not have syndromes or specific comorbid conditions that would complicate or negatively affect short- and long-term outcomes. Many are not identified until school age, when they present with learning difficulties. Within the context of a medical home, such children should receive routine monitoring of their developmental, educational, health, nutritional, dental, behavioral, and social-emotional status, as well as of acute-care needs related to typical childhood diseases, by a primary care provider (e.g., pediatrician, nurse practitioner, family practitioner). All healthy children with mild mental retardation should have, at the very least, an annual well-child physical examination and updated review of systems. Some of these children, depending on several factors, may also benefit from regular follow-up with a developmental-behavioral pediatrician, especially if challenging behaviors appear or if care coordination of multiple care systems for comorbid conditions is needed.

The three classification systems (ICF, ICD, *DSM-IV-TR*) may be much more valuable in characterizing how children with *severe* mental retardation are likely to be affected and in structuring the care that they require. Environmental factors may not be as significant as the inherent limitations already imposed on them either by the underlying cognitive disability or by the associated physical, medical, and emotional conditions. Severe mental retardation is usually diagnosed during infancy and early childhood. The management of these children is challenging, because they may be nonverbal and unable to localize symptoms or communicate pain. They often have known syndromes or historical insults that affect more than cognition, which renders management more complex as a wider array of services and subspecialists is needed. It is beyond the scope of this chapter to address specific management issues for each of the more than 200 syndromes associated with mental retardation.

ASSOCIATED DISORDERS

Specific associated disorders are commonly found in children with mental retardation, particularly children with severe mental retardation, regardless of cause. Although there is some overlap, these disorders generally fall within one of three major categories: behavioral, psychiatric, and medical.

Behavior Challenges

There are a number of behaviors that do not fit within the criteria of a diagnosable *DSM-IV-TR* disorder but cause significant disruption for families and must be addressed. As the degree of mental retardation increases, so does the prevalence of these behavioral challenges. The prevalence approaches 50% among patients with severe mental retardation.

When assessing whether a particular behavior is inappropriate, the clinician should consider the child's mental, rather than chronological, age. For example, behavior representative of the "terrible twos" in a first grader with severe mental retardation may reflect an expected challenge consistent with their developmental progress; it should not be considered "inappropriate." However, teachers may still need support managing these behaviors in the context of a "typical" classroom. In addition, incontinence should not be considered a problem in older children with mental retardation who have not yet attained a mental age of at least 2 years. Parents need not struggle with toilet training, even when the child is school aged, if the child has mastered neither the prerequisite motor and adaptive skills nor the cognitive level that would allow him or her to grasp that concept.

Although the behaviors may be obvious and well articulated by the parents, standardized tools may also be helpful. Besides detecting more subtle aspects of the behavior, they may also be useful for characterizing these problems and evaluating intervention effects. However, many have not been specifically studied in children with mental retardation, especially severe mental retardation. In two reviews, the Aberrant Behavior Checklist was singled out as the most reliable.[97,98] Other tools thought to be helpful with this population include the Behavior Scale of the Vineland Adaptive Behavior Scale, the Clinical Global Impressions, the Child Behavior Checklist, and the Reiss Screen for Maladaptive Behavior. The Nisonger Child Behavior Rating Form has also been promoted for this purpose.[99]

Problematic behaviors often appear because a nonverbal child is unable to communicate his or her frustrations. In a nonverbal child, a change in behavior can also be the first sign of a new health concern, such as dental caries, a gastrointestinal disorder, or a skin infection. In fact, a medical concern is the most likely cause of a new disturbance in routine behaviors, especially when an individual is nonverbal and unable to localize pain.[100] If a new medical condition has been ruled out and the behaviors are disrupting family functioning or preventing the child from participating in family, school, and community activities, then intervention is indicated.

The clinician should always attempt to eliminate the behavior by nonmedical means. A survey of experts rated the three most effective components of psychosocial (nonmedical) intervention to be applied behavioral analysis, patient and caregiver education, and environmental management.[98] The timely introduction of behavior management strategies, often by behavior specialists employed by EIPs and schools, by psychologists, and by other mental health professionals, and ideally before a situation gets out of control, provides the various care providers with methods to analyze, modify, and monitor behavioral concerns. Although not every situation can be anticipated, a consistent approach empowers caregivers to be consistent across various settings.

Some challenging behaviors may be refractory to behavioral interventions and/or so disruptive that medical intervention is warranted. The article by Rush and Frances revealed that "psychosocial experts" were much more likely to treat behaviors, even severely challenging ones, with nonmedical means than were the "medication experts."[98] Although the majority of "medication experts" stated that they would treat "self-injurious behaviors with the potential to cause bodily harm" and "aggressive behaviors" with medications as a first-line strategy, fewer than 30% of the "psychosocial experts" would use medication first. In these extreme situations, medical treatment should be just one component of a comprehensive behavior management plan. Even when a medication is prescribed, it is helpful to know the motivation for the challenging behavior. For example, if the child is disruptive during "circle time" at school, it would be helpful to know why. If it is because he or she is very anxious about joining the group, then a selective serotonin reuptake inhibitor (SSRI) might be appropriate. If it is because he or she also has comorbid ADHD type, then stimulant therapy might be more appropriate.

Clinical examples of behavior challenges include sleep disorders and psychogenic (self-induced) recurrent vomiting.

Sleep disorders are probably the most common and challenging example of the behavioral comorbid conditions. Poor sleep is associated with poor daytime learning, poor occupational performance, and increased daytime behavioral challenges. However, the most severe consequence of a sleep disturbance is often the resulting physical and emotional burdens on the child's family and caregivers.

As in normal children, management of sleep disorders should begin with behavioral strategies to improve sleep hygiene: avoidance of overstimulation at least one half hour before bedtime and implementation of consistent bedtime routines that include a settling ritual (television off; a bath; a bed-time story; and lights off). Zeitgebers, naturally occurring entraining factors that adjust the endogenous sleep-wake cycle, should also be incorporated into the management plan. The most powerful zeitgeber is dark; turning lights off stimulates endogenous melatonin release. Social cues (parental behaviors, noise) and certain foods also function as zeitgebers.[101] When problems persist, additional behavioral strategies may be required: sleep scheduling, gradual distancing, extinction, and bedtime fading.

On some occasions, biological interventions, such as exogenous melatonin and other medications, may be needed. Some medications (e.g., antihistamines, sedatives, clonidine) have been used on a long-term basis in children of all ages, whereas others (Ambien) are best reserved for older patients (5 years and older) for short-term use during vacations, scout camp, and sleepovers with friends and/or relatives. Exogenous melatonin is a strong zeitgeber and has been widely studied in children with disabilities; it is, however, not yet approved by the U.S. Food and Drug Administration.[102] It has been found to be very effective in both inducing and prolonging sleep.[103,104] Although there are no established guidelines, most investigators prescribed between 2 and 10 mg per dose. Short-acting preparations should be used when the child has difficulty falling asleep, and longer acting ones should be used for children with middle-of-the-night awakenings. The short-acting ones are generally in gel form and have an onset of action between 30 and 60 minutes. Drug levels remain higher than endogenous ones for 3 to 4 hours, regardless of nutritional status. The peak level of slow-release tablets is related to nutritional status; taking it on a full stomach may delay the onset of action considerably. Concentrations remain high for 5 to 7 hours. Side effects with melatonin are rare and, when they occur, are minor: headaches, nausea, and lightheadedness. Nightmares have been described, but this is believed to be a function of improved sleep. There is a report of a child with an underlying neurological condition having increased seizure frequency while taking melatonin, whereas another study demonstrated that seizure frequency actually decreased as a result of better sleep and decreased fatigue.[105] There are also reports of exogenous melatonin's having a delaying effect on the timing of puberty.[106]

Psychogenic (self-induced) recurrent vomiting is commonly seen in children with mental retardation. It may serve as a means to communicate gastrointestinal pain or as an expression of anger, frustration, or anxiety. Thus, the first challenge is to discern whether symptoms are organic or behavioral in etiology. This may require the coordinated efforts of a gastroenterologist, a developmental-behavioral pediatrician, a child psychologist, and/or a behavior specialist.

Psychiatric Disorders

The prevalence of psychiatric disorders is approximately threefold to fourfold higher in individuals with mental retardation, especially severe mental retardation, than in the general population.[5,107,108] It appears to be even higher in individuals raised in institutions than in those raised at home. The types of disorders prevalent in individuals with mental retardation are the same as those in the general populations, the most common ones being anxiety and stress disorders. In adults, these are associated primarily with trauma and incidents of abuse.[5,100] Other common disorders include ADHD, depression, obsessive compulsive disorder, and oppositional defiant disorder. Schizophrenia is rare. It has been shown that approximately 15% to 20% of children with known severe mental retardation may also meet full criteria for autism.[56] Although it was not mentioned in practice guidelines published in the mid-1990s, it is now thought that about 7% of children with Down syndrome meet criteria for autism.[109,110] In these children, social skills, particularly joint attention, and language skills are significantly more delayed than skills in other domains.

There has been a historical tendency to attribute all behavioral and mood changes to the underlying mental retardation diagnosis ("diagnostic overshadowing").[5] The term *dual diagnosis* is now used when a specific mental illness (with a specific *DSM-IV-TR* diagnosis) occurs in a person who also meets diagnostic criteria for mental retardation. It is now recognized that such comorbidity is common. When using the *DSM-IV-TR*, the newest edition of the *DSM* system, the clinician would code for mental retardation as an Axis II disorder. When the mental retardation is part of a known etiological syndrome, it is coded under Axis III as well. Diagnoses on Axis II do not necessitate psychiatric care, and they do not respond to psychotropic medications; they do improve with supports and treatment. When there is a comorbid mental illness, an appropriate Axis I diagnosis is identified.

When assessing an individual with mental retardation for psychiatric illness, the clinician must take into account the individual's developmental levels, especially their language abilities. Diagnosis is challenging when communication skills are poor. In nonverbal individuals, the clinician must be attentive to subtle behavioral cues that can lead to the appropriate comorbid psychiatric diagnosis.[100] When evaluating a child, the clinician must remember that environmental stressors (change of residence, school, or routine; loss of significant caregiver; overcrowding; noises; physical abuse; teasing, taunts, and bullying) can trigger problems and affect the child's compensatory mechanisms.

Although some standardized tools are useful for children with mild mental retardation, a comprehensive review commissioned by the National Institute of Mental Health revealed that few tools were reliable for those with more severe forms of mental retardation.[97] Aman[97] stated that it would take numerous tools to have an adequate armamentarium because those tools would have to address a number of domains while carefully considering the patient's age and level of mental retardation and the informant's status (self, caregiver, clinician). Expert consensus guidelines listed standardized rating scales as a second-line evaluation method.[98] Some standardized tools can also be useful in assessing efficacy of specific interventions; others are important in assessing side effects, such as tardive dyskinesias. It is important to constantly monitor the medication effects (and side effects) on the child's functional status and his or her ability to carry out daily activities and to participate in habilitation therapies.

The American Academy of Child and Adolescent Psychiatry's practice parameter on diagnosis of comorbid mental illness in persons with mental retardation defines key components of a comprehensive assessment: A detailed review of medical, developmental, and behavioral histories, combined with any prior assessments of cognition, adaptive functioning, communication, and social skills, may help focus the evaluation.[98,111] New or repeat evaluations may be required if the available information is incomplete or if new methods to define a cause or unusual symptoms have been developed. A functional analysis of behavior or, when not available, very specific and detailed descriptions of behaviors, antecedent events, and environmental circumstances define the specific concern. Describing what has been tried and what has been successful is also important.

Informed consent by the parents or guardian for psychotropic medications, especially those with significant side effects, is always advised.[98] The older teenager or young adult with mental retardation should be included in this process if he or she has the capacity to participate. When a medication is chosen, the patient should "start low and go slow." A poor response may be affected by variations in medication metabolism or compliance. Experts state that initial doses should be lower in children with mental retar-

dation than in the general population and that titration should occur more slowly. However, maintenance and maximum doses are no different from those for the general population.[98] The clinician should identify the specific index behavior or condition in advance to better evaluate efficacy of the treatment, especially for nonverbal children. Blood levels, if available, may be especially informative when side effects, poor response, worsening behaviors, and polypharmacy are concerns.

General recommendations from the American Academy of Child and Adolescent Psychiatry guidelines for individuals with mental retardation include using SSRIs as the first-line medication for posttraumatic stress disorder, depression, anxiety, or obsessive-compulsive disorder.[98] Neuroleptic agents, especially the newer atypical ones, which have fewer side effects, were noted to be the treatment of choice for schizophrenia and psychosis not otherwise specified. They may also be helpful in children with mental retardation and comorbid behavioral conditions not defined by the *DSM-IV-TR*, such as self-injurious behaviors, aggression, and disabling stereotypical behaviors.[99] For patients who are noncompliant with oral medication regimens, a long-acting depot antipsychotic may be needed. α-Agonists (clonidine, guanfacine) and β-blockers (propranolol) were cited as drugs of choice for disruptive behaviors. Antiepileptic drugs (e.g., valproate and carbamazepine) may be effective in treating agitation, irritability, and mood swings, especially in patients with comorbid epilepsy. Like individuals without mental retardation, those with mental retardation at risk for suicide, severe self-injury, or injury to others or with acute psychotic symptoms should be hospitalized.

The consensus guidelines recommended that patients be seen at least every 3 months and within 1 month of a drug or dosage change. They also provided guidance regarding dosing strategies (primarily in older teenagers and adults) and the duration of a medication trial before a switch to another medication is considered: 3 to 8 weeks for antipsychotics, 1 to 3 weeks for mood stabilizers, and 6 to 8 weeks for SSRIs.[98] Although interclass polypharmaceutical treatment is sometimes needed in refractory cases, intraclass polypharmaceutical treatment is rarely justified. Clinicians are advised to minimize certain prescribing practices, including the long-term use of "as needed" medication orders, of benzodiazepines for "anxiety," and of long- and short-acting sedative hypnotics. Certain antiepileptic medications (phenytoin, phenobarbital, and primidone) are not recommended as psychotropic medications.

Clinical examples of psychiatric disorders include attention deficits, impulsivity, and hyperactivity.

Attention deficits, impulsivity, and *hyperactivity* are common in school-aged children, including those with mental retardation. Although the American Academy of Pediatrics' Practice Guidelines for evaluation and treatment of ADHD do not address children with mental retardation, it is reasonable and appropriate to prescribe them to this population.[112,113] Studies have shown that questionnaires and teachers' observations are also valid and reliable in children with mental retardation.[114,115] The most challenging diagnostic dilemma is determining the degree to which the child with mental retardation is demonstrating true symptoms of ADHD or the effect the child's lower mental age is having on their clinical presentation. When the child's inability to function in class appears to result from ADHD and not his or her lower mental age, medical treatment may be indicated. Stimulant therapy has been found to be effective, especially in reducing hyperactivity; results may be less consistent in individuals with more severe forms of mental retardation.[98,116]

Medical Disorders

All children with mental retardation, especially those with severe mental retardation who are unable to express themselves, should have comprehensive physical examinations at least annually in the context of an established medical home. For the most part, children with mental retardation contract the same illnesses as do children who are developing normally. A new or evolving medical condition might manifest as a change in behavior or routine. For example, self-injurious behavior, especially head banging, might be the only way a nonverbal child can express pain associated with a headache or tooth abscess. The major causes of death are similar to those in the normal population: cardiovascular disease, stroke, and cancer. The incidence of death from respiratory disease is significantly higher in those with severe mental retardation living in institutions than in those living at home. The prevalence of the following conditions may be higher in children with mental retardation than in the general population:[5,91,107]

1. *Seizure disorders* are approximately 10 times more common in children with mental retardation, especially in those with severe impairments.[5,107] The prevalence reaches 50% among children with both mental retardation and cerebral palsy. Several epileptic syndromes are strongly associated with mental retardation and characterized by seizures that are very difficult to control (e.g., West and Lennox-Gastaut syndromes). Even seizures not associated with known syndromes can be more therapeutically challenging in persons with mental retardation caused by central nervous system disease and the coexistence of multiple seizure types in a single patient. If a child is prone to status epilepticus, an emergency protocol should be established with the family, which may include rectal administration of anticonvulsants at home and at school.

2. *Hearing and vision impairments* are also more common in children with mental retardation than in the general population, especially in those with associated craniofacial syndromes. Approximately one half of the children with severe mental retardation have visual deficits, the most common being strabismus and refractive errors.[117]

3. *Motor impairments* are seen in approximately 10% of individuals with mild mental retardation. About 20% of those with severe mental retardation have significant motor deficits consistent with a diagnosis of cerebral palsy. On the other hand, approximately 50% of children with cerebral palsy have comorbid mental retardation. Seizures are much more common when a child has both cerebral palsy and mental retardation.[118]

4. *Type 2 diabetes* may be more common in individuals with mental retardation than in the general population because of the high prevalence of obesity and inactivity in this population.[89] In one study, obesity rates were noted to be as high as 75% in girls and women with mental retardation.[90] In contrast, a survey of Special Olympic participants revealed a prevalence of Type 1 diabetes equal to that in the normal population.[91] It is imperative that physicians monitor growth and encourage healthy diets and frequent exercise in patients with mental retardation. Using high-calorie snacks as rewards for appropriate behavior should be discouraged.

5. *Gastrointestinal disorders* may occur in children with all levels of mental retardation; however, they are more difficult to diagnose and manage when a child has severe mental retardation with limited speech and the inability to localize pain. The most challenging aspect may be in trying to determine whether emesis is organic or behavioral in origin. In a nonverbal child, it may play a role in the child's expression of frustration, anger, or anxiety. Recurrent emesis may indicate a medical condition such as gastroesophageal reflux in patients with severe mental retardation, especially those with comorbid cerebral palsy, who spend most of their day in semi-recumbent positions. These individuals may have also experienced hypoxic damage to vagal nuclei and/or may be taking medications that affect lower esophageal sphincter function. Recurrent emesis may also indicate a gastric ulcer or, in rare cases, an underlying metabolic disorder.

SPECIAL HEALTH CONCERNS IN ADOLESCENTS AND YOUNG ADULTS WITH MENTAL RETARDATION

Successful social relationships foster self-esteem and contribute to better quality of life. Teenagers with severe mental retardation may experience difficulty in developing social relationships, for many reasons: stigmatizing dysmorphic features, lack of awareness of social etiquette, inappropriate sexual behavior, comorbid medical or physical disabilities, and overprotection from parents. Social development is chiefly experiential; teenagers with mental retardation, especially more severe forms of mental retardation, may have fewer opportunities to acquire social experience. Teenagers with mental retardation may need formal training in mastering social greetings, telephone skills, and proper etiquette (e.g., inhibition of sexual urges in public settings).

As in normal teenagers, the pediatrician must address issues of puberty and sexuality in teenagers with mental retardation, although explanations should be more basic. Sexuality is a fundamental human right and encompasses more than genital sex. It includes gender awareness and the needs to be liked and accepted, to feel valued and attractive, to display and receive affection, and to share thoughts and feelings. Until the 1990s, the issue of sexuality was rarely addressed in children with mental retardation; the topic was considered "taboo" for fear that the mere mentioning of the topic would unleash inappropriate desires and behaviors. There is now a growing body of literature addressing the topic.[119,120] Numerous training programs have been developed to teach appropriate behaviors to teenagers with mental retardation through the use of videos, comic book stories, and role playing. Individuals with mental retardation, especially those with more severe mental retardation, may be less aware of others' opinions and less inhibited in public settings. Maladaptive behaviors related to sexuality can be a significant barrier to the adolescent's successful inclusion in school, work, and community settings.

Girls and women with mental retardation, like other girls and women, should strive to become independent in self-care and hygiene; this may be more challenging in those with more severe levels of mental retardation. Some female patients may never accomplish independence and may experience extreme anxiety and fear during menses, being unable to comprehend the concept of periodic benign bleeding. Gynecological care may likewise be complicated by increased anxiety and lack of cooperation during a "routine" pelvic examination. Preparation aided by pictures, role playing, having a trusted caregiver present during the appointment, and the use of alternative positions other than pelvic stirrups may minimize fear and stress.[119]

Parents of girls with mental retardation often express concerns about the possibility of pregnancy, the possibility of sexual abuse, and the efficacy of available birth control methods. These issues harbor many religious and ethical beliefs. Many parents worry that their daughter would never be able to care for her child. For boys, many parents are concerned about protecting the boy from the obligation of parental support that he would probably not be able to fulfill. Finally, there is the fear that the parents themselves would be required to care for their grandchild by default.

Although involuntary sterilization was an option in the past, it is no longer permissible.[121,122] The eugenics movement of the early 20th century influenced sterilization policies and led to the passage of laws addressing sterilization in 30 states. These laws allowed, and in some cases required, sterilization of individuals with mental retardation and other disabilities. This level of intervention came about primarily as the result of a U.S. Supreme Court decision upholding Virginia's authority to involuntarily sterilize "mentally defective" persons housed in state institutions. The decision was influenced, in part, by the mistaken assumption that most, if not all, children born to parents who had mental retardation would also have mental retardation. More than 60,000 men and women were sterilized in the ensuing years. In view of the atrocities of Nazi Germany, attitudes and practices began to change toward the end of World War II; however, states did not begin repealing these sterilization laws until the 1960s. Involuntary sterilization should never be performed on anyone who possesses, or might possess in the future, the capacity to provide valid consent to marriage, the capacity for reproductive decision making, and/or the ability to raise a child. In individuals who permanently and completely lack all of those capacities, sterilization should still be the procedure of last resort. It should be used only when less invasive and temporary alternatives are not possible and when the procedure is necessary and clearly in the best interest of the person with mental retardation. In every case, all possible measures must be taken to ensure a good outcome.[122]

There are now many effective and reversible alternatives to sterilization. In addition to traditional 28-day-cycle oral contraceptives, long-term contraception is now available and may be helpful in teenagers with limited cognition, limited motivation, and/or limited physical dexterity.[123] These include weekly applied transdermal patches, monthly intramuscular injections, and implants and long-term progestin-releasing intrauterine devices that can provide protection for several years. A decision to use these interventions is between the physician, the parents, and, whenever possible, the individual. Possible side effects and drug interactions, especially when the individual is taking medications for treatment of comorbid disorders, must be carefully considered. Although parents may have legitimate concerns, the well-being and religious beliefs of the individual with mental retardation should prevail throughout the decision-making process.

On their 18th birthday, teenagers with mental retardation automatically become their own legal guardians. If parents and the professionals working with the individual do not feel that she or he is capable of making responsible decisions, a formal evaluation should be conducted to determine the need for guardianship. This should be pursued with great care, because guardianship contradicts the principles of self-determination; it is not an all-or-nothing issue, especially when the adult has milder deficits. If guardianship is in the individual's best interests, services should be sought to help the parents navigate the legal, judicial, and medical systems. The parents may consult the child's primary care provider, a developmental-behavioral pediatrician, or another specialist who knows the child well; medical information is often required. The designated guardian or guardians for the individual might be one or both parents, an adult sibling, a relative, a family friend, or a professional. For some higher functioning individuals, only a financial conservator, rather than a guardian, may be needed. The conservator helps the individual with mental retardation navigate the procedures and forms necessary to maintain the individual's public supports (SSI, Medicaid); the individual maintains the right to make all other day-to-day decisions.

DEVELOPMENTAL, EDUCATIONAL, AND VOCATIONAL SERVICES

Developmental, educational, and vocational services are the mainstays of management for children with mental retardation. Each may assume a position of primary importance, depending on the individual's age and degree of involvement. For example, health concerns and interventions may be the focus in the very young child with severe mental retardation and comorbid medical conditions. The common focus of each service system is habilitation: to provide equal opportunities so as to facilitate full participation in society for these individuals by identifying and addressing their strengths and weaknesses and to work toward a goal of "normalization."[111]

The type and intensity of supports needed are almost always determined through a multidisciplinary process. Professionals with expertise in numerous areas, most far beyond a narrow medical focus, join together to develop a support delivery plan based on the age, developmental level, and other unique char-

TABLE 11-5 ■ Comparison of Different Support Plans

Plan	Age	Services Provided
Individualized Family Support Plan (IFSP)	Children younger than 3 years	Early intervention
Individualized Education Plan (IEP)	Children aged 3 to 16 years	Educational
Individualized Transition Plan (ITP)	Adolescents aged 14-16 years through graduation	Transition, vocational, independent living
Individualized Habilitation (Support) Plan (IHP)	After graduation	Adult support

acteristics of the child. Those with mild mental retardation usually need fewer services and supports than do those with more severe mental retardation. The focus of the written document, or *Individualized Plan*, depends on the age of the child. In all cases, it represents the child's *Individualized Support Plan*; this umbrella term reflects the AAIDD support paradigm (Table 11-5).[5]

In their efforts to identify and provide the best services, a parent of a child with mental retardation may feel as if every person or agency they deal with is speaking a foreign language. A new set of terms, definitions, references to public laws, and eligibility requirements seem to make each decision more complex and the results contradictory. Social, economic, and cultural background differences also contribute to this confusion. For these reasons, disability rights advocates and advocacy organizations have assumed an important role throughout the educational and vocational support processes. At their best, advocates identify the key issues important to the family, help match those goals with available services, and propose solutions in which resources from across categorical boundaries are used. It is hoped that the need to assume and promote an adversarial position continues to decline in frequency and intensity.

Early Developmental Intervention: Part C of the Individuals with Disabilities Education Act (2004)

Severe global delays, especially in children with dysmorphic features, are usually diagnosed in infancy or shortly thereafter, and such children should be referred to an EIP as soon as their medical conditions are stabilized and they are able to participate. EIPs are government-funded developmental programs in which children with developmental delays or with known disabilities are entitled to participate. When a child receives a diagnosis of a syndrome known to be associated with mental retardation (e.g., Down syndrome), he or she becomes eligible for services at the time of diagnosis, even though delays may not yet be evident. On the other hand, a child without a recognizable syndrome is not eligible until a delay becomes evident. A specific, etiological diagnosis is not necessary to access early intervention services; in fact, it is advisable to refer the child to EIPs as soon as a delay becomes evident so that the child can receive appropriate services while the etiological workup progresses.

On referral, the child is scheduled for a multidisciplinary team evaluation to confirm eligibility. State eligibility criteria for EIPs vary; many states define a "delay" as at least a 33% lag in one developmental skill set or a 25% lag in two or more skill sets (e.g., language, gross and fine motor, social, and self-help skills). This evaluation serves as the foundation to develop an Individualized Family Service Plan (IFSP). The IFSP stresses the importance of the family as the central focus of and decision maker about individualized services for the child. The "service menu" may vary from state to state, but most programs offer case management, family support, parent training, and some direct therapy (speech, occupational, and physical). The cost is free in some states; in others, there may be a sliding fee scale based on family income. The child's health insurance company may also be billed for the direct therapies. Ideally, all of these services take place in a child's natural environment: that is, at home or in the childcare center that he or she attends. Every effort is made to schedule visits when the parents can also be present.

Evidence of the benefits of EIPs has been demonstrated best in disadvantaged children: that is, children of low-income families in which parents have less than a high school education.[124] Outcome studies vary, and the magnitude of their effect appears to depend on several factors, including the appropriateness and intensity of the interventions and on the degree of parental involvement. When surveyed about consumer satisfaction, parents rated EIP programs as having a positive effect on their family's acceptance of and caregiver abilities for the child.[125] There is less conclusive evidence regarding lasting gains from standardized measures of language and cognitive development.

Special Education

The primary focus of management in a child with idiopathic mild "global developmental delays" or mental retardation is almost always educational. Edu-

cational services should begin as soon as the delay or deficit is recognized and should be delivered in integrated settings with typically developing peers to the greatest extent possible.

PRESCHOOL

Often, children with mild to moderate mental retardation are not identified as such until after the third birthday and do not have the opportunity to benefit from early developmental services. At this point, the child should be referred to the special education department at the local school. Children aged 3 to 6 years are usually served in a Preschool Program for Children with Disabilities, although the 2004 IDEA legislation authorizes states to adopt policies that will provide families the option to remain in an EIP until the child is 5 years old.[126] Determination of eligibility is again accomplished through a multidisciplinary team. The team's evaluation serves as the basis for development of a support plan that is now called an *Individualized Education Plan* (IEP). The change in terminology from IFSP to IEP reflects a transition in focus from the family to the child.

Services described in the child's IEP include educational or instructional adaptations that the child needs in order to be academically successful and transportation methods for the child to receive those services. If appropriate, the IEP may include requirements for speech, occupational, and/or, but less frequently, physical therapy services. However, school-based therapy, unlike other therapy settings, addresses only skills that are necessary for success in academic and typical classroom activities. The specifics of how and with what frequency these services are used to provide a "free and appropriate public education" can vary widely among school districts. More often than not, the therapy is "consultative" rather than "hands-on" or "direct." This means that the therapists periodically evaluate the child's progress; reconfirm or revise (depending on the child's progress) therapy goals and objectives; and provide the parents, teachers, and aides with a new set of goals and individualized strategies to promote skill attainment.

ELEMENTARY SCHOOL

As the child ages and becomes eligible for elementary school, another evaluation is necessary to determine whether she or he is still eligible for special education services. If so, a new IEP is developed. In addition to describing the type, intensity, and frequency of supports and services recommended, the team also determines the best setting or settings for service delivery. According to the IDEA of 1990 and its subsequent re-authorizations in 1997 and 2004, the child should receive educational services in the "least restrictive environment" appropriate for that individual.[126a] Children with mental retardation, especially those with mild mental retardation, appear to have better outcomes when they are included in regular classrooms with typically developing peers. The extent of inclusion depends on the level of mental retardation and the extent of maladaptive behaviors (e.g., aggressive, self-injurious). It also depends on the school district's resources. The child should be included in the regular classroom for as many academic classes as possible and for all nonacademic activities (recess, physical education, music, art, lunch, recess). Children with mild mental retardation usually need additional supports for academic classes during elementary and junior high (middle) school years: adaptations to the classroom, subject content, teaching strategies, and so forth. This may best be accomplished with a specially trained teacher aide who might be shared among several students with special needs. Although the "least restrictive environment" principle is very important, placement in a regular classroom should never prevent a child from receiving the specialized services outlined in his or her IEP.

When service delivery is not feasible in the regular classroom, the child might be "pulled out" to attend a resource classroom for one or more academic subjects. A resource classroom is characterized by a small number of students (usually fewer than 10) who also demonstrate various learning challenges. The special education teacher, with the help of specially trained aides, provides direct individualized instruction. Such students, however, should remain with their typically developing peers for nonacademic activities. When needed, an aide may assist the child or children in the regular classroom to facilitate inclusion.

Children with severe mental retardation, especially those with challenging behaviors, may need a full-time separate or "self-contained" classroom in which they participate in life skills training (e.g., feeding, dressing, toileting, and other developmentally appropriate interventions). Nevertheless, their inclusion with typically developing peers in nonacademic activities should also be facilitated as much as possible. The most restricted environments include residential state institutions; however, with the passage of the Americans with Disabilities Act and IDEA and advocacy efforts to close these institutions, fewer children attend these segregated programs. If the Healthy People 2010 goal is met, all children with mental retardation will be served in community schools.

HIGH SCHOOL

Children with mental retardation may require fewer supports during their junior high (middle school) and senior high school years. Vocational classes targeting their interests and strengths become the focus of training, replacing academic classes. Skills needed for successful independent living and meaningful employment are targeted.[127] Although planning activities may begin as early as 14 years of age, teenagers with mental retardation should have an Individualized Transition Plan (ITP) in place by the time they are 16 years old. The ITP is different from the IEP in several specific ways:

1. The student is a member of the multidisciplinary planning team and helps determine educational goals, objectives, services, and settings.
2. The plan's emphasis changes from academic to vocational services and from remedial instruction for deficits to fostering abilities. A vocational assessment should be conducted to evaluate the teenager's interests and strengths and to determine the services needed to promote independence in the workplace and the community.
3. The team should discuss goals and recommend training that will be needed to accomplish successful independent living after graduation. The teenager's cultural, ethnic, linguistic, and economic characteristics should be always be considered.
4. Representatives from adult-oriented disability agencies (state vocational rehabilitation agencies and/or The Arc of the United States) are invited to attend the meeting and provide input and recommendations. On occasion, these agencies may provide transition services before graduation.
5. Depending on the individual's cognitive level, health condition, work habits, and behavioral challenges, preparation for one of the following types of employment is targeted. Off-campus on-the-job training may be an option. Other options include the following:
   a. Competitive employment: The individual is hired, trained, and compensated in a manner similar for those who are not disabled. The job may include unskilled, semiskilled, or, in some cases, even skilled duties. Work takes place in an integrated environment with minimal or intermittent supports.
   b. Supported employment: The individual is hired to perform specific duties for competitive wages and is provided a job coach and/or environmental or schedule modifications that are necessary for success. As the individual masters the skills needed, coaching services are phased out.
   c. Sheltered employment: The individual works under constant supervision in a segregated setting. Often the work is contracted with local businesses. Examples range from silk screening T-shirts to assembling and sealing individual packets of plastic eating utensils, napkins, salt,

and pepper for fast-food carry-out restaurants. The individual may receive a weekly stipend (rarely consistent with minimum wage standards), or he or she may be compensated per unit completed.

Children with disabilities may attend public school through 21 years of age. Usually, this continuation of services reflects prolonged training opportunities in vocational or life skills during high school years rather than actual grade retention. Most children with mild mental retardation have the potential for learning that parallels that of children and teenagers without mental retardation. However, that learning occurs at a slower rate and plateaus at a lower academic level, creating a clear deficit in comparison with typically developing peers; attending college is much less likely.

Additional Considerations

PERIODIC EVALUATIONS

By law, students must be reevaluated every 3 years. Parents, according to recommendations from health care providers, other professionals, or school personnel, may also request off-cycle evaluations if there is a new crisis affecting learning, a lack of expected progress, unexpected significant progress, or a change to a new setting or school. The goal of the reevaluation is to establish the current level of functioning, to review the services the student is receiving, and to revise, as necessary, interventions to optimize the student's outcome under the new conditions. The depth and breadth of any reevaluation should be based on specific, individualized concerns rather than adhering to a routine process or method.

Over time, it is important for educational, medical, and other professionals working with a child to discuss long-term goals with the parents and, when feasible, with that child. The developmental-behavioral pediatrician can assist the primary care provider in this endeavor, as either a resource or a facilitator. Ongoing communication with school personnel and a team approach optimize the individual's functional outcomes and chances for a better quality of life.

The following factors should be considered:

1. Are the long-term goals realistic, considering the student's cognitive level?
2. Is the student receiving the services and academic instruction necessary to reach those goals?
3. Are there additional measures that professionals can take to optimize the physical and emotional health of the student?
4. Is the student demonstrating any challenging behaviors that are impeding progress? Is medical treatment or counseling indicated?

5. Are the student and family coping well? If not, are counseling, medical, or community support services indicated?

BEHAVIORAL CHALLENGES

During the student's school career, disruptive behaviors often prevent the child from benefiting from educational services. Inappropriate behaviors may also prevent inclusion in a regular classroom or in an off-campus vocational program. These may be especially problematic if they cause the student to be a danger to himself or herself, to others, or to school property. A systematic evaluation by psychologists or other trained specialists of the antecedent-behavior-consequence behavioral paradigm in various contextual and environmental circumstances is called a *functional analysis of behavior.* The first goal of this analysis is to determine the etiology of the student's behavior: a desire to *e*scape, a need for *a*ttention or a *t*angible object (e.g., food, toy, crayon), and/or a need for an increase or a decrease in *s*ensory input (EATS). Once this is determined, a Behavior Intervention Plan (BIP) should be developed for any child with mental retardation who demonstrates challenging behaviors, in order to eliminate or decrease the behaviors so that the child can receive maximum benefit from educational/vocational services and be included in a regular classroom with typically developing peers as much as possible. For many children, this may be the most critical and frequently used aspect of the IEP. Sometimes, in order to receive maximum benefit, behavior interventions may need to be supplemented with medical interventions. (See previous "Health Care" section.)

RECREATIONAL AND SOCIAL ACTIVITIES

Children and teenagers with mild mental retardation and younger children with more severe mental retardation are not usually excluded from integrated social activities with typically developing peers; teenagers with more severe forms of mental retardation have fewer opportunities for such social interactions. Throughout the school years, it is important that students with mental retardation, regardless of severity, be included in regular school events (dances, fund raisers, pep rallies) and extracurricular activities (band, pep squad, choir) as much as possible. These promote appropriate social skills, self-worth, dignity, and friendships with nondisabled peers. Students with mental retardation often benefit from participation in school- or community-sponsored social and athletic programs, such as the Special Olympics. These programs promote physical health and fitness and improve self-esteem while also providing opportunities for socialization. Many states, with the assistance of federal funding, have contracted with community agencies to develop and implement leadership training opportunities for youths with disabilities. These usually occur during the summer and foster social, self-advocacy, and leadership skills. Developmental-behavioral pediatricians should be aware of opportunities in their state and encourage their teenage patients to participation in these to the maximum extent possible.

COMMUNITY AND PUBLIC SUPPORTS

Supports are resources and strategies that promote development, education, individual functioning, independence, and personal well-being. They are ideally delivered in a systemized manner through an Individualized Support Plan (ISP). The focus of the support plan varies, depending on the child's age: IFSP, IEP, or ITP (see Table 11-5). Of all health care professionals, the developmental-behavioral pediatrician is often the most knowledgeable about community and public supports and can be helpful to parents as they attempt to navigate a complex menu of services, each with their own unique eligibility criteria, admission procedures, and funding constraints.

The management of any chronic condition must also address the needs of the family, the child's best single resource and support. Early supports, through the IFSP, target the concerns and goals of parents; the IFSP is unique in this focus. Most support needs of children and teenagers with mental retardation are met through the educational system, especially when schools promote integration of children with mental retardation into ongoing sports, social, and extracurricular activities. Additional community-based programs can also promote integration and foster social well-being and independence. Siblings of individuals with mental retardation may require supports at any time, depending on their own age and life situation, independent of their affected sibling.

The following discussion of supports is organized in order of needs across the lifespan of the individual with mental retardation and his or her family. Thus, supports important for new parents are discussed first, followed by supports for the children themselves. Sibling issues are presented at the end of this section.

Parent-Centered Supports

Supporting parents in their caregiving roles is very important, especially for a child with severe mental retardation, who may need extensive and prolonged care and supervision within the family home. A fam-

ily's requirement for additional supports depends not only on the characteristics of the child (i.e., the degree of cognitive impairment, comorbid disorders, behavioral challenges, and degree and duration of dependence) but also on the family's characteristics: structural (e.g., single-parent household), functional (e.g., coping strategies), and external (e.g., income and work schedules).[128] There are critical periods when parents, who might otherwise be doing fairly well with a little help from extended family and friends, need extra support.[129] These times are usually ones of major life-status transitions when the child's differences are most obvious. Early in the child's life, such periods include the times when the diagnosis is first made, when a younger sibling developmentally surpasses the child with mental retardation, and when the affected child first enrolls in *special* education. Later in their child's life, critical periods might include the onset of puberty, with its escalation of behavioral problems and inappropriate sexual behaviors; the graduation from high school, especially in the absence of vocational opportunities and/or community supports; the transition from pediatric to adult providers of health care; the process of determining legal guardianship at their child's 18th birthday; and the death of a custodial parent. Parents' coping skills are also challenged when they see their adolescent child being excluded from typical rites of adolescent passage such as social and athletic events, independent dating activities, and driver education classes.

Besides the natural support systems that come from extended family members, neighbors, friends, and religious community members, there are two additional systems of supports: community (or informal) and public (or formal). Community organizations that provide information, advocacy, parent training, counseling, daycare, respite care, and recreational activities for the family can be extremely valuable. Formal family supports include publicly funded entitlement programs, eligibility for which is based on parents' income or the condition of their child. The most important such public support is an entitlement for *all* children, not just children with mental retardation: a free and appropriate public education. Other public supports are not available to all parents of a child with mental retardation; instead, they depend on the child's degree of mental retardation (those with mild mental retardation are often excluded) and on the parents' financial status.

INFORMATION AND EDUCATION

One of the most important early supports to parents is the provision of up-to-date and accurate information about their child's condition, especially if it is associated with a known syndrome.[79] Education empowers and supports parents in their caregiving roles. A survey of parents of children with chronic disorders reported that parents desired much more information than their pediatricians believed was necessary.[130] It is hoped that the clinician making the diagnosis involves appropriate subspecialists in the child's care, such as a developmental-behavioral pediatrician, or is able to provide a wider array of diagnosis-specific parent handouts. If this is not possible, the diagnosing clinician, the primary care provider, or the parents can contact the national organization that represents the disorder. National organizations, and sometimes even state and local chapters, can be found for most of the more common mental retardation–associated syndromes (e.g., the National Down Syndrome Congress). When this is not the case, the parents or physician can contact the National Organization for Rare Disorders for help. These organizations are usually governed by a professional board of directors, often with guidance from a medical advisory council. They may author, edit, or at least oversee the publications and information distributed by the staff or made available through their Web sites. This syndrome-specific information can be very helpful to both parents and professionals as they face the medical, developmental, educational, behavioral, and psychiatric challenges unique to that syndrome. Such organizations may host national conferences for parents and professionals and may assist parents of children with newly diagnosed disorders in contacting other parents of children with the same syndrome. Finally, some disorder-specific organizations maintain a national registry and sponsor bench and/or clinical research.

When there is no identifiable syndrome, the clinician should carefully explain and/or provide more generic literature regarding strategies to address the extra challenges that most children with mental retardation encounter, especially in the mastery of academic, adaptive, and social skills. In some cases, national organizations such as the AAIDD, The Arc of the United States, the Parent Advocacy Coalition for Educational Rights, and the National Dissemination Center for Children with Disabilities have developed such information for parents of a child with any disability, regardless of cause.

The Internet has rapidly become an important tool in accessing disability information, inasmuch as both local and national organizations have developed Web sites. Some Web sites include real-time "ask the expert" sessions. Listserve, message boards, and electronic discussion groups allow parents to expand their peer support network across the globe. Unfortunately, information found on Web sites may not be peer reviewed; thus, quality and validity may be questionable. Parents should be warned and advised to use caution in interpreting information from non–peer-reviewed sites. Rosenbaum and Stewart offered guidelines for parents on using the Internet as a source of information.[131] Parents should be especially warned about Web sites that offer quick "cures," usually through an alternative medicine approach. They should be referred to reputable professional sites that provide scientific critiques of alternative medicine interventions (e.g., *http://www.quackwatch.org*).

COMMUNITY (INFORMAL) SUPPORTS

As families of children with mental retardation look to community organizations for additional support, they may find that the depth and breadth of services vary from state to state and even within state boundaries. Rural areas may offer few services from a limited number of local organizations, whereas urban areas tend to have a greater variety of programs. There is rarely a single point of entry, regardless of location. Eligibility criteria, fees, and admission procedures vary, which makes navigation of these systems very challenging. The greatest impediment to access is simply the lack of knowledge that these organizations and services exist. The developmental-behavioral pediatrician should have a detailed knowledge of existing regional programs, the types of children they serve, and a method of sharing that information with the local primary care physicians. The local United Way, Part C program, and special education staff can sometimes be very helpful in both educating the clinician and assisting the individual family. "Parent-to-parent" groups (to be discussed) or a single seasoned parent who has successfully navigated the system can be the clinician's best resource, helping other parents understand the educational system, access public supports, and encourage their development of advocacy skills.

One of the earliest needs that most parents have, especially if both are employed outside the home, is dependable and affordable *childcare*. This may not be an issue for the child with mild mental retardation or even one with more severe mental retardation, as long as there are no challenging health or behavior concerns. However, for children needing specialized medical care or individual supervision, accessibility to childcare is often not possible, despite the Americans with Disabilities Act mandates. When specialized childcare is available, it is often expensive, and the cost may outweigh the potential earned income.[132] In these instances, one parent often decides to quit his or her job and remain at home to care for the child. The parent may later choose to reenter the work force when the child reaches school age.

Families of children with mental retardation are faced with added caregiving and supervision responsibilities, especially if the child has complicated health care or behavioral needs. Although many parents do well during their child's early years, their parenting journey may bring them to a point where they are "burned out" with their childrearing role. Parents of all children benefit from occasional breaks in caregiving routines. Parents often turn to extended family members or friends for these breaks. If this is not possible, especially when caregivers with special skills are needed, a family needs to seek the assistance of an agency that provides respite services. *Respite service* (temporary care of a child with a disability by a trained provider for the purpose of providing relief to the family) is often cited by parents as the most needed support.[133,134] Respite care may enable parents to face the caregiving role with renewed vigor. There are various respite care models; however, its availability, like so many other important support services, varies among communities. Respite care options include both home- and center-based care. Although center-based care, with trained caregivers and nurses in facility settings, was popular in the 1990s, newer legislation has provided increasing support for in-home options. There are advantages and disadvantages associated with both models, but a family's options are often determined by the state's funding allocation practices rather than by choice. (See the following "Public [Formal] Supports" section.) Family cooperatives, in which parents of children with similar disabilities agree to "swap" care with other families at no cost, may be more flexible because they are not dependent on public funding and are less restrictive. In extreme cases, parents may need an immediate break, or emergency respite care, to cope and, on occasion, as a measure to prevent abuse. Emergency respite care is more costly, requires around-the-clock staff, and is not always available in communities, even large urban ones.

Although not disability-specific, *parent-to-parent organizations* can assist in linking parents of children with similar disorders. Many parents derive a great deal of comfort from other parents who have encountered the same experiences. They often learn more useful and practical information from other parents than from professionals or published literature. These organizations can also provide parents with valuable information about local services and state disability legislation. Many conduct conferences and train parents in advocacy. Some organizations have become very effective in improving services for children with mental retardation at the local, state and, sometimes, even national levels. Parent Training and Information Centers are now federally mandated and exist in every state. These centers train and disseminate information to parents to help them become active collaborators, partners, decision makers, and problem solvers alongside policy makers, professionals, and agency personnel.[128]

PUBLIC (FORMAL) SUPPORTS

Most publicly funded formal supports for children with mental retardation exist because of federal legislation; that legislation exists because of the heroic efforts of parents and disability advocates. These supports include programs that provide financial assistance (e.g., SSI benefits and Food Stamps); education; and medical (Medicaid), vocational, and residential/living services. However, the implementation of these programs at the state level is frequently and significantly influenced by budgetary restrictions and the establishment of eligibility criteria. Some supports are available to all children, such as a free public education. Others are need based; access depends on financial need and/or severity of disability.

SSI benefits (distributed by the Social Security Administration since 1974) represented the first financial support for families raising children with severe disabilities, including those with mental retardation, at home. However, it was designed and continues to be a needs-based (i.e., based on income and assets) benefit for *low-income* families.[135,136] Because of this requirement, many children with idiopathic mild mental retardation are not eligible for this support. If both financial need and disability severity criteria are met, the family receives a monthly stipend. Of greater importance is the fact that in most states, the receipt of any stipend amount automatically makes the child eligible for Medicaid. The benefit amount has slowly but steadily is increased since 1974. In 2007, the maximum month subsidy is $623; however, a family might actually receive much less.

In addition to supports provided through SSI, educational, and health-care programs (Medicaid), families of children with severe mental retardation, especially those with comorbid health and/or behavior conditions may now be eligible for additional supports to assist them in raising their child. In the past, the only way a family could access these supports was to institutionalize their child. In the 1970s, most funding supported large state-operated institutions; however, legislation has subsequently shifted the preponderance of funding to community-based services.[81,137] Although funding for community-based supports has been increasing since the 1970s, the degree of funding allocated for these services varies a great deal from state to state. Some states have policies that guarantee that all children with mental retardation will live in family settings, but many states still allocate large sums to institutional settings (state facilities, nursing homes, and intermediate care facilities for individuals with mental retardation).

The most common funding mechanism for in-home supports is the home- and community-based waiver services (HCBS). HCBS funding is available to families through waiver options because consideration of the family's income and assets is waived for purposes of eligibility; thus, access is equitable across all income levels. Eligibility depends then entirely on the severity of the child's disability and the effect that the disability imposes on the family. However, many states have long waiting lists. States have developed different mechanisms to distribute their limited resources: "first come, first served" waiting lists, urgency of need, time-limited supports, and a lottery system. Once a child becomes eligible for a funded slot, the family is assigned a case manager. Case managers work collaboratively with families and providers to design an annual service plan that includes choices from a menu of possible supports, such as respite (in-home, center- or camp-based) care, medical equipment, and home modifications for accessibility. The child also typically becomes eligible for regular Medicaid, which, in itself, is a great support to most families.

In addition to HCBS waivers, many states provide direct cash subsidies that enable parents raising their child with a disability at home to purchase services from an approved menu of options similar to those listed previously through the waiver system.[132] This funding strategy is sometimes called a *voucher program.* These services vary significantly among the states and are very vulnerable to budget cuts. Annual distributions in 2000 ranged from $350 to $8500 per family. By 2002, 20 states had designed cash subsidy or voucher programs. Of all current mechanisms, this one provides the parents with the most flexibility and control. In the voucher program, parents themselves recruit, train, and enter into a formal contract with an individual (sometimes an extended family member) or a provider organization. Often, states have opted to provide families with a combination of funding strategies, including both waiver options and cash subsides. One funding stream may predominate over the other, depending on current state policy. For example, the state that provided the lowest annual cash subsidy to families also provided the highest annual waiver funding ($13,600 per family).[132]

The goal of these various programs is to provide adequate support services so that families do not feel the need for an out-of-home placement for their affected child or adult. A few states have adopted a unique "support family system" similar to shared custody arrangements between divorced couples. The birth family recruits a "support family" from extended family members or from the community, often with the assistance of a state-designated agency.[80] The two families plan, in advance, for weekends and other times in which each will care for the child. This gives the birth family scheduled times of extended respite. In this way, costly institutionalization is prevented,

and the child enjoys the benefits of growing up in a stable and nurturing family environment.

Because each state's services and access mechanisms are organized differently, clinicians and families must learn their own state's idiosyncrasies in order to efficiently access necessary supports. To do this, they can contact the state or county offices of the Departments of Health and Human Services, Mental Health, and Mental Retardation or their state's developmental disabilities organization. In addition, local parent advocacy organizations, The Arc of the United States, early intervention administrators, and/ or school district special education coordinators are often knowledgeable about various programs and their eligibility requirements.

Youth- and Adult-Centered Supports

During the school years, youth with mental retardation receive most of their public supports from the educational system through development and implementation of an IFSP, an IEP, or an ITP, depending on the age of the child. In addition to the public support that schools supply, there are a number of national and community-based organizations that support children and adults with mental retardation (see Appendix). Examples include organizations such as the Young Men's Christian Association (YMCA) that sponsor recreational and social activities, religious youth groups that provide opportunities to develop spirituality and new friendships, scouting programs that promote civic awareness, and camps that provide outdoor opportunities.[138] Other organizations promote the development of special talents and interests such as painting, acting, singing, dancing, and athletics. Some may sponsor regional, state, and national competitions and even provide opportunities for professional performances. There are also Internet peer group organizations that link teenagers with mental retardation with one another. These opportunities promote independence, self-esteem, and social and leadership skills Other supports might be considered "too simple" and of no real consequence. However, such simple solutions as Velcro fasteners, which facilitate independence in dressing and toileting, and books in which pictures instead of words provide opportunities to garden and cook for those who cannot read do make a difference.[139]

When young adults with mental retardation graduate, they lose many of the public supports previously developed for them. However, the support paradigm described by the AAIDD has made a significant difference in their management after graduation.[5,9,84] Ideally, support needs should still be determined by a multidisciplinary team and implemented as an ISP or, in some cases, an IHP. Needs should be evaluated in several areas: vocational training, home living, community living, employment, health, safety, behavior, social skills, and protection/self-advocacy. Providing necessary supports to adults is now recognized as a way to improve the functional capabilities and to enhance the social well-being of persons with mental retardation. Supports should serve to enhance independence, personal well-being, relationships, and participation in community activities. Supports may include tangible items, home modifications, accessible transportation, job coaching, attendant care, and/or crisis training. Available in all types and varieties, effective supports reduce the mismatch between environmental demands and a person's capabilities.[9,140]

Some younger teenagers with severe mental retardation may already receive SSI and Medicaid benefits because of low family income. Other adolescents with mental retardation are not eligible for these benefits until they turn 18 years old, when financial eligibility depends solely on their income rather than the incomes of their parents. Many adults with mild mental retardation have competitive jobs and are self-sufficient; they meet neither the financial nor the functional limitations of SSI criteria for eligibility.

Adults with severe mental retardation who require persistent supervision may also qualify for a HCBS waiver. Instead of funding respite services for the family, these waivers can now provide living supports for the adult child in a group home. HCBS waiver programs can also be used to pay a job coach or a houseparent to supervise the group home clients and to assist with shopping, transportation, financial matters, and medication administration. Because of these supports, adults with more severe levels of mental retardation can now live in community settings instead of large state institutions.

Unfortunately, these critical public supports may be lost if the adult with mental retardation receives a monetary gift from a well-meaning relative or an inheritance from his or her parents that causes him or her to no longer meet their specific financial criterion. However, continued access to public supports can be protected with the implementation of a "Special Needs Will and Trust."[141,142] A critical aspect of that document is a statement indicating that the inheritance is to be used only for items and services not covered by Medicaid, SSI, or other federal subsidies. Failure to include this statement will result in the loss of benefits until the amount equivalent to the value of the gift or inheritance is spent. In cases in which such statements are not in place, the individual may be required to repay the government for previously provided services. Siblings' shares of the inheritance may also be at risk. Various nonprofit advocacy organizations and large life insurance companies employ benefit advisers who are available to inform and guide parents in the preparation of this legal document (see Appendix).

PUTTING A SUPPORT PLAN IN PLACE

As noted in the "Clinical Diagnosis" section, supports may be necessary over an individual's lifespan in five dimensions: intellectual abilities, adaptive behavior, health, environmental context and participation, and interactions and social roles. Supports must be flexible and tailored to an individual's intellectual, physical, emotional, and functional needs. Identified supports are needed at varying levels of intensity: limited, intermittent, extensive, or pervasive.[5,9] They should also take into account the individual's cultural, ethnic, linguistic, and economic characteristics.[5] Preferences and progress must be monitored and revised when necessary.

For example, an older teenager with Down syndrome has recently graduated, has moved out of his parent's home, and has been placed in a supported employment program at a local fast food restaurant. He may benefit from an ISP similar to the one described in Table 11-6. The success of this ISP depends

		Methods			
Dimension	**Task**	**Support**	**Activities**	**Time Span**	**Intensity**
Intellectual abilities	Learn money concepts	Trainer/teacher	Balance checkbook	Ongoing	Limited
Adaptive behavior	Learn to make breakfast	Houseparent	Prepare food Clean up	Time limited	Limited
Health (physical, mental, etiological)	Treat depression	Counseling, medication prompts	Clinic visits, daily medication	Ongoing	Extensive
Environmental context	Live in a group home	Houseparent	Homemaking skills	Ongoing	Limited
Social (roles, interactions, participation)	Develop interpersonal relationships	Peer befriending	Social outings	Ongoing	Intermittent

TABLE 11-6 ■ Developing a Support Plan

on an array of natural, community, and public supports. Natural supports might include the assistance of family, friends, a religious organization, housemates, and peer staff at the restaurant. Community supports might include social activities sponsored by the church youth group, the Arc of the United States, or the local YMCA chapter. The success of the entire system, however, depends strongly on public supports, particularly funding resources, including SSI stipends, Food Stamps, housing subsidies, Medicaid health benefits, and HCBS waiver programs.

Sibling Supports

As with parents, the discovery that a child has mental retardation has a profound effect on siblings. The news can have both positive and negative effects.[143] Some evidence suggests that in comparison with families without a child with mental retardation, siblings of children with mental retardation may be more sensitive, helping, emotionally supportive, and accepting of people with differences.[144-146] Some have become very effective advocates for disability issues, rising even to national recognition. However, there are also some negative effects. Siblings may feel that they need to compete for their parent's attention, especially when the child with mental retardation also has significant medical or psychiatric comorbid conditions. The feelings associated with this competition are strongly associated with the parents' awareness of their actions and the sibling's cognitive understanding of the disability. Some siblings may perceive increased parental expectations and struggle to be a high achiever to compensate for the child with mental retardation. Unless the parents have adequately explained mental retardation, siblings may harbor misconceptions and fears that they will "catch" the disability as if it was an infectious process. Relationships among siblings with and without disabilities are going to be different; that does not mean that those relationships are inferior or require intervention.[147] An older or a younger sibling (if she or he has surpassed the child with mental retardation) may be expected to act as a surrogate parent and experience an accelerated passage to adulthood at the expense of beneficial childhood experiences. Such siblings often assume roles of managers and teachers of the sibling with a disability.[148] Finally, siblings, even at a young age, may harbor concerns that they are expected to care for the child with mental retardation after the parents die. Thus, pediatricians should express genuine concern about the siblings themselves and practice vigilance for their well-being. In addition, there are national organizations (Sib Shops) and electronic Web sites created just for siblings (see Appendix).

ADULT OUTCOME

Substantial variability exists in developmental/intelligence test scores from early childhood until about ages 6 to 9 years. If serial testing at that point demonstrates a consistent developmental velocity, the test's predictive value is enhanced. Although measured intelligence is very important in determining adult outcome, other factors may significantly affect functioning and foster drastically different results.[6,149] These factors include coexisting medical and sensory disorders and, more important, behavioral and psychiatric disorders. Environmental factors (degree of inclusion in integrated settings during childhood) are also important, as are parents' parenting style (i.e., the provision of opportunity, fostering of well-being, and promotion of stability). With increasing age, social and adaptive skills assume a greater importance than do intellectual skills in determining independence and the ability to successfully function in the community.[150] Despite the interaction of all of these confounding variables, some very general statements can be made regarding the degree of mental retardation and levels of functioning as an adult (Table 11-7).

It can also be very helpful to graphically correlate chronological age, mental age, and academic grade level when the "natural history" of mental retardation is explained to a family (Fig. 11-1). This graph effectively depicts the widening of the gap between individuals with mental retardation and typically developing peers over time. This may be helpful in reassuring families that their child's condition is not "getting worse." It may also be of value in demonstrating why a child with mild mental retardation (the majority of cases) may not be identified until at or near school entry, when the gap reaches a significant level of difference. Finally, it can be a source of encouragement to families as they try to predict what their child is and is not able to do.

FUTURE RESEARCH

Because mental retardation is believed to be the result of the interaction of a number of factors that significantly affect an individual across the lifespan, future research efforts must address issues of etiology, treatment of the primary condition, and the effect of associated comorbid conditions. Genetic discoveries have helped explain the biological reason for several conditions associated with mental retardation, such as fragile X and Rett syndromes. There are ongoing efforts to better understand the interaction between some of these genetic mechanisms and the environ-

TABLE 11-7 ■ Adult Outcomes of Individuals with Different Levels of Mental Retardation

Level of Mental Retardation	Learning Rate (% of Normal)	Adult Reading Level	Typical High School Program	Adult Living Situation	Social Relationships	Work Setting	Other
Mild	50%-66%	3rd-6th grades	Vocational-technical	Independent living	Often marry and parent children	Competitive job ± work habits	Independence and self-support should be the goal
Moderate	33%-50%	1st-3rd grades	Vocational Can be taught life skills	Community living in group home	Occasionally marry and parent children	Supported or sheltered employment	Comorbid conditions affect opportunities and outcomes
Severe	25%-33%	Survival sight reading ("stop," "exit")	Some assistance in completing life skills	Community living in group home, if no behavioral problems	Do not marry or parent children	Sheltered employment if no other comorbid conditions	May have coexisting medical conditions
Profound	<25%	No reading skills	Pervasive assistance in life skills Custodial care in high school	Placement depends on other medical and behavioral needs	Do not marry or parent children	None	Often have coexisting medical conditions, may have self-injurious behaviors

ment. Will there one day be a role for prenatal gene therapy for conditions responsible for some forms of mental retardation? What other discoveries may be possible with newer imaging techniques such as positron emission tomography and diffusion tensor imaging? There must also be a research focus to consider this disabling condition from its effect on different societal systems: family, health care, work. As the trend away from institutional care continues, what interventions and supports are most effective in maximizing the benefits of home or community based care and living? It is well documented that individuals with mental retardation have poorer access to routine health and preventative care. Methods to ensure appropriate access to care and the inclusion of individuals with mental retardation in health promotion efforts, although already a goal of Health People 2010, must be developed and implemented. Very often the associated comorbid conditions, especially behavior, are what severely limit the ability of an individual with mental retardation to be fully included in society. How can a natural system of supports for inclusion be implemented? For research in mental retardation to be most effective, it must move outside of the laboratory and beyond simply asking the question "Why did this happen?"

CONCLUSIONS

Making a timely diagnosis of mental retardation may depend on a high index of suspicion, especially in a child who looks normal and initially demonstrates only language delays. Diagnosis is a two-part process that includes the clinical diagnosis of mental retardation that is based on *DSM-IV-TR* and/or AAMR criteria and a systematic search for a medical cause. The diagnostic process can be facilitated by the developmental-behavioral pediatrician, ideally as part of a multidisciplinary team approach. Management begins with genetic counseling (when a cause is known), parent education, and a prompt referral to an infant intervention program or, for older children, to the public education system. Children with mental retardation should be cared for in the context of a medical home and receive ongoing quality physical, behavioral, dental, and mental health surveillance and treatment. The primary care provider should also promote fitness and discourage inactivity and obesity. It is important to consider the well-being of all family members and help them identify and access appropriate community and public supports when necessary, with the realization that those needs change over time. Regardless of the degree of mental retardation, parents should be encouraged to promote independence to the maximum extent possible throughout all stages of their child's development. If it is financially

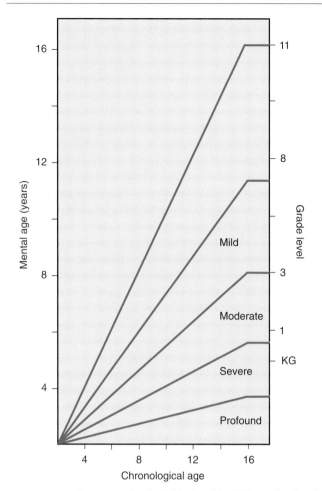

FIGURE 11-1 Outcomes for individuals with different levels of mental retardation. KG, kindergarten. (From Accardo PM, Capute AJ: Mental retardation. *In* Capute AJ, Accardo PM, eds: Developmental Disabilities in Infancy and Childhood. Baltimore: Paul Brookes, 1996, p 211.)

feasible, parents should initiate long-term planning in the form of a Special Needs Will and Trust early in the child's life. Developmental-behavioral pediatricians can play important roles as consultants and facilitators of integrated and coordinated care, especially when comorbid conditions or challenging behaviors appear. The developmental-behavioral pediatrician can also provide appropriate anticipatory guidance to prevent secondary disabilities and assist in transitioning the adolescent into adult systems of care that may include education and training of the health providers.

REFERENCES

1. Centers for Disease Control and Prevention: Economic costs associated with mental retardation, cerebral palsy, hearing loss and vision impairment—United States, 2003. MMWR Morb Mortal Wkly Rep 53(3):57-59, 2004.

2. Snyder TD, Hoffman CM: Digest of Educational Statistics and Figures (NCES 2003-060). Washington, DC: National Center for Education Statistics, 2002.

3. Finley WML, Lyons E: Rejecting the label: A social constructionist analysis. Ment Retard 43:120-134, 2005.

4. Panek PE, Smith JL: Assessment of terms to describe mental retardation. Res Dev Disabil 26:565-576, 2005.

5. American Association on Mental Retardation: Definition, theoretical model, framework for assessment, and operational Definitions. *In* Luckasson RA, Schalock RL, Spitalnik DM, et al eds: Mental Retardation: Definition, Classification, and Systems of Support, 10th ed. Washington, DC: American Association on Mental Retardation, 2002, pp 5-17.

6. American Psychiatric Association: Diagnostic and Statistical Manual of Mental Disorders, 4th ed, Text Revision. Washington, DC: American Psychiatric Association, 2000, pp 38-49.

7. Sparrow SS, Davis SM: Recent advances in the assessment of intelligence and cognition. J Child Psychol Psychiatry 41:117-131, 2000.

8. Leonard H, Wen X: The epidemiology of mental retardation: Challenges and opportunities in the new millennium. Ment Retard Dev Disabil Res Rev 8:117-134, 2002.

9. Thompson JR, Bryant BR, Campbell EM: Support Intensity Scale. Washington, DC: American Association on Mental Retardation, 2004.

10. Harries J, Guscia R, Kirby N, et al: Support needs and adaptive behaviors. Am J Ment Retard 110:393-404, 2005.

11. U.S. Public Health Service: Closing the Gap: A National Blueprint to Improve the Health of Persons with Mental Retardation: Report of the Surgeon General's Conference on Health Disparities and Mental Retardation. Washington, DC: U.S. Department of Health and Human Services, Office of the Surgeon General, 2002.

12. Larson SA, Larkin KC, Anderson L, et al: Prevalence of mental retardation and developmental disabilities: Estimates from the 1994/1995 national health interview survey disability supplements. Am J Ment Retard 106:231-252, 2001.

13. Bhasin TK, Brocksen S, Avchen RN, et al: Prevalence of four developmental disabilities children aged 8 years—Metropolitan Atlanta Developmental Disabilities Surveillance Program, 1996 and 2000. MMWR Surveill Summ 55(1):1-9, 2006 [erratum in MMWR Morb Mortal Wkly Rep 55(4):105-106, 2006].

14. Flint J: The genetic basis of cognition. Brain 122:2015-2031, 1999.

15. Plomin R: Genetics, genes, genomics and G. Mol Psychiatry 8:1-5, 2003.

16. Jellife LL, Shaw GM, Nelson V, et al: Risk of mental retardation among children born with birth defects. Arch Pediatr Adolesc Med 157:545-550, 2003.

17. Sameroff AJ, Seifer R, Baldwin A, et al: Stability of intelligence from preschool to adolescence: The influ-

ence of social and family risk factors. Child Dev 64: 80-97, 1993.

18. Gutman LM, Sameroff AJ, Cole R: Academic growth curve trajectories from 1st grade to 12th grade: Effects of multiple social risk factors and preschool child factors. Dev Psychol 39:777-790, 2003.

19. Chapman DA, Scott KG, Mason CA: Early risk factors for mental retardation: Role of maternal age and maternal education. Am J Ment Retard 107:46-59, 2002.

20. Jelliffe-Pawloski LL, Shaw GM, Nelson V, et al: Risks for severe mental retardation occurring in isolation and with other developmental disabilities. Am J Med Genet A 136:152-157, 2005.

21. van Karnebeek CDM, Jansweijer MCE, Leenders AGE, et al: Diagnostic investigation in individuals with mental retardation: A systematic literature review of their usefulness. Eur J Hum Genet 13:6-25, 2005.

22. van Karnebeek CDM, Scheper FY, Abeling NG, et al: Etiology of mental retardation in children referred to a tertiary care center: A prospective study. Am J Ment Retard 110:253-267, 2005.

23. Moog U: The outcome of diagnostic studies on the etiology of mental retardation: Consideration on the classification of the causes. Am J Med Genet A 137:228-231, 2005.

24. Lenhard W, Breitenbach E, Ebert H, et al: Psychological benefit of diagnostic certainty for mothers of children with disabilities: Lessons from Down syndrome. Am J Med Genet A 133:170-175, 2005.

25. O'Leary CM: Fetal alcohol syndrome: Diagnosis, epidemiology and developmental outcomes. J Pediatr Child Health 40:2-7, 2002.

26. Bennetto L, Pennington B: Neuropsychology. *In* Hagerman RJ, Hagerman PJ, eds: Fragile X Syndrome: Diagnosis, Treatment and Research. Baltimore: Johns Hopkins University Press, 2002, pp 206-248.

27. Pennington BF, Moon J, Edgin J, et al: The neuropsychology of Down syndrome: Evidence for hippocampal dysfunction. Child Dev 74:75-93, 2003.

28. Committee to Study Fetal Alcohol Syndrome, Institute of Medicine: Diagnosis and clinical evaluation of fetal alcohol syndrome. *In* Stratton K, Howe C, Battaglia F, eds: Fetal Alcohol Syndrome: Diagnosis, Epidemiology, Prevention and Treatment. Washington, DC: National Academies Press, 1996, pp 63-81.

29. Sokol RJ, Delaney-Black V, Nordstrom B: Fetal alcohol spectrum disorder. JAMA 290:2996-2999, 2003.

30. Hoyme HE, May PA, Kolberg WO, et al: A practical clinical approach to diagnosis of fetal alcohol spectrum disorder: Clarification of the 1996 Institute of Medicine criteria. Pediatrics 115:39-47, 2005.

31. Astley SJ, Clarren SK: Diagnosing the full spectrum of fetal alcohol exposed individuals: Introducing the 4-digit diagnostic code. Alcohol Alcohol 35:400-410, 2000.

32. Streissguth AP, Bookstein HM, Barr HM, et al: Risk factors for adverse life outcomes in fetal alcohol syndrome and fetal alcohol effects. J Dev Behav Pediatr 25:228-238, 2004.

33. Crnic LS, Hagerman R: Fragile X syndrome: Frontiers of understanding gene-brain-behavior relationships. Ment Retard Dev Disabil Res Rev 10:1-2, 2004.

34. Terracciano A, Chiurazzi P, Neri G, et al: Fragile X syndrome. Am J Med Genet C Semin Med Genet 137: 32-37, 2005.

35. Cornish K, Sudhalter V, Turk J, et al: Attention and language in fragile X. Ment Retard Dev Disabil Res Rev 10:11-16, 2004.

36. Cohen D, Pichard N, Tordjman S, et al: Specific genetic disorders and autism: Clinical contributions toward their identification. J Autism Dev Disord 35:103-116, 2005.

37. Loesch DZ, Huggins RM, Hagerman RJ, et al: Phenotypic variation and FMRP levels in fragile X. Ment Retard Dev Disabil Res Rev 10:31-41, 2004.

38. Bailey DB, Skinner D, Sparkman KL, et al: Discovering fragile X: Family experiences and perceptions. Pediatrics 111:407-416, 2003.

39. Roizen NJ: Down syndrome: Progress in research. Ment Retard Dev Disabil Res Rev 7:38-44, 2001.

40. Chapman RS, Hesketh LJ: Behavioral phenotype of individuals with Down syndrome. Ment Retard Dev Disabil Res Rev 6:84-95, 2000.

41. Chapman RS, Seung H-K, Schwartz SE, et al: Language skills of children and adolescents with Down syndrome: II. Production deficits. J Speech Lang Hear Res 41:861-873, 1998.

42. Nadel L: Down syndrome: A genetic disorder in biobehavioral perspective. Genes Brain Behav 2:156-166, 2003.

43. Brown FR, Greer MK, Aylward EH, et al: Intellectual and adaptive functioning in individuals with Down syndrome in relation to age and environmental placement. Pediatrics 85:450-452, 1990.

44. Turner S, Alborz A: Academic attainment of children with Down syndrome: A longitudinal study. Br J Educ Psychol 73:563-582, 2003.

45. Rasmussen P, Borheson O, Wentz E, et al: Autistic disorders in Down syndrome: Background factors and clinical correlates. Dev Med Child Neurol 43:750-754, 2001.

46. Roizen NJ, Patterson D: Down syndrome. Lancet 361:1281-1289, 2003.

47. Hagberg PSG: Aetiology in severe and mild mental retardation: A population based study of Norwegian children. Dev Med Child Neurol 42:76-86, 2000.

48. Xu J, Chen Z: Advances in molecular cytogenetics for the evaluation of mental retardation. Am J Med Genet C Semin Med Genet 117:15-24, 2003.

49. Winnepenninckx B, Rooms L, Kooy R, et al: Mental retardation: A review of the genetic causes. Br J Dev Disabil 49:29-44, 2003.

50. Curry CJ, Stevenson RE, Aughton D, et al: Evaluation of mental retardation: Recommendations of a consensus conference: American College of Medical Genetics. Am J Med Genet 72:468-477, 1997.

51. Shevell M, Ashwal S, Donley D, et al: Practice parameter: Evaluation of the child with global developmental delay: Report of the Quality Standards Subcommittee of the American Academy of Neurology and the Prac-

tice Committee of the Child Neurology Society. Neurology 60:367-380, 2003.

52. Murphy CC, Boyle C, Schendel D, et al: Epidemiology of mental retardation in children. Ment Retard Dev Disabil Res Rev 4:6-13, 1998.

53. Drews CD, Murphy CC, Yeargin-Allsopp M, et al: The relationship between idiopathic mental retardation and maternal smoking during pregnancy. Pediatrics 97:547-553, 1996.

54. Sampson PD, Streissguth AP, Bookstein FL, et al: Incidence of fetal alcohol syndrome and prevalence of alcohol-related neurodevelopmental disorders. Teratology 56:317-326, 1997.

55. Council on Children with Disabilities; Section on Developmental Behavioral Pediatrics; Bright Futures Steering Committee; Medical Home Initiatives for Children with Special Needs Project Advisory Committee: Identifying infants and young children with developmental disorders in the medical home: An algorithm for developmental surveillance and screening. Pediatrics 118:405-420, 2006 [erratum in Pediatrics 118:1808-1809, 2006].

56. de Bildt A, Sytoma S, Kraijer D, et al: Prevalence of pervasive developmental disorders in children and adolescents with mental retardation. J Child Psychol Psychiatry 46:275-286, 2005.

57. Poehlmann J, Clements M, Abbeduto L, et al: Family experiences associated with a child's diagnosis of fragile X or Down syndrome: Evidence for disruption and resilience. Ment Retard 43:255-267, 2005.

58. Shevell M, Majnemer A, Platt R, et al: Developmental and functional outcomes in children with global developmental delay or developmental language impairment. Dev Med Child Neurol 47:678-683, 2005.

59. Coplan J: Three pitfalls in the early diagnosis of mental retardation. Clin Pediatr 21:308-310, 1982.

60. Saye KB: Preschool intellectual assessment *In* Reynolds CR, Kamphaus RW, eds: Handbook of Psychological and Educational Assessment of Children: Intelligence, Aptitude and Achievement, 2nd ed. New York: Guilford, 2003, pp 187-203.

61. Lichtenberger EO: General measures of cognition for the preschool child. Ment Retard Dev Disabil Res Rev 11:197-208, 2005.

62. Bayley N: Bayley Scales of Infant and Toddler Development, 3rd ed. San Antonio, TX: Harcourt Assessments, 2005.

63. Roid G: Stanford-Binet Intelligence Scale, 5th ed. Toronto: Thomas Nelson Corp., 2003.

64. Kaufman A, Kaufman D: Kaufman Assessment Battery for Children, 2nd ed. Shoreview, MN: AGS, 2003.

65. Wechsler D: Wechsler Preschool and Primary Scale of Intelligence III. San Antonio, TX: Harcourt Assessment, 2002.

66. Wechsler Intelligence Scale for Children, 4th ed. San Antonio, TX: Harcourt Assessment, 2003.

67. Sparrow SS, Cicchetti DV, Balla DA, et al: Vineland Adaptive Behavior Scales, 2nd ed. Shoreview, MN: AGS, 2005.

68. Harrison P, Oakland T: Adaptive Behavior Assessment System—II. San Antonio, TX: Harcourt Assessment, 2003.

69. Bruininks RH, Woodcock RW, Weatherman RF, et al: Scales of independent behavior revised (SIB-R). Toronto: Thomas Nelson Corp., 1996.

70. Battaglia A, Carey JC: Diagnostic evaluation of developmental delay/mental retardation: An overview. Am J Med Genet C Semin Med Genet 117:3-14, 2003.

70a. Moeschler JB, Shevell M, AAP Committee on Genetics: Clinical Genetic Evaluation of the Child with Mental Retardation or Developmental Delays. Pediatrics 117:2304-2316, 2006.

71. Roberts G, Palfrey J, Bridgemohan C: A rational approach to the medical evaluation of a child with developmental delay. Contemp Pediatr 21:76-100, 2004.

72. van Karnebeek CD, Scheper FY, Abeling NG, et al: Etiology of mental retardation in children referred to a tertiary care center: A prospective study. Am J Ment Retard 110:253-267, 2005.

73. Baker E, Hinton L, Callen DF, et al: Study of 250 children with idiopathic mental retardation reveals nine cryptic and diverse subtelomeric chromosome anomalies. Am J Med Genet 107:285-293, 2002.

74. Battaglia A: Neuroimaging studies in the evaluation of developmental delay/mental retardation. Am J Med Genet C Semin Med Genet 117:25-30, 2003.

75. Williams HJ: Imaging the child with developmental delay. Imaging 16:174-185, 2004.

76. Papavasiliou AS, Bazigou H, Paraskevoulakas E, et al: Neurometabolic testing in developmental delay. J Child Neurol 15:620-622, 2000.

77. Rinaldo P, Tortorelli S, Matern D, et al: Recent developments and new applications of tandem mass spectrometry in newborn screening. Curr Opin Pediatr 16:427-433, 2004.

78. Newborn Screening: Toward a Uniform Screening Panel and System. (Available at: *ftp.hrsa.gov/mchb/genetics/screeningdraftforcomment.pdf;* accessed 11/22/06.)

79. Rahi JS, Manaras I, Tuomainen H, et al: Meeting the needs of parents around the time of diagnosis of disability among their children: Evaluation of a novel program for information, support, and liaison by key workers. Pediatrics 114:e477-e482, 2004.

80. Rosenau N: Family-Based Alternatives. Austin, TX: Every Child, 2005.

81. Braddock D, Hemp R, Rizzolo MC: State of the states in developmental disabilities. Ment Retard 42:356-370, 2004.

82. U.S. Department of Health and Human Services: Healthy People 2010, 2nd ed. With Understanding and Improving Health and Objectives for Improving Health. Washington, DC: U.S. Government Printing Office, 2000.

83. Johnson CP, Kastner TA: Helping families raise children with special health care needs at home. Pediatrics 115:507-511, 2005.

84. American Association on Mental Retardation: *In* Luckasson R, Coulter DL, Polloway EA, et al eds:

Mental Retardation: Definition, Classification and Systems of Supports, 9th ed. Washington, DC, American Association on Mental Retardation, 1992.

85. Denning CB, Chamberlain JA, Polloway EA: An evaluation of state guidelines for mental retardation: Focus on definition and classification practices. Educ Train Ment Retard Dev Disabil 35:226-232, 2000.

86. American Academy of Pediatrics, Task Force on the Medical Home: The medical home. Pediatrics 113(Suppl):1471-1458, 2002.

87. Strickland B, McPherson M, Weissman G, et al: Access to the medical home: Results of the National Survey of Children with Special Health Care Needs. Pediatrics 113:1485-1492, 2004.

88. Blum WB, ed: Improving transition for adolescents with special health care needs from pediatric to adult-centered health care. Pediatrics 110(Suppl):1301-1335, 2002.

89. Pitetti KH, Campbell KD: Mentally retarded individuals: A population at risk? Med Sci Sports Exerc 23:586-593, 1991.

90. Rimmer J: Aging, mental retardation and physical fitness. Arc Newsletter pp 1-7, November 1997. Available at *http://www.thearc.org/faqs/fitnessage.html*.

91. Horwitz SM, Kerker BD, Owens PL, et al: The Health Status and Needs of Individuals with Mental Retardation. Washington, DC: Special Olympics, 2000. Available at *http://www.specialolympics.org/Special+Olympics+ Public+Website/English/Initiatives/Research/Health_ Research/Health+Status+and+ Needs.htm*.

92. Fenton SJ, Perlman S, Turner H, eds: Oral Health Care for People with Special Needs: Guidelines for Comprehensive Care. River Edge, NJ: Exceptional Parent, Psy-Ed Corp., 2003.

93. World Health Organization: International Classification of Impairments, Disabilities, and Handicaps. A Manual of Classification Relating to the Consequences of Disease (ICIDH). Geneva, Switzerland: World Health Organization, 1980.

94. World Health Organization: International Classification of Functioning and Disability (ICIDH-2). Geneva, Switzerland: World Health Organization, 2000.

95. World Health Organization: International Classification of Functioning, Disability and Health (ICF). Geneva, Switzerland: World Health Organization, 2001.

96. World Health Organization: ICD-10: International Statistical Classification of Disease and Related Health Problems. Geneva, Switzerland: World Health Organization, 1992.

97. Aman MG: Review and evaluation of instruments for assessing emotional and behavioural disorders. Aust N Z J Dev Disabil 17:127-145, 1991.

98. Rush AJ, Frances A: Expert consensus guidelines on the treatment of psychiatric and behavioral problems in mental retardation [Special Issue]. Am J Ment Retard 105:159-228, 2000.

99. Findling RL, Aman MG, Eerdenkens M, et al: Long term, open-label study of risperidone in children with severe disruptive behaviors and below-average IQ. Am J Psychiatry 161:677-684, 2004.

100. Ryan R: Recognizing psychosis in nonverbal patients with developmental disabilities. Psychiatr Times 18(12):1-6, 2001.

101. Nir I, Meir D, Zilber N, et al: Brief report: Circadian melatonin, thyroid-stimulating hormone, prolactin and cortisol levels in serum of young adults with autism. J Autism Dev Disord 25:641-654, 1995.

102. Arendt J, Skene DJ: Melatonin as a chronobiotic. Sleep Med Rev 9(1):25-39, 2005.

103. Jan JE: Melatonin treatment of sleep-wake cycle disorders in children and adolescents. Dev Med Child Neurol 41:491-500, 1999.

104. Dodge NN: Melatonin reduces sleep latency. J Child Neurol 16:581-584, 2001.

105. Sheldon SH: Proconvulsant effects of oral melatonin in neurologically disabled children. Lancet 351:1254, 1998.

106. Cavallo A: Melatonin and human puberty: Current perspectives. J Pineal Res 15:115-121, 1993.

107. Gillberg C: Practitioner review: Physical investigations in mental retardation. J Child Psychol Psychiatry 38:889-897, 1997.

108. Dosen A, Day K, eds: Treating Mental Illness and Behavior Disorders in Children and Adults with Mental Retardation. Washington, DC: American Psychiatric Press, 2001.

109. Kent L, Evans J, Paul M, et al: Co-morbidity of autism spectrum disorder in children with Down syndrome. Dev Med Child Neurol 41:153-158, 1999.

110. Starr EM, Berument SK, Tomlins M, et al: Brief report: autism in individuals with Down syndrome. J Autism Dev Disord 35:665-673, 2005.

111. Szymanski L, King BH: Summary of the practice parameters for the assessment and treatment of children, adolescents and adults with mental retardation and comorbid mental disorders. American Academy of Child and Adolescent Psychiatry. J Am Acad Child Adolesc Psychol 38:1606-1610, 1999.

112. Clinical practice guideline: Diagnosis and evaluation of the child with attention-deficit/hyperactivity disorder. American Academy of Pediatrics. Pediatrics 105:1158-1170, 2000.

113. American Academy of Pediatrics, Subcommittee on Attention-Deficit/Hyperactivity Disorder and Committee on Quality Improvement: Clinical Practice Guideline: Treatment of the school-aged child with attention-deficit/hyperactivity disorder. Pediatrics 108:1033-1044, 2001.

114. Miller M, Fee VE, Jones CJ: Psychometric properties of ADHD rating scales among children with mental retardation. Res Dev Disabil 25:477-492, 2004.

115. Miller ML, Fee VE, Netterville AK: Psychometric properties of ADHD rating scales among children with mental retardation 1: Reliability. Res Dev Disabil 25:459-476, 2004.

116. Handen BL, McAuliffe S, Caro-Martinez L: Learning effects of methylphenidate in children with mental retardation. J Dev Phys Disabil 8:335-346, 1996.

117. Warburg M: Visual impairments in adult people with intellectual disability: Literature review. J Intellect Disabil Res 45:424-438, 2001.

118. Beckung E, Steffenberg U, Uvebrant P: Motor and sensory dysfunction in children with mental retardation and epilepsy. Seizure 6(1):43-50, 1997.

119. Murphy NA, Young P: Sexuality in children and adolescents with disabilities. Dev Med Child Neurol 47:640-644, 2005.

120. Murphy NA, Elias ER, AAP Committee/Section on Children with Disabilities: Sexuality of children and adolescents with developmental disabilities. Pediatrics 118:398-403, 2006.

121. Sterilization of minors with developmental disabilities. American Academy of Pediatrics. Committee on Bioethics. Pediatrics 104:337-340, 1999.

122. Diekema DS: Involuntary sterilization of persons with mental retardation: An ethical analysis. Ment Retard Dev Disabil Res Rev 9:21-26, 2003.

123. Blum RW: Sexual health contraceptive need of adolescents with chronic conditions. Arch Pediatr Adolesc Med 151:290-297, 1997.

124. Ramey CT, Bryan DM, Wasik BH, et al: Infant health and development for low birth weight premature infants: Program elements, family participation and child intelligence. Pediatrics 89:454-465, 1992.

125. Bailey DB, Hebbeler K, Scarborough A, et al: First experience with early intervention: A national perspective. Pediatrics 113:887-896, 2004.

126. Reiff MI: Comparison of IDEA 1997 and 2004. AAP Section on Developmental and Behavioral Pediatrics Newsletter (Autumn):15-17, 2005.

126a. Williamson P, McLeskey J, Hoppey D, Rentz T: Educating students with mental retardation in general education classrooms. Exceptional Children 72:347-361, 2006.

127. McPherson M, Weissman G, Strickland BB, et al: Implementing community-based systems of services for children and youths with special health care needs: How well are we doing? Pediatrics 113:1538-1544, 2004.

128. Johnson CP, Blasco PA: Community resources for children with special healthcare needs. Pediatr Ann 26:11-16, 1997.

129. Taanik A, Syrjala L, Kokkonen J, et al: Coping of parents with physically and intellectually disabled children. Child Care Health Dev 28:73-86, 2002.

130. Liptak GS, Revell GM: Community physician's role in case management of children with chronic illness. Pediatrics 84:465-471, 1989.

131. Rosenbaum P, Stewart D: Alternative and complementary therapies for children and youth with disabilities. Infants Young Child 14(1):51-59, 2002.

132. Parish SL, Pomeranz-Essley A, Braddock D: Family support in the United States: Financing trends and emerging initiatives. Ment Retard 41:174-187, 2003.

133. Any Baby Can: The Survey of Health Care Experiences of Family of Children with Special Health Care Needs. Austin, TX: Any Baby Can, 1994.

134. Any Baby Can: The Survey of Health Care Experiences of Family of Children with Special Health Care Needs. Austin, TX: Any Baby Can, 1999.

135. American Academy of Pediatrics, Committee on Children with Disabilities: Why Supplemental Security Income is important for children and adolescents. Pediatrics 95:603-609, 1995.

136. American Academy of Pediatrics, Committee on Children with Disabilities: The continued importance of Supplemental Security Income for children and adolescents with disabilities. Pediatrics 107:790-793, 2001.

137. Agosta J, Melda K: Supporting families who provide care at home for children with disabilities. Except Child 62:271-282, 1995.

138. Johnson CP: Camping options for children with disabilities. Pediatr News Updates 5:8-10, 1997.

139. Orth T: Teaching anyone how to cook for themselves. Except Parent 33(2):30-34, 2003.

140. Schalock RL, Stark JA, Snell ME, et al: The changing conception of mental retardation: Implication for the field. Ment Retard 32:181-193, 1994.

141. Brunetti FL: Estate planning: Getting started. Excep Parent 25(12):41-44, 1995.

142. Brunetti FL: Estate planning: Trusts for children with disabilities. Except Parent 26(12):50-51, 1996.

143. Stoneman Z: Siblings of children with disabilities: Research themes. Ment Retard 43:339-350, 2005.

144. Cleveland D, Miller C: Attitudes and life commitments of older siblings of mentally retarded adults: An exploratory study. Ment Retard 15:38-41, 1977.

145. Hannah ME, Midlarsky E: Helping by siblings of children with mental retardation. Am J Ment Retard 110(2):87-99, 2005.

146. Hannah ME, Midlarsky E: Competence and adjustment of siblings of children with mental retardation. Am J Ment Retard 104(1):22-37, 1999.

147. Stoneman Z: Supporting positive sibling relationships during childhood. Ment Retard Dev Disabil Res Rev 7:134-142, 2001.

148. Neely-Barnes S, Marcenko M: predicting impact of childhood disability on families: Results from the 1995 National Health Interview Survey Disability Supplement. Ment Retard 42:284-293, 2004.

149. Accardo PM, Capute AJ: Mental retardation. In Capute AJ, Accardo PM, eds: Developmental Disabilities in Infancy and Childhood. Baltimore: Paul Brookes, 1996, p 211.

150. O'Brien G: Adult outcome of childhood learning disability. Dev Med Child Neurol 43:634-638, 2001.

Learning Disabilities

MARCIA A. BARNES ■ LYNN S. FUCHS*

Students with learning disabilities constitute the majority of school-age individuals with disabilities; the number of students with learning disabilities increased from 1.2 million in 1979 to 1980 to 2.9 million in 2003 to 2004.[1] Learning disabilities are the most common childhood disabilities and often have lifelong consequences for health and occupational success.[2] The prevalence of learning disabilities varies, depending on how learning disabilities are defined and, in the United States, may range from about 4% to 20%.[3] In the past, much of the emphasis in medical and psychological pediatric practice has been placed on diagnosis and assessment; indeed, the most controversial issue in the field of learning disabilities currently concerns diagnostic and definitional issues, even though prevention and intervention are equally if not more important clinical issues.

This chapter begins with a brief historical overview of learning disabilities, followed by a discussion of current issues in the definitions and diagnosis of learning disability. What is known about the cognitive correlates of the two most common learning disabilities, reading disability and math disability, is presented, along with a selected review of research on the neurobiology of learning disabilities. The next section is devoted to research on prevention and evidence-based intervention/treatment programs for reading disability and math disability. A brief review of long-term outcomes follows. The chapter closes with a discussion of clinical management of learning disabilities with reference to diagnosis and assessment, comorbid conditions, and prevention and interventions. For further reading on these topics, we

suggest peer-reviewed papers and chapters on assessment and identification,[4] prevention and intervention,[5] the genetics of learning disabilities,[6] and comorbid conditions associated with learning disabilities.[7-9]

HISTORICAL OVERVIEW

Learning disabilities were defined in U.S. federal law with the Learning Disabilities Act in 1969 to address the needs of these children who were not previously well served by the education system.[10] The Association for Children with Learning Disabilities, formed by parents and educators and led by the psychologist Samuel Kirk, advocated for recognition of learning disabilities and access to special education services. Lyon and associates[5] proposed that, as with many other advancements in fields of medicine, psychology, education, and public policy, systematic scientific inquiry into learning disabilities followed from the identification of real-world problems experienced by children and from public advocacy on their behalf.

Despite the mobilizing influence on research of the recognition of learning disabilities, the scientific basis of learning disabilities has historical roots in the neurology of acquired language disorders studied in the 1800s. In these studies of aphasia, specific deficits in the comprehension and production of language in the context of otherwise spared cognitive function were noted in adults with acquired brain lesions. These observations proved important with regard to one of the central features of learning disabilities: namely, that learning difficulties could result in selective rather than general cognitive deficits.[11]

In the late 1800s and early 1900s, cases of what today would be called *reading disabilities* were reported by neurologists who observed children and adults with no known brain injuries who could not read

*Supported by grants from the National Institute of Child Health and Human Development, P01 HD46261, Cognitive, Instructional, and Neuroimaging Factors in Math, and from the Canadian Language and Literacy Research Network, Comprehension in English- and French-speaking Children: Core Processes & Predictors.

despite seemingly intact general cognitive abilities.[12] In the 1920s, Samuel Orton, a neurologist, proposed that in children who could not read, development of left hemisphere dominance for language functions was delayed or had failed. He was the first to address the heterogeneity of learning disabilities as disorders that could specifically affect reading, writing, speech, comprehension, or motor skills.[11] In collaboration with the linguist, Anne Gillingham, he devised intervention programs for children with reading difficulties, variants of which are still in use[13] and undergoing evaluation as to their efficacy.[5] Another important influence in the field of learning disabilities arose from studies in which investigators attempted to understand similarities in behavioral disorders such as hyperactivity in children with brain injuries and in children with no brain injury who had learning difficulties and normal intelligence. It was inferred that this latter group had minimal brain dysfunction.[11]

Several notions were common to these early conceptualizations of learning disability: namely, that there is a neurobiological basis for the learning difficulty; that there can be selective deficits rather than global retardation; and that processes that help or interfere with learning could be identified and remedied through interventions. The field of learning disabilities continues to be influenced by these conceptualizations, as discussed in the next section.

DIAGNOSTIC AND DEFINITIONAL ISSUES

Many policymakers and school administrators are concerned about the increasing prevalence of learning disabilities, at least in part because special education is much more costly than general education: $12,000 versus $6500 per student.[14] This is at least one reason why establishing acceptable criteria for learning disability identification has been the most controversial issue in the field of learning disability. At the heart of this controversy is the IQ-achievement discrepancy. Although not required by law, a severe discrepancy between achievement and intellectual ability is most frequently used for identification. It is easy to see how the IQ-achievement discrepancy grew out of the early observations that learning disabilities were deficits in specific skills in an otherwise cognitively intact individual. However, the IQ-achievement discrepancy is fraught with measurement and conceptual problems. After a review of current diagnostic guidelines, we describe these technical difficulties.

U.S. federal regulations governing special education refer to learning disabilities as disorders that can occur in one or more of the following: oral expression, listening comprehension, written expression, basic reading skill, reading comprehension, mathematics calculation, and mathematics reasoning. The federal definition of learning disabilities is notable for its emphasis on exclusionary factors in identification, including the idea of a discrepancy between IQ and achievement that is not caused by a sensory or motor handicap; by mental retardation; by emotional disturbance; or by social, cultural, and economic factors.[15,16] In Canada, education is under provincial, not federal, jurisdiction. However, provincial regulations governing special education are very similar to those in the United States. For example, the Ontario Ministry of Education defines learning disabilities with discrepancy and exclusionary criteria similar to those in the U.S. federal definition.[17]

The *Diagnostic and Statistical Manual of Mental Disorders, 4th Edition (DSM-IV)*,[18] and the International Classification of Diseases, 10th edition,[19] provide criteria for diagnosing specific and general learning disabilities. For example, in the *DSM-IV*, learning disorders are classified into four categories: Reading Disorder, Mathematics Disorder, Disorder of Written Expression, and Learning Disorder Not Otherwise Specified. In the *DSM-IV*, Learning Disorders are also defined in an exclusionary manner. For example, a *reading disorder* refers to a failure to achieve at expected levels for reading accuracy or reading comprehension and would be diagnosed (1) when reading achievement, measured by standardized tests of reading accuracy and/or comprehension, is substantially below what is expected on the basis of the individual's age, intelligence, and appropriate educational experiences; (2) when this failure interferes with academic achievement or activities of daily living that require reading; or, (3) if a sensory impairment is present, the reading deficit is in excess of what is typically expected for that impairment.[20]

Classification systems are fundamental in many areas of science and practice, and as such, scientific evaluation of their validity, reliability, and coverage is required in order for them to be useful.[21] Such scientific evidence was unavailable at the time learning disabilities were categorized, and despite substantial subsequent research on the validity and reliability of learning disability classification, the definition of learning disabilities and their categorization have not changed much in practice. We discuss evidence pertaining to validity and reliability in learning disability classification with regard to (1) the use of the IQ-achievement discrepancy, (2) the heterogeneity of learning disabilities, and (3) exclusionary factors. Comprehensive reviews of this literature were provided by Lyon and associates[11] and by Fletcher and colleagues.[21]

IQ-Achievement Discrepancy

The traditional learning disability diagnosis—low achievement in one or more of the learning disability domains that is significantly discrepant from intelligence—is a classification hypothesis that requires validation. Validation studies, in which groups defined by the discrepancy formula are compared with groups defined according to poor academic achievement without reference to IQ, reveal the following: First, few cognitive or affective characteristics such as memory and phonological awareness differentiate poor readers with discrepancies from those without discrepancies.[22] Second, the degree of discrepancy from IQ is not meaningfully related to the severity of the learning disability.[23] Third, the degree of discrepancy is predictive neither of rate of growth in reading over time nor the reading levels of children with or without IQ-achievement discrepancy over time.[24] Fourth, the degree of discrepancy is not predictive of whether or how well a child will respond to intervention,[25] nor does it inform instruction in important ways.[26] Fifth, differences in heritability estimates for children with and without the discrepancy, although significant, are typically small even in large samples.[27]

In addition to problems with validity, other difficulties in the reliability of the discrepancy hypothesis concern measurement error of the intelligence and achievement tests, unreliability of difference or discrepancy scores, and use of arbitrary cutoff points to partition what is a normal distribution of skills, particularly in the absence of validation studies indicating what those clinical cutoff points should be.[11] If categorization based on IQ-achievement discrepancy is reliable, then the classification of children as having a learning disability by an IQ-achievement discrepancy should be stable over time. However, there is considerable instability in classification with actual or simulated data.[28,29] In sum, evidence for the validity of the discrepancy hypothesis is weak, which raises questions about its use in assessment and identification of learning disabilities and in decision making with regard to special education services. Despite technical difficulties in traditional methods for learning disability identification, few experts disagree that the construct of learning disability is a legitimate one or that learning disabilities can have heterogeneous forms.

Heterogeneity of Learning Disabilities

Several types of learning disabilities are identified in classification systems, these types of learning disabilities frequently co-occur, and learning disabilities are often accompanied by other childhood disorders such as attention disorders and problems in social and emotional domains.[8,30]

How well do the classifications in federal law and the *DSM-IV* capture what is known about heterogeneity of learning disabilities? There is strong evidence for the existence of at least two types of reading disability—one in word reading and one in reading comprehension—and perhaps a third in reading fluency.[21] When reading decoding accuracy and fluency are intact, the deficit in reading comprehension parallels that observed in listening comprehension,[31] which suggests that disabilities in reading comprehension and listening comprehension may be indistinguishable. In a similar way, some evidence substantiates at least two forms of math disability, one in arithmetic calculations and another in word problems,[32] but there is little evidence, at present, of a disability in math reasoning.[11] Evidence of a specific learning disability in written expression in the absence of other learning disabilities is also weak.[21] In most cases, comorbidity (e.g., reading disability with math disability or reading disability with attention-deficit/hyperactivity disorder [ADHD]) is associated with greater impairment in academic domains than when disorders occur independently.[21] In addition, there is some evidence that the nature of math disabilities and their cognitive characteristics differ in some ways, depending on whether there is a comorbid reading disability.[33]

In sum, there is empirical support for some, but not all, of the learning disability classifications in federal law and in the *DSM-IV*. The issue of comorbidity in terms of symptom severity and overlap or differentiation in cognitive correlates is not addressed in current learning disability classification systems.

Exclusionary Criteria

The hypothesis that learning disability reflects "unexpected" low achievement—as opposed to low achievement as a result of emotional disturbance, social or economic disadvantage, cultural factors, or inadequate instruction—was not based on empirical validation of these factors. There is currently no evidence that children who suffer from emotional disorders such as depression or anxiety differ in any important way from children with learning disability without emotional disorders in terms of the causes of the learning disorder or their response to intervention.[21]

Environmental factors influence the developmental precursors important for learning how to read and perform math. Particularly striking are studies showing that children who are socially and economically disadvantaged have vocabularies half the size of those of nondisadvantaged children at school entry[34];

enter kindergarten knowing only one letter of the alphabet[35]; and begin school with less informal number and quantitative knowledge than do their middle-income peers.[36] However, provision of high-quality language and literacy instruction improves academic preparedness in children graduating from Head Start,[37] as do mathematical interventions with disadvantaged preschool-aged children.[38] Interventions based on phonological and alphabetical instruction also yield positive effects for older disadvantaged children.[39] In sum, socially and economically disadvantaged children develop in environments that may provide less than optimal support for the growth of cognitive skills that are important precursors for later academic skill learning, but they respond to high-quality interventions in similar ways as do their nondisadvantaged peers with learning disabilities. In view of these observations, the validity of exclusion on social and economic bases seems unwarranted.

At the time learning disabilities were defined, there was little consensus about what constituted adequate instruction. This knowledge base, at least for reading, is now substantive.[39,40] The definition implies that the child's response to adequate instruction should be assessed before the learning disability label is applied,[21] and yet the adequacy of instruction is often assumed rather than measured.

One promising model for reconceptualizing learning disability is in terms of a failure to respond to validated intervention.[41-43] Responsiveness to intervention (RTI) as an approach to identifying learning disability was first proposed in a 1982 National Research Council report.[44] Three criteria were suggested for judging the validity of a special education classification: (1) whether the quality of the general education program is such that adequate learning might be expected; (2) whether the special education is of sufficient value to improve student outcomes and thereby justify the classification; and (3) whether the assessment process used for identification is accurate and meaningful. When all three criteria are met, a special education classification is deemed valid. RTI links multiple short assessments over time to intervention and has been shown to have stronger validity and reliability than other identification models. Because identification of a learning disability under RTI is based on lack of response to high-quality instruction, intervention is attempted before the learning disability label is applied. This approach is quite different from all other models, in which diagnosis is applied before intervention.[45] However, for classification, there is still a need to be able to identify a child according to some criterion score, and this criterion score needs to be linked directly to functional outcome.[45]

How Should Learning Disabilities Be Identified?

To summarize, several of the original criteria for identification of a learning disability and classification of learning disabilities have proved to be invalid or unreliable, although these research findings are only just beginning to have an influence on assessment and diagnosis. Furthermore, none of the current classification systems takes relations between learning disabilities or between learning disabilities and other developmental disorders into account. Despite the problems with current diagnostic and classification criteria, the reality is that many jurisdictions use discrepancy formulas and exclusionary criteria to determine who has a learning disability, and this has consequences for who receives special education services. Hybrid models that take into account both low achievement and response to instruction may better identify children who truly have "unexpected" low achievement despite exposure to high-quality instruction.[28] As an example, the current means of diagnosing a learning disability is typically based on a single formal assessment point, followed by treatment (the test-and-treat model), whereas the review just presented suggests that a better model would involve the use of high-quality intervention for low academic achievement (identified by teachers and/or parents and assessed by valid and reliable achievement tests), followed by assessment of response to intervention (the treat-and-test model[4]). It is important to note that the 2004 reauthorization of the Individuals with Disabilities Education Act provides the field of learning disabilities with RTI as an option to the IQ-achievement discrepancy for identifying learning disability. The implications of the critique of current assessment and identification systems and of changes to the Individuals with Disabilities Education Act for the practice of the developmental-behavioral pediatrician are addressed in the final section of this chapter.

CORE COGNITIVE CORRELATES AND NEUROBIOLOGICAL FACTORS

Reading Disability

WORD READING: ACCURACY AND FLUENCY

Core Cognitive Characteristics

Most children who receive special education services in the learning disability category are children with reading disabilities, and these disabilities have also received the most research attention in terms of developmental, cognitive, and neurobiological studies and interventions. Two core cognitive skills have been identified as being causally connected both to the ability to acquire word reading skills and to difficulties in learning how to read: phonological awareness and rapid retrieval of names for visual symbols, or rapid naming.

Although reading requires the decoding of print, it is actually the ability to gain awareness of the sound structure of language at the level of the phoneme, which is essential for learning how to read.[46] Unlike letters, which are discrete visual symbols, phonemes in syllables and words sound undifferentiated in normally paced speech. Phonological awareness is measured by tasks that tap the ability of the child to distinguish and manipulate language at the level of the phoneme, such as the abilities to listen to a word and to match sounds in words on the basis of phonemes, to segment words on the basis of phonemes, to blend sounds to form words, and to isolate phonemes in spoken words.[47] Longitudinal studies of the reading acquisition process show that phonological awareness at school entry is a potent and unique predictor of word reading ability well into the middle elementary grades.[48,49]

Phonological measures are also quite accurate for predicting which young children are at risk for reading failure,[50] and there is a wealth of research supporting the idea that deficits in phonological processing are at the core of word reading disabilities.[51] Researchers who have attempted to identify reading disability subtypes have shown that almost all subtypes identified are characterized by deficits in phonological awareness.[52] The use of interventions that address phonological awareness and word recognition are most effective for beginning readers considered to be at high risk for reading failure, and the severity of the deficit in phonological awareness is an important predictor of how easy or difficult it is to remediate reading.[53,54]

Longitudinal studies also show that the ability to rapidly access names for series of visual symbols such as numbers, objects, and, in particular, letters at school entry is predictive of word reading independently of phonological awareness, although these skills become less predictive past the early elementary grades.[48,55] There is some evidence that performance on these rapid naming tasks is more strongly related to fluency and reading comprehension than is performance on phonological awareness tasks[56] (see Vukovic & Siegel[57] for an alternative view on rapid visual naming as a unique predictor of reading ability).

Subtyping studies show that some children with reading disability have a specific deficit in rapid naming that is not accompanied by deficits in phonological awareness.[52] Lovett and colleagues[58,59] demonstrated that children who have specific disabilities in reading rate have more circumscribed deficits in reading connected text, in spelling, and in some aspects of reading comprehension in comparison with children who have difficulty in phonological skills and word reading accuracy. Children who have deficits in both phonological awareness and rapid naming are reported to be more severely impaired in terms of their reading than are children with a deficit in only phonological awareness or rapid naming.[59,60]

The research literature on reading is replete with studies that relate reading skill to many other cognitive variables. The weakest of these predictors tends to be sensory and motor skills such as visual-perceptual processes and speech perception.[50] More contemporary studies of sensory processes and reading[61-63] have been criticized on several grounds, including the criteria used to classify children as reading disabled, the insensitivity of these measures for identifying children with reading disabilities or subtypes of reading disability, and the failure of this research to explain how sensory deficits are related to learning how to read or to difficulties in learning how to read.[11,13] It remains to be seen whether newer proposals that combine theories of visual and auditory sensory processes to argue that reading disability reflects a general deficit in neuronal timing[62] have validity.[13]

Between 15% and 40% of children identified as having a reading disability also have ADHD,[64,65] and 25% to 40% of samples with children identified as having ADHD also have reading disability.[66,67] Comorbid reading disability and ADHD leads to greater impairment in both reading-related and attention-related measures.[68] Results of a large-scale study of comorbid conditions[9] suggest that children with reading disability alone and those with ADHD alone can be distinguished by different cognitive characteristics, which is consistent with previous findings.[30] Reading disability is strongly linked to deficits in phonological awareness, whereas ADHD is not.[30] However, children with reading disability only, those with ADHD only, and those with reading disability and ADHD had a common deficit in slow and variable processing speed.[9] It remains to be seen whether this common cognitive deficit is replicated in other samples, whether it is related to shared genetic effects, and whether it has consequences for intervention.

Neurobiological Factors
Research on reading disability has revealed that (1) there are subtle differences in several brain structures between individuals with reading disability and those without reading disability; (2) the brains of individuals with reading disability show different patterns of

brain activation than those of nonaffected individuals during tasks requiring reading; and (3) intensive evidence-based reading intervention "normalizes" these patterns of activation in the brains of children with reading disability or in those at risk for reading disability. Also, genetic studies have revealed that there is a susceptibility to inherit varying levels of word reading ability. These findings are reviewed as follows.

Structural imaging studies of differences in brain structure in individuals with and without reading disability have produced mixed results. Despite difficulties associated with structural magnetic resonance imaging (MRI) studies including the use of different imaging methods, methods of analysis, and so forth, the data generally support the notion that there are subtle differences between children with and without reading disability and these differences are most likely to be found in those left hemisphere regions that support language.[11,69]

In contrast to anatomical studies with MRI, functional neuroimaging studies have yielded reliable differences in patterns of activation during phonological and reading tasks in the brains of individuals with and without reading disability that indicate impaired processing and disrupted connectivity mostly in regions of the left hemisphere, including the inferior frontal gyrus, the middle and superior temporal gyrus, and the angular gyrus.[70] In studies of children using magnetic source imaging (MSI), Simos and colleagues[71] demonstrated that children with and without reading disability did not differ in brain activation when *listening* to words but did differ when they read words. In children with no learning disability, occipital areas were activated, followed by ventral visual association cortices in both cerebral hemispheres and then particular areas in the *left* temporoparietal region (angular gyrus, Wernicke's area, and superior temporal gyrus). When children with reading disability read words, the same time course of events was observed, but the temporoparietal areas of the *right* rather than the left hemisphere were activated. Such results suggest that it is not specific areas of brain that are "damaged" in reading disability but rather that the problem resides in the functional connectivity within the left hemisphere.[72]

Perhaps the most interesting findings in the functional imaging literature concern the effects of intervention on these patterns of brain activation. Simos and colleagues[73] provided 80 hours of intensive phonologically based reading instruction to children and youth with significant word reading disabilities. MSI before intervention revealed the same pattern discussed previously for reading pronounceable nonwords. After intervention, word reading improved significantly, and there was increased activation

in left hemisphere circuits for each child, as well as some reduction in right hemisphere activity (Aylward et al[74] obtained similar findings with functional MRI and shorter intervention). Similar "normalization" of brain activation patterns have been found for young children considered at high risk for reading disability who responded to an early intervention program.[75]

Reading problems have long been observed to run in families, and the risk for a reading disability in a child with a reading-disabled parent is eight times that in the general population.[76] Twin, family studies, and linkage studies all suggest that reading skill has a strong heritable component but that environmental influences are also significant.[77] Of importance is that heritability estimates for reading skill are quite high both in individuals with and in those without reading disability[78] and for several components of reading, including phonological and orthographic skills.[79] A review of linkage findings is beyond the scope of this chapter, as is new research on unique and shared genetic effects for reading disability and ADHD, as well as other childhood disorders.[6,80,81]

READING COMPREHENSION

Core Cognitive Characteristics

The cognitive characteristics of reading comprehension have been studied in both typically developing children and in children with difficulties in reading comprehension. However, less is known about the core processes involved in learning how to comprehend what is read than about learning how to read words.[40] It is clear that word reading and comprehension are dissociable in both typical and atypical development,[82,83] although learning disabilities in both word reading and comprehension can be present simultaneously. Disabilities in word reading are easily identified before third grade, but disabilities in reading comprehension are more likely to be identified after third grade.[84] Leach and colleagues[84] showed that after third grade, of children identified with reading disability, about one third had specific word reading disability, one third had problems with both word reading and listening comprehension, and one third had problems with comprehension but not word reading. Some investigators have estimated rates of specific reading comprehension difficulties at between 5% and 10%.[85]

Studies of children with reading comprehension disabilities, but no word reading disability, suggest that phonological skills are not deficient[86] but difficulties with inference making, text integration, metacognitive skills, and verbal working memory are common.[87] In children with learning disabilities in word reading and comprehension, both phonological skills and these comprehension and memory skills may be deficient.[88] In some children, more basic language deficits in both vocabulary knowledge and understanding of syntax limit comprehension of both oral and written language.[89] Some researchers question whether children who read words well but have language comprehension problems actually have specific language impairment rather than reading comprehension disability per se. However, the majority of children with good word reading and poor comprehension do not meet the diagnostic criteria for specific language impairment.[86] Reading comprehension disabilities were reviewed by Lyon and associates[11] and Fletcher and colleagues.[90]

In sum, phonological awareness is causally related to reading acquisition and reading disabilities, and successful reading interventions include phonological instructional components. The evidence for a separate deficit in the rapid verbal retrieval of visual symbols is more controversial, but it may characterize some subtypes of reading disability, particularly one that involves deficits in reading fluency. Evidence for deficits in basic sensory processes specifically related to the acquisition of word reading and to word reading disability is weak. Although reading comprehension difficulties can exist in the absence of word reading disability, they are probably synonymous with difficulties in listening comprehension. There is relatively little information on how comprehension skills develop or fail to develop; such information is needed in order to design valid assessment tools and identify core cognitive characteristics. In accordance with newer models of gene-brain-environment interactions, what is inherited is a *susceptibility* to competency in reading, which can be moderated by the environment (e.g., instruction), the product of which has a distinct neural signature. The neurobiology of disabilities in reading comprehension has received little study.

Math Disability

Math disabilities are as common as reading disabilities, and about half of all children with reading disability also have math disability.[91] However, knowledge about the typical development of math skills, math disability, math interventions, and neurobiological factors related to math disability have not been as well studied as the same aspects of reading. One possibility for this imbalance is that reading disabilities have traditionally been considered to be of more cost to society in terms of both school achievement and general health and employment.[92] However, human resource studies show that mathematical ability is as predictive of occupational success, productivity, and wages as is literacy.[93]

CORE COGNITIVE CHARACTERISTICS

There is more uncertainty about the core cognitive processes related to math disability than about those for reading. This is compounded by the fact that, unlike reading, mathematics is composed of many different domains, including arithmetic, geometry, and algebra, each of which could have different developmental trajectories and cognitive correlates, different neural signatures, and different genetic associations. The most studied domain of mathematics is arithmetic, or computation.

The models and methods applied to the understanding of development of mathematical skills are the same models that are being applied to understand math disability, which reflects the beginning of a theoretical and methodological convergence in the field of math disabilities similar to that experienced earlier in the field of reading disabilities.[33,94] The two most prominent theoretical positions about math disability arise from very different ways of explaining the origins of mathematical abilities.

One position[95,96] arises from the view that, in contrast to reading, which is a relatively recent human achievement, an ability to understand magnitude or quantities and compare numbers is an ability that human and even nonhuman animals are born with. Although there is debate over the interpretation of some of the infant research, very young infants are sensitive to differences in the numerical values of small sets.[97] Five-month-olds also appear sensitive to changes in very small set sizes involving adding and taking away.[98] Preschoolers can judge whether one set or number is bigger or smaller than another set or number.[99] Butterworth[95] suggested that this sensitivity to number is the infant's "starter kit" for later mathematical development and that deficits in these very basic mathematical abilities that are not influenced by environment or schooling underlie math disability. Proponents of this view do not argue that this is the only source of children's difficulty in mathematics. For example, mathematical tasks that require language, such as word problem solving, would be influenced by language skills.

The second view is that mathematical skills in different domains are built from other, more basic or general cognitive systems, such as the language system,[100] the visual-spatial system,[101] and the central executive or attentional and working memory systems. Geary's framework[33,102] is the most comprehensive example of this view. In this framework, the skills that are important for the development of mathematical competence are the same ones proposed to be deficient in the development of math disabilities. According to this view, difficulties in math could arise in the language system, the visual-spatial system, the central executive system that sustains attention and inhibits irrelevant information, or any combination of these general cognitive systems. At present, there is some preliminary evidence for the framework,[102] but there is as yet no coherent body of literature that would allow researchers to fully test the model or that pits this model against another math disability model.

Despite these theoretical differences in the field of math development and math disability, consensus has begun to emerge from studies about the core math skills that are consistently deficient in children with math disability. Regardless of whether there is a comorbid reading disability or an acquired or congenital brain injury in childhood, children with math disability have difficulties in the accuracy and speed with which they can compute answers to single-digit problems.[103-105] This is often referred to as *deficit in math fact retrieval*. Before formal schooling, children learn to solve simple everyday problems through the use of counting strategies, such as adding two things to four things by counting 1, 2, 3, 4 and 5, 6 either on fingers or verbally. Practice with computing typically leads to a more developmentally sophisticated strategy in which the child counts up from the largest number (4, then 5, 6). Eventually, the child comes to associate the problem with the answer in memory such that he or she *knows* that 4 plus 2 is 6 (direct retrieval from memory). Accurate and fluent single-digit arithmetic is thought to be important for freeing cognitive resources during the learning and application of more complex procedures such as carrying and borrowing, and fluency in math fact retrieval is strongly related to accurate performance in multiple-digit arithmetic.[104] In view of the evidence of deficits in math fact retrieval in math disabilities, current research on the early identification of math disability is focusing on the developmental precursors of math fact retrieval.[106]

As noted earlier, the combination of reading disability and math disability results in more severe symptoms in some areas of mathematics than does math disability alone. Young children with both reading disability and math disability make more counting errors when computing answers to single-digit problems than do children with only math disability,[107] and they also have greater deficits in word problem solving.[108,109]

NEUROBIOLOGICAL FACTORS

Risk of math disorders in families with a child who has a math disability appears to be about 10 times that expected in the general population.[110,111] Twin and adoption studies on math disabilities have yielded heritability estimates between 0.20 and 0.90.[76] A large study of 7-year-old twins[112] revealed that monozygotic twin correlations for mathematics performance indicated both substantial genetic influence and moderate environmental influence. The genetic correlations between mathematics and reading were high, which suggests that many of the genes that are predictive of individual differences in one academic domain are also predictive of individual differences in the other. Plomin and Kovas[6] suggested a "generalist genes" theory of learning abilities and disabilities whereby genes that affect learning in an academic skill such as reading are largely, although not completely, the same genes that affect learning in mathematics. This theory is compatible with what is known about the substantial overlap in the two disorders. However, progress in understanding the cognitive phenotype of math ability and disability (e.g., similarities and differences in core cognitive correlates associated with math disability only versus both reading disability and math disability; potentially different types of math disability in different domains of mathematics), is crucial for informing behavioral genetic studies of mathematical skills.

Neuroimaging studies of math and math interventions in children with and without math disability are in the early stages. Different types of mathematical processing exhibit clear dissociations in adults with brain lesions and in functional neuroimaging studies with normal adults.[113] These studies suggest that different neural circuits are involved in different types of mathematical processing. Dehaene and colleagues[113,114] proposed that circuits in the parietal lobe are implicated in mathematical function and dysfunction: a bilateral intraparietal system for core quantitative processing, a region of the left angular gyrus for verbal processing of numbers, and a posterior superior parietal system for mathematical processing such as estimation that may require spatial attention. It is unknown whether the developing brain adheres to these same neural divisions during the acquisition of math skills, whether any or all of these neural circuits are involved in math disabilities, and whether math interventions that target different aspects of mathematical skill affect the operation of those circuits.

PREVENTION AND INTERVENTION

Prevention

As is true for many diseases and disorders, prevention is preferable to intervention or treatment in terms of costs both to individuals and to societies. Advances made in the science of learning disabilities since the 1990s have increasingly made prevention a viable and attractive option because children at high risk for reading disability (and perhaps math disability, too) can be identified in the preschool and very early school years. But are they identified? In addition to the conceptual and methodological limitations of the discrepancy method for identifying learning disabilities, the psychometric or measurement limitations of the tools used to assess discrepancies in intelligence and achievement render IQ-achievement discrepancy formulas unreliable before third grade. The consequence of these measurement limitations is that many affected children are not identified until third grade or later. Lyon and associates[10] labeled this approach to the diagnosis and treatment of learning disabilities the "Wait to Fail" model. Early identification of children at risk for learning disabilities means that prevention can also be initiated earlier to narrow the achievement gap.[5,10,115] Learning disability prevention programs have four main advantages over treatment programs that are instituted later in schooling. First, prevention can substantially reduce, although not eliminate, learning disabilities.[39,116] Second, prevention programs are *more* effective for treating some components of learning disabilities. When evidence-based reading programs are used in kindergarten for at-risk students, many children learn to read both accurately and fluently. In contrast, when intervention programs, even those of high quality, begin in or after third grade, the ability to read words accurately can improve considerably, but fluency continues to lag behind.[116] The third advantage of prevention over intervention programs is that prevention programs are less expensive because they can often be carried out in the general education classroom or in conjunction with general education programming. Fourth, prevention programs reduce the length of

time that individual children struggle academically and emotionally with learning difficulties. The developmental-behavioral pediatrician has a very important role to play in the prevention of learning disabilities; this is discussed in the final section of the chapter.

Conceptual Approaches to Remediating Learning Disabilities

Since the 1990s, six conceptual approaches for treating the academic deficits of students with learning disabilities have garnered attention (Table 12-1). Three of these approaches, however, have netted limited effects for students with learning disabilities. The *neuropsychological* approach, which incorporates concepts from medical and psychoeducational theories, shares some shortcomings with these older models, including inadequate technical features of the assessment procedures[117-119] and poor ecological validity.[118] Moreover, although neuropsychological programs have proliferated since the 1990s, with advances in basic neuroscience, their importance for education has failed to materialize because implementation has not been linked to improved outcomes.[11] The second approach with limited efficacy data focuses on *intraindividual differences in cognitive processes*, which calls for better delineation of the cognitive profiles associated with learning disabilities to inform treatment. The weaknesses of this model are its focus on test scores that describe the performance in isolation from classroom performance, its focus on behaviors that are removed from academic skills, and little empirical evidence to support utility.[11] The third

---

TABLE 12-1 ■ Conceptual Approaches to Remediating Learning Disabilities

Approach	Orientation	Strengths/Limitations for Students with Learning Disabilities
Neuropsychological	Medical Seeks to enhance processes thought to underlie learning disabilities	Inadequate assessment tools Poor ecological validity Poor outcomes
Intraindividual differences in cognitive processes	Cognitive/psychoeducational Seeks to enhance cognitive processes thought to underlie learning disabilities	Inadequate assessment tools Removal from academics Poor outcomes
Constructivism	Encourages child-centered instruction for student discovery of rules/principles	Requires sophisticated teacher Poor outcomes
Cognitive/strategy	Targets processes that are directly linked to academic skills; encourages academically strategic behavior	Strong outcomes
Cognitive-behavioral	Combines the cognitive approach with behavioral principles, with explicit, teacher-directed instruction	Strong outcomes
Task analytic (e.g., direct instruction)	Emphasizes environmental causes of learning failure, with well-specified learning objectives and detailed sequences of instructional steps	Strong outcomes

model, *constructivism*, stresses teacher empowerment, child-centered instruction, integration of listening, student interests and background, disavowal of sub-skills instruction, a view that children are naturally predisposed to learning, and reliance on unstructured activities from which learners construct their own meaning.[120] This approach is demonstrably ineffective for students with learning disabilities.

Each of the three remaining approaches, in contrast, is supported by persuasive research for remedying the academic deficits of students with learning disabilities. *Cognitive* models target information-processing abilities (e.g., memory or metacognition), as well as abilities more directly linked to academic skills (e.g., phonological awareness). Sometimes termed *strategy instruction*, these methods teach students to increase awareness of task demands, to use academic skills in a strategically optimal manner, and to apply strategies toward task completion so that content information can be acquired, manipulated, stored, retrieved, and expressed.[118] When rooted in academic content, these approaches have proved effective.[121-125]

A second and related approach is the *cognitive-behavioral* model. It combines the methods of strategy instruction with behavioral principles. For example, self-regulated strategy development[123,126] was designed to help students master higher-level cognitive processes (e.g., reading comprehension, math problem solving, narrative and expository writing) and strategies underlying effective academic performance; develop reflective, self-regulated use of these processes and strategies; and form positive attitudes about themselves and their academic capabilities. This and related approaches enhance reading, math, and writing performance.[126,127]

The third approach, the *task-analytic* model, emphasizes the influence of environment while deemphasizing underlying causal mechanisms or thought processes. The task-analytic model requires an operational learning objective, along with a detailed description and sequencing of the steps for achieving the objective.[128] The task-analytic model is exemplified by direct instruction,[129] which involves review of prerequisite learning; preview of goals; presentation of new concepts and material in small steps, with student practice after each step; provision of clear, explicit, detailed instructions and explanations; ongoing assessment of student understanding through teacher questioning; and systematic feedback and corrections. Task-analytic methods have been criticized because they control the teaching process in ways that minimize professional discretion; however, the methods have been shown to be effective.[130,131]

The most persuasive evidence for promoting academic learning among students with learning disabilities is currently provided by the task-analytic approach (e.g., direct instruction) and the cognitive or cognitive-behavioral approach (e.g., strategy instruction, like self-regulated strategy development). In a 1999 meta-analysis, for example, Swanson and colleagues[131a] classified studies into four intervention models: direct instruction, strategy instruction, direct instruction combined with strategy instruction, and "other" interventions. Direct instruction produced larger effect sizes than "other" interventions, as did strategy instruction. But combining direct instruction and strategy instruction yielded larger effect sizes in comparison with either method alone, which yielded moderate to large effects. A comprehensive review of programs within the task-analytic and cognitive/cognitive-behavioral approaches is not possible in this chapter. Instead, we illustrate the combined use of the task-analytic and strategy methods by describing one or two representative programs in each domain. The illustrative examples presented as follows are based on data from intervention research that has the following characteristics: random assignment, adequate description of interventions, adequate identification of the effective components of the intervention, long enough duration of intervention, control over prior interventions, measurement of teacher and contextual variables, and adequate generalization to real classrooms[5] (also see National Reading Panel[39] and Snow[40] for methods for identifying evidence-based interventions in education).

Practices Illustrating Effective Remediation with the Task-Analytic and Cognitive/Cognitive-Behavioral Instructional Models

WORD-LEVEL READING SKILL

The longest continuous research program on reading remediation is directed by Maureen Lovett at The Hospital for Sick Children.[132] She and her colleagues have developed and researched complementary programs that illustrate how direct instruction and strategy instruction can be combined synergistically to enhance the word-level skills of students with learning disabilities in reading. The program of phonological analysis and blending/direct instruction relies on the task-analytic method to explicitly and systematically teach children how to break apart words. Word identification strategy training (WIST) is a metacognitive program designed to teach word recognition through the application of strategies that facilitate transfer of word-level skills. Lovett's research documents superior effects for the aligned use of the two programs.

A second research program, conducted by Torgesen and colleagues at Florida State University, also shows how comprehensive and intense programs, even with somewhat different emphases promote substantial improvement for students with learning disabilities in reading, when the programs integrate task-analytic and cognitive-behavioral/strategy instruction. For example, Torgesen and colleagues[115] randomly assigned third, fourth, and fifth graders who scored below the third percentile in word recognition to one of two 8-week programs, each with 2 hours of daily instruction. Both interventions incorporated direct instruction and strategy instruction, including explicit instruction in the alphabetical principle, structured practice of new skills, and the cuing of appropriate strategies in context. Results showed significant improvement of about one standard deviation in word recognition and about two thirds of a standard deviation in comprehension; moreover, word recognition gains were maintained for 2 years. Of importance was that there was no difference in relative efficacy of the two programs (but, disappointingly, there was no improvement in fluency).

Across these and other programs of research on students with learning disabilities in reading, results show word recognition skill can be improved, with transfer to comprehension when direct instruction and strategy instruction are combined. Fluency gains, however, are limited. Various approaches are associated with improvement; gains are more impressive with greater intensity, explicitness, duration, and systematic delivery.

READING COMPREHENSION

Williams and associates also developed and assessed the efficacy of interventions that illustrate the combination of direct instruction and strategy instruction.[133-135] For example, with the Theme-Identification Program,[136] lessons are organized around a single story and include prereading discussion of the theme concept; reading the story aloud; discussing the important story information, with organizing questions as a guide (i.e., the "theme-scheme"); transfer and application of the theme to other story examples and real-life situations; review; and activity. The heart of the program is the "theme-scheme," which provides a set of questions that organize the important story components to help students follow the plot and derive the theme. The teacher models how to answer these questions, and students gradually assume increasing responsibility for asking the questions and identifying the theme. The students also rehearse and commit to memory these questions so they can apply the theme-scheme guide independently to untaught stories. Toward the end of instruction, transfer instruction is provided explicitly, with two additional questions employed to help students generalize the theme to other relevant situations.

Williams and associates[136] applied this program in second and third grade New York City classrooms, representing students with high, average, and low performance in relation to their classmates. Classrooms were assigned randomly to the Theme-Identification Program or to a more traditional comprehension program that emphasized vocabulary and plot. Students were assessed on a variety of acquisition and transfer measures. Results revealed that, as a function of the Theme-Identification Program, students acquired the concept of a theme and learned the theme-scheme questions. Of more importance was that on novel passages, students in the experimental condition were more skilled at identifying themes. Effects pertained to high-, average-, and low-achieving classmates, as well as to students with learning disabilities, in second and third grade. The methods illustrated how teachers can address a high-level comprehension skill (i.e., identification of a story's theme) even among students with serious word-reading difficulties. Across the research of Williams and associates and other researchers working on remedying the comprehension difficulties of students with learning disabilities, results highlight how programs that incorporate direct "skills" instruction in combination with strategy instruction can be effective at promoting reading comprehension skill.

MATHEMATICS FACT RETRIEVAL AND PROCEDURAL SKILL

The majority of remediation research for students with learning disabilities in math focuses on fact retrieval and procedural math (i.e., multiple-digit computation). For example, Fuchs and colleagues[137,138] cumulatively designed and tested a set of instructional components for enhancing students' math competence. Three studies conducted at second through sixth grades addressed procedural math. Two additional studies assessed fact retrieval along with procedural math (i.e., multiple-digit computation and estimation) in kindergarten[139] and first grade.[140] Effects were assessed separately for students with learning disabilities and students not identified with learning disabilities who had low, average, and high initial achievement status. Across all four types of learners throughout the primary and intermediate grades, statistically significant effects resulted from a combination of (1) explicit, procedurally clear, conceptually based explanations; (2) pictorial representations of the math; (3) verbal rehearsal with gradual fading; and (4) timed practice on mixed problem sets, which systematically provided cumulative review of previously mastered problem types. Again, explicit instruction, combining the task-analytic and cognitive/strategy approaches, shows impressive gains for students with learning disabilities.

MATHEMATICAL PROBLEM SOLVING

Less attention, however, has been focused on complex math problem solving, in which problems incorporate irrelevant information and more varied syntactic structures and in which many problems require two or more computations for solution. This lack of attention to math problem solving, especially at the primary grades, is unfortunate for three reasons. First, for students with learning disabilities, a critical outcome of schooling is real-world math problem solving. Second, research even with typical students reveals the challenges associated with effecting math problem solving. Teachers cannot assume that interventions for promoting success with simple word problems will translate into improved math problem solving. Finally, despite severe challenges with foundational math skills,[141] waiting for mastery of those foundational skills before working on math problem solving may create deficits in such work that are impossible to address later in school.

Fuchs and colleagues therefore focused on math problem solving in third grade with "Hot Math," a program that combines task-analytic instruction to teach students solutions to word problems and strategy instruction to help students transfer these skills to more contextually rich and novel word problems. In a series of studies, Fuchs and colleagues[142-144] used this framework to explicitly teach math problem solving. For example, they randomly assigned classrooms to four study conditions[143]: (1) teacher-designed instruction; (2) task-analytic solution instruction (20 sessions); (3) strategic instruction to transfer (20 sessions: half as much task-analytic solution instruction); and (4) task-analytic solution instruction with strategic instruction to transfer (30 sessions). Instruction was delivered over 16 weeks with strong fidelity, with teacher-directed and peer-mediated instructional arrangements, and effects were assessed on avariety of math problem solving measures. Results showed that task-analytic solution instruction was sufficient to improve performance on problems very similar to those used in intervention; that strategic instruction to transfer was necessary to enhance performance on less similar problems; and that for students with learning disabilities and other low-performing students, the full course of both components was most effective. For students with and without disability, the effect sizes were large. Thus, as is the case for reading and writing, effective interventions in the area of mathematics incorporate not only task-analytic skills instruction but also explicit instruction on strategies that facilitate transfer and maintenance of those skills.

Conclusions

Across reading and mathematics, research provides the basis for drawing six conclusions about how to enhance academic outcomes for students with learning disabilities:

1. Students with learning disabilities require task-analytic instruction, which is explicit, is well-organized, and provides opportunity for cumulative review of previously mastered content. This appears to represent the cornerstone of effective practice.
2. Strategy instruction, whereby students are taught strategic behavior to optimize their performance by monitoring their progress, setting goals, and transferring and maintaining skills, provides an added value over and beyond task-analytic instruction.
3. Peer mediation provides a feasible and effective method for extending task-analytic instruction and strategy instruction, by creating structured opportunities for supported practice in ways that enhance acquisition of knowledge and extend transfer of learned content.
4. It is possible to produce impressive growth on higher order processes such as reading comprehension or math problem solving even when students' foundational skills such as word reading or arithmetic are weak. This implies that teachers should provide systematic instruction on both dimensions of academic performance so that as foundational skills are strengthened, teachers simultaneously work explicitly to improve students' text comprehension, written expression, and math problem solving.
5. Gains are specific to what is taught. If interventions do not teach academic content, little academic learning will occur. Similarly, if academic content in one domain is learned, it does not necessarily lead to improvement in another domain.
6. Student progress must be frequently monitored[42] so that programs can be evaluated formatively, and the response of individual students with learning disabilities assessed continuously, so that programs can be revised in a timely manner, as needed, to ensure adequate progress over time.

LONG-TERM OUTCOMES

The Connecticut Longitudinal Study,[3,145] which monitored children from kindergarten through grade 12, demonstrated that children with reading disabilities could be identified by 6 years of age and that they remained poorer readers than their peers with no learning disabilities at every other assessment point. Of importance is that reading scores did improve over time, but the difference between the individuals with and without reading disorders was maintained throughout development, so that fully 70% of the children identified with reading disorders by third grade were still identified as having reading disorders in high school. It is worth noting that these children were identified as learning disabled, and so they had received special education services. Although the Connecticut Longitudinal Study findings underline the fact that reading difficulties can be lifelong disorders, some individuals with reading disabilities are high achieving. In university samples of young adults with childhood diagnoses of reading disability, reading comprehension is better than word recognition, but the core deficit in phonological processing remains.[146] Although many of these young adults are successful in school and in their occupations, they may continue to struggle more than their peers with reading-related tasks and may require supports into their college years (see Gerber et al[147] for a study of the employment experiences of young American and Canadian adults with learning disabilities).

In the Connecticut Longitudinal Study, youths with reading disability did not differ from their typically developing peers with regard to other outcomes such as substance abuse or legal problems.[145] In contrast, the Ottawa Language Study[148] revealed an increased risk of substance abuse in adolescents with learning disorders and an elevated risk for poor behavioral outcomes in association with social and economic disadvantage, lower intelligence, and poorer academic and occupational achievements. These differences in nonreading outcomes across studies may be related to the high rate of language impairment in the Ottawa Language Study, which itself carries high risk for behavior disorder.[149]

THE ROLE OF THE DEVELOPMENTAL-BEHAVIORAL PEDIATRICIAN IN THE CLINICAL MANAGEMENT OF LEARNING DISABILITY

Advocating an Evidence-Based Approach

For children with learning disabilities and their parents, the developmental-behavioral pediatrician is a valuable source of evidence-based information and can make important contributions to decision making with regard to assessment and intervention. Public knowledge about learning disabilities is sometimes based on folklore and strongly held beliefs that are not borne out by the research. For example, children do not outgrow learning disabilities, boys do not eventually "catch up" if they are experiencing real

difficulties in learning to read, letter reversals in reading and writing are not the defining feature of dyslexia, and there are no "quick fixes" for "curing" learning disabilities. Evidence-based practice for learning disabilities aligns the clinical management of this disorder with that practiced for other childhood medical disorders. The following section applies the research on identification, assessment, comorbidity and treatment of learning disabilities presented previously to clinical practice.

Assessment

Learning disabilities are rarely related to primary sensory deficits; however, problems in vision and hearing do need to be investigated, as does the presence of a medical condition that could contribute to lack of achievement in school (e.g., severe fatigue and school absence in association with some disorders). In beginning a discussion about a suspected learning disability, the developmental-behavioral pediatrician should obtain a family and child history that is pertinent to learning. The following are some important questions to ask, although this list is not exhaustive:

- Has any one in the family (immediate and extended) ever had difficulty in school? In what subject or subjects? What are the educational attainments of family members?
- If the child is of school age, did the child have any speech and language difficulties earlier in development? Was treatment provided? Are any assessment and treatment data available? (If the child is a preschooler or just entering the school system, the same questions apply. Children with speech and language impairment are at elevated risk for reading difficulties.[7])
- Are there any other developmental risk factors for later learning difficulties such as a neurodevelopmental or other comorbid disorder (see the later section "Understanding the Relation between Learning Disabilities and Comorbid Disorders")? Were there significant fine motor delays, severe behavior problems, and the like, necessitating referral for developmental services and/or intervention? If so, are assessment and treatment data/reports available from occupational therapy, psychology, and other disciplines?
- If the child is of school age, what are the child's grades in language arts (which includes reading, language and reading comprehension, and oral and written expression) and mathematics (which may include arithmetic or number sense and numeration and other aspects of math such as geometry, measurement, problem solving, patterning and algebra, and data management) this year

and in previous years? What are the teacher's comments?

■ If the child is just entering school, does he or she have some of the skills that are important precursors of later academic skills, such as being able to name the letters of the alphabet, knowing how to count objects by using one-to-one correspondence, and knowing some simple shapes, as well as what size words and position words (e.g., "large"; "beside") mean?

There are no medical diagnostic tests, including those that involve brain imaging, that can be used to diagnose learning disabilities or that have current practical clinical utility for assessing treatment benefits or making prognoses. For a child with a suspected learning disability, the most important tests are those that measure achievement in core academic domains. The developmental-behavioral pediatrician who is trained in psychometric measurement or the psychologist or assessment-literate teacher can assess these areas. For example, some developmental-behavioral pediatricians may employ academic screening measures, such as the Wide Range Achievement Test, 3rd Edition,[150] that are relatively brief and easy to administer. This type of academic screening measure can be used for children from kindergarten on up to assess reading (letter and word recognition), spelling (writing letters and spelling words in response to dictation), and math (counting, reading numbers, simple verbal problems, and written computations).

However, such screening tools need to be followed by academic measures that more comprehensively assess the range of skills in core academic domains that are important for school functioning. These include measures of reading decoding, reading fluency, and reading comprehension; mathematics computations and math word problems; and written expression, such as handwriting, spelling, and composition. The Woodcock-Johnson III Tests of Achievement[151] and the Wechsler Individual Achievement Test–Second Edition[152] are reliable and well-validated measures of these academic skills that also account for variations in ethnicity and socioeconomic status.[4]

Assessments that include intelligence tests and measures of cognitive domains such as memory and general problem solving do not contribute much to the choice of appropriate interventions. For example, although working memory deficits are common in children with various learning disabilities,[153] knowing about the type and level of the working memory deficit in children suspected of a learning disability does not inform the choice of intervention strategies. As discussed earlier, the choice of the intervention program needs to be based on an assessment that measures the specific academic deficit or deficits. This

is powerful knowledge for practitioners to have about the relation between cognitive and academic assessment and intervention, and it carries two important practical and ethical consequences: Children need not undergo time-consuming psychometric testing for determining learning intervention needs, and funding can be directed toward intervention rather than assessment. In keeping with the earlier section on identification of learning disabilities, academic achievement tests such as these may be all that is needed to identify academic underachievement before a program of intervention is begun. Response to intervention (assuming that intervention is of sufficient intensity and duration) can be measured at appropriate intervals, with the same tests and also monitored by the teacher with brief and fairly frequent measures of progress (e.g. curriculum based measurement tools; see www.studentprogress.org).

We are not suggesting that more comprehensive assessments that include measures of intelligence, memory, visual-motor skills, adaptive functioning, and so forth are never useful but rather that they are often not necessary before intervention is begun. They may become warranted in the following situations: (1) When other disorders such as mental retardation or ADHD are suspected, the child may qualify for special education services under a category other than learning disability and would require an assessment adequate to diagnose such disorders; (2) when a child fails to respond to high-quality interventions of sufficient duration, a more comprehensive assessment may prove useful, particularly for older children with learning disability, in terms of making classroom accommodations and adjusting the Individualized Education Plan (IEP) to best suit the student's needs; (3) when the child has a disorder with frank central nervous system involvement such as traumatic head injury or spina bifida, the contribution of other neuropsychological deficits may be important in terms of making classroom accommodations so that intervention programs for academic skills can be most effective; and (4) when publicly funded delivery of special education services mandates such assessments.

Prevention

The pediatrician is often the first person who is consulted when a child has suspected developmental difficulties, and the pediatrician is also the professional who sees the child continuously across time. This places the pediatrician in a unique position with regard to early intervention for very young children who may be at risk for later learning disabilities. This intervention might involve referrals such as that for speech and language therapy for delayed language in toddlers and preschoolers. The developmental-behavioral pediatrician has an important role to play with regard to liaison with other health professionals and can provide support and education for parents in terms of prevention strategies. For example, information about learning disabilities in neurodevelopmental disorders such as spina bifida (see the following section) that is communicated to parents of such preschool children may result in careful monitoring of learning and early interventions that could prevent or reduce learning disabilities in these high-risk groups.

Understanding the Relation between Learning Disabilities and Comorbid Disorders

An important role of the medical practitioner is in the assessment and treatment of comorbid developmental disorders. For example, ADHD co-occurs with reading disability at a rate higher than that expected for the general population.[30] This means that children presenting with any learning disability need to be thoroughly evaluated for ADHD and children with ADHD, for learning disability. Academic intervention and clinical drug trials for children with ADHD show that the learning disability and the ADHD necessitate treatments that are specific to each disorder[154]; that is, behavioral and medication treatments for the ADHD do not affect the learning disability, and academic treatments for the learning disability do not affect the behavioral symptoms of the ADHD. Whether combined treatments such as medication plus evidence-based reading interventions serve to potentiate treatment effects for children with comorbid ADHD and reading disability is a question of current research interest.[155]

Other disorders can co-occur with learning disabilities, including conduct disorder[154] and speech and language disorders. These other disorders need to be addressed in their own right. For example, a comorbid language disorder would need to be assessed by a speech and language pathologist, and combined reading and language disorders may necessitate a somewhat different approach to treatment than either disorder alone.[156]

Several investigators have reported that children and adults with learning disability have a range of social-emotional difficulties, including poor social skills[157] and substance abuse disorders,[148] as well as depression, anxiety, and low self-esteem.[158] One study revealed a reduction in depression in later grades for children who received academic interventions in first grade.[159] A meta-analysis of depression and learning disability[8] revealed that children with learning disabilities reported higher depression scores than did their nondisabled peers, but the reporting of clinical or severe depression was not elevated in students with learning disabilities. The authors cautioned that in clinical practice, diagnoses of depression are not made on the basis of depression inventories alone and that diagnoses need to be made by a qualified mental health professional and treated according to best practices for childhood depression.

It is also important to be aware of common neurodevelopmental disorders that are associated with higher than expected rates of learning disabilities. For example, very low birth weight is associated with learning disabilities even when such children have relatively spared cognitive and intellectual skills, and math may be particularly affected.[160] Spina bifida,[104] hydrocephalus from other etiologies,[161] Turner syndrome,[162] and the fragile X syndrome[162] are all associated with relatively high rates of math disability, even when, in some of these neurodevelopmental disorders, word reading develops adequately. Traumatic head injury is associated with difficulties in acquiring word reading skills and math calculation skills, particularly for children who are injured during the preschool or very early school years.[163,164] This relation of learning difficulties with an early age at injury is true for both severe and mild to moderate injuries.[164] Standard academic achievement tests tend to underestimate the difficulties that children with traumatic brain injury have with academic skills in the classroom, which may reflect the influence of deficits in other cognitive systems such as memory, attention, and executive functions that support learning.[165] Children with cancer, such as acute lymphoblastic leukemia, are also more affected by central nervous system treatment at younger ages of diagnosis. Difficulties have been found in math and in reading, and the manifestation of these learning disabilities in the classroom may be exacerbated by accompanying deficits in information processing speed, memory, attention, and visual-motor skills.[166] Children with sickle cell disease are at high risk of learning disabilities, as well as other cognitive difficulties in domains such as attention, and this is true not only of those with overt strokes but also of children with clinically silent strokes.[167] Furthermore, pain associated with the disease, medications to treat the pain, socioeconomic disadvantage, and behavioral issues may complicate how children with sickle cell disease function in the classroom, over and above the presence of learning disabilities and other cognitive deficits.

Intervention and Advocacy

An important role for the developmental-behavioral pediatrician is to convey information about evidence-based interventions for learning disabilities and, conversely, to be prepared to use professional knowledge to convey to parents which interventions are unlikely to work despite personal testimonials, advertisements, and media reports. This latter category of ineffective methods includes prosthetic devices and medications (e.g., colored lenses or colored overlays, medications for motion sickness/inner ear disease) or programs that do not directly address the academic disability (e.g., sensory integration training; learning styles or sensory modality). (See Chapter 8E.)

The developmental-behavioral pediatrician should be prepared to make referrals to a preferred roster of educational practitioners who deliver evidence-based interventions that meet the specifications of those discussed in the earlier section "Intervention and Advocacy." Programs offered by these tutors should provide explicit instruction in the areas of academic need, provide instruction in both foundational (e.g., word decoding) and higher order academic skills (e.g., reading comprehension strategies), and be of sufficient duration and intensity to assess whether the interventions are working.

Another role for the medical practitioner is to ask for and obtain reports in which academic progress is assessed. As mentioned earlier, monitoring of progress is what informs intervention and changes in intervention strategies. The need to monitor response to intervention is an idea that is second nature to medical practitioners, but it is an idea that is not always consistently applied to behavioral academic interventions for learning disabilities. The developmental-behavioral pediatrician may speak with the family and the child about progress or lack of progress and next steps. He or she may make a referral to professionals such as a psychologist to reassess the child.

In view of the importance of the school in the progress of children with learning disabilities, it is necessary for the pediatric practitioner to (1) be familiar with local school resources and guidelines/criteria for accessing special education resources and (2) be able to refer parents to resources that will familiarize them with the processes that surround identification and access to special education or to prereferral programs designed to help students who are having learning difficulties.[45] In other words, the developmental-behavioral pediatrician plays an advocacy role for children with learning disabilities and their families. One important thing to keep in mind is that identification as a student in need of special education is a legal process. This means that the developmental-behavioral pediatrician should know the legislation governing identification, as well as processes such as parent appeal. As mentioned earlier, alternatives to the traditional discrepancy formula for identifying learning disabilities have become acceptable under the Individuals with Disabilities Education Act. Because parents are often the best advocates for their children, the pediatrician may be key in educating some parents about their advocacy roles and the rules governing the process of identification.[168] Information about legislation affecting children with learning disability and advocacy tools for health professionals, parents, teachers, and individuals with learning disability can be found on the Web sites of some of the learning disability organizations (e.g., Learning Disabilities Association of America, Learning Disabilities Association of Canada, National Center for Learning Disabilities).

The developmental-behavioral pediatrician may also play a more direct role in the identification process by writing a letter for the Identification Placement Review Committee meeting or the IEP meeting.[168] The letter might include a summary of assessment and/or intervention data and pertinent developmental history information. It is also important for the medical practitioner to provide information about comorbid conditions or medical conditions such as those reviewed previously that could affect the child's learning and that might also be used to establish eligibility for special education resources through a disabilities category other than learning disability.[11] Information on the Identification Placement Review Committee and IEP can be found on several of the Web sites of the learning disability organizations listed earlier.

Finally, the developmental-behavioral pediatrician has an important role to play in terms of transition care as youths prepare to transfer from the child health system to the adult health system. As the health care professional who is often part of the child's health care team from the child's birth to adolescence, the developmental-behavioral pediatrician is well suited to transferring care to an appropriate primary care physician. The pediatrician may begin transition planning when the child is about 14 years of age, at a time when the education system is also charged with planning for transitions for further education and/or employment of youths with learning disabilities.[169] For youths with learning disabilities, the pediatrician may promote self-advocacy and awareness of legislation governing the rights and entitlements of persons with disabilities.

CONCLUSION

As knowledge about the cognitive and neurobiological correlates of typical and atypical development of academic skills and effective interventions has grown, conceptualizations of learning disabilities have also changed. The application of science into practice and public policy is not always straightforward, and the field of learning disabilities is no exception to this general rule. However, a pediatric practitioner's scientific knowledge about learning disabilities is crucial for the provision of evidence-based clinical management of children with learning disabilities.

REFERENCES

1. U.S. Department of Education, Office of Special Education Program, Data Analysis System, 2004 IDEA Part B Child Count: Twenty-sixth Annual Report to Congress on the Implementation of the Individuals with Disabilities Education Act. Washington, DC: U. S. Government Printing Office, 2004.

2. Spreen O, Risser A, Edgell D: Developmental Neuropsychology. New York: Oxford University Press, 1995.

3. Shaywitz SE, Fletcher JM, Shaywitz BA: A conceptual model and definition of dyslexia: Findings emerging from the Connecticut Longitudinal Study. *In* Beitchman JH, Cohen NJ, Konstantareas MM, et al, eds: Language, Learning, and Behavior Disorders. New York: Cambridge University Press, 1996, pp 199-223.

4. Fletcher JM, Francis, DJ, Morris R, et al: Evidence-based assessment of learning disabilities in children and adolescents. J Clin Child Adolesc Psychol 34:506-522, 2005.

5. Lyon GR, Fletcher JM, Fuchs, LS, et al: Learning disabilities. *In* Mash E, Barkley R, eds: Treatment of Childhood Disorders, 2nd ed. New York: Guilford, 2006.

6. Plomin R, Kovas Y: Generalist genes and learning disabilities. Psychol Bull 131:592-617, 2005.

7. Bishop DVM, Snowling MJ: Developmental dyslexia and specific language impairment: Same or different? Psychol Bull 130:858-886, 2004.

8. Maag JW, Reid R: Depression among students with learning disabilities: Assessing the risk. J Learn Disabil 39:3-10, 2006.

9. Willcutt EG, Pennington BF, Olsen RK, et al: Neuropsychological analysis of comorbidity between reading disability and attention deficit hyperactivity disorder: In search of the common deficit. Dev Neuropsychol 27:35-78, 2005.

10. Lyon GR, Fletcher JM, Shaywitz SE, et al: Rethinking learning disabilities. *In* Finn CE Jr, Rotherham RAJ, Hokanson, CR Jr, eds: Rethinking Special Education for a New Century. Washington, DC: Thomas B. Fordham Foundation and Progressive Policy Institute, 2001, pp 259-287.

11. Lyon GR, Fletcher JM, Barnes MA: Learning disabilities. *In* Mash EJ, Barkley R, eds: Child Psychopathology, 2nd ed. New York: Guilford, 2003, pp 520-588.

12. Hinshelwood J: Congenital Word Blindness. London: HK Lewis, 1917.

13. Lovett MW, Barron RW: Neuropsychological perspectives on reading development and developmental reading disorders. *In* Segalowitz SJ, Rapin I, eds:

14. Chambers JG, Parrish T, Harr JJ: What are we spending on special education services in the United States, 1999-2000? Advance Report #1, Office of Special Education Program. Washington, DC: American Institutes for Research, March 2002. Available at: http://www.csef-air.org/publications/seep/nationa/AdvRpt1.pdf.

15. U.S. Office of Education: Assistance to states for education for handicapped children: Procedures for evaluating specific learning disabilities. Fed Regist 42:G1082-G1085, 1977.

16. U.S. Department of Education: Assistance to the states for the education of children with disabilities: Criteria for determining the existence of a specific learning disability, Part 300.541. Fed Regist 64:12405-12454, 1999.

17. Special Education: A Guide for Educators, Ministry of Education, Ontario, 2001. Available at: http://www.edu.gov.on.ca/eng/general/elemsec/speced/handbook.pdf.

18. American Psychiatric Association: Diagnostic and Statistical Manual of Mental Disorders, 4th ed, International Version. Washington, DC: American Psychiatric Association, 1994.

19. World Health Organization: The ICD-10 Classification of Mental and Behavioral Disorders: Clinical Descriptions and Diagnostic Guidelines. Geneva: World Health Organization, 1992.

20. Rapoport JL, Ismond DR: DSM-IV Training Guide for Diagnosis of Childhood Disorders. Philadelphia: Brunner/Mazel, 1996.

21. Fletcher JM, Lyon GR, Barnes MA, et al: Classification of learning disabilities: An evidence-based evaluation. *In* Bradley R, Danielson L, Hallahan D, eds: Identification of Learning Disabilities: Research in Practice. Mahwah, NJ: Erlbaum, 2002, pp 185-250.

22. Stuebing KK, Fletcher JM, LeDoux JM, et al: Validity of discrepancy classifications of reading difficulties: A meta-analysis. Am Educ Res J 39:469-518, 2002.

23. Stanovich KE, Siegel LS: Phenotypic performance profiles of children with reading disabilities: A regression-based test of the phonological-core variable difference model. J Educ Psychol 86:24-53, 1994.

24. Francis DJ, Shaywitz SE, Stuebing KK, et al: Developmental lag versus deficit models of reading disability: A longitudinal, individual growth curves analysis. J Educ Psychol 88:3-17, 1996.

25. Vellutino FR, Scanlon DM, Lyon GR: Differentiating between difficult-to-remediate and readily remediated poor readers: More evidence against the IQ-achievement discrepancy definition for reading disability. J Learn Disabil 33:223-238, 2000.

26. Elliot SN, Fuchs LS: The utility of curriculum-based measurement and performance assessment as alternatives to traditional intelligence and achievement tests. School Psychol Rev 26:224-233, 1997.

27. Wadsworth SJ, Olson RK, Pennington BF, et al: Differential genetic etiology of reading disability as a function of IQ. J Learn Disabil 33:192-199, 2000.

Handbook of Neuropsychology, vol 8: Child Neuropsychology, Part II (Boller F, Grafman J, series eds). Amsterdam: Elsevier, 2003, pp 671-716.

28. Francis DJ, Fletcher JM, Stuebing KK, et al: Psychometric approaches to the identification of learning disabilities. Test scores are not sufficient. J Learn Disabil 38:545-552, 2005.

29. Shaywitz SE, Escobar MD, Shaywitz BA, et al: Evidence that dyslexia may represent the lower tail of a normal distribution of reading ability. N Engl J Med 326:145-150, 1992.

30. Fletcher JM, Shaywitz SE, Shaywitz BA: Comorbidity of learning and attention disorders: Separate but equal. Pediatr Clin North Am 46:885-897, 1999.

31. Shankweiler D, Lundquist E, Katz L, et al: Comprehension and decoding: Patterns of association in children with reading difficulties. Sci Stud Read 3:69-94, 1999.

32. Fuchs LS, Fuchs D, Stuebing K, Fletcher JM, et al: Calculation and problem-solving skill: Are they shared or distinct aspects of mathematical problem solving? Manuscript submitted for publication.

33. Geary DC: Mathematical disabilities: Cognitive, neuropsychological, and genetic components. Psychol Bull 114:345-362, 1993.

34. Hart B, Risley TR: Meaningful Differences in the Everyday Experience of Young American Children. Baltimore: Paul H. Brookes, 1999.

35. Whitehurst GJ, Massetti GM: How well does Head Start prepare children to learn to read? In Zigler E, Styfco SJ, eds: The Head Start Debates. Baltimore: Paul H. Brooks, 2004, pp 251-262.

36. Case R, Griffin, Kelly WM: Socioeconomic gradients in mathematical ability and their responsiveness to intervention during early childhood. In Keating DP, Hertzman C, eds: Developmental Health and the Wealth of Nations. New York: Guilford, 1999, pp 21-40.

37. Whitehurst GJ, Lonigan C: Child development and emergent literacy. Child Dev 69:848-872, 1998.

38. Starkey P, Klein A, Wakeley A: Enhancing young children's mathematical knowledge through a pre-kindergarten mathematics intervention. Early Child Res Q 19:99-120, 2004.

39. National Reading Panel: Teaching Children to Read: An Evidence-Based Assessment of the Scientific Research Literature on Reading and Its Implications for Reading Instruction. Washington, DC: National Institute of Child Health and Human Development, 2000.

40. Snow CE: Reading for Understanding: Toward an R & D Program in Reading Comprehension. Santa Monica, CA: RAND Corporation, 2002.

41. Berninger VW, Abbott RD: Redefining learning disabilities: Moving beyond aptitude achievement discrepancies to failure to respond to validated treatment protocols. In Lyon GR, ed: Frames of Reference for the Assessment of Learning Disabilities: New Views on Measurement Issues. Baltimore: Paul H. Brookes, 1994, pp 163-183.

42. Fuchs LS, Fuchs D: Treatment validity: A unifying concept for reconceptualizing the identification of learning disabilities. Learn Disabil Res Prac 13:204-219, 1998.

43. Vellutino FR, Scanlon DM: Phonological coding, phonological awareness, and reading ability: Evidence from a longitudinal and experimental study. Merrill Palmer Q 33:321-363, 1987.

44. Heller KA, Holtzman WH, Messick S, eds: Placing Children in Special Education: A Strategy for Equity. Washington, DC: National Academies Press, 1982.

45. Fletcher JM, Lyon GR: Learning disabilities. In Maria B, ed: Current Management in Child Neurology, 3rd ed. Hamilton, Ontario: BC Decker, 2005.

46. Liberman IY, Shankweiler D, Liberman AM: The alphabetic principle and learning to read. In Shankweiler D, Liberman IY, eds: Phonology and Reading Disability: Solving the Reading Puzzle. Ann Arbor, MI: University of Michigan Press, 1989, pp 1-33.

47. Adams MJ: Beginning to Read: Thinking and Learning about Print. Cambridge, MA: MIT Press, 1990.

48. Wagner RK, Torgesen JK, Rashotte CA, et al: Changing relations between phonological processing abilities and word-level reading as children develop from beginning to skilled readers: A five year longitudinal study. Dev Psychol 33:468-479, 1997.

49. Torgesen JK, Wagner RK, Rashotte CA, et al: Contributions of phonological awareness and rapid automatic naming ability to the growth of word-reading skills in second- to fifth-grade children. Sci Stud Read 1:161-185, 1997.

50. Scarborough HS: Early identification of children at risk for reading disabilities. In Shapiro BK, Accardo PJ, Capute AJ, eds: Specific Reading Disability: A View of the Spectrum. Timonium, MD: York Press, 1998, pp 75-119.

51. Stanovich KE: Explaining the differences between the dyslexic and the garden-variety poor reader: The phonological-core variable-difference model. J Learn Disabil 21:590-604, 1988.

52. Morris RD, Stuebing KK, Fletcher JM, et al: Subtypes of reading disability: Variability around a phonological core. J Educ Psychol 90:1-27, 1998.

53. Torgesen JK, Wagner RK, Rashotte CA, et al: Preventing reading failure in young children with phonological processing disabilities: Group and individual responses to instruction. J Educ Psychol 91:579-593, 1999.

54. Vellutino FR, Scanlon DM, Sipay ER, et al: Cognitive profiles of difficult-to-remediate and readily remediated poor readers: Early intervention as a vehicle for distinguishing between cognitive and experiential deficits as basic causes of specific reading disability. J Educ Psychol 88:601-638, 1996.

55. Manis FR, Seidenberg MS, Doi L: See Dick RAN: Rapid naming and the longitudinal prediction of reading subskills in first and second graders. Sci Stud Read 3:129-157, 1999.

56. Bowers PG, Sunseth K, Golden J: The route between rapid naming and reading progress. Sci Stud Read 3:31-53, 1999.

57. Vukovic RK, Siegel LS: The double deficit hypothesis: A comprehensive review of the evidence. J Learn Disabil 39:25-47, 2006.

58. Lovett MW: A developmental approach to reading disability: Accuracy and speed criteria of normal and deficit reading children. Child Dev 58:234-260, 1987.

59. Lovett MW, Steinbach KA, Frijters JC: Remediating the core deficits of developmental reading disability: A double deficit perspective. J Learn Disabil 33:334-358, 2000.

60. Wolf M, Bowers PG: The double-deficit hypothesis for the developmental dyslexias. J Educ Psychol 91:415-438, 1999.

61. Cestnick L, Coltheart M: The relationship between language-processing and visual-processing deficits in developmental dyslexia. Cognition 71:231-255, 1999.

62. Stein JF: The neurobiology of reading difficulties. In Wolf M, ed: Dyslexia, Fluency, and the Brain. Baltimore: York Press, 2001.

63. Tallal P, Miller SL, Jenkins WM, et al: The role of temporal processing in developmental language-based learning disorders: Research and clinical implications. In Blachman BA, ed: Foundations of Reading Acquisition and Dyslexia: Implications for Early Intervention. Mahwah NJ: Erlbaum, 1997, pp 49-66.

64. Shaywitz BA, Fletcher JM, Shaywitz SE: Defining and classifying learning disabilities and attention-deficit/hyperactivity disorder. J Child Neurol 10:50-57, 1995.

65. Willcutt EG, Pennington BF: Comorbidity of reading disability and attention-deficit/hyperactivity disorder: Differences by gender and subtype. J Learn Disabil 33:179-191, 2000.

66. Dykman RA, Ackerman PT: Attention deficit disorder and specific reading disability: Separate but often overlapping disorders. J Learn Disabil 24:96-103, 1991.

67. Semrud-Clikeman M, Biederman J, Sprich-Buckminster S, et al: Comorbidity between ADDH and learning disability: A review and report in a clinically referred sample. J Am Acad Child Adolesc Psychiatry 31:439-448, 1992.

68. Willcutt EG, Pennington BF, Boada R, et al: A comparison of the cognitive deficits in reading disability and attention-deficit/hyperactivity disorder. J Abnorm Psychol 110:157-172, 2001.

69. Filipek PA: Neuroimaging in the developmental disorders: The state of the science. J Child Psychol Psychiatry 40:113-128, 1999.

70. Shaywitz SE, Pugh KR, Jenner AR, et al: The neurobiology of reading and reading disability (dyslexia). In Kamil ML, Mosenthal PB, Pearson PD, et al, eds: Handbook of Reading Research, vol 3. Mahwah, NJ: Erlbaum, 2000, pp 229-249.

71. Simos PG, Breier JI, Fletcher JM, et al: Brain activation profiles in dyslexic children during nonword reading: A magnetic source imaging study. Neurosci Rep 290:61-65, 2000.

72. Pugh KR, Mencl WE, Shaywitz BA, et al: The angular gyrus in developmental dyslexia: Task-specific differences in functional connectivity within posterior cortex. Psychol Sci 11:51-56, 2000.

73. Simos PG, Fletcher JM, Bergman E, et al: Dyslexia-specific brain activation profiles becomes normal following successful remedial training. Neurology 58:1-10, 2000.

74. Aylward EH, Richards TL, Berninger VW, et al: Instructional treatment associated with changes in brain activation in children with dyslexia. Neurology 22:212-219, 2003.

75. Simos PG, Fletcher JM, Sarkari S, et al: Early development of neurophysiological processes involved in normal reading and reading disability: A magnetic source imaging study. Neuropsychology 19:787-798, 2005.

76. Pennington BB: Dyslexia as a neurodevelopmental disorder. In Tager-Flusberg H, ed: Neurodevelopmental Disorders. Cambridge, MA: MIT Press, 1999, pp 307-330.

77. Grigorenko EL: Developmental dyslexia: An update on genes, brains, and environments. J Child Psychol Psychiatry 42:91-125, 2001.

78. Alarcon M, DeFries JC: Reading performance and general cognitive ability in twins with reading difficulties and control pairs. Pers Individ Dif 22:793-803, 1997.

79. Gayan J, Olson RK: Genetic and environmental influences on orthographic and phonological skills in children with reading disabilities. Dev Neuropsychol 20:483-507, 2001.

80. Grigorenko EL, Wood FB, Golovyan L, et al: Continuing the search for dyslexia genes on 6p. Am J Med Genet B Neuropsychiatr Genet 118B:89-98, 2003.

81. Gayan J, Willcutt EG, Fisher SE, et al: Bivariate linkage scan for reading disability and attention-deficit/hyperactivity disorder localizes pleiotropic loci. J Child Psychol Psychiatry 46:1045-1056, 2005.

82. Oakhill J, Cain K, Bryant PE: The dissociation of word reading and text comprehension: Evidence from component skills. Lang Cogn Proc 18:443-468, 2003.

83. Barnes MA: The decoding-comprehension dissociation in the reading of children with hydrocephalus: A reply to Yamada. Brain Lang 80:260-263, 2002.

84. Leach JM, Scarborough HS, Rescorla L: Late-emerging reading disabilities. J Educ Psychol 95:211-224, 2003.

85. Cornoldi C, DeBeni R, Pazzaglia F: Profiles of reading comprehension difficulties: An analysis of single cases. In Cornoldi C, Oakhill J, eds: Reading Comprehension Difficulties: Processes and Intervention. Mahwah, NJ: Erlbaum, 1996, pp 113-136.

86. Nation K, Clarke P, Marshall M, et al: Hidden language impairments in children: Parallels between poor reading comprehension and speech and language impairment? J Speech Lang Hear Res 47:199-211, 2004.

87. Cain K, Oakhill JV, Bryant P: Phonological skills and comprehension failures: A test of the phonological processing deficits hypothesis. Read Write 13:31-56, 2000.

88. Barnes MA, Dennis M: Reading comprehension deficits arise from diverse sources: Evidence from readers with and without developmental brain pathology. In

Cornoldi C, Oakhill J, eds: Reading Comprehension Difficulties. Hillsdale, NJ: Erlbaum, 1996, pp 251-278.

89. Nation K, Clarke P, Snowling MJ: General cognitive ability in children with poor reading comprehension. Br J Educ Psychol 72:549-560, 2002.

90. Fletcher JM, Lyon GR, Fuchs LS, et al: Learning Disabilities: From Identification to Intervention. New York: Guilford, 2006.

91. Shalev RS, Auerbach J, Manor O, et al: Developmental dyscalculia: Prevalence and prognosis. Eur Child Adolesc Psychiatry 9:58-64, 2000.

92. Fleishner JE: Diagnosis and assessment of mathematics learning disabilities. In Lyon GR, ed: Frames of Reference for the Assessment of Learning Disabilities: New Views on Measurement Issues. Baltimore: Paul H. Brookes, 1994, pp 441-458.

93. Rivera-Batiz FL: Quantitative literacy and the likelihood of employment among young adults in the United States. J Hum Resour 27:313-328, 1992.

94. Jordan NC, Hanich LB, Kaplan D: A longitudinal study of mathematical competencies in children with specific math difficulties versus children with comorbid mathematics and reading difficulties. Child Dev 74:834-850, 2003.

95. Butterworth B: What Counts: How Every Brain is Hardwired for Math. New York: Simon & Schuster, 1999.

96. Butterworth B: Developmental dyscalculia. In Campbell JID, ed: Handbook of Mathematical Cognition. New York: Psychology Press, 2005, pp 455-467.

97. Starkey P, Spelke ES, Gelman R: Numerical abstraction by human infants. Cognition 36:97-127, 1990.

98. Wynn K: Addition and subtraction by human infants. Nature 358:749-750, 1992.

99. Ginsberg HP, Klein A, Starkey P: The development of children's mathematical thinking: Connecting research with practice. In Siegel IE, Renninger KA, eds: Handbook of Child Psychology, vol 4: Child Psychology in Practice, 5th ed (Damon W, series ed). New York: Wiley, 1998, pp 401-476.

100. Gelman R, Butterworth B: Number and language: How are they related? Trends Cogn Sci 9:6-10, 2005.

101. Rourke BP: Arithmetic disabilities, specific and otherwise: A neuropsychological perspective. J Learn Disabil 26:214-226, 1993.

102. Geary DC, Hoard MK: Learning disabilities in arithmetic and mathematics: Theoretical and empirical perspectives. In Campbell JID, ed: Handbook of Mathematical Cognition. New York: Psychology Press, 2005, pp 253-267.

103. Ashcraft MH, Yamashita TS, Aram DM: Mathematics performance in left and right brain–lesioned children and adolescents. Brain Cogn 19:208-252, 1992.

104. Barnes MA, Wilkinson M, Khemani E, et al: Arithmetic processing in children with spina bifida: Calculation accuracy, strategy use, and fact retrieval fluency. J Learn Disabil 39:174-187, 2006.

105. Jordan NC, Hanich LB, Kaplan D: Arithmetic fact mastery in young children: A longitudinal investigation. J Exp Child Psychol 85:103-119, 2003.

106. Gersten RM, Jordan NC, Flojo JR: Early identification and interventions for students with mathematical difficulties. J Learn Disabil 38:293-304, 2005.

107. Geary DC, Hamson CO, Hoard MK: Numerical and arithmetical cognition: A longitudinal study of process and concept deficits in children with learning disability. J Exp Child Psychol 77:236-263, 2000.

108. Fuchs LS, Fuchs D: Mathematical problem-solving profiles of students with mathematics disabilities with and without co-morbid reading disabilities. J Learn Disabil 35:563-573, 2002.

109. Hanich L, Jordan N, Kaplan D, et al: Performance across different areas of mathematical cognition in children with learning difficulties. J Educ Psychol 93:615-626, 2001.

110. Gross-Tsur V, Manor O, Shalev RS: Developmental dyscalculia: Prevalence and demographic features. Dev Med Child Neurol 38:25-33, 1996.

111. Shalev RS, Manor O, Kerem B, et al: Developmental dyscalculia is a familial learning disability. J Learn Disabil 34:59-65, 2001.

112. Kovas Y, Harlaar N, Petrill SA, et al: "Generalist genes" and mathematics in 7-year-old twins. Intelligence 33:473-489, 2005.

113. Dehaene S, Spelke E, Pinel P, et al: Sources of mathematical thinking: Behavioral and brain-imaging evidence. Science 284:970-974, 1999.

114. Dehaene S, Piazza M, Pinel P, et al: Three parietal circuits for number processing. In Campbell JID, ed: Handbook of Mathematical Cognition. New York: Psychology Press, 2005, pp 433-453.

115. Torgesen JK, Alexander AW, Wagner RK, et al: Intensive remedial instruction for children with severe reading disabilities: Immediate and long-term outcomes from two instructional approaches. J Learn Disabil 34:33-58, 2001.

116. Torgesen JK: Lessons learned from research on interventions for students who have difficulty learning to read. In McCardle P, Chhabra V, eds: The Voice of Evidence in Reading Research. Baltimore: Paul H. Brookes, 2004, pp 355-382.

117. Brown AL, Campione J: Psychological theory and the study of learning disabilities. Am Psychol 41:14-21, 1986.

118. Lyon GR, Moats LC: Critical issues in the instruction of the leaning disabled. J Consult Clin Psychol 56:830-835, 1988.

119. Torgesen JK: Empirical and theoretical support for direct diagnosis of learning disabilities by assessment of intrinsic processing weaknesses. In Bradley R, Danielson L, Hallahan D, eds: Identification of Learning Disabilities: Research to Practice. Mahwah, NJ: Erlbaum, 2002, pp 565-650.

120. Reid DK, Hresko WP: A Cognitive Approach to Learning Disabilities. New York: McGraw-Hill, 1981.

121. Englert CS, Hiebert EH, Stewart SR: Spelling unfamiliar words by an analogy strategy. J Spec Educ 19:291-306, 1986.

122. Fuchs LS, Fuchs D, Hamlett CL, et al: Explicitly teaching for transfer: Effects on the mathematical problem

solving performance of students with disabilities. Learn Disabil Res Prac 17:90-106, 2002.

123. Graham S, Harris K: Addressing problems in attention, memory, and executive function. *In* Lyon GR Krasnegor NA, eds: Attention, Memory, and Executive Function. Baltimore: Paul H. Brookes, 1996, pp 349-366.

124. Palinscar AS, Brown DA: Enhancing instructional time through attention to metacognition. J Learn Disabil 20:66-75, 1987.

125. Vaughn S, Klingner JK: Teaching reading comprehension to students with learning disabilities: Instructional/intervention frameworks. *In* Stone CA, Silliman ER, Apel K, Ehren BJ, et al, eds: Handbook of Language and Literacy Development and Disorders. New York: Guilford, 2004.

126. Graham S, Harris KR: Students with learning disabilities and the process of writing: A meta-analysis of SRSD studies. *In* Swanson HL, Harris KR, Graham S, eds: Handbook of Learning Disabilities. New York: Guilford, 2003, pp 323-344.

127. Case LP, Harris KR, Graham S: Improving the mathematical problem-solving skills of students with learning disabilities: Self-regulated strategy development. J Spec Educ 26:1-19, 1992.

128. Hallahan DP, Kauffman J, Lloyd J: Introduction to Learning Disabilities. Needham Heights, MA: Allyn & Bacon, 1996.

129. Rosenshine B, Stevens R: Teaching functions. *In* Wittrock MC, ed: Handbook of Research on Teaching, 3rd ed. New York: Macmillan, 1986, pp 376-391.

130. Adams G, Carnine D: Direct instruction. *In* Swanson HL, Harris KR, Graham S, eds: Handbook of Learning Disabilities. New York: Guilford, 2003, pp 403-416.

131. Gersten RM, White WA, Falco R, et al: Teaching basic discriminations to handicapped and non-handicapped individuals through a dynamic presentation of instructional stimuli. Anal Interven Dev Disabil 2:305-317, 1982.

131a. Swanson HL: Interventions for students with Learning Disabilities. New York: Guilford, 1999.

132. Lovett MW, Lacerenza L, Borden SL, et al: Components of effective remediation for developmental reading disabilities: Combining phonological and strategy-based instruction to improve outcomes. J Educ Psychol 92:263-283, 2000.

133. Wilder AA, Williams JP: Students with severe learning disabilities can learn higher-order comprehension skills. J Educ Psychol 93:268-278, 2001.

134. Williams JP: Teaching text structure to improve reading comprehension. *In* Swanson HL, Harris KR, Graham S, eds: Handbook of Learning Disabilities. New York: Guilford, 2003, pp 293-305.

135. Williams JP, Brown LG, Silverman AK, et al: An instructional program for adolescents with learning disabilities in the comprehension of narrative themes. Learn Disabil Q 17:205-221, 1994.

136. Williams JP: Using the Theme Scheme to improve story comprehension. *In* Block CC, Pressley M, eds: Comprehension Instruction: Research-Based Best Practices. New York: Guilford, 2002, pp 126-139.

137. Fuchs LS, Fuchs D, Hamlett CL, et al: Class wide curriculum-based measurement: Helping general educators meet the challenge of student diversity. Except Child 60:518-537, 1994.

138. Fuchs LS, Fuchs D, Phillips CL, et al: General educators' specialized adaptation for students with learning disabilities. Except Child 61:440, 1995.

139. Fuchs LS, Fuchs D, Karns K: Enhancing kindergartners' mathematical development: Effects of peer-assisted learning strategies. Elem Sch J 101:494-510, 2001.

140. Fuchs LS, Fuchs D, Yazdian L, et al: Enhancing first-grade children's mathematical development with peer-assisted learning strategies. Sch Psychol Rev 31:569-584, 2002.

141. Jordan NC, Hanich LB: Mathematical thinking in second-grade children with different forms of LD. J Learn Disabil 33:567-578, 2000.

142. Fuchs LS, Fuchs D, Prentice K, et al: Enhancing third-grade students' mathematical problem solving with self-regulated learning strategies. J Educ Psychol 95:306-315, 2003.

143. Fuchs LS, Fuchs D, Prentice K, et al: Explicitly teaching for transfer: Effects on third-grade students' mathematical problem solving. J Educ Psychol 95:293-304, 2003.

144. Fuchs LS, Fuchs D, Prentice K, et al: Enhancing mathematical problem solving among third-grade students with schema-based instruction. J Educ Psychol 96:635-647, 2004.

145. Shaywitz SE, Fletcher JM, Holahan JM, et al: Persistence of dyslexia: The Connecticut Longitudinal Study at adolescence. Pediatrics 104:1351-1359, 1999.

146. Bruck M: Outcomes of adults with childhood histories of dyslexia. *In* Hume C, Joshi RM, eds: Reading and Spelling: Development and Disorders. Mahwah, NJ: Erlbaum, 1998, pp 179-200.

147. Gerber PJ, Price LA, Mulligan R, et al: Beyond transition: A comparison of the employment experiences of American and Canadian Adults with LD. J Learn Disabil 37:283-291, 2004.

148. Beitchman JH, Wilson B, Douglas L, et al: Substance use disorders in young adults with and without LD: Predictive and concurrent relationships. J Learn Disabil 34:317-332, 2001.

149. Tomblin JB, Zhang X, Buckwalter P, et al: The association of reading disability, behavioral disorders, and language impairment among second-grade children. J Child Psychol Psychiatry 41:473-482, 2000.

150. Wilkinson GS: The Wide Range Achievement Test, 3rd ed. New York: Academic Press, 1993.

151. Woodcock RW, McGrew KS, Mather N: Woodcock-Johnson III Tests of Achievement. Itasca, IL: Riverside, 2001.

152. Wechsler D: Wechsler Individual Achievement Test-II, 2nd ed. Examiner's Manual. San Antonio, TX: Psychological Corporation, 2001.

153. Gathercole SE, Pickering SJ: Working memory deficits in children with low achievements in the national curriculum at 7 years of age. Br J Educ Psychol 70:177-194, 2000.

154. Rabiner DL, Malone PS, and the Conduct Problems Prevention Research Group: The impact of tutoring on early reading achievement for children with and without attention problem. J Abnorm Child Psychol 32:273-284, 2004.

155. Tannock R, Lovett M, Martinussen R, et al: Intervention for ADHD with comorbid reading disorders: Combined modality approach (Abstract, p. 46). Scientific Proceedings of the 2005 Joint Annual Meeting of the American Academy of Child & Adolescent Psychiatry and the Canadian Academy of Child & Adolescent Psychiatry, Toronto, October 18-23, 2005.

156. Bishop DVM: Uncommon Understanding: Development and Disorders of Language Comprehension in Children. Hove, East Sussex, UK: Psychology Press, 1997.

157. Kavale KA, Forness SR: Social skills deficits and learning disabilities: A meta-analysis. J Learn Disabil 29:226-237, 1996.

158. Johnson DJ, Blalock J, eds: Adults with Learning Disabilities. Orlando, FL: Grune & Stratton, 1987.

159. Kellam SG, Rebok GW, Mayer LS, et al: Depressive symptoms over first grade and their response to a developmental epidemiologically based preventive trial aimed at improving achievement. Dev Psychopathol 6:463-481, 1994.

160. Litt J, Taylor HG, Klein N, et al: Learning disabilities in children with very low birthweight: Prevalence, neuropsychological correlates, and educational interventions. J Learn Disabil 38:130-141, 2005.

161. Barnes MA, Pengelly S, Dennis M, et al: Mathematics skills in good readers with hydrocephalus. J Int Neuropsychol Soc 8:72-82, 2002.

162. Mazzocco MMM, McCloskey M: Math performance in girls with Turner or fragile X syndrome. *In* Campbell JID, ed: Handbook of Mathematical Cognition. New York: Psychology Press, 2005, pp 269-297.

163. Barnes MA, Dennis M, Wilkinson M: Reading after closed head injury in childhood: Effects on decoding, fluency, and comprehension. Dev Neuropsychol 15:1-24, 1999.

164. Ewing-Cobbs L, Barnes MA, Fletcher JM, et al: Modeling of longitudinal academic achievement scores after pediatric traumatic brain injury. Dev Neuropsychol 25:107-134, 2004.

165. Barnes MA, Ewing-Cobbs L, Fletcher JM: Mathematical disabilities in congenital and acquired neurodevelopmental disorders. *In* Berch D, Mazzocco M, eds: New York: Brookes Publishing, in press.

166. Armstrong DF, Briery BG: Childhood cancer and the school. *In* Brown RT, ed: Handbook of Pediatric Psychology in School Settings. Mahwah, NJ: Erlbaum, 2004, pp 263-281.

167. Bonner MJ, Hardy KK, Elzell E, et al: Hematological disorders: Sickle cell disease and hemophilia. *In* Brown RT, ed: Handbook of Pediatric Psychology in School Settings. Mahwah, NJ: Erlbaum, 2004, pp 241-261.

168. The pediatrician's role in development and implementation of an Individual Education Plan (IEP) and/or an Individual Family Service Plan (IFSP). American Academy of Pediatrics. Committee on Children with Disabilities. Pediatrics 104:124-127, 1999.

169. American Academy of Pediatrics Committee on Children with Disabilities: The role of the pediatrician in transitioning children and adolescents with developmental disabilities and chronic illnesses from school to work or college. American Academy of Pediatrics. Committee on Children with Disabilities. Pediatrics 106:854-856, 2000.

Language and Speech Disorders

HEIDI M. FELDMAN ■ CHERYL MESSICK

Language and speech sound disorders are a heterogeneous group of conditions that limit age-appropriate understanding and/or production of symbolic human communication. Child language disorders are defined in large part by the components of the language system adversely affected (see Chapter 7D): vocabulary, morphology, syntax, semantics, pragmatics, or combinations of these components. Speech sound disorders are conditions in which speech sounds, fluency, and/or voice and resonance are abnormal. Further differentiation of these disorders is based on detailed analysis of the characteristics: (1) underlying cause, such as hearing impairment, cognitive deficits, or genetic syndromes, and (2) prognosis. Multiple components of language and speech may be affected in a single individual.

We discuss delays in early language development that may be precursors to language disorders. We then discuss several different language and speech disorders. Each section contains a description of the condition and a discussion of possible causes of the disorders, prognosis when known, and therapy or management strategies that are used for that condition. Important areas of research or clinical issues are highlighted in each section.

DEVELOPMENTAL DELAYS IN LANGUAGE AND SPEECH

Description

The rate of language and speech development during the toddler and preschool years varies across children. A child's communication may be considered delayed when it is noticeably poorer than that of age-matched peers. However, there is no consensus on the precise degree of delay that is clinically significant. The definition depends in large part on the purpose of categorization. In research studies, the criterion for language delay consists of (1) performance 2 standard deviations or more below the population mean in one component of speech or language or (2) performance of at least 1.5 standard deviations below the population mean in two or more components. In some states, a developmental delay of at least 25% in one or more domains of functioning renders the child eligible for early intervention services. According to this definition, a 24-month-old child who is functioning at the level of a child younger than 18 months of age in at least one aspect of language development can be considered to have a significant delay.

In children in the early phases of language and speech development, performance in vocabulary is typically correlated with performance in other components of language, such as syntax. Thus, in young children with a delay in one component, other components of language and speech are likely to be delayed. For example, children with slow expressive language development have small vocabularies and immature syntax. As children grow older and become more capable, language and speech components differentiate. One component of the communication system may be delayed or disordered without corresponding adverse effects in other components. For example, in preschool- or school-aged children with language impairment, vocabulary size may be appropriate but grammatical skills remain immature. Informal and formal assessments can be used to evaluate the status of the various language components to generate a comprehensive picture of communication strengths and weaknesses for the purposes of categorization of the disorder, treatment planning, and progress monitoring.

Prognosis

The term *delay* implies that children will eventually catch up with typically developing peers. In the case of language development, approximately half of the children who have language delay at age 2 years

467

eventually function in the normal range by the time they reach ages 3 to 4 years.[1,2] Research has not identified good predictors of which children with early delays are likely to continue to exhibit later language disorders. A favorable prognosis at early stages has been loosely associated with age-appropriate receptive language skills and symbolic play.[3] Of interest is that children with the most severe initial difficulties are not necessarily those whose language delays persist. More research is needed to learn more about predictors and risk factors for long-standing communication difficulties.

Delays during the preschool period that are severe and limit age-appropriate functioning in learning, communication, and social relatedness may warrant classification as a disorder. Children with persistent language problems at school entry are likely to continue to experience difficulties throughout childhood. At that age, persistent delays may be better conceptualized as language disorders. The prevalence of such disorders has been estimated to be as high as 16% to 22%.[5] However, other estimates at early school age are approximately 7% for language disorders and approximately 4% for speech disorders.[5] Some children whose early delays in language and speech apparently resolve during the preschool years demonstrate reading disorders at school age, which implies that the initial delay was indicative of a fundamental, although subtle, long-standing disorder.[6,7]

Cause

The precise cause of early delays in language or speech development is not known. A large study of same-sex twins in the United Kingdom revealed that early delays in language development had low heritability, which was suggestive of strong environmental influences, whereas persistent delays had high heritability, suggestive of strong genetic influences.[8] Consistent with these findings are studies demonstrating that the amount and type of parental input is positively correlated with rates of language development.[9,10] In addition, children with persistent language delays are likely to have family histories positive for language and speech disorders.[11,12] How environmental factors interact with genetic predisposition has not been elucidated.

Family members or professionals sometimes assume that clinically significant language delays in toddlers and young preschoolers are temporary because they are associated with one of three factors: the child is a boy, second or third born, or being raised in a bilingual environment. None of these is an adequate explanation for clinically significant delays, nor is any reliably associated with resolution of the delays. Studies document that boys develop language more slowly than girls do in the preschool period. However, the magnitude of the difference is approximately 1 to 2 months, below the threshold of clinical significance.[13] Boys are also more likely than girls to develop speech and language disorders and therefore should be evaluated promptly if clinically significant delays are identified. The research literature is inconsistent with regard to the effect of birth order on language development. Some studies reveal modest delays in the early stages of language development on particular measures or aspects of communication.[14,15] These weak effects have been attributed to environmental factors, such as the possibility that higher birth order results in reduced child-directed adult input and/or confusion because of three-way communication. If the degree of delay is substantial, then the prudent course of action is assessment.

Finally, being raised in a bilingual environment generally does not slow the process of language learning. Some investigators who compare bilingual children with monolingual children find that bilingual children have smaller vocabularies if only one of their two languages is assessed. However, the differences between bilingual and monolingual children disappear when the total vocabulary of the bilingual children—that is, the number of words in both languages—is compared with the single vocabulary of the monolingual children.[16] Early in development, children in bilingual environments may show language mixing or code switching, a tendency to use words from both languages in a single short sentence.[17] This language mixing occurs primarily when children do not know the target word in the language of the sentence. Differentiation of the two languages is facilitated when clear environmental cues are associated with each language, such as when one parent consistently uses one language and the other parent uses the other language or when the child reliably hears one language at home and the second language at school. Children from bilingual environments may show uneven skills in the two languages, depending on the amounts of exposure to each language. Bilingualism should be conceptualized as a continuum of proficiencies.[16] Children from bilingual households may also have language and speech disorders. Significant delays or deficits in the language of children in bilingual households may signal a possible language disorder, rather than a difference in communication skills related to bilingual input, and warrant evaluation.

Management

Because it is very difficult to predict accurately which children with delays in early language skills are destined to improve and which are likely to have language disorders, children with clinically significant delays are often referred for treatment. Children may qualify for federally funded early intervention services, particularly if the language delay is substantial or accompanied by other developmental delays. For children who do not qualify for early intervention, referral to a speech and language pathologist is advisable to determine whether treatment is warranted. Children whose rate of learning increases and who catch up with typically developing peers can be discharged from treatment; children whose rate of learning remains behind their peers will have had the benefit of early treatment.

Treatment of young children with language delays is generally based on a developmental model. The therapist assesses the child's developmental level and provides the child with many opportunities to learn structures typically acquired in the following level. The child receives opportunities to demonstrate comprehension and to model and use new structures in communication. Therapists may also offer feedback to move the child to the next level of functioning. Treatment for young children also typically incorporates parent training, focusing on helping the parents to learn language facilitation techniques. In most clinical settings, children have brief sessions with a speech and language pathologist on a weekly basis. Parent training increases the potential effect of the treatment.

LANGUAGE DISORDERS

A language disorder represents impairment in the ability to understand and/or use words in context. Language disorders take many forms. Children may produce or understand only a limited number of words, relying on words that occur frequently in the language or those that are easy to produce. They may demonstrate grammatical immaturities or irregularities in the way that they compose sentences or may fail to understand or accurately produce sentences with complex structures, such as passive voice or embedded clauses. They may exhibit poor understanding of the meaning of words, sentences, or connected discourse or may use words, sentences, and discourse in idiosyncratic ways. Finally, they may use unusual intonation patterns, fail to clearly distinguish questions from statements, or violate rules of polite conversation. Such problems can result in an inability to fully comprehend or express ideas. Language assessment can be used to confirm clinical impressions of a language disorder, specify the components of language affected, determine treatment approaches, and monitor progress during treatment (see Chapter 7D).

In some situations, an underlying cause of the language disorders may be discovered. The most likely causes are hearing loss, global cognitive impairment, autistic disorders, neurological injuries, and psychosocial disorders (child abuse, child neglect, or environmental deprivation). In children with no known cause of language impairments, specific language impairment (SLI) or simply language impairment is diagnosed. We discuss the effect of the potential causes on the patterns of language and communication and then describe characteristics of SLI (Table 13-1).

Known Causes of Language Disorders

HEARING LOSS

Sounds are described in terms of intensity (decibels), which is associated with the psychological experience of loudness, and frequency (Hertz), which is associated with the psychological experience of pitch. (See Chapter 10F for more detail on hearing impairments.) Normal conversation averages 40 to 60 dB in intensity and clusters in the range of 500 to 2000 Hz in frequency. Some speech sounds, including vowel sounds and consonants /m/, /n/, and /b/, are of low frequency and high intensity, and thus they are relatively easy to hear. Other sounds, such as consonants /s/, /f/, and /th/, are of high frequency and low intensity, and thus they are relatively hard to hear.

Hearing losses vary in terms of the threshold of hearing and the cause of the disorder. In mild hearing loss, the quietest sound that a person can hear with the better ear is 25 to 40 decibels loud. At this degree of loss, some of the high-frequency speech sounds may be difficult to detect and other sounds may be distorted. In moderate hearing loss, the quietest sound that a person can hear with the better ear is typically defined as 40 to 60 or 70 decibels, depending on the specific standards used. With this degree of hearing loss, many to all speech sounds in normal conversations are difficult to detect. A severe loss is defined by a hearing threshold of 70 to 90 decibels, and a profound loss is a lower hearing threshold of more than 90 decibels. At these levels, almost all conversational language cannot be perceived. Hearing loss may be caused by problems of the outer and middle ear (conductive), the inner ear (sensorineural), a combination of both, or the central auditory pathways. Conductive hearing loss may be temporary, as in the case of otitis media, whereas sensorineural loss is generally permanent.

Language and speech development in children with hearing impairment depends on many factors, including the degree of hearing loss (mild, moderate, severe, or profound), whether the loss is unilateral or

TABLE 13-1 ■ Description, Management Strategies, and Prognosis of Selected Language Disorders

Condition	Description	Management	Prognosis
Developmental delay	Slow rate of development	Many therapeutic approaches associated with improvement	About half of delayed 2-year olds catch up by age 4 years Longer delays indicate higher likelihood that disorder will persist at school age
Hearing loss	Speech problems with mild to profound loss Language problem may occur with mild to moderate loss Speech and language problems with severe to profound loss	Amplification for mild to profound loss Cochlear implantation for bilateral severe and profound loss Decision about modality of communication for persistent severe language problems	Depends on age at onset, success of amplification, consistent use of amplification, and success of cochlear implantation
Cognitive impairment	Vocabulary and syntax typically more affected than are pragmatic skills	Increased language stimulation Improvements in environment	Depends on degree of impairment and other factors
Specific genetic and chromosomal disorders			
Down syndrome	Verbal skills delayed more than cognitive skills; speech and language difficulties	Early introduction of signs	Persistent vulnerabilities of syntax
Fragile X syndrome	Rapid bursts; phonological disorders, frequent echolalia; poor pragmatic skills	Speech & language treatment to increase communication effectiveness & improve pragmatic skills	—
Williams syndrome	Early delays in language development; limited comprehension	Early speech and language therapy Continued attention to comprehension, discourse, abstract language	Language and social skills are often areas of relative strength
Autism	Pragmatic & comprehension skills affected more than expressive vocabulary and grammar	Discrete trial learning Emphasis on social communication	Highly variable but good outcome associated with early and intense treatment Pragmatic skills, including intonation, may not normalize Prognosis influenced by cognitive level with children with stronger cognitive skills having a better outcome than those with limited cognitive abilities
Neurological disorders			
Hydrocephalus	Good vocabulary, appropriate syntax, well-articulated speech; verbose and superficial in conversation; poor pragmatic skills	Treatment for social communication	Highly variable
Landau-Kleffner seizure disorder	Abrupt disruption of language functioning in child with normal language development	Treatment of underlying seizure disorder Speech and language therapy	Seizures usually controlled with medication; variable outcomes for cognition and language
Disorders caused by child abuse and neglect	Low cognitive, receptive, and expressive language scores	Safe and nurturing environment Speech and language therapy	Highly variable
Specific language impairment	Persistent delays; gradual improvements May show deficits in receptive &/or expressive language. May have deficits in one or more components of language (e.g., phonology, syntax, morphology)	Speech and language therapy	Improvements in vocabulary and pragmatics Residual problems may be seen in syntax Language may improve and reading disorders emerge

bilateral, the age at identification, the age at receiving amplification, and the consistency of use of amplification. Since the late 1990s, most states in the United States have adopted universal neonatal hearing screening.[18,19] As a result of these policies, many cases of sensorineural hearing loss are detected in the neonatal period. The current public health standard in most states is for these children to receive amplification by 6 months of age, a dramatic improvement over the era when hearing loss was often not detected until language delays were identified at ages 2 to 3 years. An intriguing research questions is whether introduction of this public policy will result in better language and speech outcomes for children with hearing loss.

Another major advance in clinical practice for children with bilateral severe to profound hearing loss is cochlear implantation, the use of a prosthetic device to allow perception of the auditory signal. Cochlear implantation changes the prognosis for speech and language skills in many children with hearing loss, although factors such as the age at implantation and the quality of environmental input after implantation are relevant to outcomes (see Chapter 10F for more detail on hearing impairments).[20] For children with severe to profound hearing loss who are not candidates for cochlear implantation, whose parents have elected not to give them cochlear implants, or for whom cochlear implantation has not produced successful outcomes, the decision about the type of communication—oral, total communication (sign language plus verbal language), or sign language—must be made.

Children with mild to moderate hearing loss have variable outcomes in terms of language. Some have normal vocabulary skills, demonstrate sentence comprehension, and achieve literacy, whereas others have difficulty with multiple aspects of language.[21] In addition to the variables related to treatment of the hearing loss, the degree of hearing loss, the child's success at phonological discrimination, and the child's phonological memory are related to his or her language skills.[21] Children with mild to moderate sensorineural hearing loss are likely to have a speech disorder (described later in this chapter).[21]

Research on the effect of recurrent or chronic otitis media on language development has yielded conflicting results. Association studies reveal that children with fluctuating conductive hearing loss from otitis media with effusion have language and speech disorders.[22] However, prospective studies find that these associations are short-lived or caused by other factors, including the quality of the language environment.[23,24] In addition, randomized clinical trials of tympanostomy tubes for persistent middle ear effusion have not revealed that prompt tube insertion improves the outcomes for language or speech in comparison with delayed or no tube insertion. These results suggest that the associations of otitis media and unfavorable outcomes may have been spurious or that both conditions are related to common underlying factors.[25]

In terms of treatment, children with mild to profound hearing loss should be given a trial of amplification as soon as the loss is detected. Speech and language therapy is indicated for children with hearing loss in association with language or speech impairment. Children with hearing loss may require more exposure than do children with normal hearing to learn vocabulary, grammatical structures, and other aspects of language. Speech therapy for such children usually incorporates visual feedback systems. This method assists children in learning sound differentiations (such as /p/ vs. /b/ or /a/ vs./u/) that they have difficulty perceiving with their hearing loss.

COGNITIVE IMPAIRMENT

Developmental delays in language learning are often the presenting complaint for children with mild to moderate cognitive impairment. Language skills represent the earliest milestones closely tied to cognitive skills. If cognitive delays persist and affect adaptive behaviors as these children get older, they may receive a diagnosis of mental retardation. The severity of cognitive impairment and adaptive behavior is described in terms of levels of mental retardation: mild, moderate, severe, and profound.

The profile of children with mild cognitive impairment is typically a normal progression at a slow developmental rate. In terms of language development, both vocabulary and grammar are typically affected. Pragmatic skills may be preserved. Mild mental retardation in many cases is caused by a combination of biological and environmental factors. Parents of children with mild mental retardation as a group have intelligence quotients below the population mean, which is suggestive of a genetic contribution. In addition, these parents may be challenged in setting up a stimulating home environment. Early intervention services are for children with mild cognitive impairment or mild mental retardation help them by improving the quantity and quality of language input to those children. Some early intervention programs focus on providing support to parents in increasing the level of stimulation in the home. Other programs provide children with enriching environments outside the home.

Moderate, severe, and profound mental retardation are often associated with a single biological cause, such as genetic disorders, metabolic diseases, or neural malformation. With treatment services language skills can be improved; however, the prognosis for language skills is less favorable than in mild retardation. Social interactions with typically developing peers and speech and language therapy may also improve functional communication. Some chromosomal and genetic conditions that are associated with cognitive impairment are also associated with distinctive behavioral phenotypes in terms of language.

Down Syndrome

Down syndrome results from an extra copy of chromosome 21, usually manifested as a trisomy. Children with Down syndrome, whose cognitive impairment is often at the mild to moderate level of mental retardation, display more significant delays in the early phases of language development than would be predicted on the basis of their cognitive abilities or mental age.[26] The rate of language development in children with Down syndrome is often uneven, with long periods of plateau followed by spurts of change. In general, expressive skills are more severely affected than receptive skills.[27] As the children with Down syndrome grow older, receptive language and vocabulary knowledge often approach the level of nonverbal intelligence. However, children with Down syndrome have a particular vulnerability in the acquisition of grammar. For example, the mean length of sentences is shorter than what would be predicted on the basis of their mental age. The proportion of verbs is lower than expected for vocabulary size, and the children have difficulty including morphemes, such as a plural "-s" or past tense "-ed." In addition to language deficits, some children with Down syndrome also have deficits in speech skills. Even during the late school-age years and adulthood, their speech may be very unintelligible or characterized by dysfluent speech patterns.[28]

The reason for the language phenotype in children with Down syndrome is largely unknown. Although many children with Down syndrome have mild to moderate conductive or mixed conductive-sensorineural hearing losses, hearing loss contributes only a small amount to the variance in language abilities.[29] Parental language directed toward children with Down syndrome differs in some ways from that directed toward children developing typically, even those matched for language level. However, this factor alone does not explain the expressive language delays and speech dysfluency. Auditory and verbal memory deficits may also contribute to the language disorder in children with Down syndrome,[29] although such deficits may actually be the result of the language disorder. The language of children with Down syndrome resembles the language of children with SLI, described later. One interesting theoretical possibility that must be investigated in future research is whether the cause of the language disturbance in both clinical populations is related.[26]

From a clinical perspective, children with Down syndrome should be enrolled as early as possible in early intervention services. Because of the delayed development of expressive language and because of the frustration and behavioral problems that sometimes result, early intervention for many children with Down syndrome includes exposure to manual signs, as well as verbal language.[30] The goal is to launch a process of communication from which verbal language can develop. Typically developing children use brief actions associated with objects as gestural labels shortly before they express their first words, which suggests that the manual modality may be easier to comprehend or learn than the verbal modality.[31] The long-term effect of this educational strategy has not been well studied.

Fragile X Syndrome

The fragile X syndrome is a genetic syndrome caused by a trinucleotide repeat on the X-chromosome, with a resulting cascade of abnormal processes. The fragile X syndrome is associated with cognitive impairment in boys and girls. However, the cognitive and social impairment is generally more severe in boys than in girls. Boys with the fragile X syndrome also have a distinctive language profile. At a young age, the first signs of impending language difficulties include oral hypotonicity, poor sucking and chewing, and lack of control of saliva. Development of expressive language and emergence of phrase-level communication are also delayed.[32] Boys with the fragile X syndrome learn to speak late, although their vocabulary and grammatical skills eventually appear to be consistent with their level of nonverbal intelligence. The rate and rhythm of language are characterized by frequent rapid bursts. Affected children also show accompanying phonological disorders.[33] Therefore, their communication is frequently unintelligible to unfamiliar listeners. Boys with the fragile X syndrome also demonstrate echolalia, or repetition of words. The perseveration of the words or sounds at the end of sentences, called *palilalia,* can become so dramatic that they cannot complete sentences.[34]

Another characteristic feature of boys with the fragile X syndrome is poor pragmatic skills.[34] They are likely either to talk incessantly about a topic, unaware of the effect of the narrow conversational focus on the listener, or to show difficulties maintaining topic, introducing tangential topics into the conversation. Their conversation is often highly repetitive. These language problems are most dramatic in situations in which the child must make eye contact with the listener or when the child becomes anxious. From the theoretical perspective, research on why boys with the fragile X syndrome exhibit this constellation of findings must be investigated. From a clinical perspective, treatment of boys with the fragile X syndrome, like treatment of autism, focuses on improving the communication functions of language. However, more research into the efficacy and effectiveness of such treatment is necessary.

Williams Syndrome

Williams syndrome is a genetic condition caused by a deletion on chromosome 7 that is associated with moderate mental retardation; however, affected children show better expressive language skills than would be expected from their cognitive abilities. Language disorders, although also present in other genetic disorders, are not an inevitable feature of mild to moderate mental retardation. Of interest is that children with Williams syndrome may be quite delayed initially in language abilities at a young age and indistinguishable behaviorally from children with Down syndrome, but they use different communication strategies.[35] As they develop, language and social skills develop at a faster rate than visual-spatial skills.[36] The factors that allow this rapid language development after initial delays are not yet understood. From a clinical perspective, detailed assessment of language and speech in children with Williams syndrome is warranted early in life because of significant delays and differences in their developmental course. If children develop strong verbal skills as they get older, continued therapy may be advisable because their fluent language skills may mask problems with comprehension of sentences and discourse and with comprehension and use of abstract language concepts. Because expressive language abilities represent a relative strength, these children should be supported so that as adolescents and young adults, they can use these strengths for obtaining employment and participating fully in community life.

AUTISM SPECTRUM DISORDERS

Autism is a severe neurobehavioral disorder, defined in terms of a triad of behavioral symptoms: qualitative impairment of social interaction; qualitative impairments in communication; and restricted, repetitive, and/or stereotyped patterns of behavior, interests, and activities (see Chapter 15 for more information). Diagnoses of autism are increasing in prevalence, in part because of changing definitions of the disorder.[37] Accordingly, autism is in clinical practice becoming more frequently used as the explanation for language delays in children in the first 3 years of life and children with autism are becoming a larger proportion of the case load of speech/language pathologists. Autism should be considered in children with language delays or regression in the language and social domains.

Autism is currently conceptualized as a spectrum disorder.[38,39] In the most severe cases, children totally lack a means of communication, whether verbal language, sign language, or gestures. They communicate rarely and nonsymbolically. For example, they might drag a parent to a desired object and whine or cry until the parent figures out what they want. These children may eventually learn rudimentary language, but they tend to use their communicative abilities predominantly to meet their needs and wants instead of to participate in social exchanges. They do not, in the most severe manifestation, describe or comment on objects or events that have drawn their attention. This limitation has been described as a lack of joint attention. Failure of joint attention not only characterizes children with autism but can also be a prognostic indicator and a potential intervention goal.[40]

In moderately severe cases, children with autism may exhibit limited vocabulary and grammar skills; poor pragmatic skills; and stereotyped, repetitive, or idiosyncratic uses of language. In mild cases, affected children may display an inability to initiate or sustain a conversation and to participate in social exchanges with other people. The communication pattern of children with autism can be described as talking at rather than with others. Like boys with the fragile X syndrome, children with Asperger disorder, a condition on the mild end of the autistic spectrum, may talk incessantly about a topic despite attempts by others to interject comments or change the topic. They also need to be prompted to answer questions, because of their tendency to steer the conversation toward their obsessive topic of interest. These language and communication features further compromise the poor social abilities of individuals with autism and limit their ability to develop friendships.

The prognosis for language and communication for children with autism is evolving as the definition of the disorder is broadened and intensive early intervention services are provided for affected children. Some children with autism develop functional communication skills. However, even in adults with autism who have become successful communicators, pragmatic skills typically remain underdeveloped. For example, adults with autism have difficulty understanding humor or metaphor. They continue to have problems interpreting the language and social cues of their listener and modifying the topics of communication accordingly. Intonation patterns remain relatively flat or unchanging.

Prognosis has been shown to improve for children who, early in life, receive structured treatments based on the principles of applied behavioral analysis.[41] For children with moderate to severe autism, discrete trial learning is one such approach that has been used successfully as an initial strategy to promote language learning and self-help skills. The method is predicated on the observations that children with autism are poor at observational or social learning and cannot reliably differentiate important from background information. Therefore, the method breaks down complex tasks, such as understanding natural language, into short, uncomplicated activities or trials and provides tangible rewards for successful completion of a task. As the child progresses in terms of receptive and expressive communication, language expectations increase. Another teaching approache focuses on social interactions rather than on behavioral approaches to language development. A third approach utilizes picture symbols to foster communication, capitalizing on the strengths on the visual domain. Treatment features associated with favorable outcomes include intensive involvement, integrating communication goals with social and communication skills, programming for generalization, and integration with typical peers whenever possible.[42] However, more research is needed because social communication approaches have not been subjected to careful, large-scale evaluations.

NEUROLOGICAL CONDITIONS

Disorders of language and speech may be present in association with neurological conditions. Neurological disorders are typically diagnosed on the basis of abnormal physical findings, such as large head circumference or asymmetrical limb tone. Delays in language learning are an associated finding but rarely the presenting complaint in children with neurological illnesses or injuries. Nonetheless, distinctive patterns of language use have been associated with some neurological conditions.

Hydrocephalus

Hydrocephalus, or hydrocephaly, is a condition in which there is an abnormal accumulation of the cerebrospinal fluid, the watery element in and around the brain. Hydrocephalus develops for many reasons, may occur in isolation or in association with other disorders such as myelomeningocele, and may be present at or near birth or may develop as children age. It is usually suspected on the basis of enlarged head circumference and confirmed in neural imaging studies. Language and speech development of children with early hydrocephalus may be impaired as a function of sensory or neurological factors.[43] Many children with favorable outcomes of congenital or early-onset hydrocephalus develop diverse vocabularies, appropriate syntax, and well-articulated speech. However, in conversation, they are often verbose and the content of speech is superficial or repetitive. These character-

istics have been summarized as "cocktail party speech" to emphasize the impoverished content and cursory treatment of concepts in their conversation. They may also show impairments in processes important for understanding the meaning of discourse. For example, they may have difficulty in understanding abstract terms and figurative language, such as idioms. They may be weak at drawing inferences from facts presented. Thus, their language difficulties are generally in the realms of semantics and pragmatics.[43] Their profile is in some ways similar to that of children with Williams syndrome, and the treatment approaches are therefore also similar. In addition, some children with hydrocephalus have language-related academic difficulties, including difficulty with reading comprehension, despite average intelligence.[43]

Seizure Disorders

Specific seizure disorders have been associated with language disorders. It is unclear whether these are distinct disorders or related conditions. Landau-Kleffner syndrome is a rare acquired seizure disorder that manifests with an abrupt disruption of language functioning in a child who had previously exhibited normal language development. The language disorder is a severe, receptive language disorder that has been called *acquired verbal agnosia* to emphasize the poor comprehension abilities of affected children. Imaging studies typically show no clear abnormality, and the electroencephalographic (EEG) abnormalities vary.[44] Although the prognosis for seizures is generally favorable, the long-term outcomes of cognition and language are highly variable. Clearly more research on this condition is necessary.

Electrical status epilepticus in slow-wave sleep, also known as *continuous spike and wave in slow-wave sleep,* is another related and rare acquired seizure disorder that affects cognitive and language functioning.[44] Most of the children affected were previously normal, although about one third had previous neurological conditions. Age at onset is typically between 5 and 7 years. Atrophy and neural injuries are more likely to be observed on imaging studies of the brain than in Landau-Kleffner syndrome. Language abnormalities may be accompanied by memory disturbances and behavioral disorders of varying severity.

Some children with autism show regression in language, social relatedness, and behavior in association with a seizure or epileptiform EEG pattern. Abnormal EEG findings are also observed in children with autism who have not exhibited regression. Therefore, it is difficult to relate the language disturbance specifically to EEG abnormalities.[44]

Traumatic Brain Injury

Traumatic brain injury in children is very likely to manifest persistent but variable characteristics, caused by multiple factors, including the severity and location of injury. The features of communication also evolve in the period after injury, in association with additional factors such as the age at injury and the socioeconomic factors of the family. Among children with severe injury, even those who show good recovery of language skills may be left with subtle changes in speech.

Acquired Focal Left Hemisphere Injuries

Children and adults with these injuries may show disturbances in language functioning. Aphasia, a severe acquired language disorder, is associated with left hemisphere injury in about 95% of cases in adults. On this basis, it has been generally accepted that the left hemisphere is the neural substrate for language in most mature language users. Of interest is that children with congenital injuries to the left hemisphere typically do not develop aphasia.[45] Indeed, their language and speech skills are only mildly delayed in development and subtly different at older ages. Functional imaging studies of children with congenital left hemisphere injury performing language tasks typically show more activation in the right hemisphere than what is found in children developing typically.[46] These findings demonstrate the plasticity of the nervous system for language and speech when neurological injury occurs in early childhood.

CHILD ABUSE AND NEGLECT

Children who have been maltreated are at substantial risk for language delays and deficits. Children who experience physical abuse achieve substantially lower cognitive, receptive language, and expressive language scores on formal measures than do well-matched uninjured controls. Children who experienced neglect without physical abuse are indistinguishable from those who experienced only physical abuse.[47] Functional communication deficits in these children are less severe and noticeable than indicated by formal test results or analysis of conversational samples, which suggests that functional assessment measures may be insensitive in this clinical area and should be supported or supplemented by standardized measures of language.

A likely explanation for the findings in children with abuse and neglect is the poor quantity and quality of child-directed verbal language in their environment. In children developing typically and children at high social risk, differences in maternal talkativeness account for a significant proportion of the variance in the rate of vocabulary growth.[10] Similarly, the diversity of syntactic structures and the use of polite language, which is associated with longer sentences and placement of auxiliary verbs in noticeable positions at the start of sentences, are associated

with the rate of syntactic growth.[9] Some children with abuse and/or neglect may have suffered previous neural injuries, which would further contribute to developmental delays and ultimate disorders.

BEHAVIOR DISORDERS

More than half of children with persistent communication disorders develop behavioral disorders and social-emotional problems. In addition, the number of children who have social-emotional and communication deficits increases as language disorders develop across the school-age period.[48] Therefore, longitudinal follow-up of such children should include monitoring of the behavioral and emotional status. In addition, many children with behavior disorders have subtle communication difficulties, including poor comprehension and poor expression. In many cases, the communication deficits remain undiagnosed. These children may experience frustration, limited coping skills, and poor self-esteem as a function of these communication difficulties. They may struggle to interact appropriately with peers, family members, and professionals. In some cases, the communication difficulties may actually be expressed as behavioral disturbances or may exaggerate other negative behavioral characteristics. An important issue for children with behavioral disorders is early and appropriate evaluation of communication and referral for services when needed. Professionals in the mental health arena must collaborate actively with speech and language pathologists, educators, and other support staff to create an integrated and effective treatment program.

Speech and language treatment with these children with behavior disorders often focuses heavily on pragmatic skills, as well as receptive and expressive vocabulary.[49,50] Treatment incorporating emotional vocabulary for expressing feelings, improving listening skills, and using self-talk to help with self-regulation[51] can occur through collaborative exchanges between the professionals providing speech and language treatment and psychological counseling with these children.

Specific Language Impairment

Specific language impairment (SLI), also known as *language impairment,* is the term used for children with language deficits who meet the following criteria: normal nonverbal intelligence; normal hearing; normal neurological functioning, and normal structure and functioning of the oral mechanism. Although SLI is a heterogeneous disorder, most affected children have greater difficulty with expressive skills than with receptive skills. In fact, children with both receptive and expressive impairment are more severely affected than those with an isolated expressive disorder. Grammatical Skills (including syntax and morphology) are the most vulnerable part of the language system, although the precise grammatical structures that are most vulnerable vary across languages. Some affected children also have difficulty producing speech sounds.[11] The prevalence of SLI is 5% to 7% of children entering school.[5] The high rates of SLI in families suggest that genetic mechanisms are important.

The underlying processing mechanisms that give rise to SLI are not completely understood. There may be multiple causes and risk factors. In addition to the language issues, some children with SLI have difficulty identifying and discriminating speech sounds. One major theory is that the language deficits are secondary to more fundamental auditory perceptual processes that affect both nonlinguistic and linguistic stimuli.[52] A related theory is that these children have difficulty in processing rapid or brief stimuli, whether in the auditory or other sensory systems.[53] The results of this processing issue would be most dramatic in speech because discriminations require perception of multiple and rapidly changing stimuli. Results of electrophysiological and functional neuroimaging studies of auditory perception in humans have suggested that two pathways arise from the primary auditory cortex: a ventral stream, which is involved in mapping sound onto meaning, and a dorsal stream, which is involved in mapping sound onto articulation-based representations.[54] The ventral stream projects toward the inferior posterior temporal cortex and ultimately links to widely distributed conceptual representations. The dorsal stream connects posteriorly via the inferior parietal lobe or Wernicke's area and ultimately to the frontal lobes, including Broca's area. Each pathway is sensitive to different characteristics of the signal and different modes of processing. Differences in the relative balance of information processing between them may explain some of the phenomena of SLI. Most children with SLI show gradual improvement with speech, language treatment, however, language processing, reading, and writing remain areas of relative weakness as they age.

GENERAL ISSUES IN MANAGEMENT OF LANGUAGE DISORDERS

The treatment for language disorders is predicated largely on the child's language profile and level of communication rather than on cause. Children with language disorders generally benefit from therapy with a speech and language pathologist. A major focus of the therapy is to create an optimal language learning environment, capitalizing on the importance of environmental stimulation to the process of language learning. The speech and language pathologist may also focus on specific areas of deficit, such as teaching the grammatical structures, increasing

vocabulary diversity, or lengthening conversations. The techniques can involve direct engagement with the child and also coaching for parents and teachers.

Intervention with young children typically includes teaching family members how to stimulate language development so that family members can then replicate the techniques within the home. At school age, collaboration of the speech–language pathologist and classroom teachers is important to prove methods for facilitating the language skill necessary for academic performance and to continue the use of strategies used in therapy in the classroom.

Speech–language therapy for young children entails the use of techniques to facilitate learning. For example, the child may be asked to demonstrate comprehension or to produce a target structure in appropriate contexts. Modeling and imitation are other useful strategies. Drill work may be initially used to teach structures, followed by opportunities to use the structures in conversational exchanges in the clinic and in other environments (i.e., classroom, playground, and home) to increase the likelihood that the child will generalize new abilities to everyday situations. In contrast, the focus in language treatment for school-aged children shifts to developing language skills necessary to be successful in the educational setting. For example, the speech–language pathologist may work collaboratively with the classroom teacher to teach the child new vocabulary concepts that will be introduced in an upcoming curricular unit. For children with pragmatic skill deficits, social communication skills can be taught through peer interaction or peer modeling.

The outcome of therapy is highly variable. Children with mild to moderate disorders are more likely to improve than are those with severe disorders. There is currently little evidence of which treatment strategies are the most effective for which types of language disorders. It is known, however, that children who participate in speech-language treatment show better improvement than children who have no treatment.

SPEECH SOUND DISORDERS

A speech sound disorder represents impairment in the ability to produce the sounds of the words of the language. The primary symptom of speech impairment is unintelligible speech. Speech disorders are alternatively described in terms of the characteristics of the speech sound errors or the cause of the problem. Speech disorders include problems with articulating sounds, using speech rules (phonological rules), or planning and executing speech sounds. The overall prevalence of such disorders is approximately 4%

among 6-year-old children.[5] Up to approximately 15% of children with persisting speech delay have evidence of SLI, and up to 8% of children with persisting SLI have speech delays.[5] Children with speech sound disorders may also have disorders of voice and resonance or dysfluent speech.

Some speech sound disorders are the result of hearing loss; anatomical abnormalities, such as cleft palate or velopharyngeal insufficiency; or neuromotor disorders. However, in many cases, an underlying cause of the speech sound disorder cannot be identified. *Functional articulation disorder* is the term for when a child's speech fails to mature at the rate of that of age-matched peers for no apparent reason. The nature of the speech sound disorder is determined by the characteristics of the child's speech errors and his or her ability to rapidly move the mouth for nonspeech movements, as well as syllable sequences. The nature of the speech sound disorder affects the treatment process and the prognosis for improvement (Table 13-2).

Articulation Disorders

The inability to produce sounds correctly in speech is referred to as an *articulation disorder.* Children with articulation disorders typically exhibit errors on a small subset of sounds (e.g., /r/, /l/, /s/). In most cases, there is no known cause of an articulation disorder, and they are thus presumed to be the result of mistaken learning. In an articulation error, the child is unable to produce the sound correctly in all contexts (i.e., at the beginning, middle, or end of a word). Children with articulation disorders typically have mild to moderate deficits in speech intelligibility. Their difficulties may be identified as early as the preschool years or not until elementary school age.

One known cause of articulation disorders is permanent bilateral mild to moderate hearing loss. In mild hearing loss in general, the speech sounds most difficult to detect are those of relatively high frequency (2000 to 4000 Hz) and low energy (20 to 30 dB). These sounds, including /s/, /f/, and /th/ as in *thin,* are late-developing sounds in children developing typically. Because high-frequency hearing loss is more prevalent than low-frequency loss, these sounds are difficult to discriminate and to produce by individuals with mild hearing loss. Children with mild hearing loss may benefit considerably from amplification with hearing aids. They may also benefit from speech therapy to correct inaccurate speech sound productions. Children with severe to profound hearing losses have severe speech sound errors and language deficits and also show resonance difficulties characterized by hypernasal speech patterns.

Treatment for articulation disorders is based on a behavioral model. Techniques include rewarding successive approximations toward accurate production, modeling, imitation, and reinforcement. Additional strategies to establish a new sound include phonetic placement cues (e.g., "Put your tongue tip behind your front teeth" to elicit a /t/ or /d/), mirror work (providing the opportunity for the child to see how the sound is produced), and labeling the sound with its descriptive name (e.g., "make the snake sound" for /s/). Treatment progresses from simple linguistic units, such as syllables, to more complex linguistic units, such as phrases and sentences. The goal is always improvements in functional communication. Children and adults with speech disorders often experience embarrassment and poor self-esteem. Therapy is designed to reduce the negative psychological consequences of the disorder, as well as to provide direct remediation.

TABLE 13-2 ■ Description, Management Strategies, and Prognosis of Selected Speech Disorders			
Condition	Description	Management	Prognosis
Articulation disorders	Errors in a subset of sounds	Behavioral models of speech therapy	Good for normalization
Phonological disorders	Errors based on implicit rules of sound production and co-occurrence	Teaching that sound changes alter meaning	Good, but not as good as for articulation disorders
Cleft palate	Severe speech problems; maybe language problems; hypernasal speech	Surgical repair, retraining of idiosyncratic articulation processes	Fair
Hearing loss	Depends on degree of loss	Visual cuing for sounds	Highly variable
Childhood apraxia of speech	Severe speech delay followed by inconsistent production of phonemes; decreasing accuracy with increasing rate or word length	Intensive treatment, drill-based approach	Improvements in speech; maybe residual problems in speech, language comprehension, cognition, and academic skills

Phonological Disorders

Phonological errors occur when a child's speech errors are based on patterns or implicit rules, despite the ability to produce those same sounds correctly in other contexts. One example of a phonological disorder is final consonant deletion. A child may be able to say the consonant /g/ in *go,* /d/ in *doll,* and /b/ in *Ben* and yet says *pi* for *pig, fee* for *feed,* and *tuh* for *tub;* despite the ability to produce the sound at the beginning of the word, the child does not put the same consonants on the end of the word. Phonological disorders result from applying an incorrect rule (e.g., "it is permissible to drop the last sound of a word"), not an inability to produce the sound correctly. Most commonly, the child continues to use a rule that was age appropriate at an earlier time. In some situations, they produce rule-based errors that are atypical of normal development (e.g., deletion of initial consonants). Children with phonological errors typically have moderate to severe deficits in speech skills, which significantly affect their overall intelligibility and communication effectiveness. Some of these children have co-occurring deficits in language skills (receptive and/or expressive language), whereas others have normal language skills.

Treatment of phonological disorders focuses on teaching the child that differences in meaning are conveyed by changes in sound production. Minimal contrast word pairs are used to demonstrate the role of sound in meaning. For example, to treat the rule of final consonant deletion, the speech-language pathologist may engage the child in an activity in which use of the final consonant results in a specific outcome. Minimal contrast word pairs, such as "bow" versus "boat," "toe" versus "toad," and "tea" versus "team," would be incorporated in a game with pictures of these items where the child must say the words with an ending sounds in order to win. In children with severe phonological disorders, 29 treatment sessions, on average, have been shown to have a significant effect on their intelligibility.[55]

Children with cleft palate are at extremely high risk for phonological disorders, as well as language deficits. Cleft palate may occur in isolation, in conjunction with cleft lip, or in association with other structural and functional abnormalities. Cleft lip may be part of a genetic syndrome, such as velocardiofacial syndrome (deletion 22q11.2), which has a specific behavioral phenotype.[56] The outcome of cleft palate depends on the cause and the constellation of coexisting problems. In general, even after early and appropriate repair of an isolated cleft palate, the children remain at risk for problems in speech sound skills. The main problem for these children is that the velopharyngeal structures function abnormally, which results in an inability to generate intraoral air pressure for the production of consonants. Air tends to escape through the nose, which causes what is known as hypernasal speech. Moreover, children with cleft palate often have almost continuous otitis media with effusion and may experience mild to moderate conductive hearing loss. Therefore, the care of children with cleft palate usually requires an interdisciplinary team that includes audiologists and speech-language pathologists, as well as surgeons, dentists, and general pediatricians. Children with cleft lip and/or palate often exhibit unusual or idiosyncratic patterns of articulation, even when they have had surgery at a young age on the palate. For example, they may only produce consonants made in the back of the mouth (e.g., /k/, /g/, /u/) or may use consonants that do not appear in the English language (e.g., pharyngeal fricatives and nasal snorts).

Of importance is that some children experience the soft palate making adequate contact with the oropharyngeal wall during speech, a condition known as *velopharyngeal insufficiency.*[57] These children are at risk for speech sound disorders similar to those of children with cleft palate. The velum is supported in early childhood by the adenoids. As the adenoids shrink with age, the speech disorder may become more obvious. This speech problem is not amenable to the usual articulation therapy and may necessitate surgical correction. In addition, adenoidectomy might exacerbate speech problems in children with velopharyngeal insufficiency. For that reason, otolaryngologists should avoid adenoidectomy in children who have had a cleft palate repair, have a submucous cleft, or have hypernasal speech, which is suggestive of velopharyngeal insufficiency.

Dysarthria

Dysarthria is a speech disorder associated with neuromotor disorders or dysfunction. For example, children with cerebral palsy may have dysarthria. High muscle tone, poor coordination of motor movements, and dyscoordination of respiration and sound production result in slow muscular adjustments and limited range of motion. Dysarthric speech has a slurred and strained quality, often affecting not only the accuracy of speech sound production but also rate, pitch, and intonation. Velopharyngeal insufficiency may further compromise speech quality. Speech therapy for such children can help them to slow the pace of their speaking, improve respiratory control for phrase production, and improve the intelligibility of their output. For children whose speech intelligibility is severely compromised despite intact language skills, an assistive or augmentative communication device, such as a picture exchange system or a computer device, may improve their functional communication.

Childhood Apraxia of Speech

Childhood apraxia of speech, known alternatively as *developmental verbal apraxia* or *dyspraxia,* is a condition in which children have difficulty with the controlled production of speech sounds. Criteria for diagnosis vary among clinicians.[58] The first symptoms of apraxia may be a lack of expressive vocabulary despite normal hearing and language comprehension skills. As expressive language emerges, speech may consist of primarily vowel sequences, with very few consonants produced, even in babbling. In childhood apraxia of speech, children produce speech sounds with enormous variability in terms of phonemes, loudness, and related features. The inconsistency in their productions makes interpretation of the sounds very challenging. In addition, these children have difficulties varying the stress in syllables and varying their intonation.[58] They may require enormous effort to produce even short phrases. Once they are able to produce a sound correctly in a word, they are not necessarily able to produce the same sound in other words. In some children with apraxia of speech, there is an isolated speech deficit. In some children, it is associated with cognitive, motor, or behavioral abnormalities. In view of the variations in diagnosis, the precise prevalence is not known. In addition, the cause of apraxia of speech is as yet undetermined.

Treatment of childhood apraxia of speech is difficult and must include an intensive schedule of treatment (three to five sessions per week). Children with apraxia have been shown to require 151 sessions of speech treatment, on average, to have a significant effect on the intelligibility of their speech.[55] Treatment with these children requires massive amounts of practice, with drill-based activities and teaching of each phoneme and syllable. The intervention helps these children learn to produce sounds in syllables or words of increasing complexity. The preferred approach targets motor learning, multimodality input, and language enrichment. Progress is often slow. Some children with treatment develop normal speech patterns, but many affected children have residual speech sound errors as well as learning disabilities in reading and writing difficulties comprehension.

Stuttering

Dysfluency is the disruption or interruption of the ongoing flow of speech. Children between the ages of 3 and 4 years frequently demonstrate what is considered to be normal patterns of dysfluency, often repeating whole words, phrases, or sentences. This occurs as the messages they seek to convey become complex and length of their sentences increases but their proficiency in production is limited. The behavior thus appears to represent a dyscoordination of thought and language. Fluency in the normal child improves at age 4, although adults may display continued bursts of dysfluency when under stress or when trying to explain difficult material.

Stuttering is the most common cause of significant dysfluency, manifested by repetition of sounds and syllables and prolongation of vowels. Stuttering is often accompanied by inappropriate pauses, repetitive facial expressions, or other behavioral routines. Sometimes other motor mannerisms are found in conjunction with stuttering. Approximately 1% of people stutter, and the prevalence is higher in boys and men than in girls and women.[59] The degree of stuttering is highly variable across people, ranging from a mild annoyance to a severe disruption of speech. The degree of stuttering is also highly variable within individuals, subsiding in relaxed conversation and flaring on the telephone or during public speaking. Stuttering disorders may co-occur with speech sound disorders and/or language disorders. They are also not uncommon in children and adults with developmental disabilities resulting from cognitive impairments.

The cause of stuttering is not known. Some cases are associated with known neural injury, which fuels the speculation that the disorder represents a neural timing disorder. Modern structural and functional imaging studies have shown some differences in the neural structures and activation patterns between individuals with fluent speech and individuals with stuttering. However, these tests are not useful in the clinical arena at this time. Stuttering is also associated with anxiety, and it remains unclear which is the primary cause and which the effect. However, in most studies, individuals who stutter do not differ from control populations in terms of personality. Speech therapy started at very young ages has been shown to improve stuttering, with treatment typically focusing on teaching family members to provide an environment to facilitate fluent speech behaviors. For example, strategies include providing pauses for children to communicate, using a slower rate of speech consistently, and using active listening techniques so that the child does not feel pressure when trying to formulate thoughts. At older ages, treatment focuses on teaching compensatory strategies and encouraging the child to be comfortable interacting and communicating in different environments despite the disability.

Voice and Resonance

Voice disorders are abnormalities in the production of vocal tone. They include abnormalities in the volume of the voice (inordinate loudness or softness) and also abnormalities of the vibratory quality of the vocal cords (hoarseness or a raspy voice quality). Voice depends on the vibratory characteristics of the vocal folds, setting the air above the level of the larynx into vibrations as well. The intonation and stress patterns of conversation and connected discourse require rapid changes in the delicate laryngeal musculature.

A common voice problem in children is caused by stress on the laryngeal tissues from excessive screaming and shouting. Loudness can be generated without damage, as in the case of actors or opera singers. However, in young untrained children, the effect of frequently using a loud voice may be edema and inflammation of the vocal chords. In the long-term, such vocal abuse can cause polyps, necessitating surgical intervention. Speech therapy can reeducate children to vary their voice patterns and thereby prevent these complications.

CONCLUSION

Language and speech sound disorders are highly prevalent in the population. They can adversely affect several domains of functioning, including learning, communication, and social relationships. Early identification of problems is facilitated by systematic screening of young children. Certain populations of children at extremely high risk for disorders of language and speech, such as children with Down syndrome, the fragile X syndrome, traumatic brain injury, and hearing loss, should routinely be evaluated. Furthermore, children who are entering foster placement in the aftermath of child abuse or neglect should also be evaluated for communication skills.

Proper diagnosis may entail formal and informal assessments of multiple domains of communication, as well as of play/cognition, academics, social skills, and emotional characteristics. Therapy and other management strategies are predicated on the specific diagnosis and the child's level of language or speech. Intensive early treatment provides children with the best opportunities for normalization of language and speech. Close monitoring of functional improvement is necessary to refine management strategies, combat poor self-esteem, and provide children with alternative communication strategies if verbal language will not be possible.

An interdisciplinary team approach for many children with language and speech disorders is necessary to achieve optimal outcomes. Medical subspecialists, such as developmental-behavioral pediatricians or child neurologists, play an important role in the care of children with language and speech disorders. They typically conduct comprehensive evaluations to uncover other developmental delays or disorders, as well as to identify physical or neurological causes of the disorder. Their evaluations may reveal poor attentional skills, limited behavior regulation, and reading problems, which are prevalent coexisting conditions with language and speech disorders. The developmental subspecialist should refer families to community resources that provide parent-to-parent support, information, treatment, respite care, and related services and should monitor progress to reduce secondary disabilities, such as mental health disorders or learning disabilities. Primary care physicians and their team should create a medical home for children with language and speech disorders. Their distinctive contributions to care include coordinating services within the health care system and linking the health care system with the education system. In addition, they can offer support to increase families' understanding of their roles and responsibilities in facilitating language and speech development, supporting the families in their central roles as decision makers, and monitoring the child's progress over time.

REFERENCES

1. Dale PS, Price TS, Bishop DV, et al: Outcomes of early language delay: I. Predicting persistent and transient language difficulties at 3 and 4 years. J Speech Lang Hear Res 46:544-560, 2003.
2. Feldman HM, Dale PS, Campbell TF, et al: Concurrent and predictive validity of parent reports of child language at ages 2 and 3 years. Child Dev 76:856-868, 2005.
3. Thal DJ, Tobias S, Morrison D: Language and gesture in late talkers: A 1-year follow-up. J Speech Hear Res 34:604-612, 1991.
4. Beitchman JH, Nair R, Clegg M, et al: Prevalence of speech and language disorders in 5-year-old kindergarten children in the Ottawa-Carleton region. J Speech Hear Disord 51:98-110, 1986.
5. Shriberg LD, Tomblin J, McSweeny JL: Prevalence of speech delay in 6-year-old children and comorbidity with language impairment. J Speech Lang Hear Res 42:1461-1481, 1999.
6. Tomblin J, Zhang X, Buckwalter P, et al: The association of reading disability, behavioral disorders, and language impairment among second-grade children. J Child Psychol Psychiatry 41:473-482, 2000.
7. Catts HW, Fey ME, Tomblin J, et al: A longitudinal investigation of reading outcomes in children with language impairments. J Speech Lang Hear Res 45:1142-1157, 2002.
8. Bishop DV, Price TS, Dale PS, et al: Outcomes of early language delay: II. Etiology of transient and persistent language difficulties. J Speech Lang Hear Res 46:561-575, 2003.
9. Huttenlocher J, Vasilyeva M, Cymerman E, et al: Language input and child syntax. Cogn Psychol 45:337-74, 2002.

10. Huttenlocher J: Language input and language growth. Prev Med 27:195-199, 1998.

11. Tomblin JB, Zhang X: Language patterns and etiology in children with specific language impairment. *In* Tager-Flusberg H, ed: Neurodevelopmental Disorders. Cambridge, MA: MIT Press, 1999, pp 361-382.

12. Tomblin JB: Genetic and environmental contributions to the risk for specific language impairment. *In* Rice MLE, ed: Toward a Genetics of Language. Hillsdale, NJ: Erlbaum, 1996, pp 191-210.

13. Fenson L, Dale PS, Reznick J, et al: Variability in early communicative development. Monogr Soc Res Child Dev 59:5-173, 1994.

14. Bornstein MH, Leach DB, Haynes OM: Vocabulary competence in first- and secondborn siblings of the same chronological age. J Child Lang 31:855-873, 2004.

15. Hoff-Ginsberg E: The relation of birth order and socioeconomic status to children's language experience and language development. Appl Psycholinguist 19:603-629, 1998.

16. Gutierrez-Clellen VF: Language choice in intervention with bilingual children. Am J Speech Lang Pathol 8:291-302, 1999.

17. Genesee F: Early bilingual development: one language or two? J Child Lang 16:161-179, 1989.

18. Joint Committee on Infant Hearing, American Academy of Audiology, American Academy of Pediatrics, et al: Year 2000 position statement: Principles and guidelines for early hearing detection and intervention programs. Joint Committee on Infant Hearing, American Academy of Audiology, American Academy of Pediatrics, American Speech-Language-Hearing Association, and Directors of Speech and Hearing Programs in State Health and Welfare Agencies. Pediatrics 106:798-817, 2000.

19. Task Force on Newborn and Infant Hearing: Newborn and infant hearing loss: Detection and intervention. Pediatrics 103:527-530, 1999.

20. Hammes DM, Novak MA, Rotz LA, et al: Early identification and cochlear implantation: Critical factors for spoken language development. Ann Otol Rhinol Laryngol Suppl 189:74-78, 2002.

21. Briscoe J, Bishop DV, Norbury CF: Phonological processing, language, and literacy: A comparison of children with mild-to-moderate sensorineural hearing loss and those with specific language impairment. J Child Psychol Psychiatry 42:329-340, 2001.

22. Nittrouer S, Burton LT: The role of early language experience in the development of speech perception and phonological processing abilities: Evidence from 5-year-olds with histories of otitis media with effusion and low socioeconomic status. J Commun Disord 38:29-63, 2005.

23. Roberts JE, Burchinal MR, Jackson SC, et al: Otitis media in childhood in relation to preschool language and school readiness skills among black children. Pediatrics 106:725-735, 2000.

24. Roberts JE, Burchinal MR, Zeisel SA, et al: Otitis media, the caregiving environment, and language and cognitive outcomes at 2 years. Pediatrics 102:346-354, 1998.

25. Paradise JL, Campbell TF, Dollaghan CA, et al: Developmental outcomes after early or delayed insertion of tympanostomy tubes. New England Journal of Medicine 353:576-586, 2005.

26. Laws G, Bishop DV: Verbal deficits in Down's syndrome and specific language impairment: a comparison. International Journal of Language & Communication Disorders 39:423-451, 2004.

27. Chapman RS, Hesketh LJ: Language, cognition, and short-term memory in individuals with Down syndrome. Down Syndrome: Research & Practice 7:1-7, 2001.

28. Chapman RS, Hesketh LJ: Behavioral phenotype of individuals with Down syndrome. Ment Retard Dev Disabil Res Rev 6:84-95, 2000.

29. Laws G: Contributions of phonological memory, language comprehension and hearing to the expressive language of adolescents and young adults with Down syndrome. J Child Psychol Psychiatry 45:1085-1095, 2004.

30. Clibbens J: Signing and lexical development in children with Down syndrome. Down Syndrome: Research & Practice 7:101-105, 2001.

31. Bates E, Dick F: Language, gesture, and the developing brain. Developmental Psychobiology 40:293-310, 2002.

32. Spiridigliozzi GL, Lachiewicz A, Mirrett S, McConkie-Rosell A: Fragile X syndrome in young children. *In* Layton T, Crais E, Watson L, eds: Handbook of Early Language Impairment in Children: Nature. Albany, NY: Delmar, 2001, pp 258-301.

33. Kau AS, Meyer WA, Kaufmann WE: Early development in males with fragile X syndrome: A review of the literature. Microsc Res Tech 57:174-178, 2002.

34. Cornish K, Sudhalter V, Turk J: Attention and language in fragile X. Ment Retard Dev Disabil Res Rev 10:11-16, 2004.

35. Laing E, Butterworth G, Ansari D, et al: Atypical development of language and social communication in toddlers with Williams syndrome. Dev Sci 5:233-246, 2002.

36. Paterson SJ, Brown JH, Gsodl MK, et al: Cognitive modularity and genetic disorders. Science 286:2355-2358, 1999.

37. Barbaresi WJ, Katusic SK, Colligan RC, et al: The incidence of autism in Olmsted County, Minnesota, 1976-1997: Results from a population-based study [see comment]. Arch Pediatr Adolesc Med 159:37-44, 2005.

38. Volkmar F, Chawarska K, Klin A: Autism in infancy and early childhood. Annu Rev Psychol 56:315-336, 2005.

39. Volkmar FR, Lord C, Bailey A, et al: Autism and pervasive developmental disorders. J Child Psychol Psychiatry 45:135-170, 2004.

40. Bruinsma Y, Koegel RL, Koegel LK: Joint attention and children with autism: A review of the literature. Ment Retard Dev Disabil Res Rev 10:169-175, 2004.

41. Lovaas OI: The development of a treatment-research project for developmentally disabled and autistic children. J Appl Behav Anal 26:617-630, 1993.

42. Diggle T, McConachie HR, Randle VR: Parent-mediated early intervention for young children with autism spectrum disorder. Cochrane Database Syst Rev (1):CD003496, 2003.

43. Fletcher JM, Barnes M, Dennis M: Language development in children with spina bifida. Semi Pediatr Neurol 9:201-208, 2002.

44. McVicar KA, Shinnar S: Landau-Kleffner syndrome, electrical status epilepticus in slow wave sleep, and language regression in children. Ment Retard Dev Disabil Res Rev 10:144-149, 2004.

45. Feldman H: Language learning with an injured brain. Lang Learn Dev 1:265-288, 2005.

46. Booth JR, MacWhinney B, Thulborn KR, et al: Developmental and lesion effects in brain activation during sentence comprehension and mental rotation. Dev Neuropsychol 18:139-169, 2000.

47. Barlow KM, Thomson E, Johnson D, et al: Late neurologic and cognitive sequelae of inflicted traumatic brain injury in infancy. Pediatrics 116:e174-e185, 2005.

48. Baltaxe C: Emotional, behavioral, and other psychiatric disorders of childhood associated with communication disorders. *In* Layton T, Crais E, Watson L, eds: Handbook of Early Language Impairment in Children: Nature. Albany, NY: Delmar, 2001, pp 63-125.

49. Giddan J, Milling L: Language disorders and emotional disturbance. *In* Layton T, Crais E, Watson L, eds: Handbook of Early Language Impairment in Children: Nature. Albany, NY: Delmar, 2001, pp 19-36.

50. Prizant B, Meyer E: Socioemotional aspects of language and social-communication disorders in young children. Am J Speech Lang Pathol 2:56-71, 1993.

51. Brinton B, Fujiki M: Social interactional behaviors of children with specific language impairments. Topics Lang Disord 19:49-69, 1999.

52. McArthur GM, Bishop DV: Speech and non-speech processing in people with specific language impairment: A behavioural and electrophysiological study. Brain Lang 94:260-273, 2005.

53. Tallal P: Improving language and literacy is a matter of time. Nat Rev Neurosci 5:721-728, 2004.

54. Hickok G, Poeppel D: Dorsal and ventral streams: A framework for understanding aspects of the functional anatomy of language. Cognition 92:67-99, 2004.

55. Campbell TF: Functional treatment outcomes in young children with motor speech disorders. *In* Caruso AJ, Strand EA, eds: Clinical Management of Motor Speech Disorders in Children. New York: Thieme, 2001, pp 385-396.

56. Wang PP, Woodin MF, Kreps-Falk R, et al: Research on behavioral phenotypes: Velocardiofacial syndrome (deletion 22q11.2). Dev Med Child Neurol 42:422-427, 2000.

57. Willging JP: Velopharyngeal insufficiency. Curr Opin Otolaryngol Head Neck Surg 11:452-455, 2003.

58. Shriberg LD, Campbell TF, Karlsson HB, et al: A diagnostic marker for childhood apraxia of speech: the lexical stress ratio. Clin Linguist Phon 17:549-574, 2003.

59. Craig A, Tran Y: The epidemiology of stuttering: The need for reliable estimates of prevalence and anxiety levels over the lifespan. Adv Speech Lang Pathol 7:41-46, 2005.

Motor Disabilities and Multiple Handicapping Conditions

ROBERT E. NICKEL ■ MARIO C. PETERSEN

In this chapter, we will discuss two of the more common motor disabilities: cerebral palsy and spina bifida. The term *cerebral palsy* actually refers to a group of disorders that are characterized by impairments in movement or posture as a result of injury or anomaly of the developing brain. *Spina bifida* is a generic term for chronic conditions related to defects in the developing neural tube. For each, we discuss definition and classification, prevalence, etiology, strategies for prevention, evaluation, management, and associated health and developmental problems.

The National Center for Medical Rehabilitation Research of the National Institutes of Health has identified five dimensions of disability:

- Pathophysiology—interruption of normal physiological processes or structures
- Impairments—loss or abnormality at the organ system level
- Functional limitations—restriction in ability to perform an action
- Disability—limitation in performing tasks, expected roles
- Societal limitations—restrictions related to social policy or barriers.[1]

Treatment programs for children with spina bifida and cerebral palsy have evolved from an emphasis on treatment of the pathophysiology (e.g., spasticity) and impairments (e.g., joint contractures) to an emphasis on improving functional skills and facilitating active participation in typical community activities.

In general, the goal of the management of children with motor disabilities such as cerebral palsy and spina bifida is to ensure the highest possible quality of life by facilitating the child's early motor progress; improving the quality and efficiency of gait; improving the child's functional skills; preventing secondary problems; treating associated health conditions; and encouraging the development of self-determination and independence throughout the lifespan.

CEREBRAL PALSY

Definition and Classification

Cerebral palsy refers not to a single condition but to a number of different and varied chronic conditions. The traditional definition of cerebral palsy is a nonprogressive impairment in movement or posture caused by injury or anomaly of the developing brain. This definition excludes recognized progressive or degenerative brain disorders.

Classification of cerebral palsy is based on anatomical distribution of the dysfunction, type of neurological involvement, and function. Children may have monoplegia (involvement of a single extremity), hemiplegia (one side involved), diplegia (predominant involvement of legs), or quadriplegia (total body involvement). Motor dysfunction may be asymmetrical or there may be primary involvement of one arm and both legs (triplegia). Neurological type is classified as spastic, dyskinetic (includes dystonia and athetosis), ataxic, and mixed. Some clinicians also include a hypotonic or atonic type of cerebral palsy. The Gross Motor Function Classification System (GMFCS) defines functional status by categorizing children with cerebral palsy into one of five different levels of function primarily on the basis of skills in sitting and walking (Table 14-1).[2]

With the current system, it has not been clear when diplegia with significant upper extremity involvement should be classified as quadriplegia or when involvement of one upper extremity and both legs should be classified as asymmetrical quadriplegia, triplegia, or diplegia with superimposed hemiplegia.[3] It has also been unclear what various authors have meant by "mixed"; for example, how significant is the spasticity and the dystonia in a child with mixed spastic dystonic quadriplegia? Children with cerebral palsy often have significant oral motor (bulbar) and truncal involvement, and neither is

TABLE 14-1 ■ The Gross Motor Function Classification System	
Level I	Walks without restrictions; limitations in advanced skills only
Level II	Walks without assistive devices; limited outdoors/community mobility
Level III	Walks with assistive mobility devices; limited outdoors/community mobility
Level IV	Self-mobility with limitations; transported in wheelchair or use power mobility in outdoors/community
Level V	Self-mobility is severely limited, even with the use of assistive technology

From Palisano R, Rosenbaum P, Walter S, et al: Development and reliability of a system to classify gross motor function in children with cerebral palsy. Dev Med Child Neurol 39:214-223, 1997.

TABLE 14-2 ■ Components of a Proposed Classification System for Children with Cerebral Palsy
Motor abnormalities
Tone and movement abnormalities
Functional motor abilities
Associated impairments
Seizures; hearing or vision impairments; and attention, behavior, communication, and/or cognitive deficits
Anatomic and radiologic findings
Anatomic distribution
Radiologic findings
Causation and timing

From Bax M, Goldstein M, Rosenbaum P, et al: Proposed definition and classification of cerebral palsy. Dev Med Child Neurol 47:571-576, 2005.

included in the current classification system. Although the GMFCS has become a widely used and validated tool for functional classification,[4] it does not address upper extremity function. Finally, studies have varied with regard to which children with known genetic disorders and which young children with acquired brain injury to include or exclude.

In 2004, discussions at the International Workshop on Definition and Classification held in Bethesda, Maryland, led to the publication in 2005 of a proposed new definition and classification system for cerebral palsy (Table 14-2).[5] A number of cited factors supported the need for the new definition and classification system, including improved knowledge of brain development, neuroimaging techniques, and measurement tools; the increase in number and quality of outcome studies; and the need to compare children across studies. The authors also noted that the current definition and classification system did not include associated disabilities and chronic health problems, which are common and significantly affect a child's ability to participate in desired societal roles. The proposed definition is as follows:

Cerebral palsy . . . describes a group of disorders of the development of movement and posture, causing activity limitation, that are attributed to non-progressive disturbances that occurred in the developing fetal or infant brain. The motor disorders of cerebral palsy are often accompanied by disturbances of sensation, cognition, communication, perception, and/or behavior, and/or by seizure disorder.

—Bax et al, 2005, p 572[5]

The proposed classification system addresses most of these issues. The components of the proposed cerebral palsy classification are listed in Table 14-2. Classification requires identification of the predominant tone or movement abnormality and identification of any secondary tone or movement abnormalities. It also requires description of the functional motor abilities in all body areas, although the authors acknowledged the need for research validation of measurement tools for arm and hand function and for speech and oral motor function. This classification eliminates the categorization of diplegia, quadriplegia, and so forth; requires description of the distribution of the dysfunction in all body areas, including the trunk and bulbar regions, and a description of associated health and developmental conditions or deficits; and includes identification of a clearly defined cause if there is one. This addresses a key issue for parents: the cause of the child's problem. This classification does not resolve the issue of inclusion or exclusion of children with known genetic disorders or the age for inclusion of children with postnatally acquired brain injury. It may exclude some children currently classified as having cerebral palsy who have no or minimal activity limitation. Much work remains to be done to develop a reliable and useful system for both clinical and research practice.

Prevalence

The prevalence of cerebral palsy remains at 1.5 to 2.5 per 1000, and has remained essentially unchanged for a number of decades.[6-11] Studies on the prevalence of cerebral palsy have varied in whether they have included children with postnatal causes[7,9] and whether they have included children with known causation.[11] Improvement in the survival of infants with low birth weight has contributed to an increase in prevalence of cerebral palsy for these children[12,13]; however, the prevalence of cerebral palsy in children with birth weights of 2500 g or more has remained generally unchanged.[14] In one study, investigators reported an increase in the number of children born at term with dyskinetic cerebral palsy.[7] In this group, perinatal hypoxic-ischemic encephalopathy (HIE) was present in 71%.

Etiology

The brain injury or developmental defect that results in cerebral palsy may occur prenatally, perinatally, or postnatally. Table 14-3 lists representative prenatal, perinatal, and postnatal causative factors.

The use of magnetic resonance imaging (MRI) in children with cerebral palsy has expanded the identification of children with developmental defects of the central nervous system. In one study, more than half of the children with cerebral palsy who were born at term had evidence of a prenatal causative factor, and most of them had developmental defects of the brain.[15] In addition, 7% to 11% of all children with cerebral palsy who have undergone neuroimaging have been shown to have a central nervous system malformation.[16] MRI also has improved the identification of schizencephaly in children with hemiplegia or quadriplegia. Schizencephaly results from probable ischemic injury to the brain at the 10th to 12th weeks of gestation. Only a small number of children with severe bilateral schizencephaly have an apparent genetic disorder.[17] Case reports of children with hemiplegia associated with thrombophilic factors[18,19] have increased research interest in the more general association of prothrombic factors in children with cerebral palsy. To date, there has been little research support for this association, other than for children who have had neonatal stroke.[20-26] Children with identified genetic factors represent only about 1% to 5% of children with cerebral palsy.[16,17,27]

In a study that excluded postnatal causes, the relative contribution of prenatal factors was 22% and that of perinatal factors was 47%; the remainder of cases were unclassified.[9] Of infants with low birth weight in that study, 59% had a perinatal causative factor, primarily periventricular leukomalacia (PVL) and intraventricular hemorrhage. In general, preterm infants with PVL represent about 35% to 40% of children with cerebral palsy.[27] These children present with spastic diplegia, and their condition represents a common clinical type of cerebral palsy. Other common clinical types related to perinatal factors are hemiplegia and posthemorrhagic hydrocephalus after premature birth with grade IV intraventricular hemorrhage; congenital spastic hemiplegia and porencephaly visible on MRI scan (prenatal or perinatal factor); dyskinetic quadriplegia with a history of HIE; and athetoid quadriplegia with sensorineural hearing loss and a history of hyperbilirubinemia and kernicterus. Postnatal causative factors are identified in only about 10% of children with cerebral palsy.[27]

Prevention

Research into the causes of cerebral palsy in preterm infants has focused on two mechanisms of brain damage: insufficient cerebral perfusion and cytokine-mediated damage, potentially triggered by maternal or neonatal infection.[12,28] For example, a number of studies have demonstrated an association between chorioamnionitis (infection), inflammatory cytokines, and white matter damage.[29-32] Additional studies are needed in order to develop effective prevention strategies—for example, to document that chorioamnionitis actually precedes white matter damage[29]—and to clarify the role of protective factors such as thyroid hormones or glucocorticoids.[12]

Prevention strategies for full-term infants have focused on prevention of secondary or reperfusion injury in neonates with HIE. For example, MRI with diffusion-weighted imaging during the first days after birth is contributing to the early identification of full-term infants with significant HIE at high risk for subsequent cerebral palsy, so that neuroprotective strategies can be initiated.[33-36] A randomized clinical trial (RCT) of whole-body hypothermia in neonates with moderate and severe HIE has demonstrated reduction in the risk of both death and disability in the experimental group.[37]

TABLE 14-3 ■ Causative Factors Associated with Cerebral Palsy		
Prenatal	**Perinatal**	**Postnatal**
Brain malformation	Periventricular leukomalacia	Meningitis/encephalitis
Neuronal migration disorder	Intraventricular hemorrhage	Traumatic brain injury (e.g., shaken baby syndrome)
Congenital infection	Meningitis, encephalitis	Hemorrhage
Vascular events (schizencephaly, thrombophilia)	Hypoxic ischemic encephalopathy	Metabolic
Metabolic disorder (e.g., glutaric acidemia type I)	Metabolic disorder (e.g., hypoglycemia, hyperbilirubinemia)	Other mechanisms of acquired brain injury (e.g., near-drowning)
Genetic disorder	Perinatal stroke	Vascular (e.g., postcardiotomy chorea)
		Brain tumor

Identification

NEWBORN

In general, cranial ultrasonography and MRI of preterm and full-term infants are more predictive than the clinical examination of the neonate or the identification of individual or combinations of perinatal risk factors. The neurological examination of the newborn is best at demonstrating current status but is poorly predictive of subsequent neurodevelopmental disability. In addition, data from the National Collaborative Perinatal Project demonstrated that perinatal risk factors, whether present alone or in combination, are poor predictors of cerebral palsy.[38] Of children with high-risk factors, 97% did not have cerebral palsy, and high-risk factors were present in only 63% of the children with cerebral palsy.[39]

The finding of persistent ventricular dilatation, cystic PVL, and grades III and IV intraventricular hemorrhage on cranial ultrasonography are highly predictive of subsequent cerebral palsy.[40] The timing of cranial ultrasonography in the preterm infant is critical. In one study, cranial ultrasonography detected 29% of abnormalities only after 28 days after birth.[41] In the same study, 83% of the children with cerebral palsy at 2 years had major cranial ultrasonographic abnormalities on examinations that were repeated weekly to 40 weeks' postconceptual age. The practice parameter of the Child Neurology Society recommends cranial ultrasonography at 7 to 14 days and again at 36 to 40 weeks' postconceptual age.[42]

The MRI is the imaging study of choice for full-term infants with possible HIE. Diffusion-weighted imaging and magnetic resonance spectroscopy are improving the identification of full-term infants with acute ischemia who are at risk for HIE and subsequent cerebral palsy.[33,36] Abnormalities of the thalamus and basal ganglia visible on MRI are highly predictive of subsequent neurodevelopmental problems, including cerebral palsy.[38] The role of MRI in preterm infants is evolving. MRI, including diffusion-weighted imaging with attention to the myelination of the posterior limb of the internal capsule at 36 to 40 weeks' postcenceptual age, may prove to be a valuable addition to cranial ultrasonography in the early detection of PVL and subsequently cerebral palsy. It is superior to cranial ultrasonography in the detection of diffuse PVL in preterm infants[40] and may be helpful in evaluation of preterm infants with acute ischemia. The use of MRI diffusion tensor imaging to map white matter pathways and also to identify white matter injury in the neonatal period may be helpful.[33] Computed tomography has limited utility in full-term and preterm neonates.[40]

INFANT AND TODDLER

The accurate identification of infants and toddlers with cerebral palsy depends on repeating examinations at different ages and evaluating the quality of movement patterns, in addition to assessing motor milestones and completing the traditional neurological examination. Important movement patterns include primitive reflexes, such as the asymmetrical tonic neck reflex, the tonic labyrinthine reflex-supine, and the neonatal positive support reflex, which disappear with maturation; and automatic reactions, such as truncal equilibrium responses and parachute responses that appear with increasing age. In addition, it is important to observe the motor patterns used to roll, come to sit, and pull to stand. A number of screening tests incorporate some or most of these items: the Alberta Infant Motor Scale,[43,44] the Chandler Movement Assessment of Infants Screening Test,[45] the Infant Motor Screen,[46] the Milani Comparetti Motor Development Screening Test,[47] and the Primitive Reflex Profile.[48] Screening tests provide a structure for making accurate observations and can assist with referral decisions.

Other authors have emphasized making careful observations of the generalized movements of very young infants to improve the identification of cerebral palsy.[49,50] This approach is based on the work of Heinz Prechtl and involves scoring the video recording of the movement of infants from a few weeks to several months of age. The age for fidgety movements (2 to 4 months) is reported to be the best age for making predictions.[50] As with other methods, however, prediction of developmental outcomes are best made on the basis of a longitudinal series of assessments.[50]

A number of infants continue to present diagnostic challenges. Some preterm infants appear to have spasticity in their legs and a spastic diplegia pattern of cerebral palsy; however, these signs resolve after a year of age. In one study, only 118 of 229 children with a diagnosis of cerebral palsy at 1 year of age still had the diagnosis at 7 years.[51] This pattern of development is called *transient dystonia*. A few infants with mild diplegia, hemiplegia, or extrapyramidal cerebral palsy may be "missed" when examined in the first year. Athetosis and ataxia may not develop until after a year of age. Finally, a few infants present with the signs of cerebral palsy but subsequently are shown to have a progressive disorder. All these issues underline the importance of repeating examinations at different ages.

Evaluation

The diagnostic evaluation of the child with suspected cerebral palsy is best done by an experienced neurodevelopmental team. The goals of the history and physical examination are to confirm the diagnosis, clarify the type and distribution of the neuromotor impairment, review causation and timing, identify associated health issues, and plan for additional evaluations as needed. The practice parameter on the diagnostic assessment of the child with cerebral palsy formulated by the Quality Standards Subcommittee of the American Academy of Neurology and the Practice Committee of the Child Neurology Society recommends neuroimaging in all children with cerebral palsy if the etiology is not established and consideration of coagulation studies in children with hemiplegic cerebral palsy and unexplained hemorrhagic infarction.[16] Routine metabolic and genetic studies and routine electroencephalography are not recommended. The MRI is the imaging study of choice. Children who do have central nervous system malformations may benefit from further genetic testing or evaluation. An example is the child with agenesis of the corpus callosum, spastic paraplegia, and mutations in the *L1CAM* gene.[52] An accurate medical diagnosis helps clarify natural history and risk for associated problems such as seizures, helps identify potentially treatable conditions such as dopa-responsive dystonia, and helps identify progressive disorders such as ataxia-telangiectasia.

The practice parameter also recommends screening children for mental retardation, vision impairments, and hearing impairments and monitoring nutrition, growth, and swallowing dysfunction. The revised classification system for children with cerebral palsy[5] also includes evaluation of attention and behavior and potential associated impairments: for example, gastrointestinal problems. Table 14-4 lists representative tools for the evaluation of speech and language, gross and fine motor skills, functional motor abilities, overall developmental progress, and attention and behavior. Children with speech and language delay should have formal audiological testing. The results of the diagnostic evaluation form the basis for the development of the initial management plan and may include recommendations for therapy services, as well as adaptive equipment. These are discussed in greater detail later in this chapter.

DIFFERENTIAL DIAGNOSIS

A number of different disorders may be confused with cerebral palsy, particularly on initial evaluation. These include other static disorders such as habitual toe walking; disorders that manifest neurological progression or deterioration, such as familial spastic paraplegia and ataxia telangiectasia; and potentially treatable disorders, such as dopa-responsive dystonia and glutaric acidemia. The diagnosis of habitual toe walking is one of exclusion.[53] Parents of affected children typically report that the children have always

TABLE 14-4 ■ Representative Instruments for the Developmental Assessment of Children with Cerebral Palsy

Speech and Language
Preschool Language Scale IV (PLS)

Motor Skills
Peabody Developmental Motor Scale–2 (PDMS-2)[358]
Gross Motor Function Measure (GMFM)[359]

Functional Skills
Pediatric Evaluation of Disability Inventory (PEDI)[360,361]
Functional Independence Measure for Children (WeeFIM)[362,363]
Pediatric Outcomes Data Collection Instrument (PODCI)[364]

Cognitive Development
Bayley Scales of Infant Development, 2nd edition[365]
Stanford-Binet Intelligence Scales, 5th edition[366]
Wechsler Preschool and Primary Scale of Intelligence, 3rd edition (WPPSI-III)[367]
Wechsler Intelligence Scale for Children, 4th edition (WISC-IV)[368]

Attention and Behavior
Child Behavior Checklist: Parent, Teacher, and Youth forms (CBCL)[369-371]

walked on their toes. They have no evidence of spasticity, muscle weakness, or other neurological condition. They may or may not present with Achilles tendon contractures and may have a positive family history of toe walking.[54] Clinicians may confuse habitual toe walking with mild spastic diplegia; however, electromyography helps differentiate the two in difficult cases.[55]

A positive family history of cerebral palsy should raise the question of familial or hereditary spastic paraplegia and the need for further genetic evaluation. Dopa-responsive dystonia is often initially misdiagnosed as cerebral palsy. It is an autosomal dominant genetic disorder (arising from mutation in the *GCH-1* gene) that is characterized by diurnal variation in motor performance that responds dramatically to low doses of l-dopa.[56,57]

Management

The impairments of children with cerebral palsy include oral motor dysfunction, joint contractures, hip subluxation and dislocation, and spine changes (scoliosis, kyphosis, and lordosis). Functional problems include feeding dysfunction, delayed and disordered speech, limited independent mobility and written communication, and difficulty performing self-care activities. These impairments, as well as the functional problems of children with cerebral palsy, result from one or more of the following pathophysi-ological conditions: hypertonicity (spasticity and dys-tonia) and hypotonia; muscle weakness and easy fatigability; loss of selective motor control; impaired balance; and involuntary movement.

Associated health problems, such as inadequate nutrition and seizures that are difficult to manage may also significantly influence the functional abili-ties of children with cerebral palsy.

SPECIALIZED EVALUATIONS

In general, children with cerebral palsy are reevalu-ated every 6 to 12 months or as needed to monitor their motor progress and associated health problems, update the treatment plan, support the child and family, advocate for needed services, and address emerging problems related to the child's growth and development. In addition to the evaluations listed previously, children with cerebral palsy may require a number of specialized evaluations. These include measures of muscle tone, gait, and quality of life.

Muscle Tone

Hypertonia may result from rigidity, spasticity, dystonia, or a combination of all.[58] Hypertonia is defined as abnormally increased resistance to passive movement at a joint. Rigidity is typically not seen in children, and we do not further discuss it. Spasticity is the velocity-dependent increase in resistance to passive movement about a joint, so that resistance increases with increasing speed of the stretch.[58] It can be measured with the Ashworth Scale,[59] the Modified Ashworth Scale,[60] and the Tardieu Scale.[61] The Tardieu Scale specifically compares the occurrence of the "catch," or exaggerated stretch reflex, at low and high speeds. *Dystonia* refers to involuntary sustained or intermittent muscle contractions that cause twist-ing or repetitive movement, abnormal postures, or both.[58] Dystonia is typically exacerbated by voluntary movement, may vary with posture and type of attempted movement, and is often associated with athetosis. The severity of dystonia can be rated with Barry Albright Dystonia Scale.[62] The differentiation of spasticity from dystonia is crucial for treatment planning.

Gait Analysis

The objective measurement of gait parameters in the laboratory has become an essential part of the evaluation for many children with cerebral palsy. Three-dimensional computerized gait analysis can assist with preoperative planning particularly for multilevel orthopedic surgery and can document changes before and after both surgical and nonsurgi-cal treatments.[63-67] The components of gait analysis include electromyographic analysis, videotaped assessment of kinematics (joint angles and velocities) and kinetics (joint movements, powers, and ground-reaction forces), force plate analysis, and, at times, oxygen consumption. Standard gait parameters include step and stride length, gait velocity, and cadence. The laboratory gait analysis complements the clinical evaluation of the child.[63,68]

Quality-of-Life Scales

Quality-of-life measures are particularly important for the families of children with severe cerebral palsy. For example, the treatment goals for a child classified as having level V cerebral palsy on the GMFCS who is receiving intrathecal baclofen therapy may focus on improvement in ease of care and sleep and decrease in pain and discomfort, rather than improvement in functional skills. Pain is a common experience for children and adults with cerebral palsy.[69,70] Although there is increasing recognition of the importance of quality-of-life measures and the assessment of pain, there are significant limitations in current measures of quality of life and in health-related quality-of-life scales.[71-73] The Child Health Question-naire is one example of a quality-of-life measure.[74-76] Several tools to assess health-related quality of life and pain in children with cerebral palsy are under development.[34,72,77,78]

Treatment

Treatments for children with cerebral palsy may target the pathophysiological process (e.g., selective dorsal rhizotomy [SDR] for spasticity or physical therapy for muscle strengthening), the impairment (e.g., surgery for joint contractures or bracing for foot and ankle deformities), functional skills and activity participation (e.g., manual wheelchair for mobility and participation in sports), or quality-of-life issues. The treatment plan for a child with cerebral palsy may include physical and occupational therapy; braces and adaptive equipment; seating and positioning devices; oral, intramuscular, and intrathecal medications; orthopedic and neurological surgical procedures; and other therapy, such as electrical stimulation. In general, the evidence base that supports the efficacy of the various treatments for children with cerebral palsy is limited but improving.

PHYSICAL AND OCCUPATIONAL THERAPY

The roles of the physical therapist and occupational therapist with children who have cerebral palsy and their families are broad. They provide direct treat-ment, participate in diagnostic evaluations, recom-mend braces and assistive devices, and provide training and support to children and caregivers. In general, the indications for physical and occupational therapy treatment services, including regular therapy during the preschool years and subsequent interval physical and occupational therapy services, are to improve strength, endurance, and speed; gait training, particularly with new orthoses or assistive devices; to assess when there is a change in motor skills or emerging skills such as independent walking; postoperative services, when a child is removed from casts after surgery; impending joint contractures; and other situations, such as prescription of a new brace or ambulatory aide.[79]

The evidence base to support the efficacy of physical and occupational therapy treatment, however, is limited.[80,81] A systematic review of 21 studies, including 7 RCTs, by the Treatment Outcomes Committee of the American Academy for Cerebral Palsy and Developmental Medicine revealed no evidence to support the efficacy of neurodevelopmental treatment for young children with cerebral palsy.[81] In addition, many treatment studies have provided low levels of evidence of efficacy (i.e., Sackett levels III to V).[82] On the other hand, studies have reported the efficacy of physical therapy for muscle strengthening in children with cerebral palsy, including such functional improvements as increase in activity level.[83-85] Other studies have reported the benefits of constraint induced therapy, a relatively new therapy for children with hemiplegia.[86-89] In this therapy, the child's unaffected arm is constrained in a cast or by another method, in order to force the child to use the affected hand and arm. The research studies, however, have varied with regard to the method and length of constraint used and outcome measures.

BRACES, ADAPTIVE EQUIPMENT, AND POSITIONING DEVICES

In general, clinicians prescribe lower and upper extremity braces (orthoses) to maintain normal alignment at a joint, prevent deformity, and improve function. There is regional variability in the type of orthoses prescribed for children with cerebral palsy. Unfortunately, the research evidence supporting one brace over another is limited; therefore, clinical experience primarily determines choice. There is considerable evidence documenting the efficacy of ankle-foot orthoses over barefoot walking on gait parameters of children with dynamic equinus.[66,80,90-92] In addition, there is limited data on the efficacy of specific types of ankle-foot orthoses (posterior leaf spring, hinged vs. solid) in less impaired children[91] and some support for functional improvement with these braces.[93]

Adaptive seating is crucial in some children with cerebral palsy (GMFCS levels IV and V) for improving function, including feeding and speech; for improving quality of life; for preventing progression of secondary problems such as scoliosis; and for offering an opportunity for safe, independent mobility. Unfortunately, the evidence to support the efficacy of adaptive seating for any of these indications is limited. Studies have documented the benefits of power-drive wheelchairs for children as young as 2 years, who have no other choices for independent mobility.[94]

TONE MANAGEMENT

Control of hypertonicity or tone management is a significant part of the treatment program for many children with cerebral palsy. Treatment approaches include oral medications, intramuscular injections with botulinum toxin, nerve blocks with phenol or alcohol, intrathecal baclofen, and SDR. Children with marked spasticity and or dystonia are likely to benefit from a combination of these treatments. Decisions are complex and require an experienced multidisciplinary team.[95] One goal of early tone management is to prevent orthopedic complications such as flexion contractures in order to avoid the need for subsequent orthopedic surgical procedures. A population-based study from Sweden appears to confirm the appropriateness of this strategy. This study reported a reduction of orthopedic surgery for contracture or skeletal torsion deformity from 40% to 15% in children up to 8 years of age during an aggressive early tone management program.[96]

Oral Medications

Table 14-5 lists the common oral medications used for the treatment of spasticity and dystonia. These include baclofen, diazepam and other benzodiazepines, dantrolene, and tizanidine and other α_2-adrenergic agents for spasticity and levodopa-carbidopa, trihexyphenidyl, and baclofen for dystonia.[97] Side

---

TABLE 14-5 ■ Oral Medications for Tone Management in Children with Cerebral Palsy

Medication	Mechanism of Action
Spasticity	
Baclofen	GABA agonist
Benzodiazepines (diazepam, clonazepam)	GABA agonist
Dantrolene	Inhibits calcium release from muscle sarcoplasmic reticulum
α_2-Adrenergic agonists (tizanidine, clonidine)	Decrease excitatory amino acids, hyperpolarize neurons
Gabapentin	Increase brain GABA levels
Dystonia	
Levodopa-carbidopa	Dopaminergic
Trihexyphenidyl	Anticholinergic

Adapted from Krach L: Pharmacotherapy of spasticity: Oral medications and intrathecal baclofen. J Child Neurol 16:31-36, 2001.
GABA, γ-amino butyric acid.

effects, including sedation, drowsiness, and weakness, have limited the modest benefits of oral medications. A systematic review of 12 RCTs of oral antispasticity medications concluded that the evidence of efficacy is scarce and weak.[98] The authors could make no recommendations to guide clinical practice because of the low methodological quality of the studies, the limited numbers of patients, the short duration of follow-up, and the failure to include functional outcomes. In a small RCT in India, a single nighttime dose of diazepam significantly reduced tone and improved range of motion in children with cerebral palsy and thus may be of benefit in developing countries with little access to other treatments, such as botulinum toxin and intrathecal baclofen.[99] A trial of levodopa-carbidopa is indicated in children with unexplained dystonia, because of the variability in the presentation of children with dopa-responsive dystonia.

Benzodiazepines also can cause physiological addiction and potentially a withdrawal syndrome. Abrupt withdrawal of baclofen can result in serious side effects, including pruritus, increase in spasticity, confusion, hallucinations, and seizures. Use of dantrolene and tizanidine has been associated with liver dysfunction, and liver function must be tested when children are taking these medications.

Botulinum Toxin, Phenol, and Alcohol

Traditionally, phenol and alcohol have been injected into motor points or onto the motor nerves for the reduction of spasticity. These medications cause protein denaturation and axonal degeneration, have an onset of action of hours, and a duration of action of up to 12 months.[100,101] Injections may be repeated. Treatment indications include improving the ease of care, improving gait, and treating pain secondary to spasticity. The technical expertise necessary for the procedure and the risk of chronic pain or paresthesia after the procedure limit their use.

Botulinum toxin has become the procedure of choice for neuromuscular blockade because of the ease of administration, low risk of side effects, and rapid onset of action. It interferes with the release of acetylcholine at the neuromuscular junction. The primary limitations to the use of botulinum toxin are the relatively short duration of action (up to 3 months after the initial injection) and the limited number of muscles that can receive injections at one time. Two serotypes (A and B) currently are available for clinical use, and they vary in dosage and duration of action. Consensus dosing guidelines are available.[101] In individual studies, investigators have reported significant reduction in spasticity and functional improvement in both the upper and lower extremities. However, systematic reviews of use in the upper extremities and

lower extremities have revealed insufficient evidence to support or refute its use.[102,103] One group of authors recommends a cautious approach to the use of botulinum toxin injections because the data on long-term outcomes are limited.[104]

Intrathecal Baclofen

Baclofen is a GABA agonist, and its site of action is the spinal cord. It can be given intrathecally in small doses to maximize benefits with limited side effects. The effects of a single dose of intrathecal baclofen last only a few hours, and so it is given by a continuous-infusion pump. Since initial reports in the early 1990s,[105,106] intrathecal baclofen has become widely used for the management of spasticity and dystonia. The Treatment Outcomes Committee of the American Academy for Cerebral Palsy and Developmental Medicine published the results of a systematic review of 14 studies, including one RCT in 2000.[107] The review revealed evidence of decreased tone in upper and lower extremities, improved function of upper and lower extremities, improved ease of care and sleep, and decreased pain, as well as decreased truncal tone. Other studies have confirmed the benefits of intrathecal baclofen in children with both spasticity and dystonia.[108-111] Despite concerns about the relationship of intrathecal baclofen to progression of hip subluxation and scoliosis and increase in seizures, studies have demonstrated no relationship between intrathecal baclofen and change in seizure frequency[112] or hip status.[113] Both intrathecal baclofen withdrawal and overdose can be life-threatening emergencies. Table 14-6 reviews the signs and symptoms of baclofen overdose and withdrawal.

Selective Dorsal Rhizotomy

SDR is a neurosurgical procedure for the treatment of spasticity that is not effective for dystonia. It involves severing the dorsal spinal rootlets from the levels of L2 to S1 or S2. However, the number of rootlets cut and other procedural issues has varied significantly from center to center.[114] The ideal candidate for SDR

TABLE 14-6 ■ Signs and Symptoms of Baclofen Withdrawal and Overdose	
Baclofen Withdrawal	**Baclofen Overdose**
Itching (pruritus without rash)	Drowsiness
Hypertension	Dizziness, lightheadedness
Increased spasticity, rigidity	Hypoventilation
High fever	Seizures
Confusion, coma (may resemble malignant hyperthermia or autonomic dysreflexia)	Progressive hypotonia
	Somnolence, coma

appears to be a child who was born prematurely, has spastic diplegia, and is ambulatory with little or no truncal weakness. In the weeks after surgery, most children do manifest significant weakness, and maximum functional improvement does not occur until 6 to 12 months after the procedure. Three RCTs have demonstrated significant reductions in spasticity, and two revealed significant gains in functional skills as measured by the Gross Motor Function Measure, as did a subsequent meta-analysis.[115-118]

Functional changes after SDR persist over time.[119] SDR does not change the need for orthopedic surgery, especially for older children,[120] and SDR has no significant effect on the progression of hip subluxation.[121] Studies have reported conflicting data on the presence and progression of spinal deformities after SDR.[122,123] Of note, the number of children undergoing SDR has significantly fallen concomitantly with an increase in the number of children treated by intrathecal baclofen. There have been few available studies in which researchers compared SDR, intrathecal baclofen, or orthopedic interventions.

ORTHOPEDIC MANAGEMENT

The musculoskeletal problems of children with cerebral palsy include hip subluxation and dislocation, scoliosis and other spinal deformities, flexion contractures, foot and ankle deformities, hand and arm deformities, rotational deformities of the legs, leg length discrepancy, patella alta, osteopenia and fractures, joint pain, and hypertrophic ossification after surgery. Clinical gait abnormalities include the crouched gait and stiff knee gait. Orthopedic surgery is one of the treatment options for most of these issues. Orthopedic surgical procedures are either soft tissue surgical procedures, such as tendon and muscle releases, or bone surgical procedures, such as varus osteotomy of the femur or derotation osteotomy of the tibia. In general, orthopedic surgery is usually delayed until after 5 to 8 years of age, when all aspects of the deformity of the legs may be addressed at one time (multilevel surgery), unless structural issues necessitate earlier surgery to preserve function. For example, lengthening of the Achilles tendon before 8 years of age carries a higher risk for overcorrection,[124] and surgery before age 5 years carries the risk of recurrence of the plantar flexion contracture. Traditionally, investigators of surgical outcomes have reported change in the deformity and range of motion but have rarely reported change in function or activity participation.

Hip Subluxation and Dislocation

A common problem for children with spastic diplegia and spastic quadriplegia is hip subluxation and dislocation. As many as 30% of adults with cerebral

palsy and untreated hip dislocation have chronic hip pain.[125] For this reason, monitoring of the hip status of young children with cerebral palsy is important for detecting progressive hip subluxation early and preventing dislocation and possible pain in the hip. Clinicians monitor children with plain radiographs of the hip, starting at about 18 months of age. The migration percentage, or the percentage of the femoral head that is uncovered by the acetabulum, is the principal measure of hip stability. In hips with a migration percentage of 40% or greater at the time of soft tissue surgery, the migration progresses,[126] and in most hips with a preoperative migration percentage of less than 40%, the migration remains reduced. The initial surgical procedure is release of bilateral adductor tendons. Additional procedures may include varus osteotomies of the proximal femur and acetabular augmentation.

Scoliosis

Spinal deformity is a common problem in children with quadriplegia. Hip subluxation and dislocation with an asymmetrical sitting posture may contribute to progression of scoliosis. A spinal curve of 40% is likely to worsen and necessitate surgical stabilization.[127] Surgical stabilization is with posterior or combined anterior and posterior instrumentation and fusion. In general, parents and caregivers are pleased with the results of surgery for children with cerebral palsy, particularly with improvement in quality of life and ease of care.[128,129] The benefits of surgical stabilization of scoliosis in profoundly involved children, however, remain controversial.

ASSOCIATED PROBLEMS

Table 14-7 lists the associated health problems of children with cerebral palsy.

TABLE 14-7 ■ Health Problems of Children with Cerebral Palsy
Poor growth/nutrition
Oral motor dysfunction
Gastroesophageal reflux
Chronic and recurrent respiratory illnesses
Sleep disorder, including sleep apnea
Seizures
Visual impairment, strabismus, and nystagmus
Hearing impairment, persistent or recurrent otitis
Drooling
Constipation, urinary incontinence
Dental issues, including multiple caries, gingivitis, malocclusion
Pain and discomfort

Adapted from Nickel R: Cerebral palsy. *In* Nickel RE, Desch LW, eds: The Physician's Guide to Caring for Children with Disabilities and Chronic Conditions. Baltimore: Paul H. Brookes, 2000, p 146.

Osteopenia

Nonambulatory children with cerebral palsy are at risk for decreased bone mineral density, osteopenia, and recurrent fractures. In one study, 77% of 117 children with moderate and severe cerebral palsy had osteopenia (bone mineral density z-score ≤2 standard deviations), as did all of the participants who were unable to stand and older than 9 years.[130] The severity of the cerebral palsy, poor nutritional status, and the use of anticonvulsants increase the risk for osteopenia. The osteopenia in children with cerebral palsy results from the slow rate of growth in bone mineralization and not from loss of bone mineral, as in elderly adults.[131] Treatment consists of supplementation with vitamin D and calcium, standing programs,[132] and, in rare cases, the use of bisphosphonates. In a small RCT, pamidronate increased bone mineral density by 89% in the experimental group, in comparison with only 9% in the controls.[133] The authors noted no major adverse effects.

Oral Motor Dysfunction

A team approach is the most effective in the management of children with significant oral motor dysfunction. Signs of oral motor dysfunction in children with cerebral palsy include poor lip closure, drooling and inability to handle secretions, weak suck, lack of age-appropriate chewing, tonic bite and tongue thrust, coughing and gagging with feeding, and difficulty handling different textures of food and thin liquids.

Feeding problems are common in children with cerebral palsy and are highly correlated with indicators of poor health and nutrition.[134,135] In a study of 3- to 12-year-old children with moderate and severe cerebral palsy, 38% had significantly reduced fat stores; however, standard weight-to-height ratios were poor indices for the reduced fat stores.[136] Children with severe oral motor dysfunction may require enteral feeding to maintain adequate nutrition; however, limited information is available on the long-term benefits of gastrostomy feeding. In two systematic reviews, authors reported insufficient evidence for judging the effects of gastrostomy feedings in children with cerebral palsy.[137,138] A prospective multi-center cohort study of 57 children with cerebral palsy did demonstrate significant weight gain at 6 and 12 months after gastrostomy placement, and almost all parents reported decreased time in feeding and fewer hospital days.[139] The growth of children with cerebral palsy should be monitored with standard anthropomorphic measures, including length, weight, and body mass index; a measure of subcutaneous fat stores, such as the triceps skinfold; and alternative measures of linear growth, such as upper arm length and knee height, as needed.

Gastroesophageal Reflux

Gastroesophageal reflux is common in neurologically impaired children and is also associated with poor nutrition, oral motor dysfunction, and risk for aspiration. The symptoms of gastroesophageal reflux include recurrent vomiting or spitting up, choking and frequent swallowing during feeding, refusal of feedings or apparent early satiety, arching with feeding, torticollis (associated with esophagitis), recurrent respiratory symptoms, episodes of irritability, and frequent nighttime awakenings.[140]

Gastroesophageal reflux may be ameliorated with small, thickened feedings and careful positioning; however, children with persistent gastroesophageal reflux require medications to decrease gastric acidity, neutralize gastric acid, or increase intestinal motility. Infants with severe gastroesophageal reflux may require a Nissan fundoplication. Because of the risk for symptomatic gastroesophageal reflux, a current controversy is whether children who require placement of a gastrostomy for enteral feeding should undergo fundoplication at the same time. Placement of a percutaneous endoscopic gastrostomy does not appear to increase the risk for gastroesophageal reflux. In one study, 8% of children developed gastroesophageal reflux after percutaneous endoscopic gastrostomy, and it resolved in 38% of the children who had had gastroesophageal reflux preoperatively.[141] Percutaneous endoscopic gastrostomy is becoming the gastrostomy of choice because of its low cost, ease of placement, and cosmetic advantage.[142]

Incontinence, Constipation, and Drooling

The age at successful toilet training is significantly delayed for the majority of children with cerebral palsy,[143] and some children continue to have daytime urinary incontinence even though they have established independent bowel control. About one third of children with cerebral palsy have dysfunctional voiding.[144] The primary issues are urgency incontinence and, to a lesser extent, hesitancy (i.e., difficulty initiating a urinary stream).[144-146] Urodynamic findings include detrusor overactivity, detrusor-sphincter dyssynergia, and low bladder capacity.[144] Treatment is individualized and primarily involves use of anticholinergic medications and, in rare cases, intermittent catheterization.

Gastrointestinal problems are common in children with cerebral palsy, and chronic constipation is the most frequent condition identified, with a prevalence of 70% to 90%.[147,148] The factors that contribute to constipation include decreased mobility and activity, decreased fluid and fiber intake, difficulty positioning securely on the toilet, side effects of medications, and decreased colonic motility. In one study, all children with constipation and 70% of the children with cerebral palsy without constipation showed an abnormal colonic transit time in at least one segment of the colon.[149] Steps in the treatment of chronic constipation and secondary impaction include reviewing positioning/seating for toileting, addressing behavioral issues, making dietary alterations, performing a "clean-out" program for children with impaction (enemas, oral stimulants, or polyethylene glycol), and beginning a daily maintenance program (supplemental fiber and fluid, mineral oil, sorbitol or lactulose, or polyethylene glycol).

The goal of treatment is a stool of normal size and consistency at least every day or every other day. Treatment failure results primarily from the failure to treat constipation vigorously and as long as necessary. Children often require active treatment for 3 to 6 months and require supplemental fluid and fiber and dietary alterations indefinitely.

Drooling in children with cerebral palsy results from oral motor dysfunction, not from overproduction of saliva.[150] Persistent drooling can disrupt school and other day-to-day activities, cause chronic skin irritation, and interfere with social relationships. The treatment of drooling needs to be individualized and includes behavioral approaches, medications, injections of botulinum toxin, and surgical procedures. The goals of treatment are to improve the child's quality of life and social functioning. Behavioral strategies typically are ineffective when the child is focusing attention on other activities such as schoolwork. The use of medications, botulinum toxin, and possible surgery is usually considered in school-aged children with persistent drooling. In general, anticholinergic medications are the initial treatment, with consideration of botulinum toxin injections and surgery for children who do not respond to medications or who have significant side effects.

Glycopyrrolate (Robinul) is a commonly used medication because it does not appear to have the central nervous system side effects of other anticholinergic medications. A number of studies have reported significant benefit from anticholinergic medications,[151-153] including improvement in social functioning.[154] However, side effects—primarily constipation, sedation, irritability, and, less frequently, blurred vision and urinary retention—are frequent. The use of intraglandular botulinum toxin injections is a relatively new intervention for drooling. Several studies have documented the effectiveness of these injections.[155-157] However, dosage has varied across studies, and the effect persists for only a few months. A single clinical trial has been conducted to compare intraglandular botulinum toxin injections and scopolamine patches.[156] The magnitude of response to botulinum toxin was much higher (42% reduction in flow vs. 25%). However, 95% of the children responded to

scopolamine, whereas only 49% of the children responded to botulinum toxin. Surgical interventions have included salivary gland excision and salivary duct ligation or rerouting.[158-160] There is no consensus on the most appropriate surgical procedure, and postoperative complications are significant. These have included dry mouth with thick saliva, increased caries and other dental problems, and worsening of oral motor skills.[161] The data on the use of intraoral appliances to treat drooling are very limited.[162]

Seizures

In general, the prevalence of epilepsy in children with cerebral palsy varies markedly, depending on the anatomical type of cerebral palsy and whether cerebral palsy is associated with mental retardation. Epilepsy occurs in 20% to 40% of children with mental retardation and cerebral palsy.[163] It is more common in children with quadriplegia and more difficult to treat.[164] In children with cerebral palsy monitored in a neurology clinic, 60% of children with quadriplegia had intractable epilepsy, in comparison with 27.3% of children with hemiplegia and 16.7% of children with diplegia.[165] Newer antiepileptic drugs, procedures such as vagal stimulation, and epilepsy surgery have significantly improved the management of children with cerebral palsy and epilepsy.

Pain

Pain is a significant and understudied problem of children and adults with cerebral palsy. In a study of 100 adults with cerebral palsy, 67 reported one or more chronic pain problems and 19 reported daily pain.[166] Similarly, in a study of 43 families, 67% of parents reported that their children had pain within the previous month, and assisted stretching was the daily living activity most often associated with pain.[167] In a separate study, 11% of parents with children with cerebral palsy and GMFCS levels III to V reported that their children had daily pain. The pain was correlated with the severity of the motor impairment and with school days missed.[168] Assessment of pain in children with cerebral palsy can be difficult, because they may have associated communication or cognitive deficits. McKearnan and colleagues reviewed pain management in detail.[69]

COMPLEMENTARY AND ALTERNATIVE TREATMENTS

The use of complementary and alternative medicine (CAM) is frequent among children with chronic conditions and disabilities, including cerebral palsy (see Chapter 8E). Of families of children with chronic conditions who received care through a regional center in Arizona, 64% reported that their children used CAM.[169] Seventy-six percent of families reported

TABLE 14-8 ■ Representative Complementary and Alternative Medicine Treatments Used by Families of Children with Cerebral Palsy
Homeopathic medicine
Acupuncture
Hyperbaric oxygen
Threshold electrical stimulation (TES)
Craniosacral therapy
Doman-Delacato therapy (patterning)
Adeli suit
Conductive education
Massage therapy
Aquatherapy

TABLE 14-9 ■ Common Developmental and Mental Health Issues in Children with Cerebral Palsy
Speech and language disorder
Impaired written communication
Learning disability; nonverbal learning disability
Visual motor and visual perceptual dysfunction
Developmental delay and mental retardation
Attention-deficit/hyperactivity disorder
Autism spectrum disorders
Low self-esteem, social isolation, depression

that their children used CAM if their condition was noncorrectable. Similarly, 56% of families attending a cerebral palsy clinic reported that their children used one or more CAM treatments.[170] The children with quadriplegia who were nonambulatory used CAM the most often. The study reported massage therapy and aqua therapy as the most frequently used CAM treatments. Table 14-8 lists a number of CAM treatments used by children with cerebral palsy. Unfortunately, there are few rigorous scientific studies of CAM treatments for children with cerebral palsy. Collet and coworkers reported the results of a RCT on the use of hyperbaric oxygen in children with cerebral palsy.[171] The researchers reported no significant differences between the experimental and control groups.

The responsibilities of the health care provider are to be familiar with CAM treatments and providers; to provide families with information on the efficacy, safety, and cost of all treatments; and to assist families with evaluation of the effects of a CAM treatment.[172-174]

DEVELOPMENTAL AND MENTAL HEALTH ISSUES

Table 14-9 lists the common developmental and mental health issues experienced by children with cerebral palsy. Many children have both a physical disability (cerebral palsy) and one or more developmental disabilities. For example, cerebral palsy may be present in association with attention-deficit/hyperactivity disorder and learning disabilities or with mental retardation. Children with cerebral palsy and mental retardation are more likely than those without these conditions to have seizures and other chronic health problems such as gastroesophageal reflux. Adolescents with cerebral palsy are more likely than their peers to report low self-esteem and to be more socially isolated. Although they rate having friends as very important, they have limited contact with friends outside of school and rarely participate in after-school community activities.[175,176]

LIFESPAN ISSUES

A minority of adults with cerebral palsy are fully employed.[177,178] Some affected individuals lose the ability to walk, and many report a deterioration in walking ability.[177,179] Many do not have access to health insurance and regular health surveillance, although they continue to have problems with neck, back, and joint pain, as well as drooling, dental hygiene issues, constipation, urinary tract infections, and other adult health care issues. The health-related quality of life and the successful participation of individuals with cerebral palsy in all aspects of life depend as much on the treatment of associated health conditions, the development of social skills, and competency in making their own health care decisions as they do on the presence and treatment of motor impairments. It is crucial to take a lifespan approach in working with persons with cerebral palsy to maximize their successful participation and overall quality of life. Preparation for the transition to adult health care, employment, and independent living must begin early in life by encouraging self-care, independence, participation in community activities typical for the child's age, and the development of self-determination.

SPINA BIFIDA

Few medical conditions can affect so many of a child's organs and functions as spina bifida. Myelomeningocele and related neural tube defects (NTDs) are among the most frequent and complex malformations affecting children. In this section, we provide a general overview of the frequent medical problems and treatment. Although we focus on patients with open spina bifida (myelomeningocele), many of the issues, such as bowel and bladder management and neuro-orthopedic problems of the spine, are also present in patients with other types of NTDs such as lipomeningocele, tight filum terminale, spinal lipomas, or diastematomyelia.

Definition and Classification

Spinal cord malformations occur during the early stages of embryo development. They can occur during the early formation of the neural tube during week 3 and 4 or during its further development (secondary neurulation) during weeks 5 and 6. *Spinal dysphraphims* is the term for spinal cord malformations, and they are clinically categorized as open and closed, on the basis of whether the abnormal nervous tissue is exposed to the environment or covered by skin. Open spina bifida includes conditions such as meningocele, which involves the meninges but not the spinal cord, and myelomeningocele, which includes the meninges and all or part of the spinal cord. In most cases, the spinal cord below the defect is nonfunctional. In patients with spina bifida occulta, the defect is covered by skin. There are two main types of spina bifida occulta. The most common type is an isolated failure of fusion of the posterior arches of the lumbosacral spine. This is a very common finding (15% to 20% of the general population) and, in general, has no clinical consequences. The other type is a group of malformations characterized by opening of the posterior arches and involvement of other tissues. Many patients with this type have abnormalities in the skin or subcutaneous tissue in the low lumbar or sacral area, such as a deep sacral dimple, hemangiomas, a patch of hair, or a mass of fat. In lipomyelocele, the mass includes fat tissue alone; in lipomyelomeningocele, it also includes some spinal cord. Other cases of closed spina bifida can be simple dysraphic states, such as tight filum terminale, intradural lipomas, persistent terminal ventricle, and dermal sinuses, or more complex malformations, such as diastematomyelia. Other anomalies of the spine related to notochord formation include caudal agenesis and spinal segmental dysgenesis. Anencephaly is the most severe form of NTD. Newborns with anencephaly do not survive. The etiology and prevalence of anencephaly are strongly associated with those of open spina bifida.

There is limited agreement on how to classify myelomeningocele according to the anatomical or motor functional level of the defect. The relevance of the classification often has to do with the purpose of the study. All authors classify a thoracic defect as *high level.* Defects at level L1 and L2 are referred to as *high lumbar.* Most authors refer to defects at L4 and L5 as *low lumbar.* In some classifications, L3 is included with the high lumbar level; in others, with the low lumbar levels; in yet others it is grouped together with L4 defects to as *midlumbar.* Most authors agree on using *sacral level* as another categorical group. According to distribution based on level, approximately 10% to 20% of defects are thoracic, 15% to 20% are high lumbar, 26% to 37% are low lumbar, and 21% to 35% are sacral.[180]

Prevalence

In the United States, the current prevalence of myelomeningocele is 0.20 per 1000 live births. The prevalence of anencephaly is 0.09 per 1000 live birth.[181] The increased awareness of the role of folic acid in reducing the risk of spina bifida has helped to reduce the risk of NTDs. In 1992, the U.S. Public Health Service recommended that women of childbearing age increase consumption of the vitamin folic acid to reduce spina bifida and anencephaly.[181a] Mandatory fortification of enriched cereal grain products with folic acid by the U.S. Food and Drug Administration began in January 1998. The prevalence of spina bifida decreased by 20% between 1991 and 2001. The prevalence of NTDs decreases from the eastern to western United States.[182] The prevalence is lower among African Americans than in white people, and most studies find a higher risk in Hispanic/Latino families.[183] A relatively higher prevalence of NTDs in low-income populations may be related to limited access to health care, as well environmental and dietary factors.

Etiology

A combination of multiple risk factors cause NTDs, including dietary, environmental, and genetic factors (Table 14-10).[184] Detailed nutritional studies, as well as laboratory research, pointed to folic acid as a likely mediator. Randomized studies conducted in the late 1980s showed that extra intake of folic acid could reduce the risk of NTDs by 50% to 70%.[185,186] In countries that enforced enrichment of flour with folic acid, the prevalence of NTDs has declined.[183,187] There is also strong evidence for a genetic contribution to the risk of NTD. Prevalence is different among ethnic groups, even when they share a similar environment. In the United States, families of Irish origin have a higher risk of spina bifida, whereas African-American families have a lower risk.[188] The recurrence risk is 2% to 4% after a mother has a single child with a NTD. After two affected pregnancies, the risk increases to 11%-15%.[184] Studies have identified a variant form of methylenetetrahydrofolate dehydrogenase, 677C-T, as a risk factor for NTDs, but the prevalence of the genotype explains only a small portion of the protective effect of folic acid.[189,190] Researchers have found an association of homeobox genes *(PAX, PRX, HOX)* with NTDs in animals and in some patients.[191-194] The understanding of the genetic factors is expected to increase in the near future.

TABLE 14-10 ■ Risk Factors for Neural Tube Defects

Risk Factor	Evidence of Risk
Nutritional	Incidence of neural tube defects peaks after famine Seasonal variations Preventive effect of folic acid in case-controlled and randomized studies
Environmental	East-to-west trend in United States Decreased risk among Irish who migrate to United States Seasonal variations

Genetic	Familial risk
	  2%-4% recurrence after one affected child
	  11%-15% recurrence after two affected children
	Ethnic differences
	  Prevalence in U.S. populations: Hispanic > white >African American
	  Great Britain: highest risk in Celtic population
	  India: highest risk in Sikh population
	Chromosomal abnormalities
	Genetic disorders (Waardenburg syndrome; 22p11 microdeletion)
	Variant form of methylenetetrahydrofolate dehydrogenase (677C-T)

Physical	Association with maternal fever during pregnancy Association with maternal use of hot tubs or sauna during pregnancy
Maternal	Obesity Diabetes mellitus
Teratogenic	High vitamin A intake Valproic acid Alcohol

Other known risk factors during pregnancy include high fever, valproic acid, carbamazepine, exposure to high doses of vitamin A, maternal diabetes, and obesity.[184,195-198] Chromosomal abnormalities, such as trisomies 13 and 18, and a number of other syndromes can manifest with spina bifida.

Prevention Strategies

The effectiveness of folic acid supplementation to reduce the risk of NTD is now well established. Current recommendation for all women of childbearing age is to take 0.4 mg of folic acid daily, the usual dose in most multivitamins. Women with a higher risk of having a child with NTDs should take 1 to 4 mg daily. Women at high risk are those who have had a previous baby with a NTD, have a relative with a NTD, are obese, have diabetes, or are taking valproic acid or other anticonvulsant medication. Avoidance of known teratogens, such as alcohol, high doses of vitamin A, isotretinoin (Accutane), or etretinate (Tegison) is important.

Evaluation

Currently, screening of pregnant women includes a triple marker screen (α-fetoprotein combined with human chorionic gonadotropin and unconjugated estriol). Routine screening is done ideally between the 15th and 18th weeks of gestation.[199] Early diagnosis of open spina bifida or anencephaly can be suspected if the maternal α-fetoprotein level is increased. α-Fetoprotein levels change significantly with gestational age, and the most frequent reason for elevated levels is incorrect dating of the pregnancy. Twin pregnancy can also elevate the α-fetoprotein level. If the level is high, high-resolution ultrasonography should be performed. This study can help to identify other associated abnormalities, such as hydrocephalus, Chiari malformation, and abnormalities of the spine. American College of Obstetricians and Gynecologists guidelines recommend amniocentesis if α-fetoprotein level is high.[199a] High levels of α-fetoprotein and acetylcholinesterase in amniotic fluid can confirm the diagnosis of NTD. Chromosome analysis should rule out chromosomal abnormalities and aid in prenatal counseling. Routine ultrasonography can detect NTD. Analysis of fetal movements by ultrasonography is not predictive of future function, although the level of the defect is somewhat predictive.[200,201] If the spinal defect is located at the thoracic level, it is very likely that the child will have very limited or no movements in the lower extremities. Children with sacral defects have good prognosis for ambulation in most cases. When the defect is in the lumbar area, it is more difficult to determine the prognosis, because one vertebra level higher or one level lower can mean the difference between functional ambulation or no ambulation. MRI may provide a more detailed evaluation of the defect and associated malformations, although it is not recommended as a standard evaluation during pregnancy. In general, surgery for open spina bifida in the fetus has not been effective. Fetal surgery of the spinal defect does appear to reduce the prevalence of hydrocephalus, with no changes in the sensorimotor function.[202,203] Investigators are currently evaluating the risk : benefit ratio of a surgery that necessitates two cesarean sections in less than 3 months and the risk of prematurity.[204] Fetal surgery to treat hydrocephalus has not yielded satisfactory results. Whenever possible, the delivery of a fetus identified with myelomeningocele should be in a tertiary care center with a readily available experienced team. The benefit of cesarean section over vaginal delivery is controversial.[205-207] Once the diagnosis is made, a clinician experienced in myelomeningocele should provide counseling to the family.

Management

INITIAL CARE

After birth and stabilization of cardiopulmonary function, a careful examination should be performed. Sterile gauze should cover the defect, with saline solution to keep it moist. If the child requires placement in the supine position, a donut of sterile gauze may protect the defect. Avoidance of trauma to the sac is important. If the sac is open, it must be closed immediately. When the defect is intact and covered by skin, it can be closed days or weeks later. Initial assessment should include a complete neurological examination. This examination may help predict future motor function, although patients may have temporary loss of movements after the trauma of the spinal cord surgery or may have movements that originate at a spinal level and are not under the control of the cortex. This examination should include the observation of movements in upper and lower extremities and the use of pinpricks to evaluate sensation. The skeletal examination may reveal orthopedic malformations in the spine and lower extremities. These defects are frequent and are the result of the lack of innervations of some groups of muscles. Chromosome analysis and genetic consultation should be performed if the child has other physical abnormalities not related to the defect. Fluorescent in situ hybridization 22q11 analysis is indicated in children with cardiac malformations, cleft palate, or DiGeorge syndrome.[208,209] Head ultrasonography or computed tomography should be performed to evaluate for the presence of Arnold-Chiari malformation and hydrocephalus. Daily head circumference measurements should be performed to monitor for the presence of hydrocephalus, the response to shunt insertion, and early detection of shunt malfunction. Symptoms related to Arnold-Chiari malformation, such as feeding or swallowing difficulties or apnea, require special attention. Children may present with early symptoms of neurogenic bladder. The monitoring of urinary output, physical examination to detect bladder distention, and measurement of renal function with creatinine and blood urea nitrogen are important, as is consultation with the urology department. Initial evaluation must include vesicoureterography and renal ultrasonography.[210,211] Some urologists advocate the use of urodynamics in the initial evaluation.[212] However, spinal cord surgery can temporarily affect bladder dynamics. Monitoring of bowel movements and stool characteristics should include instruction of parents on the risk of constipation. The high prevalence of congenital cardiac defects among children with myelomeningocele suggests the need for echocardiography before discharge.[213]

INTERDISCIPLINARY CARE

The number and complexity of health issues that require attention underscore the need for a coordinated, multidisciplinary team. Table 14-11 suggests the types of professionals in the team caring for a child with myelomeningocele, as well as main areas of concern. These issues will affect the children at different ages. Neurosurgeons address issues such as closure of the defect and hydrocephalus during the neonatal period. Hydronephrosis necessitates urgent treatment, whereas treatment of urine and bowel incontinence can be deferred until the preschool years. Orthopedic problems rarely necessitate urgent attention, although clubfoot may necessitate early

TABLE 14-11 ■ Multidisciplinary Participation in Care of Children with Myelomeningocele	
Discipline	**Clinical Focus**
Neurosurgery	Hydrocephalus Posterior fossa compression Tethered cord
Orthopedics	Scoliosis Contractures Hip subluxation Gait abnormalities
Urology	Urinary incontinence Hydronephrosis Urinary infection
Developmental pediatrics	Growth and nutrition Endocrinological disorders Developmental problems Attention-deficit/hyperactivity disorder Allergy
Physical therapy	Ambulation Contractures Braces/orthoses Equipment Lower extremity weakness/spasticity
Occupational therapy	Visual-motor problems Functional problems Upper extremity weakness/spasticity
Psychology and special education	Learning disabilities Mental retardation Nonverbal learning disability
Nursing	Health supervision Urinary incontinence Clean intermittent catheterization Bowel incontinence/constipation Skin care
Social work	Family problems Community resources Health care access
Ophthalmology	Nystagmus Strabismus Amblyopia

treatment. Control and treatment of joint problems and scoliosis require ongoing follow-up. Developmental issues may arise at any age. Although severe developmental delay necessitates attention in infants, mild learning problems may not become apparent until adolescence.

MOTOR FUNCTION

The strength of the movements in the lower extremities allows estimation of the child's functional level (Table 14-12). Patients with thoracic-level defects have no controlled movements of the lower extremities, and their prognosis for independent ambulation is poor. They may be able to stand with the use of orthoses (parapodium; parawalker) and move with the use of a walker or crutches. Between 5% and 20% of such children may demonstrate household ambulation.[180,214] Children with high lumbar motor function of L1, L2, and some L3 have some movements of the hips. The children can ambulate with the use of orthoses: a high-level orthosis, a reciprocating-gait orthosis, or a hip-knee-ankle-foot orthosis. These children need the support of a walker or crutches, and most use a wheelchair for long-distance ambulation. Ambulation is achieved in 52% to 67% of patients with high lumbar or mid-lumbar defects.[180,214,215] The benefit of intensive treatment to achieve ambulation in children with high-level defects is controversial, because older children prefer to use a wheelchair.[216,217] Children

with L4 motor level defects need low-level braces, either a knee-ankle-foot orthosis or an ankle-foot orthosis, to support their feet; they may later need a wheelchair for long-distance and independent mobility. Children with an L5 motor level defect are functionally independent in most cases, requiring only low-level braces (ankle-foot orthoses). Children with low lumbar defects have a good prognosis; 85% to 95% are able to ambulate.[180,214] Children with sacral defects may have weakness of the intrinsic muscles of the feet and have no limitations on ambulation. Motor function can deteriorate with worsening of orthopedic problems, such as scoliosis or contractures, or with neurological injuries caused by shunt complications, such as tethered cord or spasticity.[218,219] In a study of 35 adults with sacral defects who had been community ambulators, Brinker and associates found a decline in the ability to walk in 30% of the patients, with 11% of the 35 subjects becoming nonambulators and 13% household ambulators.[220]

Treatment

PRINCIPLES IN MOTOR MANAGEMENT

The main goal for motor management is to maximize functional abilities. Independent ambulation and self-care are the primary objectives. To achieve these goals, the patient requires good range of motion and

---

TABLE 14-12 ■ Motor Level and Expected Function

Spinal Level	Movement	Muscles	Household Ambulation	Community Ambulation
Thoracic	Abdomen	Abdominal	Wheelchair; Standing with standing frame or parapodium HKAFO or RGO	Wheelchair
L1	Hip flexion	Iliopsoas	Wheelchair use indoors	Wheelchair
L2	Hip flexion Hip adductors	Iliopsoas Sartorius	High-level orthosis (HKAFO or RGO) with walking aids	
L3	Knee extension	Quadriceps	High-level orthosis (HKAFO or KAFO) and help of walking aids	With high-level orthosis and help of walking aids; wheelchair
L4	Foot dorsiflexion (inversion) Hip abduction	Tibialis anterior Tensor fascia latae		
L5	Strong abduction Foot inversion Some knee flexion	Gluteus medius and minimus Tibialis posterior Semitendinous, medial hamstring	Low-level orthosis AFO or UCBL No need for walking aids	Wheelchair may be needed for long distances
S1	Plantar flexion Great toe dorsiflexion	Gastrocnemius soleus Flexor hallucis longus	Low-level orthosis AFO or UCBL No need for walking aids	Wheelchair may be needed for long distances
S2	Intrinsic movement of the foot	Muscles of the foot	Normal or UCBL	Normal

Data from Bartonek and Saraste, 2001,[372] and from Bartonek, Saraste, and Knutson, 1999.[373]
AFO: ankle-foot orthosis; HKAFO: hip-knee-ankle-foot orthosis; KAFO: knee-ankle-foot orthosis; RGO: reciprocating gait orthosis; UCBL: University of California, Berkeley, laboratory orthosis.

an appropriate posture and may need walking aids or a wheelchair. Maintaining range of motion mandates lifelong attention. The appropriate posture depends on the functional level of the myelomeningocele and appropriate orthosis (Table 14-13). Ideally, the treatment plan follows normal developmental stages: upright position, standing, and ambulation. The use of parapodium or standers in children at 12 months with high lumbar and thoracic defects can help achieve a standing posture. Around 2 or 3 years of age, children with high lumbar defects require a high-level orthosis and gait training in order to obtain independent ambulation. The use of a wheelchair provides independent mobility. Periodic physical therapy and occupational therapy assessments should be part of the treatment of all the children with myelomeningocele. Range of motion, muscle strength, and function should be assessed. The provision of regular physical and occupational therapy evaluations of children with myelomeningocele should begin in infancy. Therapy goals include maintenance or improvement of joint range of motion; selection of an appropriate orthosis and assistive devices; monitoring strength and coordination of the upper extremities; training on ambulation and transfers in and out of a wheelchair; selection of an appropriate wheelchair and seating devices; and assisting the family and the

patient in solving activities of daily living, such as bathing, toileting, and driving. Periodic assessments must guide treatment and also detect change in function, because multiple neurological and orthopedic complications can negatively affect motor function.

ORTHOPEDIC MANAGEMENT

In general, the long-term outcomes after orthopedic surgery for correction of hip, spine, and joint contractures are better for older children, because recurrence of contractures are less likely and surgeries done on the spine in younger children can slow or arrest the growth of the spine.

Scoliosis is caused by an imbalance of muscle strength and spine malformations. It is a frequent problem, affecting about 47% to 70% of children with myelomeningocele.[221-223] The frequency of scoliosis varies with the level of the spinal defect. It can be as high as 94% among children with thoracic defects and as low as 5% among children with sacral defects.[224,225] Once the curvature in scoliosis is greater than 40 degrees, it tends to progress and necessitates surgical treatment. Rapid progression of scoliosis can be a symptom of tethered cord.

Children with thoracic or high lumbar motor function often develop hip dislocation as the strength of the iliopsoas muscle is unopposed. The risk for hip

TABLE 14-13 ■ Orthopedic Problems and Treatments		
Condition	**Indications**	**Treatment**
Scoliosis	More than 20 degrees of curvature	Bracing
	More than 40 degrees of curvature	Anterior or posterior fusion with Luque instrumentation
Kyphosis	Progression	Bracing
	Recurrent decubitus; problems with sitting, balance, or progression	Anterior or posterior fusion with Luque instrumentation
		Kyphectomy in young children (controversial)
Hip subluxation or dislocation	In an ambulating patient	Passive range of motion
		Iliopsoas or adductors transfer (controversial)
	In a nonambulating patient	Anterior release of hip contractures
Clubfoot	In a newborn	Serial casting
	In an infant	Posterior medial foot release
	In an adolescent	Triple arthrodesis
Hip flexion contractures	Lumbar to thoracic levels	Passive range of motion
	Contractures greater than 30 degrees	Anterior tendon release
Knee flexion contractures	Lumbar to thoracic levels	Passive range of motion
	Contractures greater than 20 degrees	Posterior tendon release
Equinus foot	Lumbar to thoracic levels	Passive range of motion
		Bracing (ankle-foot orthosis)
	Contractures greater than 10 degrees	Release of Achilles tendon
Calcaneus foot	In an infant	Passive range of motion
		Bracing (ankle-foot orthosis)
	Improving foot posture during ambulation for older child	Anterior tibialis transfer or anterior release

dislocation is 60% to 70% with thoracic defects, 75 to 85% with high lumbar defects, 25% with low lumbar defects, and 3% with sacral defects.[214] Children with a poor prognosis for ambulation and no pain do not require surgery.[226] Muscle transfer of the iliopsoas or adductors can stabilize the hip and prevent further migration.[227,228] Surgical treatment for hip dislocation has yielded mixed results.[226] Careful evaluation of the gait pattern, functional abilities, and resources is indicated before surgery. In addition, patients often develop joint contractures as a result of decreased mobility.[229] Treatment of contractures is based on the extent that they impair the child's functioning or interfere with caring for the child.

Some newborns with myelomeningocele have foot malformations related to the level of the defect and muscle innervations.[230] Children with sacral defects may have clawed toes and flat feet; those with paralysis below L5 may have calcaneous foot; those with defect below L4 may have equinovarus foot; and those with higher level defects may also have equinovarus.[231,232] Nonambulatory children may require surgery to facilitate care and use of shoes. Surgical treatment during infancy carries a high risk of recurrence of the malformation.[231]

OSTEOPOROSIS MANAGEMENT

Patients with myelomeningocele have decreased bone mineral density, and 22% to 40% develop fractures as a result of osteoporosis.[233-237] Although lack of weight bearing can explain osteoporosis in the lower extremities, the etiology of the osteoporosis is not yet understood. For example, investigations of the radial bone revealed significantly lower values of bone density in children with myelomeningocele that are not explained by lack of use.[234] Children who are placed in standing position have less osteoporosis and a decreased risk for fractures.[238,239] The measurement of bone mineral density can help to identify the patients at greatest risk for multiple fractures. Treatment with oral bisphosphonates can decrease osteoporosis and apparently reduces the incidence of fractures in patients with myelomeningocele.[240]

NEUROGENIC BLADDER MANAGEMENT

Neurogenic bladder is the most common problem with spina bifida. Even patients with low sacral defects and no apparent motor or sensory deficit may have impairment in bladder function. We briefly describe the physiology of the bladder: The external sphincter receives its innervation from the pudendal nerve (sacral levels S2 to S4). The bladder has a predominance of β-adrenergic receptors. The sympathetic component of the autonomic nervous system stimulates these receptors. β-Adrenergic stimulation, via fibers of the hypogastric nerve (T11 to L2), suppresses contraction of the detrusor. The detrusor contracts by the parasympathetic stimulation from fibers in the pelvic nerve. The primary receptors in the bladder neck are α-adrenergic. These receptors are stimulated by the hypogastric nerve arising at the low thoracic level. During micturition, supraspinal centers block stimulation by the hypogastric and pudendal nerves. This relaxes the internal and external sphincters and removes the sympathetic inhibition of the parasympathetic receptors. The result is contraction of the detrusor. Disruption of the relationship between autonomic and voluntary control can result in three types of urological problems: a system with increased pressure, urinary stasis, and urinary incontinence.

Ureteral Reflux and Hydronephrosis Management

The causes of increased pressure in the bladder include increased activity of the bladder, hypertonic sphincter, and uninhibited contractions of the bladder and sphincter. This increased pressure results in vesicoureteral reflux in 20% of the patients with myelomeningocele. Hydronephrosis occurs in 7% to 30% of such infants. The hyperactivity of the bladder results in poor compliance of the bladder, which can worsen during the first months of life. Between 32% and 45% of children with myelomeningocele and initial normal bladder pressures have abnormal pressures at older ages.[241,242] Therefore, normal findings of a urodynamic study after birth do not ensure normal bladder function, and such children require longitudinal monitoring. Most centers conduct periodic evaluations with renal ultrasonography, voiding cystourethrography, and/or urodynamic tests.[243] Early treatment of hydronephrosis prevents renal damage. The standard intervention is the use of clean intermittent catheterization (CIC). Some experts advocate starting with CIC in the neonatal period in all children, arguing that they will ultimately require CIC for social continence and an early start will facilitate compliance. The use of anticholinergic medication will increase bladder capacity and decrease hyperactivity of the detrusor. Intravesical instillation of oxybutynin can avoid systemic effects from the medication.[244,245] Vesicostomy can be done as a temporary surgery when medical treatment fails.[246] Vesicoureteral reflux may resolve after reducing the bladder pressure, although it often requires surgical intervention.

Urinary Infections Management

Incomplete emptying of the bladder and/or ureters results in increased risk for urinary infections. Periodic emptying with CIC helps to reduce the risk of infections. In patients with recurrent urinary tract infections (UTI), the use of prophylactic antibiotics by mouth or by local instillation can help to reduce the number of infections. Detection of UTI can be challenging since abnormal urinalysis with increased white cell or bacteriuria is common in children using CIC. The use of nitrite and leukocyte esterase chemstrip can help as screening tests.[247,248] Most centers treat bacteriuria only if the child has other clinical signs or symptoms (fever, dysuria, flank pain, changes in the urinary pattern).[243]

Social Continence Management

A combination of lack or limited sensation from the bladder, lack of voluntary control of the sphincter and bladder, hypertonic bladder, and/or hypotonic sphincter causes incontinence. Most children with myelomeningocele require an active treatment for social continence. Urinary incontinence can decrease social integration and self perception of subjects with myelomeningocele.[249-251] Medical management is usually a combination of CIC and anticholinergic medication. α-Adrenergic agonist medication can help to improve continence when the internal sphincter is hypotonic. About 50% of the children can obtain social continence with medical management.[252] Catheterizations should be sufficiently frequent to avoid accidents. Bladder augmentation can increase the bladder capacity when medical treatment fails. This procedure can assist the older child who has a well-established catheterization program, but is unable to obtain continence due to the low volume of the bladder. Augmentation uses a flap obtained from the colon, ileum, or stomach, or by detrusor myotomy to increase bladder volume. Stone formation due to mucous secretion is a frequent complication (18% to 48%) when augmentation is done with colon.[253,254] Metabolic acidosis can occur in some children after augmentation.[236,255] The use of a ureter for augmentation appears to solve some of the problems from other augmentation techniques.[256-258] For patients with weak sphincter, other surgical procedures may be helpful, including the implantation of an artificial sphincter, bladder neck wrap with muscle (sling procedure), or the injection of bulking agents around the neck.[259-261] There is no agreement on which procedure has a better outcome. Ileal conduit urinary diversion, a frequent treatment in the past, is now rarely done because of the high number of complications.[262,263] If the child is unable to perform self catheterization due to anatomical impairments, a urinary diversion using the appendix (Mitrofanoff procedure) or a tubularization of ileum or sigmoid can be effective in achieving independent continence.[264,265] The patient or a caregiver performs catheterizations through a stoma.

Caregivers perform CIC during early childhood. At the age of 6 or 7 years, children can begin performing their own catheterizations. The success of self-catheterization depends on the child's cognitive abilities and organizational skills; the absence of significant anatomical limitations such as scoliosis, contractures, or obesity; the child's fine motor coordination, balance, and trunk control; and external support.

Hydronephrosis, chronic pyelonephritis, and associated malformations can affect renal function.[266] Approximately 40% of older children and adults with these malformations have abnormal renal function.[266,267] Renal transplantation has been successful after renal failure.[268,269]

NEUROGENIC BOWEL MANAGEMENT

Along with neurogenic bladder, problems with bowel incontinence and constipation are among the most frustrating problems for children and families. The abnormal function of the sigmoid colon and rectum, the lack of sphincter control, and decreased or absent sensation result in constipation and/or incontinence in most patients with myelomeningocele. The pudendal nerve (S2 to S4) provides the voluntary innervation of the external sphincter and muscles of the pelvic floor. The hypogastric nerve (L1 to L3) supplies sympathetic innervation, which inhibits motility. Parasympathic innervations to the sigmoid colon and rectum stimulate motility and gastrointestinal secretions through the splanchnic nerves (S1 to S4).

Constipation

Constipation can manifest early in life and necessitates active treatment in most patients with myelomeningocele. When constipation is present, the treatment must be proactive, not delayed until the child has missed a bowel movement or stools for several days. Treatment includes a diet high in fiber and sufficient fluid intake. When the child's diet has insufficient fiber, it can be added to foods. Clinicians can recommend the use of foods with natural laxative effect, such as prunes, on a routine basis. Some children need laxatives such as polyethylene glycol, bisacodyl, or senna. Bowel training with timed toileting on a daily basis can be effective in achieving continence in cooperative patients who have no constipation and have sufficient abdominal muscles strength. Some patients may require digital stimulation of the rectum to initiate the defecation reflex. Some patients require routine use of suppositories and enemas. The antegrade continence enema procedure may be effective for patients with recalcitrant constipation. The original description by Malone and colleagues consists of a nonrefluxing channel in which the appendix is used to produce a catheterizable colonic stoma.[270] If the appendix is not available, options include retubularization of the sigmoid or ileum or a standard gastrostomy button placed in the cecum.[265,271,272] A few patients with myelomeningocele have an overactive colon, which results in loose stools and incontinence that is difficult to manage. The antisecretory and antimotility agent loperamide can be helpful for some of these patients. The child and family require an individualized bowel program. Although a systematic approach and a family commitment are keys to a bowel program, they do not guarantee success.

SENSORY FUNCTION AND ITS MANAGEMENT

Children with myelomeningocele lack sensation for touch, pressure, pain, and temperature below the defect. This lack of sensation can be asymmetrical and may not be at the same level as the lack of motor function. Figure 14-1 depicts the dermatomes or areas of the skin supplied by sensory fibers of single posterior spinal roots.

Pinprick examination can be used periodically to assess the sensory level. Spinal cord complications, such as tethered cord or syringomyelia, can produce loss of sensation, and the confirmation by physical examination can help with diagnosis and treatment decisions. During the sensory examination, the examiner should carefully watch the motor response of the infant. It is important to prevent older children from seeing the pinprick, because they often report positive sensation, even in areas with proven anesthesia. Lack

of sensation can result in pressure sores or injuries. In one study, McDonnell found that 35% of adults with myelomeningocele had pressure sores. The location of ulcers and pressure sores varies with the ambulatory status of the child. Children who ambulate in wheelchairs tend to have pressure sores in the gluteal area, whereas those who ambulate upright develop ulcers in the lower extremities.[217] In one study, 15% of adults with sacral motor defects lost their ability to ambulate because of complications from skin infections.[220] Children do not complain about lack of sensation. From an early age, parents must learn regular care of skin to prevent injuries produced by pressure, cold temperatures, hot temperatures, and friction. Checking the skin daily is important. Older children must learn self-examination. It is critical that patients be instructed to wear new braces and shoes for a very short period, around 20 minutes, and then inspect the skin. Once sores develop, they can take several weeks to heal. In certain situations, patients may require surgical procedures to correct pressure sores.[273,274] An estimated $2 million was the cost of the care of patients admitted for treatment of pressure sores in a single institution during a 13-year period.[275]

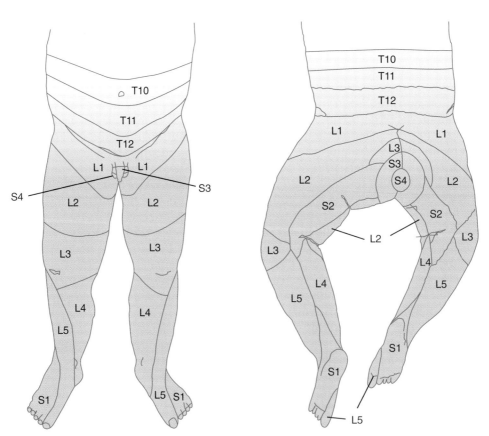

FIGURE 14-1 Dermatomes. *(Data from Foerster A, Haymaker W, Woodhall B: Peripheral Nerve Injury, 2nd ed. Philadelphia: WB Saunders, 1953.)*

NEUROLOGICAL/NEUROSURGICAL MANAGEMENT

Arnold-Chiari malformation consists of the displacement of cerebellum and brainstem through the opening in the back of the skull (foramen magnum), which often interferes with the flow of cerebral spinal fluid. Ninety-five percent of children with open spina bifida have some degree of Arnold-Chiari malformation. The most frequent problem resulting from Arnold-Chiari malformation is hydrocephalus.

Arnold-Chiari Malformation

Arnold-Chiari type II malformation consists of herniation of the tonsils and the contents of the posterior fossa into the foramen magnum. This herniation involves the brainstem, fourth ventricle, and cerebellar vermis. About 5% to 10% of the children with spina bifida present with symptoms related to compression of the brainstem caused by the Arnold-Chiari malformation.[276] Anatomopathology studies have demonstrated that compression of the brainstem results in ischemia and hemorrhages, although in some cases, abnormal anatomical findings suggest a developmental anomaly in the brainstem.[277] Symptoms include stridor, dysphagia, weakness in the upper extremities, ataxia, and nystagmus.[277-279] Mortality is high among patients with abnormal respiratory function that necessitates tracheotomy.[277] Shunt evaluation is essential before surgery for posterior fossa decompression is considered.

Some neurosurgeons recommend posterior fossa decompression on an emergency basis as soon the patient shows any symptoms of Arnold-Chiari malformation.[280,281] Patients with posterior fossa compression also may require placement of tracheostomy, ventilatory assistance, and gastrostomy. Symptomatic Arnold-Chiari malformation is the most common cause of death in children with spina bifida.

Hydrocephalus

About 85% of children with open spina bifida have hydrocephalus. The treatment is a ventricular shunt, which a neurosurgeon typically places a few days after the child's birth or simultaneously during the closure of the back during the first surgery. The presence of hydrocephalus is not predictive of future cognitive function except in severe cases, although the accumulation of shunt problems and/or infections increases the risk for cognitive limitations.[282] If the shunt is obstructed, the patient often exhibits the classic symptoms of increased intracranial pressure: bulging fontanelle in infants and lethargy, headaches, and vomiting in older children. A shunt can sometimes fail without obvious symptoms, and this failure can manifest with occasional morning headaches or the patient's awakening with headaches during the night, having occasional morning vomiting, or displaying changes in behavior or learning. Failure occurs in 45% to 60% of placed shunts.[283,284] Failure of the shunt can be caused by obstruction (70% to 80%) or infection (20% to 30%).[285] Shunt infection rates vary among centers and range from 0% to as high as 15%.[283] The shunt has fewer complications when it is placed at the time of the myelomeningocele repair.[284] Shunt infection is rare after 6 months of the shunt placement or revision.[286] Ventriculoatrial shunts are currently present only in adult patients or patients with intra-abdominal complications that necessitate the removal of a peritoneal shunt. Ventriculoatrial shunts have more complications, including thrombosis of the superior vena cava, pulmonary hypertension, and endocarditis.[287,288] Patients with ventriculoatrial shunts require prophylaxis for bacterial endocarditis. Annual monitoring is necessary for patients with hydrocephalus, because shunts can fail after several years of normal function or hydrocephalus can decompensate after many years in patients with stable, nonfunctional (i.e., disconnected) shunts.[289,290]

Tethered Cord

In patients with myelomeningocele, tethered cord can manifest with progressive scoliosis, back pain, changes in bowel or bladder function, increased spasticity, or loss of motor or sensory function.[291] The stretching of the spinal cord produces symptoms resulting from impaired oxidative metabolism on the stretched segments of the spinal cord. Spine MRI demonstrates that almost all patients with myelomeningocele have the end of the spinal cord below L2. For this reason, the low setting of the conus medullaris is not diagnostic of tethered cord.[292,293] Tethered cord is a common complication in children with spina bifida (15% to 25%). Periodic evaluation of motor and sensory function and evaluation of the spine can facilitate diagnosis. Children with high-level defects present with tethered cord at younger ages, usually before 6 years of age, whereas diagnosis is often later for children with lower level defects.[294] Surgical release is effective in reducing symptoms or stopping the progression in 47% to 80% of cases, and results are better when surgery is performed soon after presentation.[291,295,296]

Syringomyelia

Asymptomatic hydromelia or syringomyelia is found in 50% of spine MRI scans in children with myelomeningocele. On occasion, the syrinx becomes symptomatic, and patients present with complex upper limb weakness and wasting, sensory disturbance, dysphagia, or ataxia.[297] Worsening of symptoms should first prompt a careful evaluation of shunt function. Symptoms and radiological findings often improve after shunt revision. Sometimes, the release of tethered cord or posterior fossa decompression can improve the symptoms and resolve the hydromelia. Some patients require shunting of the syrinx to the subarachnoid space, the pleural space, or to the peritoneum.[298,299]

Seizures

About 16% to 20% of children with myelomeningocele have seizures at some time.[300-302] The number of shunt revisions and additional brain anomalies are associated with increased risk for seizures.[300,302] Seizures respond well to medication, and 75% of children with seizures can later discontinue treatment.[301] Seizures can be the first symptom of central nervous system complications such as infection, bleeding, or shunt malfunction. Chronic headaches affect 55% to 88% of patients with myelomeningocele and may not be caused by shunt malfunction or complications of Arnold-Chiari malformations.[303,304]

GROWTH AND NUTRITION MANAGEMENT

Evaluation of linear growth in children with spina bifida requires the use of alternative measurements. Poor growth in the lower extremities, contractures, and scoliosis make the measurement of length or height an inaccurate estimate of linear growth. The measurement of arm span is a good alternative. Clinicians may use an arm span growth chart or plot the arm span on a growth chart of height or length. The latter method is less accurate but readily available.[305-307] Periodic measurement of arm span helps identify endocrine disorders such as growth hormone deficiency or hypothyroidism.[308] The use of weight, height for weight, or body mass index measures are poor indicators of nutritional status, inasmuch as the body proportions are different for children with different levels of myelomeningocele. The use of other measurements such as arm circumference and skin fold can provide a better estimation of nutrition.[309-311] Feeding problems in infants with Arnold-Chiari type II symptoms may necessitate gastrostomy tube placement to maintain nutrition or prevent pulmonary aspiration.[312,313,221] These children may have a sensitive gag reflex with intolerance to food with texture.

Obesity

Investigators recognized obesity[309,314] as another health problem in myelomeningocele since the early 1970s. The risk for obesity has many contributing factors. Children with myelomeningocele require less energy than normal, particularly if they are nonambulatory.[315-318] Social isolation and decreased physical activity increase the risk. Sometimes, medical complications such as pressure sores or surgical procedures cause children to decrease their activity further.

In children with myelomeningocele, excessive weight has serious consequences. Obesity can result in the loss of their ability to ambulate. In severe cases, obesity may impair the ability to perform such daily life activities as self-catheterization or toileting. In older teenagers and adults, it jeopardizes their independence, as they may need help with transfers from the wheelchair to the bed or toilet. Pediatricians and parents should monitor the child's weight from infancy, and they should implement treatment as soon as the child is overweight.

Growth Hormone Deficiency

Children with spina bifida and hydrocephalus have increased risk for endocrinological disorders. Researchers estimate the prevalence of growth hormone deficiency to be between 11% and 18%.[319] Clinicians should suspect growth hormone deficiency when the arm span is below the third percentile on the growth chart. Routine evaluation of short children with insulin-like growth factor 1 and insulin-like growth factor binding protein 3 can help with early diagnosis.[319] Children treated with growth hormone show a response similar to that of children with idiopathic growth hormone deficiency.[308,320,321] With treatment, growth velocity and final height can be close to that expected for age.[322] Treatment of growth hormone deficiency can precipitate symptoms of tethered cord; therefore, children require frequent monitoring during treatment.[323] Hyperthyroidism has a prevalence of about 3%.[324]

Precocious Puberty

The prevalence of precocious puberty in children with myelomeningocele is 6% to 18%.[324-327] Children with both hydrocephalus and myelomeningocele start puberty 2 years before their peers. Careful genital examination and breast examination during the prepubertal years can assist in early diagnosis and treatment. Untreated precocious puberty can lead to short stature, particularly in women.[328]

REPRODUCTION AND SEXUAL FUNCTION

Women with myelomeningocele appear to have normal fertility. Information about the risk in individuals with myelomeningocele of having a child with NTD is limited. In one study, investigators examined the outcome of 39 pregnancies from 11 men and 11 women with spina bifida. Four offspring had NTD (two with anencephaly and two with open spina bifida).[329] Results should be interpreted cautiously, because most patients in 1975 with open spina bifida had a poor prognosis for survival. Other reported risks among pregnant women with myelomeningocele include urinary tract infections, constipation, decreased mobility, and decubitus. Cesarean section can be more challenging in women with bladder augmentation, ileal conduit, or ventriculoperitoneal shunt.

Sexual Function

Information regarding sexual function and reproduction is scant.[329a-329d] In general, patients with lower spinal defects have better outcomes. Although the percentage of adults reporting sexual activity is relatively high, study subjects are not representative of all patients with myelomeningocele. In a study by Sandler and associates, who used an objective measurement of penile rigidity, 11 of 15 young men reported erections, whereas objective documentation showed normal erections in only 2 subjects (who had sacral defects), brief and incomplete erections in 7 other subjects, and no response in 6. In this study, patients with lower motor and sensory defects had better outcomes.[330] Erection dysfunction can respond to sildenafil.[331]

CARDIOVASCULAR SYSTEM

The risk for congenital cardiovascular defects is higher in children with myelomeningocele than in a normal population. Ritter and coworkers, in a retrospective study of 105 children who underwent echocardiography before surgery, found that 37% had a cardiac malformation. In their sample, 25% had a secundum atrial septal defect, 9% had ventricular septal defect, and almost 5% had other defects (anomalous pulmonary venous return, tetralogy of Fallot, bicuspid aortic valve, coarctation, and hypoplastic left heart syndrome).[213] Kidney damage from repeated pyelonephritis, nephrolithiasis, and hydronephrosis can result in hypertension and/or renal insufficiency.[332] In a study of adults with myelomeningocele, 14% had hypertension; 46% had abnormal kidneys as a result of scarring, hydronephrosis, or nephrolithiasis; and 3% had renal failure that necessitated dialysis or kidney transplantation.[333] Blood pressure and renal function should be monitored in all patients with myelomeningocele. Patients with ventriculoatrial shunts have an increased risk for pulmonary hypertension. The cause of the pulmonary hypertension may be microembolism from the catheter or an immunological reaction of the pulmonary vessels to proteins from the cerebrospinal fluid.[334,335]

COGNITIVE AND DEVELOPMENTAL OUTCOME

In general, cognitive function is often poorer for children with high spinal lesions than in those with lower lesions. The prevalence of mental retardation is close to 40% in subjects with thoracic lesions but much lower in the population with sacral lesions. The larger number of brain malformations in children with higher defects mediates the association between level

of the lesion and cognitive function.[336,337] In the typical cognitive profile of patients with hydrocephalus, verbal skills are better than nonverbal skills.[338-340] "Cocktail party syndrome" describes some children with an exaggerated profile of nonverbal learning disability, with verbal expression that significantly exceeds cognitive skills. These children tend to be very friendly, characteristically make inappropriate comments, and appear to understand more than they really do. In clinical practice, it is important to objectively verify verbal comprehension of recommendations or explanations. The interaction between cognitive function and long-term outcome is complex. Low cognitive function is the most significant factor limiting independence.[282,341] However, reported quality of life and self-esteem are more closely associated with bowel and bladder functioning.

Attention-deficit/hyperactivity disorder is another frequent diagnosis. The prevalence varies between 34% and 39%.[337,342] Response to stimulant medication in children with spina bifida is similar to that in other children with this disorder. Cognitive or behavioral deterioration can occur after central nervous system infections or with chronic shunt malfunction.[343] It is therefore important to perform periodic neuropsychological evaluations.

OPHTHALMOLOGICAL ISSUES

Eye motor coordination disorders are very frequent. Strabismus occurs in 42% to 44% of children with spinal lesions; most of these have convergent esotropia.[344,345] Optic disc abnormalities, such as papilledema or disc atrophy, occur in 32%. In one study, only 27% of 322 children with myelomeningocele had normal results of eye examinations.[344] Not surprisingly, there is a correlation between the degree of mesencephalic abnormalities and problems with eye motor coordination.[346,347] The sudden appearance of strabismus, other ocular motility disorders, or papilledema is usually a manifestation of uncontrolled hydrocephalus. Children with myelomeningocele require regular ophthalmological evaluations.

LATEX ALLERGY

Allergy to latex can be a life-threatening condition for some patients with myelomeningocele. It was recognized as a common problem in the early 1990s, after some patients suffered anaphylactic shock during surgery.[348,349] The reported prevalence varies, depending on the criteria used to identify patients with allergy. Researchers have reported different prevalence rates of sensitized children with latex allergy, such as 32% to 55% and 15% to 34%.[350-352] The clinical manifestation may include redness after contact with objects made from rubber, such as balloons or gloves. Pinprick testing or specific immunoglobulin E or radioallergosorbent testing can help identify asymptomatic children with latex sensitivity. The number of surgical procedures is the major risk factor for latex allergy, along with a personal and family history of atopy.[353-355] Because it is important to prevent all contacts with latex products, patients who have had allergic reactions should wear an alert bracelet and carry epinephrine. Patients should be aware of cross-sensitization with fruits from trees, such as kiwi, avocado, and banana.[356] Most clinical centers currently avoid the use of latex in the operating rooms and clinics. Avoiding exposure to latex starting with the first surgery may decrease the number of patients with allergy.[357]

REFERENCES

1. National Institute of Child Health and Human Development, National Institutes of Health: Research Plan for the National Center for Medical Rehabilitation Research, NIH Publication No. 93-3509. Washington, DC: U.S. Department of Health and Human Services, Public Health Service, 1993.

2. Palisano R, Rosenbaum P, Walter S, et al: Development and reliability of a system to classify gross motor function in children with cerebral palsy. Dev Med Child Neurol 39:214-223, 1997.

3. Shapiro BK: Cerebral palsy: A reconceptualization of the spectrum. J Pediatr 145(2 Suppl):S3-S7, 2004.

4. Morris C, Bartlett D: Gross Motor Function Classification System: Impact and utility. Dev Med Child Neurol 46:60-65, 2004.

5. Bax M, Goldstein M, Rosenbaum P, et al: Proposed definition and classification of cerebral palsy, April 2005. Dev Med Child Neurol 47:571-576, 2005.

6. Prevalence and characteristics of children with cerebral palsy in Europe. Dev Med Child Neurol 44:633-640, 2002.

7. Himmelmann K, Hagberg G, Beckung E, et al: The changing panorama of cerebral palsy in Sweden. IX. Prevalence and origin in the birth-year period 1995-1998. Acta Paediatr 94:287-294, 2005.

8. Kuban KCK, Leviton A: Cerebral palsy. N Engl J Med 330:188-195, 1994.

9. Meberg A, Broch H: Etiology of cerebral palsy. J Perinat Med 32:434-439, 2004.

10. Paneth, N: Birth and the origins of cerebral palsy. N Engl J Med 315:124-126, 1986.

11. Williams K, Albermann E: The impact of diagnostic labelling in population-based research into cerebral palsy. Dev Med Child Neurol 40:182-185, 1998.

12. O'Shea TM: Cerebral palsy in very preterm infants: New epidemiological insights. Ment Retard Dev Disabil Res Rev 8:135-145, 2002.

13. Pharoah POD, Cooke T, Rosenbloom L: Acquired cerebral palsy. Arch Dis Child 64:1013-1016, 1989.

14. Munch L: Annotations: Cerebral palsy epidemiology: Where are we now and where are we going? Dev Med Child Neurol 34:547-555, 1992.

15. Truwit CL, Barkovich AJ, Koch TK, et al: Cerebral palsy: MR findings in 40 patients. AJNR Am J Neuroradiol 13:67-78, 1992.

16. Ashwal S, Russman BS, Blasco PA, et al: Practice parameter: Diagnostic assessment of the child with cerebral palsy: Report of the Quality Standards Subcommittee of the American Academy of Neurology and the Practice Committee of the Child Neurology Society. Neurology 62:851-863, 2004.

17. Granata T, Freri E, Caccia C, et al: Schizencephaly: Clinical spectrum, epilepsy, and pathogenesis. J Child Neurol 20:313-318, 2005.

18. Thorarensen O, Ryan S, Hunter J, et al: Factor V Leiden mutation: An unrecognized cause of hemiplegic cerebral palsy, neonatal stroke, and placental thrombosis. Ann Neurol 42:372-375, 1998.

19. Verdu A, Cazorla MR, Moreno JC, et al: Prenatal stroke in a neonate heterozygous for factor V Leiden mutation. Brain Dev 27:451-454, 2005.

20. Fattal-Valevski A, Kenet G, Kupfermine MJ, et al: Role of thrombophilic risk factors in children with non-stroke cerebral palsy. Thromb Res 116:133-137, 2005.

21. Gibson CS, MacLennan AH, Hague WM, et al: Associations between inherited thrombophilias, gestational age, and cerebral palsy. Am J Obstet Gynecol 193:1437, 2005.

22. Lee J, Croen LA, Backstrand KH, et al: Maternal and infant characteristics associated with perinatal arterial stroke in the infant. JAMA 293:723-729, 2005.

23. Lynch JK, Nelson KB, Curry CJ, et al: Cerebrovascular disorders in children with the factor V Leiden mutation. J Child Neurol 16:735-744, 2001.

24. Mercuri E, Cowan F, Gupte G, et al: Prothrombotic disorders and abnormal neurodevelopmental outcome in infants with neonatal cerebral infarction. Pediatrics 107:1400-1404, 2001.

25. Nelson KB, Lynch JK: Stroke in newborn infants. Lancet Neurol 3:150-158, 2004.

26. Smith RA, Skelton M, Howard M, et al: Is thrombophilia a factor in the development of hemiplegic cerebral palsy? Dev Med Child Neurol 43:724-730, 2001.

27. Paneth N: Etiologic factors in cerebral palsy. Pediatr Ann 15:193-201, 1986.

28. Back SA, Rivkees SA: Emerging concepts in periventricular white matter injury. Semin Perinatol 28:405-414, 2004.

29. Dammann O, Leviton A: Inflammatory brain damage in preterm newborns—Dry numbers, wet lab, and causal inferences. Early Hum Dev 79:1-15, 2004.

30. Hagberg H, Mallard C, Jacobsson B: Role of cytokines in preterm labour and brain injury. BJOG 112(Suppl 1):16-18, 2005.

31. Kent A, Lomas F, Hurrion E, et al: Antenatal steroids may reduce adverse neurological outcome following chorioamnionitis: Neurodevelopmental outcome and chorioamnionitis in premature infants. J Paediatr Child Health 41:186-190, 2005.

32. Willoughby RE Jr, Nelson KB: Chorioamnionitis and brain injury. Clin Perinatol 29:603-621, 2002.

33. Accardo J, Kammann H, Hoon AH Jr: Neuroimaging in cerebral palsy. J Pediatr 145:S19-S27, 2004.

34. Hunt A, Goldman A, Seers K, et al: Clinical validation of the paediatric pain profile. Dev Med Child Neurol 46:9-18, 2004.

35. Khong PL, Tse C, Wong IY, et al: Diffusion-weighted imaging and proton magnetic resonance spectroscopy in perinatal hypoxic-ischemic encephalopathy: Association with neuromotor outcome at 18 months of age. J Child Neurol 19:872-881, 2004.

36. Perlman J: Brain injury in the term infant. Semin Perinatol 28:415-424, 2004.

37. Shankaran S, Laptook AR, Ehrenkranz RA, et al: Whole-body hypothermia for neonates with hypoxic-ischemic encephalopathy. N Engl J Med 353:1574-1584, 2005.

38. Palmer F: Strategies for the early diagnosis of cerebral palsy. J Pediatr 145:S8-S11, 2004.

39. Nelson KB, Ellenberg JH: Antecedents of cerebral palsy. Multivariate analysis of risk. N Engl J Med 315:81-86, 1986.

40. Neil JJ, Inder TE: Imaging perinatal brain injury in premature infants. Semin Perinatol 28:433-443, 2004.

41. De Vries LS, Van Haastert IL, Rademaker KJ, et al: Ultrasound abnormalities preceding cerebral palsy in high-risk preterm infants. J Pediatr 144:815-820, 2004.

42. Ment LR, Bada HS, Barnes P, et al: Practice parameter: Neuroimaging of the neonate: Report of the Quality Standards Subcommittee of the American Academy of Neurology and the Practice Committee of the Child Neurology Society. Neurology 58:1726-1738, 2002.

43. Darrah J, Piper M, Watt MJ: Assessment of gross motor skills of at-risk infants: Predictive validity of the Alberta Infant Motor Scale. Dev Med Child Neurol 40:485-491, 1998.

44. Piper MC, Pinnell LE, Darrah J, et al: Construction and validation of the Alberta Infant Motor Scale (AIMS). Can J Public Health 83(Suppl 2):S46-S50, 1994.

45. Chandler L: Screening for movement dysfunction in infancy. Phys Occup Ther Pediatr 6:171-190, 1986.

46. Nickel RE, Renken CA, Gallenstein JA: The Infant Motor Screen. Dev Med Child Neurol 31:35-42, 1989.

47. Ellison PH, Browning CA, Larson B, et al: Development of a scoring system for the Milani-Comparetti and Gidoni method of assessing neurologic abnormality in infancy. Phys Ther 63:1414-1423, 1983.

48. Capute AJ, Palmer FB, Shapiro BK, et al: Primitive Reflex Profile: A quantitation of primitive reflexes in infancy. Dev Med Child Neurol 26:375-383, 1984.

49. Groen SE, de Blecourt AC, Postema K, et al: General movements in early infancy predict neuromotor development at 9 to 12 years of age. Dev Med Child Neurol 47:731-738, 2005.

50. Hadders-Algra M: General movements: A window for early identification of children at high risk for developmental disorders. J Pediatr 145(2 Suppl):S12-S18, 2004.

51. Nelson KB, Ellenberg JH: Children who "outgrew" cerebral palsy. Pediatrics 69:529-536, 1982.

52. Silan F, Ozdemir I, Lissens W: A novel *L1CAM* mutation with L1 spectrum disorders. Prenat Diagn 25:57-59, 2005.

53. Furrer F, Deonna T: Persistent toe-walking in children. A comprehensive clinical study of 28 cases. Helv Paediatr Acta 37:301-316, 1982.

54. Katz M, Mubarak SJ: Hereditary tendo Achillis contractures. J Pediatr Orthop 4:711-714, 1984.

55. Policy JF, Torburn L, Rinsky LA, et al: Electromyographic test to differentiate mild diplegic cerebral palsy and idiopathic toe-walking. J Pediatr Orthop 21:784-789, 2001.

56. Jan M: Misdiagnoses in children with dopa-responsive dystonia. Pediatr Neurol 31:298-303, 2004.

57. Segawa M, Nomura Y, Nishiyama N: Autosomal dominant guanosine triphosphate cyclohydrolase I deficiency (Segawa disease). Ann Neurol 54(Suppl 6):S32-S45, 2003.

58. Sanger TD, Delgado MR, Gaebler-Spira D, et al: Classification and definition of disorders causing hypertonia in childhood. Pediatrics 111(1):e89-e97, 2003.

59. Ashworth B: Preliminary trial of carisoprodol in multiple sclerosis. Practitioner 192:540-542, 1964.

60. Bohannon R, Smith MB: Interrater reliability of a modified Ashworth scale of muscle spasticity. Phys Ther 67:206-207, 1987.

61. Boyd RN, Graham HK: Objective measurement of clinical findings in the use of botulinum toxin type A for the management of children with cerebral palsy. Eur J Neurol 6(Suppl 4):S23-S35, 1999.

62. Albright AL, Barry MJ, Painter MJ, et al: Infusion of intrathecal baclofen for generalized dystonia in cerebral palsy. J Neurosurg 88:73-76, 1998.

63. Cook RE, Schneider I, Hazlewood ME, et al: Gait analysis alters decision-making in cerebral palsy. J Pediatr Orthop 23:292-295, 2003.

64. Graham HK, Baker R, Dobson F, et al: Multilevel orthopaedic surgery in group IV spastic hemiplegia. J Bone Joint Surg Br 87:548-555, 2005.

65. Postans NG, Granat MH: Effect of functional electrical stimulation, applied during walking, on gait in spastic cerebral palsy. Dev Med Child Neurol 47:46-52, 2005.

66. Radtka SA, Skinner SR, Johanson ME: A comparison of gait with solid and hinged ankle-foot orthoses in children with spastic diplegic cerebral palsy. Gait Posture 21:303-310, 2005.

67. Saraph V, Zwick EB, Steinwender G, et al: Leg lengthening as part of gait improvement surgery in cerebral palsy: An evaluation using gait analysis. Gait Posture 23:83-90, 2006.

68. Desloovere K, Molenaers G, Feys H, et al: Do dynamic and static clinical measurements correlate with gait analysis parameters in children with cerebral palsy? Gait Posture 24:302-313, 2006.

69. McKearnan KA, Kieckhefer GM, Engel JM, et al: Pain in children with cerebral palsy: A review. J Neurosci Nurs 36:252-259, 2004.

70. Schwartz L, Engel JM, Jensen MP: Pain in persons with cerebral palsy. Arch Phys Med Rehabil 80:1243-1246, 1999.

71. McCarthy ML, Silberstein CB, Atkins EA, et al: Comparing reliability and validity of pediatric instruments for measuring health and well-being of children with spastic cerebral palsy. Dev Med Child Neurol 44:468-476, 2002.

72. Morris C, Kurinczuk JJ, Fitzpatrick R: Child or family assessed measures of activity performance and participation for children with cerebral palsy: A structured review. Child Care Health Dev 31:397-407, 2005.

73. Waters E, Maher E, Salmon L, et al: Development of a condition-specific measure of quality of life for children with cerebral palsy: Empirical thematic data reported by parents and children. Child Care Health Dev 31:127-135, 2005.

74. Landgraf JM, Abetz L, Ware JE: The Child Health Questionnaire Users Manual. Boston: Health Institute, New England Medical Center, 1996.

75. Vargus-Adams J: Health-related quality of life in childhood cerebral palsy. Arch Phys Med Rehabil 86:940-945, 2005.

76. Vitale MG, Roye EA, Choe JC, et al: Assessment of health status in patients with cerebral palsy: What is the role of quality-of-life measures? J Pediatr Orthop 25:792-797, 2005.

77. Hadden KL, von Baeyer CL: Global and specific behavioral measures of pain in children with cerebral palsy. Clin J Pain 21:140-146, 2005.

78. Schneider JW, Gurucharri LM, Gutierrez AL, et al: Health-related quality of life and functional outcome measures for children with cerebral palsy. Dev Med Child Neurol 43:601-608, 2001.

79. Nickel R: Cerebral palsy. *In* Nickel RE, Desch LW, eds: The Physician's Guide to Caring for Children with Disabilities and Chronic Conditions. Baltimore: Paul H. Brookes, 2000, pp 141-184.

80. Boyd RN, Morris ME, Graham HK: Management of upper limb dysfunction in children with cerebral palsy: A systematic review. Eur J Neurol 8(Suppl 5): 150-166, 2001.

81. Butler C, Darrah J: Effects of neurodevelopmental treatment (NDT) for cerebral palsy: An AACPDM evidence report. Dev Med Child Neurol 43:778-790, 2001.

82. Harris SR, Roxborough L: Efficacy and effectiveness of physical therapy in enhancing postural control in children with cerebral palsy. Neural Plast 12:229-243, 2005.

83. Dodd KJ, Taylor NF, Damiano DL: A systematic review of the effectiveness of strength-training programs for people with cerebral palsy. Arch Phys Med Rehabil 83:1157-1164, 2002.

84. Dodd KJ, Taylor NF, Graham HK: A randomized clinical trial of strength training in young people with cerebral palsy. Dev Med Child Neurol 45:652-657, 2003.

85. McBurney H, Taylor NF, Dodd KJ, et al: A qualitative analysis of the benefits of strength training for young people with cerebral palsy. Dev Med Child Neurol 45:658-663, 2003.

86. Eliasson AC, Krumlinde-Sundholm L, Shaw K, et al: Effects of constraint-induced movement therapy in young children with hemiplegic cerebral palsy: An adapted model. Dev Med Child Neurol 47:266-275, 2005.

87. Naylor CE, Bower E: Modified constraint-induced movement therapy for young children with hemiplegic cerebral palsy: A pilot study. Dev Med Child Neurol 47:365-369, 2005.

88. Taub E, Ramey SL, DeLuca S, et al: Efficacy of constraint-induced movement therapy for children with cerebral palsy with asymmetric motor impairment. Pediatrics 113:305-312, 2004.

89. Willis JK, Morello A, Davie A, et al: Forced use treatment of childhood hemiparesis. Pediatrics 110(1 Pt 1): 94-96, 2002.

90. Buckon CE, Thomas SS, Jakobson-Huston S, et al: Comparison of three ankle-foot orthosis configurations for children with spastic diplegia. Dev Med Child Neurol 46:590-598, 2004.

91. Morris C: A review of the efficacy of lower-limb orthoses used for cerebral palsy. Dev Med Child Neurol 44:205-211, 2002.

92. White H, Jenkins J, Neace WP, et al: Clinically prescribed orthoses demonstrate an increase in velocity of gait in children with cerebral palsy: A retrospective study. Dev Med Child Neurol 44:227-232, 2002.

93. Russell DJ, Gorter JW: Assessing functional differences in gross motor skills in chidlren with cerebral palsy who use an ambulatory aid or orthoses: Can the GMFM-88 help? Dev Med Child Neurol 47:462-467, 2005.

94. Butler C: Powered tots: Augmentative mobility for locomotor disabled youngsters. Tot Line 4:18-19, 1988.

95. Gormley ME Jr, Krach LE, Piccini L: Spasticity management in the child with spastic quadriplegia. Eur J Neurol 8(Suppl 5):127-135, 2001.

96. Hagglund G, Andersson S, Duppe H, et al: Prevention of severe contractures might replace multilevel surgery in cerebral palsy: Results of a population-based health care programme and new techniques to reduce spasticity. J Pediatr Orthop B 14:269-273, 2005.

97. Krach L: Pharmacotherapy of spasticity: Oral medications and intrathecal baclofen. J Child Neurol 16:31-36, 2001.

98. Montane E, Vallano A, Laporte JR: Oral antispastic drugs in nonprogressive neurologic diseases: A systematic review. Neurology 63:1357-1363, 2004.

99. Mathew A, Mathew MC, Thomas M, et al: The efficacy of diazepam in enhancing motor function in children with spastic cerebral palsy. J Trop Pediatr 51:109-113, 2005.

100. Gracies JM, Elovic E, McGuire J, et al: Traditional pharmacological treatments for spasticity: Part I. Local treatments. Muscle Nerve Suppl 6:S61-S91, 1997.

101. Tilton A: Injectable neuromuscular blockade in the treatment of spasticity and movement disorders. J Child Neurol 18(Suppl 1):S50-S66, 2003.

102. Ade-Hall RA, Moore AP: Botulinum toxin type A in the treatment of lower limb spasticity in cerebral palsy. Cochrane Database Syst Rev (2):CD001408, 2000.

103. Wasiak J, Hoare B, Wallen M: Botulinum toxin A as an adjunct to treatment in the management of the upper limb in children with spastic cerebral palsy. Cochrane Database Syst Rev (4):CD003469, 2004.

104. Gough M, Fairhurst C, Shortland AP: Botulinum toxin and cerebral palsy: Time for reflection? Dev Med Child Neurol 47:709-712, 2005.

105. Albright AL, Barron WB, Fasick MP, et al: Continuous intrathecal baclofen infusion for spasticity of cerebral origin. JAMA 270:2475-2477, 1993.

106. Albright AL, Cervi A, Singletary J: Intrathecal baclofen for spasticity in cerebral palsy. JAMA 265:1418-1422, 1991.

107. Butler C, Campbell S: Evidence of the effects of intrathecal baclofen for spastic and dystonic cerebral palsy. ACPDM Treatment Outcomes Committee Review Panel. Dev Med Child Neurol 42:634-645, 2000.

108. Albright AL, Barry MJ, Shafton DH, et al: Intrathecal baclofen for generalized dystonia. Dev Med Child Neurol 43:652-657, 2001.

109. Bjornson KF, McLaughlin JF, Loeser JD, et al: Oral motor, communication, and nutritional status of children during intrathecal baclofen therapy: A descriptive pilot study. Arch Phys Med Rehabil 84:500-506, 2003.

110. Krach LE, Kriel RL, Gilmartin RC, et al: GMFM 1 year after continuous intrathecal baclofen infusion. Pediatr Rehabil 8:207-213, 2005.

111. Murphy NA, Irwin MC, Hoff C: Intrathecal baclofen therapy in chidlren with cerebral palsy: Efficacy and complications. Arch Phys Med Rehabil 83:1721-1725, 2002.

112. Buonaguro V, Scelsa B, Curci D, et al: Epilepsy and intrathecal baclofen therapy in children with cerebral palsy. Pediatr Neurol 33:110-113, 2005.

113. Krach LE, Kriel RL, Gilmartin RC, et al: Hip status in cerebral palsy after one year of continuous intrathecal baclofen infusion. Pediatr Neurol 30:163-168, 2004.

114. Steinbok P, Kestle JR: Variation between centers in electrophysiologic techniques used in lumbosacral selective dorsal rhizotomy for spastic cerebral palsy. Pediatr Neurosurg 25:233-239, 1996.

115. McLaughlin J, Bjornson K, Temkin N, et al: Selective dorsal rhizotomy: Meta-analysis of three randomized controlled trials. Dev Med Child Neurol 44:17-25, 2002.

116. McLaughlin JF, Bjornson KF, Astley SJ, et al: Selective dorsal rhizotomy: Efficacy and safety in an investigator-masked randomized clinical trial. Dev Med Child Neurol 40:220-232, 1998.

117. Steinbok P, Reiner AM, Beauchamp R, et al: A randomized clinical trial to compare selective posterior rhizotomy plus physiotherapy with physiotherapy alone in children with spastic diplegic cerebral palsy. Dev Med Child Neurol 39:178-184, 1997.

118. Wright FV, Sheil EM, Drake JM, et al: Evaluation of selective dorsal rhizotomy for the reduction of spasticity in cerebral palsy: A randomized controlled trial. Dev Med Child Neurol 40:239-247, 1998.

119. Mittal S, Farmer JP, Al-Atassi B, et al: Long-term functional outcome after selective posterior rhizotomy. J Neurosurg 97:315-325, 2002.

120. O'Brien DF, Park TS, Puglisi JA, et al: Effect of selective dorsal rhizotomy on need for orthopedic surgery for spastic quadriplegic cerebral palsy: Long-term outcome analysis in relation to age. J Neurosurg 101 (1 Suppl):59-63, 2004.

121. Hicdonmez T, Steinbok P, Beauchamp R, et al: Hip joint subluxation after selective dorsal rhizotomy for spastic cerebral palsy. J Neurosurg 103(1 Suppl):10-16, 2005.

122. Spiegel DA, Loder RT, Alley KA, et al: Spinal deformity following selective dorsal rhizotomy. J Pediatr Orthop 24:30-36, 2004.

123. Steinbok P, Hicdonmez T, Sawatzky B, et al: Spinal deformities after selective dorsal rhizotomy for spastic cerebral palsy. J Neurosurg 102(4 Suppl):363-373, 2005.

124. Borton DC, Walker K, Pirpiris M, et al: Isolated calf lengthening in cerebral palsy. Outcome analysis of risk factors. J Bone Joint Surg Br 83:364-370, 2001.

125. Knapp DR Jr, Cortes H: Untreated hip dislocation in cerebral palsy. J Pediatr Orthop 22:668-671, 2002.

126. Cornell MS, Hatrick NC, Boyd R, et al: The hip in children with cerebral palsy. Predicting the outcome of soft tissue surgery. Clin Orthop Relat Res 340:165-171, 1997.

127. Saito N, Ebara S, Ohotsuka K, et al: Natural history of scoliosis in spastic cerebral palsy. Lancet 351:1687-1692, 1998.

128. Jones KB, Sponseller PD, Shindle MK, et al: Longitudinal parental perceptions of spinal fusion for neuromuscular spine deformity in patients with totally involved cerebral palsy. J Pediatr Orthop 23:143-149, 2003.

129. Tsirikos AI, Chang WN, Dabney KW, et al: Comparison of parents' and caregivers' satisfaction after spinal fusion in children with cerebral palsy. J Pediatr Orthop 24:54-58, 2004.

130. Henderson RC, Lark RK, Gurka MJ, et al: Bone density and metabolism in children and adolescents with moderate to severe cerebral palsy. Pediatrics 110(1 Pt 1):e5, 2002.

131. Henderson RC, Kairella JA, Barrington JW, et al: Longitudinal changes in bone density in children and adolescents with moderate to severe cerebral palsy. J Pediatr 146:769-775, 2005.

132. Caulton JM, Ward KA, Alsop CW, et al: A randomized controlled trial of standing programme on bone mineral density in non-ambulant children with cerebral palsy. Arch Dis Child 89:131-135, 2004.

133. Henderson RC, Lark RK, Kecskemethy HH, et al: Bisphosphonates to treat osteopenia in children with quadriplegic cerebral palsy: a randomized, placebo-controlled clinical trial. J Pediatr 141:644-651, 2002.

134. Fung EB, Samson-Fang L, Stallings VA, et al: Feeding dysfunction is associated with poor growth and health

status in children with cerebral palsy. J Am Diet Assoc 102:361-373, 2002.

135. Samson-Fang L, Fung E, Stallings VA, et al: Relationship of nutritional status to health and societal participation in children with cerebral palsy. J Pediatr 141:637-643, 2002.

136. Samson-Fang LJ, Stevenson RD: Identification of malnutrition in children with cerebral palsy: poor performance of weight-for-height centiles. Dev Med Child Neurol 42:162-168, 2000.

137. Sleigh G, Brocklehurst P: Gastrostomy feeding in cerebral palsy: A systematic review. Arch Dis Child 89:534-539, 2004.

138. Sleigh G, Sullivan PB, Thomas AG: Gastrostomy feeding versus oral feeding alone for children with cerebral palsy. Cochrane Database Syst Rev (2): CD003943, 2004.

139. Sullivan PB, Juszczak E, Bachlet AME, et al: Gastrostomy tube feeding in children with cerebral palsy: A prospective, longitudinal study. Dev Med Child Neurol 47:77-85, 2005.

140. Jepsen C, Nickel RE: Nutrition and growth. *In* Nickel RE, Desch LW, eds: The Physician's Guide to Caring for Children with Disabilities and Chronic Conditions. Baltimore: Paul Brookes, 2000, pp 78-99.

141. Saitua F, Acuna R, Herrera P: Percutaneous endoscopic gastrostomy: The technique of choice? J Pediatr Surg 38:1512-1515, 2003.

142. Wadie GM, Lobe TE: Gastroesophageal reflux disease in neurologically impaired children: The role of the gastrostomy tube. Semin Laparosc Surg 9:180-189, 2002.

143. Roijen LE, Postema K, Limbeek VJ, et al: Development of bladder control in children and adolescents with cerebral palsy. Dev Med Child Neurol 43:103-107, 2001.

144. Karaman MI, Kaya C, Caskurlu T, et al: Urodynamic findings in children with cerebral palsy. Int J Urol 12:717-720, 2005.

145. Mayo M: Lower urinary tract dysfunction in cerebral palsy. J Urol 147:419-420, 1992.

146. Reid CJ, Borzyskowski M: Lower urinary tract dysfunction in cerebral palsy. Arch Dis Child 68:739-742, 1993.

147. Agnarsson U, Warde C, McCarthy G, et al: Anorectal function of children with neurological problems. II: Cerebral palsy. Dev Med Child Neurol 35:903-908, 1993.

148. Del Giudice E, Staiano A, Capano G, et al: Gastrointestinal manifestations in children with cerebral palsy. Brain Dev 21:307-311, 1999.

149. Park ES, Park CI, Cho SR, et al: Colonic transit time and constipation in children with spastic cerebral palsy. Arch Phys Med Rehabil 85:453-456, 2004.

150. Senner JE, Logemann J, Zecker S, et al: Drooling, saliva production, and swallowing in cerebral palsy. Dev Med Child Neurol 46:801-806, 2004.

151. Bachrach SJ, Walter RS, Trzcinski K: Use of glycopyrrodate and other anticholinergic medications for sialorrhea in children with cerebral palsy. Clin Pediatr (Phila) 37:485-490, 1998.

152. Blasco PA: Glycopyrrolate treatment of chronic drooling. Arch Pediatr Adolesc Med 150:932-935, 1996.

153. Stern L: Preliminary study of glycopyrrolate in the management of drooling. J Pediatr Child Health 33:52-54, 1997.

154. van der Burg JJ, Jongerius PH, van Limbeek J, et al: Social interaction and self-esteem of children with cerebral palsy after treatment for severe drooling. Eur J Pediatr 165:37-41, 2006.

155. Jongerius PH, Joosten F, Hoogen FJ, et al: The treatment of drooling by ultrasound-guided intraglandular injections of botulinum toxin type A into the salivary glands. Laryngoscope 113:107-111, 2003.

156. Jongerius PH, R.J, van Limbeek J, Gabreels FJ, van Hulst K, van den Hoogen, FJ, Botulinum toxin effect on salivary flow rate in children with cerebral palsy. Neurology 63:1371-1375, 2004.

157. Suskind DL, Tilton A: Clinical study of botulinum-A toxin in the treatment of sialorrhea in children with cerebral palsy. Laryngoscope 112:73-81, 2002.

158. Blasco PA: Management of drooling: 10 years after the Consortium on Drooling, 1990. Dev Med Child Neurol 44:778-781, 2002.

159. Hockstein NG, Samadi DS, Gendron K, et al: Sialorrhea: A management challenge. Am Fam Physician 69:2628-2634, 2004.

160. McAloney N, Kerawala CJ, Stassen LF: Mnagement of drooling by transposition of the submandibular ducts and excision of the sublingual glands. J Ir Dent Assoc 51:126-131, 2005.

161. Hallett KB, Lucas JO, Johnston T, et al: Dental health of children with cerebral palsy following sialodochoplasty. Spec Care Dentist 15:234-238, 1995.

162. Johnson HM, Reid SM, Hazard CJ, et al: Effectiveness of the Innsbruck Sensorimotor Activator and Regulator in improving saliva control in children with cerebral palsy. Dev Med Child Neurol 46:39-45, 2004.

163. Pellock JM, Morton LD: Treatment of epilepsy in the multiply handicapped. Ment Retard Dev Disabil Res Rev 6:309-323, 2000.

164. Kulak W, Sobaniec W, Smigielska-Kuzia J, et al: A comparison of spastic diplegic and tetraplegic cerebral palsy. Pediatr Neurol 32:311-317, 2005.

165. Kulak W, Sobaniec W: Risk factors and prognosis of epilepsy in children with cerebral palsy in northeastern Poland. Brain Dev 25:499-506, 2003.

166. Engel JM, Jensen MP, Hoffman AJ, et al: Pain in persons with cerebral palsy: Extension and cross validation. Arch Phys Med Rehabil 84:1125-1128, 2003.

167. Hadden KL, von Baeyer CL: Pain in children with cerebral palsy: Common triggers and expressive behaviors. Pain 99:281-288, 2002.

168. Houlihan CM, O'Donnell M, Conaway M, et al: Bodily pain and health-related quality of life in children with cerebral palsy. Dev Med Child Neurol 46:305-310, 2004.

169. Sanders H, Davis MF, Duncan B, et al: Use of complementary and alternative medical therapies among children with special health care needs in southern Arizona. Pediatrics 111:584-587, 2003.

170. Hurvitz EA, Leonard C, Ayyangar R, et al: Complementary and alternative medicine use in families of children with cerebral palsy. Dev Med Child Neurol 45:364-370, 2003.

171. Collet JP, Vanasse M, Marois P, et al: Hyperbaric oxygen for children with cerebral palsy: A randomized multicentre trial. HBO-CP Research Group. Lancet 357:582-586, 2001.

172. Liptak G: Complementary and alternative therapies for cerebral palsy. Ment Retard Dev Disabil Res Rev 11:156-163, 2005.

173. Nickel R: The use of complementary and alternative medicine by families of children with disabilities. *In* Oken B, ed: Complementary Therapies in Neurology: An Evidence-Based Approach. Boca Raton, FL: Parthenon, 2004, pp 371-389.

174. Rosenbaum P: Controversial treatment of spasticity: Exploring alternative therapies for motor function in children with cerebral palsy. J Child Neurol 18(Suppl 1):S89-S94, 2003.

175. Blum RW, Resnick MD, Nelson R, et al: Family and peer issues among adolescents with spina bifida and cerebral palsy. Pediatrics 88:280-285, 1991.

176. Wadsworth JS, Harper DC: The social needs of adolescents with cerebral palsy. Dev Med Child Neurol 35:1019-1022, 1993.

177. Andersson C, Mattsson E: Adults with cerebral palsy: A survey describing problems, needs, and resources, with special emphasis on locomotion. Dev Med Child Neurol 43:76-82, 2001.

178. Michelsen SI, Uldall P, Kejs AM, et al: Education and employment prospects in cerebral palsy. Dev Med Child Neurol 47:511-517, 2005.

179. Bottos M, Feliciangeli A, Sciuto L, et al: Functional status of adults with cerebral palsy and implications for treatment of children. Dev Med Child Neurol 43:516-528, 2001.

180. Williams EN, Broughton NS, Menelaus MB: Age-related walking in children with spina bifida. Dev Med Child Neurol 41:446-449, 1999.

181. Spina bifida and anencephaly before and after folic acid mandate—United States, 1995-1996 and 1999-2000. MMWR Morb Mortal Wkly Rep 53:362-365, 2004.

181a. CDC. Recommendations for the use of folic acid to reduce the number of cases of spina bifidal and other neural tube defects. MMWR 1992; 14 (No. RR-14).

182. Greenberg F, James LM, Oakley GP Jr: Estimates of birth prevalence rates of spina bifida in the United States from computer-generated maps. Am J Obstet Gynecol 145:570-573, 1983.

183. Williams LJ, Rasmussen SA, Flores A, et al: Decline in the prevalence of spina bifida and anencephaly by race/ethnicity: 1995-2002. Pediatrics 116:580-586, 2005.

184. Elwood JM, Little J, Elwood J: Epidemiology and control of neural tube defects. *In* Vessey M, ed: Monographs in Epidemiology and Biostatistics, vol 20. Oxford, UK: Oxford University Press, 1992.

185. Czeizel AE, Dudas I: Prevention of the first occurrence of neural-tube defects by periconceptional vitamin supplementation. N Engl J Med 327:1832-1835, 1992.

186. Prevention of neural tube defects: Results of the Medical Research Council Vitamin Study. MRC Vitamin Study Research Group. Lancet 338:131-137, 1991.

187. Lopez-Camelo JS, Orioli IM, da Graca Dutra M, et al: Reduction of birth prevalence rates of neural tube defects after folic acid fortification in Chile. Am J Med Genet A 135:120-125, 2005.

188. Chatkupt S, Skurnick JH, Jaggi M, et al: Study of genetics, epidemiology, and vitamin usage in familial spina bifida in the United States in the 1990s. Neurology 44:65-70, 1994.

189. van der Put NM, Steegers-Theunissen RP, Frosst P, et al: Mutated methylenetetrahydrofolate reductase as a risk factor for spina bifida. Lancet 346:1070-1071, 1995.

190. van der Put NM, van den Heuvel LP, Steegers-Theunissen RP, et al: Decreased methylene tetrahydrofolate reductase activity due to the 677C→T mutation in families with spina bifida offspring. J Mol Med 74:691-694, 1996.

191. Epstein DJ, Vekemans M, Gros P: Splotch (Sp2H), a mutation affecting development of the mouse neural tube, shows a deletion within the paired homeodomain of *Pax-3*. Cell 67:767-774, 1991.

192. Goulding M, Paquette A: *Pax* genes and neural tube defects in the mouse. Ciba Found Symp 181:103-113, 1994 [discussion, Ciba Found Symp 181:113-117, 1994].

193. Hol FA, Geurds MP, Chatkupt S, et al: *PAX* genes and human neural tube defects: An amino acid substitution in *PAX1* in a patient with spina bifida. J Med Genet 33:655-660, 1996.

194. Martin JF, Olson EN: Identification of a *prx1* limb enhancer. Genesis 26:225-229, 2000.

195. Anderson JL, Waller DK, Canfield MA, et al: Maternal obesity, gestational diabetes, and central nervous system birth defects. Epidemiology 16:87-92, 2005.

196. Layde PM, Edmonds LD, Erickson JD: Maternal fever and neural tube defects. Teratology 21:105-108, 1980.

197. Martinez-Frias ML, Garcia Mazario MJ, Caldas CF, et al: High maternal fever during gestation and severe congenital limb disruptions. Am J Med Genet 98:201-203, 2001.

198. Watkins ML, Rasmussen SA, Honein MA, et al: Maternal obesity and risk for birth defects. Pediatrics 111(5 Part 2):1152-1158, 2003.

199. Muller F: Prenatal biochemical screening for neural tube defects. Childs Nerv Syst 19:433-435, 2003.

199a. ACOG practice bulletin neural tube defects. Number 44 July 2003 Int. J. Gynaecol Obstet 83:122-133, 2003.

200. Coniglio SJ, Anderson SM, Ferguson JE 2nd: Functional motor outcome in children with myelomeningocele: Correlation with anatomic level on prenatal ultrasound. Dev Med Child Neurol 38:675-680, 1996.

201. Sival DA, Begeer JH, Staal-Schreinemachers AL, et al: Perinatal motor behaviour and neurological outcome

in spina bifida aperta. Early Hum Dev 50:27-37, 1997.

202. Bruner JP, Tulipan N, Paschall RL, et al: Fetal surgery for myelomeningocele and the incidence of shunt-dependent hydrocephalus. JAMA 282:1819-1825, 1999.

203. Tulipan N, Bruner JP, Hernanz-Schulman M, et al: Effect of intrauterine myelomeningocele repair on central nervous system structure and function. Pediatr Neurosurg 31:183-188, 1999.

204. Chescheir NC, D'Alton M: Evidence-based medicine and fetal treatment: How to get involved. Obstet Gynecol 106:610-613, 2005.

205. Lewis D, Tolosa, JE, Kaufmann M, et al: Elective cesarean delivery and long-term motor function or ambulation status in infants with meningomyelocele. Obstet Gynecol 103:469-473, 2004.

206. Merrill DC, Goodwin P, Burson JM, et al: The optimal route of delivery for fetal meningomyelocele. Am J Obstet Gynecol 179:235-240, 1998.

207. Shurtleff DB, Luthy DA, Nyberg DA, et al: Meningomyelocele: Management in utero and post natum. Ciba Found Symp 181:270-280, 1994 [discussion, Ciba Found Symp 181:280-286, 1994].

208. Nickel RE, Magenis RE: Neural tube defects and deletions of 22q11. Am J Med Genet 66:25-27, 1996.

209. Nickel RE, Pillers DA, Merkens M, et al: Velo-cardio-facial syndrome and DiGeorge sequence with meningomyelocele and deletions of the 22q11 region. Am J Med Genet 52:445-449, 1994.

210. Hopps CV, Kropp KA: Preservation of renal function in children with myelomeningocele managed with basic newborn evaluation and close followup. J Urol 169:305-308, 2003.

211. Wu HY, Baskin LS, Kogan BA: Neurogenic bladder dysfunction due to myelomeningocele: Neonatal versus childhood treatment. J Urol 157:2295-2297, 1997.

212. Snodgrass WT, Adams R: Initial urologic management of myelomeningocele. Urol Clin North Am 31:427-434, viii, 2004.

213. Ritter S, Tani LY, Shaddy RE, et al: Are screening echocardiograms warranted for neonates with meningomyelocele? Arch Pediatr Adolesc Med 153:1264-1266, 1999.

214. Iborra J, Pages E, Cuxart A: Neurological abnormalities, major orthopaedic deformities and ambulation analysis in a myelomeningocele population in Catalonia (Spain). Spinal Cord 37:351-357, 1999.

215. Charney EB, Melchionni JB, Smith DR: Community ambulation by children with myelomeningocele and high-level paralysis. J Pediatr Orthop 11:579-582, 1991.

216. Gerritsma-Bleeker CL, Heeg M, Vos-Niel H: Ambulation with the reciprocating-gait orthosis. Experience in 15 children with myelomeningocele or paraplegia. Acta Orthop Scand 68:470-473, 1997.

217. Liptak GS, Shurtleff DB, Bloss JW, et al: Mobility aids for children with high-level myelomeningocele: Parapodium versus wheelchair. Dev Med Child Neurol 34:787-796, 1992.

218. Bartonek A, Saraste H, Samuelsson L, et al: Ambulation in patients with myelomeningocele: A 12-year follow-up. J Pediatr Orthop 19:202-206, 1999.

219. Schiltenwolf M, Carstens C, Rohwedder J, et al: Results of orthotic treatment in children with myelomeningocele. Eur J Pediatr Surg 1(Suppl 1):50-52, 1991.

220. Brinker MR, Rosenfeld SR, Feiwell E, et al: Myelomeningocele at the sacral level. Long-term outcomes in adults. J Bone Joint Surg Am 76:1293-1300, 1994.

221. Bowman RM, McLone DG, Grant JA, et al: Spina bifida outcome: A 25-year prospective. Pediatr Neurosurg 34:114-120, 2001.

222. Piggott H: The natural history of scoliosis in myelodysplasia. J Bone Joint Surg Br 62:54-58, 1980.

223. Trivedi J, Thomson JD, Slakey JB, et al: Clinical and radiographic predictors of scoliosis in patients with myelomeningocele. J Bone Joint Surg Am 84:1389-1394, 2002.

224. Muller EB, Nordwall A: Prevalence of scoliosis in children with myelomeningocele in western Sweden. Spine 17:1097-1102, 1992.

225. Parsch D, Geiger F, Brocai DR, et al: Surgical management of paralytic scoliosis in myelomeningocele. J Pediatr Orthop B 10:10-17, 2001.

226. Sherk HH, Uppal GS, Lane G, et al: Treatment versus non-treatment of hip dislocations in ambulatory patients with myelomeningocele. Dev Med Child Neurol 33:491-494, 1991.

227. Lorente Molto FJ, Martinez Garrido I: Retrospective review of L3 myelomeningocele in three age groups: Should posterolateral iliopsoas transfer still be indicated to stabilize the hip? J Pediatr Orthop B 14:177-184, 2005.

228. Tosi LL, Buck BD, Nason SS, et al: Dislocation of hip in myelomeningocele. The McKay hip stabilization. J Bone Joint Surg Am 78:664-673, 1996.

229. Wright JG, Menelaus MB, Broughton NS, et al: Natural history of knee contractures in myelomeningocele. J Pediatr Orthop 11:725-730, 1991.

230. Omeroglu S, Peker T, Omeroglu H, et al: Intrauterine structure of foot muscles in talipes equinovarus due to high-level myelomeningocele: A light microscopic study in fetal cadavers. J Pediatr Orthop B 13:263-267, 2004.

231. Frischhut B, Stockl B, Landauer F, et al: Foot deformities in adolescents and young adults with spina bifida. J Pediatr Orthop B 9:161-169, 2000.

232. Hesz N, Wolraich M.: Myelodysplasia. In Wolraich M, ed: The Practical Assessment and Management of Children with Disorders of Development and Learning, Chicago: Year Book Medical, 1987, pp 194-221.

233. Hafez AT, McLorie G, Gilday D, et al: Long-term evaluation of metabolic profile and bone mineral density after ileocystoplasty in children. J Urol 170(4 Pt 2):1639-1641, 2003.

234. Quan A, Adams R, Ekmark E, et al: Bone mineral density in children with myelomeningocele. Pediatrics 102(3):E34, 1998.

235. James CC: Fractures of the lower limbs in spina bifida cystica: A survey of 44 fractures in 122 children. Dev Med Child Neurol (Suppl 22):88+, 1970.

236. Koch MO, McDougal WS, Hall MC, et al: Long-term metabolic effects of urinary diversion: A comparison of myelomeningocele patients managed by clean intermittent catheterization and urinary diversion. J Urol 147:1343-1347, 1992.

237. Kumar SJ, Cowell HR, Townsend P: Physeal, metaphyseal, and diaphyseal injuries of the lower extremities in children with myelomeningocele. J Pediatr Orthop 4:25-27, 1984.

238. Anschuetz RH, Freehafer AA, Shaffer JW, et al: Severe fracture complications in myelodysplasia. J Pediatr Orthop 4:22-24, 1984.

239. Rosenstein BD, Greene WB, Herrington RT, et al: Bone density in myelomeningocele: The effects of ambulatory status and other factors. Dev Med Child Neurol 29:486-494, 1987.

240. Sholas MG, Tann B, Gaebler-Spira D: Oral bisphosphonates to treat disuse osteopenia in children with disabilities: A case series. J Pediatr Orthop 25:326-331, 2005.

241. Roach, MB, Switters DM, Stone AR: The changing urodynamic pattern in infants with myelomeningocele. J Urol 150:944-947, 1993.

242. Sillen U, Hansson E, Hermansson G, et al: Development of the urodynamic pattern in infants with myelomeningocele. Br J Urol 78:596-601, 1996.

243. Elliott SP, Villar R, Duncan B: Bacteriuria management and urological evaluation of patients with spina bifida and neurogenic bladder: A multicenter survey. J Urol 173:217-220, 2005.

244. Greenfield SP, Fera M: The use of intravesical oxybutynin chloride in children with neurogenic bladder. J Urol 146(2 Pt 2):532-534, 1991.

245. Zerin JM, DiPietro MA, Ritchey ML, et al: Intravesical oxybutinin chloride in children with intermittent catheterization: Sonographic findings. Pediatr Radiol 24:348-350, 1994.

246. Lee MW, Greenfield SP: Intractable high-pressure bladder in female infants with spina bifida: clinical characteristics and use of vesicostomy. Urology 65:568-571, 2005.

247. Anderson JD, Chambers GK, Johnson HW: Application of a leukocyte and nitrite urine test strip to the management of children with neurogenic bladder. Diagn Microbiol Infect Dis 17(1):29-33, 1993.

248. Schlager TA, Dilks SA, Lohr JA, et al: Periurethral colonization and urinary leukocytes as markers for bacteriuria in children with neurogenic bladder. Urol Res 20:361-363, 1992.

249. Edwards M, Borzyskowski M, Cox A, et al: Neuropathic bladder and intermittent catheterization: Social and psychological impact on children and adolescents. Dev Med Child Neurol 46:168-177, 2004.

250. Moore C, Kogan BA, Parekh A: Impact of urinary incontinence on self-concept in children with spina bifida. J Urol 171:1659-1662, 2004.

251. Verhoef M, Lurvink M, Barf HA, et al: High prevalence of incontinence among young adults with spina bifida: Description, prediction and problem perception. Spinal Cord 43:331-340, 2005.

252. Knoll M, Madersbacher H: The chances of a spina bifida patient becoming continent/socially dry by conservative therapy. Paraplegia 31:22-27, 1993.

253. Hensle TW, Bingham J, Lam J, et al: Preventing reservoir calculi after augmentation cystoplasty and continent urinary diversion: The influence of an irrigation protocol. BJU Int 93:585-587, 2004.

254. Zhang H, Yamataka A, Koga H, et al: Bladder stone formation after sigmoidocolocystoplasty: Statistical analysis of risk factors. J Pediatr Surg 40:407-411, 2005.

255. Mingin G, Maroni P, Gerharz EW, et al: Linear growth after enterocystoplasty in children and adolescents: A review. World J Urol 22:196-199, 2004.

256. Bellinger MF: Ureterocystoplasty: A unique method for vesical augmentation in children. J Urol 149:811-813, 1993.

257. Bellinger, MF: Ureterocystoplasty update. World J Urol 16:251-254, 1998.

258. Wolf JS Jr, Turzan CW: Augmentation ureterocystoplasty. J Urol 149:1095-1098, 1993.

259. Godbole P, Bryant R, MacKinnon AE, et al: Endourethral injection of bulking agents for urinary incontinence in children. BJU Int 91:536-539, 2003.

260. Godbole P, Mackinnon AE: Expanded PTFE bladder neck slings for incontinence in children: The long-term outcome. BJU Int 93:139-141, 2004.

261. Spiess PE, Capolicchio JP, Kiruluta G, et al: Is an artificial sphincter the best choice for incontinent boys with spina bifida? Review of our long term experience with the AS-800 artificial sphincter. Can J Urol 9:1486-1491, 2002.

262. Crooks KK, Enrile BG: Comparison of the ileal conduit and clean intermittent catheterization for myelomeningocele. Pediatrics 72:203-206, 1983.

263. Heath AL, Eckstein HB: Ileal conduit urinary diversion in children. A long term follow-up. J Urol (Paris) 90:91-96, 1984.

264. Harris CF, Cooper CS, Hutcheson JC, et al: Appendicovesicostomy: The Mitrofanoff procedure—A 15-year perspective. J Urol 163:1922-1926, 2000.

265. Lemelle JL, Simo AK, Schmitt M: Comparative study of the Yang-Monti channel and appendix for continent diversion in the Mitrofanoff and Malone principles. J Urol 172(5 Pt 1):1907-1910, 2004.

266. Brown S, Marshall D, Patterson D, et al: Chronic pyelonephritis in association with neuropathic bladder. Eur J Pediatr Surg 9(Suppl 1):29-30, 1999.

267. Chan YL, Chan KW, Yeung CK, et al: Potential utility of MRI in the evaluation of children at risk of renal scarring. Pediatr Radiol 29:856-862, 1999.

268. Hamdi M, Mohan P, Little DM, et al: Successful renal transplantation in children with spina bifida: Long term single center experience. Pediatr Transplant 8:167-170, 2004.

269. Mendizabal S, Estornell F, Zamora I, et al: Renal transplantation in children with severe bladder dysfunction. J Urol 173:226-229, 2005.

270. Malone PS, Ransley PG, Kiely EM: Preliminary report: The antegrade continence enema. Lancet 336:1217-1218, 1990.

271. Duel BP, Gonzalez R: The button cecostomy for management of fecal incontinence. Pediatr Surg Int 15:559-561, 1999.

272. Herndon CD, Cain MP, Casale AJ, et al: The colon flap/extension Malone antegrade continence enema: An alternative to the Monti-Malone antegrade continence enema. J Urol 174:299-302, 2005.

272a. McDonnell GV, McCann JP: Issues of medical management in adults with spina bifida. Childs Nerv Syst 16:222-227, 2000.

273. Krupp S, Kuhn W, Zaech GA: The use of innervated flaps for the closure of ischial pressure sores. Paraplegia 21:119-126, 1983.

274. Thomson HG, Azhar Ali M, Healy H: The recurrent neurotrophic buttock ulcer in the meningomyelocele paraplegic: A sensate flap solution. Plast Reconstr Surg 108:1192-1196, 2001.

275. Harris MB, Banta JV: Cost of skin care in the myelomeningocele population. J Pediatr Orthop 10:355-361, 1990.

276. Verhoef M, Barf HA, Post MW, et al: Secondary impairments in young adults with spina bifida. Dev Med Child Neurol 46:420-427, 2004.

277. McLone DG, Dias MS: The Chiari II malformation: Cause and impact. Childs Nerv Syst 19:540-550, 2003.

278. Dyste GN, Menezes AH, VanGilder JC: Symptomatic Chiari malformations. An analysis of presentation, management, and long-term outcome. J Neurosurg 71:159-168, 1989.

279. Hoffman HJ, Hendrick EB, Humphreys RP: Manifestations and management of Arnold-Chiari malformation in patients with myelomeningocele. Childs Brain 1:255-259, 1975.

280. Pollack IF, Pang D, Albright AL, et al: Outcome following hindbrain decompression of symptomatic Chiari malformations in children previously treated with myelomeningocele closure and shunts. J Neurosurg 77:881-888, 1992.

281. Vandertop WP, Asai A, Hoffman HJ, et al: Surgical decompression for symptomatic Chiari II malformation in neonates with myelomeningocele. J Neurosurg 77:541-544, 1992.

282. Hetherington R, Dennis M, Barnes M, et al: Functional outcome in young adults with spina bifida and hydrocephalus. Childs Nerv Syst 22:117-124, 2006.

283. Albright AL, Pollack IF, Adelson PD, et al: Outcome data and analysis in pediatric neurosurgery. Neurosurgery 45:101-106, 1999.

284. Caldarelli M, Di Rocco C, La Marca F: Shunt complications in the first postoperative year in children with meningomyelocele. Childs Nerv Syst 12:748-754, 1996.

285. Tuli S, Drake J, Lamberti-Pasculli M: Long-term outcome of hydrocephalus management in myelomeningoceles. Childs Nerv Syst 19:286-291, 2003.

286. Enger PO, Svendsen F, Wester K: CSF shunt infections in children: Experiences from a population-based study. Acta Neurochir (Wien) 145:243-248, 2003.

287. Kuffer F: Prophylactic long-term anticoagulant treatment of hydrocephalic patients with ventriculo-atrial shunts. Dev Med Child Neurol (Suppl 37):74-77, 1976.

288. Sleigh G, Dawson A, Penny WJ: Cor pulmonale as a complication of ventriculo-atrial shunts reviewed. Dev Med Child Neurol 35:74-78, 1993.

289. Lorber J, Pucholt V: When is a shunt no longer necessary? An investigation of 300 patients with hydrocephalus and myelomeningocele: 11-22 year follow up. Z Kinderchir 34:327-329, 1981.

290. Tomlinson P, Sugarman ID: Complications with shunts in adults with spina bifida. BMJ 311:286-287, 1995.

291. Hudgins RJ, Gilreath CL: Tethered spinal cord following repair of myelomeningocele. Neurosurg Focus 16(2):E7, 2004.

292. Naik DR, Emery JL: The position of the spinal cord segments related to the vertebral bodies in children with meningomyelocele and hydrocephalus. Dev Med Child Neurol (Suppl 16):62-18, 1968.

293. Oi S, Yamada H, Matsumoto S: Tethered cord syndrome versus low-placed conus medullaris in an over-distended spinal cord following initial repair for myelodysplasia. Childs Nerv Syst 6:264-269, 1990.

294. Petersen MC: Tethered cord syndrome in myelodysplasia: Correlation between level of lesion and height at time of presentation. Dev Med Child Neurol 34:604-610, 1992.

295. Haberl H, Tallen G, Michael T, et al: Surgical aspects and outcome of delayed tethered cord release. Zentralbl Neurochir 65:161-167, 2004.

296. Sarwark JF, Weber DT, Gabrieli AP, et al: Tethered cord syndrome in low motor level children with myelomeningocele. Pediatr Neurosurg 25:295-301, 1996.

297. Craig JJ, Gray WJ, McCann JP: The Chiari/hydrosyringomyelia complex presenting in adults with myelomeningocoele: An indication for early intervention. Spinal Cord 37:275-278, 1999.

298. Chapman PH, Frim DM: Symptomatic syringomyelia following surgery to treat retethering of lipomyelomeningoceles. J Neurosurg 82:752-755, 1995.

299. Park TS, Cail WS, Broaddus WC, et al: Lumboperitoneal shunt combined with myelotomy for treatment of syringohydromyelia. J Neurosurg 70:721-727, 1989.

300. Klepper J, Busse M, Strassburg HM, et al: Epilepsy in shunt-treated hydrocephalus. Dev Med Child Neurol 40:731-736, 1998.

301. Noetzel MJ, Blake JN: Prognosis for seizure control and remission in children with myelomeningocele. Dev Med Child Neurol 33:803-810, 1991.

302. Talwar D, Baldwin MA, Horbatt CI: Epilepsy in children with meningomyelocele. Pediatr Neurol 13:29-32, 1995.

303. Clancy CA, McGrath PJ, Oddson BE: Pain in children and adolescents with spina bifida. Dev Med Child Neurol 47:27-34, 2005.

304. Edwards RJ, Witchell C, Pople IK: Chronic headaches in adults with spina bifida and associated hydrocephalus. Eur J Pediatr Surg 13(Suppl 1):S13-S17, 2003.

305. Charney EB, Rosenblum M, Finegold D: Linear growth in a population of children with myelomeningocele. Z Kinderchir 34:415-419, 1981.

306. Rosenblum MF, Finegold DN, Charney EB: Assessment of stature of children with myelomeningocele, and usefulness of arm-span measurement. Dev Med Child Neurol 25:338-342, 1983.

307. Rotenstein D, Adams M, Reigel DH: Adult stature and anthropomorphic measurements of patients with myelomeningocele. Eur J Pediatr 154:398-402, 1995.

308. Satin-Smith MS, Katz LL, Thornton P, et al: Arm span as measurement of response to growth hormone (GH) treatment in a group of children with meningomyelocele and GH deficiency. J Clin Endocrinol Metab 81:1654-1656, 1996.

309. Hayes-Allen, MC, Tring FC: Obesity: Another hazard for spina bifida children. Br J Prev Soc Med 27:192-196, 1973.

310. Mita K, Akataki K, Itoh K, et al: Assessment of obesity of children with spina bifida. Dev Med Child Neurol 35:305-311, 1993.

311. Roberts D, Shepherd RW, Shepherd K: Anthropometry and obesity in myelomeningocele. J Paediatr Child Health 27:83-90, 1991.

312. Fernbach SK, McLone DG: Derangement of swallowing in children with myelomeningocele. Pediatr Radiol 15:311-314, 1985.

313. Hesz N, Wolraich M: Vocal-cord paralysis and brainstem dysfunction in children with spina bifida. Dev Med Child Neurol 27:528-531, 1985.

314. Hayes-Allen MC: Obesity and short stature in children with myelomeningocele. Dev Med Child Neurol Suppl 27:59-64, 1972.

315. Grogan CB, Ekvall SM: Body composition of children with myelomeningocele, determined by 40K, urinary creatinine and anthropometric measures. J Am Coll Nutr 18:316-323, 1999.

316. Littlewood RA, Trocki O, Shepherd RW, et al: Resting energy expenditure and body composition in children with myelomeningocele. Pediatr Rehabil 6:31-37, 2003.

317. Shepherd K, Roberts D, Golding S, et al: Body composition in myelomeningocele. Am J Clin Nutr 53:1-6, 1991.

318. van den Berg-Emons HJ, Bussmann JB, Meyerink HJ, et al: Body fat, fitness and level of everyday physical activity in adolescents and young adults with meningomyelocele. J Rehabil Med 35:271-275, 2003.

319. Trollmann R, Strehl E, Wenzel D, et al: Arm span, serum IGF-1 and IGFBP-3 levels as screening parameters for the diagnosis of growth hormone deficiency in patients with myelomeningocele—Preliminary data. Eur J Pediatr 157:451-455, 1998.

320. Hochhaus F, Butenandt O, Ring-Mrozik E: One-year treatment with recombinant human growth hormone of children with meningomyelocele and growth hormone deficiency: A comparison of supine length and arm span. J Pediatr Endocrinol Metab 12:153-159, 1999.

321. Rotenstein D, Breen TJ: Growth hormone treatment of children with myelomeningocele. J Pediatr 128(5 Pt 2):S28-S31, 1996.

322. Rotenstein D, Bass AN: Treatment to near adult stature of patients with myelomeningocele with recombinant human growth hormone. J Pediatr Endocrinol Metab 17:1195-1200, 2004.

323. Trollmann R, Strehl E, Wenzel D, et al: Does growth hormone (GH) enhance growth in GH-deficient children with myelomeningocele? J Clin Endocrinol Metab 85:2740-2743, 2000.

324. Hochhaus F, Butenandt O, Schwarz HP, et al: Auxological and endocrinological evaluation of children with hydrocephalus and/or meningomyelocele. Eur J Pediatr 156:597-601, 1997.

325. Meyer, S, Landau H: Precocious puberty in myelomeningocele patients. J Pediatr Orthop 4:28-31, 1984.

326. Perrone L, Del Gaizo D, D'Angelo E, et al: Endocrine studies in children with myelomeningocele. J Pediatr Endocrinol 7:219-223, 1994.

327. Trollmann R, Dorr HG, Strehl E, et al: Growth and pubertal development in patients with meningomyelocele: A retrospective analysis. Acta Paediatr 85:76-80, 1996.

328. Galluzzi F, Bindi G, Poggi G, et al: [Precocious puberty, Gh deficiency and obesity can affect final height in patients with myelomeningocele: Comparison of males and females]. Pediatr Med Chir 21:73-78, 1999.

329. Laurence KM, Beresford A: Continence, friends, marriage and children in 51 adults with spina bifida. Dev Med Child Neurol (Suppl 35):123-128, 1975.

329a. Cass AS, Bloom BA, Luxenberg M: Sexual function in adults with myelomeningocele. J Urol 136:425-426, 1986.

329b. Sawyer SM, Roberts KV: Sexual and reproductive health in young people with spina bifida. Dev Med Child Neurol 41:671-675, 1999.

329c. Decter RM, Furness PD 3rd, Nguyen TA, et al: Reproductive understanding, sexual functioning and testosterone levels in men with spina bifida. J Urol 157:1466-1468, 1997.

329d. Verhoef M, Barf HA, Vroege JA, et al: Sex education, relationships, and sexuality in young adults with spina bifida. Arch Phys Med Rehabil 86:979-987, 2005.

330. Sandler AD, Worley G, Leroy EC, et al: Sexual function and erection capability among young men with spina bifida. Dev Med Child Neurol 38:823-829, 1996.

331. Palmer JS, Kaplan WE, Firlit CF: Erectile dysfunction in patients with spina bifida is a treatable condition. J Urol 164(3 Pt 2):958-961, 2000.

332. Muller T, Arbeiter K, Aufricht C: Renal function in meningomyelocele: Risk factors, chronic renal failure, renal replacement therapy and transplantation. Curr Opin Urol 12:479-484, 2002.

333. McDonnell GV, McCann JP: Issues of medical management in adults with spina bifida. Childs Nerv Syst 16:222-227, 2000.

334. Milton CA, Sanders P, Steele PM: Late cardiopulmonary complication of ventriculo-atrial shunt. Lancet 358:1608, 2001.

335. Vernet O, Rilliet B: Late complications of ventriculoatrial or ventriculoperitoneal shunts. Lancet 358:1569-1570, 2001.

336. Beeker TW, Scheers MM, Faber JA, et al: Prediction of independence and intelligence at birth in meningomyelocele. Childs Nerv Syst 22:33-37, 2006.

337. Fletcher JM, Copeland K, Frederick JA, et al: Spinal lesion level in spina bifida: A source of neural and cognitive heterogeneity. J Neurosurg 102(3 Suppl):268-279, 2005.

338. Brookshire BL, Fletcher JM, Bohan TP, et al: Verbal and nonverbal skill discrepancies in children with hydrocephalus: A five-year longitudinal follow-up. J Pediatr Psychol 20:785-800, 1995.

339. Fletcher JM, Bohan TP, Brandt ME, et al: Morphometric evaluation of the hydrocephalic brain: relationships with cognitive development. Childs Nerv Syst 12:192-199, 1996.

340. Rendeli C, Salvaggio E, Sciascia Cannizzaro G, et al: Does locomotion improve the cognitive profile of children with meningomyelocele? Childs Nerv Syst 18:231-234, 2002.

341. Schoenmakers MA, Uiterwaal CS, Gulmans VA, et al: Determinants of functional independence and quality of life in children with spina bifida. Clin Rehabil 19:677-685, 2005.

342. Davidovitch M, Manning-Courtney P, Hartmann LA, et al: The prevalence of attentional problems and the effect of methylphenidate in children with myelomenigocele. Pediatr Rehabil 3:29-35, 1999.

343. Kawamura T, Nishio S, Morioka T, et al: Callosal anomalies in patients with spinal dysraphism: Correlation of clinical and neuroimaging features with hemispheric abnormalities. Neurol Res 24:463-467, 2002.

344. Gaston H: Ophthalmic complications of spina bifida and hydrocephalus. Eye 5(Pt 3):279-290, 1991.

345. Pinello L, Bortolin C, Drigo P: [Visual motor and visual defects in spina bifida]. Pediatr Med Chir 25:437-441, 2003.

346. Lennerstrand G, Gallo JE, Samuelsson L: Neuro-ophthalmological findings in relation to CNS lesions in patients with myelomeningocele. Dev Med Child Neurol 32:423-431, 1990.

347. Tubbs RS, Soleau S, Custis J, et al: Degree of tectal beaking correlates to the presence of nystagmus in children with Chiari II malformation. Childs Nerv Syst 20:459-461, 2004.

348. Merguerian PA, Klein RB, Graven MA, et al: Intraoperative anaphylactic reaction due to latex hypersensitivity. Urology 38:301-303, 1991.

349. Moneret-Vautrin DA, Mata E, Gueant JL, et al: High risk of anaphylactic shock during surgery for spina bifida. Lancet 335:865-866, 1990.

350. Niggemann B, Buck D, Michael T, et al: Latex provocation tests in patients with spina bifida: Who is at risk of becoming symptomatic? J Allergy Clin Immunol 102(4 Pt 1):665-670, 1998.

351. Obojski A, Chodorski J, Barg W, et al: Latex allergy and sensitization in children with spina bifida. Pediatr Neurosurg 37:262-266, 2002.

352. Shah S, Cawley M, Gleeson R, et al: Latex allergy and latex sensitization in children and adolescents with meningomyelocele. J Allergy Clin Immunol 101(6 Pt 1):741-746, 1998.

353. Buck D, Michael T, Wahn U, et al: Ventricular shunts and the prevalence of sensitization and clinically relevant allergy to latex in patients with spina bifida. Pediatr Allergy Immunol 11:111-115, 2000.

354. Mazon A, Nieto A, Pamies R, et al: Influence of the type of operations on the development of latex sensitization in children with myelomeningocele. J Pediatr Surg 40:688-692, 2005.

355. Pires G, Morais-Almeida M, Gaspar A, et al: Risk factors for latex sensitization in children with spina bifida. Allergol Immunopathol (Madr) 30:5-13, 2002.

356. Machado M, Sant'anna C, Aires V, et al: [Latex and banana allergies in children with myelomeningocele in the city of Rio de Janeiro]. Rev Assoc Med Bras 50:83-86, 2004.

357. Cremer R, Kleine-Diepenbruck U, Hering F, et al: Reduction of latex sensitisation in spina bifida patients by a primary prophylaxis programme (five years experience). Eur J Pediatr Surg 12(Suppl 1):S19-S21, 2002.

358. Folio MR, Fewell R: Peabody Developmental Motor Scales and Activity Cards (PDMS). Itasca, IL: River Side, 1983.

359. Russell DJ, Rosenbaum PL, Avery LM, et al: Gross Motor Function Measure (GMFM-66 and GMFM-88) User's Manual (Clinics in Developmental Medicine). London: Mac Keith Press, 2002.

360. Fedman AB, Haley SM, Coryell J: Concurrent and constructive validity of the pediatric evaluation of disability inventory. Phys Ther 70:602-610, 1990.

361. Haley SM, Coster WJ, Ludlow LH, et al: Pediatric Evaluation of Disability Inventory (PEDI) Version 1.0: Developmental, Standardization, and Administration Manual. Boston: New England Medical Center Hospitals, 1992.

362. Hamilton BB, Granger CV: WeeFIM. Buffalo: Research Foundation of the State University of New York, 1991.

363. Ottenbacher KJ, Msall ME, Lyon NR, et al: Interrater agreement and stability of the Functional Independence Measure for Children (WeeFIM): Use in children with developmental disabilities. Arch Phys Med Rehabil 78:1309-1315, 1997.

364. Damiano DL, Gilgannon MD, Abel MF: Responsiveness and uniqueness of the pediatric outcomes data collection instrument compared to the gross motor function measure for measuring orthopaedic and neurosurgical outcomes in cerebral palsy. J Pediatr Orthop 25:641-645, 2005.

365. Bayley N: Bayley Scales of Infant Development, 2nd ed. San Antonio, TX: The Psychological Corporation, 1993.

366. Roid G: Stanford-Binet Intelligence Scales, 5th ed. Itasca, IL: Riverside, 2003.

367. Weschsler Preschool and Primary Scale of Intelligence, 3rd ed, Record Form. San Antonio, TX: The Psychological Corporation, 2002.

368. Wechsler Intelligence Scale for Children, 4th ed, Response Booklet 1. San Antonio, TX: The Psychological Corporation, 2003.

369. Achenbach T: Manual for the Child Behavior Checklist and Revised Child Behavior Profile. Burlington: University of Vermont, 1991.

370. Achenbach T: Manual for the Child Behavior Checklist and Youth Self-Report. Burlington: University of Vermont, 1991.

371. Achenbach T: Manual for the Teacher Report Form and the Child Behavior Profile. Burlington: University of Vermont, 1991.

372. Bartonek A, Saraste H: Factors influencing ambulation in myelomeningocele: A cross-sectional study. Dev Med Child Neurol 43:253-260, 2001.

373. Bartonek A, Saraste H, Knutson LM: Comparison of different systems to classify the neurological level of lesion in patients with myelomeningocele. Dev Med Child Neurol 41:796-805, 1999.

Autism Spectrum Disorders

CHRIS PLAUCHÉ JOHNSON ■ SCOTT M. MYERS

Before the 1990s, autism was thought to be a rare disorder with a dismal prognosis whose victims rarely achieved independent living and enduring relationships. Instead, most affected adults lived with their parents or in state institutions.[1] Most individuals in whom autism as diagnosed were nonverbal and assumed to have some degree of mental retardation even when standardized measurements of intelligence were not available. Treatment programs, if existent, were usually housed in facilities serving segregated populations. There were no published autism guidelines, and there was little interest in research outside a relatively small circle of dedicated investigators. The media, lay public, and members of Congress were generally not even aware of the term *autism,* much less concerned about it.

The 1990 decade was proclaimed "the decade of the brain,"[2] partly because of advances in neuroimaging and expanding knowledge about how the central nervous system worked. However, the 1990s might also be called the "the decade of autism" because of the rapidly expanding body of knowledge in the field. The 1990s also marked a period of significantly heightened public awareness, attributable at least in part to the 1988 release of the Academy Award–wining movie "Rainman." Although some advocates expressed concern about how autism was portrayed, the movie nevertheless brought autism to public awareness. Public attention has remained high because autism has been and continues to be engulfed in a sea of controversy. Concerns about a possible "epidemic" relating to vaccines and toxins and the media's frenzy regarding miraculous cures (auditory integration therapy, facilitated communication, secretin injections, and mercury chelation) have made *autism* a household term. Furthermore the media, motivated by dedicated advocates, has played an important role in capturing the attention of Congress, which in turn has resulted in autism-specific activities mandated by

national legislation: the Children's Health Act of 2000,[3] the New Freedom Initiative of 2001,[4] and the Combating Autism Act of 2005.[5]

Because of mandated federal support, autism "centers of excellence" emerged and contributed to a rapidly expanding body of knowledge. Thus, interest in autism within professional circles paralleled that of the lay public; this attention is illustrated by the exponential growth of training activities and published articles during the 1990s. Whereas before 2000 professional organizations such as the American Academy of Pediatrics (AAP) offered no stand-alone course in autism at its national conferences, since then autism has been at the top of the AAP list of "hot topics" and now consistently appears as a topic on conference agendas. Similarly, approximately 3000 autism-related articles were published in scientific peer-reviewed journals between 1943 (when it was first described by Kanner[6]) and 1990, whereas more than 4000 appeared in the 1990s alone.[7] Beginning at the end of the 20th century, the first policy statements and practice guidelines were published.[8-13] In spite of this, the cause of autism is still not known, and there is no known cure.

In light of the increased public and professional attention and the resulting demands this has placed upon pediatricians, particularly those specializing in child development, the goals of this chapter are as follows:

- To increase awareness and understanding of the broad spectrum of disorders related to autism.
- To facilitate earlier recognition and diagnosis.
- To provide information on the expanding menu of existing autism-related interventions.
- To assist with training of primary care providers.
- To provide a scholarly foundation on which the clinician can develop research and advocacy initiatives.

It is impossible to discuss the voluminous literature surrounding the autistic spectrum disorders (ASDs) in a single chapter. The ambitious reader is referred to *Handbook of Autism and Pervasive Developmental Disorders* (Volumes 1 and 2),[14] *Neurobiology of Autism*,[15] *Autism Spectrum Disorders in Children*,[16] and *Autism Spectrum Disorders*.[17]

TERMINOLOGY

Terminology, definitions, and diagnostic criteria have changed over the years. The concept of "autism" before the 1990s apparently represented only a small proportion of ASDs. Although frequently used by European investigators in the 1990s, the term *autistic spectrum disorder* did not become popular in the United States until about 2000.[18] It has become an "umbrella term" that includes three of the five pervasive developmental disorders (PDDs) listed in the most recent revisions of *The Diagnostic and Statistic Manual of Mental Disorders* (*DSM*) of the American Psychiatric Association[19,20] and the *Diagnostic and Statistical Manual for Primary Care, Child and Adolescent Version*[21]: autistic disorder, Asperger disorder (referred to as *Asperger syndrome* in this chapter), and pervasive developmental disorder, not otherwise specified (PDD-NOS). The remaining two PDDs, Rett syndrome and childhood disintegrative disorder, are not discussed in this chapter.

The ASDs are neurodevelopmental conditions characterized by one or a combination of the following: significant social skill deficits, both qualitative and quantitative language abnormalities, restricted interests, and repetitive motor mannerisms. Although ASDs appear to have a strong genetic basis,[22,23] the precise cause is unknown; thus, there is no pathognomonic physical sign or laboratory test. Instead, the diagnosis is made by determining the presence of characteristic developmental and behavioral criteria described in the fourth edition of the *DSM* (*DSM-IV*)[19] or in the text revision (*DSM-IV-TR*).[20] Many clinicians use a standardized evaluation tool that operationalizes the *DSM* criteria. Nevertheless, considerable subjectivity still exists in making this diagnosis, largely because of the wide range of symptoms included within the scope of the spectrum.

Autism Disorder

Autism was first described in the third edition of the *DSM* (*DSM-III*) in 1980[24] as "Infantile Autism"; the current term, "Autistic Disorder" replaced "Infantile Autism" in the revised version of the *DSM-III* (*DSM-III-R*) in 1987.[25] Although clinical patterns vary in regard to severity, age at onset, underlying cognitive

deficits, and other features, diagnosis of "classic" autistic disorder is dependent on the presence of at least half (six) of the criteria (Table 15-1).[20] Symptoms in at least one of these areas must have been present before the age of 3.

Asperger Syndrome

Asperger syndrome is characterized by the same impairment in social interaction and restricted interests as in autistic disorder; however, language skills are relatively normal (defined as use of single words by age 2 years and phrases by 3 years) (Table 15-2).[20] Later language is characterized by pragmatic deficits (problems with the social use of language). In addition, cognitive and adaptive skills are normal. Depending on the child's age, it is sometimes quite challenging to distinguish between children with Asperger syndrome and children with autistic disorder and normal intelligence. Because of this, controversy exists as to whether Asperger syndrome represents a high-functioning form of autism or a separate entity.[26,27] Children with Asperger syndrome are usually not recognized until after 4 years of age, when social interactions with peers in preschool settings become a concern.

Pervasive Developmental Disorder, Not Otherwise Specified

Pervasive Developmental Disorder, Not Otherwise Specified is a subthreshold term that is used when a child demonstrates some but not all of the criteria necessary to make a diagnosis of one of the specific PDDs. Unfortunately, there was an error in the *DSM-IV* text[19]: It stated that PDD-NOS should be used when there was an "impairment in . . . social interaction" *or* in verbal and nonverbal skills. This allowed clinicians to apply the PDD-NOS label in the absence of social skill deficits, thus broadening the definition of PDD-NOS and causing loss of specificity. This error was corrected in the *DSM-IV-TR*.[20] The PDD-NOS label is reserved for persons who demonstrate "severe and pervasive impairment in the development of reciprocal social interaction" *and* either communication deficits or restricted interests/repetitive behaviors. Confusion still exists regarding the actual *number* of criteria that are necessary to apply the PPD-NOS label; by convention, at least two but not more than five should be present. PDD-NOS also includes "atypical autism," which refers to persons with at least one feature that is dissonant with traditional autism, such as later onset or absence of stereotypies.[28,29]

Throughout this chapter, *ASD* refers to all three disorders as a group. When a specific ASD is dis-

TABLE 15-1 ■ Diagnostic Criteria for 299.00 Autism Disorder

A. A total of six (or more) items from (1), (2), and (3), with at least two from (1), and one each from (2) and (3):

(1) qualitative impairment in social interaction, as manifested by at least two of the following:

   (a) marked impairment in the use of multiple nonverbal behaviors such as eye-to-eye gaze, facial expression, body postures, and gestures to regulate social interaction

   (b) failure to develop peer relationships appropriate to developmental level

   (c) a lack of spontaneous seeking to share enjoyment, interests, or achievements with other people (e.g., by a lack of showing, bringing, or pointing out objects of interest)

   (d) lack of social or emotional reciprocity

(2) qualitative impairments in communication as manifested by at least one of the following:

   (a) delay in, or total lack of, the development of spoken language (not accompanied by an attempt to compensate through alternative modes of communication such as gesture or mime)

   (b) in individuals with adequate speech, marked impairment in the ability to initiate or sustain a conversation with others

   (c) stereotyped and repetitive use of language or idiosyncratic language

   (d) lack of varied, spontaneous make-believe play or social imitative play appropriate to developmental level

(3) restricted repetitive and stereotyped patterns of behavior, interests, and activities, as manifested by at least one of the following:

   (a) encompassing preoccupation with one or more stereotyped and restricted patterns of interest that is abnormal either in intensity or focus

   (b) apparently inflexible adherence to specific, nonfunctional routines or rituals

   (c) stereotyped and repetitive motor mannerisms (e.g., hand or finger flapping or twisting, or complex whole-body movements)

   (d) persistent preoccupation with parts of objects

B. Delays or abnormal functioning in at least one of the following areas, with onset prior to age 3 years: (1) social interaction, (2) language as used in social communication, or (3) symbolic or imaginative play.

C. The disturbance is not better accounted for by Rett's Disorder or Childhood Disintegrative Disorder.

Reprinted with permission from the Diagnostic and Statistical Manual of Mental Disorders, 4th ed, Text Revision. Washington, DC: American Psychiatric Association, 2000, p 75.

TABLE 15-2 ■ Diagnostic Criteria for 299.80 Asperger Disorder*

A. Qualitative impairment in social interaction, as manifested by at least two of the following:

   (1) marked impairment in the use of multiple nonverbal behaviors such as eye-to-eye gaze, facial expression, body postures, and gestures to regulate social interaction

   (2) failure to develop peer relationships appropriate to developmental level

   (3) a lack of spontaneous seeking to share enjoyment, interests, or achievements with other people (e.g., by a lack of showing, bringing, or pointing out objects of interest to other people)

   (4) lack of social or emotional reciprocity

B. Restricted repetitive and stereotyped patterns of behavior, interests, and activities, as manifested by at least one of the following:

   (1) encompassing preoccupation with one or more stereotyped and restricted patterns of interest that is abnormal either in intensity or focus

   (2) apparently inflexible adherence to specific, nonfunctional routines or rituals

   (3) stereotyped and repetitive motor mannerisms (e.g., hand or finger flapping or twisting, or complex whole-body movements)

   (4) persistent preoccupation with parts of objects

C. The disturbance causes clinically significant impairment in social, occupational, or other important areas of functioning.

D. There is no clinically significant general delay in language (e.g., single words used by age 2 years, communicative phrases used by age 3 years).

E. There is no clinically significant delay in cognitive development or in the development of age-appropriate self-help skills, adaptive behavior (other than in social interaction), and curiosity about the environment in childhood.

F. Criteria are not met for another specific Pervasive Developmental Disorder or Schizophrenia.

Reprinted with permission from the Diagnostic and Statistical Manual of Mental Disorders, 4th ed, Text Revision. Washington, DC: American Psychiatric Association, 2000, p 75.
Asperger syndrome is the term used in this text to distinguish the abbreviation AD (autism disorder) from AS (Asperger syndrome).

cussed, the appropriate term is used. *Autism* is used in reference to older literature published before the concept of a spectrum of autistic disorders emerged. A broad spectrum does appear to exist, although its external and internal boundaries are hazy.[30,31] Family studies have shown that the entire spectrum may be expressed in the same pedigree. Sometimes the term *broader autism phenotype* is used for individuals with isolated social deficits, particularly in the context of extended-family relatives of probands with autism.[32,33]

HISTORY

In 1943, Leo Kanner, a psychiatrist at the Johns Hopkins University School of Medicine, first defined autism as it is known today.[6] About the same time, Hans Asperger, an Austrian pediatrician, unaware of Kanner's work, published an article in German[34] describing four children who demonstrated symptoms similar to those described by Kanner with the exception of better verbal and cognitive skills. Asperger syndrome escaped recognition until it was popularized by Wing's translation into English.[35,36] In 1978, Rutter[37] published the first set of "essential criteria" for autism. These were incorporated into the next edition of the *DSM* (*DSM-III*),[24] and autism became recognized as a separate entity within the newly created category of Pervasive Developmental Disorders.

New criteria were developed for the *DSM-III-R*,[25] published in 1987, and were criticized for being too inclusive and thus promoting overidentification of autistic disorder.[38] The criteria still in use today were published in 1994 in the *DSM-IV*[19]; Asperger syndrome criteria appeared for the first time in this version. The *DSM-IV* Autistic Disorder criteria were the result of years of analyses to reduce the overinclusiveness of *DSM-III-R*. Furthermore, collaboration with European groups working on the manual for the revised International Classification of Diseases, 10th edition (ICD-10),[39] promoted conformity between the two classification systems. Studies have revealed that the *DSM-IV* criteria have better specificity (0.87) than do *DSM-III-R* criteria.[40] Criteria for autistic disorder and Asperger syndrome have not changed in the *DSM-IV-TR*.[20]

Although Kanner initially hypothesized that autism was an inborn, biological condition,[41] misconceptions based on psychodynamic theory soon became prevalent. Probably the most important one was the mistaken concept that autism might be caused by cold and unnurturing parents ("the refrigerator theory"). Bettelheim[42] promoted this concept in his book, *The Empty Fortress: Infantile Autism and the Birth of Self*. The refrigerator theory remained popular until the 1960s when Rimland hypothesized a neurological cause.[43]

This hypothesis was later supported by the demonstration of neuropathological abnormalities on magnetic resonance imaging (MRI)[44] and documentation of a high rate of coexisting seizures.[45]

The science of ASD has advanced a great deal. Collaborative research centers and multidisciplinary diagnostic teams proliferated during the late 1990s and continue to do so with even greater momentum in the new millennium. Since the 1990s, there have been a number of rapid developments: the debut of the first screening tools, the development of evaluation tools that operationalize *DSM-IV* criteria, neuropathic studies that revealed an early prenatal onset, identification of multiple genetic susceptibility genes, recognition of the relative importance of social skill deficits in defining ASDs, and evidence that early and appropriate intervention is effective in improving outcomes.[7,13]

PREVALENCE

The apparent dramatic rise in prevalence of ASDs has become a focus for parent advocacy groups and the media and may well be one of the most controversial topics in the field of autism (Table 15-3). More than 30 studies documented an apparent increase in prevalence of these diagnoses.[46-55c] In 2000, the Centers for Disease Control and Prevention organized the Autism and Developmental Disabilities Monitoring (ADDM) Network, a multisite, records-based surveillance program, to study the prevalence of ASDs. The ADDM Network employs systematic screening of developmental evaluation records for autistic behaviors rather than depending on a medical or educational diagnostic label of an ASD. In 2007, the ADDM Network reported ASD rates ranging from 1 in 303 to 1 in 94 8-year-old children for two time periods (2000, 2002) in a total of 14 sites in the United States; the average rate was 1 in 150 or 6.6 per 1000 8-year-olds.[56] Studies varied in methods, definition, and case ascertainment strategies, but overall there appeared to have been up to a 10-fold increase worldwide since the 1950s.

Several factors complicate the interpretation these data, making it very difficult to discern whether there has been a true rise in prevalence or simply an apparent one. Most investigators have demonstrated that the apparent rise in prevalence is attributable, at least in part, to changing broader criteria and increased public and professional awareness.[51,54,57] This is supported by a greater increase in the numbers of milder cases (i.e., PDD-NOS and Asperger syndrome). Other factors contributing to the apparent rise include the emergence of screening tools in the 1990s, which resulted in improved ascertainment, and the development of better diagnostic tools that can more reliably

TABLE 15-3 ■ Prevalence of Autism and Autism Spectrum Disorder over a Half-Century

Dates of Studies	Rate	Published Criteria	Terminology	Estimated % with Coexisting Mental Retardation
1960-1980	0.4 to 0.5 per 1000	Kanner criteria	Autism	
1980s	Up to 1.5 per 1000	*DSM-III* criteria	Autistic Disorder	90%
1990s	0.7 to 1.1 per 1000	*DSM-III-R* criteria	Autistic Disorder	75%
2000s	4.0 to 6.0 per 1000	*DSM-IV* criteria	Autistic Spectrum Disorder	26%-68%

DSM, Diagnostic and Statistical Manual of Mental Disorder (III, 3rd edition; III-R, 3rd edition revised; IV, 4th edition).

identify children at younger ages. The media (e.g., the National Broadcasting Company's Autism Speaks Campaign, April 2006) and advocacy groups have been successful in raising public awareness so that parents are now recognizing ASD symptoms in their children and voicing their concerns earlier to physicians. There has also been an increase in recognition of ASDs among children who have disorders unrelated to ASD, such as Down syndrome[58] and the syndrome of coloboma, heart anomaly, choanal atresia, retardation, genital lesions, and ear abnormalities (CHARGE association).[59] Autistic features can also be detected in some children with congenital sensory disorders, especially when severe vision and/or hearing deficits are not detected and intervention is not implemented early.[60,61]

Finally, public policies have also made a significant effect on reported prevalence rates obtained from public administrative data. The Education of All Handicapped Children Act (Public Law 94-142) of 1975[62] made schools accessible to children with some disabilities. Many children with more severe disabilities, such as those with both autism and severe mental retardation, continued to live in segregated state institutions. Later laws such as the Americans with Disabilities Act of 1990[63] promoted closure of institutions; which caused more children with disabilities to live at home and attend community schools. Autism first became a diagnostic category for which children could receive services with passage of the Individuals with Disabilities Education Act (IDEA) in 1991.[64] Before 1991, children with autism were most likely to be served under categories established by older laws, such as "mental retardation," "learning disabled," "speech delayed," "or emotionally disturbed."[65] Since the passage of IDEA,[64] school eligibility diagnoses have usually conformed to medical diagnoses of an ASD. This phenomenon of "diagnostic substitution" may account for a substantial proportion of the apparent rise in prevalence; however, educational administrative data may not be completely reliable.[66-71] IDEA amendments[72,73] have made supplementary services

available to children with ASD that are not available to children with other disabilities, such as "year-around school." When criteria for ASD are marginal, professionals may be tempted to apply the label in order to secure these supplementary services, which often also provide additional support for the parents. Such strategies tend to inflate the "prevalence" when values are obtained solely from educational sources.

The reasons for the reported 10-fold rise in prevalence of ASD remain controversial.[50,51,74-82] However, there is broad agreement that more boys than girls are consistently found to be affected with ASD; sex ratios range from 2 : 1 to 4 : 1.[50,53,79,83-86] The male : female ratio is even higher for high-functioning autism and Asperger syndrome, ranging from 6 : 1 to 15 : 1.[87] A 2006 study, in which most affected children (53.3%) had normal intelligence, demonstrated a male : female ratio of 9 : 1.[55]

ETIOLOGY

ASDs are now believed to be biologically based neurodevelopmental disorders that are highly heritable.[88] Because of the wide phenotypic spectrum, most experts believe that many genes are involved.[89] In a minority of cases, ASDs may be associated with a medical condition or a known syndrome characterized by dysmorphic features and some degree of comorbid mental retardation.[47,48] Although ASDs are believed to be mainly genetic in origin, the lack of 100% concordance in monozygotic twins indicates that environmental factors may modulate the phenotypic expression.[22,88] Thus it has become increasingly apparent that the cause is multifactorial, with a variety of genetic and, to a lesser extent, environmental factors playing a role.

Genetic Underpinnings

Studies of twins have revealed concordance rates of classic autism in 60% of monozygotic pairs and in 0% to 3% of dizygotic pairs.[22,88,90] When the broader phenotype was taken into consideration, the rates were 60% to 92% and 0% to 10%, respectively. In addition, family studies have demonstrated a rapid decrease in prevalence among first-, second-, and third-degree relatives. Using these data, Bailey and colleagues[22] calculated that the predisposition for autism was more than 90% heritable, with multiple interacting genetic influences and strong family clustering.[91] In spite of these strong genetic underpinnings, the exact cause or causes are still unknown. The task has been daunting because of genetic complexity and phenotypic variation. First, ASDs appear to be complex heritable disorders involving multiple genes; estimates based on family studies range from 5 to 20 genes.[89] Each gene or gene combination may result in somewhat different subtype but often with overlapping behavioral phenotypes. The number of genes contributing to the disorder and the relative prevalence of each will increase or decrease the probability of identifying the cause; that is, success is more likely if there are relatively few genes that are somewhat common than if there are many genes that are rarer.[91] A second factor making gene identification more challenging is the variability in the ASD phenotype. The wide spectrum of symptoms sometimes promotes inclusion of participants in a study with various ASDs, sometimes even including individuals with disorders falsely categorized to be in the spectrum. This imprecise diagnosis contaminates the study group and makes identification of a unifying etiological agent elusive.[92,93]

Two major strategies have been used in the search for the ASD susceptibility genes: targeted cytogenetic studies and whole genome screens of families of children with ASD.[91,94] The first strategy depends on developing a hypothesis regarding the pathogenesis of ASD, focusing on one or more potential candidate genes and testing them genetically for an association with ASD. Candidate genes in ASD include, among others, those that appear to play a role in brain development (e.g., cerebellar Purkinje cell proliferation)[15,95] or in neurotransmitter function (e.g., serotonin transmitter).[96] The second strategy entails an indirect method and does not require investigators to make assumptions regarding the mechanism of inheritance. Instead, families with multiple members demonstrating an ASD (multiplex families) are studied to identify recurring DNA markers (breakpoints, translocations, duplications, and deletions) present in affected, but not in unaffected, members. Unfortunately, progress has been limited because the phenotypic endpoints of ASD are not well defined. Changes in *DSM* criteria and inconsistency in ascertainment strategies, resulting in a hazy delineation between "affected" and "unaffected" family members, contaminate outcomes and challenge interpretation of results.

This phenotypic heterogeneity has challenged molecular searches for the ASD gene or genes in spite of several genome-wide screens (International Molecular Genetic Study of Autism Consortium [IMGSAC]) and multicenter collaborative efforts since the 1980s.[93,97-99] The results are very enlightening; however, rather than providing conclusions based on replicated findings from multiple labs, these studies have often produced confusion and uncertainty as more susceptibility loci are described. Although at least one autism-linked abnormality has been found on almost every chromosome, few sites have been identified with any frequency. Table 15-4 provides a summary of some of the more consistent findings; however, the reader is advised to consult more extensive reviews.[7,92,100-104] Large study samples with pooled data from multiple populations (maximizing homogeneous samples) are needed to confirm the validity of reported candidate genes and susceptibility sites in ASD.[93]

Table 15-4 describes findings of genetic investigations that have, for the most part, targeted etiological possibilities for "idiopathic ASD," which represents most cases of ASD. Although the literature provides multiple systems for characterizing ASDs, it is perhaps most helpful in a discussion of etiology to subtype ASDs as either idiopathic or secondary.[103] For the purposes of this discussion, patients with idiopathic ASD are those who do *not* have a coexisting associated medical condition or syndrome known to cause an ASD. Most individuals with ASD (perhaps almost all of those with Asperger syndrome) have the idiopathic subtype. Children with idiopathic ASD demonstrate variable behavioral phenotypes, are less likely to have coexisting mental retardation, and do not have dysmorphic features heralding a recognizable syndrome. Nevertheless, twin and family studies have revealed that idiopathic ASD is very heritable, with a recurrence rate of 3% to 7%,[22] although phenotypic expression may be modified by other variables.[92]

Patients with "secondary" ASD are children with a known identifiable syndrome or medical disorder believed to play an etiological role in ASD; this occurs in only 2% to 10% of cases.[23,66,103-113] In a meta-analysis of 23 epidemiological studies, Chakrabarti and Fombonne[47] reported that a recognizable condition was identified in an average of 6% of those with a confirmed ASD. The rate of coexisting mental retardation was 26%, the lowest reported prevalence to date. The presence of severe mental retardation, especially when associated with dysmorphic features, increases the likelihood of identifying a genetic etiology.[10,104,110,114] Genetic syndromes associated with ASD and coexisting mental retardation include

TABLE 15-4 ■ Selected Autism Spectrum Disorder (ASD) Genetic Markers

The high male : female ratio and the discovery of genes for both fragile X syndrome and Rett syndrome on the X-chromosome made it a plausible target.[116,362,553] Investigators have targeted a variety of possible roles for the X-chromosome in ASD:

Skewed X-chromosome inactivation is known to occur in X-linked mental retardation carriers[554] and to be responsible for most of the phenotypic variability seen in Rett syndrome.[362] X-chromosome inactivation patterns in female patients with ASD and controls (from the AGRE database) were studied to determine whether skewness might account for expression of possible autism genes on the X-chromosome.[553] Indeed, statistically greater skewness was found in those with classic Autism disorder than in controls (33% vs. 11%). Furthermore, of 10 asymptomatic mothers of Autism daughters demonstrating skewness, 5 also had highly skewed X-chromosome inactivation; of the mothers of the four control daughters showing skewness, none showed skewed inactivation. These results warrant further study to determine the possibility of skewed X-chromosome inactivation and/or X-linked candidate genes in the etiology of ASD in both male and female patients.

An epigenetic phenomenon similar to the one occurring in Rett syndrome has been proposed because of overlapping clinical presentations (i.e., stereotypies and regression in social and communication skills) and the discovery that a few individuals with ASD also demonstrated Rett syndrome–like mutations.[362,363,361a] A mutation in a regulator gene on the X-chromosome may cause the inappropriate activation or inactivation of otherwise normal genes that affect brain development and, in turn result in ASD. Between 2% and 7% of children with Angelman syndrome and a rare child with ASD also have been found to have MECP2 mutations.[124,361a]

Imprinting on the X-chromosome has been offered as a possible explanation for the high male : female ratio. Investigations of girls with either Turner syndrome or partial deletions of the X-chromosome revealed an increase risk for social skill deficits similar to those seen in ASD.[97,100,555,556] Paternally rather than maternally derived deletions were more strongly associated with poor social cognition. Thus, it appears the paternal X-chromosome is important for development of this skill, and because boys do not receive X-chromosomes from their fathers, they might be at higher risk for social deficits as a result of imprinting (parental origin effect).

Isolated findings of Xp22 deletions or duplications have been reported in a few individuals with ASD.[557]

Genome screens have found a linkage to the Xq13-21 region that contains the genes that code for neuroligin, a cell-adhesion molecule that is thought to be involved with synaptogenesis.[558]

Mutations of the angiotensin II receptor gene on the Xq22-23 region have been implicated in one of the X-linked mental retardation syndromes in which almost 20% also meet criteria for ASD.[559]

Chromosome 2

A site on 2q, which appears to contain a susceptibility gene for autism and language delay (2q37), was identified in several studies, including two IMGSAC screens[92,96,97,559]; however, a more recent screen entailing a different database failed to confirm this.[93]

Chromosome 3

In a genome screen of pooled data from two countries, the 3p24-26 region emerged as the most promising.[93] This locus contains the oxytocin receptor gene (OXTR). The possible link between ASD and oxytocin regulation of social behavior has been noted since the mid-1990s,[96,561,562] and oxytocin receptors have been found throughout the limbic system. Social deficits in oxytocin knockout mice[563] reduced oxytocin plasma levels,[564] and some evidence that synthetic oxytocin ameliorated repetitive behaviors in adults with ASD[565] have all pointed toward a contributing role for oxytocin.

Chromosome 7

Genome screens of this chromosome have resulted in the most consistent findings.[97,98,566] Researchers have postulated a susceptibility site, called the AUTSI locus (7q31-33), where mutations in one or more of the involved genes can potentially increase the risk of an ASD.[198] The RELN (7q22-33) gene and its secretory glycoprotein, reelin, appear to play a role in migration and cell lamination in the brain, especially in the cerebellum, where some of the most consistent neuropathological abnormalities occur.[198,567] Other genes also occur at this site and may play a role. The FOXP2 gene (7q31-35) appears to play a role in the embryonic development of neural pathways involved in the acquisition of expressive language. Several mutations have been found in patients with speech disorders.[568] Finally, the WNT2 gene on chromosome 7 appears to play a role in social skills.[569]

Chromosome 15

A variety of cytogenetic abnormalities occur at the 15q11-13 locus (duplications, deletions, translocations). In regard to ASD, 1% to 4% of study cohorts may demonstrate a duplication, usually maternally derived, at this site.[100,122,123,570,571] A "chromosome 15 phenotype" has begun to emerge that is characterized by hypotonia, joint laxity, global (especially motor) developmental delays, seizures, speech delay, social deficits, stereotypies, and a variable pattern of mild facial dysmorphisms.[123] Other abnormalities (deletions) also occur at the site and produce either Angelman or Prader-Willie syndrome, depending on the parent of origin. A GABA receptor gene (coding for a neurotransmitter highly implicated in ASD) also occurs at this site.[92,100]

Chromosome 17

Because serotonin is pivotal during brain development[213,572] and platelet serotonin is one of the most common laboratory abnormalities in children with ASD,[96,573,574] the serotonin transporter gene (17q11-12) has become a popular target for study. A susceptibility site at 17p12-q21 was noted to be the second most promising one in a comprehensive genome screen involving two databases from different countries.[93]

TABLE 15-4 ■ Selected Autism Spectrum Disorder (ASD) Genetic Markers—cont'd

Chromosome 22

Terminal deletions at 22q13 have been associated with hypotonia, developmental delay, autistic-like behavior, and subtle physical features (ear anomalies, short nose, smooth philtrum, and full lips).[366] Another study reported that 14% of patients with a confirmed microdeletion of 22q11.2 also met criteria for an ASD.[367] Two other well-known syndromes (velocardiofacial [Shprintzen] syndrome and DiGeorge syndrome) are also associated with microdeletions at this site.[113,575]

Other Chromosomes

Older IMGSAC studies have consistently revealed possible sites on 2q, 7q, and 17q; a more recent combined analysis of two primary genome scans from AGRE (United States) and Finnish populations (314 autism-affected families) revealed the best loci to be 3p24-26 and 17p12-q21 with additional promising sites at 1p12-q25, 4q21-31; 5p15-q12; 6q14-21, 7q33-36; 8q22-24; and 19p13-q13.[93] Larger samples and more homogeneous samples are needed in order to narrow the focus and promote eventual success in identifying the autism gene or genes.

AGRE, Autism Genetic Resource Exchange; GABA, γ-amino butyric acid; IMGSAC, International Molecular Genetic Study of Autism Consortium.

- the fragile X syndrome[115-117]
- tuberous sclerosis[118-120]
- phenylketonuria[121]
- Angelman syndrome[122-125]

Of these four entities, the fragile X syndrome is the most common known genetic cause for the autistic phenotype, present in 1% to 5% of children with ASD, whereas 30% to 50% of those with genetically confirmed fragile X syndrome demonstrate some characteristics of ASD.[117,126] The presence of a known disorder does not automatically imply causation. A few children with genetic syndromes characterized by features quite different from ASD may also meet full *DSM* criteria. For example, investigators have reported that that 6% to 7% of children with Down syndrome (usually characterized by relatively good social skills and obvious physical stigmata)[58,127,128] and almost 50% of children with the CHARGE association[59,129] meet criteria for a diagnosis of either autistic disorder or PDD-NOS. Children with severe congenital sensory impairments (visual and/or auditory) are also at risk for the development of symptoms consistent with ASD, especially when appropriate early intervention is not provided.[60,61] Advancing paternal age has been shown to be associated with an increased risk of ASD possibly due to de novo spontaneous mutations and/or alterations in genetic imprinting.[129a]

A variety of immunological abnormalities in T cells, immunoglobulins, and anti–brain autoantibodies have all been reported in retrospective case studies,[130-134] but systematic studies have confirmed neither their existence nor their relevance.[102,135] Prospective studies have revealed that, except for a few individuals with recurrent infections, healthy children with ASD generally have normal immune function.[135] Epidemiological data revealed clustering of autoimmune disorders in ASD families; however there was no increase in autoimmune disorders of the central nervous system and the patients with

ASD did not themselves exhibit autoimmune disorders.[136] Food allergies have also been implicated to play an etiological role in a few case reports,[137,138] but, again, this has not been confirmed with rigorous studies.[12,102,139]

Environmental Factors

Regardless of the mechanism, a review of studies published since the 1950s reveals convincing evidence that most cases of ASD result from genetic factors with possible interacting environmental factors.[22,92,140,141] Environmental influences may represent a "second hit" or "trigger" phenomenon; that is, they may modulate/stimulate preexisting genetic factors to result in the manifestation of ASD in an individual child.

Environmental factors should have their greatest effect during the *prenatal* period, especially early in gestation, because the developmental brain abnormalities associated with ASD occur during the first and second trimesters.[141-144] Factors already identified to play a role include maternal rubella[145] or cytomegalovirus infections[146,147] and treatment with valproate[148,149] or thalidomide.[144,150] An isolated report[150] indicated that fetal exposure to thalidomide during days 20 to 24 of gestational age was associated with ASD symptoms; later exposure resulted in the more characteristic limb abnormalities but no ASD characteristics. Nelson and associates[151] reported increased cord blood levels of brain-derived neurotrophic factor and other neurotrophins in newborns in whom ASD was later diagnosed, which may have implications regarding the mechanism of the characteristic early brain overgrowth. Some investigators feel that fetal toxin exposure might be implicated by studies that have demonstrated higher rates of ASD in offspring of mothers who resided in urban settings during pregnancy[152,153]; however, other factors such as better access to diagnostic services in urban areas may be operative.

PERINATAL

Perinatal events have also been investigated, but findings have not been consistent and need replication.[154-157] Among other factors, the strongest associations have been with threatened abortion and advanced maternal age.[158] An association has been suggested between full-term neonatal encephalopathy and later diagnoses of ASD.[159] In one study, ASD were diagnosed in 5% of survivors, which represented an almost sixfold increase in comparison with matched controls. This association, if replicated and confirmed, may represent a genetically derived predisposition making the infants vulnerable to both encephalopathy and ASD or a causative mechanism.

POSTNATAL

Postnatal causes of ASD are less likely possibilities. Moderate environmental deprivation has not been found to play an etiological role in ASD.[152,160] One study of Romanian orphanages revealed that severe environmental deprivation could lead to something resembling at least "quasi-autism"; however, most symptoms disappeared if the children were adopted into nurturing homes during early childhood.[161] A causal association between the measles, mumps, and rubella (MMR) vaccine and the development of ASD was proposed in a controversial case series study of 12 children with autistic regression and colitis.[162] The onset of autistic behavior reportedly occurred shortly after receipt of the MMR vaccination. The Institute of Medicine,[163] the AAP,[164] the British Medical Research Council,[165] and the Cochrane Collaboration[166] reviewed epidemiological studies and other published and unpublished evidence and concluded that there is no evidence of a causal association. In 2004, 10 of the 13 authors of the original article stated in a retraction that they did not believe the data supported the conclusions regarding a possible causal relationship.[167] Most recently, a multisite Collaborative Programs of Excellence in Autism study of 351 children with ASD failed to reveal any evidence of a causal association between ASD symptoms and the MMR vaccine.[168]

Questions have been raised repeatedly[80,81,153] about the possible effects of environmental mercury exposure and mercury-containing vaccines on the development of ASD and other developmental disabilities. From large data sets from the United States, Sweden, and Denmark, no consistent association has been found between vaccines containing thimerosal (the mercury-based preservative) and ASD or other neurodevelopmental outcomes.[169-171] Statements that the neuropathological and clinical presentations of ASD and mercury poisoning are similar were also refuted by Nelson and Bauman.[172]

Although scientific evidence[170] of no association between vaccines (specifically MMR and thimerosal- or mercury-containing vaccines) and ASD continues to accumulate, many parents, as well as some professionals, remain unconvinced of the validity of the evidence.[81a] In a best seller (*Evidence of Harm,* 2005), Kirby[82] hypothesized that various governmental agencies and medical organizations have conspired to cover up the possible harmful effects of thimerosal. The disbelief in the scientific evidence regarding mercury and vaccines remains one of the most challenging public heath problems faced by pediatricians in the United States today.

Although the preceding discussion reveals the wide variety of coexisting conditions known to be associated with ASD, a thorough etiological investigation in the individual child with ASD rarely identifies a known cause, especially in the absence of mental retardation, dysmorphic features, a positive family history, and/or positive results of a focal neurological examination.[10,12,47,104,107] Multicentered collaborative studies are needed and are currently being designed to systematically evaluate children with ASD for comorbid conditions.[173] The inclusion of controls with mental retardation and/or other disabilities is important in determining whether the conditions are unique to ASD or equally prevalent among children with significant neurodevelopmental disabilities in general.

NEUROLOGICAL CORRELATES

A neurobiological basis for autism was first suspected in the 1970s when it was noted that approximately one third of persons with autism had epilepsy.[174] The neurological basis was further supported by evidence that autism was associated with tuberous sclerosis, a neurocutaneous disorder.[118] Since that time, a growing body of evidence has revealed that brain growth and organization are different between normal children and those with ASD and that the onset of these abnormalities begins early in prenatal brain development, in some cases as early as days 20 to 24 of gestation.[15,95,144,150,175] Information regarding brain development, cytoarchitecture, and functioning has been accessed through a variety of methods, including evoked potentials, electroencephalography (EEG) and magnetoencephalography, structural and functional MRI (sMRI and fMRI), positron emission tomography, neurotransmitter levels, neuropsychological testing, and postmortem examination of brain tissue. Many findings have been nonspecific and inconsistent; neuroimaging studies sometimes reveal results that are disparate from those of microscopic tissue examinations. Study samples have been characterized by a wide spectrum of behavioral heterogeneity and IQ scores. The presence or absence of coexisting mental retardation has often confounded the interpretation of reports and has been responsible for conflicting results. The highly variable and complex ASD phenotype, coupled with changing *DSM* criteria, has prevented the recognition of a cohesive neurological mechanism to explain all core symptoms. Research has been further impeded by the dearth of available specimens, lack of an animal model, and logistical challenges in studying children who are nonverbal with behavioral challenges.

Although individuals have been evaluated with clinical neuroimaging since the 1960s, the first rigorous research-quality neuroimaging studies did not begin to appear in the literature until the 1980s.[176] The first systematic postmortem study of tissue in an individual with known autism was reported in 1985.[177] In 1988, the first MRI abnormality (hypoplasia of the cerebellum) was reported.[44] Since then, studies describing neurophysiological and neuropathological abnormalities, as well as theories regarding their effect on behavior and learning, have mushroomed. For a more thorough review of the neurological aspects of ASD, the reader is referred to related chapters by Volkmar and colleagues[14] (see also Anderson and Hoshino[178]) and reviews by Bauman and Kemper[15] and Polleux and Lauder.[179] In 2006, the neurological findings supported by the greatest degree of evidence included the following:

- Increased prevalence of epilepsy and abnormal electroencephalograms.
- Accelerated brain growth during childhood associated with macrocephaly (occipitofrontal circumference >98 percentile) and megalencephaly (increased brain volume per sMRI, primarily in young children).
- Decreased number of Purkinje cells in the cerebellar hemispheres.
- Decreased neuronal cell size, increased cell number, and increased packing density in limbic structures.
- Abnormal minicolumns in the cerebral cortex.
- Hypoactivity in the fusiform gyrus during face recognition tasks.
- Increased peripheral serotonin levels.

Although early investigators occasionally reported slightly enlarged ventricles, the changes were therapeutically insignificant.[176] Studies of the cingulated gyrus, basal ganglia, thalamus, and brainstem are fewer in number and less conclusive. There are many additional findings and theories, but these are not as well studied, more controversial, or confounded by comorbid medical conditions and/or intellectual deficits.

Seizures and Electroencephalographic Data

Electrophysiological studies were among the earliest used to probe differences in the autistic brain and provided the first evidence that autism was a neurological rather than a behavioral disorder. Abnormal electroencephalographic results are more prevalent in autism than is frank epilepsy (50% vs. 30%, respectively)[176,180] and reflect the disruption of balance between inhibition and excitation, which in turn can negatively affect attention and sensory processing.[179,181]

Brain Growth

Kanner[6] himself noted that 5 of his 11 original patients had large heads, but it was not until the1990s that brain size/volume in ASD was systematically studied through both indirect methods (occipitofrontal circumference measurements) and direct methods (sMRI and postmortem examinations). Although these early studies revealed increased brain size[182] and volume,[183] the mechanisms and changes in growth velocity over the developmental period in children were not recognized until the late 1990s. Head size does not appear to be large at birth; in fact, it is sometimes reported as somewhat smaller than average.[184] Acceleration of growth, as evidenced by serial occipitofrontal circumference measurements and confirmed with volumetric studies, begins to occur around 6 months and peaks between 2 and 4 years of age, thus occurring in concert with (or even before) the appearance of ASD symptoms.[185-188] Approximately one third of children with ASD meet criteria for macrocephaly, and 90% have greater than average brain volumes.[185] Growth appears to level off in late childhood in the majority; thus, brain volume is not significantly different from that in controls by age 12 years, although macrocephaly (as measured by occipitofrontal circumference) may persist.[186,189,190] Furthermore, increased cortical folding resulting in abnormal gyral patterns, reflecting increased volume, has been noted in affected children but not adolescents or adults.[191] These findings appear very consistent, especially when study subjects are matched for intelligence. The main contribution to increased size lies in nonuniform changes in the hippocampus, amygdala, and cerebral white matter and, less consistently, gray matter.[185,192-194] Although several theories have been proposed for the abnormal growth pattern (e.g., increased neurogenesis, glial cell proliferation, abnormal myelin, and/or decreased apoptosis/pruning), it seems most likely that it is the outer radiate zone, related to intrahemispheric synaptogenesis and connectivity, that matures postnatally and produces the rapid growth in ASD. Interestingly, parents of children with ASD can have macrocephaly in the absence of ASD symptoms. Thus, macrocephaly might be caused by a susceptibility gene that works in concert with other genes to produce ASD.

Although there are numerous published sMRI studies, no consistent abnormalities have been reported with regard to the gross anatomy or growth of other brain structures such as the brainstem, basal ganglia, and cerebellum.[44,182,183,192,193] Several studies have consistently shown impaired growth (caused by hypoplasia, not atrophy) in the body and posterior regions of the corpus callosum. Only one study has correlated these anatomical findings with deficits in interhemispheric cognitive tasks.[195] Rather than a focal neurological abnormality, ASD seems to be characterized by abnormalities of neural distribution and connectivity with excessive intrahemispheric connectivity and deficient interhemispheric connections (corpus callosum).[176]

Cerebellar Purkinje Cells

Although comparisons of sMRI and volumetric studies of the cerebellum have been controversial, one of the most consistent findings over time has been the marked decrease in Purkinje cells noted in postmortem microscopic studies.[15,95,196] The absence of empty baskets suggests that the process is one of hypoplasia rather than atrophy after a noxious event, but some authorities disagree.[197] Reductions in reelin may contribute abnormal regulation of neuronal layering and microscopic abnormalities found in the cerebellum.[198] The absence of glial hyperplasia indicates the pathological process occurs early in brain development, before the time when the brain is able to initiate a reaction to neuronal injury. Furthermore, the number of olivary neurons is preserved, which provides additional evidence that the process must occur before weeks 28 to 30 of gestation. After this time, tight neuronal unions form between the two areas, and cell loss in the cerebellum would prompt an obligatory retrograde cell loss in the ascending olivary neurons.[15,95,143,175] Although it has long been known that the cerebellum played a role in motor learning, modulation, and coordination, there is growing evidence that it also plays a role in verbal processing, affective behavior, and shifting of attention.[199] Bauman and Kemper[175] suggested that early in embryological life, the climbing olivary neurons might form primitive unions with collateral cells in the lamina dessicans (which disappears at 28 to 30 weeks) of the cerebellar peduncles. These neural units are not as efficient as the primary pathways and cease to function after a brief period. An intriguing question is whether this process may contribute to "autistic regression."

Decreased Cell Size, Increased Cell Number, and Increased Packing Density in Limbic Structures

Investigators have targeted the limbic system because it plays an important role in social behavior/cognition (amygdala) and associative social memory, especially relationships among the emotional aspects of an experience (hippocampus). Postmortem microscopic studies have consistently revealed abnormalities in cell number and size and packing density in both the amygdala and hippocampus. However, sMRI and volumetric data have been inconsistent, diverse, and often contradictory.[193,200,201]

Abnormal Minicolumns in the Cerebral Cortex

Abnormal cortical minicolumns (defined as the most basic unit of neural organization) have been added to the growing number of neuropathological abnormalities found in ASD. Although Bailey and colleagues[202] described several abnormalities of pyramidal neuronal migration (ectopic neurons in white matter zones, misoriented apical dendrites, and disorganized cellular layers) in the superior temporal gyrus. Casanova and coworkers[203] more recently introduced "minicolumn" terminology into ASD literature. Minicolumns in some areas of the autistic frontal cortex were found to be smaller (representing an underdeveloped system) and had abnormal patterning. Both findings are consistent with deviant processes that occur very early in the second trimester. These anatomical abnormalities may result in deficient neuronal "insulation" and serve as the structural basis for increased neuronal "cross-talk" and overstimulation. This, in turn, may cause the sensory gating and processing difficulties found in some individuals with ASD.[203,204] Other autistic symptoms then might be explained by a disregulation of axonal outgrowth, dendritic arborization, and synaptic connectivity.[179] Abnormalities described in cortical frontostriatal circuits may be associated with ritualistic and repetitive behaviors.[204] Volumetric sMRI studies of cortical systems serving language functions have revealed the absence of the usual left hemispheric hypertrophy (representing left brain dominance and language specialization). Instead of a larger left hemisphere (specifically, the Wernicke receptive language processing area), the planum temporale volumes were equal in subjects with ASD.[205] Furthermore, decreased gray matter in the left inferior prefrontal gyrus or Broca's area (expressive language center) resulted in actual reversal of the typical hemispheric asymmetry (left larger than right) in language-impaired subjects with ASD.[206]

Hypoactivity in the Fusiform Gyrus during Face Recognition Tasks

Functional neuroimaging techniques, primarily positron emission tomography and fMRI, have confirmed clinical and neuroanatomical data depicting ASD as a disorder characterized by uneven rather than generalized deficits.[207] The most consistent fMRI finding has been hypoactivity in the fusiform gyrus, particularly in the fusiform facial area, confirming the clinical impression that deficits in facial recognition are characteristic of ASD.[208,209] fMRI has also demonstrated associated deficits in related areas of the "social brain," such as the amygdala, which plays a critical role in emotional arousal and integration of emotional data.[210] Persons with ASD appear to be less motivated to look at faces or to follow the point of conversational partners.[208] Computerized eye tracking techniques have also revealed that they pay less attention to faces and more attention to inanimate details in the background.[209,211,212] When they do look at the face, they target the mouth rather than the eyes. Because oral expressions provide less information about emotional states than the eyes, persons with ASD often fail to detect meaningful social information during interactions.[208]

Neurochemical Testing

Neurochemical abnormalities may also be present in children with ASD.[178] Increased levels of 5-hydroxytryptamine in whole blood, chiefly platelets, has been a fairly consistent finding. Although 5-hydroxytryptamine is an important neurotransmitter for brain development and modulation of sleep, mood, body temperature, appetite, and hormone release, no consistent abnormalities have been found in central nervous system levels. Age-related differences in serotonin synthesis capacity have also been demonstrated between children with autism and nonautistic controls.[213]

In conclusion, it is widely accepted that ASD is a "neurodevelopmental disorder," although the specific underlying abnormalities have not been identified. ASD may actually represent a disorder of neural distribution rather than frank structural abnormalities.[176] A project to create the first ever atlas of the autistic brain at several ages is well under way.[214] Newer functional brain studies have provided some intriguing links between the neuroanatomical substrate and characteristic clinical features. Well-designed studies with participants matched for IQ levels and with the most sophisticated technology (e.g., diffusion tensor imaging) are needed to unravel the mystery of anatomical differences and white matter "connectivity" and associated discrepancies in learning and neuropsychological functioning. Such studies may provide valuable information that can be used to design, implement, and evaluate new and effective intervention strategies.

CLINICAL SIGNS

Although emphasis has historically been placed on language deficits, they are not specific to ASD and are commonly also the presenting feature of children with mental retardation, hearing loss, and communication disorders. Stereotypies may be obvious and easily recognized, but they also occur in other conditions, primarily severe mental retardation and blindness. Furthermore, they often do not appear until after 3 years of age,[215] and some forms (e.g., hand flapping) can be normal in certain situations (e.g., in an excited toddler). Thus, language deficits and stereotypies do not clearly distinguish ASD from other childhood disorders. During the 1990s, it became apparent that the social deficits, specifically those relating to "social communication," were the most consistent and characteristic symptoms of ASD. The diagnosis of classic autistic disorder currently requires that at least one criterion be met in each of the language and restricted interests domains and that two criteria be met in the social skills domain.[19,20] Several early recognizable social communication deficits (e.g., joint attention) appear to be fairly specific for ASD. The severity of these deficits varies significantly from patient to patient, thus creating diagnostic challenges.

Most parents first become concerned about their children's development when they are between 15 and 18 months of age[216,217]; their first concerns usually focus on speech delays. Indeed, this has been the historical hallmark of ASD and will probably continue to be so because these deficits are easily recognized. However, with heightened public awareness about the early signs that occur before development of vocal speech, parents are beginning to voice concerns about more subtle receptive language skills (the child's not responding to his or her name being called) and social skills (e.g., decreased eye contact, unusual attachments to objects, not caring whether parent is nearby). Studies have demonstrated that symptoms can appear before 1 year of age, although these may be subtle.[218] Some infants appear to develop normally until approximately the second year of life, when they demonstrate regression in speech and social skills, withdraw, and become indifferent to their surroundings.[219,220] Subtle abnormalities in social communication may be evident on careful examination of 1-year-old birthday video recordings.[221-223] Expanded discussions can be found in chapters and reviews dedicated solely to early clinical characteristics.[224-227]

Social Skills Deficits

As noted previously, abnormalities in social communication skills are the most unique and consistent findings in infants with ASD. They appear earlier than identifiable speech deficits but are often more subtle. Children with ASD universally demonstrate deficits in social relatedness, defined as the inherent drive to connect with others and share complementary emotional states.[228] Children with other types of disabilities (e.g., mental retardation, sensory disabilities) still attempt to connect with others: Those with hearing deficits compensate with eye gaze and gestures, and those with vision deficits compensate with voice and touch. Children with ASD do not appear to seek this connectedness; they are usually content with being alone, rarely make eye contact or bids for others' attention with gestures or vocalizations, and react little to praise or bids for attention from others. In later years, they have difficulty in sharing the emotional state of others in cooperative games and group settings and have few, if any, friends.

DEFICITS IN JOINT ATTENTION AND SHARING OF INTERESTS

One of the most distinguishing characteristics of very young children with ASD is a deficit in "joint attention."[229-235] Joint attention is the desire coupled with the ability (facial expressions, gestures and/or speech) to draw another's attention to objects, events, or other persons simply for the enjoyment of sharing experiences. Like other developmental skills, joint attention appears to develop in graduated stages, usually between 8 and 16 months. At approximately 8 months of age, a typically developing infant may participate in "gaze monitoring": that is, when a parent looks away (e.g., to check the time), the infant follows the parent's gaze and looks in the same direction. This social skill should be differentiated from simple auditory orienting, in which both the infant and the parent are stimulated by an environmental stimulus (e.g., clock alarm) at the same time. Children begin to "follow a point" at about 10 to 12 months of age. If a parent points in the direction of an interesting object or event and says, "Look," the typically developing child looks in the direction that the parent is pointing. Upon seeing the object/event, the child looks back at the parent and smiles, frowns, or shows fear, whichever emotion is appropriate to the situation. An infant with ASD does not follow a point even when a parent tries repeatedly, calling the child's name in a loud voice or with physical prompts such as touching the child's shoulder before pointing.[218]

Subsequently, joint attention milestones involve the child's, rather than the caregiver's, initiating the interaction. At approximately 12 to 14 months of age, the typically developing child begins to point. At first, he or she may point to a desired object that is out of reach. The child looks alternatively at the desired object and at the parent during the bid for attention. Depending on his or her speech skills, the child may utter simple sounds ("uh") or actual words while pointing. Pointing to request an object is often called *protoimperative pointing* and may not actually represent true joint attention, inasmuch as in this triad, the object is the goal and the caregiver is the means by which the child is able to obtain that goal. Alternating eye contact between the object and the caregiver is critical in designating this as a quasi–joint attention skill. A child with ASD is more likely to take the caregiver's hand and lead him or her to the object.

At 14 to 16 months of age, the typically developing child begins to point simply to "comment" about, or "share," an interesting object/event (*protodeclarative pointing*). As the child points, he or she looks alternatively between the object/event of interest and the caregiver. The same triad exists (child, caregiver, object), but the goal is reversed. It is the shared social experience, not the object, that the child seeks. Children with ASD consistently fail to point to "comment" at age-appropriate times. If and when they do start to point, they are less likely to show positive affect and connectedness during the act. About the same time, typical children also begin to "show" items of interest to parents. This bid for attention is distinct from asking for help (e.g., bringing a jar of bubbles to the parent as a request to open it). Mastery of joint attention appears to be a reliable predictor of functional language development.[13,236-238]

The ability to disengage and shift focus of attention from one stimulus to a novel one is a very basic skill that can be measured in normally developing 6-month-olds. The inability to shift attention was proposed as a characteristic deficit in autism that possibly contributed to deficits in joint attention, inasmuch as it relies on shifting attention between an object/event and a partner.[44,199] Multicenter studies of infant siblings of older children with ASD have revealed that the inability to shift one's attention (from parent to object of interest and back to parent again) is measurable and perhaps the first reliable sign of ASD.[218]

POOR SOCIAL AND EMOTIONAL RECIPROCITY

One of the earliest developmental milestones is the ability to orient to social stimuli—in particular, turning to respond to one's own name.[239] At about 8 to 10 months of age, most children turn preferentially when their name is called. Like children with hearing impairments, those with ASD often fail to orient to their name. In fact, an early concern of parents of children later diagnosed with ASD is about their infant's hearing. Parents are often puzzled because such children seem to attend to environmental sounds better than to human voices.[240] Retrospective studies of 1-year-old birthday video recordings in children who later received diagnoses of ASD have demonstrated that failure to orient to one's name being called is one of the most consistent deficits in affected children at that age.[221,222] Reciprocal social interaction includes ongoing back-and-forth bids for attention and social interactions with multiple emotional expressions, sounds, and other gestures. Social referencing[241] is the ability to recognize the emotional states of others as they respond to various stimuli. When faced with a novel situation, a normal infant might look to his or her caregiver for an indication of delight, anger, or fear in her facial expression. His or her facial expression will then usually mimic the caregiver's, although he or she may not fully understand the situation. A child with ASD engages in less social referencing and less imitation.[242]

DIFFICULTY IN MAKING AND KEEPING FRIENDS

Because children with ASD lack the fundamental social skill building blocks described previously, they are less likely to develop appropriate peer relationships. They may have few or no friends, and they tend to relate better with either much younger children or adults. These relationships, when present, usually evolve around the child's own special interests. Later developing skills may be deficient and also impair friendships. Many authorities believe that impaired central coherence is a basic characteristic of children with ASD, especially older ones. Central coherence is the ability to interpret stimuli in a relatively global way, taking context into account.[243,244] Persons with ASD tend to focus on parts and to make less use of context; their processing is more piecemeal. They have difficulty integrating component features into a cohesive unit and seeing the "big picture." Although central coherence is not a true social skill, deficits in central coherence can impair social interactions, because this type of information processing is very different from that of typically developing peers. Theory-of-mind skills enable a person to take the perspective of another person and are based on the realization that others have thoughts and emotions that are independent from one's own.[245-247] Theory-of-mind skills include the ability to infer states of mind on the basis of external behavior. This inability to take the perspectives of other people is another impediment to forming and maintaining friendships. Although the deficit itself is not unique to patients with ASD, the degree of the deficit is much more severe than has been noted in other disorders. Because of deficits in perspective taking, children with ASD have difficulties with social-emotional behaviors such as empathy, sharing, and comforting. It is now gener-

ally accepted that in the course of typical development, children have a sense of the mental states of others by 4 years of age.[248,249] Although not helpful in the early diagnosis of autistic disorder, lack of theory-of-mind skills is critical in the early diagnosis of later recognized Asperger syndrome. Unlike deficits in joint attention, theory-of-mind deficits are not specific for ASD; similar findings can be seen in children with cognitive impairments and are consistent with their general level of developmental functioning.[250]

Communication Deficits

Most children in whom autistic disorder and PPD-NOS are later diagnosed present initially with "speech delay," although this trend is slowly changing as parents become more aware of social milestones and sense that something is wrong before the child is 18 months old.[230,249] Although lack of or severe deficits in speech without any effort to compensate with gestures has long been thought to be characteristic of autistic disorder, more children who now receive diagnoses of autistic disorder do have some speech. Vocabulary deficits are often the focus of concern, but there are typically earlier communication deficits that, if detected, could promote earlier diagnosis.[241,249] For example,

- Lack of the alternating to-and-fro pattern of vocalizations between baby and parent that usually occurs at approximately 5 months (i.e., babies with ASD usually continue vocalizing without regard for the parent's speech).
- Lack of recognition of mother's (or father's or consistent caregiver's) voice.
- Disregard for vocalizations but keen awareness of environmental sounds.
- Delayed onset of babbling (past 9 months of age).
- Decreased or no use of prespeech gestures (waving, pointing, showing).
- Lack of expressions such as "oh oh" and "huh."
- Lack of interest or response of any kind of neutral statements (e.g., "Oh, no, it's raining!").

Parents are often unaware of these deficits unless the milestones are brought to their attention.

Approximately 25% to 30% of children with autistic disorder and PDD-NOS begin to say words at 12 to 18 months but then stop using them. "Autistic regression" characteristically takes place between 15 and 24 months of age after the child has mastered 5 to 10 words.[219,251] Many such children become completely nonverbal and cease to gesture (wave, point, and so forth). Although this regression is seemingly dramatic, some parents are able to rationalize the regression and attribute the loss of skills to a family event such as the birth of a new sibling or a move to a new house. Home videos recorded before the onset of regression have revealed that, in at least some children, mild delays and subtle early signs were present before the apparent regression, although there is a subset of children who were apparently normal.[168,220]

Some children use "pop-up words": that is, words that are verbalized inconsistently and with no apparent communicative intent. These words are said out of context for a short period of time (days or weeks) and then, as suddenly as they might pop up for no apparent reason, they also disappear.[17,238,249] On occasion, these utterances may be phrases or entire sentences, also said out of context. Spontaneously uttered pop-up words should be distinguished from "echolalia." Echolalia, sometimes called "parroting" by lay individuals, is the repetition of another's speech. It is classified as "immediate" when the child repeats another's words right after they are heard or as "delayed" when repeated at distant time later. Normal children pass through a brief developmental stage ("vocabulary burst stage") in which they imitate other's speech, particularly the last one or two words of a sentence. Autistic echolalia can persist throughout the lifespan with little or no apparent communicative function. It often occurs long after the utterance (delayed echolalia) and is also qualitatively different in that the utterances are more exact, have a monotone quality and consist of larger verbal "chunks" (e.g., TV advertisement jingles, video re-enactments, or nursery rhymes). These verbalizations often exceed the child's functional language skills and may be misinterpreted as "advanced" when in fact the child has difficulty following a simple one-step command. Some children with ASD become quite obsessed with labeling colors, shapes, numbers, and letters of the alphabet, and yet they cannot point to them on request or incorporate the labels into functional language. Later they may develop hyperlexia or advanced oral reading without corresponding comprehension skills.

Children with Asperger syndrome may have mild or very limited speech delays and thus escape recognition until around 3 to 4 years of age, when their inability to make friends becomes a concern. Although unnoticed, language development is atypical in that children are often quite verbal about some subjects (usually things or events), but unable to express simple feelings or recognize the feelings and viewpoints of others. Speech may be fluent but limited to only a few topics, typically those that hold a strong, all-consuming interest for the child. It can also be overly formal (pedantic), a reason why they are sometimes described as "little professors."[247] Children with Asperger syndrome also have deficits in the *social use* of language (pragmatics): how to choose a topic of conversation; understanding and producing appropriate tempo, facial expression, and body language during conversation; turn-taking; recognizing when the partner has lost interest in a topic; knowing when to start, sustain, and end a conversation on the basis of listener cues; knowing when and how to repair a communication breakdown; and using the appropriate degree of formality and politeness. Language may seem odd, pedantic, self-centered, and not listener-responsive and often results in a monotone monologue. These children may demonstrate unique delivery of speech (prosody) in regard to intonation, volume, rhythm, pitch, and personal space, and they tend to disregard listener needs. Children with Asperger syndrome and high-functioning autism have difficulty with abstract reasoning and with discussion of thoughts and opinions of others. Inability to discern and judge the conversational intents of others, especially when their conversation includes words or phrases with ambiguous meanings impairs their ability to understand metaphors, humor, sarcasm, teasing, metaphors, irony, lies, jokes, faux pas, and deception.[245,246]

Play Skill Deficits

Play has many attributes. It can be sensorimotor, functional, constructive, pretend, or imaginary. Play can take place in isolation of, in parallel with, or through interaction with other children. It can also be pathological (i.e., ritualistic play). Mastery of pretend play, especially during interaction with others, builds on both communication and social skills. Lack of or significantly delayed pretend play, coupled with persistent sensorimotor and/or ritualistic play, is very characteristic of ASD and serves as a discriminating feature of both screening and evaluation ASD tools. Some children with severe ASD may never progress past the sensorimotor play stage. They mouth, twirl, bang, and manipulate objects in a stereotypic or ritualistic manner. Often they prefer to play with common objects (string, sticks, rocks, or ballpoint pens) rather than store-bought toys. One exception is puzzles, especially shape-matching ones and computerized "puzzle games." These represent a form of "constructive play" (i.e., using objects in combination to create a product).[241] Children with ASD are often content to play alone for hours, requiring little attention or supervision. Often this "play" is either constructive (puzzles, computer games, and blocks), ritualistic (lining objects up or sorting/matching shapes or colors), or sensorimotor (mouthing, banging, twirling) in nature. Children with ASD may seem to enjoy chase games and roughhousing, but it is actually the games' sensorimotor aspects rather than the social aspects that the child enjoys. Even when symbolic play does develop, it may not advance to more sophisticated social play such as role-playing with a peer. These children have trouble interacting in groups and cooperating in the social rules of games. Often they are left out, ignored, and at high risk of being bullied by peers.

Atypical Behaviors

Children with ASD often manifest repetitive, non-functional, atypical behaviors or stereotypies (e.g., hand flapping, finger movements, rocking, twirling).[19,20,227] Although most such behaviors are harmless by themselves, they are problematic in that they may prevent the child from accomplishing tasks and learning new skills and may interfere with inclusion in natural environments with typically developing peers. Although stereotypies are very distinctive and obvious, they are not specific to children with ASD. Children with severe mental retardation and/or severe visual deficits also commonly demonstrate stereotypies. Even normal toddlers, especially before the onset of fluent language, may flap their arms briefly when they are excited or frustrated. True autistic stereotypies often do not appear until after age 3 years and may include some behaviors such as habitual toe walking and/or sensory stereotypies (persistent sniffing and licking of nonfood items) that are less common in children with other disorders.

Although most children, at some time during their early development, form attachments with a stuffed animal, special pillow, or blanket, children with ASD often prefer hard items (ballpoint pens, flashlight, keys, action toys). Moreover, the attachment is much more robust; they may even insist on holding the object most of the day, even during meals, and protest violently when the object is removed. On a similar note, children with ASD may insist on "sameness," again protesting when forced to make a transition from one activity to the next or to perform some activity out of order from the usual routine. Without warning, these protests may quickly escalate to severe and prolonged temper tantrums characterized by aggression or self-injurious behaviors.

Children with ASD, especially those with cognitive deficits, may demonstrate various forms of self-injurious behavior.[252] Such behaviors (e.g., head banging, skin picking, eye poking, hand biting) represent a class of stereotypies that, unlike those described previously, may cause bodily harm. Reasons for self-injurious behavior include those that may cause any child, with or without ASD, to display inappropriate behavior. These may include frustration during unsuccessful communication attempts to procure a desired object, protest against transitions, anxiety in new environments, boredom, pain, depression, fatigue,

and sleep deprivation. In rare cases, it may result from an endogenous neurochemical abnormality in dopa, serotonin, opioid, or γ-amino butyric acid neural transmitter systems and/or a part of a behavioral phenotype associated with a known genetic syndrome such as the finger and lip biting characteristic in Lesch-Nyhan syndrome.

Additional Clinical Features That Are Common but Are Not Core Features

MENTAL RETARDATION

In the past, cognitive deficits were thought to be extremely common in autism, and in fact, in most studies published before 1990, investigators reported the estimated prevalence of coexisting mental retardation as 90%.[83] Reviews and guidelines published from the late 1990s generally reported the prevalence as approximately 75%.[8,10-12,92,114] This statistic dropped with more recent prevalence studies,[52,53] with a low of 26% in England[47,48] and 47% in the United States.[55-55b] Better ascertainment of children with milder disorders, improved professional training, and more effective strategies/tools for evaluating cognitive abilities in children with ASD have all been cited as possible reasons for the decreasing prevalence of coexisting mental retardation.

SPLINTER AND SAVANT SKILLS

A unique characteristic of ASD is the unevenness of skills. Abilities may be significantly delayed in many areas of development but advanced in others, often because of exceptional memory, calculation, music, or art abilities.[253] These advanced skills are often called *splinter skills* when they serve little or no purpose in day-to-day life and do not improve the ultimate prognosis. For some patients, they may lead to a career that provides financial independence and even widespread recognition[254,255] and thus may be called "savant skills."

ABNORMAL SENSORY PROCESSING

Children with ASD may demonstrate deficits in multisensory integration and processing.[256] They may demonstrate simultaneous hyposensitivities and hypersensitivities for different stimuli even within the same sensory modality.[257] Although a child may seem not to hear his or her name being called, he or she is annoyed by the sound of dripping water in a distant room. In the visual modality, a child may explore toys while holding them very close to his or her eyes (as if visually impaired) and yet be exceptionally sensitive to the subtle flickering of fluorescent lights. Children with ASD may have oral aversions and/or overall "tactile defensiveness" to soft touch but no apparent response to injuries and other painful stimuli. The dichotomy may arise from an abnormal arousal level or an abnormal sensory gating system.

MOTOR ABNORMALITIES

In addition to the peculiar motor stereotypies that serve as a defining characteristic of the ASD, some affected children also demonstrate poor coordination and even frank delays, usually in the context of global developmental delay (GDD) or severe mental retardation. Others actually appear to have advanced motor skills; still others may have deficits in praxis (the planning, execution, and sequencing of movements).[228] Apraxia (severe deficits) and dyspraxia (milder deficits) affect the imitation of speech, facial expressions, play, and/or motor patterns of the extremities. Some investigators believe that, although not a defining characteristic by *DSM* or ICD-10 standards, motor clumsiness is a distinguishing characteristic of Asperger syndrome.[101,258] Some children with ASD may appear to be "hyperactive" and "motor-driven" with an exterior focus of attention, whereas others may be hypoactive and withdrawn and move little.[257]

In summary, ASD is characterized by a broad array of clinical features, which make distinct boundaries impossible. A thorough knowledge of the early social and preverbal communication deficits provides opportunities to encourage earlier diagnosis and intervention that, in turn, promote improved outcomes.

IDENTIFICATION AND DIAGNOSIS

Screening

The importance of screening for ASD has been emphasized because early identification allows early intervention that can potentially improve outcome and also leads to etiological investigation and counseling with regard to recurrence risk.[13] Although the clinical practice of developmental-behavioral pediatricians is more likely to involve comprehensive diagnostic evaluations than screening, training of general pediatricians and other primary health care providers in effective autism-specific screening strategies has become a primary obligation. Developmental-behavioral pediatricians may also be in a position to train or advise early intervention multidisciplinary teams with regard to screening for ASD.

Historically, the initial concerns of parents of children who later received diagnoses of ASD were dismissed, and diagnosis and intervention were therefore delayed.[216,217,259] In spite of increased public and professional awareness, the diagnosis of ASD is still often delayed. In a 2006 Centers for Disease Control and Prevention Atlanta-based study, Wiggins and col-

leagues[55] reported that the average age at the first documented ASD diagnosis was 60 months (range, 17 to 105 months). The average age at diagnosis was significantly younger (i.e., 41 months) in children with overall impairments. An average delay of 13 months occurred between the first evaluation by a qualified professional and the first ASD diagnosis. To address these ongoing challenges, the AAP now recommends administering a standardized autism-specific screening tool at the 18-month evaluation[260] and, perhaps additionally at the 24-month health supervision visits[261,262] and at any age when ASD concerns are raised spontaneously by parents or as a result of clinicians' observations or surveillance questions about social, communicative, and play behaviors.

ASD-specific screening tools are sometimes described as level 1 or level 2 screens.[263] Level 1 screening measures are administered to all children and are designed to differentiate children at risk for an ASD from the general population, especially those with typical development. Level 2 screening measures are more often used in settings such as early intervention programs or developmental clinics that serve children with a variety of developmental problems; they help differentiate children at risk for ASD from those at risk for other developmental disorders such as mental retardation or specific language impairment. Level 2 screening tools generally require more time and training to administer, score, and interpret than do level 1 measures, and there is considerable overlap between the concept of a level 2 screening tool and that of a diagnostic instrument.[263,264] Level 2 screening measures may be used as part of a diagnostic evaluation, but they should not be used in isolation to make a diagnosis. It is important for developmental-behavioral pediatricians to be familiar with the array of ASD screening tools available in order to train primary care providers and to conduct or assist with advanced level 2 screening.

Properties of some level 1 and level 2 ASD screening tools designed for use with very young children are reviewed in Table 15-5.[263,265-276] Several level 1 tools, such as the Checklist for Autism in Toddlers (CHAT) and the Modified Checklist for Autism in Toddlers (M-CHAT), are available to the clinician at no cost. Wong and associates[276] translated the M-CHAT into Chinese, modified the response choices and the scoring system, and combined it with the five observational items from the CHAT to form the CHAT-23. The Screening Tool for Autism in Two-Year-Olds (STAT) is an interactive measure developed for use as a level 2 screening measure in children between the ages of 24 and 36 months; investigation of its utility with younger and older children is under way.[263] Completion of a training workshop is required before use of the STAT. Tools such as the Autism Behavior

TABLE 15-5 ■ Autism Spectrum Disorder: Specific Early Childhood Screening Measures

Screening Tool	Sensitivity	Specificity	Ages	Format	Time to Complete
Level 1					
Checklist for Autism in Toddlers (CHAT)	0.18-0.38[†]	0.98-1.0[†]	18 months	Interview and interactive	5 minutes
Checklist for Autism in Toddlers (CHAT), Denver Modifications	0.65-0.85*	1.0*	18 months	Interview and interactive	5 minutes
Checklist for Autism in Toddlers–23 (CHAT-23)	Part A: 0.84-0.93* Part B: 0.74*	Part A: 0.77-0.85* Part B: 0.91*	16-86 months, but all had mental ages of 18-24 months[†]	Parent questionnaire	10 minutes
Modified Checklist for Autism in Toddlers (M-CHAT)	0.85[‡]	0.93[‡]	16-30 months	Parent questionnaire	5-10 minutes
Pervasive Developmental Disorders Screening Test–II (PDDST-II), Primary Care Screener (PCS)	0.92*	0.91*	18-48 months	Parent questionnaire	10-15 minutes
Level 2					
Autism Behavior Checklist (ABC)	0.38-0.58*	0.76-0.97*	18 months and older	Behavioral checklist completed by interviewer	10-20 minutes
Childhood Autism Rating Scale (CARS)	0.92-0.98*	—	Older than 2 years	Behavioral checklist completed by interviewer	Untimed
Gilliam Autism Rating Scale (GARS)	0.48-0.80[‡]	—	3-22 years	Behavioral checklist completed by parent or teacher	5-10 minutes
Pervasive Developmental Disorders Screening Test–II (PDDST-II), Developmental Clinic Screener (DCS)	0.73*	0.49*	18-48 months	Parent questionnaire	10-15 minutes
Pervasive Developmental Disorders Screening Test–II (PDDST-II), Autism Clinic Severity Screener (ACSC)	0.58*	0.60*	18-48 months	Parent questionnaire	10-15 minutes
Screening Tool for Autism in Two-Year-Olds (STAT)	0.92[‡]	0.853	24-36 months	Interactive, requires specific training	20 minutes
Social Communication Questionnaire (SCQ)	0.85-0.96*	0.67-0.80*	4 years and older	Parent questionnaire	5-10 minutes

Adapted from Coonrod EE, Stone WL: Screening for autism in young children. *In* Volkmar FR, Paul R, Klin A, et al, eds: Handbook of Autism and Pervasive Developmental Disorders. Hoboken, NJ: Wiley, 2005, pp 707-729.
*Clinical sample. [†]Population-based sample, [‡]Clinical and population-based samples.
[†]Wang et al: Pediatrics, 2004.

Checklist,[277] the Childhood Autism Rating Scale (CARS),[278-281] the Gilliam Autism Rating Scale (GARS),[282] and the Social Communication Questionnaire[283] can be used to screen for risk of ASD over a wide age range, including the preschool age group (see Table 15-5). Significant concerns about the psychometric properties of the Autism Behavior Checklist, GARS, and Pervasive Developmental Disorders Screening Test–II have been raised.[263,284,285] The Social Communication Questionnaire was derived from the Autism Diagnostic Interview–Revised and has fairly strong psychometric properties.[283,286] The Social Communication Questionnaire is recommended for use in children older than 4 years and is currently being evaluated to determine the most appropriate cutoff scores for 2- and 3-year-old children.

Many of the ASD-specific screening measures are currently being revised or further evaluated, and new tools are being developed to address some of the weaknesses of existing instruments. Attempts are being made to design instruments capable of detecting ASDs at younger ages. For example, the Early Screening for Autism[287,288] is being developed as a level 1 ASD screen for 14-month-old children, and the Systematic Observation of Red Flags for Autism Spectrum Disorders in Young Children,[289] which is based on the Communication and Symbolic Behavior Scales Developmental Profile Behavior Sample, may be a valuable level 2 screening tool for use in the second year of life.

Comprehensive Evaluation

The developmental-behavioral pediatrician, acting either alone or as a member of a multidisciplinary or interdisciplinary developmental team, is ideally suited for making the definitive diagnosis of an ASD. Although other pediatric subspecialists are quite capable of making the diagnosis, especially with the assistance of an experienced psychologist who can perform psychometric testing, the developmental components may be challenging for the younger child. The developmental-behavioral pediatrician is specifically trained to evaluate child's overall level of functioning, as well as strengths and limitations in specific domains, a task that is critical in providing the framework for evaluating results of ASD-specific tools, in guiding the etiological workup, in planning intervention strategies, and assessing prognosis.

Because there can be a long waiting period for a subspecialty evaluation, the developmental-behavioral pediatrician or clinic staff should ensure at the time of the initial referral that the child has already been referred for an audiological evaluation and to an early intervention program or a school program (depending on the child's age) by the primary care provider.[260,262] If the child has not, then this should be done immediately so that intervention strategies can be implemented in a timely manner. Immediately available services should address the child's individual pattern of developmental deficits; strategies can be revised to be more ASD-specific, if necessary, after the definitive diagnosis is made.

There are three major diagnostic challenges in the comprehensive assessment of a child with suspected ASD: determining the child's overall level of functioning, making the definitive diagnosis of an ASD, and determining the extent of the search for an associated etiological syndrome. To accomplish these three goals, a comprehensive evaluation should include the following components:

1. Health, developmental, behavioral, and family histories, including a review of systems.
2. Thorough physical examination.
3. Developmental and/or psychometric evaluation (depending on mental age).
4. Determination of the presence/absence of *DSM-IV-TR* criteria.
5. Assessment of family functioning and available resources.
6. Laboratory investigation, guided by information obtained in steps 1 to 5.

When appropriate, the evaluation includes information from multiple sources, because the child's performance may vary among settings and care providers. The entire process may require several appointments or, in the context of an interdisciplinary team evaluation, it may consist of a single arena-style evaluation or a series of individual evaluations by team members over the course of a day. The child's developmental level or mental age, capacity for cooperation (especially relating to fatigue in an all-day evaluation), severity of autistic symptoms, family characteristics, and local insurance policies and procedures all play a role in the selection of the most appropriate strategy. Regardless of whether the evaluation is made by a team or an individual clinician, the etiological search usually takes place over a period of time in collaboration with the child's primary care provider. Referrals to a neurologist and/or a geneticist may be helpful in further evaluating abnormal neurological findings, seizures, regression, dysmorphic features, and/or a complex family history.

For a comprehensive discussion regarding the rationale and strategies for accomplishing these tasks, the reader is referred to published neurology guidelines[10]; pediatric guidelines[11,12]; the American Speech and Hearing Association Position Statement[290] and Technical Report[291]; and chapters in two books, *Autism*

Spectrum Disorders: A Transactional Developmental Perspective[17] and *Handbook of Autism and Pervasive Developmental Disorders*[14] particularly Chapter 20 (on medical workup), 21 (on diagnostic instruments), 29 (on evaluation components), 30 (on communication assessment), 31 (on behavior assessment), and 32 (on sensorimotor assessment).

COMPREHENSIVE HISTORY

A comprehensive evaluation should begin with thorough health (including neonatal events),[159] family, developmental, emotional, and behavioral histories. A three-generation family history especially targeting ASD and its broader phenotype—mental retardation, language delays, and psychiatric and learning disorders—can be very helpful in guiding the etiological workup. A review of systems may be more challenging with the nonverbal child who cannot vocalize symptoms (e.g., depression) or localize pain (e.g., abdominal). Conditions that occur with a higher frequency in children with ASD (e.g., seizures[292]) should be targeted, as should conditions (e.g., lead toxicity) that result from predisposing ASD-related behaviors (e.g., prolonged mouthing or pica).[293] Symptoms of other *DSM* conditions (e.g., anxiety, obsessive-compulsive disorder, and/or attention-deficit/hyperactivity [ADHD] disorder) may overlap with those of ASD, making diagnosis more difficult. ASD-specific surveys and behavioral interview tools (see discussion in the section "Determination of the Presence or Absence of *DSM-IV-TR* Criteria") may assist the developmental-behavioral pediatrician in obtaining pertinent developmental, behavioral and emotional information relating to *DSM* criteria.

THOROUGH PHYSICAL EXAMINATION

Although a thorough physical examination may be challenging, it is important in identifying syndromes and medical conditions known to be associated with ASD. Measurement of head circumference, a neurodevelopmental examination, and a meticulous search for dysmorphic features, including a Wood's lamp examination for early subtle neurocutaneous lesions, are especially relevant components of the examination. As previously noted, approximately one third of affected children meet criteria for macrocephaly.[184-188] Gillberg and Coleman[294] found posteriorly rotated ears in 30%, but this finding has not been replicated in subsequent studies. Mild hypotonia has been noted in some children with idiopathic ASD.[295] Positive findings are important in determining the type and extent of an etiological workup; however, because most children have "idiopathic ASD," the physical examination is chiefly noteworthy for its *lack* of positive findings.

DEVELOPMENTAL AND/OR PSYCHOMETRIC EVALUATION

Determining the child's overall level of functioning can be the most challenging component of the evaluation because of the child's inability or unwillingness to cooperate with testing. On occasion, children have been inappropriately labeled by default as having severe mental retardation when they were "untestable." Severe intellectual deficits may not be the cause of low scores; rather, tester inexperience, environmental factors (overstimulation, absence of structure), the choice of inappropriate tools (too advanced), and/or other child factors (e.g., fatigue, illness, oppositional behavior) may be the reason. Parents play a critical role in the evaluation process by providing information about developmental skills that cannot be easily assessed in a clinical environment and by judging the validity of the child's performance in clinic in comparison with his or her typical behavior in naturalistic settings.

Young children with ASD, especially those with high-functioning autism, often demonstrate a significant discrepancy among domains; that is, motor, cognitive and adaptive skills are generally more advanced than language and social (in particular, joint attention) skills.[235,296-298] Individual scores for each domain that reveal the child's relative strengths and deficits are often more valuable than a summarized score in describing the child and in planning intervention. Often multiple tools are needed to address all domains. High "outlier" scores may represent splinter skills that do not necessarily reflect the child's ability to function in natural settings.[7,235] In fact, the discrepancy between scores on standardized tests and real-life functioning is a relatively common finding.

Although the Bayley Scales of Infant Development–II has excellent properties and has been the most widely used developmental assessment tool[299] in infant research and many clinical settings, it has not been as helpful in the evaluation of ASD. The Mental Development Index score summarizes nonverbal problem-solving, language, and social skills into a single numerical value, thus obscuring the discrepancies that characterize the profile scatter in ASD.[235] The newer Bayley scales, third edition,[300] offers promise because they do provide individual scores; however, further study is needed in this population. The Mullen Scales of Early Learning[301] have often been used in research endeavors because individual domain scores are possible; however, additional tools are needed to assess adaptive and social skills. Deficits in adaptive ability are critical in the diagnosis of comorbid GDD/mental retardation, and deficits in social skills in relation to general functioning are critical in the diagnosis of ASD.[20,37,235] Voigt and associates[297] used the

Cognitive Adaptive Test/Clinical Linguistic and Auditory Milestone Scale (CAT-CLAMS)[303-305] to illustrate discrepant scores in children with ASD, although this measure is not regarded as a comprehensive evaluation tool. All study children demonstrated significant discrepancies in that the developmental quotient for visual-motor problem-solving (CAT) skills averaged 36.4 points above that for language (CLAMS) skills ($SD = 15.9$; $p < 0.00001$). In general, the higher the general level of functioning (overall developmental quotient) was, the more significant was the discrepancy ($p < 0.0001$). A more comprehensive language-specific tool may be helpful with fluent children in order to assess both the quantitative and qualitative differences characteristic of high-functioning autism and Asperger syndrome. Although some rating scales and checklists have been developed to facilitate the assessment process,[306] the speech and language pathologist must draw from clinical expertise to detect and describe samples of atypical language such as echolalia, pronoun reversal, pop-up words, neologisms, and pragmatic deficits.[290,291] A more comprehensive measure of sensorimotor function may be helpful in supplementing the information gained from a neurological examination.[307]

Measurement of abilities across all domains can be more challenging and time consuming in older, higher functioning children. The menu of instruments is more extensive, and some knowledge of the child's verbal abilities is necessary to make appropriate choices.[235] Regardless of the tool or tools chosen, subtest scores are again often more helpful than the composite score in making a diagnosis and in planning intervention. Although the Wechsler Preschool and Primary Scale of Intelligence and the Wechsler Intelligence Scale for Children (depending on the child's age) are "gold standards" for assessment of intelligence, the behavioral challenges and language deficits characteristic of this population may preclude their use. Thus, the clinician must be flexible and able to quickly and skillfully transition to alternative strategies and/or tools while, at the same time, maintaining the child's interest and attention. The Leiter Scales of Nonverbal Intelligence[308] can be helpful in children who have little speech and/or who are noncompliant with tasks that require pointing responses.[309-311] This tool uses manipulatives that seem to foster cooperation in children who are otherwise difficult to test; however, it measures only nonverbal skills, and thus the resulting IQ score may not represent the child's ability to problem solve in real-life situations. The original Leiter scales contained relatively few items in each age category, and some stimulus drawings are now outdated; in addition, the IQ score is calculated. The revised Leiter scales[312] are an attempt to ameliorate these disadvantages; however, rather than a manipulative paradigm, it uses the more standard pointing response, which decreases its utility in some difficult-to-test children. Distinguishing between children with severe GDD/mental retardation and stereotypies from those with primary ASD and coexisting GDD/mental retardation can be challenging especially in children with mental ages less than 18 months who are unable to participate optimally in standardized testing. The Pervasive Developmental Disorder in Mental Retardation Scale (PDD-MRS) was developed to assist in this task, but a standardized measure of cognition is necessary to implement the tool.[313] Although not a routine component of the evaluation, a more extensive battery of neuropsychological tests can sometimes be helpful in the evaluation of additional deficits (e.g., executive function, central coherence, theory of mind, memory, and shifting of attention) that are characteristic of older and higher-functioning children with ASD.

Knowing whether a child has coexisting mental retardation is critical in determining the type and extent of the etiological search, the optimal school placement, and eligibility for additional financial and support services. In addition to an IQ score below 70 to 75, a measurement of adaptive ability is necessary.[314] Adaptive skills can be assessed with the Vineland Adaptive Behavior Scales,[315] a semistructured interview technique that addresses motor, social, communication, and daily living skills. Several versions exist for use in different settings. Children with ASD usually demonstrate relative strengths in daily living and motor skills in comparison with communication and social skills.[235,316] New norms have been developed for specific application to persons with ASD.[317] In addition, a new version, the Vineland Social Emotional Early Childhood Scales,[318] contains more early-emerging social skills applicable to ASD. Although not as informative as direct testing of actual skills, the composite Vineland Adaptive Behavior Scales score can be compared with the social and communication subscale scores to demonstrate whether there is a discrepancy between general functioning and these skills.[235,319,320]

DETERMINATION OF THE PRESENCE OR ABSENCE OF DSM-IV-TR CRITERIA

Since the 1980s, the *DSM-IV* and *DSM-IV-TR* criteria have served as the "gold standard" for the diagnosis of an ASD. However, very young children who later receive diagnoses of autistic disorder may not demonstrate full *DSM* criteria. For example, "failure to form age-appropriate peer relationships" is really not applicable in very young children. In addition, in a preverbal child, it is difficult to demonstrate abnormal conversational skills and stereotypic language. As noted previously, ritualistic behaviors, a need for routines, and stereotypies are often not present or at least not recognized in children younger than 3 years. Thus, even children appearing to have severe autism may not meet full criteria at very young ages. Instead, they usually receive the "subthreshold" provisional diagnosis of PDD-NOS or "speech delay with autistic tendencies" and then, if additional signs appear and full criteria are met, the diagnosis is revised to one of the ASDs. Realizing this diagnostic dilemma, especially because earlier diagnosis is being promoted, Stone[215] recommended a modified *DSM* strategy for children younger than 3 years whereby the clinician consider only three *DSM* criteria from the social skills domain and one from the communication domain:

1 a: Decreased use of nonverbal behavior (eye-to-eye gaze, facial expression, body posture, gestures).
  c: Lack of social and emotional reciprocity.
  d: Lack of seeking to share enjoyment, interests, or achievements with other people (absence of showing, bringing, or pointing to objects of interest).
2 a: Delayed or absent language skills.

When all four criteria are unequivocally present, the "provisional" diagnosis of ASD can be made. The provisional ASD diagnosis may facilitate earlier access to ASD-specific intervention strategies such as those that target joint attention skills. Ideally, the experienced therapist should recognize the child's unique configuration of strengths and deficits and implement appropriate individualized intervention services, regardless of whether a child does or does not have a medically derived diagnostic label. Unfortunately, a formal diagnosis is sometimes necessary to access reimbursement mechanisms.

Although the *DSM* criteria are still regarded as the "gold standard," a significant amount of subjectivity exists when they are used alone, especially when clinicians are inexperienced. In addition, observation of the child during a brief unstructured encounter may fail to reveal *DSM*-related deficits (e.g., joint attention and/or pretend play) but amplify atypical behaviors (i.e., stereotypies associated with boredom and lack of stimulation in a typical examination room). Ideally, an evaluation should include observation of the child in free play to determine whether he or she engages in spontaneous bids for joint attention, imitative play, and/or engagement with the parents, coupled with a more structured session in which the tester attempts to elicit *DSM*-related behaviors by using a standardized format.[235]

Standardized tools have been developed to assist the clinician in operationalizing *DSM* criteria and in making the diagnosis of ASD. Although several tools have been in existence since the 1980s, a 2006 Atlanta study revealed that only 30% of practitioners actually used one to make the ASD diagnosis.[55] A few of the more widely used tools are briefly discussed in the next section; however, the reader is advised to refer to much more detailed descriptions of these tools and their properties in excellent reviews.[114,249,264,322,323] Knowledge of the child's verbal skills is often important in choosing the appropriate ASD-specific tool (e.g., the most appropriate Autism Diagnostic Observation Schedule [ADOS] module). Tools include those that support a DSM-IV diagnosis and are used in clinical settings, or those that are considered "gold standard" diagnostic instruments and are required for NIH-funded research endeavors.

Standardized Tools That Support a Clinical DSM-IV-TR Diagnosis

1. *Psychoeducational Profile, Third Edition* (PEP-3): The original PEP was developed in 1979 and revised in 1990 as the PEP-R[324] and again in 2005 as the PEP-3.[325] It is a systematic observational tool used to determine the severity (on a 3-point scale) of autistic behaviors in the area of tool play, language, affect, relationships and sensory modalities. It is highly correlated with the CARS (listed later).[264]

2. *Autism Behavior Checklist*[277]: This measure was developed in 1980 and is a behavior checklist containing 57 items divided into five categories: sensory, body and object use, language, social, and self-help. Little training is needed for scoring the measure, but interrater reliability is variable. It is not an attempt to operationalize *DSM* criteria and has low sensitivity, which makes it less useful as a diagnostic tool.[263]

3. *Childhood Autism Rating Scale*[280]: The CARS was published in 1988 and aligned with *DSM-III* criteria. Rellini and associates[326] revealed that there was a 100% agreement between diagnoses made with the CARS and those made by clinicians with ASD expertise who used clinical judgment based on *DSM-IV* criteria. This measure consists of a 15-item structured interview, with each item scored according to seven levels of severity. The scale was designed for use with children older than 2 years, requires training to administer, and takes about 20 to 30 minutes to complete. It may overidentify very young children or those with severe mental retardation and may underidentify older patients with high-functioning autism. It is still "the strongest, best-documented, and most widely used clinical rating scale for autism."[264] Of the 30% of practitioners using a tool for the initial evaluation of a child for ASD in the Atlanta study discussed previously, 68% of them used the CARS.[55]

4. *Gilliam Autism Rating Scale:* The GARS[282] was developed in 1995 and revised in 2005[263] and is a parent-completed checklist based on *DSM-IV* criteria. The 56 items are grouped into four categories address-

ing social development, communication, stereotypic behaviors, and developmental disturbances. Each item is scored on a 4-point scale, and all scores from each category are summed into an autism quotient that indicates the probability of autism. It was designed for use in children older than 3 years. Although reliability is reportedly high, it has not been confirmed.[284,285]

5. *Diagnostic Interview for Social and Communication Disorders*[327]: This measure is a standardized, semistructured interview tool based on diagnostic criteria of both the *DSM-IV* and ICD-10[39]; in addition, it includes developmentally based items from the Vineland Behavior Scales.[315] It can be used appropriately with children of all ages and levels of ability and has become a popular clinical tool in Europe. Algorithms have been developed for use in research endeavors.[328]

"Gold Standard" Diagnostic Tools Necessary for Research Endeavors

1. *Autism Diagnostic Interview–Revised*[329]: This measure was originally developed as a research tool in 1989 but was revised into a shortened clinical one in 1994. Both versions operationalize criteria from the *DSM-IV* and the ICD-10.[39] Depending on whether the interview is done within a clinical or research context, it may take $1^{1}/_{2}$ to 3 hours to complete. Training workshops are required for researchers and highly recommended for clinicians (although training video materials may be used). The Autism Diagnostic Interview–Revised has been translated into several languages.

2. *Autism Diagnostic Observation Schedule*[330]: The ADOS is a standardized protocol for observing social behavior in natural communicative contexts, with four different modules that target children demonstrating various levels of language development. Children are guided through a series of standardized "presses" to simulate samples of social interaction, communication, and play that are then coded and scored. Modules 3 and 4 are useful in the evaluation of verbal, higher functioning children with suspected ASD, including Asperger syndrome. The current ADOS (originally named the ADOS–Generic) is actually a revision of its two precursors (the original ADOS[331] and the Pre-linguistic ADOS[332] for children with little or no speech) and addresses a broader range of ages and developmental levels than its precursors. It takes about 30 to 45 minutes to complete. It has excellent sensitivity (90% to 97%) and specificity (87% to 93%).[330] There have been some concerns that it might overidentify very young children with GDD or older ones with severe mental retardation. Again, training is required for researchers and recommended for clinicians.

Knowledge of the child's overall developmental or mental age is important for interpreting results, because some of these ASD tools tend to overidentify ASD in children with severe GDD/mental retardation.[264] For a more detailed discussion of these and additional tools, the reader is referred to the multidisciplinary panel review[114] and practice parameter[10] and to Volkmar and colleagues.[14]

SPECIFIC ASSESSMENTS FOR ASPERGER SYNDROME

Diagnosis of Asperger syndrome usually occurs after 4 years of age. Deficits in social skills without accompanying language delays often go unnoticed until children attend school and demonstrate difficulties in classroom activities with peers. For this reason, school personnel, rather than parents or pediatricians, often initiate the Asperger syndrome evaluation. Targeted level 2 screening when symptoms are recognized, rather than universal screening, has been suggested by published guidelines[10-12,114]; this remains the current suggestion.[262] Teachers, parents, and, depending on the age, the students themselves may be asked to complete an Asperger syndrome checklist as a first step in the evaluation process. Although many checklists are currently available for level 2 screening, none is ideal. Of the level 2 tools, the Australian Scale for Asperger Syndrome is perhaps the most popular, mainly because it is easily accessed[333] (see *www.aspergersyndrome.org*). However, it has not been standardized, and the Web site reports low specificity. Like many of the other level 2 surveys, it queries the parents/teachers about abnormalities in social, emotional, communication, cognitive, and movement skills and the presence of unusual interests and rigid routines/rituals. Campbell[334] evaluated five of the rating scales. The scales reviewed included the Asperger Syndrome Diagnostic Scale,[335] Autism Spectrum Screening Questionnaire,[336] Childhood Asperger Syndrome Test,[337] Gilliam Asperger's Disorder Scale,[338] and Krug Asperger's Disorder Index.[339] All five measures fell short of current standards, but the Krug measure showed the strongest properties. None of these surveys should ever be used in isolation; however, they can be helpful as a component of a multidisciplinary evaluation.

Pediatric and neurology guidelines did not address the comprehensive evaluation of a child with Asperger syndrome.[10-12,114] Some guidance can be found in two other consensus-driven protocols: the California Practice Guidelines for children older than 6 years[323] and the ASHA guidelines.[290,291] Developing a consensus statement may be more challenging for several reasons: (1) There remains controversy about whether Asperger syndrome is a distinct entity versus a subtype of high-functioning autism[27]; (2) there are several sets of criteria for Asperger syndrome[36,340]; (3) because these children's skills are more complex and differentiated, a wider variety of tests is necessary to quantify the skills[323]; and (4) most instruments lack sensitivity in identifying more subtle social communication deficits.[290,291]

For these reasons, the process necessary to make an accurate diagnosis of Asperger syndrome is challenging and almost always involves a team approach. The Autism Diagnostic Interview–Revised and Module 3 or 4 of the ADOS are ideally suited for higher functioning verbal children such as those with Asperger syndrome. In addition to historical aspects of the child's early development (particularly language development), a complete battery of standardized tests is needed to differentiate Asperger syndrome from learning disorders with overlapping characteristics (e.g., nonverbal learning disability, pragmatic disorder, semantic-pragmatic language disorder, hyperlexia). Asperger syndrome is even less often associated with a known medical condition than is autistic disorder[18]; nevertheless, a number of mental health conditions (i.e., schizophrenia, schizoid personality, anxiety disorder, obsessive-compulsive disorder, oppositional defiant disorder, and selective/elective mutism) may mimic Asperger syndrome or coexist with it. Thus, a physician with expertise in

ASD and mental health conditions should be involved in the diagnostic process. Table 15-6 lists similar and contrasting characteristics of some of these learning and mental health disorders.

ASSESSMENT OF FAMILY FUNCTIONING AND AVAILABLE RESOURCES

An important part of the comprehensive evaluation of a child with a suspected ASD is the assessment of the family. It should begin with an assessment of the parents' current understanding of ASD in order to determine both the family's ability to advocate effectively for their child and the appropriate level of training activities needed. Sometimes parents may need assistance in evaluating the information they already have, especially if it is not peer reviewed and has been accessed from the Internet. The developmental-behavioral pediatrician should also assess the family's coping strategies, resources (financial, childcare, health insurance), and support systems, including family, friends, neighbors, and religious and local community agencies. On the basis of these considerations, the developmental-behavioral pediatrician or, when available, a team social worker or nurse coordinator can formulate a family support plan.[341-343] Referrals to local or Internet-based sources of information, advocacy, and support should be provided. Sleep deprivation, depression, physical well-being,

TABLE 15-6 ■ Differential Diagnosis of Asperger Syndrome

	HFA	Asperger	NV-LD	OCD	Semantic-Pragmatic	Schizoid	Schizophrenia
Social skills	↓↓	↓↓	↓	NL	NL	↓	↓
Pragmatic deficits	++	++	+	NL	++	−	−
Delayed language	+	−	−	−	+	−	−
Echolalia	++	−	−	−	−	−	−
Verbal memory	↓	NL	↑	NA			
Stereotypies and rituals	+	+	−	+*	−	−	−
Restricted interests	+	++	−	−	−	−	−
Hallucinations and delusions	†	†	−	−	−	−	+
Intelligence Quotient (IQ)	NL	NL to high	NL	NA	NA	NA	NA
Verbal/performance IQ	PIQ ≥ VIQ	VIQ > PIQ	VIQ > PIQ	NA	NA	NA	NA
Learning disability	−	−	Math	NA	−	NA	NA
Motor skills	NL	↓	↓	NL	NA	NA	NA
Visual memory skills	↑	↓	↓	NA	NA	NA	NA
Onset of true symptoms	<3 years	>3 years	>3 years	>3 years	<3 years	>3 years	>>3 years

↓↓, Severely deficient; ↓, deficient; ↑, increased; −, not present; +, present; ++, consistently present; >>, much higher/older than normal.
HFA, high-functioning autism; NA, not applicable; NL, normal; NV-LD, nonverbal learning disability; OCD, obsessive-compulsive disorder; PIQ, Performance IQ; VIQ, Verbal IQ.
*Driven by thoughts and worries; unlike persons with HFA and Asperger syndrome, individuals with OCD have insight into and concern for their unrealistic nature.
†Patients with HFA and Asperger syndrome may reenact favorite movies, advertisements, and so forth, and these behaviors should be differentiated from true hallucinations and delusions.

and emotional conditions resulting from stress are more likely to occur in members of families with children with ASD.[344-347] These problems should be considered and referrals made when appropriate.

LABORATORY INVESTIGATION

The final challenge in the evaluation of ASD, and perhaps the most controversial, is determining the extent of the etiological "search." Published etiological yields vary and generally are more highly correlated with the presence or absence of coexisting mental retardation rather than with ASD itself. The majority of reports describe finding an underlying cause in 2% to 10% of patients.[47,48,104,107-110,348] These yields are lower than the 10% to 81% reported in studies of GDD/mental retardation without coexisting ASD.[349,350] Unfortunately, the extent and sophistication of the laboratory investigations vary a great deal among ASD-specific studies and even within the same study. Patient factors such as the presence of coexisting GDD/mental retardation, dysmorphic features, and/or a positive family history are often not addressed. Some investigators report a "positive yield," whereas, in fact, the identified abnormality is non-specific, is not related to a known autism-related etiology, and does not affect counseling and/or management (e.g., delayed mylinization on MRI). In other studies, positive test results indicate coexisting conditions that, although they may be common in children with ASD (e.g., gastrointestinal disorders), are not known to play an etiological role. Thus, a positive laboratory test result does *not* necessarily mean a positive "yield."

There are certainly many advantages in having a formal diagnosis, such as genetic counseling and information regarding recurrence risks of known syndromes, possibility of a specific treatment strategy, counseling about the natural history of a known disorder, anticipation of a later associated comorbid disorder, prevention of secondary disorders, availability of prenatal diagnosis, access to public supports, access to syndrome-specific parent support groups, and, in some cases, empowering parents to "move on" and to focus on habilitative interventions.

In view of the heterogeneity of ASD and the absence of evidence to support extensive workups in all patients with ASD, the laboratory search should be guided by clinical judgment based on history (e.g., health, birth, developmental, behavioral, family) and clinical presentation (e.g., coexisting mental retardation, regression, seizures, neurodevelopmental findings, dysmorphic features, comorbid medical conditions). Family characteristics (e.g., lack of insurance, concern about the child's discomfort, interest in pursuing a "no-stone-left-unturned" etiological workup) may also influence parental decisions about the extent of the workup. Finally, the local availability of subspecialists and sophisticated technology, the need for and feasibility of sedation, managed care cost-benefit guidelines, and physicians' beliefs may each play a role in decisions about the appropriate extent of the diagnostic workup.

The fields of genetic testing and neuroimaging are rapidly becoming more sophisticated. In fact, clinicians caring for children participating in multisite collaborative studies may pursue more extensive laboratory investigations according to standardized research protocols. Many of the tests are investigational, have unknown utility, and are not currently clinically available. Although they may be very valuable in the future in determining the cause or causes of ASD and defining specific subtypes, they do not currently have a role in the routine workup of ASD.

The emergence of new technology and the lack of overall consensus among subspecialty expert panels presents a formidable challenge when clinicians attempt to develop a consistent search strategy for children with ASD, especially those with comorbid GDD/mental retardation. The American College of Medical Genetics[349,351] and the American Academy of Neurology and Child Neurology Society (AAN-CNS)[350] have published guidelines for the evaluation of children with GDD/mental retardation that are based on a considerable body of evidence in this population; however, their recommendations are somewhat discordant. Additional recommendations are anticipated in the future from the AAP Committee on Genetics because they will be based on the availability of newer technology (Brad Schaefer, personal communication, March 2006). In the period 2000 to 2001, the first ASD guidelines were published both by the AAN-CNS[10] and by the AAP.[11,12] Because there was some overlap of the authoring panels, there is much agreement between the two documents. Although implied, neither of the ASD guidelines specifically addresses the laboratory investigation of children with high functioning autism or Asperger syndrome. Prevalence studies suggest that the yield is extremely low in the absence of GDD/mental retardation and perhaps even lower in Asperger syndrome.[36,47,104,107,352,353] Etiological yield tends to be highest in isolated GDD/mental retardation (10% to 81%), moderate in ASD with coexisting GDD/mental retardation (2% to 10%), and lowest in isolated ASD with normal intelligence (<5%).

In view of comorbidity, discordant guidelines, limitations in current evidence, and emerging technology, we support a practical approach such as a tiered strategy. The AAP Committees on Children with Disabilities and Genetics are in the process of developing ASD guidelines that will be published at a future date and may deviate somewhat from the following recommendations. The proposed strategy advocates for informed clinical judgment and decision making that is based on the presence or absence of coexistent GDD/mental retardation and/or clinical indicators.

Proposed Strategy for a Tiered Etiological Search

Level 1: studies that should be considered in all children with ASD.

Level 2: studies that should be considered in children with ASD *and* coexisting GDD/mental retardation.

Level 3: targeted studies that should be considered when specific clinical findings are identified by history or physical examination.

LEVEL 1 SEARCH

All children with language delays, including those with ASD, should have an audiology evaluation. Published ASD-specific guidelines for young children presenting with symptoms of ASD reinforce this recommendation.[10-12,114,262] School-based hearing screening may be adequate in older children with Asperger syndrome who have no significant language deficits, especially in the absence of any academic concerns.

LEVEL 2 SEARCH

The workup of a child with ASD with coexisting GDD/mental retardation should be guided by published guidelines for both conditions. As noted previously, the etiological yield rates are typically lower in children with both ASD and GDD/mental retardation than in those with isolated GDD/mental retardation, especially those with severe GDD. For children who have both conditions, ASD guidelines recommend (1) a high-resolution karyotype and (2) a molecular study for the fragile X syndrome, unless the child has a known etiology to explain the GDD/mental retardation or presents with characteristics of a disorder that can be confirmed by a specific targeted laboratory test (e.g., MECP2 in a girl with classic Rett symptoms).[10-12,114,262] These guidelines also suggest that the tests just described may be helpful in the absence of GDD/mental retardation if there is a family history of mental retardation (especially mental retardation caused by the fragile X syndrome), but it is recognized that the yield will be extremely low. The presence of more than two dysmorphic features increases the likelihood of a positive yield; however, this finding is more highly correlated with GDD/mental retardation than with ASD.[294,350,354] The relative importance of the fragile X syndrome in the cause of ASD has been somewhat controversial and, depending on the study, the prevalence of a positive DNA assay varies between 1.6% and 16%.[355] In a review of 40 studies,[356] identical pooled proportions of the fragile X syndrome were found in boys with autism and in boys with isolated mental retardation; this raises concern about the rela-

tive causative role of the fragile X syndrome in ASD. If the karyotype and fragile X test are negative (as most are), but a recognizable cause is still suspected, then the clinician should consider level 3 tests and/or consultation with a clinical geneticist and/or neurologist, depending on indicators from the history and/or physical examination.

Although the 2003 AAN-CNS practice parameter[350] recommends additional "screening" laboratory tests (e.g., MRI, subtelomere fluorescent in situ hybridization [FISH] studies) for all children with GDD/mental retardation, it has not been endorsed by the AAP for GDD/mental retardation or ASD. Published genetic GDD/mental retardation guidelines have recommended fewer "screening" tests and a more targeted approach that is based on clinical judgment.[349,351,354] Although more sophisticated and effective screening techniques may be on the horizon, there are currently no existing data to support more extensive laboratory evaluation in children with ASD. As the apparent prevalence of coexisting GDD/mental retardation continues to decrease, the need to consider GDD/mental retardation guidelines will occur less often.[47,55-55b,348]

No etiological laboratory tests are recommended in the evaluation of high-functioning children with ASD, including Asperger syndrome, in the absence of suggestive clinical findings. If a child demonstrates regression or new symptoms consistent with a syndrome known to be associated with ASD (e.g., seizures and/or the appearance of an ash leaf or facial angiofibromas characteristic of tuberous sclerosis), then a laboratory investigation becomes necessary. Laboratory recommendations might also change for this population as research reveals more consistent genetic markers in idiopathic ASDs and as more advanced cytogenetic techniques become clinically available and more cost effective.

LEVEL 3 SEARCH

Level 3 investigations include additional subspecialty evaluations and/or additional laboratory investigations that are indicated by specific clinical indicators. On the basis of local availability and the developmental-behavioral pediatrician's level of confidence in these evaluations, she or he should consider referrals to a clinical geneticist and/or to a child neurologist.

A geneticist can assist with an extended pedigree history and a more meticulous dysmorphic examination. Expensive, more sophisticated laboratory tests may require the assistance of a geneticist for authorization (especially when they are not yet clinically available) and interpretation. When the child's evaluation includes profound mental retardation, consanguinity, a complex family history, or a vague dysmorphic gestalt, the geneticist may order subtelomere testing.[356b] Yields for subtelomere studies are extremely low in those with mild mental retardation and usually zero in studies that target individuals with ASD.[104,112] The geneticist may order single-locus studies (e.g., 15q or 22q) or newer macroarray FISH studies; however, the latter are expensive and may not be clinically available in all settings. When specific indicators are present, the geneticist is also helpful in ordering and interpreting the level 3 targeted tests listed in nos. 1 to 9 below.

A child neurologist can be very helpful in assisting with the evaluation of a child with regression, seizures, or specific neurological examination findings. The neurologist is able to address certain aspects of the history and physical examination in more detail and thus may identify indicators for level 3 laboratory studies. A high index of suspicion and meticulous monitoring is recommended to identify subtle seizures.[10-12,114,350] Some neurologists may recommend "screening" EEG and MRI. Although nonspecific abnormalities have been found in the majority of children, the significance of these abnormalities is not clear, treatment has not been of any proven value,[357] and there is currently insufficient evidence to recommend or discourage the use of screening EEG.[358,359] Furthermore, MRI has not been recommended for all children with isolated macrocephaly associated with idiopathic ASD.[10,321]

The clinician (developmental-behavioral pediatrician, geneticist, neurologist, neurodevelopmental disabilities specialist, or other qualified specialist) should pursue level 3 tests when clinical findings characteristic of one or more specific disorders become apparent. Identification of these clinical indicators depends, in part, on the thoroughness of the history and physical examination. The following recommendations for a targeted etiological search in the individual child are relatively consistent with the original ASD guidelines.[10-12,114] Level 3 testing should be individualized according to the following specific clinical findings:

1. *Dysmorphic features:* Although children with coexisting GDD/mental retardation should have undergone high-resolution karyotype and DNA testing for the fragile X syndrome, even more thorough dysmorphic examination to identify indicators for targeted testing at this level may be helpful, especially if the screening test results are negative. Children without GDD/mental retardation should also be examined carefully for abnormal physical findings to discern whether a high-resolution karyotype and/or DNA testing for the fragile X syndrome would be helpful, especially when there is a positive family history of mental retardation or genetic disorders.

2. *Characteristic behavioral phenotype:* When a child manifests a constellation of behaviors that are classic for a known syndrome (e.g., Angelman syndrome, Smith-Magenis syndrome) that can be confirmed by a specific laboratory test (e.g., targeted FISH or methylation studies), the child should be referred to a laboratory capable of performing and interpreting the appropriate test.

3. *Regression:* There is some controversy whether every child with regression needs an in-depth workup. Clinical judgment should be exercised for a child with idiopathic ASD who demonstrates "typical autism regression" between the ages of 18 and 36 months, especially if he or she is being evaluated after the regression has subsided and developmental progress has resumed, albeit usually at a slower pace.[359] On the other hand, those with regression characteristic of Landau-Kleffner syndrome or other acquired epileptic aphasias should always be studied, especially in the presence of seizures.[219] Studies will probably include MRI and electrencephalography (sleep or 24-hour). Girls with ASD symptoms who exhibit regression, show deceleration of head growth, develop seizures, and/or demonstrate other features of the Rett phenotype should be evaluated for MECP2 mutations.

4. *Seizures:* Children with known seizures or suspected of having subclinical seizures should be referred to child neurologist for an evaluation, MRI, and prolonged sleep electrencephalography.[219] There is currently insufficient evidence to recommend the use of screening EEG,[358] but a high index of suspicion and meticulous monitoring are recommended for subtle signs of seizures. Functional neuroimaging is not indicated for clinical use, although it has been quite informative from a research perspective with regard to neural processing in higher functioning individuals with ASD.

5. *Abnormal neurological examination:* Children with microcephaly, a midline facial abnormality, neurocutaneous findings, or focal neurological signs should be referred for an MRI study and to a child neurologist. Isolated macrocephaly is not in itself an indication for MRI.[10,18,114,321]

6. *Metabolic symptoms:* Children with cyclic vomiting, hypotonia, lethargy (especially when associated with mild illnesses), poor growth, unusual odors, multiple organ involvement, ataxia or other movement disorder, or evidence of a storage disease (e.g., coarse features) are probably best referred to a geneticist and/or a neurologist for an evaluation of a possible metabolic disorder, including mitochondrial and storage diseases.[349,360] One study[361] revealed some support for a limited metabolic battery (lactate,

pyruvate, ammonia and free/total carnintine), but replication studies are needed.

7. *Lack of confirming evidence of a negative result of a neonatal screening test for phenylketonuria:* Children should undergo a quantitative plasma amino acid assay to rule out phenylketonuria when it is suspected and neonatal screening results are not available.

8. *Indicators of the association of toxoplasmosis, other infections, rubella, cytomegalovirus, and herpes simplex infections (TORCH):* Children with a history and/or chronic symptoms consistent with one of the intrauterine infections (e.g., rubella syndrome) should have a TORCH titer drawn.[145]

9. *Pica:* Although lead toxicity is not believed to cause ASD, it can have a detrimental effect on learning and cognition, which may indirectly intensify ASD symptoms. Children with pica, especially when they live in at-risk environments, should be monitored with blood lead levels as long as the behavior persists.[293]

Additional tentative suggestions for a level 3 targeted search that were based on new data since the original ASD guidelines were published include the following:

- Because Rett mutations can sometimes occur in boys (especially those with Klinefelter syndrome), MECP2 assays should also be considered in boys who present with regressive ASD. Universal screening as part of a research protocol has revealed that MECP2 mutations are present in a few ASD children without evidence of the Rett phenotype; if these findings are replicated, universal screening of all children with ASD may be recommended in the future.[361a,362,363]

- Because an association has been found between Angelman syndrome and assisted reproductive techniques,[364] methylation testing for Angelman syndrome should be considered if children conceived by assisted reproductive techniques present with ASD features, because some overlap with the Angelman phenotype.

- Because an association between ASD and a mild variant of Smith-Lemli-Opitz syndrome has been described, 7-dehydrocholesterol testing might be considered when a child with ASD presents with hypotonia and syndactyly of the second and third toes. This suggestion is important for genetic counseling because Smith-Lemli-Opitz syndrome is an autosomal recessive disorder.[365]

Reviews[18] continue to support the recommendations published in previous guidelines[10-12,114] that the following tests are *not* indicated in the typical workup of a child with ASD: hair analysis for trace elements, vitamin levels, celiac antibodies, immunological

workup, allergy testing, intestinal permeability studies, stool analysis, urinary peptide measurements, thyroid function tests, or erythrocyte glutathione perioxidase level measurements.

Patients enrolled in one of several multicenter research studies may also undergo a number of additional tests (e.g., functional imaging, immunological studies, fibroblast karyotypes, neuroligan gene testing, mitochondrial gene sequencing, and additional metabolic studies)[173] that may not currently be universally available or clinically indicated in most children with idiopathic ASD, especially those with Asperger syndrome and high-functioning autism. Insurers rarely pay for such tests, evidence does not support doing these routinely, and the results may promote unrealistic expectations. As information regarding genetic markers for ASD expands and technology continues to become more sophisticated, the yield of complex genetic and laboratory investigations may increase in children with idiopathic ASD and eventually become clinically useful as part of the routine ASD workup. Currently the most promising probes are those that target 15q duplications, 22q deletions, and abnormalities on the X-chromosome and chromosomes 2, 3, 7, and 17. Some investigators have already suggested screening FISH for the 15q and 22q abnormalities[111] (Brad Schaefer, personal communication, March 2006); however, more evidence is needed before this becomes standard of care. Testing for 22q deletions, may be particularly important for genetic counseling purposes because about half of the cases in one study were caused by balanced translocations.[366-367]

SUMMARY

In conclusion, developmental-behavioral pediatricians play an important role in teaching primary care providers to recognize the early signs of ASD, conduct ongoing developmental surveillancem and use an ASD-specific screening tool at the 18- and 24-month well-child visits. They should also encourage primary care providers to listen to parents' concerns relating to language and social skills and to act on them. Such action should include simultaneous referrals for audiological testing, an appropriate intervention program, and a pediatric subspecialist/developmental team with expertise in the evaluation of children with ASD. Depending on the clinical presentation, referrals to neurology and/or genetics may also be indicated. Either acting alone or as a member of a developmental assessment team, the developmental-behavioral pediatrician should evaluate the child's health, developmental, and behavioral status; apply *DSM-IV-TR* criteria, preferably through the use of a standardized ASD-specific evaluation tool; and decide on the extent of the etiological laboratory workup, sometimes with guidance from genetic and/or neurology colleagues. The entire process should be done in a collaborative manner and communicated with a concise summary report. The developmental-behavioral pediatrician should interpret the results of the clinical and laboratory evaluations with the parents in an unhurried, sensitive, and compassionate manner that is culturally appropriate. The evaluation process should include appropriate follow-up because genetic and neuroimaging technology is constantly evolving, manifestations of the *DSM* criteria may evolve with development, and children may present with additional comorbid symptoms and/or challenging behaviors at any point in their lives.

MANAGEMENT

ASDs, like other neurodevelopmental disabilities, are generally not curable. The primary goals of treatment are to maximize functional independence and quality of life and to alleviate family distress by facilitating development and learning, promoting socialization, and reducing interfering maladaptive behaviors. Ideally, interventions should address the core features of these disorders: impairment in social reciprocity, deficits in communication, and restricted, repetitive behavioral repertoire. Educational interventions, including behavioral strategies and habilitative therapies, are the cornerstones of management of ASD. These interventions address communication, social skills, daily living skills, play and leisure skills, academic achievement, and aberrant behaviors.

Optimization of medical care is also likely to have a positive effect on habilitative progress and quality of life. Management of sleep dysfunction, coexisting psychiatric conditions, and associated deficits such as seizures may be particularly important. Medications have not been proved to correct the core deficits of ASD, and there are no pharmacological agents with U.S. Food and Drug Administration–approved labeling specific for the treatment of these disorders in children. If associated maladaptive behaviors or psychiatric comorbidities interfere with educational progress, socialization, health or safety, and quality of life, these behaviors may be amenable to psychopharmacological intervention or, in some cases, to treatment of underlying medical conditions that are causing or exacerbating the behaviors. Effective medical management is likely to allow an individual to benefit more optimally from other interventions.

Educational Interventions

In the late1960s and the 1970s, when the psychogenic theory of causation faded and Section 504 of the Rehabilitation Act of 1973 (Public Law 93-112)[368] and the Education of All Handicapped Children Act of 1975 (Public Law 94-142)[62] mandated appropriate public education for all children with disabilities, education of the child began to replace psychodynamic treatment of the parents as the primary intervention for autism. Education has been defined as fostering of acquisition of skills and knowledge to assist a child in developing independence and personal responsibility; it encompasses not only academic learning but also socialization, adaptive skills, communication, amelioration of interfering behaviors, and generalization of abilities across multiple environments.[13] Teachers, behavior therapists, speech and language therapists, occupational therapists, paraprofessional staff, parents, and other experts commonly play key roles in the education of children with ASD. Physicians and other clinicians are often in a position to guide families to empirically supported practices and help them evaluate the appropriateness of the educational services that are being offered.

PROGRAMS FOR PRESCHOOL- AND EARLY SCHOOL-AGED CHILDREN

Since the 1980s, autism education research and program development have focused disproportionately on very young children as a result of earlier identification and evidence that early intensive intervention may result in substantially better outcomes.[369] Model programs have been described,[13,370,371] and selected examples are summarized in Table 15-7. Although these programs may differ in philosophy and relative emphasis on particular strategies, they share many common goals, and there is a growing consensus that important principles and components of effective early childhood intervention for children for with ASD include the following[13,369,372,373,374]:

1. Entry into intervention as soon as an autism diagnosis is seriously considered, rather than delaying until a definitive diagnosis is made.
2. Provision of intensive intervention, with active engagement of the child at least 25 hours per week, 12 months per year, in systematically planned, developmentally appropriate educational activities designed to address identified objectives.
3. Low student : teacher ratio to allow sufficient amounts of 1 : 1 and very small group instruction to meet specific individualized goals.
4. Inclusion of a family component, including parent training when appropriate.
5. Promotion of opportunities for interaction with typically developing peers to the extent that these opportunities are helpful in addressing specified educational goals.
6. Ongoing measurement and documentation of the individual child's progress toward educational

TABLE 15-7 ■ Model Intervention Programs for Young Children with Autism Spectrum Disorder			
Program	Primary Intervention Location	Primary Philosophy Description	Special Emphasis or Features
Children's Unit for Treatment and Evaluation, State University of New York at Binghamton	Center-based	Applied behavior analytic	Individualized goal setting curriculum, extensive computerized monitoring system
Denver Model, University of Colorado	Public school-based	Developmental	Use of play, interpersonal relationships, and activities to foster symbolic thought and teach the power of communication
Developmental, Individual-Difference, Relationship-Based Model, George Washington University	Home-based	Developmental	"Floor-time" child-directed play techniques
Douglass Developmental Disabilities Center, Rutgers University	Center-based	Applied behavior analytic	Staged preschool program systematically moves children from intensive 1 : 1 applied behavior analysis experiences to small group instruction and then integrated instruction
Learning Experiences, an Alternative Program for Preschoolers and Their Parents (LEAP)	Center-based and public school-based	Applied behavior analytic and developmental	Inclusion of typically developing peers
Pivotal Response Training, University of California at Santa Barbara	Home-based	Applied behavior analytic	Naturalistic approach, focus on teaching key behaviors, especially self-initiation responses
Princeton Child Development Institute	Center-based	Applied behavior analytic	Activity schedules to foster independence, promote generalization, and teach social interaction
Treatment and Education of Autistic and Related Communication Handicapped Children, University of North Carolina	Public school-based	Structured teaching	Structure, environmental modification, behavioral approach to communication
Walden Early Childhood Programs, Emory University	Center-based	Applied behavior analytic	Incidental teaching strategies to increase the application of learned skills to more natural environments
Young Autism Project, University of California at Los Angeles	Home-based	Applied behavior analytic	Emphasis on discrimination learning early in the curriculum, discrete trial training, massed trials

objectives, resulting in adjustments in programming when indicated.

7. Incorporation of a high degree of structure through elements such as predictable routine, visual activity schedules, and clear physical boundaries to minimize distractions.
8. Implementation of strategies to generalize learned skills to new environments and situations.
9. Use of assessment-based curricula addressing the following:
   a. Functional, spontaneous communication.
   b. Social skills, including joint attention, imitation, reciprocal interaction, initiation, and self-management.
   c. Functional adaptive skills that prepare the child for increased responsibility and independence.
   d. Reduction of disruptive or maladaptive behavior through empirically supported strategies, including functional assessment.
   e. Cognitive skills, such as symbolic play and perspective-taking.
   f. Traditional readiness skills and academic skills.

PROGRAMS FOR OLDER CHILDREN

Some model programs, such as the Princeton Child Development Institute[375] and the Treatment and Education of Autistic and Related Communication-

Handicapped Children (TEACCH) program,[376] provide programming throughout childhood and into adulthood. More commonly, the focus of specialized programs is on early childhood; there have been few evaluations of comprehensive educational programs for older children and adolescents with ASD. There is empirical support for the use of certain strategies, especially those based on applied behavior analysis (ABA), across all age groups to increase and maintain desirable adaptive behaviors, reduce interfering maladaptive behaviors or narrow the conditions in which they occur, teach new skills, and generalize behaviors to new environments or situations.[377-379]

When children with ASD move beyond preschool and early elementary programs, educational intervention continues to involve assessment of existing skills, formulation of individualized goals and objectives, selection and implementation of appropriate intervention strategies and supports, assessment of progress, and adaptation of teaching strategies as necessary to enable students to acquire target skills. The focus on achieving social communication competence, emotional and behavioral regulation, and functional adaptive skills necessary for independence continues. Intervention programs should not be based solely on a given diagnosis. Instead, educational programs should be individualized to address the specific impairments and needs while capitalizing on the child's assets.

The specific goals and objectives in the Individualized Education Plan and the supports required to achieve them should be the driving force behind decisions regarding the most appropriate, least restrictive educational settings. Appropriate setting may range from self-contained special education classrooms to regular classrooms. Often a mix of specialized and inclusion experience is appropriate. Even high-functioning students with ASD often require accommodations and other supports such as provision of explicit directions, modification of classroom and homework assignments, organizational supports, access to a computer and word processing software for writing tasks, and social communication skills training. When a paraprofessional aide is assigned, it is important that there is an infrastructure of expertise and support for the child beyond the immediate presence of the aide.[380] The specific duties of the aide should be outlined, the strategies to be used should be defined, and the aide should receive adequate training.

SPECIFIC STRATEGIES

A variety of specific methods are used in educational programs for children with ASD. Detailed reviews of intervention strategies to enhance communication[13,377,381-387] and reduce interfering maladaptive behaviors[377,388,389] are available. A few specific strate-

gies are briefly reviewed as follows because of their importance, based on empirical support in the literature or popularity.

Applied Behavior Analysis

ABA is the process of applying interventions according to the principles of learning derived from experimental psychology research to systematically change behavior. ABA methods are used to increase and maintain desirable adaptive behaviors, reduce interfering maladaptive behaviors or narrow the conditions under which they occur, teach new skills, and generalize behaviors to new environments or situations. ABA focuses on the reliable measurement and objective evaluation of observable behavior within relevant settings, including the home, school, and community.

Highly structured comprehensive early intervention programs for children with ASD such as the Young Autism Project at the University of California, Los Angeles,[390,391] rely heavily on discrete trial training methods, but this is only one of dozens of techniques used within the realm of ABA. Discrete trial training methods are very useful in establishing learning readiness by teaching foundation skills such as attention, compliance, imitation, and discrimination learning, as well as a variety of other skills. However, discrete trial training has been criticized because of problems with generalization of learned behaviors to spontaneous use in natural environments and because the highly structured teaching environment is not representative of natural adult-child interactions. Traditional ABA techniques have been modified to address these issues. Naturalistic behavioral interventions such as incidental teaching and natural language paradigm/pivotal response training are more child centered and take place in more loosely structured environments.[379]

Functional behavior analysis, or functional assessment, is an important aspect of ABA-based treatment of unwanted behaviors. Most problem behaviors serve an adaptive function of some type and are reinforced by their consequences, such as (1) attainment of adult attention; (2) attainment of a desired object, activity, or sensation; or (3) escape from an undesired situation or demand. Functional assessment is a rigorous, empirically based method of gathering information that can be used to maximize the effectiveness and efficiency of behavioral support interventions.[392] It includes formulating a clear description of the problem behavior (including frequency and intensity); identifying the antecedents, consequences, and other environmental factors that maintain the behavior; developing hypotheses specifying the motivating function of the behavior; and collecting direct observational data to test the hypothesis. Functional analysis is also useful in identifying antecedents and consequences that are associated with increased frequency of desirable behaviors so that these can be used to evoke new adaptive behaviors.

Empirically validated behavioral methods for the treatment of problem behaviors include antecedent interventions, consequence-based interventions, and some classical or respondent conditioning procedures.[377] Antecedent interventions focus on preventing the occurrence of problem behaviors and include strategies such as (1) providing optimal levels of environmental stimulation, predictable schedules and routines, favorable staffing patterns, antecedent physical exercise, personal choices, and balanced task difficulty and (2) utilizing errorless learning, behavioral momentum, stimulus change, functional communication training, social skills training, and self-management procedures. Adaptive skill acquisition is a vital component of antecedent interventions. Consequence-based interventions include interruption and redirection, reinforcement-based interventions, extinction procedures, and sometimes noncontingent reinforcement and punishment procedures. Classical conditioning procedures sometimes used in clinical practice include desensitization and relaxation techniques.

Speech and Language Therapy

Individuals with ASD have deficits in social communication, and treatment by a speech and language pathologist is almost always warranted. Most children with ASD can develop useful speech. Chronological age, lack of typical prerequisite skills, failure to benefit from previous language intervention, and lack of discrepancy between language and IQ scores should not preclude speech and language services.[290,291] Speech and language therapists are likely to be most effective when they train and work in close collaboration with teachers, support personnel, families, and the child's peers to promote functional communication in natural settings throughout the day; traditional, low-intensity pull-out service delivery models are often ineffective.

Augmentative and alternative communication modalities, including gestures, sign language, and picture communication programs, often are effective in enhancing communication.[381,384] The picture exchange communication system[393,394] is widely used. The picture exchange communication system method incorporates ABA and developmental-pragmatic principles, by which the child is taught to initiate a picture request and persist with the communication until the partner responds. There is also evidence that some nonverbal individuals with ASD benefit from exposure to voice output communication devices.[384] Introduction of augmentative and alternative

communication systems to nonverbal children with ASD does not keep them from learning to talk, and there is some evidence that they may be more stimulated to learn speech if they already understand something about symbolic communication.[393,395]

Social Skills Instruction

There is some objective evidence to support various approaches to teaching social skills.[385-387,396-399,404] Joint attention training may be especially beneficial in young, preverbal children with ASD, because joint attention behaviors precede and are predictive of social language development.[400,401] Families can facilitate joint attention and other reciprocal social interaction experiences throughout the day in the course of the child's regular activities. Examples of these techniques are described in the AAP parent booklet *Understanding Autism Spectrum Disorders*[402] (pp 27 to 30).

A social skills curriculum should focus on responding to the social overtures of other children and adults, initiating social behavior, minimizing stereotyped perseverative behavior while using a flexible and varied repertoire of responses, and self-managing new and established skills.[369] Social skills groups, social stories, visual cuing, social games, video modeling, scripts, peer-mediated techniques, and play and leisure curricula are supported primarily by descriptive and anecdotal literature, but the quantity and quality of research is increasing.[369,373,398] Relationship Development Intervention focuses on activities that elicit interactive behaviors with the goal of engaging the child in a social relationship so that he or she discovers the value of positive interpersonal activity and becomes more motivated to learn the skills necessary to sustain these relationships.[403]. However, the evidence of efficacy of Relationship Development Intervention is anecdotal; published empirical scientific research is lacking at this time. A number of social skills curricula and guidelines are available for use in school programs and at home.[369,396,404]

Sensory Integration Therapy

Sensory integration therapy is often used alone or as part of a broader program of occupational therapy for children with ASD. The goal of sensory integration therapy is not to teach specific skills or behaviors but to remediate deficits in neurological processing and integration of sensory information to allow the child to interact with the environment in a more adaptive manner. Unusual sensory responses are common in children with ASD, but there is no strong evidence that these symptoms differentiate ASD from other developmental disorders, and the efficacy of sensory integration therapy has not been objectively demonstrated.[405-407] Available studies are plagued by methodological limitations, but proponents have noted that higher quality sensory integration research is forthcoming.[408]

COMPARATIVE EFFICACY OF EDUCATIONAL INTERVENTIONS

All treatments, including educational interventions, should be based on sound theoretical constructs, rigorous methods, and empirical studies of efficacy.[373] Proponents of behavior-analytic approaches have been the most active in using scientific methods to evaluate their work, and most research studies of comprehensive treatment programs that meet minimal scientific standards involve treatment of preschoolers with behavioral approaches.[374] The effectiveness of ABA-based intervention in autism is well documented, primarily through five decades of research through single-subject methods[77,388,378,409] but also in controlled studies of comprehensive early intensive behavioral interventions.[390,410-415]

There is limited empirical evidence of efficacy for non-ABA early intervention models such as the Denver model,[416-418] TEACCH,[376,419-422] and the responsive teaching curriculum developed by Mahoney and colleagues.[423,424] Greenspan and Wieder's developmental, individual-difference, relationship-based model ("Floor Time") is supported in the literature only by an unblinded review of case records with comparison to an inappropriate control group and use of a questionable primary outcome measure[425] and a descriptive follow-up study of 8% of the original group of patients.[426]

Although categorization by philosophical orientation (e.g., behavior analytic, developmental, structured teaching) has some meaning, there is also overlap among the different approaches. For example, contemporary comprehensive behavioral curricula borrow from ideas that were introduced from a developmental or cognitive orientation (such as addressing joint attention, reciprocal imitation, symbolic play, and theory of mind and using indirect language stimulation and contingent imitation techniques), and in developmental models such as the Denver model and the structured teaching approach of the TEACCH program, behavioral techniques are used to fulfill their curriculum goals.[369,379]

Most educational programs available to young children with ASD are based in their communities, and often an "eclectic" treatment approach is used. This approach draws from a combination of methods, including ABA methods such as discrete trial training, TEACCH-based procedures, speech and language therapy (with or without the picture exchange communication system or related augmentative or alternative communication strategies), sensory integration therapy, and typical preschool activities. In three studies in which intensive ABA programs (25 to 40 hours per week) were compared with equally intensive "eclectic" approaches, results have suggested that the ABA programs were significantly more effective.[410,411,427] Although the groups of children achieved very similar scores on key dependent measures before treatment began, parent-determined rather than random assignment to treatment group was a limitation of these studies. Additional comparisons of educational treatment approaches are warranted.

PROGRAM FOR ADOLESCENTS: TRANSITION ISSUES

Transition is defined as the movement from child-centered activities to adult-oriented activities. The major transitions are from the school environment to the workplace and from home to community living. In schools, transition planning activities may begin as early as age 14, and by age 16 the Individualized Education Plan typically becomes an Individualized Transition Plan. The emphasis may shift from academic to vocational services and from remediating deficits to fostering abilities. A vocational assessment is conducted to evaluate the teenager's interests and strengths and to determine the services needed to promote independence in the workplace and the community.

Adolescents with ASD, especially those with comorbid mental retardation, may attend public school through 21 years of age. Usually, opportunities are provided for prolonged training opportunities in vocational or life skills during the high school years rather than actual grade retention. Comprehensive transition planning involves the student, parents, teachers, and representatives from all concerned community agencies. Depending on the individual's cognitive level, social skills, health condition, work habits, and behavioral challenges, preparation for competitive, supported, or sheltered employment is targeted. Regardless of the type of employment, attention to skill development should never stop.

At some point, depending on the adolescent's cognitive level, communication and social skills, and comorbid behavior challenges, the adolescent with ASD may decide to move out from the family home into the community. The school transition process, if properly executed, should help in facilitating this. Skills necessary for independent living should be taught to the degree possible with the abilities of the individual. A growing body of literature addresses sexuality education for individuals with developmental disabilities,[428-430] as well as training regarding leisure skills.. During the final school years, assessments should be conducted to determine whether the individual is capable of living independently or whether some degree of supervision and daily support, such as that typically provided in government subsidized group homes, is needed. As with decisions regarding educational placement settings, the least restrictive environment should be sought in order to ensure maximum possible autonomy and self-determination.

Some comprehensive programs, such as the Princeton Child Development Institute and TEACCH, have curricula for adults with ASD that extend many of the same approaches offered for children while increasing the emphasis on self-care and community-living skills. A self-determination program designed specifically for individuals with ASD who want to have more control over financial and other important decisions has been described,[431] and the emphasis on self-determination will probably continue to grow.

Medical Aspects of Habilitation

Children with ASD have the same basic health care needs as children without disabilities and benefit from the same health promotion and disease prevention activities, including immunizations. In addition, they may have unique health care needs related to underlying etiological conditions, such as fragile X syndrome or tuberous sclerosis, or to other conditions, such as epilepsy, that are often associated with ASD.

GENETIC COUNSELING

Genetic counseling regarding recurrence risk in siblings is very important even when the etiological workup results are negative. Parents need to understand that such results do not mean that future siblings are without risk; the recurrence risk is approximately 5% to 6% (range, 2% to 8%) in idiopathic ASD.[92,432] The prevalence of abnormality in siblings is even higher, perhaps 20%, when the broader phenotype or milder constellation of similar social, communication, and behavioral abnormalities is considered.[432] If there are already two siblings with ASD in a family, it is likely that the recurrence risk for strictly defined ASD in subsequent pregnancies is well above 8% and may approach 25%, but there is insufficient evidence to be more precise.[432] It is important to discuss the recurrence risk promptly after diagnosis in order to provide parents with the opportunity to consider this information before they conceive another child.[92] If a specific cause is determined, the recurrence risk may be lower or higher than the risk in idiopathic ASD, depending on the syndrome or other etiological condition identified. In addition, in some conditions (e.g., fragile X syndrome), prenatal diagnosis may be possible.

SEIZURES

The reported prevalence of epilepsy among individuals with ASD ranges from 11% to 39%.[292] Coexisting severe mental retardation and motor deficits are associated with a high prevalence of seizures (42%),[433] whereas the prevalence of seizures is only 6% to 8% in children with ASD but without severe mental retardation, motor deficit, associated etiological medical disorder, or positive family history of epilepsy.[433,434] The prevalence of epilepsy is also higher in studies that include adolescents and young adults because the onset of epilepsy in ASD has two peaks: one before age 5 and another in adolescence. Anticonvulsant treatment in children with ASD is based on the same criteria that are used for other children with epilepsy, including accurate diagnosis of the particular seizure type.

Epileptiform abnormalities on EEG are more common than full-blown epilepsy in children with ASD; reported frequencies range from 10% to 72%.[358] Some studies have suggested that epileptiform abnormalities on EEG[219] and/or epilepsy[435] is more common in the subgroup of children with ASD who have a history of regression, whereas other studies have not demonstrated this association.[357,436] Autistic regression with epileptiform findings on EEG has been compared by analogy to Landau-Kleffner syndrome and electrical status epilepticus in sleep, but there are important differences between these conditions, and the treatment implications are unclear.[180,292] Whether subclinical seizures have adverse effects on language, cognition, and behavior is debated, and there is no evidence-based recommendation for treatment of children with ASD and epileptiform findings on EEG, with or without regression.[180]

GASTROINTESTINAL PROBLEMS

The prevalence of gastrointestinal problems is unclear, because most investigators have not examined representative groups of children with ASD in comparison with appropriate controls.[437,438] In some published studies, researchers have found that gastrointestinal problems such as chronic constipation or diarrhea occur in 46% to 70% of children with ASD,[439-441] whereas lower rates, in the range of 9% to 24%, have been reported in several other studies.[442-445]

In children with ASD undergoing endoscopy, high rates of lymphoid nodular hyperplasia and often histologically subtle esophagitis, gastritis, duodenitis, and colitis have been described, and preliminary evidence suggests that some immunohistochemical features may be unique to inflammation associated with ASD.[437,446,447] The existing literature does not support routine specialized gastroenterological testing for asymptomatic children with ASD.[437] However, if a child with ASD presents with symptoms such as chronic or recurrent abdominal pain, vomiting, diarrhea, or constipation, it is reasonable to evaluate the gastrointestinal tract. Occult gastrointestinal discomfort should also be considered in a child presenting with outbursts of aggression or self-injury.

Standard acid-inhibiting therapy for the symptomatic child with reflux esophagitis or gastritis is probably warranted, as is treatment of identified *Helicobacter pylori* infection, although there are no data specific to ASD. The role of immune modulators for mucosal inflammation associated with ASD has not been studied, although there are anecdotal reports of response in the literature.[447] Radiographic evidence of constipation has been found to be more common in children with ASD than in controls with abdominal pain (36% vs. 10%),[448] and effective management may provide some benefit.

PSYCHOPHARMACOLOGY

Surveys indicate that approximately 45% of children and adolescents[449-451] and up to 75% of adults[452] with ASD are treated with psychotropic medication. Older age, poorer adaptive skills and social competence, and higher levels of challenging behavior are associated with likelihood of medication use.[451]

The Decision to Initiate Medical Treatment

Discussion of potential pharmacological intervention often arises in the setting of problematic aggression, self-injurious behavior, repetitive behaviors (e.g., perseveration, obsessions, compulsions, and stereotypic movements), sleep disturbance, mood lability, irritability, anxiety, hyperactivity, inattention, destructive behavior, or other disruptive behaviors.

Before initiating a trial of psychotropic medication, it is important to search for medical factors that may be causing or exacerbating the maladaptive behaviors. Recognition and treatment of medical conditions may eliminate the need for psychopharmacological agents in some cases. For example, in the case of an acute onset or exacerbation of aggressive or self-injurious behavior, an occult source of pain such as otitis media, otitis externa, pharyngitis, sinusitis, dental abscess, constipation, urinary tract infection, fracture, headache, esophagitis, gastritis, colitis, or allergic rhinitis may be identified and treated. When behavioral deterioration is temporally related to menstrual cycles in an adolescent girl, use of an analgesic or an oral or injectable contraceptive may be helpful. Obstructive sleep apnea may contribute to behavioral deterioration and may be ameliorated by weight reduction, tonsillectomy and adenoidectomy, or continuous positive airway pressure. Extreme food selectivity has the

potential to lead to malnutrition or vitamin or mineral deficiencies; however, most evaluations of nutritional status in children with ASD suggest that despite dietary selectivity, malnutrition is uncommon.[437,453] Although the prevalence in ASD is unknown, pica related to iron or zinc deficiency may respond to supplementation.

It is also important to consider environmental factors that may be precipitating challenging behaviors. Parents, teachers, or other caregivers may inadvertently reinforce maladaptive behaviors, and in such cases, the most appropriate and effective interventions are behavioral. In some instances, a mismatch between educational or behavioral expectations and cognitive ability of the child is responsible for disruptive behavior (e.g., when mental retardation is present but has not been diagnosed), and adjustment of the expectations is the most appropriate intervention. In both situations, a functional analysis of behavior, completed by a behavior specialist in the settings in which the problems occur, identifies factors in the environment that exacerbate or maintain the problematic behavior. A strategy for intervention through behavioral techniques and environmental manipulations can then be formulated and tested.

After treatable medical causes and modifiable environmental factors have been ruled out, a therapeutic trial of medication may be considered if the behavioral symptoms are causing significant impairment in functioning. In some cases, a coexisting disorder such as major depression, bipolar disorder, or an anxiety disorder can be reasonably diagnosed, and the patient can be treated with the medications that are useful for treating these conditions in otherwise typically developing children and adolescents. Modifications of diagnostic criteria may be necessary to account for clinical presentations of psychiatric conditions in individuals with developmental disabilities.[454,455] In other cases, clinicians opt to treat interfering maladaptive behaviors in the absence of a clear comorbid psychiatric diagnosis.

Choice of Medication

The evidence regarding the efficacy of psychopharmacological interventions in ASD has been detailed in reviews.[139,456-458] Although most psychotropic medications have been used in children with ASD, there is currently insufficient literature to establish a consensus-based, evidence-based approach to pharmacological management. Fortunately, there has been an increase in publication of randomized, double-blind, placebo-controlled clinical trials to guide clinical practice. A summary of selected target symptoms, potential psychiatric diagnoses, and medication options is provided in Table 15-8.

TABLE 15-8 ■ Selected Medication Options for Common Target Symptoms or Comorbid Diagnoses in Children with Autism Spectrum Disorder

Target Symptom Cluster	Possible Comorbid Diagnosis	Suggested Medications
Repetitive behavior, behavioral rigidity, obsessive-compulsive symptoms	Obsessive-compulsive disorder	SSRI (fluoxetine, fluvoxamine, citalopram, escitalopram, paroxetine, sertraline) Clomipramine Atypical antipsychotic (risperidone, aripiprazole, olanzapine, quetiapine, ziprasidone)
Hyperactivity, impulsivity, inattention	Attention-deficit/hyperactivity disorder	Stimulant (methylphenidate, dextroamphetamine, mixed amphetamine salts) α_2 Agonist (clonidine, guanfacine) Atomoxetine Atypical antipsychotic (risperidone, aripiprazole, olanzapine, quetiapine, ziprasidone)
Aggression, explosive outbursts, self-injury	Intermittent explosive disorder	Atypical antipsychotic (risperidone, aripiprazole, olanzapine, quetiapine, ziprasidone) α_2 Agonist Anticonvulsant mood stabilizer (levetiracetam, topiramate, valproate) Lithium SSRI (fluoxetine, fluvoxamine, citalopram, escitalopram, paroxetine, sertraline) β Blocker
Sleep dysfunction	Circadian rhythm sleep disorder, dyssomnia not otherwise specified	Melatonin Antihistamine (diphenhydramine, hydroxyzine) Clonidine Trazodone Zolpidem Mirtazapine
Anxiety	Generalized anxiety disorder, anxiety disorder not otherwise specified	SSRI (fluoxetine, fluvoxamine, citalopram, escitalopram, paroxetine, sertraline) Buspirone
Depressive phenotype (marked change from baseline, including symptoms such as social withdrawal, irritability, sadness or crying spells, decreased energy, anorexia, weight loss, sleep dysfunction)	Major depressive disorder, depressive disorder not otherwise specified	SSRI (fluoxetine, fluvoxamine, citalopram, escitalopram, paroxetine, sertraline) Venlafaxine Mirtazapine
Bipolar phenotype (behavioral cycling with rages and euphoria, decreased need for sleep, maniclike hyperactivity, irritability, aggression, self-injury, sexual behaviors)	Bipolar I disorder, bipolar disorder not otherwise specified	Anticonvulsant mood stabilizer (levetiracetam, topiramate, valproate) Atypical antipsychotic (risperidone, aripiprazole, olanzapine, quetiapine, ziprasidone) Lithium

Adapted from Myers SM, Challman TD: Psychopharmacology: An approach to management in autism and intellectual disabilities. *In* Accardo PJ, ed: Capute & Accardo's Neurodevelopmental Disabilities in Infancy and Childhood, 3rd ed. Baltimore: Paul H. Brookes, in press.
SSRI, selective serotonin reuptake inhibitor.

STIMULANTS, α_2 AGONISTS, AND ATOMOXETINE

Although early studies of the effects of stimulants yielded negative results, more recent double-blind, placebo-controlled trials of methylphenidate have demonstrated improvement in hyperactivity, impulsivity, and inattention in children with ASD.[459-461] Methylphenidate is effective in some children with ASD, but the response rate is lower than in children with isolated ADHD, adverse effects are more fre-

quent, and it is unclear whether the results can be generalized to other stimulants.[461,462] Two very small, double-blind, placebo-controlled trials have documented modest benefits of clonidine in reducing hyperarousal symptoms, including hyperactivity, irritability and outbursts, impulsivity, and repetitive behaviors in children with ASD.[463,464] A retrospective record review study revealed that open-label treatment with guanfacine was effective in 19 (24%) of 80 children with ASD.[465] Patients without mental retardation were more likely to show improvement in target symptoms, including hyperactivity, inattention, insomnia, and tics. Atomoxetine has not been evaluated in controlled trials in children with ASD, but a retrospective study suggested that it might be effective for ADHD-like symptoms in this population.[466]

ATYPICAL ANTIPSYCHOTIC AGENTS

Atypical antipsychotic medications currently available in the United States include clozapine, risperidone, olanzapine, quetiapine, ziprasidone, and aripiprazole. There is evidence that atypical antipsychotics are efficacious in the treatment of children and adolescents with severe disruptive behaviors associated with intellectual disability,[467-469] in addition to those with psychosis, bipolar disorder, Tourette syndrome, and, potentially, conduct disorder and severe ADHD.[470] Two large, multisite, randomized controlled trials have confirmed the short-term efficacy of risperidone for severe disruptive behaviors such as tantrums, aggression, and self-injurious behavior in youths with ASD.[471-474] Results of two open-label studies, each with a double-blind discontinuation component, have suggested long-term benefits and tolerance.[475,476] The effect of risperidone on core symptoms of ASD is less dramatic. The Research Units on Pediatric Psychopharmacology Autism Network trial revealed that treatment with risperidone improved the restricted, repetitive, and stereotyped patterns of interests and behavior but did not significantly affect impairments in social interaction or communication.[473]

SELECTIVE SEROTONIN REUPTAKE INHIBITORS

Selective serotonin reuptake inhibitors (SSRIs) include fluoxetine, sertraline, fluvoxamine, paroxetine, citalopram, and escitalopram. Double-blind, placebo-controlled trials have demonstrated efficacy of fluoxetine[477] and fluvoxamine[478,479] in the treatment of repetitive and other maladaptive behaviors in patients with ASD. Open-label trials of various serotonin reuptake inhibitors in children and adults with ASD report response rates in the range of 50% to 75% but are susceptible to publication bias and other shortcomings of uncontrolled studies.[480] Improvements in target symptoms, including repetitive behaviors, irritability, depressive symptoms, tantrums, anxiety, aggression, difficulty with transitions, social interaction, and language, have been reported.[477-480]

ANTICONVULSANT MOOD STABILIZERS AND LITHIUM

In small open-label trials, valproate,[481] levetiracetam,[482] and topiramate[482a] were effective in reducing symptoms such as aggression, impulsivity, hyperactivity, conduct problems, and mood lability in children with ASDs. In an open-label valproate trial[481] and several case reports,[483,484] improvements in language and social skills were also described. A small double-blind, placebo-controlled trial[485] demonstrated significant improvement in repetitive behavior in children with ASDs who were treated with valproate. Valproate may also be associated with significant improvement in electrencephalographic recordings and subjective clinical status.[486] Uvebrant and Bauziene[487] reported a decrease in "autistic symptoms" in 8 of 13 patients treated with lamotrigine for intractable epilepsy, regardless of efficacy in controlling the seizures. However, in a double-blind, placebo-controlled study, Belsito and coworkers[488] did not find significant differences between lamotrigine and placebo. Several case reports describe children with ASD and atypical bipolar disorder or mania who responded well to open-label treatment with lithium.[489-491]

General Clinical Principles of Medication Management

Principles to guide the approach to psychopharmacological management of ASD in clinical practice have been proposed by several authors.[139,457,458] It is important to identify the coexisting psychiatric diagnosis or formulate a hypothesis regarding the origin of the target behaviors in order to select the medication that might be most effective (see Table 15-8). In addition, medication-specific issues, such as side effects, preparations available, dosing schedules, cost, and monitoring requirements should be considered. Potential benefits and side effects should be explained, informed consent obtained, baseline data regarding behaviors and somatic complaints collected, and potential strategies for dealing with treatment failure or partial response reviewed.

It is important to have some quantifiable means of assessing the efficacy of the medication and to obtain input from a variety of sources, such as parents, teachers, therapists, and aides. Consistent use of validated, treatment-sensitive rating scales and medication side effect scales is desirable. A wide variety of outcome measures have been used in research trials and in clinical practice to measure maladaptive behavior treatment effects.[492] Among the most common are the Clinical Global Impression scale, Aberrant Behavior Checklist, and Nisonger Child Behavior Rating Form.

In general, only one medication change should be made at a time in order to be able to judge the treatment effect. It is usually best to begin with a low dose and gradually titrate upwards to the target effect to minimize the risk of treatment-emergent adverse events. If a particular medication is found to be ineffective after appropriate titration (i.e., adequate dose and duration to expect therapeutic effect) or associated with intolerable side effects, the medication should be discontinued. Gradual tapering may be warranted, depending on the medication. This is particularly important with certain agents (e.g., antipsychotics) because of the risk of withdrawal dyskinesias.

In the case of partial or suboptimal response, the clinician and family must decide whether to substitute another agent or add a second medication. Although monotherapy is desirable, augmentation or combination strategies are sometimes found to be necessary, particularly in the setting of significant mood instability and severe aggression or self-injury. When multiple medications are necessary, the clinician must be aware of potential interactions among drugs and monitor accordingly.

Periodic setbacks or exacerbations are to be expected, and it is wise to avoid quickly changing or adding medications to treat each behavior that arises. Careful withdrawal of a medication should be considered after 6 to 12 months of stability so that it is possible to determine whether the medication is still necessary.

SLEEP DISTURBANCE

Sleep problems are common in children and adolescents with ASD at all levels of cognitive functioning.[493-497] Sleep problems are associated with family distress and may have significant impact on daytime functioning and quality of life in children with ASD. Behavioral interventions, including sleep hygiene measures, restriction of daytime sleep, positive bedtime routines, and extinction procedures, are often effective.[493,498,499]

Relatively little empirical information regarding pharmacological management of sleep problems in children with ASD or other developmental disabilities is available. Recommendations are typically based on case reports and open-label trials, extrapolation from the adult literature, and expert consensus.[498] There is some evidence of abnormality of melatonin regulation in ASD,[500,501] and melatonin may be effective for improving sleep onset in children with ASD, as well as in children with other developmental disabilities, although there have been few randomized placebo-controlled trials.[502-504] Antihistamines, α_2 agonists, benzodiazepines, chloral hydrate, trazodone, and newer non-benzodiazepine hypnotics such as zolpidem and zaleplon are also sometimes utilized to treat pediatric insomnia.[498] In some cases, other conditions or symptoms such as epilepsy, depression, anxiety, or aggressive outbursts warrant pharmacological treatment, and an agent that may also assist with sleep can be chosen.[493]

COMPLEMENTARY AND ALTERNATIVE MEDICINE

Complementary and alternative medicine (CAM) use is common in children with ASD[449,505] Detailed reviews of general CAM issues in developmental disabilities are available in this volume (see Chapter 8E) and elsewhere,[506] and ASD-specific CAM reviews have also been published.[506a,507] The boundary between therapies considered conventional and those viewed as complementary and alternative is often poorly delineated, and a therapy initially considered to fall within the realm of CAM may later be supported by sufficient evidence to become part of standard, "conventional" practice.

CAM therapies used to treat ASD have been categorized as biological or nonbiological.[507] Nonbiological interventions include treatments such as auditory integration training, behavioral optometry, craniosacral manipulation, dolphin-assisted therapy, and facilitated communication. Biological therapies include immunoregulatory interventions (e.g., dietary restriction of food allergens, intravenous immune globulin, and antiviral agents), detoxification therapies (e.g., chelation), gastrointestinal treatments (e.g., digestive enzymes, antifungal agents, probiotics, "yeast-free diet," gluten-free/casein-free diet, and vancomycin), and supplemental therapies purported to act by modulating neurotransmission (e.g., vitamin A, vitamin C, vitamin B_6 and magnesium, folic acid, folinic acid, vitamin B_{12}, dimethylglycine and trimethylglycine, carnosine, omega-3 fatty acids, inositol, and various minerals).[506a,507]

For most of these CAM interventions, there is little or no scientific evidence of efficacy. Some interventions have been appropriately studied and their efficacy or validity has been disproved. For example, more than a dozen randomized, double-blind, placebo-controlled trials involving more than 700 patients have demonstrated that secretin is not an effective treatment for ASD, and it should not be used for this purpose.[508,509] There is also a substantial body of research indicating that facilitated communication lacks credibility.[510-512] This technique is used by a trained facilitator to provide physical support to a nonverbal person's hand or arm while that person uses a computer keyboard or other device to spell. The evidence suggests that the communications produced actually originate from the facilitator.[513,514]

Evidence-based recommendations regarding additional CAM therapies are not possible because they have been evaluated inadequately as a result of methodological flaws, insufficient numbers of patients, or lack of replication. The most recent and most appropriately designed trials have demonstrated no significant benefit of dimethylglycine,[515,516] vitamin B_6

and magnesium,[517,518] or auditory integration training.[519,520] Both positive[520a] and negative[521,522] results have been described in small, methodologically flawed studies of intravenous immune globulin. Although the gluten-free/casein-free diet is popular, there is little evidence to support or refute this intervention. In 2004, a Cochrane review found that meaningful conclusions could not be drawn from the existing literature[523] and the only double-blind clinical trial subsequently published demonstrated no statistically significant differences between the patients following the gluten-free/casein-free diet and the control groups.[524] Larger double-blind, placebo-controlled challenge studies are in progress.[507] Many popular interventions such as chelation of heavy metals, hyperbaric oxygen, antifungal agents to decrease yeast overgrowth, antiviral agents to modulate the immune system, and omega-3 fatty acids to modulate intracellular second messengers or cellular membranes have not yet been studied in ASD; their popularity is based on unproven theories and anecdotes.

Health care practitioners who diagnose ASDs and treat children with with these conditions should recognize that many of their patients will use nonstandard therapies. It is wise and practical to become somewhat knowledgeable about CAM therapies, inquire about current and past CAM use, provide balanced information and advice about treatment options, identify risks or potential harmful effects, avoid becoming defensive or dismissing CAM in ways that convey a lack of sensitivity or concern, maintain open communication, and continue to work with families even if there is disagreement about treatment choices[525] (see Chapter 8E). It is also essential to evaluate the scientific merits of specific therapies critically and share this information with families, educate families about how to evaluate information and recognize pseudoscience, and insist that studies of CAM be held to the same scientific and ethical standards as all clinical research.[507,525a]

Parents of children with ASD will understandably pursue interventions that they believe may present some hope of helping their child, particularly if the therapies are viewed as being unlikely to have any adverse effects. Unfortunately, families are often exposed to unsubstantiated, pseudoscientific theories and related clinical practices that at best are ineffective and at worst compete with validated treatments or lead to physical, emotional, or financial harm. Time, effort, and financial resources wasted on ineffective therapies can create an additional burden on already overwhelmed families. Unfortunately, widespread use of the Internet has promoted the rapid dissemination of an increasing number of questionable theories and practices. Without guidance, parents may have considerable difficulty distinguishing between pseudoscientific interventions and empirically validated treatment approaches.

Family Support

Management should focus not only on the child but also on the family. It has been recognized that parents, who were once viewed as the cause of their child's ASD, actually play a key role in effective treatment.[13] A child with an ASD has a substantial effect on the family. Although most family members recognize benefits of living with their child with an ASD, such as finding greater meaning in their own lives, experiencing delight in the child's accomplishments, and feeling enhanced empathy for others,[526] parents of children with ASD experience more stress and depression than do parents of children who are typically developing or who have certain other disabilities.[527-529] Supporting the family and ensuring its emotional and physical health is an extremely important aspect of overall management of ASD.

PARENT/CAREGIVER SUPPORT

Physicians and other professionals can provide support to parents by educating them about ASD, providing anticipatory guidance and training, involving them as cotherapists, assisting them in obtaining access to resources, providing emotional support through traditional strategies such as empathic listening and talking through problems, and assisting them in advocating for their child's needs.[526] In some cases, referral of parents for counseling or other appropriate mental health services may be required. These families need ongoing support, with the specific constellation of needs varying through the family life cycle.

One of the chief strategies in helping families raise children with ASD is providing them with access to needed ongoing supports, as well as additional services during critical periods and/or crises. Natural supports include spouses, extended family members, neighbors, religious institutions, and friends who can help with caregiving and who can provide psychological and emotional support. Informal supports include social networking with other families of children with ASD and community agencies that provide training, respite, social events, and recreational activities. Formal supports include publicly funded, state-administered programs such as early intervention, special education, vocational and residential/living services, respite services, Medicaid, In-Home and Community-Based Waiver Services, Supplemental Security Income (SSI) benefits, and other financial subsidies. The breadth and depth of services vary, even within the same state or region. Few services exist in many rural areas, and public programs may have long waiting lists.

SIBLING SUPPORT

The impact of ASD on a family is not limited to the parents or primary caregivers. Depression and psychosocial problems are also common in siblings of children with ASD,[530,531] who often are plagued by questions and concerns about the reason for their sibling's disability, how to cope with embarrassment or the reaction of peers to the sibling's behavior, and what the future holds with regard to their role in long-term care.[526] Family financial difficulties and lack of knowledge about the disability may exacerbate adjustment problems in the unaffected sibling, and the relationship may be influenced by a number of other external factors, including the availability of support services, especially respite services.

Sibling support groups offer the opportunity to learn important information and skills while sharing experiences and connecting with other siblings of children with ASD.[526] Although the research on support groups for siblings of children with disabilities is difficult to interpret because of study design problems and inconsistent outcome effects on sibling adjustment, these groups have generally been evaluated positively by participating siblings and parents.[526,532]

FINANCIAL SUPPORT AND RELATED ISSUES

Several publicly funded programs provide financial assistance (e.g., SSI benefits, Food Stamps, Medicaid, and In-Home and Community-Based Waiver Services). Access to some public benefits, such as SSI, depends on financial need. Because eligibility depends on the financial status of the family, need-based supports such as SSI can be lost, if, for example, a well-meaning family member bequeaths the child a monetary gift. However, the government has established rules allowing assets to be held in trust for SSI and Medicaid recipients through a Supplemental Needs or Special Needs Trust. The Special Needs Trust can be used to fund needs that go beyond the bare necessities of food, clothing, and shelter provided by SSI and the medical supports and services covered by Medicaid. The laws governing such trusts are complex, and the help of an attorney knowledgeable in special needs planning is usually required. More information about Special Needs Trust can be found at *http://www. nichcy.org/pubs/outprint/nd18.pdf.*

In addition to supports provided through SSI and health-care programs (Medicaid), families of children with ASD, especially those with coexisting mental retardation, may be eligible for additional supports to assist them in raising their child. Although funding for community-based supports has been increasing

since the 1970s, the degree of funding allocated for these services varies a great deal among states. The most common funding mechanism for families, Home and Community-Based Waiver Services, is called a "waiver option" because the family's income and assets are waived, which makes access equitable across all income levels. Eligibility depends entirely on the severity of the child's disability and the circumstances it imposes upon the family. Unfortunately, many states have long waiting lists (e.g., 5 to 7 years) before the child becomes eligible for this funding. Once the child becomes eligible, a case manager works collaboratively with the family to design an annual service plan that may include various types of respite, medical equipment, home modifications for safety reasons, and other needed supports.

Because each state's services and access mechanisms are organized differently, physicians and families must learn their own state's idiosyncrasies to access supports by contacting the state or county offices of the Department of Health and Human Services, the Department of Mental Health and Mental Retardation, or the state developmental disabilities organization. In addition, local parent advocacy organizations, national organizations such as the Autism Society of America and The Arc, Early Intervention Program administrators, and school district special education coordinators are often knowledgeable about various programs and their respective eligibility requirements.

At the age of 18, teenagers with ASD (with or without coexisting mental retardation) automatically become their own legal guardians. If parents and the professionals working with such a teenager do not believe that he or she is capable of making responsible decisions, a formal evaluation should be conducted to determine the need for guardianship. The parents should consult the child's primary physician or a developmental-behavioral pediatrician who knows the child well, because medical forms are often necessary to initiate the evaluation process. If guardianship turns out to be in the individual's best interests, then legal services can be sought to help the parents navigate the judicial system and to designate a legal guardian for the individual.

PROGNOSIS

Although prognosis is one of the parents' most pressing concerns at the time of diagnosis, it is dependent on many things and cannot usually be predicted during infancy or early childhood, especially in children younger than 3 years.[533] Important early predictors include functional play skills, responsiveness to others' bids for joint attention, and the frequency of requesting behaviors.[534] In fact, several variables are especially important: cognitive abilities, level of adaptive functioning, severity of autistic symptoms, and acquisition of functional language by age 5 years.[452,535-543] Throughout the lifespan, these variables interact. The prognosis for any given child depends on his or her place on the spectrum for each of these interacting trajectories.

Prognosis for independence as an adult may be better correlated with level of cognitive-adaptive functioning than with the severity of autistic symptoms. Children with normal intelligence and adaptive functioning and milder autistic symptoms generally have better outcomes; conversely, those with mental retardation and severe autistic symptoms usually have the worst prognosis. Those with normal cognitive-adaptive skills but severe autistic symptoms general do better than those with mental retardation and mild autistic symptoms. Coplan and colleagues[538,541,544] reaffirmed the contribution of intelligence rather than degree of atypicality (autistic symptoms) to better outcomes, although among children with normal intelligence, the degree of atypicality is important in determining prognosis. It generally appears that approximately one third of autistic children with normal intelligence and functional language tend to improve with time to the extent that they are able to participate fully in the community.

Persons with Asperger syndrome may have better outcomes than those with other disorders on the autistic spectrum, perhaps because of their normal intelligence. One study evaluated short-term outcomes in 46 children with high-functioning autism and 20 with Asperger syndrome. All were 4 to 6 years old and had normal intelligence. Tests of cognition, language, and behavior at onset and 2 years later revealed that the children with Asperger syndrome had better social skills and fewer autistic symptoms than did the children with high-functioning autism. Some of the latter group became verbally fluent and demonstrated posttest scores indistinguishable from those of the groups with Asperger syndrome. On the other hand, an adult outcome study revealed that although those with Asperger syndrome tend to have a greater likelihood of earning a college degree, the college education did not significantly affect employment or marital status.[543,545]

Additional factors associated with poorer outcomes include no joint attention by 4 years and no functional speech by 5 years of age[13]; seizures, especially when onset occurred during adolescence; coexisting medical (e.g., tuberous sclerosis) or psychiatric (e.g., schizophrenia) disorders; and extreme "aloofness" with very little interaction with others. Female gender tends to be a risk factor for poorer prognosis because

of a higher incidence of mental retardation and a lower incidence of savant skills. Factors associated with better outcomes include early identification resulting in early enrollment in appropriate intervention programs,[13,546] and inclusion in regular educational and community settings with typically developing peers.[131]

Although all of these factors have statistical significance in ASD in general, each individual is affected by a myriad of variables in the course of her or his lifetime that will help shape her or his future. A good outcome generally means that the child matures into an adult who is able to live independently and be gainfully employed. Most, if not all, such individuals retain some degree of social skill deficit. Many choose highly technical occupations that require few social interactions and gravitate to social circles that include individuals with similar characteristics. As the generation of individuals who received diagnoses early and enrolled in effective intervention programs mature and reach adulthood, more of them are marrying and having families. There is a growing number of published autobiographies and biographies now available that describe success stories, often to the credit of understanding and supportive parents and spouses.[547-551]

Life expectancy is reduced in persons with ASD associated with severe mental retardation because of seizures, respiratory disease, and accidents; however, even those with mild mental retardation were found to have shorter lifespans, generally because of accidents such as suffocation and drowning, as well as seizures.[552]

FUTURE DIRECTIONS

The developmental-behavioral pediatrician is ideally suited to train and support primary care providers, within the context of the medical home, in surveillance, screening, and management of children with ASD. The developmental-behavioral pediatrician is often the most experienced pediatric subspecialist in the health field and thus should provide leadership for a comprehensive evaluation within the context of a team or by coordinating independent evaluations by subspecialists, psychologists, and therapists. The developmental-behavioral pediatrician's services can be valuable in the management of both the coexisting medical conditions and the challenging behavioral issues associated with ASD; in assisting intervention and school personnel with developing individualized plans for effective interventions; and in training parents, caregivers, and nonmedical professionals. On the basis of their expertise and involvement in clinical care of children with ASD, developmental-behavioral pediatricians, among others, can guide clinical research so that hypotheses tested have a significant effect on the quality of life for children with ASD, their families, and/or the professionals who care for them. It is an exciting field, one in which the fund of knowledge is mushrooming on a daily basis. It is hoped that in the near future, new research findings will uncover the causes and point to interventions that will have greater efficacy than do those available currently. Continued research may help to resolve controversial issues and clarify treatment and prognostic conundrums. It is hoped that autism "specialists" across all disciplines can unite with families as one voice in the interest of children with ASD.

FAMILY RESOURCES

The reader is referred to the American Academy of Pediatrics (AAP) publications for parents and families. See the booklet entitled "Understanding Autism Spectrum Disorders" (2005) and "Autism: Caring for Children with Autism Spectrum Disorders: A Resource Toolkit for Clinicians" (in press).

REFERENCES

1. Lockyer L, Rutter M: A five to fifteen year follow-up study of infantile psychosis. IV. Patterns of cognitive ability. Br J Soc Clin Psychol 31:152-163, 1970.
2. Ball W: Dissecting the living brain: Applications for neuroimaging in the decade of the brain. J Pediatr 129:779-781, 1996.
3. The Children's Health Act of 2000. (Available at: *http://alt.samhsa.gov/legislate/Sept01/childhealth_toc.htm.*)
4. The New Freedom Initiative of 2001. (Available at: *www.hhs.gov/newfreedom/init.html* and *http://www.whitehouse.gov/news/releases/2001/06/20010619.html;* accessed 12/22/06.)
5. The Combating Autism Act of 2005, H.R. 2421. (Available at: *http://olpa.od.nih.gov/tracking/109/house_bills/session1/hr-2421.asp;* accessed 12/22/06.)
6. Kanner L: Autistic disturbances of affective contact. Nerv Child 2:217-250, 1943.
7. Volkmar FR, Lord C, Bailey A, et al: Autism and pervasive developmental disorders. J Child Psychol Psychiatry 45:135-170, 2004.
8. Volkmar F, Cook EH JR, Pomeroy J, et al: Practice parameters for the assessment and treatment of children, adolescents, and adults with autism and other pervasive developmental disorders. J Am Acad Child Adolesc Psychiatry 38:32S-54S, 1999.
9. Clinical Practice Guideline: Autism/Pervasive Developmental Disorders: Assessment and Intervention for Young Children (Age 0-3 years): The Guideline Technical Report. Albany: New York State Department of Health, Early Intervention Program, 1999.
10. Filipek PA, Accardo PJ, Ashwal S, et al: Practice parameter: Screening and diagnosis of autism: Report of the Quality Standards Subcommittee of the American Academy of Neurology and the Child Neurology Society. Neurology 55:468-479, 2000.
11. American Academy of Pediatrics, Committee on Children with Disabilities: The pediatrician's role in the diagnosis and management of autistic spectrum disorder in children. Policy Statement (RE060018). Pediatrics 107:1221-1226, 2001.
12. American Academy of Pediatrics, Committee on Children with Disabilities: The pediatrician's role in the diagnosis and management of autistic spectrum disorder in children. Technical Report. Pediatrics 107(5):85, 2001.
13. Lord C, McGee JP, eds, Committee on Educational Interventions for Children with Autism: Educating Children with Autism. National Research Council, Division of Behavioral and Social Sciences and Education. Washington, DC: National Academies Press, 2001.
14. Volkmar FR, Paul R, Klin A, et al, eds: Handbook of Autism and Pervasive Developmental Disorders, 3rd ed, vols 1 and 2. Hoboken, NJ: Wiley, 2005.
15. Bauman ML, Kemper TL, eds: The Neurobiology of Autism, 2nd ed. Baltimore: Johns Hopkins University Press, 2005.
16. Gupta VB, ed: Autism Spectrum Disorder in Children. New York: Marcel Dekker, 2004.
17. Wetherby AM, Prizant BM, eds: Autism Spectrum Disorders: A Developmental Transactional Perspective. Baltimore: Paul H. Brookes, 2000.
18. Filipek PA: Medical aspects of autism. *In* Volkmar FR, Paul R, Klin A, et al, eds: Handbook of Autism and Pervasive Developmental Disorders, 3rd ed, vol 1. Hoboken, NJ: Wiley, 2005, pp 534-582.
19. American Psychiatric Association: Diagnostic and Statistical Manual of Mental Disorders, 4th ed. Washington, DC: American Psychiatric Association, 1994.
20. American Psychiatric Association: Diagnostic and Statistical Manual of Mental Disorders, 4th ed, Text Revision. Washington, DC: American Psychiatric Association, 2000.
21. Wolraich ML, ed: The Classification of Child and Adolescent Mental Diagnoses in Primary Care: Diagnostic and Statistical Manual for Primary Care, Child and Adolescent Version. Elk Grove Village, IL: American Academy of Pediatrics, 1996.
22. Bailey A, Le Courteur A, Gottesman I, et al: Autism as a strongly genetic disorder: Evidence from a British twin study. Psychol Med 25:63-77, 1995.
23. Rutter M: Genetic studies of autism from the 1970s into the millennium. J Abnorm Child Psychol 28:3-14, 2000.
24. American Psychiatric Association: Diagnostic and Statistical Manual of Mental Disorders, 3rd ed. Washington, DC: American Psychiatric Association, 1980.
25. American Psychiatric Association: Diagnostic and Statistical Manual of Mental Disorders, 3rd ed, revised. Washington, DC: American Psychiatric Association, 1987.

26. Macintosh K, Dissanayake C: Annotation: The similarities and differences between autistic disorder and Asperger's disorder: A review of the empirical evidence. J Child Psychol Psychiatry 45:421-434, 2004.

27. Schopler E, Mesibov G, Kunce L: Asperger Sydrome or High Functioning Autism? New York: Plenum Press, 1998.

28. Tanguay PE: Commentary: Categorial versus spectrum approaches to classification in Pervasive Developmental Disorders. J Am Acad Child Adolesc Psychiatry 43:181-182, 2004.

29. Walker DR, Thompson A, Zwaigenbaum L, et al: Specifying PDD-NOS: A comparison of PDD-NOS, Asperger syndrome, and autism. J Am Acad Child Adolesc Psychiatry 43:172-180, 2004.

30. Cosgrove PV: Diagnosis of autism: Use of autistic spectrum shows undisciplined thinking [Comment]. BMJ 328:226, 2004.

31. Timimi S: Diagnosis of autism: Current epidemic has social context [Comment]. BMJ 328:226, 2004.

32. Bishop DVM, Maybery M, Wong D, et al: Characteristics of the broader phenotype in autism. Am J Med Genet B Neuropsychiatr Genet 141:117-122, 2006.

33. Rutter M: Incidence of autism spectrum disorders: Changes over time and their meaning. Acta Paediatr 94:2-15, 2005.

34. Asperger H: Die "Autistischen Psychopathen" im Kindesalter ["Autistic psychopathy" in childhood]. Arch Psychiatr Nervenkr 117:76-136, 1944.

35. Wing L: Asperger's syndrome: A clinical account. Psychol Med 11:115-129, 1981.

36. Klin A, McPartland J, Volkmar FR: Asperger syndrome. In Volkmar FR, Paul R, Klin A, et al, eds: Handbook of Autism and Pervasive Developmental Disorders, 3rd ed, vol 1. Hoboken, NJ: Wiley, 2005, pp 88-125.

37. Rutter M: Diagnosis and definition. In Rutter M, Schopler E, eds: Autism: A Reappraisal of Concepts and Treatment. New York: Plenum Press, 1978, pp 1-25.

38. Factor DC, Freeman NL, Kardash A: A comparison of *DSM-III* and *DSM-IIIR* criteria for autism. J Autism Dev Disord 19:637-640, 1989.

39. International Classification of Diseases, 10th ed. Geneva, Switzerland: World Health Organization, 1994.

40. Volkmar FR, Klin A, Siegel B, et al: Field trial of autistic disorders in *DSM-IV*. Am J Psychiatry 151:1361, 1994.

41. Kanner L: Problems of nosology and psychodynamics of early infantile autism. J Am Acad Orthop Surg 19:416-426, 1949.

42. Bettelheim B: The Empty Fortress: Infantile Autism and the Birth of Self. New York: Free Press, 1967.

43. Rimland B: Infantile Autism: The Syndrome and Its Implications for a Neural Theory of Behavior. New York: Appleton-Century-Crofts, 1964.

44. Courchesne E, Yeung-Courchesne R, Press GA, et al: Hypoplasia of cerebellar vermal lobules VI and VII in autism. N Engl J Med 318:1349-1354, 1988.

45. Minshew NJ: Indices of neural function in autism: Clinical and biologic implications. Pediatrics 87:774-780, 1991.

46. Karapurkar-Bhasin T, Lee N, Curran K, et al: The epidemiology of autism and autism spectrum disorders. In Gupta VB, ed: Autism Spectrum Disorder in Children. New York: Marcel Dekker, 2004, pp 17-42.

47. Chakrabarti S, Fombonne E: Pervasive developmental disorders in preschool children. JAMA 285:3093-3099, 2001.

48. Chakrabarti S; Fombonne E: Pervasive developmental disorders in preschool children: Confirmation of high prevalence. Am J Psychiatry 162:1133-1141, 2005.

49. Charman T: The prevalence of autism spectrum disorders. Recent evidence and future challenges. Eur Child Adolesc Psychiatry 11:249-256, 2002.

50. Fombonne E: Epidemiological surveys of autism and other pervasive developmental disorders: An update. J Autism Dev Disord 33:365-382, 2003.

51. Fombonne E, Zakarian R, Bennett A, et al: Pervasive developmental disorders in Montreal, Quebec, Canada: Prevalence and links with immunizations. Pediatrics 118(1):e139-e150, 2006.

52. Bertrand J, Mars A, Boyle C, et al: Prevalence of autism in a United States population: The Brick Township, New Jersey, investigation. Pediatrics 108:1155-1161, 2001.

53. Yeargin-Allsopp M, Rice C, Karapurkar T, et al: Prevalence of autism in a US metropolitan area. JAMA 289:49-55, 2003.

54. Barbaresi WJ, Katusic SK, Colligan RC, et al: The incidence of autism in Olmsted County, Minnesota, 1967-1997. Arch Pediatric Adolesc Med 159:37-44, 2005.

55. Wiggins L, Baio J, Rice C: Examination of the time between first evaluation and first autism spectrum diagnosis in a population-based sample. J Dev Behav Pediatr 2006; 27:79-87.

55a. Autism and Developmental Disabilities Monitoring Network: Prevalence of autism spectrum disorders—Autism and Developmental Disabilities Monitoring Network, six sites, United States, 2000. Morb Mort Wkly Rep 56(SS-1):1, 2007.

55b. Autism and Developmental Disabilities Monitoring Network: Prevalence of autism spectrum disorders—Autism and Developmental Disabilities Monitoring Network, 14 sites, United States, 2002. Morb Mort Wkly Rep 56(SS-1):12, 2007.

55c. Van Naarden Braun K, Pettygrove S, Daniels J, et al: Evaluation of a methodology for a collaborative multiple source surveillance network for autism spectrum disorders—Autism and Developmental Disabilities Monitoring Network, 14 sites, United States, 2002. Morb Mort Wkly Rep 56(SS-1):29, 2007.

56. Centers for Disease Control and Prevention: Mental health in the United States: Parental report of diagnosed autism in children aged 4-17 years—United States, 2003-2004. Morb Mort Wkly Rep 55 (17): 481-486, 2006.

57. Williams JG, Higgins JPI, CEG Brayne: Systematic review of prevalence studies of autism spectrum disorders. Arch Dis Child 91:8-15, 2006.

58. Starr EM, Berument SK, Tomlins M, et al: Brief report: Autism in individuals with Down syndrome. J Autism Dev Disord 35:665-673, 2005.

59. Johansson M, Rastam M, Billstedt E, et al: Autism spectrum disorders and underlying brain pathology in CHARGE association. Dev Med Child Neurol 48:40-50, 2006.

60. Brown R, Hobson RP, Lee A, et al: Are there "autistic-like" features in congenitally blind children? J Child Psychol Psychiatry 38:693-703, 1997.

61. Hobson RP, Lee A, Brown R: Autism and congenital blindness. J Autism Dev Disord 29:45-56, 1999.

62. Education of All Handicapped Children Act, Public Law 94-142, 1975.

63. Americans with Disabilities Act of 1990, Public Law 101-336, 1990.

64. Individuals with Disabilities Education Act Amendments, Public Law 101-476, 1991.

65. Eagle RS: Commentary: Further commentary on the debate regarding increase in autism in California. J Autism Dev Disord 35:87, 2004.

66. Croen LA, Grether JK, Hoogstrate J, et al: The changing prevalence of autism in California. J Autism Dev Disord 32:207-215, 2002.

67. Palmer RF, Blanchard S, Carlos RJ, et al: School district resources and identification of children with autistic disorder. Am J Public Health 95:125-130, 2005.

68. Shattuck PT: The contribution of diagnostic substitution to the growing administrative prevalence of autism in US special education. Pediatrics 117:1028-1037, 2006.

69. Newschaffer CJ: Investigating diagnostic substitution and autism prevalence trends. Pediatrics 117:1436-1437, 2006.

70. MIND Institute: Report to the Legislature on the Principal Findings from the Epidemiology of Autism in California: A Comprehensive Pilot Study. Davis, CA: MIND Institute, University of California, 2002.

71. Blaxill MF, Baskin DS, Spitzer WO: Commentary: Blaxill, Baskin, and Spitzer on Croen et al (2002), The changing prevalence of autism in California. J Autism Dev Disord 33:223-226, 2003.

72. Individuals with Disabilities Education Act Amendments, Public Law 105-117, 1997.

73. Individuals with Disabilities Education Act Amendments, Public Law 108-446, 2004.

74. Wing L, Potter D: The epidemiology of autistic spectrum disorders: Is the prevalence rising? Ment Retard Dev Disabil Res Rev 8:151-161, 2002.

75. Autism mysteries: New clues. Harv Ment Health Lett 20(6):1-2, 2003.

76. Lingam R, Simmons A, Andrews N, et al: Prevalence of autism and parentally reported triggers in a north east London population. Arch Dis Child 88:666-670, 2003.

77. Gillberg C, Steffenburg S, Schaumann H: Is autism more common now than ten years ago? Br J Psychiatry 158:403-409, 1991.

78. Fombonne E: Is the prevalence of autism increasing? J Autism Dev Disord 6:672-676, 1996.

79. Fombonne E: The epidemiology of autism: a review. Psychol Med 29:769-786, 1999.

80. Blaxill MF, Redwood L, Bernard S: Thimerosal and autism? A plausible hypothesis that should not be dismissed. Med Hypotheses 62:788-794, 2004.

81. Geier DA, Geier MR: Early downward trends in neurodevelopmental disorders following removal of thimerosal-containing vaccines. J Am Physicians Surg 11:8-13, 2006.

81a. Geier DA, Geier MR: A comparative evaluation of the effects of MMR immunization and mercury doses from thimerosal-containing childhood vaccines on the population prevalence of autism. Med Sci Monit 10:PI33-PI39, 2004.

82. Kirby D: Mercury in vaccines and the autism epidemic: A medical controversy. *In* Kirby D, ed: Evidence of Harm. New York: St. Martin's Press, 2005.

83. Lotter V: Epidemiology of autistic conditions in young children: I. Prevalence. Soc Psychiatry 1:124-137, 1966.

84. Gillberg C, Wing L: Autism: Not an extremely rare disorder. Acta Psychiatr Scand 99:399-406, 1999.

85. Lord C, Schopler E: Differences in sex ratios in autism as a function of measured intelligence. J Autism Dev Disord 15:185-193, 1985.

86. Nordin V, Gillberg C: Autism spectrum disorders in children with physical or mental disability or both: Screening aspects. Dev Med Child Neurol 38:314-324, 1996.

87. Volkmar F, Chawarska K, Klin A: Autism in infancy and early childhood. Annu Rev Psychol 56:315-336, 2005.

88. Bailey A, Phillips W, Rutter M: Autism: Towards an integration of clinical, genetic, neuropsychological, and neurobiological perspectives. J Child Psychol Psychiatry 37:89-126, 1996.

89. Risch N, Spiker D, Lotspeich L, et al: A genomic screen of autism: Evidence for a multilocus etiology. Am J Hum Genet 65:493-507, 1999.

90. Le Courteur A, Rutter M, Lord C, et al: Autism diagnostic interview: A standardized investigator -based instrument. J Autism Dev Disord 19:363-387, 1989.

91. Monaco AP, Bailey AJ: Autism The search for susceptibility genes. Lancet 358:S3, 2001.

92. Muhle R, Trentacoste SV, Rapin I: The genetics of autism. Pediatrics 113:e472-e486, 2004.

93. Ylisaukko-oja T, Alarcon M, Cantor RM, et al: Search for autism loci by combined analysis of Autism Genetic Resource Exchange and Finnish families. Ann Neurol 59:145-155, 2006.

94. Goldson E: Autism spectrum disorders: An overview. Adv Pediatr 51:63-109, 2004.

95. Bauman ML, Kemper TL: Neuroanatomic observations of the brain in autism: A review and future directions. Int J Dev Neurosci 23:183-187, 2005.

96. McDougle CJ, Erickson CA, Stigler KA, et al: Neurochemistry in the pathophysiology of autism. J Clin Psychiatry 10:9-18, 2005.

97. A full genome screen for autism with evidence for linkage to a region on chromosome 7q. International

Molecular Genetic Study of Autism Consortium. Hum Mol Genet 7:571-578, 1998.

98. International Molecular Genetic Study of Autism Consortium (IMGSAC): A genomewide screen for autism: Strong evidence for linkage to chromosomes 2q, 7q, and 16p. Am J Hum Genet 69:570-581, 2001.

99. Cook EH: Genetics of autism. Child Adolesc Psychiatr Clin North Am 10:333-350, 2001.

100. Cook EH Jr, Courchesne RY, Cox NJ, et al: Linkage-disequilibrium mapping of autistic disorder, with 15q11-13 markers. Am J Hum Genet 62:1077-1083, 1998.

101. Gillberg C: Asperger syndrome and high functioning autism. Br J Psychiatry 172:200-209, 1998.

102. Korvatska, E, Van de Water J, Anders TF, et al: Genetic and immunologic considerations in autism. Neurobiol Dis 9:107-125, 2002 [erratum in Neurobiol Dis 10:69, 2002].

103. Buxbaum JD: The genetics of autism spectrum disorders. Medscape Psychiatry and Mental Health 10(2), 2005.

104. Battaglia A, Bonaglia MC: The yield of subtelomeric FISH analysis in the evaluation of autistic spectrum disorders. Am J Med Genet C Semin Med Genet 142:8-12, 2006.

105. Barton M, Volkmar F: How commonly are known medical conditions associated with autism? J Autism Dev Disord 28:273-278, 1998.

106. Fombonne E: Epidemiological trends in rates of autism. Mol Psychiatry 7:S4-S6, 2002.

107. Battaglia A, Carey JC: Etiologic yield of autistic spectrum disorders: A prospective study. Am J Med Genet C Semin Med Genet 142:3-7, 2006.

108. Rutter M, Bailey A, Bolton P, et al: Autism and known medical conditions: Myth and substance. J Child Psychol Psychiatry 35:311-322, 1994.

109. Challman TD, Barbaresi WF, Katusic SK, et al: The yield of the medical evaluation of children with pervasive developmental disorders. J Autism Dev Disord 33:187-192, 2003.

110. Shevell MI, Majnemer, A, Rosenbaum P, et al: Etiologic yield of autistic spectrum disorders: A prospective study. J Child Neurol 16:509-512, 2001.

111. Abdul-Rahman O, Hudgins L: The diagnostic utility of a genetics evaluation in children with pervasive developmental disorders. Genet Med 8:50-54, 2006.

112. Keller K, Williams C, Wharton P et al: Routine cytogenetic and FISH studies for 17p11/15q11 duplications and subtelomeric rearrangement studies in children with autistic spectrum disorders. Am J Med Genet 117A:105-111, 2003.

113. van Karnebeek CD, van Gelderen I, Nijof GJ, et al: An aetiological study of 25 mentally retarded adults with autism. J Med Genet 39:205-213, 2002.

114. Filipek PA, Accardo PJ, Baranek GT, et al: The screening and diagnosis of autistic spectrum disorders. J Autism Dev Disord 29:439-484, 1999.

115. Watson MS, Leckman JF, Annex B, et al: Fragile X in a survey of 75 autistic males. N Engl J Med 310:1462, 1984.

116. Hagerman PJ, Hagerman RJ: The fragile X premutation: A maturing perspective. Am J Med Genet 74:805-816, 2004.

117. Rogers SJ, Wehner DE, Hagerman R: The behavioral phenotype in fragile X: Symptoms of autism in very young children with fragile X syndrome, idiopathic autism, and other developmental disorders. J Dev Behav Pediatr 22:409-417, 2001.

118. Smalley SL: Autism and tuberous sclerosis. J Autism Dev Disord 28:407-414, 1998.

119. Baker P, Piven J, Sato Y: Autism and tuberous sclerosis complex: Prevalence and clinical features. J Autism Dev Disord 28:279-285, 1998.

120. Wiznitzer M: Autism and tuberous sclerosis. J Child neurol l19:675-679, 2004.

121. Baieli S, Pavone L, Meli C, et al: Autism and phenylketonuria. J Autism Dev Disord 33:201-204, 2003.

122. Wolpert CM, Menold MM, Bass MP, et al: Three probands with autistic disorder and isodicentric chromosome 15. Am J Med Genet 96:365-372, 2000.

123. Bolton PF, Dennis NR, Browne CE: The phenotypic manifestations of interstitial duplications of proximal 15q with special reference to the autistic spectrum disorders. Am J Med Genet 105:675-685, 2001.

124. Thatcher KN, Peddada S, Yasui DH, et al: Homologous pairing of 15q11-13 imprinted domains in brain is developmentally regulated but deficient in Rett and autism samples. Hum Mol Genet 14:785-797, 2005.

125. Lopez-Rangel E, Lewis ME: Do other methyl-binding proteins play a role in autism? Clin Genet 69:25, 2006.

126. Denmark JL, Feldman MA, Holden JA: Behavioral relationship between autism and fragile X syndrome. Am J Ment Retard 108:314-326, 2003.

127. Howlin P, Wing L, Gould J: The recognition of autism in children with Down syndrome—Implications for intervention and some speculations about pathology. Dev Med Child Neurol 37:406-414, 1995.

128. Kent L, Evans J, Paul M, et al: Comorbidity of autistic spectrum disorders in children with Down syndrome. Dev Med Child Neurol 41:153-158, 1999.

129. Fernell E, Olsson VA, Karlgren-Leitner C, et al: Autistic disorders in children with CHARGE association. Dev Med Child Neurol 41:270-272, 1999.

129a. Reichenberg A, Gross R, Weiser M, et al: Advancing paternal age and autism. Arch Gen Psychiatry 63:1026-1032, 2006.

130. Warren RP, Margaretten NC, Pace NC, et al: Immune abnormalities in patients with autism. J Autism Dev Disord 16:189-197, 1986.

131. Gupta S, Aggarwal S, Rashanravan B, et al: Th1- and Th2-like cytokines in CD4+ and CD8+ T cells in autism. J Neuroimmunol 85:106-109, 1998.

132. Plioplys AV, Greaves A, Kazemi K, et al: Lymphocyte function in autism and Rett syndrome. Neuropsychobiology 29:12-16, 1994.

133. Singh AB, Hiehle K, Singh M, et al: The host response in graft versus host disease. I. Radiosensitive T cells of host origin inhibit parental anti-F1 cytotoxicity in murine chronic graft versus host disease. Cell Immunol 151:24-38, 1993.

134. Rumsey JM, Ernst M: Functional neuroimaging of autistic disorders. Ment Retard Dev Disabil Res Rev 6:171-179, 2000.

135. Stern L, Francoeur MJ, Primeau MN, et al: Immune function in autistic children. Ann Allergy Asthma Immunol 95:558-565, 2005.

136. Comi AM, Zimmerman AW, Frye VH, et al: Familial clustering of autoimmune disorders and evaluation of medical risk factors in autism. J Child Neurol 14:388-394, 1999.

137. Bidet B, Leboyer M, Descours B, et al: Allergic sensitization in infantile autism. J Autism Dev Disord 23:419-420, 1993.

138. Renzoni E, Beltrami V, Sestini P, et al: Brief report: Allergological evaluation of children with autism. J Autism Dev Disord 25:327-333, 1995.

139. Myers SM, Challman TD: Psychopharmacology: An approach to management in autism and mental retardation. *In* Accardo PJ, ed: Capute & Accardo's Neurodevelopmental Disabilities in Infancy and Childhood, 3rd ed. Baltimore: Paul H. Brookes, in press.

140. Asherson PJ, Curran S: Approaches to gene mapping in complex disorders and their application in child psychiatry and psychology. Br J Psychiatry 179:122-128, 2001.

141. London EA: The environment as an etiologic factor in autism: A new direction for research. Environ Health Perspect 108:401-404, 2000.

142. Bristol MM, Cohen DJ, Costello EJ, et al: State of the science in autism: Report to the National Institutes of Health. J Autism Dev Disord 26:121-154, 1996.

143. Kemper TL, Bauman M: Neuropathology of infantile autism. J Neuropathol Exp Neurol 57:645-652, 1998.

144. Rodier PM: The early origins of autism. Sci Am 282:56-63, 2000.

145. Chess S, Korn SJ, Fernandez PB: Psychiatric Disorders of Children with Congenital Rubella. New York: Brunner Mazel, 1971.

146. Stubbs EG, Ash E, Williams CP: Autism and congenital cytomegalovirus. J Autism Dev Disord 14:183-189, 1984.

147. Yamashita Y, Fujimoto C, Nakajima E, et al: Possible association between congenital cytomegalovirus infection and autistic disorder. J Autism Dev Disord 33:455-459, 2003.

148. Moore SJ, Turnpenny P, Quinn A, et al: A clinical study of 57 children with fetal anticonvulsant syndrome. J Med Genet 37:489-497, 2000.

149. Williams G, King J, Cunningham M, et al: Fetal valproate syndrome and autism: Additional evidence of an association. Dev Med Child Neurol 43:202-206, 2001.

150. Stromland K, Nordin V, Miller M, et al: Autism in thalidomide embryopathy: A population study. Dev Med Child Neurol 36:351-356, 1994.

151. Nelson KB, Grether JK, Croen LA, et al: Neuropeptides and neurotrophins in neonatal blood of children with autism or mental retardation. Ann Neurol 49:597-606, 2001.

152. Lauritsen MB, Pedersen CB, Mortensen PB: Effects of familial risk factors and place of birth on the risk of autism: A nationwide register-based study. J Child Psychol Psychiatry 46:963-971, 2005.

153. Palmer RF, Blanchard S, Stein Z, et al: Environmental mercury release, special education rates, and autism disorder: An ecological study of Texas. Health Place 12:203-209, 2006.

154. Badawi N, Kurinczuk U, Keogh JM, et al: Antepartum risk factors for newborn encephalopathy: The Western Australian case-control study. BMJ 317:1549-1553, 1998.

155. Badawi N, Kurinczuk U, Keogh JM, et al: Intrapartum risk factors for newborn encephalopathy: The Western Australian case-control study. BMJ 317:1554-1558, 1998.

156. Juul-Dam N, Townsend J, Courchesne E: Prenatal, perinatal, and neonatal factors in autism, pervasive developmental disorder–not otherwise specified, and the general population. Pediatrics 107:e63, 2001.

157. Klug MG, Burd L, Kerbeshian J, et al: A comparison of the effects of parental risk markers on pre- and perinatal variables in multiple patient cohorts with fetal alcohol syndrome, autism, Tourette syndrome and sudden death syndrome: An enviromic analysis. Neurotoxicol Teratol 25:707-717, 2003.

158. Glasson FJ, Bower C, Petterson B, et al: Perinatal factors and the development of autism: A population study. Arch Gen Psychiatry 61:618-627, 2004.

159. Badawi N, Dixon G, Felix JF, et al: Autism following a history of newborn encephalopathy: More than a coincidence? Dev Med Child Neurol 48(2):85-89, 2006.

160. Tsai L, Stewart MA, Faust M, et al: Social class distribution of fathers of children enrolled in the Iowa Autism Program. J Autism Dev Disord 12:211-221, 1982.

161. Rutter M, Anderson-Wood L, Beckett C, et al: Quasi-autistic patterns following severe early global privation. English and Romanian Adoptees (ERA) Study Team. J Child Psychol Psychiatry 40:537-549, 1999.

162. Wakefield AJ, Murch SH, Anthony A, et al: Ileal-lymphoid-nodular hyperplasia, non-specific colitis, and pervasive developmental disorder in children. Lancet 351:637-641, 1998.

163. Stratton K, Gable A, Shetty P, et al, eds: Immunization Safety Review: Measles-Mumps-Rubella Vaccine and Autism. Washington, DC: Institute of Medicine, National Academies Press, 2001.

164. Halsey NA, Hyman SL, the Conference Writing Panel: Measles-mumps-rubella vaccine and autistic spectrum disorder: Report from the New Challenges in Childhood Immunizations Conference convened in Oak Brook, Illinois, June 12-13, 2000. Pediatrics 107(5):e84, 2001. (Available at: *http://www.pediatrics.org/cgi/content/full/107/5/e84;* accessed 12/29/06.)

165. British Medical Research Council: Review of Autism Research: Epidemiology and Causes. London: British Medical Research Council, 2001.

166. Demicheli V, Jefferson T, Rivetti A, et al: Vaccines for measles, mumps and rubella in children. Cochrane Database Syst Rev (4):CD004407, 2005.

167. Horton R: A statement by the editors of The Lancet. Lancet 363:820-824, 2004.

168. Richler J, Luyster R, Risi S, et al: Is there a "regressive phenotype" of autism spectrum disorder associated with the measles-mumps-rubella vaccine? A CPEA study. J Autism Dev Disord 36:299-316, 2006.

169. Stehr-Green P, Tull P, Stellfeld M, et al: Autism and thimerosal-containing vaccines: Lack of consistent evidence for an association. Am J Prevent Med 25:101-106, 2003.

170. Institute of Medicine, Board on Health Promotion and Disease Prevention, Immunization Safety Review Committee: Immunization Safety Review: Vaccines and Autism. Washington, DC: National Academies Press, 2004.

171. DeStefano F, Bhasin TK, Thompson WW, et al: Age at first measles-mumps-rubella vaccination in children with autism and school matched control subjects: A population-based study in metropolitan Atlanta. Pediatrics 113:259-266, 2004.

172. Nelson KB, Bauman ML: Thimerosal and autism? Pediatrics 111:674-679, 2003.

173. Bauman M, Perrin J: Emerging Medical Practices in Autism Care and Treatment (EMPACT). Presented at conference sponsored by Autism Network Conference, Chicago, IL, September 2005.

174. Deykin EY, MacMahon B: The incidence of seizures among children with autistic symptoms. Am J Psychiatry 136:1312-1313, 1979.

175. Bauman ML, Kemper TL: Is autism a progressive process? Neurology 48:285, 1997.

176. Minshew NJ, Sweeney JA, Bauman ML, et al: Neurologic aspects of autism. *In* Volkmar FR, Paul R, Klin A, et al, eds: Handbook of Autism and Pervasive Developmental Disorders, 3rd ed, vol 1. Hoboken, NJ: Wiley, 2005, pp 473-514.

177. Bauman ML, Kemper TL: Histoanatomic observations of the brain in early infantile autism. Neurology 35:866-874, 1985.

178. Anderson GM, Hoshino Y: Neurochemical studies of autism. *In* Volkmar FR, Paul R, Klin A, et al, eds: Handbook of Autism and Pervasive Developmental Disorders, 3rd ed, vol 1. Hoboken, NJ: Wiley, 2005, pp 453-472.

179. Polleux F, Lauder JM: Toward a developmental neurobiology of autism. Ment Retard Dev Disabil Res Rev 10:303-317, 2004.

180. Tuchman R, Rapin I: Epilepsy in autism. Lancet Neurol 1:352-358, 2002.

181. Belmonte MK, Cook EH, Anderson GM, et al: Autism as a disorder of neural information processing: Directions for research and targets for therapy. Mol Psychiatry 9:646-663, 2004.

182. Piven J, Nehme E, Simon J, et al: Magnetic resonance imaging in autism: Measurement of the cerebellum, pons, and fourth ventricle. Biol Psychiatry 31:491-504, 1992.

183. Filipek PA, Richelme C, Kennedy DN, et al: Morphometric analysis of the brain in developmental language disorders and autism. Ann Neurol 32:475, 1992.

184. Lainhart JE, Piven J, Wzorek H, et al: Macrocephaly in children and adults with autism. J Am Acad Child Adolesc Psychiatry 36:282-290, 1997.

185. Courchesne E, Karns CM, Davis HR, et al: Unusual brain growth patterns in early life in patients with autistic disorder: An MRI study. Neurology 57:245-254, 2001.

186. Courchesne E, Carper R, Akshoomoff N: Evidence of brain overgrowth in the first year of life in autism. JAMA 290:337-344, 2003 [comment, JAMA 290:393-394, 2003].

187. Tuchman R: Autism. Neurol Clin North Am 21:915-932, 2003.

188. Dementieva YA, Vance DD, Donnelly SL, et al: Accelerated head growth in early development of individuals with autism. Pediatr Neurol 32:102-108, 2005.

189. Aylward EH, Minshew NJ, Field K, et al: Effects of age on brain volume and head circumference in autism. Neurology 59:175-183, 2002 [comment, Neurology 59:158-159, 2002].

190. Redcay E, Courchesne E: When is the brain enlarged in autism? A meta-analysis of all brain size reports. Biol Psychiatry 58:1-9, 2005.

191. Hardan AY, Jou RJ, Keshavan MS, et al: Increased frontal cortical folding in autism: A preliminary MRI study. Psychiatry Res 131:263-268, 2004.

192. Herbert MR, Ziegler DA, Deutsch CK, et al: Dissociations of cerebral cortex, subcortical and cerebral white matter volumes in autistic boys. Brain 126:1182-1192, 2003.

193. Herbert MR, Ziegler DA, Makris, et al: Localization of white matter volume increase in autism and developmental language disorder. Ann Neurol 55:530-540, 2004.

194. Palmen SJMC, van Engeland H, Hof PR, et al: Neuropathological findings in autism. Brain 127:2572-2583, 2004.

195. Nyden A, Carlsson M, Carlsson A, et al: Interhemispheric transfer in high-functioning children and adolescents with autism spectrum disorders: A controlled pilot study. Dev Med Child Neurol 46:448-454, 2004.

196. Ritvo ER, Freeman BJ, Scheibel AB, et al: Lower Purkinje cell counts in the cerebella of four autistic subjects: Initial findings of the UCLA-NSAC Autopsy Research Report. Am J Psychiatry 143:862-866, 1986.

197. Kinnear KJ: Purkinje cell vulnerability and autism: A possible etiological connection. Brain Dev 25:377-382, 2003.

198. Scherer SW, Cheung J, MacDonald JR, et al: Human chromosome 7: DNA sequence and biology. Science 300:767-772, 2003.

199. Courchesne E, Townsend JP, Akshoomoff NA, et al: Impairment in shifting attention in autistic and cerebellar patients. Behav Neurosci 108:848-865, 1994.

200. Schumann CM, Hamstra J, Goodlin-Jones BL, et al: The amygdala is enlarged in children but not adults

with autism: The hippocampus is enlarged at all ages. J Neurosci 24:6392-6401, 2004.

201. Sparks BF, Friedman SD, Shaw DW, et al: Brain structural abnormalities in young children with autism spectrum disorder. Neurology 59:184-192, 2002.

202. Bailey A, Luthert P, Dean A, et al: A clinicopathological study of autism. Brain 121:889-905, 1998.

203. Casanova MF, Buxhoeveden DP, Switala AE, et al: Minicolumnar pathology in autism. Neurology 58:428-432, 2002.

204. Buxhoeveden DP, Semendeferi K, Schenker N, et al: Decreased Cell Column Spacing in Autism [Abstract 582.6]. Presented at the 34th annual meeting of the Society for Neuroscience, San Diego, California, October 23-27, 2004.

205. Rojas DC, Bawn SD, Benkers TL, et al: Smaller left hemisphere planum temporale in adults with autistic disorder. Neurosci Lett 328:237-240, 2002.

206. Escalante-Mead PR, Minshew NJ, Sweeney JA: Abnormal brain lateralization in high-functioning autism. J Autism Dev Disord 33:539-543, 2003.

207. Schultz RT, Robins DL: Functional neuroimaging studies of autism spectrum disorders. *In* Volkmar FR, Paul R, Klin A, et al, eds: Handbook of Autism and Pervasive Developmental Disorders, 3rd ed, vol 1. Hoboken, NJ: Wiley, 2005, pp 515-533.

208. Klin A, Jones W, Schultz R, et al: The enactive mind, or from actions to cognition: Lessons from autism. Philos Trans R Soc Lond B Biol Sci 358:345-360, 2003.

209. Schultz RT, Grelotti DJ, Klin A, et al: The role of the fusiform face area in social cognition: Implications for the pathobiology of autism. Philos Trans R Soc Lond B Biol Sci 358:415-427, 2003.

210. Wang TA, Dapretto M, Hariri AR, et al: Neural correlates of facial affect processing in children and adolescents with autism spectrum disorder. J Am Acad Child Adolesc Psychiatry 43:481-490, 2004.

211. Klin A, Jones W, Schultz R, et al: Defining and quantifying the social phenotype in autism. Am J Psychiatry 159:895-908, 2002.

212. Klin A, Jones W, Schultz R, et al: Visual fixation patterns during viewing of naturalistic social situations as predictors of social competence in individuals with autism. Arch Gen Psychiatry 59:809-816, 2002.

213. Chugani DC, Muzik O, Behen M, et al: Developmental changes in brain serotonin synthesis capacity in autistic and nonautistic children. Ann Neurol 45:287-295, 1999.

214. Pickett J: Mapping the neuropathology of autism: The Brain Atlas Project. NAAARATIVE (Summer):4-5, 2003.

215. Stone WL: Can autism be diagnosed accurately in children under 3 years? J Child Psychol Psychiatry 40:219-226, 1999.

216. Howlin P, Moore A: Diagnosis in autism. A survey of over 1200 patients in the UK. Autism 1:135-162, 1997.

217. Howlin P, Asgharian A: The diagnosis of autism and Asperger syndrome: Findings from a survey of 770 families. Dev Med Child Neurol 41:834-839, 1999.

218. Zwaigenbaum L, Bryson S, Rogers T, et al: Behavioral manifestations of autism in the first year of life. Int J Dev Neurosci 23:143-152, 2005.

219. Tuchman RF, Rapin I: Regression in pervasive developmental disorders: Seizures and epileptiform electroencephalogram correlates. Pediatrics 99:560-566, 1997.

220. Werner E, Dawson G: Validation of the phenomenon of autistic regression using home videotapes. Arch Gen Psychiatry 62:889-895, 2005.

221. Osterling J, Dawson G: Early recognition of children with autism: A study of first birthday home videotapes. J Autism Dev Disord 24:247-257, 1994.

222. Baranek GT: Autism during infancy: A retrospective video analysis of sensory-motor and social behaviors at 9-12 months of age. J Autism Dev Disord 29:213-224, 1999.

223. Maestro S, Muratori F, Cristina M, et al: Attentional skills during the first 6 months of age in autism spectrum disorder. J Am Acad Child Adolesc Psychiatry 41:1239-1245, 2002.

224. Johnson CP: Early Clinical characteristics of children with autism: *In* Gupta VB, ed: Autism Spectrum Disorders in Children. New York: Marcel Dekker, 2004, pp 85-123.

225. Johnson CP: Very early signs of autism spectrum disorders. Pediatr Rev, in press.

226. Sigman M, Dijamco A, Gratier M, et al: Early detection of core deficits in autism. Ment Retard Dev Disabil Res Rev 10:221-233, 2004.

227. Chawarska K, Volkmar FR: Autism in infancy and early childhood. *In* Volkmar FR, Paul R, Klin A, et al, eds: Handbook of Autism and Pervasive Developmental Disorders, 3rd ed, vol 1. Hoboken, NJ: Wiley, 2005, pp 223-246.

228. Rogers SJ, Benneto L: Intersubjectivity in autism. *In* Wetherby AM, Prizant BM, eds: Autism Spectrum Disorders. Baltimore: Paul H. Brookes, 2000, pp 84-97.

229. Wetherby A, Watt N, Morgan L, et al: Social communication profiles of children with autism spectrum disorders late in the second year of life. J Autism Dev Disord Oct 26, 2006 [Epub ahead of print].

230. Mundy P, Markus J: On the nature of communication and language impairment in autism. Ment Retard Dev Disabil Res Rev 3:343-349, 1997.

231. Turner LM, Stone WL, Pozdol SL, et al: Follow-up of children with autism spectrum disorders from age 2-9. Autism 10:257-279, 2006.

232. Charman T: Why is joint attention a pivotal skill in autism? Philos Trans R Soc Lond B Biol Sci 358:315-324, 2003.

233. Chawarska K, Klin A, Volkmar FR: Automatic attention cueing through eye movement in 2-year-old children with autism. Child Dev 74:1108-1122, 2003.

234. Dawson G, Munson J, Estes A, et al: Neurocognitive function and joint attention ability in young children with autism spectrum disorder versus developmental delay. Child Dev 73:345-358, 2002.

235. Klin A, Saulnier C, Tsatsanis K, et al: Clinical evaluation in autism spectrum disorders: Psychological

assessment within a transdisciplinary framework. *In* Volkmar FR, Paul R, Klin A, et al, eds: Handbook of Autism and Pervasive Developmental Disorders, 3rd ed, vol 2. Hoboken, NJ: Wiley, 2005, pp 772-798.

236. Mundy P, Card J, Fox N: EEG correlates of the development of infant joint attention skills. Dev Psychobiol 36:325-338, 2000.

237. Paparella T, Kasari C: Joint attention skills and language development in special needs populations: Translating research to practice. Infants Young Child 17:269-280, 2004.

238. Lord C: Follow-up of two year-olds referred for possible autism. J Child Psychol Psychiatry 36:1365-1382, 1995.

239. Mundy P: Joint attention, social-emotional approach in children with autism. Dev Psychopathol 7:63-82, 1995.

240. Leekam S, Lopez B: Attention and joint attention in preschool children with autism. Dev Psychol 36:261-273, 2000.

241. Wetherby AM, Prizant BM, Hutchinson TA: Communicative, social/affective and symbolic profiles of young children with autism and pervasive developmental disorders. Am J Speech Lang Pathol 7:79-91, 1998.

242. Dawson G, Hill D, Spencer A, et al: Affective exchanges between young autistic children and their mothers. J Abnorm Child Psychol 18:335-345, 1990.

243. Happé F: Studying weak central coherence at log levels: Children with autism do not succumb to visual illusions. A research note. J Child Psychol Psychiatry 37:873-877, 1996.

244. Briskman J, Happé F: Exploring the cognitive phenotype of autism: Weak "central coherence" in parents and siblings of children with autism: II. Real life skills and preferences. J Child Psychol Psychiatry 42:309-316, 2001.

245. Baron-Cohen S, Leslie AM, Frith U: Does the autistic child have a "theory of mind"? Cognition 21:37-46, 1985.

246. Baron-Cohen S: Mindblindness. Cambridge, MA: MIT Press, 1995.

247. Twachtman-Cullen D: More able children with autism spectrum disorders. *In* Wetherby AM, Prizant BM, eds: Autism Spectrum Disorders. Baltimore: Paul H. Brookes, 2000, pp 225-246.

248. Astington JW, Barriault T: Children's theory of mind: How young children come to understand that people have thoughts and feelings. Infants Young Child 13:1-12, 2001.

249. Wetherby AM, Prizant BM, Schuler AL: Understanding the nature of communication and language impairments. *In* Wetherby AM, Prizant BM, eds: Autism Spectrum Disorders: A Developmental Transactional Perspective. Baltimore: Paul H. Brookes, 2000, pp 109-141.

250. Yirmiya N, Erel O, Shaked M, et al: Meta-analysis comparing theory of mind abilities of individual with autism, individuals with mental retardation, and normally developing individuals. Psychol Bull 124:283-307, 1998.

251. Lord C, Shulman C, DiLavore P: Regression and word loss in autism spectrum disorders. J Child Psychol Psychiatry 45:1-21, 2004.

252. Schroeder SR: Self-injurious behavior. Ment Retard Dev Disabil Res Rev 7:3-11, 2001.

253. Williams DL, Goldstein G, Carpenter PA, et al: Verbal and spatial working memory in autism. J Autism Dev Disord 35:1-10, 2005.

397. Grandin T, Scariano M: Emergence: Labeled Autistic. Novato, CA: Arena, 1986.

255. Hartman S, reporter: "Autistic player scores 20 points in 4 minutes." CBS News, March 2006. (Available at: *http://thatvideosite.com/video/1688;* accessed 12/29/06.)

256. Iarocci G, McDonald J: Sensory integration and the perceptual experience of persons with autism. J Autism Devel Disorders 36:77-90, 2006.

257. Anzalone ME, Williamson G: Sensory processing and motor performance in autism spectrum disorders. *In* Wetherby AM, Prizant BM, eds: Autism Spectrum Disorders. Baltimore: Paul H. Brookes, 2000, pp 143-166.

258. Gillberg C, Kadesjo B: Why bother about clumsiness? The implications of having developmental coordination disorder (DCD). Neural Plast 10:59-68, 2003.

259. Siegel B, Pliner C, Eschler J, et al: How children with autism are diagnosed: Difficulties in identification of children with multiple developmental delays. J Dev Behav Pediatr 9:199-204, 1988.

260. Council on Children with Disabilities, Section on Developmental Behavioral Pediatrics, Bright Futures Steering Committee, Medical Home Initiatives for Children with Special Needs Project Advisory Committee: Identifying infants and young children with developmental disorders in the medical home: An algorithm for developmental surveillance and screening. Pediatrics 118:405-420, 2006 [erratum in Pediatrics 118:1808-1809, 2006].

261. Gupta VB, Hyman SL, Plauché Johnson C: Identifying children with autism early? Pediatrics 119:152-153, 2007.

262. Johnson CP, Myers S, for AAP Council on Children with Disabilities and the AAP Autism Expert Panel: Identification and evaluation of children with autism spectrum disorders. Pediatrics, in press.

262a. Myers S, Johnson CP, for AAP Council on Children with Disabilities and the AAP Autism Expert Panel: Management of children with autism spectrum disorder. Pediatrics, in press.

263. Coonrod EE, Stone WL: Screening for autism in young children. *In* Volkmar FR, Paul R, Klin A, et al, eds: Handbook of Autism and Pervasive Developmental Disorders, 3rd ed, vol 2. Hoboken, NJ: Wiley, 2005, pp 707-729.

264. Lord C, Corsello C: Diagnostic instruments in autistic spectrum disorders. *In* Volkmar FR, Paul R, Klin A, et al, eds: Handbook of Autism and Pervasive Developmental Disorders, 3rd ed, vol 2. Hoboken, NJ: Wiley, 2005, pp 730-771.

265. Baird G, Charman T, Baron-Cohen S: A screening instrument for autism at 18 months of age: A 6-year

follow-up study. J Am Acad Child Adolesc Psychiatry 39:694-702, 2000.

266. Baron-Cohen S, Allen J, Gillberg C: Can autism be detected at 18 months? The needle, the haystack, and the CHAT. Br J Psychiatry 161:839-843, 1992.

267. Baron-Cohen S, Cox A, Baird G: Psychological markers in the detection of autism in infancy in a large population. Br J Psychiatry 168:158-163, 1996.

268. Baron-Cohen S, Wheelwright S, Hill J, et al: The "Reading the Mind in the Eyes" revised version: A study with normal adults, and adults with Asperger syndrome or high-functioning autism. J Child Psychol Psychiatry 42:241-251, 2001.

269. Charman T, Baird G: Practicioner review: Diagnosis of autism spectrum disorder in 2- and 3-year-old children. J Child Psychol Psychiatry 43:289-305, 2002.

270. Dumont-Mathieu T, Fein D: Screening for autism in young children: The Modified Checklist for Autism in Toddlers (M-CHAT) and other measures. Ment Retard Dev Disabil Res Rev 11:253-262, 2005.

271. Robins D, Fein D, Barton M, et al: The Modified-Checklist for Autism in Toddlers (M-CHAT): An initial investigation in the early detection of autism and pervasive developmental disorders. J Autism Dev Disord 31:131-144, 2001.

272. Scambler D, Rogers SJ, Wehner EA: Can the Checklist for Autism in Toddlers differentiate young children with autism from those with developmental delays? J Am Acad Child Adolesc Psychiatry 40:1457-1463, 2001.

273. Siegel B: The Pervasive Developmental Disorders Screening Test II (PDDST-II). San Antonio, TX: Harcourt Assessment, 2004.

274. Stone WL, Coonrod EE, Ousley OY: Screening Tool for Autism in Two-Year-Olds (STAT): Development and preliminary data. J Autism Dev Disord 30:607-612, 2000.

275. Stone WL, Coonrod EE, Turner LM, et al: Psychometric properties of the STAT for early autism screening. J Autism Dev Disord 34:691-701, 2004.

276. Wong V, Hui L, Lee W, et al: A modified screening tool for autism (Checklist for Autism in Toddlers [CHAT-23]) for Chinese children. Pediatrics 114:166-176, 2004.

277. Krug DA, Arick JR, Almond PJ: Behavior checklist for identifying severely handicapped individuals with high levels of autistic behavior. J Child Psychol Psychiatry 21:221-229, 1980.

278. Eaves RC, Milner B: The criterion-related validity of the Childhood Autism Rating Scale and the Autism Behavior Checklist. J Abnorm Child Psychol 21:481-491, 1993.

279. Schopler E: A new approach to autism. Soc Sci 7:2-3, 1986.

280. Schopler E, Reichler RJ, Rochen-Renner B: The Childhood Autism Rating Scale (CARS). Los Angeles: Western Psychological Services, 1988.

281. Sevin JA, Matson JL, Coe DA, et al: A comparison and evaluation of three commonly used autism scales. J Autism Dev Disord 21:417-432, 1991.

282. Gilliam JE: Gilliam Autism Rating Scale (GARS). Austin, TX: Pro-Ed, 1995.

283. Berument S K, Rutter M, Lord C, et al: Autism Screening Questionnaire: Diagnostic validity. Br J Psychiatry 175:444-451, 1999.

284. Lecavalier L: An evaluation of the Gilliam Autism Rating Scale. J Aut Devel Disord 35:795-805, 2005.

285. South M, Williams BJ, McMahon WM, et al: Utility of the Gilliam autism rating scale in research and clinical populations. J Autism Dev Disord 32:593-599, 2002.

286. Bishop DVM, Norbury CF: Exploring the borderlands of autistic disorder and specific language impairment: A study using standardized diagnostic instruments. J Child Psychol Psychiatry 43:1-13, 2002.

287. Dietz C, Willemsen-Swinkels SHN, Buitelaar JK, et al: Early detection of autism: Population screening. Poster presented at the biennial meeting of the Society for Research in Child Development, Albuquerque, NM, April 1999.

288. Willemsen-Swinkels SHN, Buiitelaar JK, Dietz C, et al: Screening instrument for the early detection of autism at 14 months. Poster presented at the biennial meeting of the Society for Research in Child Development, Albuquerque, NM, April 1999.

289. Wetherby AM, Woods J, Allen L, et al: Early indicators of autism spectrum disorders in the second year of life. J Autism Dev Disord 34:473-493, 2004.

290. American Speech-Language-Hearing Association: Roles and Responsibilities of Speech-Language Pathologists in Diagnosis, Assessment, and Treatment of Autism Spectrum Disorders across the Life Span: Position Statement. 2006. (Available at: *http://www.asha. org/NR/rdonlyres/4C2593BF-6920-4B44-BD0D-6067A65AEDDB/0/v3PS_autismLSpan.pdf;* accessed 12/30/06.)

291. American Speech-Language-Hearing Association: Principles for Speech-Language Pathologists in Diagnosis, Assessment, and Treatment of Autism Spectrum Disorders across the Life Span: Technical Report. 2006. (Available at: *http://www.asha.org/NR/rdonlyres/ D0370FEA-98EF-48EE-A9B6-952913FB131B/0/v3TR_ autismLSpan.pdf;* accessed 12/30/06.)

292. Ballaban-Gil K, Tuchman R: Epilepsy and epileptiform EEG: Association with autism and language disorders. Ment Retard Dev Disabil Res Rev 6:300-308, 2000.

293. Shannon M, Graef JW: Lead intoxication in children with pervasive developmental disorders. J Toxicol Clin Toxicol 34:177-182, 1997.

294. Gillberg C, Coleman M: Autism and medical disorder: A review of the literature. Dev Med Child Neurol 38:191-202, 1996.

295. Rapin I: Preschool children with inadequate communication: Developmental language disorder, autism, low IQ. *In* Rapin I, ed: Neurological Examination. London: Mac-Keith Press, 1996, pp 98-122.

296. Freeman BJ, Pegeen C: Diagnosing autism spectrum disorder in young children: An update. Infants Young Child 14(3):1-10, 2002.

297. Voigt RG, Childers D, Dickerson CL, et al: Early pediatric neurodevelopmental profile of children with autistic spectrum disorders. Clin Pediatr 39:663-668, 2000.

298. Tervo RC: Identifying patterns of developmental delays can help diagnose neurodevelopmental disorders. Clin Pediatr 45:509-517, 2006.

299. Bayley N: Bayley Scales of Infant Development—2nd ed. San Antonio, TX: Psychological Corporation, 1997.

300. Bayley N: Bayley Scales of Infant Development—3rd ed. San Antonio, TX: Psychological Corporation, 2003.

301. Mullen EM: Mullen Scales of Early Learning, AGS Edition. Bloomington, MN: American Guidance Service, 1995.

302. Voigt RG, Dickerson CL, Reynolds AM, et al: Laboratory evaluation of children with autistic spectrum disorders: A guide for primary care pediatricians. Clin Pediatr 39:669-671, 2000.

303. Hoon AH, Pulsifer MB, Gopalan R, et al: Clinical adaptive test/clinical linguistic and auditory milestone scale in early cognitive assessment. J Pediatr 123:S1-S8, 1993.

304. Capute AJ, Accardo PJ: The Infant Neurodevelopmental Assessment: A clinical interpretive manual for CAT-CLAMS in the first two years of life, part 2. Curr Prob Pediatr 26:279-306, 1996.

305. Allen MC: Neurodevelopmental assessment of the young child: The state of the art. Ment Retard Dev Disabil Res Rev 11:274-275, 2005.

306. Paul R: Assessing communication in autism spectrum disorders. *In* Volkmar FR, Paul R, Klin A, et al, eds: Handbook of Autism and Pervasive Developmental Disorders, 3rd ed, vol 2. Hoboken, NJ: Wiley, 2005, pp 799-816.

307. Baranek GT, Parham LD, Bodfish JW: Sensory and motor features in autism: Assessment and intervention. *In* Volkmar FR, Paul R, Klin A, et al, eds: Handbook of Autism and Pervasive Developmental Disorders, 3rd ed, vol 2. Hoboken, NJ: Wiley, 2005, pp 831-862.

308. Leiter RG: Leiter International Performance Scale. Chicago: Stoelting, 1948.

309. Shah A, Holmes N: Brief report: The use of the Leiter International Performance Scale with children. J Autism Dev Disord 15:195-203, 1985.

310. Tsatsanis KD, Dartnall N, Cicchetti D, et al: Concurrent validity and classification accuracy of the Leiter and Leiter-R in low-functioning children with autism. J Autism Dev Disord 33:23-30, 2003.

311. Lichtenberger EO: General measures of cognition for the preschool child. Ment Retard Dev Disabil Res Rev 11:197-208, 2005.

312. Roid GM, Miller LJ: Leiter International Performance Scale–Revised: Examiner's manual, Wood Dale, IL: Stoelting, 1997.

313. Vig S, Jedrysek E: Autistic features in young children with significant cognitive impairment: Autism or mental retardation? J Autism Dev Disord 29:235-248, 1999.

314. American Association on Mental Retardation (*In* Luckasson RA, Schalock RL, Spitalnik DM, et al, eds): Mental Retardation: Definition, Classification, and Systems of Support, 10th ed. Washington, DC: American Association on Mental Retardation, 2002, pp 73-93.

315. Sparrow SS, Balla D, Cicchetti D: Vineland Adaptive-Behavior Scales. Bloomington, MN: American Guidance Service, 1984.

316. Volkmar FR, Carter A, Sparrow SS, et al: Quantifying social development in autism. J Am Acad Child Adolesc Psychiatry 32:627-632, 1993.

317. Carter A, Volkmar FR, Sparrow SS, et al: The Vineland Adaptive Behavior Scales: Supplementary norms for individuals with autism. J Autism Dev Disord 28:287-302, 1998.

318. Sparrow SS, Falla DA, Cicchetti DV: Vineland Social Emotional Early Childhood Scales. Cirle Pines, NM: American Guidance Service, 1998.

319. Volkmar FR, Sparrow SS, Goudreau D, et al: Social deficits in autism: An operational approach using the Vineland Adaptive Behavior Scales. J Am Acad Child Adolesc Psychiatry 26:156-161, 1987.

320. Freeman BJ, Del'Homme M, Guthrie D, et al: Vineland Adaptive Behavior Scale scores as a function of age and initial IQ in 210 autistic children. J Autism Dev Disord 29:379-384, 1999.

321. Filipek PA: Neuroimaging in the developmental disorders: The state of the science. J Child Psychol Psychiatry 40:113-128, 1999.

322. O'Brien G, Pearson J, Berney T, et al: Measuring behaviour in developmental disability: A review of existing schedules. Dev Med Child Neurol Suppl 87:1-72, 2001.

323. California Department of Developmental Services: Autistic Spectrum Disorders: Best Practice Guidelines for Screening, Diagnosis and Assessment. 2002. (Available at: *http://www.ddhealthinfo.org/pdf/ASD-Guidelines1.pdf;* accessed 12/30/06.)

324. Schopler E, Reichler RJ, Bashford A, et al: The Psychoeducational Profile Revised (PEP-R). Austin, TX: Pro-Ed, 1990.

325. Schopler E, Lansing MD, Reichler RJ, et al: Pyschoeducational Profile—Third Edition. Austin, TX: Pro-Ed, 2005.

326. Rellini E, Tortolani D, Trillo S, et al: Childhood Autism Rating Scale (CARS) and Autism Behavior Checklist (ABC) correspondence and conflicts with *DSM-IV* criteria in diagnosis of autism. J Autism Dev Disord 6:703-708, 2004.

327. Wing L, Leekam SR, Libby SJ, et al: The diagnostic interview for social and communication disorders: Background, inter-rater reliability and clinical use. J Child Psychol Psychiatry 43:307-325, 2002.

328. Leekam SR, Libby SJ, Wing L, et al: The Diagnostic Interview for Social and Communication Disorders: Algorithms for ICD-10 childhood autism and Wing and Gould autistic spectrum disorder. J Child Psychol Psychiatry 43:327-342, 2002.

329. Lord C, Rutter M, Le Couteur A: Autism Diagnostic Interview–Revised: A revised version of a diagnostic interview for caregivers of individuals with possible pervasive developmental disorders. J Autism Dev Disord 24:659-685, 1994.

330. Lord C, Risi S, Lambrecht L: The Autism Diagnostic Observation Schedule–Generic: A standard measure

of social and communication deficits associated with the spectrum of autism. J Autism Dev Disord 30:205-223, 2000.

331. Lord C, Rutter M, Goode S: Autism Diagnostic Observation Schedule: A standardized observation of communicative and social behavior. J Autism Dev Disord 19:185-212, 1989.

332. DiLavore PC, Lord C, Rutter M: The Pre-linguistic Autism Diagnostic Observation Schedule. J Autism Dev Disord 25:355-379, 1995.

333. Attwood T: Asperger's Syndrome: A Guide for Parents and Professionals. London: Jessica Kingsley, 1998.

334. Campbell JM: Diagnostic assessment of Asperger's disorder: A review of five third-party rating scales. J Autism Dev Disord 35:25-35, 2005.

335. Myles B, Bock S, Simpson R: Asperger Syndrome Diagnostic Scale. Los Angeles: Western Psychological Services, 2001.

336. Ehlers S, Gillberg C, Wing L. et al: A screening questionnaire for Asperger syndrome and other high-functioning autism spectrum disorders in school age children. J Autism Dev Disord. 29:129-141, 1999.

337. Scott FJ, Baron-Cohen S, Bolton P, et al: The CAST (Childhood Asperger Syndrome Test): Preliminary development of a UK screen for mainstream primary-school-age children. Autism 6(1):9-31, 2002.

338. Gilliam J: Gilliam Asperger Disorder Scale. Austin, TX: Pro-Ed, 2001.

339. Krug D, Arick J: Krug Asperger Disorder Index. Austin, TX: Pro-Ed, 2003.

340. Klin A, Pauls D, Schultz R, et al: Three diagnostic approaches to Asperger syndrome: Implications for research. J Autism Dev Disord 35:221, 2005.

341. Blasco PA, Johnson CP: Supports for families of children with disabilities. In Capute AJ, Accardo PJ, eds: Developmental Disabilities in Infancy & Childhood, 2nd ed. Baltimore: Paul H. Brooks, 1996, pp 443-472.

342. Johnson CP, Blasco PA: Community resources for children with special health care needs. Pediatr Ann 26:279-286, 1997.

343. Blasco PA, Johnson CP, Palomo-Gonzalez S: Supports for families of children with disabilities. In Accardo PJ, ed: Capute & Accardo's Developmental Disabilites in Infancy and Childhood, 3rd ed. Baltimore: Paul H. Brookes, in press.

344. Allik H, Larrson JO, Smedje H: Health-related quality of life in parents of school-age children with Asperger syndrome or high-functioning autism. Health Qual Life Outcomes 4:1, 2006.

345. Dyson LL: Fathers and mothers of school-age children with developmental disabilities: Parental stress, family functioning, and social support. Am J Ment Retard 102:267-279, 1997.

346. Hastings RP: Child behavior problems and partner mental health as correlates of stress in mothers and fathers of children with autism. J Intellect Disabil Res 47:231-237, 2003.

347. Weiss SJ: Stressors experienced by family caregivers of children with pervasive developmental disorders. Child Psychiatry Hum Dev 21:203-216, 2001.

348. Fombonne E: Epidemiology of autistic disorder and other pervasive development disorders. J Clin Psychiatry 66 (Suppl 10):3-8, 2005.

349. Curry CJ, Stevenson RE, Aughton D, et al: Evaluation of mental retardation: Recommendations of a consensus conference: American College of Medical Genetics. Am J Med Genet 72:468-477, 1997.

350. Shevell M, Ashwal S, Donley D et al: Practice parameter: Evaluation of the child with global developmental delay: Report of the Quality Standards Subcommittee of the American Academy of Neurology and the Practice Committee of the Child Neurology Society. Neurology 60:367, 2003.

351. Roberts G, Palfrey J, Bridgemohan C: A rational approach to the medical evaluation of a child with developmental delay. Contemp Pediatr 21:76-100, 2004.

352. Fombonne E, Simmons H, Ford T, et al: Prevalence of developmental disorders in the British nationwide survey of child mental health. J Am Acad Child Adolesc Psychiatry 40:820-827, 200l.

353. Honda H, Shimizu Y, Rutter M: No effect of MMR withdrawal on the incidence of autism: A total population study. J Child Psychol Psychiatry 46:572-579, 2005.

354. van Karnebeek CD, Scheper FY, Abeling NG, et al: Etiology of mental retardation in children referred to a tertiary care center: A prospective study. Am J Ment Retard 110:253-267, 2005.

355. Bailey A, Bolton P, Butler L, et al: Prevalence of the fragile X anomaly amongst autistic twins and singletons. J Child Psychol Psychiatry 34:673-688, 1993.

356. Fisch G: Is autism associated with the fragile X syndrome? Am J Med Genet 43(l/2):4755, 1992.

356a. van Karnebeek CD, Jansweijer MC, Leenders AG, et al: Diagnostic investigations in individuals with mental retardation: A systematic literature review of their usefulness. Eur J Hum Genet 13:6-25, 2005.

356b. de Vries BB, White SM, Knight SJ, et al: Clinical studies on submicroscopic subtelomeric rearrangements: A checklist. Am J Med Genet 38:145-150, 2001.

357. Chez MG, Chang M, Krasne V, et al: Frequency of epileptiform EEG abnormalities in a sequential screening of autistic patients with no known clinical epilepsy from 1996 to 2005. Epilepsy Behavr 8:267-271, 2006.

358. Kagan-Kushnir T, Roberts SW, Snead OC 3rd: Screening electroencephalograms in autism spectrum disorders: Evidence-based guideline. J Child Neurol 20:197-206, 2005.

359. Mantovani J: Regression and seizures. Paper presented at Johns Hopkins Spectrum of Developmental Disabilities XXVIII, Baltimore, March 2006.

360. Lerman-Sagie T, Leshinsky-Silver E, Watemberg N, et al: Should autistic children be evaluated for mitochondrial disorders? J Child Neurol 19:379-381, 2004.

361. Filipek PA, Juranek J, Nguyen MT, et al: Relative carnitine deficiency in autism. J Autism Dev Disord 34:615-623, 2004.

361a. Lopez-Rangel E, Lewis MES: HotSpots. Loud and clear evidence for gene silencing by epigenetic mechanisms in autism spectrum and related neurodevelopmental disorders. Clin Genet 69:21-25, 2006.

362. Kerr A: Rett syndrome: Recent progress and implications for research and clinical practice. J Child Psychol Psychiatry 45:277, 2002.

363. Samaco RC, Nagarajan RP, Braunschweig D, et al: Multiple pathways to regulate MeCP2 expression in normal brain development and ASD. Hum Mol Genet 13:629-639, 2004.

364. Niemitz EL, Feinberg AP: Epigenetics and assisted reproductive technology: A call for investigation. Am J Hum Genet 74:599-609, 2004.

365. Elias ER, Giampietro P: Autism May Be Caused by Smith-Lemli-Opitz Syndrome (SLOS). Abstract presented at the meeting of the American College of Medical Genetics, Dallas, TX, March 2005.

366. Manning MA, Cassidy SB, Clericuzio C, et al: Terminal 22q deletion syndrome: A newly recognized cause of speech and language disability in the autism spectrum. Pediatrics 114:451-457, 2004.

367. Fine SE, Weissman A, Gerdes M, et al: Autism spectrum disorders and symptoms in children with molecularly confirmed 22q11.2 deletion syndrome. J Autism Dev Disord 35:461-470, 2005.

368. Rehabilitation Act of 1973, Public Law 93-112, 1973.

369. Olley JG: Curriculum and classroom structure. In Volkmar FR, Paul R, Klin A, et al, eds: Handbook of Autism and Pervasive Developmental Disorders, 3rd ed, vol 2. Hoboken, NJ: Wiley, 2005, pp 863-881.

370. Handleman JS, Harris SL: Preschool Education Programs for Children with Autism, 2nd ed. Austin, TX: Pro-Ed, 2001.

371. Harris SL, Handleman JS, Jennett HK: Models of educational intervention for students with autism: Home, center, and school-based programming. In Volkmar FR, Paul R, Klin A, et al, eds: Handbook of Autism and Pervasive Developmental Disorders, 3rd ed, vol 2. Hoboken, NJ: Wiley, 2005, pp 1043-1054.

372. Dawson G, Osterling J: Early intervention in autism. In Guralnick MJ, ed: The Effectiveness of Early Intervention: Second Generation Research. Baltimore: Paul H. Brookes, 1997, pp 307-326.

373. Mastergeorge AM, Rogers SJ, Corbett BA, et al: Nonmedical interventions for autism spectrum disorders. In Ozonoff S, Rogers SJ, Hendren RL, eds: Autism Spectrum Disorders: A Research Review for Practitioners. Washington, DC: American Psychiatric Press, 2003, pp 133-160.

374. Rogers SJ: Empirically supported comprehensive treatments for young children with autism. J Clin Child Psychol 27:168-179, 1998.

375. McClannahan LE, MacDuff GS, Krantz PJ: Behavior analysis and intervention for adults with autism. Behav Modif 26:9-26, 2002.

376. Mesibov GB, Shea V, Schopler E: The TEACCH Approach to Autism Spectrum Disorders. New York: Kluwer Academic/Plenum, 2005.

377. Bregman JD, Zager D, Gerdtz J: Behavioral interventions. In Volkmar FR, Paul R, Klin A, et al, eds: Handbook of Autism and Pervasive Developmental Disorders, 3rd ed, vol 2. Hoboken, NJ: Wiley, 2005, pp 897-924.

378. Matson JL, Benavidez DA, Compton LS, et al: Behavioral treatment of autistic persons: A review of research from 1980 to the present. Res Dev Disabil 17:433-465, 1996.

379. Schreibman L, Ingersoll B: Behavioral interventions to promote learning in individuals with autism. In Volkmar FR, Paul R, Klin A, et al, eds: Handbook of Autism and Pervasive Developmental Disorders, 3rd ed, vol 2. Hoboken, NJ: Wiley, 2005, pp 882-896.

380. Klin A, Volkmar FR: Treatment and intervention guidelines for individuals with Asperger syndrome. In Klin A, Volkmar FR, Sparrow SS, eds: Asperger Syndrome. New York: Guilford Press, 2000, pp 340-366.

381. Goldstein H: Communication intervention for children with autism: A review of treatment efficacy. J Autism Dev Disord 32:373-396, 2002.

382. Koegel LK: Interventions to facilitate communication in autism. J Autism Dev Disord 30:383-391, 2000.

383. Marans WD, Rubin E, Laurent A: Addressing social communication skills in individuals with high-functioning autism and Asperger syndrome: Critical priorities in educational programming. In Volkmar FR, Paul R, Klin A, et al, eds: Handbook of Autism and Pervasive Developmental Disorders, 3rd ed, vol 2. Hoboken, NJ: Wiley, 2005, pp 946-976.

384. Paul R, Sutherland D: Enhancing early language in children with autism spectrum disorders. In Volkmar FR, Paul R, Klin A, et al, eds: Handbook of Autism and Pervasive Developmental Disorders, 3rd ed, vol 2. Hoboken, NJ: Wiley, 2005, pp 946-976.

385. Lorimer PA, Simpson RL, Myles BS, et al: The use of social stories as a preventative behavioral intervention in a home setting with a child with autism. J Posit Behav Interv 4:53-60, 2002.

386. Taylor BA: Teaching peer social skills to children with autism. In Maurice C, Green G, Foxx RM, eds: Making a Difference: Behavioral Intervention for Autism. Austin, TX: Pro-Ed, 2001, pp 83-96.

387. Weiss MJ, Harris SL: Teaching social skills to people with autism. Behav Modif 25:785-802, 2001.

388. Campbell JM: Efficacy of behavioral interventions for reducing problem behavior in persons with autism: A quantitative synthesis of single-subject research. Res Dev Disabil 24:120-138, 2003.

389. Horner RH, Carr EG, Strain PS, et al: Problem behavior interventions for young children with autism: A research synthesis. J Autism Dev Disord 32:423-446, 2002.

390. Lovaas OI: Behavioral treatment and normal educational and intellectual functioning in young autistic children. J Consult Clin Psychol 55:3-9, 1987.

391. Lovaas OI, ed: Teaching Individuals with Developmental Delays: Basic Intervention Techniques. Austin, TX: Pro-Ed, 2003.

392. O'Neill R, Horner R, Albin R, et al: Functional Assessment and Program Development for Problem Behav-

ior: A Practical Handbook. Pacific Grove, CA: Brookes/Cole, 1996.

393. Bondy A, Frost L: The picture exchange communication system. Focus Autistic Behav 9:1-19, 1994.

394. Bondy A, Frost L: The picture exchange communication system. Semin Speech Lang 19:373-389, 1998.

395. Yoder PJ, Layton T: Speech following sign language training in autistic children with minimal verbal language. J Autism Dev Disord 18:217-229, 1988.

396. Krasny L, Williams BJ, Provencal S, et al: Social skills interventions for the autism spectrum: Essential ingredients and a model curriculum. Child Adolesc Psychiatr Clin North Am 12:107-122, 2003.

397. McConnell S: Interventions to facilitate social interaction for young children with autism: Review of available research and recommendations for educational intervention and future research. J Autism Dev Disord 32:351-372, 2002.

398. Reynhout G, Carter M: Social stories for children with disabilities. J Autism Devel Disord 36:445-469, 2006.

399. Rogers SJ: Interventions that facilitate socialization in children with autism. J Autism Dev Disord 30:399-409, 2000.

400. Bruinsma Y, Koegel RL, Koegel LK: Joint attention and children with autism: A review of the literature. Ment Retard Dev Disabil Res Rev 10:169-175, 2004.

401. Whalen C, Schreibman L: Joint attention training for children with autism using behavior modification procedures. J Child Psychol Psychiatry 44:456-468, 2003.

402. American Academy of Pediatrics: AAP Parent Booklet: Understanding Autism Spectrum Disorder (ASD). Washington, DC: American Academy of Pediatrics, 2006, pp 27-30.

403. Guttstein S, Sheely R: Relationship Development Intervention with Children, Adolescents, and Adults. London: Jessica Kingsley, 2002.

404. Taylor BA, Jasper S: Teaching programs to increase peer interaction. *In* Maurice C, Green G, Foxx RM, eds: Making a Difference: Behavioral Intervention for Autism. Austin, TX: Pro-Ed, 2001, pp 97-162.

405. Baranek GT: Efficacy of sensory and motor interventions for children with autism. J Autism Dev Disord 32:397-422, 2002.

406. Dawson G, Watling R: Interventions to facilitate auditory, visual, and motor integration in autism: A review of the evidence. J Autism Dev Disord 30:415-421, 2000.

407. Rogers SJ, Ozonoff S: Annotation: What do we know about sensory dysfunction in autism? A critical review of the empirical evidence. J Child Psychol Psychiatry 46:1255-1268, 2005.

408. Schaaf RC, Miller LJ: Occupational therapy using a sensory integrative approach for children with developmental disabilities. Ment Retard Dev Disabil Res Rev 11:143-148, 2005.

409. DeMyer MK, Hingtgen JN, Jackson RK: Infantile autism reviewed: A decade of research. Schizophr Bull 7:388-451, 1981.

410. Eikseth S, Smith T, Jahr E, et al: Intensive behavioral treatment at school for 4-7-year-old children with autism: A 1-year comparison controlled study. Behav Modif 26:49-68, 2002.

411. Howard JS, Sparkman CR, Cohen HG, et al: A comparison of intensive behavior analytic and eclectic treatments for young children with autism. Res Dev Disabil 26:359-383, 2005.

412. McEachin JJ, Smith T, Lovaas OI: Long-term outcome for children with autism who received early intensive behavioral treatment. Am J Ment Retard 97:359-372, 1993.

413. Smith T: Outcome of early intervention for children with autism. Clin Psychol Sci Pract 6:33-49, 1999.

414. Smith T, Groen AD, Wynne JW: Randomized trial of intensive early intervention for children with pervasive developmental disorder. Am J Ment Retard 105:269-285, 2000.

415. Weiss M: Differential rates of skill acquisition and outcomes of early intensive behavioral intervention for autism. Behav Interv 14:3-22, 1999.

416. Rogers SJ, DiLalla DL: A comparative study of the effects of a developmentally based instructional model on young children with autism and young children with other disorders of behavior and development. Top Early Child Spec Educ 11:29-47, 1991.

417. Rogers SJ, Lewis H: An effective day treatment model for young children with pervasive developmental disorders. J Am Acad Child Adolesc Psychiatry 28:207-214, 1988.

418. Rogers SJ, Lewis HC, Reis K: An effective procedure for training early special education teams to implement a model program. J Div Early Child 11:180-188, 1987.

419. Lord C, Schopler E: The role of age at assessment, developmental level, and test in the stability of intelligence scores in young autistic children. J Autism Dev Disord 19:483-499, 1989.

420. Ozonoff S, Cathcart K: Effectiveness of a home program intervention for young children with autism. J Autism Dev Disord 28:25-32, 1998.

421. Schopler E, Mesibov GB, Baker A: Evaluation of treatment for autistic children and their parents. J Am Acad Child Adolesc Psychiatry 21:262-267, 1982.

422. Venter AC, Lord C, Schopler E: A follow-up study of high-functioning autistic children. J Child Psychol Psychiatry 33:489-507, 1992.

423. Mahoney G, McDonald J: Responsive Teaching: Parent Mediated Developmental Intervention. Cleveland, OH: Case Western Reserve University, 2004.

424. Mahoney G, Perales F: Relationship-focused early intervention with children with pervasive developmental disorders and other disabilities: A comparative study. J Dev Behav Pediatr 26:77-85, 2005.

425. Greenspan SI, Wieder S: Developmental patterns and outcomes in infants and children with disorders in relating and communicating: A chart review of 200 cases of children with autistic spectrum diagnoses. J Dev Learn Disord 1:87-141, 1997.

426. Wieder S, Greenspan SI: Can children with autism master the core deficits and become empathetic, cre-

ative, and reflective? A Ten to fifteen year follow-up of a subgroup of children with autism spectrum disorders (ASD) who received a comprehensive developmental, individual-difference, relationship-based (DIR) approach. J Dev Learn Disord 9:39-61, 2005.

427. Cohen H, Amerine-Dickens M, Smith T: Early intensive behavioral treatment: Replication of the UCLA model in a community setting. J Dev Behav Pediatr 27:145-155, 2006.

428. Konstantareas MM, Lunsky YJ: Sociosexual knowledge, experience, attitudes, and interests of individuals with autistic disorder and developmental delay. J Autism Dev Disord 27:397-413, 1997.

429. Murphy N: Sexuality in children and adolescents with disabilities. Dev Med Child Neurol 47:640-644, 2005.

430. Murphy NA, Elias ER, AAP Committee/Section on Children with Disabilities: Sexuality of children and adolescents with developmental disabilities. Pediatrics 118:398-403, 2006.

431. Fullerton A, Coyne P: Developing skills and concepts for self-determination in young adults with autism. Focus Autism Other Dev Disab 14:42-52, 1999.

432. Rutter M: Genetic influences and autism. *In* Volkmar FR, Paul R, Klin A, et al, eds: Handbook of Autism and Pervasive Developmental Disorders, 3rd ed, vol 1. Hoboken, NJ: Wiley, 2005, pp 425-452.

433. Tuchman R, Rapin I, Shinnar S: Autistic and dysphasic children II: Epilepsy. Pediatrics 88:1219-1225, 1991.

434. Pavone P, Incorpora G, Flumara A, et al: Epilepsy is not a prominent feature of primary autism. Neuropediatrics 35:207-210, 2004.

435. Hrdlicka M, Komarek V, Propper L, et al: Not EEG but epilepsy is associated with autistic regression and mental functioning in childhood autism. Eur Child Adolesc Psychiatry 13:209-213, 2004.

436. Canitano R, Luchetti A, Zappella M: Epilepsy, electroencephalographic abnormalities, and regression in children with autism. J Child Neurol 20:27-31, 2005.

437. Erickson CA, Stigler KA, Corkins MR, et al: Gastrointestinal factors in autistic disorder: A critical review. J Autism Dev Disord 35:713-727, 2005.

438. Kuddo T, Nelson KB: How common are gastrointestinal disorders in children with autism? Curr Opin Pediatr 15:339-343, 2003.

439. Horvath K, Perman JA: Autism and gastrointestinal symptoms. Curr Gastroenterol Rep 4:251-258, 2002.

440. Lightdale JR, Siegel B, Heyman MB: Gastrointestinal symptoms in autistic children. Clin Perspect Gastroenterol 1:56-58, 2001.

441. Valicenti-McDermott M, McVicar K, Rapin I, et al: Frequency of gastrointestinal symptoms in children with autistic spectrum disorders and association with family history of autoimmune disease. J Dev Behav Pediatr 27:128-136, 2006.

442. Black C, Kaye JA, Jick H: Relation of childhood gastrointestinal disorders to autism: Nested case control study using data from the UK General Practice Research Database. BMJ 325:419-421, 2002.

443. Fombonne E, Chakrabarti S: No evidence for a new variant of measles-mumps-rubella-induced autism. Pediatrics 108:e58, 2001.

444. Molloy CA, Manning-Courtney P: Prevalence of chronic gastrointestinal symptoms in children with autism and autistic spectrum disorders. Autism J Res Pract 7:165-171, 2003.

445. Taylor B, Miller E, Lingam R, et al: Measles, mumps, and rubella vaccination and bowel problems or developmental regression in children with autism: Population-based study. BMJ 324:393-396, 2002.

446. Horvath K, Papadimitriou JC, Rabsztyn A, et al: Gastrointestinal abnormalities in children with autistic disorder. Pediatrics 135:559-563, 1999.

447. Torrente F, Anthony A, Heuschkel RB, et al: Focal-enhanced gastritis in regressive autism with features distinct from Crohn's and *Helicobacter pylori* gastritis. Am J Gastroenterol 99:598-604, 2004.

448. Afzal N, Murch S, Thirrupathy K, et al: Constipation with acquired megarectum in children with autism. Pediatrics 112:939-942, 2003.

449. Aman MG, Lam KS, Collier-Crespin A: Prevalence and patterns of use of psychoactive medicines among individuals with autism in the Autism Society of Ohio. J Autism Dev Disord 33:527-534, 2003.

450. Langworthy-Lam KS, Aman MG, Van Bourgondien ME: Prevalence and patterns of use of psychoactive medicines in individuals with autism in the Autism Society of North Carolina. J Child Adolesc Psychopharmacol 12:311-321, 2002.

451. Witwer A, Lecavalier L: Treatment incidence and patterns in children and adolescents with autism spectrum disorders. J Child Adolesc Psychopharmacol 15:671-681, 2005.

452. Seltzer MM, Shattuck P, Abbeduto L, et al: Trajectory of development in adolescents and adults with autism. Ment Retard Dev Disabil Res Rev 10:234-247, 2004.

453. Bowers L: An audit of referrals of children with autistic spectrum disorder to the dietetic service. J Hum Nutr Diet 15:141-144, 2002.

454. Perry DW, Marston GM, Hinder SA: The phenomenology of depressive illness in people with a learning disability and autism. Autism 5:265-275, 2001.

455. Syzmanski LS, King B, Goldberg B, et al: Diagnosis of mental disorders in people with mental retardation. *In* Reiss S, Aman MG, eds: Psychotropic Medications and Developmental Disabilities: The International Concensus Handbook. Columbus, OH: Ohio State University Nisonger Center, 1998, pp 3-17.

456. Posey DJ, McDougle CJ: The pharmacotherapy of target symptoms associated with autistic disorder and other pervasive developmental disorders. Harvard Rev Psychiatry 8:45-63, 2000.

457. Steingard RJ, Connor DF, Au T: Approaches to psychopharmacology. *In* Bauman ML, Kemper TL, eds: The Nerobiology of Autism, 2nd ed. Baltimore: Johns Hopkins University Press, 2005, pp 79-102.

458. Towbin KE: Strategies for pharmacologic treatment of high functioning autism and Asperger syndrome. Child Adolesc Psychiatr Clin North Am 12:23-45, 2003.

459. Quintana H, Birmaher B, Stedge D, et al: Use of methylphenidate in the treatment of children with autistic disorder. J Autism Dev Disord 25:283-294, 1995.

460. Handen BL, Johnson CR, Lubetsky, M: Efficacy of methylphenidate among children with autism and symptoms of attention-deficit hyperactivity disorder. J Autism Dev Disord 30:245-255, 2000.

461. Research Units on Pediatric Psychopharmacology (RUPP) Autism Network: Randomized, controlled, crossover trial of methylphenidate in pervasive developmental disorders with hyperactivity. Arch Gen Psychiatry 62:1266-1274, 2005.

462. Aman MG: Management of hyperactivity and other acting-out problems in patients with autism spectrum disorder. Semin Pediatr Neurol 11:225-228, 2004.

463. Fankhauser MP, Karumanchi VC, German ML, et al: A double-blind, placebo-controlled study of the efficacy of transdermal clonidine in autism. J Clin Psychol 53:77-82, 1992.

464. Jaselskis CA, Cook EH, Fletcher E, et al: Clonidine treatment of hyperactive and impulsive children with autistic disorder. J Clin Psychopharmacol 12:322-327, 1992.

465. Posey DJ, Puntney JI, Sasher TM, et al: Guanfacine treatment of hyperactivity and inattention in pervasive developmental disorders: A retrospective analysis of 80 cases. J Child Adolesc Psychopharmacol 14:233-241, 2004.

466. Jou RJ, Handen BL, Hardan AY: Retrospective assessment of atomoxetine in children and adolescents with pervasive developmental disorders. J Child Adolesc Psychopharmacol 15:325-330, 2005.

467. Aman MG, De Smedt G, Derivan A, et al: Double-blind, placebo-controlled study of risperidone for the treatment of disruptive behaviors in children with subaverage intelligence. Am J Psychiatry 159:1337-1346, 2002.

468. Croonenberghs J, Fegert JM, Findling RL, et al: Risperidone in children with disruptive behavior disorders and subaverage intelligence: A 1-year, open-label study of 504 patients. J Am Acad Child Adolesc Psychiatry 44:64-72, 2005.

469. Snyder R, Turgay A, Aman M, et al: Effects of risperidone on conduct and disruptive behavior disorders in children with subaverage IQs. J Am Acad Child Adolesc Psychiatry 41:1026-1036, 2002.

470. Cheng-Shannon J, McGough JJ, Pataki C, et al: Second-generation antipsychotic medications in children and adolescents. J Child Adolesc Psychopharmacol 14:372-394, 2004.

471. McCracken JT, McGough J, Shah B, et al: Risperidone in children with autism and serious behavioral problems. N Engl J Med 347:314-321, 2002.

472. Arnold LE, Vitiello B, McDougle C, et al: Parent-defined target symptoms respond to risperidone in RUPP autism study: Customer approach to clinical trials. J Am Acad Child Adolesc Psychiatry 42:1443-1450, 2003.

473. McDougle CJ, Scahill L, Aman MG, et al: Risperidone for the core symptom domains of autism: Results from the study by the autism network of the Research Units on Pediatric Psychopharmacology. Am J Psychiatry 162:1142-1148, 2005.

474. Shea S, Turgay A, Carroll A, et al: Risperidone in the treatment of disruptive behavioral symptoms in children with autistic and other pervasive developmental disorders. Pediatrics 114:e634-e641, 2004.

475. Research Units on Pediatric Psychopharmacology Autism Network: Risperidone treatment of autistic disorder: Longer-term benefits and blinded discontinuation after 6 months. Am J Psychiatry 162:1361-1369, 2005.

476. Troost PW, Lahuis BE, Steenuis M-P, et al: Long-term effects of risperidone in children with autism spectrum disorders: A placebo discontinuation study. J Am Acad Child Adolesc Psychiatry 44:1137-1144, 2005.

477. Hollander E, Phillips A, Chaplin W, et al: A placebo controlled crossover trial of liquid fluoxetine on repetitive behaviors in childhood and adolescent autism. Neuropsychopharmacology 30:582-589, 2005.

478. McDougle CJ, Naylor ST, Cohen DJ, et al: A double-blind, placebo-controlled study of fluvoxamine in adults with autistic disorder. Arch Gen Psychiatry 53:1001-1008, 1996.

479. Sugie Y, Sugie H, Fukuda T, et al: Clinical efficacy of fluvoxamine and functional polymorphism in a serotonin transporter gene on childhood autism. J Autism Dev Disord 35:377-385, 2005.

480. Moore ML, Eichner SF, Jones JR: Treating functional impairment of autism with selective serotonin-reuptake inhibitors. Ann Pharmacother 38:1515-1519, 2004.

481. Hollander E, Dolgoff-Kaspar R, Cartwright C, et al: An open trial of divalproex sodium in autism spectrum disorders. J Clin Psychol 62:530-534, 2001.

482. Rugino TA, Samsock TC: Levetiracetam in autistic children: An open-label study. J Dev Behav Pediatr 23:225-230, 2002.

482a. Hardan AY, Jou RJ, Handen BL: A retrospective assessment of topiramate in children and adolescents with pervasive developmental disorders. J Child Adolesc Psychopharmacol 14:426-432, 2004.

483. Childs JA, Blair JL: Valproic acid treatment of epilepsy in autistic twins. J Neurosci Nurs 29:244-248, 1997.

484. Plioplys AV: Autism: Electroencephalogram abnormalities and clinical improvement with valproic acid. Arch Pediatr Adolesc Med 148:220-222, 1994.

485. Hollander E, Soorya L, Wasserman S, et al: Divalproex sodium vs. placebo in the treatment of repetitive behaviours in autism spectrum disorder. Int J Neuropsychopharmacol 9:209-213, 2006.

486. Chez MG, Memon S, Hung PC: Neurologic treatment strategies in autism: An overview of medical intervention strategies Semin Pediatr Neurol 11:229-235, 2004.

487. Uvebrant P, Bauziene R: Intractable epilepsy in children. The efficacy of lamotrigine treatment, including non–seizure-related benefits. Neuropediatrics 25:284-289, 1994.

488. Belsito KM, Law PA, Kirk KS, et al: Lamotrigine therapy for autistic disorder: A randomized, double-

blind, placebo-controlled trial. J Autism Dev Disord 31:175-181, 2001.

489. DeLong R: Children with autistic spectrum disorder and a family history of affective disorder. Dev Med Child Neurol 36:674-687, 1994.

490. Kerbeshian J, Burd L, Fisher W: Lithium carbonate in the treatment of two patients with infantile autism and atypical bipolar symptomatology. J Clin Psychopharmacol 7:401-405, 1987.

491. Steingard R, Biederman J: Lithium responsive manic-like symptoms in two individuals with autism and mental retardation. J Am Acad Child Adolesc Psychiatry 26:932-935, 1987.

492. Aman MG, Novotny S, Samango-Sprouse C, et al: Outcome measures for clinical drug trials in autism. CNS Spectr 9:36-47, 2004.

493. Malow BA: Sleep disorders, epilepsy, and autism. Ment Retard Dev Disabil 10:122-125, 2004.

494. Oyane NM, Bjorvatn B: Sleep disturbances in adolescents and young adults with autism and Asperger syndrome. Autism 9:83-94, 2005.

495. Polimeni MA, Richdale AL, Francis AJ: A survey of sleep problems in autism, Asperger's disorder and typically developing children. J Intellect Disabil Res 49:260-268, 2005.

496. Wiggs L, Stores G: Sleep patterns and sleep disorders in children with autistic spectrum disorders: Insights using parent report and actigraphy. Dev Med Child Neurol 46:372-380, 2004.

497. Williams G, Sears LL, Allaed A: Sleep problems in children with autism. J Sleep Res 13:265-268, 2004.

498. Owens JA, Babcock D, Blumer J, et al: The use of pharmacotherapy in the treatment of pediatric insomnia in primary care: Rational approaches. A consensus meeting summary. J Clin Sleep Med 1:49-59, 2005.

499. Weiskop S, Richdale A, Matthews J: Behavioral treatment to reduce sleep problems in children with autism or fragile X syndrome. Dev Med Child Neurol 47:94-104, 2005.

500. Kulman G, Lissoni P, Rovelli F, et al: Evidence of pineal endocrine hypofunction in autistic children. Neuroendocrinol Lett 21:31-34, 2000.

501. Tordjman S, Anderson GM, Pichard N, et al: Nocturnal excretion of 6-sulphatoxymelatonin in children and adolescents with autistic disorder. Biol Psychiatry 57:134-138, 2005.

502. Jan JE, Freeman RD: Melatonin therapy for circadian rhythm sleep disorders in children with multiple disabilities: What have we learned in the last decade? Dev Med Child Neurol 46:776-782, 2004.

503. Phillips L, Appleton RE: Systematic review of melatonin treatment in children with neurodevelopmental disabilities and sleep impairment. Dev Med Child Neurol 46:771-775, 2004.

504. Turk J: Melatonin supplementation for severe and intractable sleep disturbance in young people with genetically determined developmental disabilities: Short review and commentary. J Med Genet 40:793-796, 2003.

505. Levy SE, Mandell DS, Merhar S, et al: Use of complementary and alternative medicine among children recently diagnosed with autistic spectrum disorder. J Dev Behav Pediatr 24:418-423, 2003.

506. Challman TD, Voigt RG, Myers SM: Nonstandard therapies in developmental disabilities. *In* Accardo PJ, ed: Capute & Accardo's Neurodevelopmental Disabilities in Infancy and Childhood, 3rd ed. Baltimore: Paul H. Brookes, in press.

506a. Gupta VB: Complementary and alternative treatments for autism. *In* Gupta VB, ed: Pediatric Habilitation Series, Volume 12: Autistic Spectrum Disorders in Children. New York: Marcel Dekker, 2004, pp 239-254.

507. Levy SE, Hyman SL: Novel treatments for autistic spectrum disorders. Ment Retard Dev Disabil Res Rev 11:131-142, 2005.

508. Sturmey P: Secretin is an ineffective treatment for pervasive developmental disabilities: A review of 15 double-blind randomized controlled trials. Res Dev Disabil 26:87-97, 2005.

509. Williams KW, Wray JJ, Wheeler DM: Intravenous secretin for autism spectrum disorder. Cochrane Database Syst Rev (3):CD003495, 2005.

510. American Academy of Pediatrics, Committee on Children with Disabilities: Auditory integration training and facilitated communication for autism. Pediatrics 102:431-433, 1998.

511. Jacobson JW, Mulick JA, Schwartz AA: A history of facilitated communication: Science, pseudoscience, and antiscience. Science Working Group on Facilitated Communication. Am Psychol 50:750-765, 1995.

512. Mostert MP: Facilitated communication since 1995: A review of published studies. J Autism Dev Disord 31:287-313, 2001.

513. Smith MD, Haas PJ, Belcher RG: Facilitated communication: The effects of facilitator knowledge and level of assistance on output. J Autism Dev Disord 24:357-367, 1994.

514. Cardinal DA, Hanson D, Wakeham J: Investigation of authorship in facilitated communication. Ment Retard 34:231-242, 1996.

515. Bolman WM, Richmond JA: A double-blind, placebo controlled pilot trial of low dose dimethylglycine in patients with autistic disorder. J Autism Dev Disord 29:191-194, 1999.

516. Kern JK, Miller VS, Cauller PL, et al: Effectiveness of *N,N*-dimethylglycine in autism and pervasive developmental disorder. J Child Neurol 16:169-173, 2001.

517. Findling RL, Maxwell K, Scotese-Wojtila L, et al: High-dose pyridoxine and magnesium administration in children with autistic disorder: An absence of salutary effects in a double-blind, placebo-controlled study. J Autism Dev Disord 27:467-478, 1997.

518. Nye C, Brice A: Combined vitamin B_6–magnesium treatment in autism spectrum disorder. Cochrane Database Syst Rev (4):CD003497, 2002.

519. Mudford OC, Cross BA, Breen S, et al: Auditory integration training for children with autism: No behav-

ioral benefits detected. Am J Ment Retard 105:118-129, 2000.

520. Sinha Y, Silove N, Wheeler D, et al: Auditory integration training and other sound therapies for autism spectrum disorders. Cochrane Database Syst Rev (1): CD003681, 2004.

520a. Gupta S, Aggarwal S, Heads C: Dysregulated immune system in children with autism: Beneficial effects of intravenous immune globulin on autistic characteristics. J Autism Dev Disord 26:439-452, 1996.

521. DelGiudice-Asch G, Simon L, Schmeidler J, et al: Brief report: A pilot open clinical trial of intravenous immunoglobulin in childhood autism. J Autism Dev Disord 29:157-160, 1999.

522. Plioplys AV: Intravenous immunoglobulin treatment of children with autism. J Child Neurol 13:79-82, 1998.

523. Millward C, Ferriter M, Calver S, et al: Gluten- and casein-free diets for autistic spectrum disorder. Cochrane Database Syst Rev (2):CD003498, 2004.

524. Elder JH, Shankar M, Shuster J, et al: The gluten-free, casein-free diet in autism: Results of a preliminary double blind clinical trial. J Autism Dev Disord 36:413-420, 2006.

525. American Academy of Pediatrics, Committee on Children with Disabilities: Counseling families who choose complementary and alternative medicine for their child with chronic illness or disability. Pediatrics 107:598-601, 2001.

525a. Hyman SL, Levy SE: Introduction: Novel therapies in developmental disabilities—hope, reason, and evidence. Ment Retard Dev Disabil Res Rev 11:107-109, 2005.

526. Marcus LM, Kunce LJ, Schopler E: Working with families. In Volkmar FR, Paul R, Klin A, et al, eds: Handbook of Autism and Pervasive Developmental Disorders, 3rd ed, vol 1. Hoboken, NJ: Wiley, 2005, pp 1055-1086.

527. Bouma R, Schweitzer R: The impact of chronic childhood illness on family stress: A comparison between autism and cystic fibrosis. J Clin Psychol 46:722-730, 1990.

528. Dumas JE, Wolf LC, Fisman SN, et al: Parenting stress, child behavior problems, and dysphoria in parents of children with autism, Down syndrome, behavior disorders, and normal development. Exceptionality 2:97-110, 1991.

529. Gray DE: Ten years on: A longitudinal study of families of children with autism. J Intellect Dev Disabil 27:215-222, 2002.

530. Bagenholm A, Gillberg C: Psychosocial effects on siblings of children with autism and mental retardation: a population-based study. J Ment Defic Res 35:291-307, 1991.

531. Gold N: Depression and social adjustment in siblings of boys with autism. J Autism Dev Disord 23:147-163, 1993.

532. Smith T, Perry A: A sibling support group for brothers and sisters of children with autism. J Dev Disabil 11:77-88, 2005.

533. Charman T, Taylor E, Drew A, et al: Outcome at 7 years of children diagnosed with autism at age 2: Predictive validity of assessments conducted at 2 and 3 years of age and pattern of symptom change over time. J Child Psychol Psychiatry 46:500-513, 2005.

534. Sigman M, McGovern CW: Improvement in cognitive and language skills from preschool to adolescence in autism. J Autism Dev Disord 35:15-23, 2005.

535. Lotter V: Follow-up studies. In Rutter M, Schopler E, eds: Autism: A Reappraisal of Concepts and Treatment. New York: Plenum Press, 1978, pp 475-495.

536. Gillberg C, Steffenburg S: Outcome and prognostic factors in infantile autism and similar conditions: A population-based study of 46 cases followed through puberty. J Autism Dev Disord 17:273-287, 1987.

537. Stevens MC, Fein DA, Dunn M, et al: Subgroups of children with autism by cluster analysis: A longitudinal examination. J Am Acad Child Adolesc Psychiatry 39:346-352, 2000.

538. Coplan J: Counseling parents regarding prognosis in autistic spectrum disorder. Pediatrics 105:65, 2000.

539. Szatmari P, Merette C, Bryson SE, et al: Quantifying dimensions in autism: A factor analysis study. J Am Acad Child Adolesc Psychiatry 41:467-474, 2002.

540. Seltzer MM, Krauss MW, Shattuck PT, et al: The symptoms of autism spectrum disorders in adolescence and adulthood. J Autism Dev Disord 33:565-558, 2003.

541. Coplan J: Atypicality, intelligence, and age: A conceptual model of autistic spectrum disorder. Dev Med Child Neurol 45:712-716, 2003.

542. Howlin P, Goode S, Hutton J, et al: Adult outcome for children with autism. J Child Psychol Psychiatry 45:212-229, 2004.

543. Howlin P, Goode S: Outcome in adult life for people with autism and Asperger's syndrome. In Volkmar FR, ed: Autism and Pervasive Developmental Disorders. New York: Cambridge University Press, 2005, pp 209-241.

544. Coplan J, Jawad AB: Modeling clinical outcome of children with autistic spectrum disorders. Pediatrics 116:117-122, 2005.

545. Howlin P: Outcome in high-functioning adults with autism with and without early language delays: Implications for the differentiation between autism and Asperger syndrome. J Autism Dev Disord 33:3-13, 2003.

546. Szatmari P, Bryson SE, Boyle MH, et al: Predictors of outcome among high functioning children with autism and Asperger syndrome. J Child Psychol Psychiatry 44:520-528, 2003.

546a. Lord C, Risi S, DiLavore, et al: Autism from 2 to 9 years of age. Arch Gen Psychiatry 63:670-694, 2006.

547. Osborne L: American normal: The culture of Asperger's syndrome. New York: Springer, 2002.

548. Jackson L, Attwood T: Freaks, Geeks and Asperger Syndrome: A User's Guide to Adolescence. London: Jessica Kingsley, 2002.

549. Stanford A, Willey A: Asperger Syndrome and Long-Term Relationship. London: Jessica Kingsley, 2002.

550. Shore S: Beyond the wall: Personal experiences with autism and Asperger syndrome. Shawnee Mission, KS: Autism Asperger Publishing, 2003.

551. McKean TA: Soon will come the light: A view from inside the autism puzzle. Arlington, TX: Future Horizons, 1994.

552. Shavelle RM, Strauss DJ, Pickett J: Causes of death in autism. J Autism Dev Disord 31:569-576, 2001.

553. Talebizadeh Z, Bittel DC, Veatch OJ, et al: Brief report: non-random X chromosome inactivation in females with autism. J Autism Dev Disord 35:675-681, 2005.

554. Plenge RM, Stevenson RA, Lubs HA, et al: Skewed X-chromosome inactivation is a common feature of X-linked mental retardation disorders. Am J Hum Genet 71:168-173, 2002.

555. Skuse DH, James RS, Bishop DV, et al: Evidence from Turner's syndrome of an imprinted X-linked locus affecting cognitive function. Nature 387:705-708, 1997.

556. Skuse DH: Imprinting, the X-chromosome, and the male brain: Explaining sex differences in the liability to autism. Pediatr Res 47:9-16, 2000.

557. Thomas NS, Sharp AJ, Browne CE, et al: Xp deletions associated with autism in three females. Hum Genet 104:43-48, 1999.

558. Shao Y, Wolpert CM, Raiford KL, et al: Genomic screen and follow-up analysis for autistic disorder. Am J Med Genet 114:99-105, 2002.

559. Vervoort R, Beachern MA, Edwards PS, et al: AGTR2 mutations in X-linked mental retardation. Science 296:2401-2403, 2002.

560. Veenstra-Vanderweele J, Cook EH: Genetics of childhood disorders: XLVI. Autism, part 5: Genetics of autism. J Am Acad Child Adolesc Psychiatry 42:116-118, 2003.

561. Modahl C, Fein D, Waterhouse L, et al: Does oxytocin deficiency mediate social deficits in autism? J Autism Dev Disord 22:449-451, 1992.

562. Insel TR, O'Brien DJ, Leckman JF: Oxytocin vasopressin, and autism: Is there a connection? Biol Psychiatry 45:145-157, 1999.

563. Winslow AJT, Insel TR: The social deficits of the oxytocin knockout mouse. Neuropeptides 36:221-229, 2002.

564. Modahl C, Green L, Fein D, et al: Plasma oxytocin levels in autistic children. Biol Psychiatry 43:270-277, 1998.

565. Hollander E, Novotny S, Hanratty M, et al: Oxytocin infusion reduces repetitive behaviors in adults with autistic and Asperger's disorders. Neutropsychopharmacology 28:193-198, 2003.

566. International Molecular Genetic Study of Autism Consortium (IMGSAC): Further characterization of the autism susceptibility locus AUTSI on chromosome 7q. Hum Mol Genet 10:973-982, 2001.

567. Gillberg C, Ehlers S: High functioning people with autism and Asperger syndrome: A literature review. *In* Scholpler E, Mesibov GB, Kunce LJ, eds: Asperger Syndrome or High-Functioning Autism? New York: Plenum Press, 1998, pp 79-106.

568. Folstein SE, Mankoski RE: Chromosome 7q: Where autism meets language disorder? Am J Hum Genet 67:278-281, 2000.

569. Wassink TH, Pivin J, Vieland VJ, et al: Evidence supporting WNT2 as an autism susceptibility gene. Am J Med Genet 105:406-413, 2001.

570. Koochek M, Harvard C, Hildebrand MJ, et al: 15q duplication associated with autism in a multiplex family with a familial cryptic translocation (14;15)(q11.2;q13.3) detected using array-CGH. Clin Genet 69:124-134, 2006.

571. Sutcliffe JS, Nurmi EL, Lombroso PJ: Genetics of childhood disorders: XLVII autism, part 6: Duplication and inherited susceptibility of chromosome 15q11-q13 genes in autism. J Am Acad Child Adolesc Psychiatry 42:253-256, 2003.

572. Chugani DC: Role of altered brain serotonin mechanisms in autism. Mol Psychiatry 7:S16-S27, 2002.

573. Anderson CM: Genetics of childhood disorders: XLV. Autism, part 4: Serotonin in autism. J Am Acad Child Adolesc Psychiatry 41:1513-1516, 2002.

574. Cook EH Jr, Courchesne R, Lord C, et al: Evidence of linkage between the serotonin transporter and autistic disorder. Mol Psychiatry 2:247-250, 1997.

575. Tezenas DU, Montcel S, Mendizibal H, et al: Prevalence of 22q11 microdeletion. J Med Genet 33:719, 1996.

Attention-Deficit/Hyperactivity Disorder

THOMAS M. LOCK ■ KIM A. WORLEY ■ MARK L. WOLRAICH

Attention-deficit/hyperactivity disorder (ADHD) is the most common neurobehavioral health condition among children. Although it has been the subject of great controversy, it is also the most studied neurobehavioral condition of childhood with the greatest empirical basis for evaluation and treatment. Affected children usually present with behavioral problems or academic difficulties. It is important to determine whether these concerns arise from true ADHD, from a condition that mimics ADHD, from ADHD complicated with by a comorbid diagnosis, or from normal activity for the child's age. Understanding the current recommendations for the evaluation, diagnosis, treatment, and management is imperative to provide these children the best care possible. Guidelines have been published by experts in pediatrics[1,2] and mental health[3,3a] for the diagnosis and treatment of ADHD. These recommendations, along with the criteria set forth in the *Diagnostic and Statistical Manual of Mental Disorders,* 4th edition (DSM-IV),[4] provide for greater uniformity of the diagnosis, treatment, and management processes in the care of children with this complicated symptom complex.

HISTORY

In the media, ADHD is often represented as a newly discovered entity. In reality, the core symptoms of ADHD have been puzzling health care providers since the mid-1800s. The first literary description was provided in a children's book written in 1848 by a German physician, Heinrich Hoffmann[5]:

> But fidgety Phil,
> He won't sit still;
> He wriggles
> And giggles,
> And then, I declare
> Swings backwards and forwards
> And tilts up his chair

The poem continues, giving a description of Fidgety Phil's antics, which resemble hyperactive/impulsive symptoms. Hoffmann also described inattentive symptoms in another character, Johnny Head-In-Air. Johnny was watching the birds and the sun and never knew what hit him when he fell headlong into the river and had to be fished out.[5]

A perhaps more parent-friendly description appeared soon after in 1851 in a story by George Sand. In this story, a mother dies young, leaving three children in the care of their father and grandparents. The woman's father encourages the father to remarry because the grandparents cannot keep up with the care of the children, particularly "Sylvain, who is not four years old, and who is never quiet day or night. He has a restless disposition like yours; that will make a good workman of him, but it makes a dreadful child, and my old wife cannot run fast enough to save him when he almost tumbles into the ditch, or when he throws himself in front of the tramping cattle."[6] This description highlights the familial nature of the disorder, its early onset, and the burden of care that it places upon families.

At first, in dealing with this disorder, the primary focus was on conduct. In 1902, Still described children with ADHD symptoms and believed these children had a "defect in moral control."[7] He stated the "problem resulted in a child's inability to internalize rules and limits, and additionally manifested itself in patterns of restlessness, inattentive, and over-aroused behaviors."[7] This stress on control of behavior has returned, renamed as *response inhibition* or *executive dysfunction.*[8] In 1937, a stimulant, racemic amphetamine (Benzedrine), was noted to improve the behaviors in children affected with these core symptoms.[9] Methylphenidate, whose effects were similar to those of the amphetamines, was released for general use in 1957.[10]

As research has revealed more about this troubling symptom complex of inattention, hyperactivity, and impulsivity, there have been many causal theories and name changes. The cause of the disorder was first thought to be brain damage when some of the children recovering from encephalitis caused by the worldwide influenza epidemic in 1917 exhibited symptoms of restlessness, inattention, impulsivity, easy arousability, and hyperactivity[11,12] When brain damage was found to be less evident in many children exhibiting symptoms, the name was changed to *minimal brain damage* and *minimal cerebral dysfunction.* It shifted from an etiological name to a behavioral descriptive name in the late 1960s. In the *Diagnostic and Statistical Manual of Mental Disorders,* 2nd edition (*DSM-II*), it was labeled *Hyperkinetic Impulse Disorder,*[13] which reflected a focus on the hyperactive symptoms. In the third edition (*DSM-III*),[14] the name underwent further change as the focus shifted from hyperactive symptoms to inattention, with the name *Attention Deficit Disorder,* on the basis of research by Douglas that demonstrated deficiencies in continuous performance and similar vigilance tasks.[15] The name *Attention-Deficit/Hyperactivity Disorder* was introduced in the revision of the third edition (*DSM-III-R*).[16] The latest terminology is defined in the fourth edition (*DSM-IV*),[4] in which Attention-Deficit/Hyperactivity Disorder is divided into three subtypes: primarily inattentive type, primarily hyperactive-impulsive type, and combined type.[4]

The confusion over the causes and even the specific definition of this symptom complex is demonstrated by the frequent name changes. This is perhaps not surprising, inasmuch as the intimate interrelationship between attention and intention was pointed out as early as 1890 by William James: "The essential achievement of the will, in short, when it is most 'voluntary,' is to *attend* to a difficult object and hold it fast before the mind. The so-doing is the *fiat;* and it is a mere physiological incident that when the object is thus attended to, immediate motor consequences should ensue."[17]

PREVALENCE

Researchers have identified individuals with ADHD symptoms in every nation and culture studied,[18] but determining the true prevalence rate of ADHD has been a challenging task. Prevalence estimates for ADHD vary, depending on the diagnostic criteria used, the population studied, and the number of sources necessary to make the diagnosis.[2] Several features of the disorder are major contributors to the challenge. First, there are no known specific biological markers (laboratory tests or image studies) that can discriminate children with ADHD from children with another neurobehavioral disorder or from

normal controls. Second, the behaviors observed in ADHD differ in quantity, not quality, from those of typical children. This contrasts to disorders such as schizophrenia, in which the presence of auditory hallucinations is qualitatively distinct from normal experience, or conduct disorder, in which a child may willfully engage in criminal activity. Third, the frequency of these behaviors is observed and reported by the child's caregivers; therefore, the diagnosis must rely on the judgment of persons who do not share any uniform training or view of child development and whose interrater reliability is unknown. Fourth, there is no consensus about what frequency of any given behavior is normal at any given age; for example, in assessing intelligence, there are clear normative guidelines for which tasks can be accomplished at which age. Fifth, the behaviors are context specific; in situations of stress, most people exhibit inattention, overactivity, and impulsive behaviors.[18a] Sixth, the ADHD core symptoms and signs are not specific to ADHD; for example, the continuous performance task that was used to establish the attentional component of ADHD was first developed to study subjects with schizophrenia.

The modifications in diagnostic criteria over time have further complicated the process of determining the true prevalence of ADHD. The most recent change, from only one subtype in *DSM-III-R* to three subtypes in *DSM-IV,* has increased the prevalence rates. In addition to the challenges to making accurate diagnoses, studies of prevalence rates are dependent on the sample studied. The rates are different in a sample referred to a mental health clinic from those in a primary care sample or from a community/school sample. In view of these challenges, it is not surprising that varying rates have been reported. The prevalence has ranged from 4% to 12% (median, 5.8%).[2] Rates are higher in community samples (10.3%) than in school samples (6.9%), and higher among male subjects (9.2%) than among female subjects (3.0%).[2] This effect also seems to extend even into population-based studies. One population-based survey in which identical interview strategies were used in four different communities revealed prevalence rates that varied from 1.6% to 9.4 % (pooled mean, 5.1%).[19]

As with other neurodevelopmental disorders, ADHD is more common in boys and men, and male : female ratios are 5 : 1 for predominantly hyperactive/impulsive type and 2 : 1 for predominantly inattentive type.[20,21] Many experts believe this gender difference exists partially because boys commonly present with the externalizing hyperactive/impulsive symptoms such as aggression and overactivity, whereas girls often present with internalizing inattentive symptoms such as underachievement and daydreaming.[20,21] This difference is thought to lead to an earlier referral for boys and a later referral and, possibly, underdiagnosis for girls.

ETIOLOGY

Despite extensive research, no single causative factor has been identified. The cause of ADHD remains unclear. It is currently thought to have a multifactorial origin. Many theories exist, but research has not consistently shown that food allergies, too much television, poor home life, poor parenting, or poor schools cause ADHD, although these issues may exacerbate ADHD symptoms and impairment.

Approximately 20% to 25% of children who have ADHD also have a diagnosis that can be associated with an organic cause. Prenatal exposure to some substances may be dangerous to the developing fetal brain. For example, children born with fetal alcohol syndrome may exhibit the same hyperactivity, inattention, and impulsivity as do children with ADHD[22] (see Chapter 11). Exposure to other toxins, including cocaine, nicotine, and lead, or the occurrence of trauma or infection that leads to central nervous system damage may produce the ADHD symptom complex.[22] In the other 75% to 80% of affected children, ADHD is thought to have a polygenic basis. Genetic evidence of ADHD has been provided by studies involving adoption, twins, siblings, and parents. In twin studies, the heritability of ADHD has been estimated at 0.75 (75% of the variance in phenotype can be attributed to genetic factors). If a child with ADHD has an identical twin, the twin has a greater than 50% chance of developing ADHD.[23] Family studies have also demonstrated that adoptive relatives of children with ADHD are less likely to have the disorder[24,25] and that first-degree relatives have a greater risk than do controls.[26-28]

Neuroimaging studies with magnetic resonance imaging, positron emission tomography, and single photon emission computed tomography have demonstrated differences in brain structure and function between individuals with ADHD and controls in the basal ganglia, cerebellar vermis, and frontal lobes. These areas are thought to regulate attention: The basal ganglia help inhibit automatic responses, the vermis is thought to regulate motivation, and the prefrontal cortex helps filter out distractions.[23,29,30] Investigations of the brain's response to stimulants have implicated the dopaminergic system as a possible contributor to the disorder. Dopamine can inhibit or intensify the activity of other neurons. It is also possible that the norepinephrine receptors may be involved; however, this has yet to be confirmed. Specific gene associations have been identified in a small proportion of individuals with ADHD. These include the dopamine transporter gene (DAT1), the D4 receptor gene (DRD4), and the human thyroid receptor–β gene.[31-34] Currently, imaging and genetic analysis are not helpful on a clinical basis because of the wide variation of size and function of the brain in individuals with ADHD and those without ADHD and the small numbers who have identified gene abnormalities.

PROGNOSIS

It was once thought that children outgrew ADHD. It is now known that 70% to 80% of children who have ADHD continue to have difficulty through adolescence and adulthood.[35] The manifestation of symptoms usually changes through a child's lifetime. In general, hyperactive core symptoms decrease over time, whereas inattentive symptoms persist.[35] Some children learn to adapt and are able to build on their strengths and minimize their impairment. The majority continues to struggle, with their impairment manifesting in different ways. The true outcome depends on the severity of symptoms, presence or absence of coexisting conditions, social circumstances, intelligence, socioeconomic status, and treatment history.[35] Adolescents with ADHD have higher rates of school failure, motor vehicle accidents, substance abuse, and encounters with law officials than do the general population.[36] Adults with ADHD may achieve lower socioeconomic status and have more marital problems than do the general population.[36]

EVALUATION AND DIAGNOSIS

Despite extensive research into the disorder, there is no single test to diagnose ADHD. The symptoms reflect a spectrum; that is, they can be seen in many children at some time or another without causing difficulty, and some symptoms may be more prominent in some children with ADHD and other symptoms in others. It is only when symptoms are persistent, are pervasive (they are present in multiple environments), cause impairment greater than that expected for the child's developmental age, and cannot be accounted for by another disorder that ADHD is established as the diagnosis.

To establish the degree of symptoms and their functional significance, and to rule out alternative causes, information must be gathered from many sources. This includes obtaining a thorough history and physical examination, reviewing ADHD-specific behaviors in multiple settings, and determining the presence of any comorbid conditions. For children, the sources must include, at a minimum, their parents and teachers.[1] Teachers observe children for up to 6 hours a day. They see them in comparison with a group of same-age peers and in situations that require the children to pay attention, control their activity level, and resist their impulses. When possible, it is also helpful to obtain information from other observers, such as coaches, scout leaders, and grandparents. Direct observation of a child's behavior in the classroom can provide some of the most objective information, if it is available, but this is labor intensive and therefore has to be limited to small samples of time.[1,4] Observations in the pediatric office are frequently not useful because they may not be well correlated with the child's behavior in the home, classroom, and community.

ADHD remains a clinical diagnosis based on specific criteria and clinical impression. It is important to use a structured, systematic approach in evaluating children with behavioral problems and not to rely on clinical judgment alone. Table 16-1 is a general overview of the recommended guidelines for diagnosing ADHD.[1,3,3a,37] Depending on the situation, many health care providers obtain information from behavioral rating scales before proceeding to an office evaluation. Scales in which *DSM-IV* criteria are used are helpful[1] (e.g., the Vanderbilt Assessment Scales,[21] DuPaul and associates' ADHD Rating Scale-IV[38]; the Revised Conners Rating Scales[39]). Broadband scales (e.g., Child Behavior Checklist[40] and Behavior Assessment System for Children[41]) were not found to

---

TABLE 16-1 ■ Evaluation Process

1. During phone call or office visit, a 6- to 12-year-old child is identified by parent/caregiver, teacher, or clinician with concerns of academic underachievement or behavioral problems (e.g., cannot sit still, cannot concentrate, does not listen, is impulsive).
2. Office staff gives parent/caregiver
   a. Parent packet, which gathers information about
      Current concerns
      Development milestones
      Family history
      Medical history
      Birth history
      Social history
   b. Teacher packet, which gathers information about
      Current concerns
      Past school reports, problems, concerns at each grade level
3. Parent/caregiver
   a. Fills out forms and returns them to pediatrician's office in person, by mail, or by fax
   b. Gives teacher packet to schoolteacher
4. Schoolteacher fills out forms and returns them to pediatrician's office in person, by mail or by fax
5. Office staff or physician determines whether child has had a complete history and physical examination in past 6 months, to include the following:
   a. History
      Current concerns
      Development milestones
      Family history
      Medical history
      Birth history
      Social history
   b. Physical examination
      Vital signs and growth
        Height
        Weight
        Pulse
        Blood pressure
      Full physical examination
      Neurological examination

   c. Screening
      Hearing screen (in past 12 months)
      Vision screen (in past 12 months)
6. As determined by office protocol, staff person may make appointment to update information just listed or may wait for all documentation and allow clinician to update information at the follow-up/education visit.
7. Once parent/teacher information has been received in the pediatric office, a staff person checks to see whether all forms are complete.
   a. If they are complete, staff person gives them to clinician to review and makes appointment for return visit.
   b. If they are not complete, staff person calls parent/teacher to gather information and, once it is complete, makes appointment for return visit.
8. The clinician
   a. Reviews parent packet and teacher packet, making note of pertinent positive and negative information.
   b. At the follow-up visit, updates and reviews history and physical examination as necessary and determines whether child meets *DSM-IV* criteria for ADHD:
      Were some symptoms present before age 7?
      Do symptoms cause impairment in 2 or more settings?
      Has impairment been present at least 6 months?
      Is *DSM-IV* symptom count met?
         Parent/caregiver Behavior Rating Scale:
            ADHD-Inattentive (/9)
            ADHD-Hyperactive (/9)
            ADHD-Combined (/9 inattentive and /9 hyperactive)
         Teacher Behavior Rating Scale:
            ADHD-Inattentive (/9)
            ADHD-Hyperactive (/9)
            ADHD-Combined (/9 inattentive and /9 hyperactive)
9. Does child have symptoms of comorbid conditions?
10. In meeting with family and child, clinician
    a. Discusses presence or absence of ADHD diagnosis.
    b. Addresses comorbid symptoms as necessary.
    c. Educates parent and child and proceeds to treatment.

ADHD, attention-deficit/hyperactivity disorder; *DSM-IV*, *Diagnostic and Statistical Manual of Mental Disorders*, 4th edition.[4]

be as helpful in making an ADHD diagnosis but do help screen for co-occurring conditions.[1] Other clinicians are more comfortable gathering information from an office visit to gain a clearer picture of the problems before proceeding to the next step. In evaluation of a child for ADHD, the differential diagnosis and common comorbid diagnoses are quite extensive (Tables 16-2 and 16-3). Keeping these in mind when the history and physical examination are updated is important because many conditions can mimic or coexist with ADHD. The correct diagnosis dictates the proper treatment and prognosis for patients. Young children most commonly have comorbid complications of developmental delays, communication disorders, developmental coordination disorder, reading and writing problems, tic disorder, oppositional

---

TABLE 16-2 ■ Differential and/or Comorbid Diagnoses

Developmental Disorders	Prenatal insult	Williams syndrome
Developmental coordination disorder	Prenatal alcohol/drug use	Neurofibromatosis type I
Language disorder	Prematurity	Inborn errors of metabolism
Learning disability	Low birth weight	
Mental retardation	Birth complications	**Psychiatric Disorders**
Motor dysfunction	Seizure disorder	Adjustment disorder
Normal variant	Sensory deficits	Mood disorder
Pervasive developmental disorder	Hearing	Depression
	Vision	Bipolar disorder
Medical Disorders	Sleep apnea/disorder	Negative/antisocial behaviors
Anemia	Substance abuse	Oppositional defiant disorder
Central nervous system damage	Thyroid disease	Conduct disorder
Trauma		Psychotic disorder
Infection	**Genetic Disorders**	Anxiety
Lead intoxication	Klinefelter syndrome	Tourette syndrome
Medications	Turner syndrome	
Asthma	Fragile X syndrome	
Antiepileptic		
Allergy		

TABLE 16-3 ■ Comorbid Protocol: Does Child Have Symptoms of Comorbid Conditions?

Learning disorder or
  language disorder
	If symptoms indicate some effect of behavior problems on learning, consider referral to
	  school study team for Section 504 classroom accommodations
	If history suggests a learning problem, instruct parents on how to request psychoeducational
	  testing or Individualized Education Program (IEP)

Mental health disorder
  Oppositional defiant disorder
  Conduct disorder
  Anxiety
  Depression
  Autistic spectrum disorder
  Pervasive developmental delay
  Bipolar
  Psychosis
  Obsessive-compulsive disorder
  Post-traumatic stress disorder
  Tics
	If yes:
	Confirm diagnosis in office *or* refer to mental health services

Medical condition
  Neurological problem
  Seizure disorder
  Tourette syndrome
  Genetic syndrome
	If yes:
	Confirm diagnosis in office *or* refer to required specialty

Psychosocial issues
  Environmental Stressors
  Family stressors
	If yes:
	Provide anticipatory guidance in office *or* refer to mental health or social work services

defiant disorder, anxiety, or autistic behaviors, whereas older children and adults may have comorbid symptoms related to depression, anxiety, substance abuse disorder, or conduct disorder. One extensive review revealed the following percentages of comorbid diagnoses: 35%, oppositional defiant disorder; 26%, conduct disorder; 18%, depression; 26%, anxiety; and 12%, learning disorders.[2]

DSM-IV Criteria

The *DSM-IV*[4,4a] provides the diagnostic criteria currently used in the United States. It contains a description of 18 core symptoms focusing on the main problems of inattention, hyperactivity, and impulsivity (Table 16-4). The child must exhibit at least six of nine inattentive behaviors inappropriately often to meet the criteria for ADHD, inattentive subtype; at least six of nine hyperactive/impulsive behaviors

inappropriately often to meet the criteria for ADHD, hyperactive/impulsive subtype; and six of nine behaviors in both dimensions to meet the criteria for ADHD, combined subtype. In addition to the presence of the core symptoms:

1. *Symptoms occur to a degree inconsistent with the child's developmental age.* Attention span increases, and activity levels decrease with age. This aspect of development may be delayed in children with other developmental delays.
2. *The symptoms must have been present for at least 6 months.* The requirement of at least 6 months' duration reflects the chronic nature of the condition.
3. *The symptoms must have started before the age of 7 years.* This age was not based on strong empirical evidence, but a search for symptoms that may have been present at a younger age, but not disabling, is usually fruitful. For example, some children with

---

TABLE 16-4 ■ DSM-IV Symptom Checklist*

DSM-IV–Defined Inattentive Symptoms	Never	Sometimes	Often	Very Often
1. Makes careless mistakes	☐	☐	☐	☐
2. Has difficulty sustaining attention	☐	☐	☐	☐
3. Does not seem to listen	☐	☐	☐	☐
4. Does not follow through on tasks	☐	☐	☐	☐
5. Is not organized	☐	☐	☐	☐
6. Avoids sustained mental effort	☐	☐	☐	☐
7. Loses things	☐	☐	☐	☐
8. Is easily distracted	☐	☐	☐	☐
9. Is forgetful	☐	☐	☐	☐
DSM-IV–Defined Hyperactive-Impulsive Symptoms	**Never**	**Sometimes**	**Often**	**Very Often**
10. Fidgets or squirms	☐	☐	☐	☐
11. Inappropriately leaves seat	☐	☐	☐	☐
12. Inappropriately runs or climbs	☐	☐	☐	☐
13. Has difficulty playing quietly	☐	☐	☐	☐
14. Is "on the go"	☐	☐	☐	☐
15. Talks excessively	☐	☐	☐	☐
16. Blurts out answers	☐	☐	☐	☐
17. Has difficulty waiting for his or her turn	☐	☐	☐	☐
18. Interrupts or intrudes on others	☐	☐	☐	☐
To Be Positive, the Symptoms Must Meet the Following Criteria	**Yes**	**No**		
1. Do symptoms occur often, to a degree inconsistent with child's developmental age?	☐	☐		
2. Have symptoms been present for at least 6 months?	☐	☐		
3. Were some symptoms present before the age of 7 years?	☐	☐		
4. Are some symptoms present in two or more settings (home, school, leisure or legal areas)?	☐	☐		
5. Is there clear evidence of significant impairment in those settings?	☐	☐		
6. Have you determined that the symptoms are not solely attributed to another condition (e.g., pervasive developmental disorder, sensory impairment, child abuse, mental retardation, schizophrenia, mood disorder, anxiety disorder)?	☐	☐		

DSM-IV, Diagnostic and Statistical Manual of Mental Disorders, 4th edition.[4]
*To be considered positive, the symptoms must be present often or very often in comparison to other children of the same developmental level.

the inattentive subtype may not come to attention until an older age, when they have a greater need to concentrate, but frequently a review of old report cards or teacher notes reveals comments on problems with following directions or organization skills. However, the onset of symptoms after the age of 7 increases the probability that symptoms may be secondary to depression or trauma, and increased care is needed to rule out these possibilities.

4. *The impairment must be present in more than one setting*, because if it is present in only one setting, the problem is more likely a property of that environment than of the child. However, this criterion is also not empirically based.

5. *The symptoms must cause significant impairment in more than one setting (e.g., school and home).* The most important aspect of the diagnosis is the concept that the core symptoms impair the patient's ability to function. There are individuals who have many of the core symptoms, but because of their strengths (such as above-average intelligence), they are able to compensate well enough to prevent the symptoms from causing significant dysfunction. In other cases, caretakers may be overrating the frequency of essentially normal behaviors, and the absence of impairment provides a check against overdiagnosis.

6. *The symptoms should not be the result of another mental disorder.* As noted previously, the symptoms of ADHD are not specific to this disorder. If symptoms of another disorder such as depression, mania, or schizophrenia predominate, the other diagnosis is made.

It is important to remember that attention is inherently an interaction between child and environment. A child's behavior varies with setting, situation, and stimulus. It is typical for symptoms to be minimal when there is novelty, immediate reinforcement, or increased stimulus salience involved (such as a movie, video game, or doctor visit). Symptoms are often most intense when the situation is less interesting or unstructured and requires concentration, such as listening to instructions, doing homework, or sitting in religious services.[36,42]

Associated problems can increase the attentional demands of a situation. Cognitive or learning disabilities, family disruption, or dysfunctional classrooms can all increase inattentive behaviors. For these differences, it is important to obtain information from multiple sources. Parent and teacher behavioral rating scales specific for ADHD can effectively provide information required to make a specific diagnosis. Broadband scales are less useful for establishing specific diagnoses but can be useful in screening for comorbid conditions.[2] This can also be achieved by verbal inter-

view, if the clinician has the time, and is systematic in the interview process. The interview can sometimes reveal biases of some reporters: for example, teachers who believe that ADHD does not exist or parents who resist accepting diagnoses of learning disorders. Sometimes a child has few symptoms in a very structured special education setting but exhibits impairment in typical settings such as regular education, in the community, and at home.

Common Noncore Symptoms of Attention-Deficit/Hyperactivity Disorder

In addition to the *DSM-IV* core symptoms, there are a number of symptoms that are frequently seen in ADHD, but do not imply an additional comorbid diagnoses. These include social skills dysfunction, problems with self-esteem, motor coordination, and sleep. Social skills deficits have been documented in preschool, middle childhood, and adolescent children with ADHD.[42a,42b] In long-term follow-up studies of hyperactive children, investigators have reported reduced numbers of friends, low measures of self-esteem , and an increase in antisocial behavior.[43] Results of one study suggested that some of these difficulties may arise from an inappropriately high level of self-esteem or "positive illusory self-concept" on the basis of sociometric analyses of child, peer, and teacher ratings of social competence.[44]

Sleep disturbances are common in children with ADHD[45-47] but may not come to the attention of the clinician until after the presenting behavioral crisis has resolved. There may then be confusion as to whether the sleep disturbance is secondary to the ADHD or is a side effect of stimulant medication. In most placebo-controlled studies of stimulant medication, investigators have reported an increase in sleep problems, although several sleep laboratory studies have not demonstrated worsening of sleep disturbance with stimulant therapy.[48,49] Reports of increased rates of inattention in children referred for sleep evaluations and improvement after tonsillectomy and adenoidectomy[50-52] underscore the importance of a good sleep history in an initial ADHD evaluation. In one comparison of children with "significant" ADHD symptoms with those with "mild" symptoms, findings suggested that obstructive apnea was uncommon in "significant" ADHD but caused a syndrome of "mild" inattention and distractibility.[53]

TREATMENT

It is important to understand that ADHD is a chronic illness for which there is no cure. However, even though there is no curative treatment for the condition, ongoing management can minimize the extent of impairment. First, it is important to educate the parents and patients about the condition and its treatment. This education can help to demystify the condition and clarify many misconceptions raised in the popular press or prevalent in the community. Educated families are better able to work as partners with the clinician in establishing and maintaining an effective treatment program. The treatment plan should be carefully tailored for each individual patient (Table 16-5). When a family is invested in the treatment plan, there is an increased chance of adherence to the regimen.[3] This investment can be maximized by educating the family about their options and by taking individual needs, family preferences, opinions, and lifestyle into account in designing the regimen. For the most favorable outcomes, it is necessary to develop a multidisciplinary approach involving the child, caregiver, educators, and clinician. Communication between home, school, and clinician is needed for monitoring outcomes and making quick changes when needed. Three treatment strategies have been studied and shown effective in treating ADHD: medication, behavioral modification, and a combination of both.[54,55]

TABLE 16-5 ■ Treatment

1. With input from information gathered from parent, teacher, and child, main problem areas are identified at home and school
2. Target goals are identified on the basis of the main problem areas
3. An individualized comprehensive treatment plan is developed on the basis of the problem areas and target goals
4. Behavioral therapy
   Positive reinforcement
   Time out
   Response cost
   Token economy
   Daily report cards
5. School plan
   Informal classroom modifications
   IEP meeting (IDEA)
   Section 504 plan
6. Social skills training
7. Stimulant medication
8. Other interventions if indicated
   Physical therapy evaluation/therapy
   Occupational therapy evaluation/therapy
   Speech evaluation/therapy
   Sensory integration evaluation/therapy
   Hearing/audiological evaluation
   Vision evaluation
   Educational/cognitive testing

IDEA, Individuals with Disabilities Education Act of 2004; IEP, Individualized Education Plan.

Family Education

Educating the caregivers and child about ADHD is essential to good treatment outcomes. Education can help the family come to grips with the diagnosis (Table 16-6). Understanding that ADHD is a brain-based problem and not caused by poor parenting or that it is not intentional misbehavior by the child can relieve guilt and help alleviate stress and frustration that have been present for many years. Raising, teaching, or being a child who has difficulty sustaining attention, filtering out stimuli, learning from past mistakes, and regulating activity level can be very challenging. Being able to change the focus on helping the child improve function instead of always pointing out bad behaviors will improve satisfaction with the child's response to treatment. ADHD runs in families, and many parents of affected children had difficult school experiences themselves. A physician or other medical personnel moderating interaction between home and school can help build trust and cooperation.

As a chronic condition, the symptoms and impairment change throughout the child's life and developmental stages (Table 16-7). Providing updated information to the child and family as these developmental stages approach helps the family face new challenges and anticipate and prepare for the future. This information can be provided through a variety of resources, including trained staff, handouts, suggested reading lists, Internet Web sites, local and national support groups, and community resources. (See Appendix: Helpful Internet Resources)[56]

Medication

Medications used for ADHD include stimulants, norepinephrine reuptake inhibitors, antihypertensives, bupropion, and modafinil. Common medications are listed in Table 16-8.

TABLE 16-6 ■ Education for Child, Parents/Caregivers, and Teacher

1. Discuss effect of ADHD on learning, behavior, social skills, family function, effects on daily life
2. Discuss current knowledge of causes of ADHD
3. Discuss treatment options and side effects
4. Periodically review child's and family's understanding of discussions 1-3
5. Offer to link family/child to other families who have a child with ADHD, to ADHD associations (e.g. CHADD), and to community resources

CHADD, Children and Adults with Attention Deficit/Hyperactivity Disorder.

TABLE 16-7 ■ Symptoms and Manifestation of Attention-Deficit/Hyperactivity Disorder through a Lifetime

Symptoms	Life Stage	Possible Presentation
Hyperactivity	Preschool-aged child	Motoric hyperactivity
Impulsivity		Aggressiveness
Inattention	Elementary school–aged child	Underachievement
Distractibility		Lack of motivation
Frustration		Reputation as class clown
Boredom		Difficulty following class rules
Poor social skills		
Poor organizational skills	Older school-aged child	Difficulty completing homework independently
Difficulty learning from mistakes	Teenager/college student	Increased social problems
		Trouble with long-term projects
		Car accidents
	Adults	Trouble juggling demands of marriage/family and work
		Trouble interacting with colleagues
		Difficulty keeping a job
		Difficulty managing money

TABLE 16-8 ■ Medication

Medication (Generic Name)	Brand Name	Starting Dosage Recommendations	Dosing Intervals	Onset of Action	Duration of Action (Hours)	Maximum Dose
Stimulants						
Mixed salts of amphetamine	Adderall	2.5-5 mg	q.d.-b.i.d.	20-60 minutes	6	40 mg
	Adderall XR	10 mg	q.d.	20-60 minutes	12	30 mg
Dextroamphetamine	Dexedrine/Dextrostat	2.5-5 mg	b.i.d.-t.i.d.	20-60 minutes	4-6	40 mg
	Dexedrine Spansules	5 mg	q.d.-b.i.d.	≥60 minutes	≥6	40 mg
Methylphenidate (D,L-threo-methylphenidate)	Concerta	18 mg	q.d.	20-60 minutes	12	72 mg
	Methylin	5 mg	b.i.d.-t.i.d.	20-60 minutes	3-5	60 mg
	Methylin SR	20 mg	q.d.-b.i.d.	1-3 hours	2-6	60 mg
	Ritalin	5 mg	b.i.d.-t.i.d.	20-60 minutes	3-5	60 mg
	Ritalin-SR	20 mg	q.d.-b.i.d.	1-3 hours	3-8	60 mg
	Ritalin-LA	10-20 mg	q.d.	20-60 minutes	>8	60 mg
	Metadate ER	10 mg	q.d.	1-3 hours	3-8	60 mg
	Metadate CD	20 mg	q.d.	20-60 minutes	8	60 mg
Methylphenidate transdermal	Daytrana	10 mg	q.d. (9 hr)	2-3 hours	12	30 mg
D-Methylphenidate	Focalin	2.5 mg	q.d.-b.i.d.	20-60 minutes	4-6	20 mg
	Focalin XR	5 mg	q.d.	1 hour	12	20 mg
Norepinephrine Reuptake Inhibitors						
Atomoxetine	Strattera	0.5 mg/kg/d	q.d.	4-8 weeks	continuous	1.5 mg/kg/d
Tricyclic antidepressants (require baseline ECG); e.g., imipramine, desipramine	Tofranil Norpramin	2 mg/kg/day	b.i.d.-t.i.d.	4 weeks	continuous	5 mg/kg/day
α₂-Adrenergic Agonists						
Clonidine	Catapres	0.05 mg	q.d.-q.i.d.	20-60 minutes	3-4	0.6 mg 0.3 q.d.
Guanfacine	Tenex	***	***	***	***	***
Novel Agents						
Bupropion	Wellbutrin	50 mg t.i.d.	q.d.-t.i.d.	4 weeks	***	100 mg t.i.d.
	Wellbutrin SR	100 mg b.i.d.	b.i.d.	4 weeks	***	150 mg b.i.d.
Modafinil	Provigil	100 mg q.d.	q.d.	1 week	continuous	400 mg q.d.

ECG, electrocardiography.

STIMULANTS

The stimulants have been the most extensively studied and are considered the first choice of pharmacological management for ADHD because of both their efficacy and safety.[2] The stimulant medications include dextroamphetamine, methylphenidate, and mixed salts of amphetamine. More than 300 studies with 6000 subjects have demonstrated the short-term efficacy of stimulants.[57] Most researchers have studied the effects of stimulants on elementary school–aged children. The medications often offer immediate and dramatic improvement to a child's symptom complex. Improvements are present only as long as medication is taken. Stimulants are effective in 70% to 80% of affected children.[36] The stimulant medications reduce the core symptoms of inattention, hyperactivity, and impulsivity. They also improve academic productivity (e.g., the number of problems completed on a math sheet), although they do not improve cognitive abilities or performance on standardized academic testing. Furthermore, in some children, they reduce oppositional and aggressive behaviors. Although the evidence for the short-term efficacy of stimulant medications is quite strong, the evidence for long-term efficacy is not as clear.[35] Evidence from the National Institute of Mental Health Multimodal Treatment Study of ADHD (MTA)[55] supports efficacy for 72 months; this has been the longest careful follow-up of children on stimulant medications.

Unlike most pediatric medications, stimulant dosing is not based on milligrams per kilogram.[3,37] Instead, current recommendations are to start at the lowest dosage possible and titrate up according to information gathered from parents and teachers about treatment effectiveness. For titrating, it is important to warn parents that there may be many changes in dosage and that the initial dosage has been selected to be low; otherwise, they may interpret the need for changes as evidence that the medication is ineffective or that excessive dosages are being reached. Depending on the child's daily schedule, multiple doses each day may be required. In most studies of methylphenidate since 2000, three-times-a-day dosing has been used, and some adolescents with evening activities or homework, or children who have a return of severe disruptive behaviors in the evening, may require a fourth dose. Many families and practitioners have experienced a phenomenon referred to as "rebound" in which returning symptoms are worse than baseline for a short time as medication wears off. In behavioral studies in which behaviors over the day are observed and counted, no true rebound has been identified, but a return of symptoms has been documented. This has been treated with half a dose of stimulant, given just before the rebound is antici-

pated. Initial medication titration necessitates follow-up at least weekly by phone or office visit. The best dosage is that at which the child has maximum success reaching individualized target goals and has the fewest side effects. Once response is stable, monitoring can be stretched to monthly and eventually quarter-yearly office visits. Table 16-9 lists monitoring guidelines.

Although most of the studies of medication efficacy have been performed on children with ADHD and normal intelligence, stimulant medications also are effective for many children with mental retardation.[58,59] Stimulant medication is reportedly used by 3.4% of children with moderate mental retardation[60] and 15% of children with mild mental retardation.[61] Although individuals with mild mental retardation respond in essentially the same way as individuals without intellectual impairments, those with severe intellectual impairment are much less likely to respond.[62]

Dextroamphetamine, methylphenidate, and mixed salts of amphetamine have similar effects, side effects, and safety. Although methylphenidate may increase the probability of a seizure in a person with a seizure disorder[63,64] and dextroamphetamine does not, both medications have been used to treat children with ADHD and seizure disorders with no recurrence of seizures as long as the children's seizure disorder

---

TABLE 16-9 ■ Monitoring

1. Weekly contact with parents and teachers until optimal response is determined from information gathered from parent and teacher:
   18 Core symptom count
   Measurement of impairment
   Target goal outcomes
   Side effects screen (if patient is taking medication)
2. Is response adequate?
   If yes, monitor the following monthly and, once patient is stable, quarter-yearly with parent and teacher:
   18 Core symptom count
   Measurement of impairment
   Target goal outcomes
   Side effects screen (if on medication)
   If no, and if patient is not taking stimulant medication, reinforce behavioral therapy, and consider stimulant medication
3. If response is poor despite an individualized plan, check the following:
   Are family, child, and school adhering to treatment?
   Is diagnosis correct?
   Is there an undiagnosed comorbid problem?
   Are target goals inappropriate?
4. If no response or intolerable side effects are present:
   Try different stimulant medication/formulation
   Consider clinical consultations for other options, including alternative medications and treatment

is adequately treated.[63,64] Even in children with other comorbid conditions such as anxiety or mood disorders, it is preferable to treat the ADHD first, because the mood disorder or depressive symptoms may diminish significantly if the stress caused by the ADHD is reduced.

There are several misconceptions about stimulant medications. The effects of the medications are not paradoxical: the same effects are seen in children without ADHD and in adults. Therefore, a response to medication cannot be used as a diagnostic test. Children with ADHD do not find stimulant medications pleasurable and do not commonly abuse them. In the more usual clinical situation, an adolescent for whom stimulants have had documented benefit refuses to take medication. There is some suggestion that children with ADHD who are appropriately managed have a lower risk of substance abuse disorders than do those who are not appropriately managed.[65]

Stimulant medications act as dopamine and norepinephrine reuptake inhibitors, increasing norepinephrine and dopamine activity primarily in the caudate nucleus and prefrontal cortex.[66] Methylphenidate is a piperidine derivative that is a racemic compound. The levo isomer is rapidly metabolized and essentially inactive.[39] Short-acting methylphenidate has a half-life of 2 to 3 hours and a duration of action of about 4 hours.[67] D-Methylphenidate has become available under the brand name Focalin; the manufacturers suggest that it may have fewer side effects but there is little reason to believe that l-methylphenidate contributes to side effects or efficacy of methylphenidate.[68a] One randomized, double-blind, placebo-controlled, comparison study of D-methylphenidate and D,L-methylphenidate found similar efficacy at half of the milligram dose of D-methylphenidate and suggested a longer duration of action in twice daily dosing.[68] Amphetamine is also active in the dextro isomer. D-Amphetamine has a similar half-life and duration of action to methylphenidate. However, L-amphetamine is converted to D-amphetamine in vivo, lengthening the duration of action. This conversion, combined with the slower dissociation and absorption of the saccharate and aspartate salts, accounts for the slightly increased duration of action of mixed amphetamine salt.[69]

Extended-Release Preparation

A number of longer acting stimulant medications have become available. There has been an interest in longer acting medications because, although short-acting stimulants have been shown to be safe and effective, their administration is more challenging.[70] Appreciation that ADHD affects important nonacademic functions has resulted in a desire for "coverage" of longer periods of time each day. When short-acting stimulants are used, symptoms return at the end of each 3- to 6-hour period, often at the most unstructured times of the day (while getting up and ready for school, at lunchtime, and on the bus ride home).[71] The need to take medication at school presents difficulties with remembering to take the dose, stigmatization of students who take medication, refusal to take medication at school, school policies that discourage the taking of medication at school, opportunities for diversion of controlled substances, and personnel costs for schools. After school, the problems of taking a third dose at the end of the school day or at daycare also cause difficulties for many families. The unevenness of the effect over the 3- to 4-hour course, repeated two to three times each day, is problematic for children with ADHD and their caretakers. The cost of medication goes up with the number of pills used, which often results in costs for generic preparations that would rival those of a once-a-day branded preparation. A medication that can be taken once daily offers many potential benefits. Two reports of stimulant medication use patterns, one in a Medicaid population and the other in a managed care population, demonstrated increased continuity of treatment with use of extended-release preparations in clinical practice.[72,73]

On the other hand, there are concerns that covering too much of the day with medication that may suppress appetite or interfere with sleep limits the utility of longer acting medications. There is also concern that the development of new medications may be driven more by profit motives of drug manufacturers than by the clinical needs of children.

The evidence of the efficacy of long-acting medications is derived almost entirely from studies financed by their manufacturers. The older preparations, developed before the advent of advertising and the U.S. Food and Drug Administration's (FDA's) "pediatric rule,"[73a] have almost no published support. Since 1998, as the market for ADHD medication has become more competitive, a number of studies assessing the newer preparations have been published. There are no large federally funded studies, such as the MTA,[55] of long-acting medications.

Criteria for the adoption of longer-acting medications should include

1 Consistent effect over the course of the day.
2 No clinically significant increase in side effects.
3 No major increase in cost.

Older Medications

Three medications with longer duration of action than immediate-release methylphenidate have been available for a number of years. These are Ritalin SR (methylphenidate in a wax matrix) and Dexedrine

Spansules (dextroamphetamine in small beads that release an initial immediate dose and release the remainder of the dose slowly over about 8 hours). Pemoline (Cylert), a third longer acting medication, has been removed from the market because of a potentially severe side effect of liver toxicity. The published literature on these medications is limited. Ritalin SR has not been as effective as expected. The onset of action is slow, often necessitating the coadministration of immediate-release methylphenidate in the morning, and afternoon efficacy requires higher drug levels not achieved by this slow-release preparation. In the one small double-blind comparison of methylphenidate, 10 mg twice a day, and methylphenidate SR 20 mg once a day, twice a day methylphenidate was comparable with the slow-release preparation on measures of cognition and social performance and superior on measures of disruption.[74] In other small studies there were no differences.[75,76] Diagnostic criteria and outcome measures employed in these studies were much different from those of recent studies of stimulants in ADHD. In one small ($N = 22$) crossover trial in a summer treatment program, Dexedrine Spansules and pemoline were more frequently recommended than methylphenidate SR or twice-a-day methylphenidate, on the basis of behavioral observations.

Newer Sustained-Release Stimulants

Since 1998, there has been a proliferation in the number of clinical trials of longer acting medications for ADHD. There have been at least 11 published studies on modified-release stimulants and 9 studies of a novel norepinephrine reuptake inhibitor, atomoxetine. All of these studies were funded by the manufacturers. There were also a number of pharmacokinetic studies that demonstrated that the desired drug levels are delivered after fasting, after a high-fat meal, or when the beaded capsules are sprinkled onto food.

In general, the stimulant studies reveal efficacy and side effects similar to those previously reported for the immediate-acting preparations of the same pharmaceuticals. The individual preparations are formulated by different approaches to the shortcomings of Ritalin SR: the need for sufficient immediate release and the need for higher blood levels in the afternoon to achieve equal effectiveness.

The first of the reformulated stimulant medications was OROS methylphenidate (Concerta). OROS methylphenidate is an osmotically active capsule with an overcoat of methylphenidate. The overcoat is delivered rapidly, and the osmotic capsule delivers medication at a rate that produces a gradually increase in blood levels over the day. The capsules are designed so that 18 mg of OROS methylphenidate should mimic the effect of

5 mg of immediate-release methylphenidate given three times a day. In an analogue classroom, double-blind, crossover situation, it has been shown to have effects comparable to three-times-a-day methylphenidate for over 12 hours.[77] In another large ($N = 282$), multisite, short-term (4 weeks), parallel group design, OROS methylphenidate was again shown to be comparable to three-times-a-day methylphenidate.[78] The reported effect sizes for both OROS methylphenidate and three-times-a-day methylphenidate were about the same. In another report, the open-label long-term follow-up of children previously studied in short-term double-blind studies ($N = 407$) revealed that 71% of patients remained on the medication for at least 1 year with maintenance of behavior ratings and a modest average increase in average dosage.[79] In a study of simulated driving in adolescents, positive effects on driving performance persisted longer into the evening with OROS methylphenidate than with three-times-a-day methylphenidate.[80]

There are two preparations now available in which delayed-release beads simulate twice-a-day administration of methylphenidate. Methylphenidate extended-release capsules (Metadate CD) are divided into 30% immediate-release and 70% delayed-release doses, and methylphenidate extended release capsules (Ritalin LA) are divided into 50% immediate-release and 50% delayed-release doses. Methylphenidate extended-release capsules (Metadate CD), 20, 40, or 60 mg, was compared with OROS methylphenidate, 18, 36, or 54 mg (in a trial funded by the manufacturer of Metadate CD); methylphenidate extended-release capsules had a quicker onset of morning action, was comparable in strength in the afternoon, and wore off sooner in the evening.[81] In a postmarketing, uncontrolled study of 308 children, 65% had significant improvement on the Clinical Global Impressions scale, and 87% of parents reported satisfaction with the treatment. In a double-blind, placebo-controlled study, methylphenidate extended-release capsules (Ritalin LA) was shown safe and effective, as expected.[82] In a double-blind crossover comparison with OROS methylphenidate, methylphenidate extended-release capsules (Ritalin LA) was shown, as expected, to have a quicker onset.[83]

The comparison studies are designed to highlight competitive advantages of one preparation over the others. For example, when a preparation designed to simulate 10 mg twice-a-day dosing is compared with a preparation designed to simulate 5 mg three-times-a-day dosing, the manufacturer of the first medication reports outcomes that stress faster onset of effect, and the manufacturer of the second reports outcomes that stress evening function.

The longer acting preparation of mixed amphetamine salts (Adderall XR) has also been shown to last more than 12 hours and to be safe and effective in a large parallel-group, double-blind, multisite study.[84] The children in this study were followed in an open-label extension for 2 years, and the medication was well tolerated.[85] A later analysis of cardiovascular effects revealed minimal effects (increased systolic blood pressure of 3.5 mm Hg, increased pulse of 3.4 beats per minute, and no change in corrected Q-T interval).[86] However, there have been reports of sudden death in adolescents taking mixed amphetamine salts. These events have been rare, and the baseline rate of sudden death in an equivalent number of untreated adolescents is unknown. The FDA has revised its recommendations to include an encouragement of physicians to identify existing cardiac conditions in patients before initiating treatment and to monitor cardiac conditions closely, but a more stringent warning (Black Box) was not believed to be warranted.[87]

A transdermal D-methylphenidate patch (Daytrana) has been approved by the FDA. Only preliminary data have been published. Results of one dose-ranging study of 36 children,[88] a study of the patch in combination with behavior modification in 27 children,[89] and a 1-week placebo-controlled crossover study of 80 children[90] all suggest efficacy and tolerability similar to those with oral treatments.

The D-threo enantiomer of methylphenidate has also been isolated in a new medication, dexmethylphenidate (Focalin). It has properties similar to those of the racemic compound but is twice as potent. It is rapidly absorbed, reaching a maximum level in the fasting state after 1 to 1.5 hours. The levels obtained were similar to those of the racemic compound. The mean elimination half-life is 2.7 hours. The metabolism, like that for the racemic compound, is principally a deesterification to ritalinic acid. In children with ADHD, it produced significant improvement in comparison with a placebo.[91] It does not appear to provide benefits or risks different from those of racemic methylphenidate.[68a] It is also available in an extended-release formulation that utilizes microbead technology (Focalin XR).

In summary, the newer generation stimulant preparations have been shown safe and effective at a standard that was not met for previous long-acting medications. However, the research is still limited by drug company sponsorship and short duration of follow-up.

Cost

Newer, patented preparations of generically available medications cost more per pill than the generic preparations that are often preferred by third-party payer pharmacy committees. However, if fewer pills are taken and other costs are taken into account,

long-acting medications may be less expensive than short-acting generic medications. In an econometric study funded by the makers of Metadate CD, the investigators attempted to factor in cost of medication, cost of school personnel to store and distribute medication, and the cost of physician evaluations for combined methylphenidate immediate-release/extended-release, methylphenidate immediate-release three times daily, extended-release methylphenidate (Metadate CD) once daily, OROS methylphenidate once daily, methylphenidate (Ritalin) three times daily, and mixed amphetamine salts (Adderall) twice daily. (Mixed amphetamine salts [Adderall XR] and extended-release methylphenidate [Ritalin LA] were not yet available at the time.)[91a] Costs ranged from $639 to $1124 per year for medication alone. However, when costs for in-school administration by school secretarial staff (estimated at $531 per year) were added, the total costs of once-a-day medication were less than those of generic methylphenidate. The savings are higher if more highly trained school personnel (nurses rather than secretaries) dispense medication at school. The analysis did not account for the costs of disruptive behavior if medication wears off at midday.

Side Effects

The most common side effects of all the stimulant medications are anorexia, headache, and sleep disturbance. The anorexia frequently diminishes after several months. In most placebo-controlled studies, the mean weight of the treated group has begun at higher than the 50th percentile and has decreased but not gone below the 50th percentile. For most patients, monitoring of weight is all that is necessary. If a patient has problematic weight loss, use of calorie-enriched food may be helpful. It is important to determine the patient's current and previous history of sleep and headaches. Sleep problems are frequently present in patients with ADHD before they begin treatment, and in prospective studies, stimulants do not appear to worsen sleep patterns in most children with ADHD.[48,49,53] However, in placebo-controlled trials, there is an increased rate of reports of sleep disturbance in the treated group. According to clinical anecdotes, in some children, increased activity as the medication is wearing off interferes with bedtime routine. In these cases, a later dose of medication may actually improve sleep. Headaches usually improve with a decrease in dose, but a change in medications may be required. The effects on growth have been ambiguous; some studies have demonstrated no effect,[92-94] and some have demonstrated some effect.[95,96]

Less common side effects include dysphoria (in extreme cases, psychotic symptoms), "overfocusing" (usually manifested by the patient's becoming listless or what parents refer to as "appearing like a zombie"), and tics. These side effects can often be resolved by lowering the dosage. Dysphoria is a feeling of being unwell, similar to depression. This may necessitate a change in medications. It is important not to confuse this side effect with worsening of the primary symptoms, because an increase in dosage can worsen these symptoms. Stimulant use has been associated with an increase in tics in some children, but because transient tics are common in children, and because the usual course of tic disorders is for the tics to wax and wane, it can be difficult to determine the relationship between the stimulant medications and the tics. In the OROS methylphenidate clinical trials, there was no significant difference between the rates of tics in the children taking OROS methylphenidate, those taking methylphenidate three times a day, and the controls taking placebo.[97] Of the children who have tics and require treatment with stimulant medication, about one fourth to one third have an increase in the tics and about a fourth have a decrease.[98] In these cases, it is important to weigh the degree of impairment caused by the ADHD symptoms against the impairment attributable to the tics when therapeutic decisions are made.

In summary, although side effects are common, most are mild, and they can be managed by careful monitoring and by slight alterations in dosage and times given. It is rarely necessary to discontinue medication because of side effects. Table 16-10 lists simple strategies for minimizing side effect complications.

Several studies have demonstrated benefits when behavioral therapy was given in addition to stimulant medication. This combined treatment plan has produced greater satisfaction in treatment, according to child, parent, and teacher report.[99,100] In the MTA,[55] combined treatment and medication-only treatment did not differ significantly in decreasing core ADHD symptoms. However, the combined treatment did produce more improvement in oppositional and internalizing symptoms, as well as in teacher-rated social skills, parent-child relations, and reading achievement. This improvement was accomplished with a lower daily dosage of medication than when medication was used alone.

If, after appropriate trials of two or three stimulants or stimulant preparations, an optimal dosage is not obtained, the diagnosis and management plan should be reexamined (see Table 16-9).[37] If the questions in Table 16-9 have been adequately addressed, it is appropriate to prescribe second-line medications, including norepinephrine reuptake inhibitors and α_2-adrenergic agents. These medications may be appropriate in some cases but should be used carefully.

TABLE 16-10 ■ Possible Regimen Modifications to Minimize Side Effects	
Side Effect	**Regimen Modifications**
Decreased appetite	Give medication after meals Change diet (calorie-dense food for breakfast) Allow brief drug holidays
Sleep problems	Reduce/eliminate afternoon dose Change to short-acting drug if patient is taking long-acting one Establish bedtime routine If response is accompanied by rebound, consider adding later dose
Irritability	Decrease dosage Try another stimulant
Headaches	Decrease dosage Try another stimulant
Stomachaches	Decrease dosage Try another stimulant
Dysphoria	Decrease dosage Try another stimulant
Behavioral rebound	Decrease afternoon dose Add later dose at half strength of previous earlier dose Try sustained- and extended-release preparation Combine sustained-release with a short-acting preparation
Growth suppression	Monitor height and weight Determine parental height history Allow drug holidays
Tics	Observe at lower dosage and with no medication to determine whether tics are truly drug related If tics are mild, discuss risks and benefits with parents and child Switch stimulants If tics occur after a sore throat, consider *Streptococcus* association
Psychosis/mania	Stop stimulant

Note: If stimulant is not working or side effects are intolerable, another stimulant or preparation should be tried. If other stimulants do not work or create intolerable side effects, the clinician should consider second-line drugs or referral to a mental health or developmental-behavioral specialist.

They can have more serious side effects and tend to necessitate more monitoring.

NOREPINEPHRINE REUPTAKE INHIBITORS

Tricyclic Antidepressants

The tricyclic antidepressants imipramine, and desipramine have been used in children with ADHD. Their mechanism of action is believed to be the inhibition of the reuptake of norepinephrine, but they also inhibit the reuptake of serotonin and have anticholinergic and quinidine-like effects. Their efficacy in the treatment of ADHD has been supported by approximately 20 randomized control trial studies. They have a much longer half-life than do stimulants; thus, they can be taken once daily, and they have no rebound effect. They also pose minimal risk for abuse. However, side effects are much more serious and include cardiovascular, neurological, and anticholinergic difficulties. Baseline electrocardiography is required before the medication is started, because of the quinidine-like cardiac effects. Acceptable parameters include a heart rate of less than 130, a P-R interval of less than 200 milliseconds, a QRS interval not increased more than 30% from baseline, and a corrected Q-T interval of less than 480 milliseconds.[3] Electrocardiography and measurement should be repeated at each major dosage change.[3] Once the maintenance dosage is determined, a serum level should be obtained, because levels higher than 150 ng/mL have been associated with electrocardiographic changes.[3] High dosages have also resulted in several sudden deaths from cardiac arrhythmias. Because of the greater side effects, particularly cardiac side effects, and the narrow margin of safety, tricyclic antidepressants are currently used only infrequently to treat ADHD.

Atomoxetine

Atomoxetine is the first new nonstimulant agent developed specifically for the treatment of ADHD in children. There are a number of studies in children and adults of various designs (parallel-group, crossover, placebo-controlled, methylphenidate controlled, double-blind, open-label, daily dosing, twice-daily dosing, faster and slower dose escalation).[101-108] Reported effect sizes are moderate (about 0.7 in children and 0.4 in adults, in comparison with the usual 1.0 in stimulant trials). Advantages of atomoxetine are its low abuse/diversion potential, its activity early in the morning before stimulants become effective (time-course, placebo-controlled trials of stimulants often show symptoms are worse with stimulants than with placebo for the first interval after a dose). In contrast to stimulants, dosing is on a milligram-per-kilogram basis. The starting dosage is about 0.5 mg/kg each morning, increasing every 4 to 7 days to a maximum dosage of 1.4 mg/kg. If side effects are excessive, the dosage can be divided to twice a day. Disadvantages are the probably mildly lower effect size and the slow onset of effect (weeks). The slow onset and round-the-clock effects of atomoxetine necessitate closer, more quantitative monitoring of symptom changes than is usual with stimulants to determine their effects, because these gradual, consistent changes are less evident to caretakers than are the rapid, daily changes observed with stimulants. This is especially true with children who have previ-

ous experience with stimulant medications whose parents may view some of the quick changes seen with stimulants as evidence that "the medication is working" and conclude that there is no medication effect with atomoxetine, even if there is a decrease in core ADHD symptoms that is demonstrable in behavior ratings. Side effects include appetite suppression, sedation if the dosage is escalated too rapidly, and irritability. A rare (probably less than 1 per 1,000,000 prescriptions) complication of reversible liver failure has been reported. Such complications are much less common and less severe than what was found with pemoline. In both reported cases, enzyme levels returned to normal after the medication was stopped, and the lack of any elevation in liver function test results before development of this syndrome suggest that routine monitoring of liver function is not useful. There have also been rare reports of suicidal ideation, although no cases of suicide have been reported.

α₂-ADRENERGIC AGONISTS

The α_2-adrenergic medications used to treat patients with ADHD are clonidine and guanfacine. They were developed as antihypertensive agents. However, they affect the central nervous system more broadly. In a meta-analysis of 11 studies of clonidine treatment of ADHD, the effect size of clonidine treatment was estimated at 0.58 (stimulants usually produce an effect size of about 1.0; atomoxetine, 0.7).[109] The side effects of the α_2-adrenergic medications include sedation, fatigue, anorexia, dry mouth, and hypotension. There have been several cases of sudden death in patients treated with a combination of clonidine and methylphenidate, but it could not be confirmed that these deaths were caused by the medications.[109,110] Because of the potential side effects and the limited evidence for efficacy, the α_2-adrenergic medications should be prescribed only if stimulant medications and noradrenergic reuptake inhibitors have failed after an adequate trial and behavioral alternatives are not effective, available, or acceptable to the family.[3] Blood pressure and pulse measurements, supine and standing, should be obtained weekly during the titration phase.[3]

Clonidine had also been used as a treatment for delayed onset of sleep in children with ADHD. One chart review of a pediatric psychopharmacology clinic showed reported that of children taking clonidine for ADHD-associated sleep disturbances, 85% experienced much or very much improvement,[111] but no properly controlled studies have been published.

BUPROPION

Bupropion is an antidepressant medication whose mechanism of action is mostly unclear. It is a weak dopamine agonist, and it decreases whole body norepinephrine levels, but neither of these effects explains its clinical results. Its reputation for efficacy in treating patients with ADHD is based on one multisite study in which it was significantly better than the placebo but not as potent as stimulant medications.[112] The side effects of bupropion include agitation, reduction in the seizure threshold, anorexia, insomnia, and nausea/vomiting.[113] Because bupropion has more sedative effects and there is sparse evidence of its efficacy, it should be prescribed only if stimulant medications, atomoxetine, and behavioral interventions have failed after adequate trials. It may take as long as 4 weeks to demonstrate effectiveness.[3]

MODAFINIL

Modafinil, which is marketed for excessive daytime sleepiness in adults, has been studied as a treatment for ADHD. Modafinil has a different chemical structure than stimulants and is believed to activate cortex directly without causing widespread central nervous system stimulation. In the largest study published to date, investigators reported an effect size between 0.6 and 0.7 for core ADHD symptoms reported by parents and teachers. These investigators used specially prepared film-coated tablets, not currently available, at dosages from 85 to 425 mg, titrated by clinical effect.[114] Modafinil has not been approved by the FDA for use in children and is a Schedule IV drug. The manufacturer has stopped development because some patients developed Stevens-Johnson syndrome in clinical trials.

Psychosocial Interventions

Psychosocial interventions include all of the interventions in which counseling or behavior management is used. The intervention most frequently employed and with the strongest scientific evidence for its efficacy is behavior modification training performed by the significant caretakers in the child's environment. Techniques shown to be effective involve contingency reinforcement, including token economies, timeouts, and response cost (earning or losing privileges).[54] Social skills therapy is an attempt to address the deficit that many children with ADHD have in social situations; however, because of the difficulty that the children have in generalizing what they learn, there is limited evidence for its efficacy unless the training takes place in actual situations with other children. Family therapy may be helpful, particularly for issues such as sibling relationships, but the evidence for its efficacy is weak. Play and cognitive therapy have not been found to be efficacious treatments for children with ADHD.[54]

Parent training occurs in different forms, depending on the severity of the behavioral problems. With children whose behavioral problems are mild and with parents who are adept at behavior management, simple advice from their primary care clinician, combined with reading material, may suffice, although this limited intervention has not been studied to determine its efficacy. Most parents are likely to require more intensive instruction that is available in many communities and consists of training groups of parents in behavior modification techniques.[115] When parents find it difficult to understand or implement the techniques and/or their children demonstrate more severe behavior problems, individualized training tailored to their needs, such as parent-child interaction therapy, is required.[116] The most severe situations, short of removing a child from the home, may require implementing the parent training directly in the home or using a day treatment situation that can train the parent and at the same time shape the child's behavior.

Parent training usually consists of three elements: (1) providing clear commands and rules to the children and then keeping them aware of those rules, (2) providing positive attention and reinforcing the children for positive behaviors, and (3) providing punishment and the removal of the positive attention for rule violations and inappropriate behaviors.[117] It is essential for caregivers (e.g., parents, teachers, child-care workers) to provide positive attention and reinforcement to children. Many times, because of the child's difficult behaviors, caregivers of children with ADHD get into a cycle in which most of their interactions are negative and involve punishment for unwanted behaviors. Unless they are able to develop a systematic method for providing quality time in the form of positive attention and for reinforcing appropriate behaviors, the punishments are ineffective, and the desired goals will not be achieved. Positive attention requires providing undivided attention to the child for activities that are mutually enjoyed by both parties. The caregivers also need to learn to recognize and reward appropriate behaviors.

One systematic method for providing reinforcement is a token system. A token system consists of identifying the appropriate behaviors that parents want their child to increase. The three or four most salient behaviors are targeted, and the child can earn points for performing the appropriate behavior. For example, if the parents want their child to say, "Please" when the child requests something, the child earns points every time he or she uses "please" appropriately. For young children between 3 and 6 to 7 years of age, tangible tokens may work better than the point system. The parents need to set up a system such as a chart to keep track of the points, and the child needs to know how many points he or she needs to achieve a reward. The target behaviors and the number of points necessary to earn rewards can be revised as the child progresses or if the system does not seem to be working. The rewards can be special privileges, such as increased television time or increased time with a parent, or they can be tangible, such as baseball cards. Rewards are most effective when the child participates in selection of the reward. Immediate praise for earning points can help enhance the effects.

A positive system alone is sometimes not sufficient to control the behavior of a child with ADHD. A punishment system may also be required for rule violations and inappropriate behaviors. Effective forms of punishment include timeouts for younger children and removal of privileges for older children. With a token system, a cost response, in which points are removed for rule violations and inappropriate behaviors, can also be employed. The child requires clear messages about the rules and what constitutes inappropriate behaviors. It is important to stress that punishment loses its effectiveness when it becomes too frequent. It has been estimated that punishment is most effective when at least four or five rewards are achieved for each punishment. Therefore, goals should be set so that from the beginning, the child is more likely to be considered successful (earns rewards) than unsuccessful (is not rewarded or is punished). Once the child perceives that he or she can achieve success (rewards), behaviors can be shaped toward the long-term goals by gradually tightening the criteria for success.

School Interventions

Children with ADHD can receive services from their public schools on the basis of Section 504 of the Rehabilitation Act for milder cases and the Individuals with Disabilities Education Act (IDEA) for more severe cases.[118] The Rehabilitation Act (Section 504) requires schools to provide accommodations so that the child can function in his or her class. All children with the diagnosis of ADHD are eligible. However, the act does not provide any added compensation to the school. Therefore, the adaptations provided are of a limited nature, and the procedures are not well defined or scrutinized. Adaptations include preferential class seating, assignment and homework reduction, and consultation with the teacher in helping her or him set up a behavioral program.

The IDEA is a much more comprehensive program, but it is available only to children with ADHD in which the ADHD interferes with their ability to learn or to those with cognitive comorbid conditions such as learning disabilities. The school system is required to provide comprehensive testing, including intellectual, achievement, speech and language, and motor evaluation if appropriate. Testing provided by an external source such as a private psychologist can be used in place of school testing if school personnel believe it is accurate; however, most frequently, outside testing has to be obtained at the parents' expense. On the basis of the test results, the school system is required to develop an Individualized Education Plan (IEP) with clearly measurable goals. Services must be provided so that the child is placed as close to the mainstream as possible (least restrictive environment). As a result, most children with ADHD spend a small portion of the day in a resource room with a teacher trained in special education or with help from an aid in the classroom. Psychological, speech/language and occupational therapy services are also provided as necessary. In cases in which behavior problems are refractory, a functional behavior analysis can be requested. This entire process, from obtaining the testing through providing the services, must be accomplished with informed parental consent. The IDEA is able to put in place such specific guidelines and services because the schools are provided with increased funding that is based on the number of students in special education that they serve and the severity of the students' needs that they address. However, the additional funds rarely cover the full cost of the services. More detailed information about Section 504 and IDEA can be found on several Web sites (see Appendix: Table of Helpful Internet Resources).

Daily report cards are an adaptation of behavioral therapy to the school setting and are an excellent way of monitoring a child's functioning over time. An example of a report card and an explanation of how to establish one can be downloaded from the Comprehensive Treatment for Attention Deficit Disorder Web site.[119] By selecting two to three specific goals to work on at home and at school and by establishing an appropriate reward system, parents and teachers can provide immediate feedback to the child concerning his or her behavior. This feedback can be very motivating for the child and the caregivers as they are able to see target goals met. Once established, they take little time from the teacher and caregiver but provide ongoing monitoring of progress, important daily communication between the teacher and parent, and discovery of problem behaviors early. This is also a good method for monitoring therapy and medication management. In general, a 20% improvement over baseline is targeted for each goal, and the child should have a success rate of 66%.[100] If the success rate target is lower, it does not provide enough encouragement, and if it is close to 100%, the tasks are too easily accomplished. As the child's behavior improves, the requirements for success should be modified to maintain the same level of success. Positive report cards should be rewarded with reinforcements that are of value to the child, such as increased privileges or tangible prizes.[100]

Behavioral interventions do have some limitations. Behavioral interventions alone are frequently insufficient to bring a child with ADHD to a normal range of functioning and are not effective for all children.[55] However, some families are uncomfortable beginning treatment with stimulants and wish to start with behavioral treatment. Beginning with behavioral therapy can also provide baseline measures that allow more precise evaluations of medication effects. In children younger than 6 years, for whom stimulant therapy is not approved by the FDA, an initial period of behavior therapy has been advocated. In addition, parental satisfaction is usually high when behavioral therapy is used. The effects of combining both stimulant medications and behavioral intervention can also lower the dose of medication required, and a less intense behavioral intervention may be needed to reach optimal treatment outcomes.[89,120]

Alternative Treatments

A number of treatments besides stimulant medications and behavioral interventions have been advocated for patients with ADHD, but there is little or no evidence of their efficacy. They can be categorized into the broad groups of diets, dietary supplements, alternative medications, biofeedback, and exercise.

DIETS

The three diets recommended to treat children with ADHD have been the Feingold diet; the oligoantigenic, or elimination, diet; and a restricted sugar diet. The Feingold diet was proposed by an allergist, Dr. Ben Feingold, who suggested that some children with ADHD have an allergic-type reaction to certain dietary elements.[121] The elements included additives, preservatives, food dyes, and salicylate compounds. His clinical impression was that a number of children with hyperactivity had this problem. However, subsequent blinded studies revealed that very few children (approximately 1% of the children studied) responded adversely when challenged with dyes or additives.[122] In addition, a strict adherence to this diet can result in inadequate vitamin C intake. Current recommendations have dropped the natural salicylate restrictions, so that the low vitamin C intake should no longer be a problem.

Similar to the Feingold diet, the oligoantigenic, or elimination, diet is based on the hypothesis that some children with ADHD are responding adversely to specific foods and dietary ingredients. This diet also restricts additives, dyes, and preservatives, but it also initially limits the patient's diet to two meats, two vegetables, two fruits, and two carbohydrates. If a positive response is seen after several weeks, other foods are gradually reintroduced, one at a time, in order to determine which foods adversely affect the patient's behavior. The hypothesis is that affected individuals have sensitivity to certain foods that adversely affect their behavior. About five studies have been performed to examine this intervention with blinded and controlled conditions.[123] Although some effects were demonstrated, methodological weaknesses, such as problems with blinding, preclude making a definitive conclusion about its efficacy.

Sugar was first believed to adversely affect behavior according to several studies in which an association was found between worse behavior and increased sugar intake. Authors discussing sugar have usually referred to refined and added sugars as the offending agents. These sugars are usually sucrose or fructose. However, 23 rigorous studies have demonstrated no association between sugar and behavior.[124] The main complication of trying to modify sugar intake is the difficulty in having the children comply, because pursuing compliance usually increases the parent-child conflicts. A further drawback is that it further stigmatizes the child with behavior and social skills problems as "different."

DIETARY SUPPLEMENTS

The dietary supplements recommended for treating children with ADHD include essential fatty acids, megavitamins, zinc, antioxidants, and herbs. The two primary essential fatty acids under consideration are linoleic and linolenic acids. There is no clear evidence that these supplements benefit any children, and it is not known whether there is any physical risk.[125] Megavitamins consist of large quantities (at least 10 times the recommended daily allowance) of most vitamins. There is no clear evidence of their efficacy, and there is the physical side effect of elevated liver function test findings.[126,127] Zinc has been recommended for the treatment of some patients with ADHD because some children were found to have zinc deficiency on the basis of hair analysis. This treatment with zinc has not been studied rigorously; therefore, there is no information about its benefits or risks. Antioxidants include melatonin, ginkgo biloba, and pycnogenol. There have been no scientific studies of their effects on patients with ADHD; thus, their potential benefits and side effects remain unknown.[125] Herbal compounds have been recommended for treating patients with ADHD mainly because of their sedative properties. The herbal compounds recommended are chamomile, kava hops, lemon balm, valerian root, and passionflower. There have not been any rigorous studies of their efficacy in patients with ADHD, and their potential side effects remain unknown.

ALTERNATIVE MEDICATIONS

The hypothesis behind antifungal therapy is that children treated on multiple occasions with broad-spectrum antibiotics, such as for otitis media, have alterations in their intestinal flora that make them susceptible to the growth of *Candida* and the absorption of candidal toxins. These toxins then produce behavioral disturbances. The treatment consists of using antifungal agents such as nystatin or ketoconazole and eliminating sugar and foods made with molds and yeast from the diet.[125] No studies have been completed to assess efficacy, and the risks are those of the side effects of the medication and the stigma of requiring a diet different from everybody else's, as noted previously. Nootropic medications are cerebral metabolic enhancers that stave off aging. Those recommended for individuals with ADHD are piracetam and dimethylaminoethanol. There have been no rigorous studies of their efficacy, and there are no reported significant side effects, although the side effects have also not been studied systematically in children.[125]

BIOFEEDBACK

Electroencephalographic biofeedback is based on the premise that the electroencephalographic pattern reflects the behavior of individuals; thus, if their electroencephalographic pattern could be changed with suppression of θ activity and enhancement of β wave production, their behavior would change. Furthermore, individuals can be trained to control these activities. Although there have been a number of positive nonrandomized studies and a few with wait-list comparison groups, there have been no randomized controlled trials.[128]

EXERCISE

Sensory integration, developed by Dr. Jean Ayres, is based on the theory that improvement in the ability to integrate the senses improves the ability to behave and pay attention. It consists of exercises to improve the integration of the senses. Although there have been a number of positive nonrandomized or methodologically flawed studies, there have been no randomized control trials demonstrating its efficacy.[128] The potential harm is the expense and time required to perform the intervention and parent-child conflicts in children who are unwilling to cooperate.

REFERENCES

1. Diagnosis and evaluation of the child with attention-deficit/hyperactivity disorder. American Academy of Pediatrics. Pediatrics 105:1158-1170, 2000.
2. Brown RT, Freeman WS, Perrin JM, et al: Prevalence and assessment of attention-deficit/hyperactivity disorder in primary care settings. Pediatrics 107(3):E43, 2001.
3. Pliszka SR, Greenhill LL, Crismon ML, et al: The Texas Children's Medication Algorithm Project: Report of the Texas Consensus Conference Panel on Medication Treatment of Childhood Attention-Deficit/Hyperactivity Disorder. Part II: Tactics. Attention-deficit/hyperactivity disorder. J Am Acad Child Adolesc Psychiatry 39:920-927, 2000.
3a. American Academy of Child and Adolescent Psychiatry. Practice parameter for the use of stimulant medication in the treatment of children, adolescents and adults. J Am Acad Child Adolesc Psychiatry: 41(2 Supplement):26S-49S, 2002.
4. American Psychiatric Association: Diagnostic and Statistical Manual of Mental Disorders, 4th ed. Washington, DC: American Psychiatric Association, 1994.
4a. American Psychiatric Association: Diagnostic and Statistical Manual of Mental Disorders, Fourth Edition, Text Revision. Washington, DC: American Psychiatric Association, 2000.
5. Hoffman H: Der Struwwelpeter. Leipzig: Imsel Verlag, 1848, pp 11-15.
6. Sand G: The devil's pool. *In* Eliot CW, ed: The Harvard Classics Shelf of Fiction: French Fiction. New York: PF Collier, 1917, p 289.
7. Still GF: The Coulstonian lectures on some abnormal physical conditions in children. Lancet 1:1008-1012, 1902.
8. Barkley R: Response inhibition in attention-deficit hyperactivity disorder. Ment Retard Dev Disabil Res Rev 5:177-184, 1999.
9. Bradley C: The behavior of children receiving Benzedrine. Am J Psychiatry 94:577-585, 1937.
10. Laufer M, Denhoff E: Hyperkinetic behavior syndrome in children. J Pediatr 50:463-474, 1957.
11. Hohman LB: Post-encephalitic behavior disorder in children. Johns Hopkins Hosp Bull 33:372-375, 1922.
12. Ebaugh FG: Neuropsychiatric sequelae of acute epidemic encephalitis in children. Am J Dis Child 25:89-97, 1923.
13. American Psychiatric Association: Diagnostic and Statistical Manual of Mental Disorders, 2nd ed. Washington, DC: American Psychiatric Association, 1967.
14. American Psychiatric Association: Diagnostic and Statistical Manual of Mental Disorders, 3rd ed. Washington, DC: American Psychiatric Association, 1980.
15. Douglas V: Stop, look and listen: The problem of sustained attention and impulse control in hyperactive and normal children. Can J Behav Sci 4:259-282, 1972.
16. American Psychiatric Association: Diagnostic and Statistical Manual of Mental Disorders, 3rd ed, revised. Washington, DC: American Psychiatric Association, 1987.

17. James W: The Principles of Psychology. Cambridge, MA: Harvard University Press, 1983, p 1166. (Originally published 1890.)

18. Scahill L, Schwab-Stone M: Epidemiology of ADHD in school-age children. Child Adolesc Psychiatr Clin North Am 9:541-555, 2000.

18a. de Fockert JW, Rees G, Frith CD, LaVie N: The role of working memory in visual selective attention. Science 291:1803-1806, 2001.

19. Jensen PS, Kettle L, Roper MT, et al: Are stimulants overprescribed? Treatment of ADHD in four U.S. communities. J Am Acad Child Adolesc Psychiatry 38:797-804, 1999.

20. Baumgaertel A, Wolraich ML, Dietrich M: Comparison of diagnostic criteria for attention deficit disorders in a German elementary school sample. J Am Acad Child Adolesc Psychiatry 34:629-638, 1995.

21. Wolraich ML, et al: Comparison of diagnostic criteria for attention deficit hyperactivity disorder in a county-wide sample. J Am Acad Child Adolesc Psychiatry 35:319-323, 1996.

22. Swanson JM, Castellanos FX. Biological bases of ADHD: Neuroanatomy, genetics and pathophysiology. Paper presented at: NIH Consensus Development Conference on Diagnosis and Treatment of Attention Deficit Hyperactivity Disorder, 1998; Bethesda, MD.

23. Barkley RA: Attention-deficit hyperactivity disorder. Sci Am 279:66-71, 1998.

24. Alberts-Corush J, Firestone P, Goodman JT: Attention and impulsivity characteristics of the biological and adoptive parents of hyperactive and normal control children. Am J Orthopsychiatry 56:413-423, 1986.

25. Morrison JR, Stewart MA: The psychiatric status of the legal families of adopted hyperactive children. Arch Gen Psychiatry 28:888-891, 1973.

26. Biederman J, Faraone SV, Keenan K, et al: Family-genetic and psychosocial risk factors in DSM-III attention deficit disorder. J Am Acad Child Adolesc Psychiatry 29:526-533, 1990.

27. Morrison JR, Stewart MA: A family study of the hyperactive child syndrome. Biol Psychiatry 3:189-195, 1971.

28. Cantwell DP: Psychiatric illness in the families of hyperactive children. Arch Gen Psychiatry 27:414-417, 1972.

29. Zametkin AJ, Ernst M: Problems in the management of attention-deficit–hyperactivity. N Engl J Med 340:40-46, 1999.

30. Shaywitz BA, Fletcher JM, Pugh KR, et al: Progress in imaging attention deficit hyperactivity disorder. Ment Retard Dev Disabil Res Rev 5:185-190, 1999.

31. Hauser P, Zametkin AJ, Martinez P, et al: Attention deficit–hyperactivity disorder in people with generalized resistance to thyroid hormone. N Engl J Med 328:997-1001, 1993.

32. Cook EH Jr, Stein MA, Krasowski MD, et al: Association of attention-deficit disorder and the dopamine transporter gene. Am J Hum Genet 56:993-998, 1995.

33. Gill M, Daly G, Heron S, et al: Confirmation of an association between attention deficit hyperactivity disorder and a dopamine transporter polymorphism. Mol Psychiatry 2:311-313, 1997.

34. Swanson JM, Sunohara GA, Kennedy JL, et al: Association of the dopamine receptor D4 (DRD4) gene with a refined phenotype of attention deficit-hyperactivity disorder (ADHD): A family-based approach. Mol Psychiatry 3:38-41, 1998.

35. Ingram S, Hechtman L, Morgenstern G: Outcome issues in ADHD: Adolescent and adult long-term outcome. Ment Retard Dev Disabil Res Rev 5:243-250, 1999.

36. Miller A, Lee S, Raina P, et al: A review of therapies for attention-deficit/hyperactivity disorder. Vancouver: Research Institute for Children's and Women's Health and University of British Columbia, 1998.

37. American Academy of Pediatrics, Subcommittee on Attention-Deficit/Hyperactivity Disorder and Committee on Quality Improvement: Clinical practice guideline: Treatment of the school-aged child with attention-deficit/hyperactivity disorder. Pediatrics 108:1033-1044, 2001.

38. DuPaul GJ, Power TJ, Anastopoulos AD, et al: Teacher ratings of attention deficit hyperactivity disorder symptoms: Factor structure and normative data. Psychol Assess 9:436-444, 1997.

39. Conners CK, Pliszka SR, Wolraich ML: Paying Attention to ADHD: Accurate Diagnosis, Effective Treatment. Philadelphia: Medical Education Systems, 1999.

40. Achenbach TM, Edelbrock L: Manual for the Child Behavior Checklist 4-18 and 1991 Profile. Burlington: University of Vermont, Department of Psychiatry, 1991.

41. Reynolds C, Kamphaus RW: The Clinician's Guide to the Behavior Assessment System for Children (BASC). New York: Guilford, 2002.

42. Wolraich M: Attention deficit hyperactivity disorder: The most studied yet most controversial diagnosis. Ment Retard Dev Disabil Res Rev 5:163-168, 1999.

42a. Du Paul GJ, McGoey KE, Eckert TL, Van Brakle J: Preschool children with attention-deficit/hyperactivity disorder: Impairments in behavioral, social and school functioning. J Am Acad Child Adolesc Psychiatry 49:508-515, 2001.

42b. Bagwell CL, Molina BSG, et al: Attention-deficit hyperactivity disorder and problems with peer relations: Predictions from childhood to adolescence. J Am Acad Child Adolesc Psychiatry 40:1285-1292, 2001.

43. Hechtman L, Weiss G, Perlman T: Self-esteem and social skills. Can J Psychiatry 25:478-483, 1980.

44. Hoza B, Pelham WE, et al: Do boys with attention-deficit/hyperactivity disorder have positive illusory self-concepts? J Abnorm Psychol 111:268-278, 2002.

45. Crabtree V, Ivenenki A, Gozal D: Clinical and parental assessment of sleep in children with attention-deficit/hyperactivity disorder referred to a pediatric sleep medicine center. Clin Pediatr 42:807-813, 2003.

46. Marcotte AC, Thacher PV, Butters M, et al: Parental report of sleep problems in children with attentional and learning disorders. J Dev Behav Pediatr 19:178-186, 1998.

47. Lebourgeois M, Avis K, Mixon M, et al: Snoring, sleep quality, and sleepiness across attention-deficit/hyperactivity disorder subtypes. Sleep 27:520-525, 2004.

48. O'Brien L, Ivanenko A, Crabtree VM, et al: The effect of stimulants on sleep characteristics in children with attention deficit/hyperactivity disorder. Sleep Med 4:309-316, 2003.

49. Tirosh E, Sadeh A, Munvez R, et al: Effects of methylphenidate on sleep in children with attention-deficit hyperactivity disorder. Am J Dis Child 147:1313-1315, 1993.

50. Avior G, Fishman G, Leor A, et al: The effect of tonsillectomy and adenoidectomy on inattention and impulsivity as measured by the Test of Variables of Attention (TOVA) in children with obstructive sleep apnea. Otolaryngol Head Neck Surg 131:367-371, 2004.

51. Mazza S, Pepin JL, Naegele B, et al: Most obstructive sleep apnoea patients exhibit vigilance and attention deficits on an extended battery of tests. Eur Respir J 25:75-80, 2005.

52. Schechter M and Section on Pediatric Pulmonology, Subcommittee on Obstructive Sleep Apnea Syndrome: Technical report: Diagnosis and management of childhood obstructive apnea syndrome. Pediatrics 109(4): e69, 2002.

53. O'Brien LM, Holbrook CR, Mervis CB, et al: Sleep and neurobehavioral characteristics of 5- to 7-year-old children with parentally reported symptoms of attention-deficit/hyperactivity disorder. Pediatrics 111:554-563, 2003.

54. Pelham WEJ, Wheeler T, Chronis A: Empirically supported psycho-social treatments for attention deficit hyperactivity disorder. J Clin Child Psychol 27:190-205, 1998.

55. Jensen PS, Hinshaw SP, Swanson JM, et al: Findings from the NIMH Multimodal Treatment Study of ADHD (MTA): Implications and applications for primary care providers. J Dev Behav Pediatr 22:60-73, 2001.

56. Children and Adults With Attention-Deficit/Hyperactivity Disorders. Ment Retard Dev Disabil Res Rev 5:215, 2001. http://www.chadd.org/

57. Wigal T, Swanson JM, Regino R, et al: Stimulant medications for the treatment of ADHD: Efficacy and l224, 1999.

58. Handen BL, Breaux AM, Janosky J, et al: Effects and noneffects of methylphenidate in children with mental retardation and ADHD. J Am Acad Child Adolesc Psychiatry 31:455-461, 1992.

59. Handen BL, Breaux AM, Gosling A, et al: Efficacy of methylphenidate among mentally retarded children with attention deficit hyperactivity disorder. Pediatrics 86:922-930, 1990.

60. Gadow KD: Prevalence and efficacy of stimulant drug use with mentally retarded children and youth. Psychopharmacol Bull 21:291-303, 1985.

61. Cullinan D, Gadow KD, Epstein MH: Psychotropic drug treatment among learning-disabled, educable mentally retarded, and seriously emotionally disturbed students. J Abnorm Child Psychol 15:469-477, 1987.

62. Aman MG, Marks RE, Turbott SH, et al: Clinical effects of methylphenidate and thioridazine in intellectually subaverage children. J Am Acad Child Adolesc Psychiatry 30:246-256, 1991.

63. Feldman H, Crumrine P, Handen BL, et al: Methylphenidate in children with seizures and attention-deficit disorder. Am J Dis Child 143:1081-1086, 1989.

64. Gross-Tsur V, Manor O, van der Meere J, et al: Epilepsy and attention deficit hyperactivity disorder: Is methylphenidate safe and effective? J Pediatr 130:670-674, 1997.

65. Biederman J, Wilens T, Mick E, et al: Psychoactive substance use in adults with attention deficit hyperactivity disorder (ADHD): Effects of ADHD and psychiatric comorbidity. Am J Psychiatry 52:1652-1658, 1995.

66. Solanto MV: Neuropsychopharmacological mechanisms of stimulant drug action in attention-deficit hyperactivity disorder. Behav Brain Res 94:127-152, 1998.

67. [Ritalin (methylphenidate) product information.] East Hanover, NJ: Novartis Pharmaceuticals, 1998. (Available at: http://www.pharma.us.novartis.com/ product/pi/pdf/ritalin_sr.pdf; accessed 1/8/06.)

68. Wigal S, Swanson JM, Feifel D, et al: A double-blind, placebo-controlled trial of dexmethylphenidate hydrochloride and D,L-threo-methylphenidate hydrochloride in children with attention-deficit/hyperactivity disorder. J Am Acad Child Adolesc Psychiatry 43:1406-1414, 2004.

68a. Heal DJ, Pierce CM. Methylphenidate and its isomers: their role in the treatment of attention-deficit hyperactivity disorder using a transdermal delivery system. CNS Drugs. 20:713-738, 2006.

69. Swanson JM, Wigal S, Greenhill L, et al: Objective and subjective measures of the pharmacodynamic effects of Adderall in the treatment of children with ADHD in a controlled laboratory classroom setting. Psychopharmacol Bull 34:55-60, 1998.

70. Greenhill LL, Pliszka S, Dulcan MK, et al: Practice parameter for the use of stimulant medications in the treatment of children, adolescents, and adults. J Am Acad Child Adolesc Psychiatry 41:26S-49S, 2002.

71. Pelham WE, Gnagy EM, Burrows-Maclean L, et al: Once-a-day Concerta methylphenidate versus three-times-daily methylphenidate in laboratory and natural settings: Safety and efficacy. Pediatrics 107(6):E105, 2001.

72. Marcus S, Wan GJ, Kemner JE, et al: Continuity of methylphenidate treatment for attention-deficit/hyperactivity disorder. Arch Pediatr Adolesc Med 159:572-578, 2005.

73. Lage M, Hwang P: Effect of methylphenidate formulation for attention deficit hyperactivity disorder on patterns and outcomes of treatment. J Child Adolesc Psychopharmacol 14:575-581, 2004.

73a. Regulations Requiring Manufacturers to Assess the Safety and Effectiveness of New Drugs and Biological Products in Pediatric Patients, 21 C.F.R. §§ 201, 312, 314, 601. Fed Register 63:66632, 1998.

74. Pelham WE, Hoza J: Behavioral assessment of psychostimulant effects on ADD children in a summer day treatment program. Adv Behav Assess Child Fam 3:3-34, 1987.

75. Whitehouse D, Shah U, Palmer FB: Comparison of sustained-release and standard methylphenidate in the treatment of minimal brain dysfunction. J Clin Psychiatry 41:282-285, 1980.

76. Fitzpatrick P, Klorman R, Brumaghim JT, et al: Effects of sustained-release and standard preparations of methylphenidate on attention deficit disorder. J Am Acad Child Adolesc Psychiatry 31:226-234, 1992.

77. Pelham W, Gnagy EM, Burrows-Maclean L, et al: Once-a-day Concerta methylphenidate versus three-times-daily methylphenidate in laboratory and natural settings: Safety and efficacy. Pediatrics 107(6):E105, 2001.

78. Wolraich ML, Greenhill LL, Pelham W, et al: Randomized controlled trial of OROS methylphenidate once a day in children with attention-deficit/hyperactivity disorder. Pediatrics 108:883-892, 2001.

79. Wilens T, Pelham W, Stein M, et al: ADHD treatment with once-daily OROS methylphenidate: Interim 12-month results from a long-term open-label study. J Am Acad Child Adolesc Psychiatry 42:424-433, 2003.

80. Cox DJ, Humphrey JW, Merkel RL, et al: Controlled-release methylphenidate improves attention during on-road driving by adolescents with attention-deficit/hyperactivity disorder. J Am Board Fam Pract 17:235-239, 2004.

81. Swanson JM, Wigal SB, Wigal T, et al: A comparison of once-daily extended-release methylphenidate formulations in children with attention-deficit/hyperactivity disorder in the laboratory school (the Comacs Study). Pediatrics 113(3 Part 1):e206-e216, 2004.

82. Biederman J, Quinn D, Weiss M, et al: Efficacy and safety of Ritalin LA, a new, once daily, extended-release dosage form of methylphenidate, in children with attention deficit hyperactivity disorder. Paediatr Drugs 5:833-841, 2003.

83. Lopez F, Silva R, Pestreich L, et al: Comparative efficacy of two once daily methylphenidate formulations (Ritalin LA and Concerta) and placebo in children with attention deficit hyperactivity disorder across the school day. Paediatr Drugs 5:545-555, 2003.

84. Biederman J, Lopez FA, Boellner SW, et al: A randomized, double-blind, placebo-controlled, parallel-group study of SLI381 (Adderall XR) in children with attention-deficit/hyperactivity disorder. Pediatrics 110:258-266, 2002.

85. McGough JJ, Biederman J, Wigal SB, et al: Long-term tolerability and effectiveness of once-daily mixed amphetamine salts (Adderall XR) in children with ADHD. J Am Acad Child Adolesc Psychiatry 44:530-538, 2005.

86. Findling R, Biederman J, Wilens TE, et al: Short- and long-term cardiovascular effects of mixed amphetamine salts extended release in children. J Pediatr 147:348-354, 2005.

87. Bridges A: Advisers Reject Strong ADHD Warnings. Associated Press, March 23, 2006.

88. Pelham WE Jr, Manos MJ, Ezzell CE, et al: A dose-ranging study of a methylphenidate transdermal system in children with ADHD. J Am Acad Child Adolesc Psychiatry 44:522-529, 2005.

89. Pelham WE, Burrows-Maclean L, Gnagy EM, et al: Transdermal methylphenidate, behavioral, and combined treatment for children with ADHD. Exp Clin Psychopharmacol 13:111-126, 2005.

90. McGough JJ, Wigal SB, Abikoff H, et al: A randomized, double-blind, placebo-controlled, laboratory classroom assessment of methylphenidate transdermal system in children with ADHD. J Atten Disord 9:476-485, 2006.

91. Keating GM, Figgitt DP: Dexmethylphenidate. Drugs 62:1899-1908, 2002.

91a. Marchetti A, Magar R, Lan H, Murphy EL, Jensen PS, Connors CK, Findling R, Wineburg E, Carotenuto I, Einarson TR, Iskedjian M: Pharmacotherapies for attention-deficit/hyperactivity disorder: expected-cost analysis. Clinical Therapeutics 23:1904-1921, 2001.

92. Kramer JR, Loney J, Ponto LB, et al: Predictors of adult height and weight in boys treated with methylphenidate for childhood behavior problems. J Am Acad Child Adolesc Psychiatry 39:517-524, 2000.

93. Sund AM, Zeiner P: Does extended medication with amphetamine or methylphenidate reduce growth in hyperactive children? Nord J Psychiatry 56:53-57, 2002.

94. Spencer T, Biederman J, Wilens T, et al: Pharmacotherapy of attention-deficit hyperactivity disorder across the life span. J Am Acad Child Adolesc Psychiatry 35:409-432, 1996.

95. Lisska MC, Rivkees SA: Daily methylphenidate use slows the growth of children: A community based study. J Pediatr Endocrinol Metab 16:711-718, 2003.

96. Poulton A, Cowell CT: Slowing of growth in height and weight on stimulants: A characteristic pattern. J Paediatr Child Health 39:180-185, 2003.

97. Palumbo D, Spencer T, Lynch J, et al: Emergence of tics in children with ADHD: Impact of once-daily OROS methylphenidate therapy. J Child Adolesc Psychopharmacol 14:185-194, 2004.

98. Gadow K, Sverd J: Stimulants for ADHD in child patients with Tourette's syndrome: The issue of relative risk. J Dev Behav Pediatr 11:269-271, 1990.

99. Jensen P: Behavioral and medication treatments for ADHD: Comparisons and combinations. Presented at the NIH Consensus Conference on Diagnosis and Treatment of Attention Deficit Hyperactivity Disorder, Washington, DC, November 16-18, 1998.

100. Pelham WE, Gnagy EM: Psychosocial and combined treatments for ADHD. Ment Retard Dev Disabil Res Rev 5:225-236, 1999.

101. Biederman J, Heiligenstein JH, Faries DE, et al: Efficacy of atomoxetine versus placebo in school-age girls with attention-deficit/hyperactivity disorder. Pediatrics 110(6):e75, 2002.

102. Kratochvil C, Bohac D, Harrington M, et al: An open-label trial of tomoxetine in pediatric attention deficit hyperactivity disorder. J Child Adolesc Psychopharmacol 11:167-170, 2001.

103. Kratochvil C, Heiligenstein JH, Dittmann R, et al: Atomoxetine and methylphenidate treatment in children with ADHD: A prospective, randomized, open-label trial. J Am Acad Child Adolesc Psychiatry 41:776-784, 2002.

104. Michelson D, Faries D, Wernicke J, et al: Atomoxetine in the treatment of children and adolescents with attention-deficit/hyperactivity disorder: A randomized, placebo-controlled, dose-response study. Pediatrics 108(5):E83, 2001.

105. Michelson D, Allen AJ, Busner J, et al: Once-daily atomoxetine treatment for children and adolescents with attention deficit hyperactivity disorder: A randomized, placebo-controlled study. Am J Psychiatry 159:1896-1901, 2002.

106. Michelson D, Adler L, Spencer T, et al: Atomoxetine in adults with ADHD: Two randomized, placebo-controlled studies. Biol Psychiatry 53:112-120, 2003.

107. Spencer T, Biederman J, Heiligenstein J, et al: An open-label, dose-ranging study of atomoxetine in children with attention deficit hyperactivity disorder. J Child Adolesc Psychopharmacol 11:251-265, 2001.

108. Spencer T, Heiligenstein JH, Biederman J, et al: Results from 2 proof-of-concept, placebo-controlled studies of atomoxetine in children with attention-deficit/hyperactivity disorder. J Clin Psychiatry 63:1140-1147, 2002.

109. Connor D, Fletcher KE, Swanson JM: A meta-analysis of clonidine for symptoms of attention-deficit hyperactivity disorder. J Am Acad Child Adolesc Psychiatry 38:1551-1559, 1999.

110. Wilens TE, Spencer TJ: A clinically sound medication option. J Am Acad Child Adolesc Psychiatry 38:5, 1999.

111. Prince J, Wilens TE, Biederman J, et al: Clonidine for sleep disturbances associated with attention-deficit hyperactivity disorder: A systematic chart review of 62 cases. J Am Acad Child Adolesc Psychiatry 35:599-605, 1996.

112. Conners CK, Casat CD, Gualtieri CT, et al: Bupropion hydrochloride in attention deficit disorder with hyperactivity. J Am Acad Child Adolesc Psychiatry 35:1314-1321, 1996.

113. Physicians' Desk Reference, 54th ed. Montvale, NJ: Medical Economics, 2000, pp 1301-1308.

114. Biederman J, Swanson JM, Wigal SB, et al: Efficacy and safety of modafinil film-coated tablets in children and adolescents with attention-deficit/hyperactivity disorder: Results of a randomized, double-blind, placebo-controlled, flexible-dose study. Pediatrics 116(6):e777-e784, 2005.

115. Cunningham C, Bremner R, Boyle M: Large group community-based parenting programs for families of preschoolers at risk for disruptive behaviour disorders: Utilization, cost, effectiveness, and outcome. J Child Psychol Psychiatry 36:1141-1159, 1995.

116. Herschell AD, Calzada E, Eyberg SM, et al: Parent-child interaction therapy: New directions in research. Cogn Behav Pract 9:9-16, 2002.

117. Hannah JN: Parenting a child with attention-deficit/hyperactivity disorder. Austin, TX: Pro-Ed, 1999.

118. Davila RR, Williams ML, MacDonald JT: Memorandum on clarification of policy to address the needs of children with attention deficit disorders within general and/or special education. *In* Parker HC, ed: The ADD Hyperactivity Handbook for Schools. Plantation, FL: Impact Publications, 1991, pp 261-268.

119. Pelham WE: How to Establish a Daily Report Card. Center for Treatment of Attention Deficit Disorder, 2005. (Available at: *http://ccf.buffalo.edu/defoul.php;* accessed 5/27/07.)

120. Pelham W, Gnagy EM, Greiner AR, et al: Behavioral versus behavioral and pharmacological treatment in ADHD children attending a summer treatment program. J Abnorm Child Psychol 28:507-525, 2000.

121. Feingold B: Why Your Child Is Hyperactive. New York: Random House, 1975.

122. Wender EH: The food additive-free diet in the treatment of behavior disorders: A review. J Dev Behav Pediatr 7:35-42, 1986.

123. Wolraich M: Attention Deficit Hyperactivity Disorder: Current Diagnosis and Treatment. Presented at the annual meeting of the American Academy of Pediatrics, Chicago, October 28, 2000. (Available at: *http://medscape.com/viewarticle/420198;* accessed 5/27/07.)

124. Wolraich ML, Wilson DB, White JW: The effect of sugar on behavior or cognition in children: A meta-analysis. JAMA 274:1617-1621, 1995.

125. Baumgaertel A: Alternative and controversial treatments for attention-deficit/hyperactivity disorder. Pediatr Clin North Am 46:977-992, 1999.

126. Arnold LE: Megavitamins for MBD: A placebo-controlled study. JAMA 20:24, 1978.

127. Haslam R, Dalby J, Rademaker A: Effects of megavitamin therapy on children with attention deficit disorders. Pediatrics 74:103-111, 1984.

128. Goldstein S, Goldstein M: Managing Attention Deficit Hyperactivity Disorder in Children: A Guide for Practitioners, 2nd ed. New York: Wiley, 1998.

Externalizing Conditions

JOHN E. LOCHMAN ▨ TAMMY D. BARRY ▨ NICOLE R. POWELL
▨ CAROLINE L. BOXMEYER ▨ KHIELA J. HOLMES

Externalizing problems in children represent the most common reasons for referral for behavioral intervention.[1] However, these behaviors undergo many changes in form and frequency during childhood and adolescence, and without an understanding of normal developmental trends, it may be difficult to determine whether a given child's behavior is typical or problematic. Therefore, clinicians must have background knowledge in the normal development of externalizing behaviors. We begin this chapter by describing how compliant/noncompliant behaviors, anger, and aggression change in expression and frequency through childhood and adolescence. In subsequent sections, we explore how externalizing behavior manifests in problematic forms, how various biopsychosocial factors contribute to the development of children's problems with aggression and conduct, and how aggression and conduct problems can be assessed. We conclude by discussing how these problems can be effectively treated with psychosocial methods.

NORMAL VARIATIONS IN EXTERNALIZING BEHAVIORS AND RELATED EMOTIONAL CHARACTERISTICS

Compliance Behaviors

All children at every age exhibit both compliant and noncompliant behaviors. Therefore, noncompliant behaviors, by themselves, are not cause for concern; however, the frequency, intensity, form, and effects of such behaviors distinguish normal and abnormal expressions of noncompliance. Clinical manifestations of noncompliance are categorized as externalizing disorders and are described in a later section. In this section, we outline patterns and contributing factors in normal compliant and noncompliant behaviors.

Although most people involved in the care of children have an idea of what is meant by compliance and noncompliance, these behaviors often prove difficult to define operationally. In their treatment manual for noncompliant children, McMahon and Forehand[2] used the definition "appropriate following of an instruction within a reasonable and/or designated time" to operationalize compliance, noting that it is important to distinguish between the initiation of compliance and the completion of the specified task.[3] Five to 15 seconds was suggested as a reasonable period for the initiation of compliance. McMahon and Forehand[2] defined noncompliance as "the refusal to initiate or complete a request" and/or "failure to follow a previously stated rule that is currently in effect" (p 2). In defining compliance and noncompliance, clinicians must also recognize that these are not stand-alone behaviors but are interactional processes between adult and child. Parenting behaviors can affect a child's likelihood of compliance, and child characteristics and responses can, in turn, affect parenting behaviors.

Children first begin to understand the consequences of their own behavior between 6 and 9 months of age and may also learn to recognize the word "no" during this time. Increasing physical development, cognitive abilities, social skills, and receptive language skills lead to improved abilities to respond to verbal directions, and children are generally able to follow simple instructions by age 2 years. Nonetheless, noncompliance with commands is very common for 2- and 3-year-old children, possibly because of parental expectations of resistance (i.e., "the terrible twos") and parents' resulting failure to train their young children to comply.[4]

Compliance levels are expected to increase with age in typically developing children.[5] However, the collection of normative data has proved to be complex and elusive because of sample characteristics and measurement issues.[2,4] A number of investigators have found the expected progression of compliant behaviors in young children as they age. Vaughn and colleagues[6] reported increases in compliance with maternal requests between 18 and 30 months of age, and Kochanska and associates[7] reported an upward trend in one form of compliance from 14 to 33 months of age. Brumfield and Roberts[4] reported that whereas 2- and 3-year-old children complied with only 32.2% of maternal commands, the compliance rate for 4- and 5-year-olds reached 77.7%. However, Kuczynski and Kochanska[8] reported no change in compliance to maternal requests between toddler age ($1^1/_2$ to $3^1/_2$ years) and age 5 years. Kuczynski and Kochanska[8] did find that direct defiance and passive noncompliance decreased with age, although simple refusal and negotiation (an indirect form of noncompliance) increased. Another longitudinal study reported stable rates of noncompliance from ages 2 to 4 years.[9]

By the time they reach school age, children are expected to comply with adult requests the majority of the time. In a review of studies, McMahon and Forehand[2] suggested that compliance rates are approximately 80% for normally developing children. Patterson and Forgatch,[10] however, reported lower compliance rates in a sample of "non-problem 10- and 11-year-old boys": 57% in response to maternal requests and 47% in response to paternal requests.

In adolescence, noncompliant behaviors often increase above childhood levels in typically developing youths. Developmental changes in cognition and social skills, combined with adolescents' growing independence and need to establish their own identity, may lead to increased parent-adolescent conflict. However, developmental research suggests that typical levels of parent-adolescent conflict are manageable and do not constitute the period of severe "storm and stress" described in early models of family relations.[11,12] Conflict tends to be at its most extreme during early adolescence and to decline from early adolescence to mid-adolescence and from mid-adolescence to late adolescence.[13]

Boys and girls differ in their normative rates of oppositional, noncompliant behaviors; boys demonstrate higher rates than do girls during childhood. However, the gender difference closes with age, and boys and girls demonstrate increasingly similar rates as they progress through adolescence.[14]

Anger and Aggression

Like compliance and noncompliance, angry and aggressive behaviors are common to all children, representing clinically significant problems only when frequent and severe enough to disrupt a child's or family's daily life. Anger is often, but not always, a precursor to aggression in children. In fact, the presence or absence of anger is often a defining factor in the classification of aggression. Anger is a key feature of *hostile aggression,* which carries the intent to harm and is accompanied by emotional arousal, but not of *instrumental aggression,* which is motivated by external reward rather than by emotional arousal. Similarly, *reactive aggression* is emotionally driven and takes the form of angry outbursts, whereas *proactive aggression* is instrumentally driven and takes the form of goal-driven behaviors (e.g., domination of others or obtaining a desired object).[15]

Another classification of aggression differentiates between physical aggression and relational aggression. Girls may be more likely to engage in acts of relational aggression, which cause harm by damaging relationships or threatening to do so (e.g., spreading rumors, social exclusion).[16]

Not surprisingly, children who are identified as angry by parents and teachers are more likely to display externalizing behaviors.[17-19] Relations have also been reported between anger in children and internalizing problems[20] and between anger in children and being victimized by peers.[21]

Anger and Development

Anger is one of the earliest emotions to appear in infancy. Between ages 2 and 6 months, infants engage in recognizable displays of anger, including a characteristic cry, and by 7 months, facial expressions of anger can be reliably detected.[22] Caregivers tend to respond to infants' anger expressions by ignoring them or reacting negatively, thus beginning the socialization process against anger.[23,24] As children learn what is socially acceptable, their displays of anger may diminish. For example, one study demonstrated that by 24 months of age, toddlers are able to modulate their expression of anger and are more likely to display sadness, which is more likely to elicit a supportive response from a caregiver.[25]

Anger is likely to be accompanied by physically aggressive behavior in very young children, but with increasing age and developmental level, expressions of anger change in typically developing children. Dunn,[26] for example, found that physical aggression and teasing were equally prevalent in 14-month-old children, but by age 24 months, children were much more likely to tease. During early childhood, children are expected to learn appropriate ways to manage and express their anger. Young children demonstrate progressive increases in their vocabulary of emotional terms and increased understanding of the causes and consequences of emotions.[27,28] By the time they reach elementary school age, children have generally developed a sophisticated understanding of the types of emotional displays that are appropriate and functional in a given context.[29] Shipman and colleagues[29] reported that children in the first through fifth grades identified verbalization of feelings as the most appropriate means of expression of anger, followed by facial displays. The children identified sulking, crying, and aggression as equally inappropriate ways of expressing anger. These findings are consistent with those of other research demonstrating that, with age, children become increasingly less likely to engage in expressive displays of anger as they come to recognize that their ability to maintain emotional control is important to their social functioning.[30]

The types of circumstances that elicit anger in children also change with developmental level. Very young children are likely to react angrily when someone or something interferes with their attempts to reach a goal, whereas anger in older children is more often precipitated by a threat to self-esteem. This change is accompanied by increases in older children's self-awareness, understanding of social norms, and the importance they place on others' perceptions of them.

Aggression and Development

An understanding of normal developmental trends in aggressive behavior is an important starting point in identifying clinically significant problems for children of a given age. In typically developing children, aggressive behaviors follow a declining trend with age during childhood and adolescence. Large-scale longitudinal and cross-sectional studies have demonstrated that rates of aggression decline during childhood and adolescence; aggressive behavior occurs at the highest levels in the youngest children and at the lowest levels in late adolescence.[14,31-33]

Declining trajectories of aggression over time hold for children of both genders; however, at any given point in childhood, boys tend to display higher rates of aggressive behavior than do girls. In fact, boys may display twice as much aggression as girls do during childhood. These gender differences appear to be present very early on, before 4 years of age, and therefore are unlikely to be caused by socialization effects associated with school attendance. Aggressive behavior declines more quickly for boys, and by late adolescence, the rates of aggression in boys and girls are indistinguishable.[14,31] Aggressive acts are nearly nonexistent in typically developing late adolescent–aged youths of both genders.

Aggressive Behavioral Problems

Because of a number of factors that are further elaborated upon later in this chapter, some children display externalizing behaviors that exceed the normal amounts or typical variations. Within this group of disruptive children, aggression is a frequent and particularly concerning complaint. Aggression is one of the most stable problem behaviors in childhood, with a developmental trajectory toward negative outcomes in adolescence, such as drug and alcohol use, truancy and dropout, delinquency, and violence.[34] Additional studies indicate that children's aggressive behavior patterns may escalate to include a wide range of severe antisocial behaviors in adolescence.[35] The negative trajectory may even continue into adulthood, as demonstrated by Olweus's finding that of adolescents identified as bullies, 60% had their first criminal conviction by age 24.[36]

These findings highlight the fact that aggressive behavior can have serious and negative implications for a child's future. The negative effects are not, however, limited to the aggressive individual, inasmuch as aggressive behavior, by definition, has the potential to cause harm or injury to others. In today's schools, aggressive bullying, which may be verbal, physical, or psychological, is increasingly recognized as a serious problem.[37] Bullying is a deliberate act with the intent of harming the victims.[38] Examples of direct bullying include hitting and kicking, charging interest on goods and stealing, name calling and intimidation, and sexual harassment. Other forms of bullying that are more indirect in nature (i.e., relational bullying) include spreading rumors about peers and gossiping.[39] The victims of bullies usually tend to be shy and likely to seek help.[40]

Children who display high levels of aggressive behavior often exhibit additional externalizing behaviors and may meet criteria for a disruptive behavior disorder diagnosis such as Oppositional Defiant Disorder (ODD) or Conduct Disorder.[41] Although not an explicit part of the diagnosis, aggression may accompany the characteristic pattern of negativistic, hostile, and defiant behavior associated with a diagnosis of ODD. More severe disruptive behaviors, including aggression toward people or animals, destruction of property, theft, and deceit, are associated with conduct disorder. Prevalence rates for these diagnoses are estimated to be from 2% to 16% of the general population for ODD and from 1 to more than 10% for conduct disorder.[41] ODD is mostly closely associated with "aggressive/oppositional behaviors" under the category of "negative/antisocial behaviors" in the *Diagnostic and Statistical Manual of Mental Disorders— Primary Care: Child and Adolescent Version*.[41a] The features of conduct disorder are similar to "secretive antisocial behaviors" under the same category. Some researchers are beginning to identify psychological features that are linked to subsequent psychopathy.[42] Youths who have psychopathic features display manipulation, impulsivity, and remorseless patterns of interpersonal behavior, are usually referred to as "callous" or "unemotional," and are considered to be conceptually different from youths with a diagnosis of Conduct Disorder.[43,44]

Symptoms associated with ODD are age inappropriate, usually appearing before 8 years of age and no later than adolescence.[41] These symptoms include angry, defiant, irritable, and oppositional behaviors and are usually first manifested in the home environment. The diagnosis of ODD should be made only if these behaviors occur more frequently than what would be typically expected of same-aged peers with a similar developmental level. Conduct disorder symptoms such as setting fires, breaking and entering, and running away from home are more severe and may become evident as early as the preschool years, but these behaviors usually begin in middle childhood to middle adolescence. Less severe symptoms (e.g., lying, shoplifting, and physical fighting) are observed initially, followed by intermediate behaviors such as burglary; the most severe behaviors (e.g., rape, theft while confronting a victim) usually emerge last.[41] Professionals who provide services to children and adolescents must be aware of the symptoms of ODD and provide intervention, because ODD is a common antecedent to conduct disorder. Furthermore, a significant subset of individuals who receive a diagnosis of Conduct Disorder, particularly those with an early onset, subsequently develop antisocial personality disorder.[41] Table 17-1 lists diagnostic criteria for ODD and Conduct Disorder from the *Diagnostic and Statistical Manual of Mental Disorders,* 4th edition, text revision (*DSM-IV-TR*).[41]

With regard to gender features, ODD is more prevalent in boys than in girls before puberty, but the rates are fairly equal after puberty. ODD symptoms are typically similar in boys and girls, except that boys exhibit more confrontational behavior and have more persistent symptoms.[41] Diagnoses of Conduct Disorder, particularly the childhood-onset type, are more common in boys than in girls. According to the American Psychiatric Association,[41] boys with conduct disorder usually display symptoms such as "fighting, stealing, vandalism, and school discipline problems," and girls with conduct disorder usually engage in "lying, truancy, running away, substance use, and prostitution."

Childhood disorders rarely occur in isolation, and comorbidity issues are important to consider in treating children within clinical populations.[45] ODD and conduct disorder are often observed in conjunction with attention-deficit/hyperactivity disorder (ADHD), academic underachievement and learning disabilities, and internalizing disorders (e.g., depression and anxiety disorders). Among youth with conduct disorder and ODD, 50% also have a diagnosis of ADHD.[45]

Furthermore, the hyperactive-impulsive subtype of ADHD is more closely associated with aggression than is the inattentive subtype. ODD in conjunction with ADHD increases the likelihood for the development of early-onset conduct disorder symptoms.[46,47] Children with disruptive behaviors are at a greater risk for dropping out of school and thus becoming part of a deviant peer group in their neighborhood. Moreover, children with both conduct problems and depressive symptoms are more likely to engage in substance abuse as adolescents than are children with conduct problems alone.

With regard to differential diagnoses, ODD should not be diagnosed if the symptoms occur exclusively during a mood or psychotic disorder. As previously noted, ADHD often co-occurs with ODD, warranting two separate diagnoses. Furthermore, the oppositional behavior associated with ODD and the impulsive and disruptive behaviors associated with ADHD should be distinguished when a diagnosis is made.[41] The diagnosis of ODD should not be made if the individual meets criteria for diagnosis of an adjustment disorder, conduct disorder, or, if the individual is aged 18 years or older, antisocial personality disorder. Last, the behaviors associated with ODD must be more frequent and severe than what is typically expected and lead to significant impairment in social, academic, or occupational functioning.[41] As with ODD, a diagnosis of Conduct Disorder should not be made if the behaviors occur exclusively during the course of a psychotic disorder, mood disorder, or ADHD. Furthermore, Conduct Disorder should not be diagnosed when the individual meets criteria for an adjustment disorder or, if the individual is 18 years of age or older, antisocial personality disorder. According to the *DSM-IV-TR,* when an individual meets criteria for both ODD and Conduct Disorder, a diagnosis of Conduct Disorder should be made.

ETIOLOGY: RISK AND CAUSAL FACTORS WITHIN A CONTEXTUAL SOCIAL-COGNITIVE MODEL

The contextual social-cognitive model,[48] which is derived from etiological research on childhood aggression, indicates that certain family and community background factors (neighborhood problems, maternal depression, poor social support, marital conflict, low socioeconomic status) have both a direct effect on children's externalizing behavior problems and an indirect effect through their influence on key mediational processes (parenting practices, children's social cognition and emotional regulation, children's peer relations). A child's developmental course is set within

TABLE 17-1 ■ *DSM-IV-TR* Diagnostic Criteria for Oppositional Defiant Disorder and Conduct Disorder	
Oppositional Defiant Disorder	**Conduct Disorder**

A pattern of negativistic, hostile, and defiant behavior lasting at least 6 months, during which four (or more) of the following occur:
1. Often loses temper
2. Often argues with adults
3. Often actively defies refuses or to comply with adults' requests or rules
4. Often deliberately annoys people
5. Often blames others for his or her mistakes or misbehavior
6. Is often touchy or easily annoyed by others
7. Is often angry and resentful
8. Is often spiteful or vindictive
	A repetitive and persistent pattern of behavior in which the basic rights of others or major age-appropriate societal norms or rules are violated, as manifested by the presence of three (or more) of the following criteria in the past 12 months, with at least one criterion present in the past 6 months:
	Aggression to people and animals
	  1. Often bullies, threatens, or intimidates others
	  2. Often initiates physical fights
	  3. Has used a weapon that can cause serious physical harm to others (e.g., a bat, brick, broken bottle, knife, gun)
	  4. Has been physically cruel to people
	  5. Has been physically cruel to animals
	  6. Has stolen while confronting a victim (e.g., mugging, purse snatching, extortion, armed robbery)
	  7. Has forced someone into sexual activity
	Destruction of property
	  8. Has deliberately set fires with the intention of causing serious damage
	  9. Has deliberately destroyed others' property (other than by setting fires)
	Deceitfulness or theft
	  10. Has broken into someone else's house, building, or car
	  11. Often lies to obtain goods or favors or to avoid obligations (i.e., "cons" others)
	  12. Has stolen items of nontrivial value without confronting a victim (e.g., shoplifting, but without breaking and entering; forgery)
	Serious violation of rules
	  13. Often stays out at night despite parental prohibitions, beginning before age 13 years
	  14. Has run away from home overnight at least twice while living in parental or parental surrogate home (or once without returning for a lengthy period)
	  15. Is often truant from school, beginning before age 13 years

There are no separate codes based on age at onset	*Conduct Disorder, Childhood-Onset Type:* Onset of at least one criterion characteristic of Conduct Disorder before age 10 years *Conduct Disorder, Adolescent-Onset Type:* Absence of any criteria characteristic of Conduct Disorder before age 10 years *Conduct Disorder, Unspecified Onset:* Age at onset is not known
There are no specified levels of severity	*Mild:* Few if any conduct problems in excess of those necessary to make the diagnosis *and* conduct problems cause only minor harm to others *Moderate:* Number of conduct problems and effect on others intermediate between "mild" and "severe" *Severe:* Many conduct problems in excess of those necessary to make the diagnosis *or* conduct problems cause considerable harm to others

DSM-IV-TR, Diagnostic and Statistic Manual of Mental Disorder, 4th edition, text revision.

the child's social ecology, and an ecological framework is required.[49] Risk factors that are biologically related are noted first, followed by contextual factors in the model, and, finally, by their effect on children's developing social-cognitive and emotional regulation processes.

Biological and Temperament Factors

With regard to biological and temperamental child factors, some prenatal factors such as maternal exposure to alcohol, methadone, cocaine, and cigarette smoke and severe nutritional deficiencies[50-53] have been found to have direct effects on childhood aggression. However, aggression is more commonly the result of interactions between the child's risk factors and environmental factors, in diathesis-stress models.[54] Thus, risk factors such as birth complications, genes, cortisol reactivity, testosterone, abnormal serotonin levels, and temperament all contribute to children's conduct problems but only when environmental factors such as harsh parenting or low socioeconomic status are present.[55-59]

Examples of these diathesis-stress models abound in the literature on children's risk factors. Birth complications such as preeclampsia, umbilical cord prolapse, forceps delivery, and fetal hypoxia increase the risk of later violence among children but only when the infants subsequently experience adverse family environments or maternal rejection.[55,58] Higher levels of testosterone among adolescents and higher cortisol reactivity to provocations are associated with more violent behavior but only when the children or adolescents live in families in which they experience high levels of abuse by parents or low socioeconomic status.[57,60] Children who have a gene that expresses only low levels of monoamine oxidase A have a higher rate of adolescent violent behavior but only when they have experienced high levels of maltreatment by parents.[61] Similar patterns of findings are found when children's temperament characteristics are examined as child-level risk factors. Highly active children,[62] children with high levels of emotional reactivity,[63] and infants with difficult temperament[56] are at risk for later aggressive and conduct problem behavior but only when they have parents who provide poor monitoring or harsh discipline. The children's family context can serve as a key moderator of children's underlying propensity for an antisocial outcome.

Contextual Family Factors

A wide array of factors in the family, ranging from poverty to more general stress and discord, can affect childhood aggression and conduct problems. Children's aggression has been linked to family background factors such as parent criminality, substance use, and depression[64-66]; low socioeconomic status and poverty[67]; stressful life events[64,68]; single and teenage parenthood[69]; marital conflict[70]; and insecure, disorganized attachment.[71] All of these family factors are intercorrelated, especially with socioeconomic status,[72] and low socioeconomic status assessed as early as the preschool years has been predictive of teacher- and peer-rated behavior problems at school.[73] These broad family risk factors can influence child behavior through their effect on parenting processes.

Starting as early as the preschool years, marital conflict probably causes disruptions in parenting that contribute to children's high levels of stress and consequent aggression.[74] Both boys and girls from homes in which marital conflict is high are especially vulnerable to externalizing problems such as aggression and conduct disorder; this is found even after age and family socioeconomic status are controlled.[74]

Parenting Practices

Parenting processes linked to children's aggression[75,76] include (1) nonresponsive parenting at age 1, in which pacing and consistency of parent responses do not meet children's needs; (2) coercive, escalating cycles of harsh parental interactions and child's noncompliance, starting in the toddler years, especially for children with difficult temperaments; (3) harsh, inconsistent discipline; (4) unclear directions and commands; (5) lack of warmth and involvement; and (6) lack of parental supervision and monitoring as children approach adolescence.

Parental physical aggression, such as spanking and more punitive discipline styles, has been associated with oppositional and aggressive behavior in both boys and girls. Poor parental warmth and involvement contribute to parents' use of physically aggressive punishment practices. Weiss and colleagues[77] found that parent ratings of the severity of parental discipline were positively correlated with teachers' ratings of aggression and behavior problems. In addition to higher aggression ratings, children experiencing harsh discipline practices exhibited poorer social information processing; this was found even when the possible effects of socioeconomic status, marital discord, and child temperament were controlled. Of importance is that although such parenting factors are associated with childhood aggression, child temperament and behavior also affect parenting behavior.[78]

Poor parental supervision has also been associated with childhood aggression. Haapasalo and Tremblay[79] found that boys who fought more often with their peers reported having less supervision and more punishment than did boys who did not fight. Interestingly, the boys who fought reported having more rules than the boys who did not fight, which suggests the possibility that parents of aggressive boys may have numerous strict rules that are difficult to follow.

Contextual Peer Factors

Children with disruptive behaviors are at risk for being rejected by their peers.[80] Childhood aggressive behavior and peer rejection are independently predictive of delinquency and conduct problems in adolescence.[81,82] Aggressive children who are also socially rejected tend to exhibit more severe behavior problems than do children who are either only aggressive or only rejected. As with bidirectional relations evident between the degree of parental positive involvement with their children and children's aggressive behavior over time,[83] children's aggressive behavior and their rejection by their peers affect each other reciprocally.[84] Children who have overestimated perceptions of their actual social acceptance can be at particular risk for aggressive behavior problems in some settings.[85]

Despite the compelling nature of these findings, race and gender may moderate the relation between peer rejection and negative adolescent outcomes. For example, Lochman and Wayland[81] found that peer rejection ratings of African American children in a mixed-race classroom were not predictive of subsequent externalizing problems in adolescence, whereas peer rejection ratings of white children were associated with future disruptive behaviors. Similarly, whereas peer rejection can be predictive of serious delinquency in boys, it can fail to be so with girls.[86]

As children with conduct problems enter adolescence, they tend to associate with deviant peers. We believe that many of these teenagers are continually rejected from more prosocial peer groups because they lack appropriate social skills and, as a result, they turn to antisocial cliques as their only sources of social support.[86] The tendency for aggressive children to associate with one another increases the probability that their aggressive behaviors will be maintained or will escalate, because of modeling effects and reinforcement of deviant behaviors.[87] The relation between childhood conduct problems and adolescent delinquency is at least partially mediated by deviant peer group affiliation.[88]

Contextual Community and School Factors

Neighborhood and school environments have also been found to be risk factors for aggression and delinquency beyond the variance accounted for by family characteristics.[89] Exposure to neighborhood violence increases children's aggressive behaviors,[90,91] reinforces their acceptance of aggression,[91] and begins to have heightened effects on the development of antisocial behavior during the middle childhood, preadolescent years.[92] Neighborhood problems disrupt parents' ability to supervise their children adequately[93] and have a direct effect on children's aggressive, antisocial behaviors[94,95] beyond the effects of poor parenting practices. Early onset of aggression and violence has been associated with neighborhood disorganization and poverty, partly because children who live in lower socioeconomic status and disorganized neighborhoods are not well supervised, engage in more risk-taking behaviors, and experience the deviant social influences that are apparent in problematic crime-ridden neighborhoods.

Schools can further exacerbate children's conduct problems through frustration with academic demands caused, in part, by their children's learning problems and by peer influences. The density of aggressive children in classroom settings can increase the amount of aggressive behavior exhibited by individual students.[96,97]

Social Information Processing

Children begin to form stable patterns of processing social information and of regulating their emotions on the basis of (1) their temperament and biological dispositions and (2) their contextual experiences with family, peers, and community.[98] Children's emotional reactions, such as anger, can contribute to later substance use and other antisocial behavior, especially when children have not developed good inhibitory control.[99] The contextual social-cognitive model[48] stresses the reciprocal, interactive relationships among children's initial cognitive appraisal of problem situations, their efforts to think about solutions to the perceived problems, their physiological arousal, and their behavioral response. The level of physiological arousal depends on the individual's biological predisposition to become aroused and varies according to the interpretation of the event.[100] The level of arousal further influences the social problem solving, operating either to intensify the fight-or-flight response or to interfere with the generation of solutions. Because of the ongoing and reciprocal nature of interactions, children may have difficulty extricating themselves from aggressive behavior patterns.

Aggressive children have cognitive distortions at the appraisal phases of social-cognitive processing because of difficulties in encoding incoming social information and in accurately interpreting social events and others' intentions. They also have cognitive deficiencies at the problem solution phases of social-cognitive processing, as evidenced by their generating maladaptive solutions for perceived problems and having nonnormative expectations for the usefulness of aggressive and nonaggressive solutions to their social problems. In the appraisal phases of information processing, aggressive children recall fewer relevant cues about events,[101] base interpretations of events on fewer cues,[102] selectively attend to hostile rather than neutral cues,[103] and recall the most recent cues in a sequence, with selective inattention to earlier presented cues.[104] At the interpretation stage of appraisal processing, aggressive children have a hostile attributional bias: They tend to infer excessively that others are acting toward them in a provocative and hostile manner.[101,102] These attributional biases tend to be more prominent in reactively aggressive children than in proactively aggressive children.[105]

The problem solving stages of information processing begin with the child accessing the goal that the individual chooses to pursue, thereby affecting the responses generated for resolving the conflict in the next processing stage. Aggressive children have social goals that are more dominance and revenge oriented, and less affiliation oriented, than those of nonaggressive children.[106] In the fourth information-processing stage, potential solutions for coping with a perceived problem are recalled from memory. At this stage, aggressive children demonstrate deficiencies in both the quality and the quantity of their problem-solving solutions. These differences are most pronounced in the quality of offered solutions: Aggressive children offer fewer verbal assertion solutions,[107,108] fewer compromise solutions,[101] more direct action solutions,[108] a greater number of help-seeking or adult intervention responses,[109] and more physically aggressive responses[110] to hypothetical vignettes describing interpersonal conflicts. The nature of the social problem-solving deficits for aggressive children varies, depending on their diagnostic classification. Boys with Conduct Disorder diagnoses produce more aggressive/antisocial solutions in vignettes about conflicts with parents and teachers and fewer verbal/nonaggressive solutions in peer conflicts than do boys with ODD.[111] Thus, children with conduct disorder have broader problem-solving deficits in multiple interpersonal contexts than do children with ODD.

The fifth processing step involves two components: (1) identifying the consequences for each of the solutions generated and (2) evaluating each solution and consequence in terms of the individual's desired outcome. In general, aggressive children evaluate aggressive behavior as more positive[112] than do children without aggressive behavior difficulties. Children's beliefs about the utility of aggression and about their ability to successfully enact an aggressive response can increase the likelihood of displayed aggression, because children with these beliefs are more likely to also believe that this type of behavior will help them achieve the desired goals, which then influences response evaluation.[101] Deficient beliefs at this stage of information processing are especially characteristic of children with proactive aggressive behavior patterns[105] and for youths who have callous-unemotional traits consistent with early phases of psychopathy.[113] Researchers have demonstrated that these beliefs about the acceptability of aggressive behavior lead to deviant processing of social cues, which in turn leads to children's aggressive behavior[114]; this indicates that these information-processing steps have recursive effects rather than strictly linear effects on each other.

The final information-processing stage involves behavioral enactment, or displaying the response that was chosen in the preceding steps. Aggressive children are less adept at enacting positive or prosocial interpersonal behaviors.[102] This interpretation suggests that improving the ability to enact positive behaviors may influence aggressive children's beliefs about their ability to engage in these more prosocial behaviors and thus change the response evaluation.

Schemas within the Social-Cognitive Model

Schemas have been proposed to have a significant effect on the information-processing steps within the contextual social-cognitive model underlying cognitive-behavioral interventions with aggressive children.[115,116] Schemas can involve children's expectations and beliefs of others[115] and of themselves, including their self-esteem and narcissism.[117] Early in the information-processing sequence, when the individual is perceiving and interpreting new social cues, schemas can have a clear, direct effect by narrowing the child's attention to certain aspects of the social cue array.[118] A child who believes it essential to be in control of others and who expects that others will try to dominate him or her, often in aversive ways, will attend particularly to verbal and nonverbal signals about someone else's control efforts, easily missing accompanying signs of friendliness or attempts to negotiate. Schemas can also have indirect effects on information processing through their influence on children's expectations for their own behavior and for others' behavior in specific situations. Lochman and Dodge[119] found that aggressive boys' perceptions of their own aggressive behavior was affected primarily by their prior expectations, whereas nonaggressive boys relied more on their actual behavior to form their perceptions.

ASSESSMENT OF EXTERNALIZING BEHAVIOR PROBLEMS

When a child is referred for an evaluation for externalizing behavioral problems, mental health specialists use an array of assessment tools to gather comprehensive information about the child. It is important that the assessment battery include data from multiple informants across multiple domains of functioning. It is also helpful if the informants observe the child in various settings, so that the clinician can draw conclusions about the consistency of the behaviors. For example, parents may be the best reporters of a child's behavior at home and with siblings, whereas teachers provide insight into the child's behavior at school and with peers. Child mental health professionals commonly use behavioral rating scales and structured interviews in their assessment of externalizing behaviors. In addition, direct behavioral observation by the clinician can supply objective data about the child's behaviors in various contexts. In planning an assessment battery for a child presenting with externalizing behavior problems, it is important to assess also for comorbid problems and associated features, such as attentional difficulties, social skills deficits, and depressive symptoms. In a comprehensive assessment, it is important to have the child complete self-report rating scales (e.g., related to self-esteem, attitudes) if the child is old enough to be a reliable informant. Most children over the age of 8 years can provide valuable assessment data.[120]

Although teachers often have insight into peer relationship problems and the social functioning of children with externalizing behavior problems, it is also helpful for clinicians to obtain peer reports whenever possible. Vignettes and hypothetical situations are also used to assess social-cognitive processes, whereas intellectual and academic achievement tests are utilized to conduct a psychoeducational assessment.[121] Table 17-2 contains examples of assessment instruments often included in a comprehensive diagnostic battery.

In addition to making a differential diagnosis, the use of a comprehensive assessment battery is important in determining which symptoms are primary and which are secondary.[121] Identification of primary and secondary symptoms is an important first step in formulating an effective treatment plan. Once all assessment data are collected, the clinician compiles the information into a clinical assessment report, in which the data from various sources are integrated, the findings interpreted, the case formulation and diagnostic impressions outlined, and the treatment plan and recommendations for the child described. In the assessment report, the clinician should document clinically significant findings, including convergent findings across sources and methods, as well as explain any existing discrepancies among sources and methods.[120] The report should provide a profile of the child that includes not only a discussion of any exist-

TABLE 17-2 ■ Recommended Battery of Assessment Tools

Type	Respondent	Examples[120,121]	Advantages	Disadvantages
Omnibus rating scales			Ease of administration Time-efficient (administering) Similar information from multiple informants Detects low-frequency behaviors Screens for comorbid disorders Normative data Interpretive flexibility Computer-based scoring	May not provide enough coverage of core symptoms to differentiate among subtypes Rarely includes information regarding the severity, age at onset, and situational variables related to the problem behaviors Not always tied to diagnostic criteria Sometimes involves excessive item overlap
	Child	Behavior Assessment System for Children–Self Report of Personality, 2nd Edition (BASC-2-SRP) Minnesota Multiphasic Personality Inventory–Adolescent (MMPI-A) Youth Self Report (YSR)		
	Parent	Behavior Assessment System for Children–Parent Rating Scale, 2nd Edition (BASC-2-PRS) Child Behavior Checklist (CBCL) Conners' Parent Rating Scales–Revised		
	Teacher	Behavior Assessment System for Children-2nd Edition-Teacher Rating Scale (BASC-2-TRS) Teacher Report Form (TRF) Conners' Teacher Rating Scales-Revised		

TABLE 17-2 ■ Recommended Battery of Assessment Tools—cont'd				
Type	**Respondent**	**Examples**[120,121]	**Advantages**	**Disadvantages**
Domain-specific rating scales			Ease of administration Time-efficient (administering) Similar information from multiple informants Normative data	May not provide enough coverage of core symptoms to differentiate among subtypes Rarely includes information regarding the severity, age at onset, comorbidity, and situational variables related to the problem behaviors Not always tied to diagnostic criteria
	Child	Reynolds Child Depression Scale (RCDS) Child Depression Inventory (CDI) Revised Child Manifest Anxiety Scale (RCMAS) Harter's Perceived Competence Scale for Children		
	Parent	Attention Deficit Disorders Evaluation Scales, 3rd Edition (ADDES-3)–Home Version Social Skills Rating System (SSRS)		
	Teacher	Attention Deficit Disorders Evaluation Scales, 3rd Edition (ADDES-3)–School Version Social Skills Rating System (SSRS)		
Structured interviews	Both child and parent	Diagnostic Interview Schedule for Children (DISC) Diagnostic Interview for Children and Adolescents (DICA) Child Assessment Schedule for Children (CAS)	Similar information from multiple informants Detailed information Can differentiate among subtypes of disorders Screens for comorbid disorders Information regarding the severity, age of onset, and situational variables related to problem behaviors Tied to diagnostic criteria	Time-consuming (administering and scoring) Requires specialized interviewer training Often does not include normative data
Direct observation	Clinician	Behavior Assessment System for Children–Student Observation System, 2nd Edition (BASC-2-SOS) Child Behavior Checklist–Direct Observation Form (CBCL-DOF) Dodge's Observation of Peer Interactions Structured Observation of Academic and Play Settings Clinician-designed systematic observation schedule	Objective; not biased by informant perception In-depth information Can collect same data across various settings and/or multiple time periods Sensitive to treatment effects Assessment of antecedents and consequences of behaviors	Time-consuming (administering) No normative data Reliability can be low (avoided by evaluation by well-trained observers) May not be standardized Does not detect low-frequency behaviors

TABLE 17-2 ■ Recommended Battery of Assessment Tools—cont'd

Type	Respondent	Examples[120,121]	Advantages	Disadvantages
Peer-referenced assessment	Peers	Sociometric data for which classmates rate other classmates (including target child) on variables such as "Liked most" and "Liked least" Supplemental variables (e.g., "Fights most," "Can't pay attention") may be included Peer Nomination Inventory of Depression (PNID)	Information for subtyping socialized versus undersocialized children with conduct problems Data about peers' perceptions are more accurate than data from teacher ratings or self-report ratings	Time-consuming (administering and scoring) Informed consent typically must be obtained from the peer group Requires teacher participation and sometimes raises teachers' concerns Must ensure client identity is not revealed to other students Little normative data
Vignettes	Child	Problem Solving Measure for Conflict (PSM-C) Child Attribution Measure	Insight into the child's problem-solving strategies	Time-consuming to administer and score (may involve elaborate coding techniques)
Intellectual tests	Child tested	*Full batteries:* Wechsler Intelligence Scale for Children, 4th edition (WISC-IV); Stanford-Binet Intelligence Scales, 5th edition; Kaufman Assessment Battery for Children, 2nd edition (K-ABC-II) *Abbreviated batteries:* Wechsler Abbreviated Scales of Intelligence (WASI); Kaufman Brief Intelligence Test, 2nd edition (K-BIT-2)	Allow interpretation of externalizing behaviors in the context of cognitive functioning Normative data	Time-consuming (administering and scoring)
Academic achievement tests	Child tested	*Full batteries:* Wechsler Individual Achievement Test, 2nd edition (WIAT-II); Woodcock-Johnson III Tests of Academic Achievement (WJ-III) *Abbreviated batteries:* WIAT-II-Screener; Mini Battery of Achievement (MBA)	Assess academic functioning, an area often negatively affected by externalizing behaviors Normative data	Time-consuming (administering and scoring)

ing deficits and problems but also information about his or her strengths.

TREATMENT OF EXTERNALIZING CONDITIONS

Preadolescent children who exhibit disruptive and aggressive behavior are at increased risk for a host of negative outcomes, including severe delinquency, violence, substance abuse, school dropout, and co-occurring psychiatric disorders.[122,123] Pediatricians can play a critical role in identifying such children and making appropriate treatment recommenda-

tions. There are numerous evidence-based interventions in which children with externalizing behavior disorders are treated effectively,[124-126] and early intervention and prevention can significantly improve affected children's developmental trajectory.[116] However, young children with conduct problems are a chronically underserved population. Brestan and Eyberg[127] found that only about 30% of children with conduct problems received any treatment and even fewer received treatments that had been empirically validated in randomized controlled trials. Pediatricians are often the first professionals to learn of disruptive behavior in children; thus, they can play a critical role in identifying children in need and providing appropriate treatment recommendations.

Systematic reviews of the treatment literature have identified a number of intervention programs with well-established therapeutic effects for children with externalizing behavior disorders.[126,127] All of the programs shown to effectively reduce disruptive and aggressive behavior in children involve the use of cognitive and behavioral treatment techniques. These treatment programs vary in their emphasis on parents and/or children; interventions for preschool-aged children focus on parent behavioral training, and interventions for school-aged children and adolescents entail teaching skills, including social problem solving, coping with anger, perspective taking, and relaxation. Multicomponent interventions that target parents and children, as well as teachers and other key adults, consistently produce stronger therapeutic effects and better maintenance of improvements over time than do interventions that focus on either the child or parent alone.[126]

Two treatment approaches are considered "well established" because of their extensive empirical support. Both originated as parent training programs and were subsequently expanded to include child-focused intervention components. The first is behavioral parent training based on Patterson and Gullion's manual *Living with Children: New Methods for Parents and Teachers.*[128] This approach is designed to teach parents operant conditioning techniques to increase prosocial behaviors in children and decrease aggressive and disruptive behaviors. These techniques include attending to and reinforcing prosocial and compliance behaviors; ignoring minor disruptive behaviors; implementing negative consequences after inappropriate behaviors (such as timeout and privilege removal); and giving effective commands. Kazdin[129] developed a parent management training program based on Patterson and Gullion's work and paired it with a child-focused problem-solving skills training program, which teaches children social problem-solving skills through modeling, role-play, and practice. Although both parent management training and problem-solving skills training can be used as stand-alone interventions, combined treatment tends to be more effective than either treatment alone.[130]

The second "well-established" treatment approach is a similar behavioral parent training program developed by Webster-Stratton[131,132] known as the *Incredible Years Training Series.* It includes video segments that model parent training, typically viewed in a therapist-led group. During these group sessions, parents view and discuss video vignettes demonstrating social learning and child development principles and how parents can use child-directed techniques—interactive play, praise, and incentive programs—and non-violent discipline techniques. An advanced version of the program incorporates video vignettes promoting parents' personal self-control, communication skills, problem-solving skills, social support, and self-care. Webster-Stratton also developed a child videotape modeling program and teacher training curriculum, which have been shown to enhance outcome effects of the original *Incredible Years* parent training program.[133,134]

Another evidence-based intervention, *parent-child interaction therapy,* was specifically designed to target the parent and child dyad, with the therapist serving as a coach during in-person encounters to improve the parent and child's interaction patterns.[135] Operant conditioning parenting techniques similar to those described previously are taught by this coaching method, including a specific system for implementing timeout after a child disobeys a command. Parent-child interaction therapy is used most often with families of preschool-aged children (i.e., between the ages of 3 and 6). Significant improvements in children's behavior, parenting stress, and parents' perceptions of control are found in families receiving parent-child interaction therapy in relation to families in a waitlist control group. Moreover, these gains are maintained after treatment completion and generalize to children's classroom behavior.[135]

More comprehensive family and community-based treatments are often needed when multiple risk factors are present (e.g., child maltreatment, marital discord, parental psychopathology, poverty, exposure to neighborhood violence) and for adolescents with serious behavior problems. *Multisystemic therapy* is an intensive family and community-based treatment program that has been implemented with chronic and violent juvenile offenders, substance-abusing juvenile offenders, adolescent sexual offenders, youths in psychiatric crisis (i.e., homicidal, suicidal, psychotic), and maltreating families.[136] The *Oregon Multidimensional Treatment Foster Care program* is also a comprehensive and systemic intervention designed to treat adolescent juvenile offenders in nonrestrictive, family-style, community-based settings.[137] Both multisystemic therapy and the Oregon program have demonstrated effectiveness in treating chronically delinquent youth and, in many cases, in changing youths' behavior and creating safer and more positive family living environments.[125]

With any intervention program for children and adolescents with externalizing behavior problems, treatment is most effective when modifications are consistent across settings. Consultation with teachers and other school personnel is crucial for tailoring interventions to children's individual needs and ensuring that they receive appropriate academic and behavioral services at school. Under the Individuals with Disabilities Education Act, children with externalizing behavior problems that adversely affect their school performance are eligible for an Individualized Education Plan or a Section 504 Plan that establishes target behavioral goals and needed interventions (e.g., classroom behavior chart, home-to-school notebook for daily behavior tracking). Pediatricians can play a critical role in educating parents about their child's right to school-based services and encouraging them to work closely with their child's school to ensure that he or she is obtaining the behavioral supports necessary to learn.

Coping Power Program

Many of the evidence-based intervention programs just described incorporate similar cognitive and behavioral treatment techniques. To provide a more detailed description of these intervention elements, we now describe the *Coping Power* program. Coping Power is a comprehensive, multicomponent intervention program that is based on the contextual social-cognitive model of risk for youth violence.[138] Coping Power draws upon many of the cognitive and behavioral techniques of well-established parent training programs and also incorporates novel techniques that target malleable, child-level social-cognitive risk factors for externalizing behavior problems. We describe the content of the Coping Power program in detail to illustrate the structure and skills taught in a comprehensive, multicomponent, evidence-based intervention for preadolescent children exhibiting disruptive and aggressive behavior.

Coping Power includes a child component, which consists of a 34-session group intervention, and a coordinated 16-session parent component, both of which are designed to be delivered over a 16- to 18-month period. Session-by-session treatment manuals are available for both the child and parent components. A teacher curriculum is also available and is typically administered during in-service teacher workshops. The Coping Power program can be implemented by mental health professionals in clinical practice settings or by school guidance counselors and related school personnel. Coping Power was originally designed to be implemented with fourth- to sixth-grade children but has been successfully adapted for younger and older children. It has also been successfully adapted for other languages (e.g., Dutch, Spanish) and cultures. An abbreviated version that can be completed in one academic year (24 child sessions, 10 parent sessions) has also been developed.

COPING POWER CHILD COMPONENT

The Coping Power Child Component includes 34 group sessions, each lasting 45 to 60 minutes. The optimal number of children per group is 4 to 6, with two coleaders. Group sessions are held approximately once a week and are supplemented by monthly individual meetings with each child. The primary aims of the one-to-one sessions are to monitor and reinforce each child's progress toward personal social behavior goals (e.g., avoiding fights with peers; resisting peer pressure) and to encourage generalization of intervention effects to other settings. The Coping Power Child Component is an expanded version of the original 18-session Anger Coping Program.[139]

The sequence and objectives of the Coping Power Child Component group sessions are detailed in Table 17-3. The foci of the child group sessions include (1) establishing group rules and a reinforcement contingency; (2) personal behavioral goal setting; (3) awareness of anger arousal and learning to use coping self-statements, relaxation, and distraction techniques to cope with arousal; (4) practicing accurate problem identification and social perspective taking with pictured and actual social problem situations; (5) generating alternative solutions to social problems, considering the consequences of each solution, and selecting and enacting the optimal solution; (6) viewing modeling videotapes of children becoming aware of physiological arousal when angry, using self-statements ("Stop! Think! What should I do?"), and using the complete set of problem-solving skills to effectively solve social problems; (7) facilitating the children's production of a videotape demonstrating effective problem solving with social problems of their own choosing; (8) enhancing social skills and methods for identifying and entering positive peer networks (focusing on cooperation and negotiation skills during structured and unstructured peer interactions); and (9) learning and rehearsing strategies for resisting peer pressure.

Several activities are repeated at the beginning and end of each session. Sessions begin with a review of each child's behavioral goal from the previous week and end with the selection of a goal for the following week. At the beginning of each session, the children are also asked to recall one of the main topics discussed or skills learned during the previous session. The goal of this activity is to foster children's recall and generalization of skills from week to week. At the end of each group meeting, the children are asked to give positive feedback to one another and are given an opportunity make purchases from a menu of reinforcers (e.g., walkie talkies, Nerf basketball, markers, lip gloss), using points earned for meeting personal behavior goals, following group rules, and positive participation. During each session, role-plays, structured activities, and homework assignments are also used to facilitate transfer of skills outside of the group setting.

TABLE 17-3 ■ Coping Power Child Sessions	
Session and Topic	**Session Goals**
Session 1	
Getting acquainted/group cohesion	To explain the general idea and purpose of the group
	To help students feel comfortable with each other and leaders
Establish structure of group and behavioral goal setting procedure	To establish a defined group structure
	To define a "goal" and to have students choose one goal to work on during the week
Sessions 2 and 3	
Setting long-term and short-term	To introduce the concept of setting and realizing goals
	To help students identify goals that they want to achieve
Personal goals	To help students understand the importance of setting long-range goals and the steps (short-term goals) needed to attain them
	To help students identify barriers to achieving goals and how to overcome them
Sessions 4 and 5	
Awareness of physiological arousal and feelings related to anger	To help students identify different feeling states in themselves and others
	To help students be in touch with their own physiological "cues" related to anger and other feeling states
	To help students identify various levels of anger
	To help students generate a list (via brainstorming) of anger triggers and coping strategies used at various levels of anger
Sessions 6 to 8	
Practice the use of prosocial self-statements when taunted	To review concepts of anger coping/self-control
	To help students practice ways of maintaining self-control
	To introduce the concept of self-talk or self-statements
	To practice using self-statements
Session 9	
Organizational and study skills	To help students identify areas of strength and weakness in school performance
	To facilitate activities related to organizational and study skills
	To practice newly learned skills
Sessions 10 and 11	
Practice use of coping self-statements and ways of defusing anger	To help students understand the importance of what people tell themselves in problematic situations
	To help students generate multiple strategies (coping statements) to use when confronted with problematic situations
	To practice using statements while being provoked in a role-play situation
	To help students identify barriers and obstacles in using coping statements and to try to solve problems around them
Session 12	
Problem identification	To explain the purpose of the problem identification, choices, and consequences (PICC) model
	To demonstrate the use of the PICC model with a problem situation chart
	To learn how to "pick apart" the problem by using the PICC model
Sessions 13 to 15	
Perspective taking with peers and teachers	To explain to students the concept of perspective taking by using illustration activities
	To "PICC apart" a social problem situation
	To help students apply the PICC model to a social situation
	To demonstrate how individuals can have different views of the same situation
	To help students understand that ambiguous social situations have unclear attributes
	To develop perspective-taking questions for the teacher interview
	To prepare students to conduct an interview with selected teacher

TABLE 17-3 ■ Coping Power Child Sessions—cont'd

Sessions 16 to 19

Social problem-solving training | To illustrate how to generate a range of solutions to a problem, and to reinforce positive verbal solutions
To illustrate, with the PICC model, how consequences follow from choices
To illustrate levels of consequences and how decisions are made on the basis of the potential outcomes
To demonstrate how automatic thinking can produce choices with poorer consequences than can deliberate thinking
To practice using PICC on problems identified by students

Sessions 20 to 22

Student-led videotape activity on PICC | To provide a model for videotaping of a problem-solving session
To develop a script for the videotape by using the PICC model
To begin the process of videotaping
To make a series of videotapes with alternative solutions that show consideration of various consequences and outcomes
To complete and review the video and reinforce the problem-solving process

End-of-year review | To review and evaluate progress on personal goals worked on during the year (by using *The Coping Power Review Game*) in order to assess retention and generalization of skills taught
To plan for goals to be worked on during year 2 of the program
To plan for and schedule with students a celebration party to bring closure to year 1 of the program

Session 23

Review of year 1 and introduction to year 2 | To review basic structure of group and program
To review with students curriculum material from year 1 and assess their recall of key points
To assess students' use of strategies during summer vacation
To engage group members in a "get acquainted" activity
To have students choose a goal to work on for the coming week

Supplementary Meeting

Organizational and study skills | Review of material from session 9

Session 24

Teacher expectations and conflict | To review material from year 1 on teacher perspectives of students' behavior
To review the most frequently given teacher responses from interviews (in the format of a TV game show)
To use the PICC model to discuss common areas of concern between teachers and students

Sessions 25 and 26

Social skills training: entering a new group and negotiating with peers | To review the PICC model and use it as a means of entering new situations and assessing appropriateness of new peers
To have group members identify important attributes in positive peers
To use the PICC model as a means of negotiating with peers

Session 27

Sibling conflict | To discuss and role-play how the PICC model can be used to address conflicts with siblings
To discuss perspective taking and how it applies to problems with siblings

Sessions 28 and 29

Peer pressure and refusal skills | To illustrate (with video) what peer pressure is and its effect on students
To brainstorm ways that peer pressure can be resisted
To have students practice using refusal skills in role-play situations

Session 30

Neighborhood problems | To review completed neighborhood survey (previously given out in individual sessions by group leader)
To use the PICC model to identify situations in neighborhoods that could produce pressure and temptation in group members
To discuss positive neighborhood resources that can serve as protective factors

TABLE 17-3 ■ Coping Power Child Sessions—cont'd	
Sessions 31 and 32	
Peer groups and group membership	To discuss how groups form and to identify groups known to students
Resisting peer pressure and joining positive peer groups	To discuss attributes of groups that get in trouble and attributes of positive groups
	To identify one's own role (place) in a group as a central or peripheral member
	To create a poster relating to peer pressure (for later display in the school)
	To have students identify strategies they can use to become members of prosocial groups
Sessions 33 and 34	
Review and termination	To use *strength bombardment* activity with group members on unique individual qualities
	To allow students to review personal qualities that have enabled them to be positive role models
	To use the *Coping Power Review Game* to bring closure to what they have learned from the process
	To celebrate successes and say good-bye to group members and leaders

COPING POWER PARENT COMPONENT

The Coping Power Parent Component includes 16 group sessions, each lasting approximately 90 minutes. Parents meet in groups of up to 12 parents (or parent dyads) with two coleaders. Parent group sessions are held within the same time period in which the child group sessions occur. The content of the Coping Power Parent Component is derived from social learning theory–based parent training programs such as those described previously.[2,128] Specifically, the parents learn skills for (1) identifying prosocial and disruptive target behaviors in their children; (2) rewarding appropriate child behaviors; (3) giving effective instructions and establishing age-appropriate rules and expectations for their child in the home; (4) applying effective nonphysical consequences to negative child behaviors; (5) managing child behavior outside the home; and (6) establishing ongoing family communication structures in the home (such as weekly family meetings).

In addition to these "standard" parent training skills, parents in Coping Power also learn skills that support the social-cognitive and problem-solving skills that their children are learning in the Coping Power child groups. Parent and child group sessions are scheduled in such a way that parent skills are introduced at the same time that the respective child skills are introduced, so that parents and children can work together at home on what they are learning. For example, parents learn to set up homework support structures and to reinforce organizational skills at the same time that children are learning study skills and organization in the Coping Power child group. Parents also learn techniques for managing sibling conflict in the home as children are addressing peer and sibling conflict resolution skills in the child groups. Finally, parents learn the problem identification, choices, and consequences (PICC) problem-solving model and

practice applying it to family problems, so that that the children's problem-solving skills are practiced and reinforced at home.

The sequence and objectives of the Coping Power Parent Component group sessions are detailed in Table 17-4. Each session follows a similar format, opening with discussion, reactions, and questions about the previous session; presentation of new session content; discussion with parents about their reactions to the new content; eliciting parents' ideas about how to adapt content to their particular situation; and homework assignment. Similar to the child groups, role-plays and in-session activities, as well as homework assignments, are used to facilitate transfer of skills learned to the home environment and other settings.

COPING POWER TEACHER COMPONENT

The Coping Power teacher curriculum is typically provided during in-service workshops. During the workshops, didactic presentations are combined with teacher discussion and problem solving around the presentation topic. The foci of the teacher meetings include (1) critical challenges that arise at the time of the middle school transition and ways in which parents and teachers can help children prepare to make this transition successfully; (2) methods for promoting positive parent involvement in the school setting and in their child's education; (3) enhancing children's study skills, ability to organize work, and completion of homework, including a focus on children's self control, the parent-teacher communications regarding homework, and children's social bond to school; (4) enhancing children's social competence by emphasizing teacher facilitation of children's emerging social problem-solving strategies; and (5) enhancing children's self-control and self-regulation through conflict management strategies involving

TABLE 17-4 ■ Coping Power Parent Sessions

Session and Topic	Session Goals
Session 1 Program orientation	To orient parents to intensive parent training To introduce basic principles of social learning To explain the ABC (antecedent, behavior, consequence) chart To complete the parent report of positive and negative behavior To introduce the concept of positive and negative consequences To introduce the concepts of labeled and unlabeled praise To present homework assignments
Session 2 Academic support at home	To review reactions to last session To offer a rationale for the timing of this session To discuss steps to set up homework assignment check To provide a structure and monitoring routine wherein parents can supervise homework
Session 3 Ignoring minor disruptive behavior	To use the concept of "catching your child being good" to lead to the concept of planned ignoring To use the ABC chart to discuss ignoring To role-play ignoring To process with parents their reactions to the concept of ignoring
Session 4 Giving instructions to children	To discuss the importance of "following instructions" as an adaptive behavior To discuss how to use an already learned parenting skill to improve compliance To discuss the importance of giving good instructions To use the ABC chart to discuss following instructions To present instructions that do and do not work
Session 5 Rules and expectations	To discuss the importance of having clear rules for children To use the ABC chart to discuss rules To role-play discussing behavior rules at home To discuss expectations for chores and other appropriate behavior To role-play negotiating chores with children
Sessions 6 and 7 Discipline and punishment	To introduce the concept of punishment To provide a working definition of punishment To teach why physical punishment is often ineffective To solicit ideas from parents about punishments To instruct in the use of timeout for noncompliance with an effective instruction To use the ABC chart to discuss timeout To discuss use of timeout for behavioral rule violations To discuss other punishment procedures such as response cost and work chores To help parents choose an effective punishment strategy
Sessions 8 and 9 Stress management	To introduce topic of stress management To present a working definition of stress To use the ABC chart to discuss stress and stress management To talk about stress in parenting To introduce the concept of "taking care of yourself" as the beginning of stress management To discuss how to operationalize "taking care of yourself" To introduce active relaxation To practice relaxation in the session To present a cognitive model of stress and mood management To role-play a stressful situation and parental overreaction
Termination for the year	To celebrate progress for year 1 and make tentative plans for reconvening at the beginning of the next school year To review and share plans for the summer

TABLE 17-4 ■ Coping Power Parent Sessions—cont'd	
Session 10	
Family cohesion building	To introduce the concept of family cohesion building
	To introduce rationale for family cohesion building
	To use the ABC chart to discuss family cohesion
	To discuss family cohesion experiences at home (e.g., family night activities)
Session 11	
Family problem solving: sibling conflict and parent-child conflict	To introduce rationale for family problem solving
	To introduce steps of family problem solving by using the PICC model from child intervention
	To show video from child group or present completed PICC forms
	To present parents' role in sibling conflict
	To use ABC chart to discuss sibling conflict
	To show videotape on family problem solving
	To role-play with a triad (parent, two children)
	To discuss implementation of problem-solving model
Session 12	
Family communication: structure and long-term plans for managing behavior outside of the home	To create or define a current structure for family communication
	To ask each parent to select a family communication structure
	To discuss managing child behavior outside of the home
	To discuss structure and positive reinforcement strategies outside of the home
	To discuss punishment procedures outside of the home
	To discuss use of ABC chart for behavior outside of the home
Session 13	
Long-term planning	To discuss the ending of the parent training program
	To introduce long-term planning
	To discuss school-based resources for the child
	To discuss family-based resources for the child
	To discuss community-based (nonschool) resources for the child
	To discuss long-term maintenance of parenting skills
	To use ABC chart to discuss long-term parenting skills
Session 14	
Parent orientation to middle school	To prepare parents for curricular, social, and organizational demands of middle school environment.
Session 15	
Getting ready for summer	To offer suggestions for structuring summer time in a productive and prosocial way (e.g., summer camps, volunteer opportunities, academic enrichment)
Session 16	
Termination	To present overview of the parent training program
	To elicit parent reactions and feelings about the program
	To give general recommendations to the group
	To share final observations and say goodbye

peer negotiation and teacher's use of proactive classroom management.

Outcome Effects of Coping Power and Anger Coping Programs

In efficacy and effectiveness studies, the Coping Power program has been found to produce lower rates of parent-reported youth substance abuse and self-reported delinquent behavior after intervention and at a 1-year follow-up, in comparison with a randomly assigned control group,[48] and lower self-reported substance abuse, reductions in proactive aggression, improvements in social competence, and greater teacher-rated behavioral improvement at the end of the intervention, in comparison with children who had not received Coping Power.[140] The Anger Coping Program from which the Coping Power Child Component was derived has also been shown to produce lasting social-cognitive gains and to prevent substance abuse into adolescence[141]; however, the adjunctive parent intervention component appears to be necessary in order to have longer term effects on children's delinquent behavior. This is consistent with similar studies that have revealed that multicomponent interventions (i.e., with both parent and child intervention components) can be the most effective for children with externalizing behavior problems.[130,133]

Follow-up by the Pediatrician

A wealth of developmental research makes it clear that without intervention, preadolescent children exhibiting disruptive behavior and aggression are at significant risk for a host of negative outcomes, as described previously.[122,123] The pediatrician should therefore remain actively involved with families once conduct problems are identified. Roles of the pediatrician can include monitoring parents' motivation to seek assessment and treatment, reinforcing parents and children for their effort to learn positive parenting and coping skills, recognizing individual differences that may affect the selection and course of treatment, collaborating with multidisciplinary service providers, and determining whether medication treatment for coexisting psychiatric conditions is warranted. It is important for pediatricians, when making treatment recommendations and referrals, to consider the developmental trajectory of aggressive and oppositional behaviors, including determining whether specific behaviors are age appropriate.

RESEARCH IMPLICATIONS AND SUMMARY

The active series of basic and intervention research studies with children with externalizing behavior problems since the 1960s has contributed to a clearer picture of the risk factors contributing to the development of children's conduct problems, as well as effective, evidence-based interventions to reduce these problems. However, there is still much to learn. Clinicians' understanding of how genetic and biological risk factors interact with contextual factors is still in very early stages. Existing studies suggest that this is an exceptionally important area to develop further and that these studies can help identify critical buffering factors that protect against children's inherent risk factors. Researchers also need to better articulate the mechanisms of action that lead to the development of serious antisocial behavior and conduct problems. Research on mediating factors is essential in this regard. Finally, investigators must examine how interventions can more effectively address children with comorbid problems, how parents can more actively engage in interventions, and how to adapt and disseminate empirically based interventions to a variety of clinical and school settings. A most important direction of research is an examination of how to pursue assessment and intervention usefully and effectively in primary care settings. Pediatricians' roles are pivotal in these efforts.

REFERENCES

1. Achenbach TM, Howell CT: Are American children's problems getting worse? A 13-year comparison. J Am Acad Child Adolesc Psychiatry 32:1145-1154, 1993.
2. McMahon RJ, Forehand RL: Helping the Noncompliant Child: Family-Based Treatment for Oppositional Behavior, 2nd ed. New York: Guilford Press, 2003.
3. Schoen SF: The status of compliance technology: Implications for programming. J Spec Educ 17:483-496, 1983.
4. Brumfield BD, Roberts MW: A comparison of two measurements of child compliance with normal preschool children. J Clin Child Psychol 27:109-116, 1998.
5. Lahey BB, Schwab-Stone M, Goodman SH, et al: Age and gender differences in oppositional behavior and conduct problems: A cross-sectional household study of middle childhood and adolescence. J Abnorm Psychol 109:488-503, 2000.
6. Vaughn BE, Kopp CB, Krakow JB: The emergence and consolidation of self-control from eighteen to thirty months of age: Normative trends and individual differences. Child Dev 55:990-1004, 1984.
7. Kochanska G, Coy KC, Murray KT: The development of self-regulation in the first four years of life. Child Dev 72:1091-1111, 2001.
8. Kuczynski L, Kochanska G: Development of children's noncompliance strategies from toddlerhood to age 5. Dev Psychol 26:398-408, 1990.
9. Smith CL, Calkins SD, Keane SP, et al: Predicting stability and change in toddler behavior problems: Contributions of maternal behavior and child gender. Dev Psychol 40:29-42, 2004.
10. Patterson GR, Forgatch M: Parents and Adolescents: Living Together. Eugene, OR: Castalia, 1987.
11. Collins WA, Laursen B: Changing relationships, changing youth: Interpersonal contexts of adolescent development. J Early Adolesc 24:55-62, 2004.
12. Steinberg L: We know some things: Parent-adolescent relationships in retrospect and prospect. J Res Adolesc 11:1-19, 2001.
13. Laursen B, Coy KC, Collins WA: Reconsidering changes in parent-child conflict across adolescence: A meta-analysis. Child Dev 69:817-832, 1998.
14. Bongers IL, Koot HM, Van der Ende J, et al: Developmental trajectories of externalizing behaviors in childhood and adolescence. Child Dev 75:1523-1537, 2004.
15. Dodge KA: The structure and function of reactive and proactive aggression. In Pepler DJ, Rubin KH, eds: Development and Treatment of Childhood Aggression. Hillsdale, NJ: Erlbaum, 1991, pp 201-218.

16. Crick NR, Grotpeter JK: Relational aggression, gender, and social-psychological adjustment. Child Dev 66:710-722, 1995.

17. Bohnert AM, Crnic KA, Lim KG: Emotional competence and aggressive behavior in school-age children. J Abnorm Child Psychol 31:79-91, 2003.

18. Denham SA, Caverly S, Schmidt M, et al: Preschool understanding of emotions: Contributions to classroom anger and aggression. J Child Psychol Psychiatry 43:901-916, 2002.

19. Rydell A, Berlin L, Bohlin G: Emotionality, emotion regulation, and adaptation among 5- to 8-year-old children. Emotion 3:30-47, 2003.

20. Eisenberg N, Sadovsky A, Spinrad TL, et al: The relations of problem behavior status to children's negative emotionality, effortful control, and impulsivity: Concurrent relations and prediction of change. Dev Psychol 41:193-211, 2005.

21. Hanish LD, Eisenberg N, Fabes RA, et al: The expression and regulation of negative emotions: Risk factors for young children's peer victimization. Dev Psychopathol 16:335-353, 2004.

22. Stenberg CR, Campos JJ, Emde RN: The facial expression of anger in seven-month-old infants. Child Dev 54:178-184, 1983.

23. Huebner RR, Izard CE: Mothers' responses to infants' facial expressions of sadness, anger, and physical distress. Motiv Emotion 12:185-196, 1988.

24. Malatesta CZ, Grigoryev P, Lamb C, et al: Emotion socialization and expressive development in preterm and full-term infants. Child Dev 57:316-330, 1986.

25. Buss KA, Kiel EJ: Comparison of sadness, anger, and fear facial expressions when toddlers look at their mothers. Child Dev 75:1761-1773, 2004.

26. Dunn JF: Sibling influences on childhood development. J Child Psychol Psychiatry 29:119-127, 1988.

27. Denham SA: Emotional Development in Young Children. New York: Guilford, 1998.

28. Ridgeway D, Waters E, Kuczaj SA: Acquisition of emotion-descriptive language: Receptive and productive vocabulary norms for ages 18 months to 6 years. Dev Psychol 21:901-908, 1985.

29. Shipman KL, Zeman J, Nesin AE, et al: Children's strategies for displaying anger and sadness: What works with whom? Merrill Palmer Q 49:100-122, 2003.

30. Underwood M, Coie J, Herbsman CR: Display rules for anger and aggression in school-aged children. Child Dev 63:366-380, 1992.

31. Bongers IL, Koot HM, Van der Ende J, Verhulst FC: The normative development of child and adolescent problem behavior. J Abnorm Psychol 112:179-192, 2003.

32. Keiley MK, Bates JE, Dodge KA, et al: A cross-domain growth analysis: Externalizing and internalizing behaviors during 8 years of childhood. J Abnorm Child Psychol 28:161-179, 2000.

33. Stanger C, Achenbach TM, Verhulst FC: Accelerated longitudinal comparisons of aggressive versus delinquent syndromes. Dev Psychopathol 9:43-58, 1997.

34. Lochman JE, Whidby JM, Fitzgerald DP: Cognitive-behavioral assessment and treatment with aggressive children. In Kendall PC, ed: Child and Adolescent Therapy: Cognitive-Behavioral Procedures, 2nd ed. New York: Guilford, 2000, pp 31-87.

35. Loeber R: Development and risk factors of juvenile antisocial behavior and delinquency. Clin Psychol Rev 10:1-41, 1990.

36. Olweus D: Bully/victims problems among schoolchildren: Basic facts and effects of a school based intervention program. In Pepler DJ, Rubin KH, eds: Development and Treatment of Childhood Aggression. Hillsdale, NJ: Erlbaum, 1991, pp 411-448.

37. Rigby K: Bullying in Schools and What to Do about It. London: Jessica Kingsley, 1996.

38. Farrington DP: Understanding and preventing bullying. In Tonry M, ed: Crime and Justice, vol 17. Chicago: University of Chicago Press, 1993, pp 381-458.

39. Ireland JL, Archer J: Association between measures of aggression and bullying among juvenile and young offenders. Aggress Behav 30:29-42, 2004.

40. Nabuzoka D, Smith PK: Sociometric status and social behavior of children with and without learning difficulties. J Child Psychol Psychiatry 34:1435-1448, 1993.

41. American Psychiatric Association: Diagnostic and Statistical Manual of Mental Disorders, 4th ed, Text Revision. Washington, DC: American Psychiatric Press, 2000.

41a. Wolraich M, Felice ME, Drotar D: The Classification of Child and Adolescent Mental Diagnoses in Primary Care: Diagnostic and Statistical Manual for Primary Care (DSM-PC) Child and Adolescent Version. Elk Grove Village, IL: American Academy of Pediatrics, 1996.

42. Barry CT, Frick PJ, DeShazo TM, et al: The importance of callous-unemotional traits for extending the concept of psychopathy to children. J Abnorm Psychol 109:335-340, 2000.

43. Cleckley H: The Mask of Insanity, 5th ed. St. Louis: CV Mosby, 1976.

44. Hart RD, Hare RD: Psychopathy: Assessment and association with criminal conduct. In Stoff DM, Breiling J, Maser JD, eds: Handbook of Antisocial Behavior. New York: Wiley, 1997, pp 22-35.

45. Hinshaw SP, Lee SS: Conduct and oppositional defiant disorders. In Mash EJ, Barkley RA, eds: Child Psychopathology, 2nd ed. New York: Guilford Press, 2003, pp 144-198.

46. Hinshaw SP, Lahey BB, Hart EL: Issues of taxonomy and comorbidity in the development of conduct disorder. Dev Psychopathol 5:31-49, 1993.

47. Loeber R, Green SM, Keenan K, et al: Which boys will fare worse?: Early predictors of the onset of conduct disorder in a six-year longitudinal study. J Am Acad Child Adolesc Psychiatry 34:499-509, 1995.

48. Lochman JE, Wells KC: Contextual social-cognitive mediators and child outcome: A test of the theoretical model in the Coping Power Program. Dev Psychopathol 14:971-993, 2002.

49. Lochman JE: Contextual factors in risk and prevention research. Merrill Palmer Q 50:311-325, 2004.

50. Brennan PA, Grekin ER, Mednick SA: Maternal smoking during pregnancy and adult male criminal outcomes. Arch Gen Psychiatry 56:215-219, 1999.

51. Delaney-Black V, Covington C, Templin T, et al: Teacher-assessed behavior of children prenatally exposed to cocaine. Pediatrics 106:782-791, 2000.

52. Kelly JJ, Davis PO, Henschke PN: The drug epidemic: Effects on newborn infants and health resource consumption at a tertiary perinatal centre. J Paediatr Child Health 36:262-264, 2000.

53. Rasanen P, Hakko H, Isobarmi M, et al: Maternal smoking during pregnancy and risk of criminal behavior among male offspring in the northern Finland 1996 birth cohort. Am J Psychiatry 156:857-862, 1999.

54. Masten AS, Best KM, Garmezy N: Resilience and development: Contributions from the study of children who overcome adversity. Dev Psychopathol 2:425-444, 1990.

55. Arseneault L, Tremblay RE, Boulerice B, et al: Obstetric complications and adolescent violent behaviors: Testing two developmental pathways. Child Dev 73:496-508, 2002.

56. Coon H, Carey G, Corley R, et al: Identifying children in the Colorado adoption project at risk for conduct disorder. J Am Acad Child Adolesc Psychiatry 31:503-511, 1992.

57. Dabbs JM, Morris R: Testosterone, social class, and antisocial behavior in a sample of 4,462 men. Psychol Science 1:209-211, 1990.

58. Raine A, Brennan P, Mednick SA: Interactions between birth complications and early maternal rejection in predisposing individuals to adult violence: Specificity to serious, early onset violence. Am J Psychiatry 154:1265-1271, 1997.

59. Scarpa A, Bowser FM, Fikretoglu D, et al: Effects of community violence II: Interactions with psychophysiologic functioning. Psychophysiology 36(Suppl):102, 1999.

60. Scarpa A, Raine A: Violence associated with anger and impulsivity. In Borod JC, ed: The Neuropsychology of Emotion. London: Oxford University Press, 2000, pp 320-339.

61. Caspi A, McClay J, Moffitt T, et al: Role of genotype in the cycle of violence in maltreated children. Science 297:851-854, 2002.

62. Colder CR, Lochman JE, Wells KC: The moderating effects of children's fear and activity level on relations between parenting practices and childhood symptomatology. J Abnorm Child Psychol 25:251-263, 1997.

63. Scaramella LV, Conger RD: Intergenerational continuity of hostile parenting and its consequences: The moderating influence of children's negative emotional reactivity. Soc Dev 12:420-439, 2003.

64. Barry TD, Dunlap ST, Cotton SJ, et al: The influence of maternal stress and distress on disruptive behavior problems in children. J Am Acad Child Adolesc Psychiatry 44:265-273, 2005.

65. Loeber R, Stouthamer-Loeber M: Development of juvenile aggression and violence: Some common misconceptions and controversies. Am Psychol 53:242-259, 1998.

66. McCarty CA, McMahon RJ, Conduct Problems Prevention Research Group: Mediators of the relation between maternal depressive symptoms and child internalizing and disruptive behavior Disorders. J Fam Psychol 17:545-556, 2003.

67. Sampson JH, Laub RJ: Crime in the Making: Pathways and Turning Points through Life. Cambridge, MA: Harvard University Press, 1993.

68. Guerra NG, Huesmann LR, Tolan PH, et al: Stressful events and individual beliefs as correlates of economic disadvantage and aggression among urban children. J Consult Clin Psychol 63:513-528, 1995.

69. Nagin D, Pogarsky G, Farrington D: Adolescent mothers and the criminal behavior of their children. Law Soc 31:137-162, 1997.

70. Erath SA, Bierman KL, Conduct Problems Prevention Research Group: Aggressive marital conflict, maternal harsh punishment, and child aggressive-disruptive behavior: Evidence for direct and indirect relations. J Fam Psychol 20:217-226, 2006.

71. Shaw DS, Vondra JI: Infant attachment security and maternal predictors of early behavior problems: A longitudinal study of low-income families. J Abnorm Child Psychol 26:407-414, 1995.

72. Luthar SS: Children in Poverty: Risk and Protective Factors in Adjustment. Thousand Oaks, CA: Sage Publications, 1999.

73. Dodge KA, Pettit GS, Bates JE: Socialization mediators of the relation between socioeconomic status and child conduct problems. Child Dev 65:649-665, 1994.

74. Dadds MR, Powell MB: The relationship of interparental conflict and global marital adjustment to aggression, anxiety, and immaturity in aggressive and nonclinic children. J Abnorm Child Psychol 19:553-567, 1992.

75. Patterson GR, Reid JB, Dishion TJ: Antisocial Boys. Eugene, OR: Castalia, 1992.

76. Shaw DS, Keenan K, Vondra JI: The developmental precursors of antisocial behavior: Ages 1-3. Dev Psychol 30:355-364, 1994.

77. Weiss B, Dodge KA, Bates JE, et al: Some consequences of early harsh discipline: Child aggression and maladaptive social information processing style. Child Dev 63:1321-1335, 1992.

78. Fite PJ, Colder CR, Lochman JE, et al: The mutual influence of parenting and boys' externalizing behavior problems. J Appl Dev Psychol 27:151-164, 2006.

79. Haapasalo J, Tremblay R: Physically aggressive boys from ages 6 to 12: Family background, parenting behavior, and prediction of delinquency. J Consult Clin Psychol 62:1044-1052, 1994.

80. Cillessen AH, Van IJzendoorn HW, Van Lieshout CF, et al: Heterogeneity among peer-rejected boys: Subtypes and stabilities. Child Dev 63:893-905, 1992.

81. Lochman JE, Wayland KK: Aggression, social acceptance and race as predictors of negative adolescent

outcomes. J Am Acad Child Adolesc Psychiatry 33:1026-1035, 1994.

82. Miller-Johnson S, Coie, JD, Maumary-Gremaud A, et al: Peer rejection and aggression and early starter models of conduct disorder. J Abnorm Child Psychol 30:217-230, 2002.

83. Bry BH, Catalano RF, Kumpfer K, et al: Scientific findings from family prevention intervention research. In Ashery R, ed: Family-Based Prevention Interventions. Rockville, MD: National Institute of Drug Abuse, 1999, pp 103-129.

84. Conduct Problems Prevention Research Group: The Fast Track experiment: Translating the developmental model into a prevention design. In Kupersmidt JB, Dodge KA, eds: Children's Peer Relations: From Development to Intervention. Washington, DC: American Psychological Association, 2004, pp 181-208.

85. Pardini DA, Barry TD, Barth JM, et al: Self-perceived social acceptance and peer social standing in children with aggressive-disruptive behaviors. Soc Dev 15:46-64, 2006.

86. Miller-Johnson S, Coie JD, Maumary-Gremaud A, et al: Relationship between childhood peer rejection and aggression and adolescent delinquency severity and type among African American youth. J Emot Behav Disord 7:137-146, 1999.

87. Dishion TJ, Andrews DW, Crosby L: Antisocial boys and their friends in early adolescence: Relationship characteristics, quality, and interactional process. Child Dev 66:139-151, 1995.

88. Vitaro F, Brendgen M, Pagani L, et al: Disruptive behavior, peer association, and conduct disorder: Testing the developmental links through early intervention. Dev Psychopathol 11:287-304, 1999.

89. Kupersmidt JB, Griesler PC, DeRosier ME, et al: Childhood aggression and peer relations in the context of family and neighborhood factors. Child Dev 66:360-375, 1995.

90. Colder CR, Mott J, Levy S, et al: The relation of perceived neighborhood danger to childhood aggression: A test of mediating mechanisms. Am J Comm Psychol 28:83-103, 2000.

91. Guerra NG, Huesmann LR, Spindler A: Community violence exposure, social cognition, and aggression among urban elementary school children. Child Dev 74:1561-1576, 2003.

92. Ingoldsby EM, Shaw DS: Neighborhood contextual factors and early-starting antisocial pathways. Clin Child Fam Psychol 5:21-55, 2002.

93. Pinderhughes EE, Nix R, Foster EM, et al: Parenting in context: Impact of neighborhood poverty, residential stability, public services, social networks and danger on parental behaviors. J Marriage Fam 63:941-953, 2001.

94. Greenberg MT, Lengua LJ, Coie JD, et al: Predicting developmental outcomes at school entry using a multiple-risk model: Four American communities. Dev Psychol 35:403-417, 1999.

95. Schwab-Stone ME, Ayers TS, Kasprow W, Voyce C, Barone C, Shriver T, Weissberg RP: No safe haven: A study of violence exposure in an urban community. J Am Acad Child Adolesc Psychiatry 34:1343-1352, 1995.

96. Barth JM, Dunlap ST, Dane H, et al: Classroom environment influences on aggression, peer relations, and academic focus. J School Psychol 42:115-133, 2004.

97. Kellam SG, Ling X, Mersica R, et al: The effect of the level of aggression in the first grade classroom on the course of malleability of aggressive behavior into middle school. Dev Psychopathol 10:165-185, 1998.

98. Dodge KA, Laird R, Lochman JE, et al: Multi-dimensional latent construct analysis of children's social information processing patterns: Correlations with aggressive behavior problems. Psychol Assess 14:60-73, 2002.

99. Pardini D, Lochman JE, Wells KC: Negative emotions and alcohol use initiation in high-risk boys: The moderating effect of good inhibitory control. J Abnorm Child Psychol 32:505-518, 2004.

100. Williams SC, Lochman JE, Phillips NC, et al: Aggressive and nonaggressive boys' physiological and cognitive processes in response to peer provocations. J Clin Child Adolesc Psychol 32:568-576, 2003.

101. Lochman JE, Dodge KA: Social-cognitive processes of severely violent, moderately aggressive, and nonaggressive boys. J Consult Clin Psychol 62:366-374, 1994.

102. Dodge KA, Pettit GS, McClaskey CL, et al: Social competence in children. Monogr Soc Res Child Dev 51:1-85, 1986.

103. Gouze KR: Attention and social problem solving as correlates of aggression in preschool males. J Abnorm Child Psychol 15:181-197, 1987.

104. Milich R., Dodge KA: Social information processing in child psychiatric populations. J Abnorm Child Psychol 12:471-489, 1984.

105. Dodge KA, Lochman JE, Harnish JD, et al: Reactive and proactive aggression in school children and psychiatrically impaired chronically assaultive youth. J Abnorm Psychol 106:37-51, 1997.

106. Lochman JE, Wayland KK, White KJ: Social goals: Relationship to adolescent adjustment and to social problem solving. J Abnorm Child Psychol 21:135-151, 1993.

107. Joffe RD, Dobson KS, Fine S, et al: Social problem-solving in depressed, conduct-disordered, and normal adolescents. J Abnorm Child Psychol 18:565-575, 1990.

108. Lochman JE, Lampron LB: Situational social problem-solving skills and self-esteem of aggressive and non-aggressive boys. J Abnorm Child Psychol 14:605-617, 1986.

109. Rabiner DL, Lenhart L, Lochman JE: Automatic vs. reflective social problem solving in relation to children's sociometric status. Dev Psychol 26:1010-1026, 1990.

110. Pepler DJ, Craig WM, Roberts WI: Observations of aggressive and nonaggressive children on the school playground. Merrill Palmer Q 44:55-76, 1998.

111. Dunn SE, Lochman JE, Colder CR: Social problem-solving skills in boys with conduct and oppositional disorders. Aggress Behav 23:457-469, 1997.

112. Crick NR, Werner NE: Response decision processes in relational and overt aggression. Child Dev 69:1630-1639, 1998.

113. Pardini DA, Lochman JE, Frick PJ: Callous/unemotional traits and social cognitive processes in adjudicated youth. J Am Acad Child Adolesc Psychiatry 42:364-371, 2003.

114. Zelli A, Dodge KA, Lochman JE, et al: The distinction between beliefs legitimizing aggression and deviant processing of social cues: Testing measurement validity and the hypothesis that biased processing mediates the effects of beliefs on aggression. J Pers Soc Psychol 77:150-166, 1999.

115. Lochman JE, Magee TN, Pardini D: Cognitive behavioral interventions for children with conduct problems. *In* Reinecke M, Clark D, eds: Cognitive Therapy over the Lifespan: Theory, Research and Practice. Cambridge, UK: Cambridge University Press, 2003, pp 441-476.

116. Lochman JE, Wells KC: The Coping Power program for preadolescent aggressive boys and their parents: Outcome effects at the one-year follow-up. J Consult Clin Psychol 72:571-578, 2004.

117. Barry TD, Thompson A, Barry CT, et al: The importance of narcissism in predicting proactive and reactive aggression in moderately to highly aggressive children. Aggress Behav, in press.

118. Lochman JE, Nelson WM III, Sims JP: A cognitive behavioral program for use with aggressive children. J Clin Child Psychol 10:146-148, 1981.

119. Lochman JE, Dodge KA: Distorted perceptions in dyadic interactions of aggressive and nonaggressive boys: Effects of prior expectations, context, and boys' age. Dev Psychopathol 10:495-512, 1998.

120. Kamphaus RW, Frick PJ: Clinical Assessment of Child and Adolescent Personality and Behavior, 2nd ed. Needham Heights, MA: Allyn & Bacon, 2001.

121. Lochman JE, Dane HE, Magee TN, et al: Disruptive behavior disorders: Assessment and intervention. *In* Vance B, Pumareiga A, eds: The Clinical Assessment of Children and Youth: Interfacing Intervention with Assessment. New York: Wiley, 2001, pp 231-262.

122. Loeber R, Farrington DP: The significance of child delinquency. *In* Loeber R, Farrington DP, eds: Child Delinquents: Development, Intervention, and Service Needs. Thousand Oaks, CA: Sage Publications, 2001, pp 1-22.

123. Patterson GR, Dishion TJ, Yoerger K: Adolescent growth in new forms of problem behavior: Macro- and micro-peer dynamics. Prev Sci 1:3-13, 2000.

124. Hibbs ED, Jensen PS: Psychosocial Treatments for Child and Adolescent Disorders: Empirically Based Strategies for Clinical Practice, 2nd ed. Washington, DC: American Psychological Association, 2005.

125. Kazdin AE, Weisz JR: Evidence-Based Psychotherapies for Children and Adolescents. New York: Guilford, 2003.

126. Lochman JE, Salekin RT: Prevention and intervention with aggressive and disruptive children: Next steps in behavioral intervention research. Behav Ther 34:413-419, 2003.

127. Brestan EV, Eyberg SM: Effective psychosocial treatments of conduct-disordered children and adolescents: 29 years, 82 studies, and 5,272 kids. J Clin Child Psychol 27:180-189, 1998.

128. Patterson GR, Gullion ME: Living with Children: New Methods for Parents and Teachers. Champaign, IL: Research Press, 1968.

129. Kazdin AE: Problem-solving skills training and parent management training for conduct disorder. *In* Kazdin AE, Weisz JR, eds: Evidence-Based Psychotherapies for Children and Adolescents. New York: Guilford, 2003, pp 241-262.

130. Kazdin AE, Siegel T, Bass D: Cognitive problem-solving skills training and parent management training in the treatment of antisocial behavior in children. J Consult Clin Psychol 60:733-747, 1992.

131. Webster-Stratton C: Randomized trial of two parent-training programs for families with conduct-disordered children. J Consult Clin Psychol 52:666-678, 1984.

132. Webster-Stratton C: Advancing videotape parent training: A comparison study. J Consult Clin Psychol 62:583-593, 1994.

133. Webster-Stratton C, Hammond M: Treating children with early-onset conduct problems: A comparison of child and parent training interventions. J Consult Clin Psychol 65:93-109, 1997.

134. Webster-Stratton C, Reid MJ: The Incredible Years Parents, Teachers, and Children Training Series. *In* Kazdin AE, Weisz JR, eds: Evidence-Based Psychotherapies for Children and Adolescents. New York: Guilford, 2003, pp 224-240.

135. Brinkmeyer MY, Eyberg SM: Parent-child interaction therapy for oppositional children. *In* Kazdin AE, Weisz JR, eds: Evidence-Based Psychotherapies for Children and Adolescents. New York: Guilford, 2003, pp 204-223.

136. Henggeler SW, Lee T: Multisystemic treatment of serious clinical problems. *In* Kazdin AE, Weisz JR, eds: Evidence-Based Psychotherapies for Children and Adolescents. New York: Guilford, 2003, pp 301-322.

137. Chamberlain P, Smith DK: Antisocial behavior in children and adolescents: The Oregon Multidimensional Treatment Foster Care Model. *In* Kazdin AE, Weisz JR, eds: Evidence-Based Psychotherapies for Children and Adolescents. New York: Guilford, 2003, pp 282-300.

138. Lochman JE, Wells KC, Murray, M: The Coping Power program: Preventive intervention at the middle school transition. *In* Tolan, P, Szapocznik J, Sambrano S, eds: Preventing Substance Abuse: 3 to 14. Washington, DC: American Psychological Association, 185-210, 2007.

139. Larson J, Lochman JE: Helping Schoolchildren Cope with Anger: A Cognitive-Behavioral Intervention. New York: Guilford, 2002.

140. Lochman JE, Wells KC: The Coping Power program at the middle school transition: Universal and indicated prevention effects. Psychol Addict Behav 16: S40-S54, 2002.

141. Lochman JE: Cognitive-behavioral intervention with aggressive boys: Three year follow-up and preventive effects. J Consult Clin Psychol 60:426-432, 1992.

Internalizing Conditions

18A.
Mood Disorders

NICOLE M. KLAUS ▪ MARY A. FRISTAD

There is a growing emphasis on psychosocial problems in pediatric care, and pediatricians are in a unique position to monitor children over time to prevent, identify, and address psychosocial concerns.[1] Primary care visits account for an increasing portion of mental health visits, and pediatricians play an important role in the management of childhood mood disorders.[2,3] Mood disorders in childhood and adolescence have received increased clinical and research attention. Mood disorders include those characterized by depressed or irritable moods (major depressive disorder (MDD), dysthymic disorder, and depressive disorder not otherwise specified) and those characterized by fluctuations between depressed and manic or hypomanic moods (bipolar I disorder, bipolar II disorder, cyclothymic disorder, and bipolar disorder not otherwise specified). This chapter summarizes how depression and bipolar disorder in childhood and adolescence are currently understood, focusing on research concerning the significance, causes, diagnosis, and treatment of these disorders. Current practice standards, as well as issues necessitating further research, are discussed.

SIGNIFICANCE

Prevalence

The incidence of depression in adolescents is similar to that found in adults, ranging from 0.4% to 8.3%. Rates are lower in preadolescents, ranging from 0.4% to 2.5%.[4] Epidemiology studies rarely include preschool-aged children; however the available data suggest that depression occurs in approximately 1% of preschool children.[5,6] Gender ratios in rates of depression also change with age. Among preadolescents, similar rates of depression are found in boys and girls. In adolescence, the rate of depression in girls increases dramatically, resulting in a gender ratio of 2 : 1, similar to that found among adults.[4]

Estimation of the prevalence of bipolar disorder in childhood and adolescence is complicated by the general lack of agreement concerning the core characteristics of the disorder, which are discussed further in the diagnosis section of this chapter.[7] No epidemiological studies currently exist for children. In a study of 14- to 18-year-olds, Lewinsohn and colleagues[8] found lifetime prevalence rates for a diagnosis of bipolar disorder to be approximately 1%; an additional 5.7% reported subthreshold symptoms. Adolescents with subsyndromal symptoms of bipolar disorder experienced functional impairments similar to those in adolescents with bipolar disorder, which continued into young adulthood. This study was based solely on interviews with adolescents, however, and more recent research has emphasized the importance of including parent report in diagnosing bipolar disorder.[9]

These incidence rates indicate that a significant proportion of children and adolescents suffer from mood disorders. In addition, the overall rates of depression in children and adolescents appear to be increasing.[5]

Course

Mood disorders often have a chronic or relapsing course, associated with continuing impairment. Episodes of MDD last 7 to 9 months on average, with relapse rates of 40% within 2 years and 70% within 5 years.[4] Weissman and colleagues[10] monitored adolescents with MDD into adulthood and found that

63% had additional depressive episodes within the following 10 to 15 years. These adolescents had a fivefold risk of suicide in comparison with control participants who had no psychiatric diagnosis in adolescence. Those with MDD also experienced continuing impairment in family, work, and social functioning. Dysthymic disorder lasts an average of 4 years and is associated with a high risk of developing MDD within 2 to 3 years, which results in double depression.[4] Bipolar disorder has a particularly chronic course in childhood, as evidenced by the findings of Geller and colleagues[11] in their 4-year follow-up of children with bipolar disorder, in which they reported that children met criteria for a mood episode, on average, for two thirds of the follow-up period.

Effect on Child and Family

Mood disorders can affect several aspects of a child's development, including social and academic development. Children accomplish many developmental tasks through normal interactions with their environment, such as interpersonal relationships and academic tasks. Mood disorders interrupt these normal interactions. For example, social interaction may be disrupted when a child experiences social withdrawal or is rejected by peers because of unusual behaviors. Similarly, a child may miss considerable instructional time in the classroom because of impaired concentration or behavioral problems related to irritability or disruptive manic behaviors. Once a child has fallen behind in social or academic development, catching up can be extremely difficult. When children experience long mood episodes and frequent relapses, the effect on development is dramatic. As one example, U.S. Department of Education statistics indicate that only 29% of children with an "emotional disturbance" graduated with a standard high school diploma in 2001, whereas 65% dropped out, in comparison to an 86% high school completion rate for all students in the same year.[12,13] Teachers rate children with depression as having more withdrawn and disruptive social behaviors than do nondepressed peers.[14] Adolescents with MDD also experience impairments in social, family, and academic functioning.[15] In comparison with children with attention-deficit/hyperactivity disorder (ADHD), children with bipolar disorder have been found to have impaired relationships with parents and peers, higher rates of placements in special education classes, and higher rates of hospitalization.[16,17]

A child's mood disorder can affect the entire family. Symptoms of irritability and mood lability can increase conflict in the child's family interactions. Parenting stress also increases because parents are faced with a child's mood and behavior problems that do not respond to typical parenting strategies.[18] Besides the stress associated with managing the child's symptoms, families can also suffer from the financial burden associated with the cost of medication and other treatments and lost time from work for doctor appointments. With more severe cases of mood disorders, multiple hospitalizations and legal difficulties related to the child's behavior further disrupt family life.

Effect on Society

Beyond the direct effect of these conditions on the child and family, there is also a significant effect on society in terms of both human and financial costs. These costs are difficult to estimate, because they include the amount of money invested in treatment and educational services, reduced productivity, lost employment, mortality, and juvenile justice services.[19] Ringel and Sturm[3] estimated a national annual expenditure of $11.68 billion on child mental health services (inpatient treatment, outpatient treatment, and psychotropic medications) in the United States, with average costs of $293 per adolescent, $163 per child, and $35 per preschooler. In addition, in 2001, more than 475,000 students aged 6 to 21 received educational services for emotional disturbance under the Individuals with Disabilities Education Act (IDEA); this population constituted 8.1% of all students served under IDEA.[13] The risk of death or physical injury related to mood disorders is also substantial. Approximately 2000 adolescents in the United States die from suicide every year, many of whom suffer from mood disorders, and an additional 700,000 require medical attention after a suicide attempt.[20] According to World Health Organization estimates, MDD is the first and bipolar disorder is the fifth leading cause of years of living with a disability among 15- to 44-year-olds worldwide.[19]

CAUSES

Genetics

There is considerable evidence for the heritability of mood disorders in adult populations, with bipolar disorder more strongly influenced by genetics than is unipolar depression. Meta-analyses of adult studies have attributed approximately 60% of the variance in bipolar disorder and 37% of the variance in MDD to genetic factors.[21,22] More recent research, using family and twin studies, has focused on the genetic influences on child and adolescent mood disorders. There is some evidence that earlier onset of a mood disorder is associated with increased prevalence of mood disorders in family members in comparison with later onset, which suggests that earlier onset may signify a more substantial genetic basis.[21]

Studies of the offspring of depressed parents have clearly demonstrated a familial association in childhood and adolescent depression, which could be the result of genetic influences, parent-child interactions, or other environmental influences. Having a parent with depression is one of the strongest predictors of depression in childhood and adolescence.[5] Several twin studies have been conducted to explore heritability; results have varied widely, depending on measurement strategy, informant, age, and gender. Heritability estimates of parent-rated depressive symptoms range from 30% to 80%.[23] Twin studies have been based on questionnaire reports of depressive or more general internalizing symptoms, and further research is needed with clinical interviews to establish diagnosis.[23]

Studies of parents with bipolar disorder have indicated that their offspring are at increased risk for mood disorders in general and bipolar disorder specifically. Among children of parents with bipolar disorder in a meta-analysis, 52% developed some type of mental disorder (2.7 times the risk in comparison with parents without bipolar disorder), 26.5% developed a mood disorder (4 times the risk in comparison with parents without bipolar disorder), and 5.4% developed bipolar disorder (in comparison with none of the control group).[24] Studies have consistently demonstrated that for children with bipolar disorder, the rates of bipolar disorder in family members are higher, and younger age at onset is related to stronger family statistical loading of bipolar disorder.[7,21] Children with psychotic depression also tend to have a family history of bipolar disorder and have a higher chance of going on to develop bipolar disorder.[7] Twin studies of childhood-onset bipolar disorder have yet to be conducted, but the evidence available from family studies suggests that early-onset bipolar disorder may have a particularly strong genetic basis, and young patients may be good candidates for molecular genetic studies.[21,25] Investigators are beginning to explore the molecular genetics of childhood-onset bipolar disorder, but consistent findings have yet to emerge.[7,21]

Biological Factors

Research in adults has identified several neurobiological correlates of mood disorders, including abnormalities in basal cortisol, cortisol regulation, corticotropin-releasing hormone, thyroid hormones, growth hormone regulation, and electroencephalographic sleep measures. Research in children and adolescents has been relatively sparse and has inconsistently replicated adult patterns.[26,27]

A review by Kaufman and colleagues[26] indicates that consistency among child, adolescent, and adult studies has been found only in response to the dexamethasone suppression test and to selective serotonin reuptake inhibitors (SSRIs). Across the lifespan, patients with depression demonstrate nonsuppression of cortisol after the dexamethasone suppression test, which is suggestive of dysregulation of the body's stress response system. There is also evidence that children and adolescents with depression respond to some SSRI medications in similar ways as do adults, which is discussed in more detail later in this chapter. However, responses to serotonergic probes in children have generally opposed findings in the adult literature, which indicates that there may be developmental differences in the dysregulation of the serotonergic system.[26]

Other neurobiological studies have yielded inconsistent findings. Studies in children with depression indicate that they show blunted response to agents that trigger growth hormone release, which is similar to adults' responses; however, results have not been as consistent in adolescents.[26] Blunted responsiveness to growth hormone has also been found in nondepressed children who are at increased risk for depression because of family history; this finding indicates that this response may reflect a predisposition to depression.[5] Sleep studies have shown that adolescents with depression may demonstrate some electroencephalographic sleep responses similar to those of adults with depression, including reduced rapid-eye-movement latency and increased rapid-eye-movement density; however, these patterns have typically not been found in children.[26] In contrast to the adult literature, abnormalities in basal levels of thyroid hormones, basal cortisol levels, and corticotropin-releasing hormone have not been consistently observed in children and adolescents.[26]

Investigators have only begun to examine the brain anatomy and functioning of children and adolescents with mood disorders; therefore, many results are preliminary. Neuroimaging studies with adults can be confounded by long duration of illness and the effects of treatment. Studies with children hold particular promise for identifying brain regions associated with the pathogenesis of mood disorders.[28]

The prefrontal cortex is influential in mood regulation and has been the focus of much of the neuroimaging research in adult depressive disorders.[5,29] A growing series of child and adolescent studies have also focused on this area. One study revealed patients with MDD who had no family history of mood disorder had larger prefrontal cortical volume than did control patients and patients with MDD who did have a positive family history of mood disorder.[28] In another study, glutamatergic concentrations in the anterior cingulate cortex were shown to be decreased by approximately 19% in patients with MDD in comparison with matched controls.[30,31] In addition, significant increases in choline compounds have been found in the left dorsolateral prefrontal cortex of child and adolescent patients with MDD.[32,33] Together, these studies reveal anatomical and biochemical anomalies in the prefrontal cortex in childhood and adolescent MDD. Furthermore, within a group of patients with MDD, Ehilich and colleagues[34] found that white matter hyperintensities were associated with history of suicide attempts. Replication and extension of these findings are necessary to establish a clearer understanding of the role of the prefrontal cortex in childhood mood disorders.

In at least 11 studies, children and adolescents with bipolar disorder have been studied with magnetic resonance imaging.[35] As reviewed by Frazier and associates,[35] these studies collectively show that early-onset bipolar disorder is associated with a variety of functional, anatomical, and biochemical abnormalities in brain regions associated with emotional regulation and processing, including the limbic-thalamic-prefrontal circuit and the limbic-striatal-pallidal-thalamic circuit.

Environmental Factors

The strong familial association in early-onset mood disorders, discussed earlier, probably reflects a combination of genetic influences and family environment influences. Parental mood disorders can affect parent-child interaction, as well as events in the home. In comparison with control families, parent-child interaction in families with depressed children is characterized by higher levels of criticism, less warmth, more conflict, and poorer communication.[15,36-39] Research on expressed emotion has suggested that a low level of parental criticism is predictive of recovery from depressive symptoms, whereas a high level of criticism is associated with the persistence of the mood disorder.[40] The depressed child's behavior also plays a role in evoking more negative interactions from parents.[41] Disruptions in the family environment, such as marital discord, abuse, and poor support, can also affect parent-child interaction and the child's risk for depressive symptoms.[4,42] Furthermore, life stressors in general have been found to precede and exacerbate depressive symptoms.[5]

The mechanisms by which environmental factors are associated with depressive symptoms have been the focus of more recent research. Diathesis-stress models suggest that depression results from an interaction between an internal predisposition and environmental stressors. This predisposition can take the form of a genetic or biological tendency or may be related to cognitive factors, such as poor coping skills or depressive cognitive style. According to the review by Hammen and Rudolph,[5] several investigators have tested the diathesis-stress model as it pertains to cognitive vulnerabilities and have found significant interactions between cognitive style and stressful events.

The association between family or psychosocial factors and depressive disorders has been clearly demonstrated across the lifespan.[4,5] In a few studies, Researchers have also begun to examine those factors in childhood bipolar disorder. In Geller and colleagues' long-term follow-up of children with bipolar disorder, children experiencing poor maternal warmth were about four times more likely to suffer relapse after recovery than were children with high maternal warmth.[11,43] Children and adolescents with bipolar disorder have also been found to experience more life stressors than children with ADHD and children with no psychiatric diagnosis.[44] These stressors included those clearly caused by the child's symptoms or behavior (e.g., hospitalization), those possibly related to the child's symptoms or behavior (e.g., removal from the home), and those unrelated to the child's symptoms or behavior (e.g., death of a parent).

DIAGNOSIS

Accurate diagnosis of mood disorders in children is important, because underdiagnosis and misdiagnosis can lead to delays in the delivery of appropriate treatment or to the selection of treatments that may be harmful.[45] For example, some research findings suggest that the use of SSRIs or stimulants can induce mania in children and adolescents with bipolar disorder; although not all researchers have replicated these findings.[7,46]

Barriers to Identification

The rate of recognition and treatment for children with psychological disorders in general is quite low. Data suggest that approximately 20% to 50% of children with a psychological problem are identified and only a portion of those cases are referred for evaluation and treatment.[1,47,48] Internalizing problems, such as mood disorders, are identified much less frequently than are externalizing problems and are more likely to be identified when they are accompanied by a comorbid externalizing condition.[49] In view of the negative effects of mood disorders on the child's school, social, and family functioning, as well as the suicidal behaviors that can accompany mood disorders, the low rate of identification and treatment is a significant concern. Because of low rates of identification and treatment, outcomes in community settings have not kept pace with advances in the development of effective treatments for mood disorders in children and adolescents.[50]

Primary care pediatricians are in an ideal position to identify mental health conditions in general and mood disorders in particular. Most children have at least one primary care visit per year, and children with psychological problems are likely to have more frequent visits.[49] Many children, particularly those from families of low socioeconomic status, receive care from only a primary care pediatrician.[1] Several factors can prevent accurate identification in a primary care setting, including pediatricians' limited training in mental health issues, parents' failure to report mental health concerns without direct questioning, limited time available for screening of nonsomatic concerns, limited referral resources, and limited availability and use of screening instruments.[1] Pediatricians can play a very important role in improving identification of mood disorders but may require education and resources to support them in this role.[1,49] The development of screening instruments and the availability of onsite support and treatment options are promising strategies for removing these barriers to identification and treatment.[1,2,50]

Symptom Manifestation

The same criteria used for adults are used to diagnose childhood mood disorders. There is consensus that childhood depressive disorders have the same clinical features as the adult form of the disorders, with a couple of differences as outlined in the *Diagnostic and Statistical Manual of Mental Disorders,* 4th edition, text revision *(DSM-IV-TR)*[51] (i.e., irritability can take the place of depressed mood; considering failure to make expected weight gains; 1- rather than 2-year duration for dysthymia). The child's cognitive and emotional development can affect symptom manifestation and profile over time, but the clinical features of depressive disorders remain fairly consistent over time.[52]

There is controversy, however, over the definition of bipolar disorder in children. The core symptoms necessary for diagnosis, the necessity of discrete episodes, and the definitions of cycling in children all continue to be points of debate in the literature, and definitions of bipolar disorder have varied across studies.[7] *DSM-IV-TR* diagnostic criteria for a manic episode include "a distinct period of persistently elevated, expansive, or irritable mood."[51] However, because irritability is so pervasive across childhood disorders, some investigators have required hallmark criteria of expansive/elated mood or gran-

diosity to help distinguish mania in children. In addition, many children meet symptom criteria for mania, with the exception of the duration criterion. These children may have intense rapid mood swings and often receive a diagnosis of Bipolar Disorder Not Otherwise Specified.

To help clarify the various conceptualizations of childhood mania, Leibenluft and colleagues[53] proposed definitions for narrow, intermediate, and broad phenotypes of mania. In the most narrow phenotype, children meet strict *DSM-IV-TR* criteria for mania or hypomania, with the hallmark symptoms of elevated mood and/or grandiosity, and meet full duration criteria. Two intermediate phenotypes were identified: mania not otherwise specified (hallmark symptoms present, but symptoms do not meet duration criteria) and irritable mania (irritability without hallmark symptoms; full duration criteria met). The broad phenotype includes symptoms of severe mood and behavioral dysregulation without the hallmark symptoms or episodic cycling. Further research is needed to determine how these various phenotypes are related and whether there are differences in terms of etiology, treatment, and prognosis among the types.

Diagnosis of mood disorders in children and adolescents can evolve and change over time. Seventy percent of children with dysthymic disorder eventually experience a major depressive episode, and 20% to 40% of children who initially present with MDD eventually experience a manic episode.[4] It is important to monitor the progression of symptoms over time to ensure that appropriate treatment strategies are used. Children who have early-onset depression, depression with psychotic features or psychomotor retardation, a family history of bipolar disorder, or a very strong family history of any mood disorders are at increased risk for developing mania.[4]

The clinical symptoms of mood disorders in children are often different from those typically seen in adults. Depressed affect, low self-esteem, and somatic complaints are more common in children than in adults, whereas anhedonia, diurnal variation, hopelessness, psychomotor retardation, and delusions increase with age.[54] Children with bipolar disorder are more likely than adults to display continuous cycling (<365 cycles per year), mixed episodes, irritable mood swings with an insidious and chronic course beginning in early childhood, and high rates of comorbidity.[16,45,55]

It is important to consider developmentally relevant symptom manifestations in diagnosis in children. Cognitive maturation influences the ways children experience and express emotion.[56] Children may be less able to express symptoms such as hopelessness, which require abstract thought until around puberty, when children begin to develop more abstract cognitive abilities.[56] As another example, during their early school years, children become cognitively capable of comparing and evaluating themselves with regard to others; thus, the symptom of low self-esteem is more relevant than in younger years.[56] In diagnosing childhood mania, it is particularly important to consider how *DSM-IV-TR* symptoms such as grandiosity, "increase in goal-directed activity," and "excessive involvement in pleasurable activities" may manifest at different ages and how they differ from typical childhood behaviors. Children have certain constraints on their behavior by virtue of being monitored by adults, being required to attend school and other activities regularly, and not having resources such as credit cards or independent transportation to engage in the types of behaviors that adults may display.

DEPRESSION: CASE ILLUSTRATION

Eight-year-old Sara often states that nobody loves her, and she wishes she could run away and be adopted by a new family. Several days per week, she is irritable and uncooperative for most of the day. Her parents describe a "look in her eye" that indicates she is having a bad day. She was brought for assessment after an episode when she tried to run away from school and ran into traffic. She no longer initiates play dates with friends but does play when asked. Sara has episodes of tearfulness three to four times per week and sometimes reports that she is crying because she misses her dog, which ran away 3 years ago. When asked what she is good at, Sara has difficulty thinking of a response. Her parents report that she takes 1 to 2 hours to fall asleep at night. She has visited her pediatrician five times over the past year because of persistent stomachaches, which have caused her to miss school. Her parents have also recently asked Sara's pediatrician about ways to help her sleep.

Sara experiences a mixture of irritability and depressed mood, which is common among children with depressive disorders. Parents of children with mood disorders commonly describe a different look in their child when the child's mood is at an extreme level, such as a "look in her eye," even if the child is not able to report feeling different. Although Sara does not report suicidal ideation, she clearly conveys a desire to escape her current life and distress by running away, which is an age-typical response. Sara's grief over the loss of her dog is prolonged and perseverative and appears to be part of her depressive disorder rather than a typical grief reaction. Sara's case also illustrates the increased use of health care services because of somatic complaints. Often children with mood disorders do not present for mental health treatment until symptoms become severe or cause significant distress to others. Sara's pediatrician would be in a good position to screen for and identify

mood problems at an earlier stage when she presented with somatic complaints and sleep problems.

BIPOLAR DISORDER: CASE ILLUSTRATION

David is 10 years old. His predominant mood state is irritability; however, he also experiences daily periods of elevated mood, lasting 30 to 60 minutes, when he becomes unusually silly and goofy and cannot settle down. According to his mother, David thinks that he "knows everything" about a variety of topics and picks fights with peers and adults if his knowledge is challenged. David has also become fearless on his bicycle and tries stunts that his peers do not attempt. David has recently decided to expand his lemonade stand to a restaurant in his mother's kitchen so that he can earn more money, and he has started advertising his new restaurant to his neighbors. In the past week, David has been sleeping approximately 5 hours per night. When he cannot sleep, he stays up making menus for his restaurant and making lists of various things he wants to do the next day. When he gets bored, David builds webs with string. He recently filled his entire bedroom with an intricate web of string in a short time. His mother additionally reports that David has been making inappropriate sexual comments and recently got into trouble for taking pictures of his genitals in his bedroom, pictures that were later found on the family camera.

Pretend play is normal in childhood, but the child who describes elaborate scenarios and cannot readily identify the play as pretend may be experiencing grandiosity, particularly if the play becomes inappropriate for the situation and impairs functioning.[57] In David's case, grandiose thoughts that are causing interference can be seen in his elaborate plans to run a restaurant to make money. He also provides several examples of increased goal-directed activity. His intense focus on making plans for his restaurant and creation of string webs that fill his bedroom reflect his increased energy and goal-directed activity. Children are not able to display typical adult pleasurable activities, such as spending sprees, but may instead display excessive "daredevil" behaviors without considering the dangerous consequences, or they may become hypersexual; David exhibits both behaviors.

Normal Variations in Mood

All children undergo development in their understanding of and ability to regulate emotions. Children begin to understand and use basic emotional terms around ages 2 to 3; however, the understanding of more complex emotions and mixed emotions continues to develop through childhood. Toddlers and preschool-aged children tend to display tantrums in response to frustration but become better able to regulate their emotional expression by the time of school entry. Children begin to regulate their subjective feeling of negative emotions first through problem-focused coping strategies and later become able to use emotion-focused coping to tolerate situations that they cannot change.[58] During puberty, hormone changes can lead to an increase in mood lability. There are also temperamental differences among children in general levels of reactivity. These normal developmental processes and individual differences should be considered in the evaluation of mood disorders.

Response to Bereavement

When a child or adolescent has experienced a loss, such as the death of a loved one or pet, a family move, or a broken relationship, symptoms of depression are common. Children's reactions to the death of a loved one can vary and may include dysphoria, crying spells, clinging to familiar routines and caregivers, impairments in school functioning, behavior problems, bedwetting, loss of interest in activities, sleep problems, and psychosomatic symptoms.[59] These symptoms are usually transient and can be differentiated from a mood disorder on the basis of the duration and associated impairment.[60] According to *DSM-IV-TR* criteria, symptoms of bereavement should not be diagnosed as a mood disorder unless they last longer than 2 months or are associated with significant functional impairment, worthlessness, suicidal ideation, psychotic symptoms, or psychomotor retardation.

In children who have experienced parental death, grief or sadness lasting a year or more is common.[61] In the largest prospective study to date of children after parental death, Cerel and colleagues[62] found that bereaved children demonstrated more impairment over a 2-year period than did a control group but less impairment than did a comparison group of nonbereaved children with a diagnosis of a depressive disorder. Overall impairment and depressive symptoms improved significantly in the bereaved group over 2 years, and this improvement was more rapid than that seen in the depressed group. Level of impairment and coping skills should be carefully monitored after parental death, because up to 20% of children display symptoms serious enough to warrant specialized treatment.[61] A child is more likely to display clinical levels of disturbance after parental death when he or she had a psychiatric disorder before the death, when the surviving parent displays high levels of depression before or after the death, or when the family has fewer socioeconomic resources.[61,62] The presence of multiple stressors in the child's life is associated with slower improvement in depressive symptoms and overall impairment.[62] Parental death by suicide is also related to higher levels of overall psychopathology.[63]

When children witness elements of a traumatic death, such as parental murder or suicide, they are at risk for post-traumatic stress disorder.[61]

After the death of a parent, many children experience suicidal ideation; however they are less likely to attempt suicide than are children with depressive disorder.[64] The suidical ideation expressed by bereaved children more often reflects a desire to be with the deceased parent rather than a wish to end their lives.[61,64] As with all reports of suicidal ideation, bereaved children who report such thoughts should be carefully assessed for risk factors, development of a suicide plan, and access to means of harming themselves.

ASSESSMENT

As with all childhood mental health concerns, a thorough assessment is necessary to establish an accurate diagnosis. Mood problems can reflect underlying medical conditions or drug reactions; therefore, medical causes for symptoms should be explored and ruled out as part of the assessment process.[45] Gathering data from multiple informants is important, because agreement between parent and child report is often low.[65] Children are generally better reporters of internal mood states, whereas parents tend to be more accurate in reporting behavioral symptoms and symptom history, although exceptions to this generalization are readily found in clinical settings.[66] Teachers also have a unique perspective, inasmuch as they see children in a structured setting where behavior can differ from home and have experience with a same-age comparison group. If possible, data from teachers, such as questionnaires, notes, and report cards, should also be integrated into the clinical assessment process.

A clinical interview with the child and at least one parent is a critical component of the assessment process. The clinical interview should cover several main topics, including an evaluation of a broad spectrum of childhood conditions to establish a differential diagnosis and identify comorbid conditions, the gathering of detailed information about mood symptom severity, reconstruction of the history of mood symptom evolution and treatment, and family history data. Questionnaires may also be used to complement the interview process.

Differential Diagnosis

Cross-sectionally, the symptoms of mood disorders can appear similar to other childhood disorders and may be misdiagnosed as ADHD, anxiety disorders, developmental disorders, or behavior disorders. Furthermore, differential diagnosis among the mood disorders can present a challenge when only current symptoms are considered. Examination of the evolution of symptoms over time can help establish the presence of episodic mood changes and whether other symptoms fluctuate with mood. For example, symptoms of social withdrawal and self-doubt may reflect depression or social anxiety, which can be difficult to distinguish with a cross-sectional assessment. A history of social anxiety preceding the development of other symptoms of depression would signify the presence of an anxiety disorder. If the symptoms developed at the same time or became significantly worse along with other mood symptoms, then they could be considered symptoms of depression.

Irritability is frequently a symptom of childhood mood disorders, but it can also be prominent in ADHD, behavior disorders, anxiety disorders, and pervasive developmental disorders, as well as in children without psychopathology who are hot, hungry, tired, or stressed.[45] Manic irritability often can be distinguished by its episodic, intense, and prolonged nature.

Children with ADHD also tend to experience difficulties with emotional regulation related to general impairments in behavioral inhibition, which can lead to quick expressions of emotional reactions that change easily.[67] Children with mood disorders also have difficulty with emotional regulation; however, they can be differentiated by their intensity, duration, associated symptoms, and environmental triggers. Children with ADHD typically experience emotional overarousal in response to environmental disorganization and overstimulation. Children with depressive disorders, on the other hand, experience depression or irritability as their predominant mood state, and their mood does not change as much in response to environmental triggers. Bipolar disorder can be distinguished from the emotional overarousal of ADHD by the episodic, intense, and prolonged nature of emotional reactions, which are accompanied by associated symptoms not typically seen in ADHD.

Because of the symptom overlap between mania and ADHD, differential diagnosis can be particularly difficult. Distractibility, rapid speech, and increased energy are symptoms of mania that overlap with those of ADHD. Geller and colleagues[55] identified five symptoms of mania that provide the best discrimination between mania and ADHD: elated mood, grandiosity, racing thoughts, decreased need for sleep, and hypersexuality. In assessment for bipolar disorder, the clinician should pay careful attention to these distinguishing symptoms, as well as symptom fluctuation with mood changes over time. In children with comorbid ADHD, distractibility, rapid speech, and

increased energy should be considered symptoms of mania only when they increase beyond the child's unique baseline level as his or her mood changes.

Hypersexual symptoms, such as those demonstrated by the example of David previously, are common in childhood-onset bipolar disorder. In Geller and colleagues' sample,[55] 43% of children displayed hypersexuality. Children who display hypersexual behaviors should be carefully assessed for evidence of sexual abuse or exposure to sexual content inappropriate for the child's age.[68] Sexual behavior with a pleasure-seeking quality that fluctuates with other mood symptoms may be a symptom of mania.[69]

Psychosis is common in both MDD and bipolar disorder in childhood and may be incorrectly diagnosed as a schizophrenia spectrum disorder.[5,70] Psychotic symptoms that are congruent with mood and fluctuate with mood symptom severity are more likely to be an associated symptom of the mood disorder.[70]

Mood Symptoms

Specific information should be gathered during the clinical interview about severity of mood symptoms. Mood symptoms should be evaluated in the context of an understanding of normal variations in children's mood. Frequency, intensity, number, and duration (FIND) guidelines can be used to assist in establishing the presence or absence of mood symptoms[45]: Individual symptoms should fluctuate with mood and occur most days of the week (frequency), at a level that causes impairment (intensity), several times per day (number), and should last a significant portion of the day (duration).[45]

Prospective mood charting can be helpful in making a diagnosis, as well as monitoring progress. Daily mood logs completed by parents or adolescents can provide valuable information about situational variables that trigger mood symptoms and response to treatment. Examples of mood logs can be found at *www.bpkids.org/site/PageServer?pagename=lrn_mood* or can be individually tailored to meet the needs of a particular child and family.

Clinician-rated mood scales can also be helpful in summarizing mood symptom severity and in tracking progress. The Children's Depression Rating Scale–Revised has been shown to be a reliable, valid, and sensitive measure of depressive symptoms in both inpatient and outpatient samples.[71] The Young Mania Rating Scale, which was developed for adult populations, has been shown to have acceptable reliability and validity in child samples.[72,73] Although widely used, this scale has several limitations, including a lack of published developmentally appropriate anchor criteria for interview-based ratings.[69] The Kiddie

Schedule for Affective Disorders and Schizophrenia (KSADS) Mania Rating Scale and Depression Rating Scale are promising new instruments developed for child and adolescent populations and are based on *DSM-IV-TR* criteria.[74] Preliminary studies have found that these instruments have good psychometric properties, and further validation with larger samples is under way.[69,74]

Mood History

The clinical interview should also gather information about history of mood symptoms. Mood disorders tend to wax and wane in manifestation, and a thorough history is thus necessary to fully understand the mood disorder. To understand how mood symptoms have evolved and fluctuated over time, it is necessary to construct a timeline of symptoms, reconstructing their onset and discontinuation in relation to significant life events, treatment history, and functioning at school, at home, and with peers. In children who initially present with symptoms of MDD, a thorough history is needed to determine whether the child has ever experienced a manic or hypomanic episode.

Family History

Information about family history can further help establish the probability of mood disorder.[69] Although a family history of mood disorders is not diagnostic of mood disorders per se, it does add additional information about the child's risk for the disorder.[69] Furthermore, because data suggest that children with MDD who have a family history of bipolar disorder are at increased risk for developing a manic episode in the future, this information may guide treatment decisions and follow-up strategies.[4]

Structured Interviews

It is important to assess for behavior, anxiety, mood, and other symptoms as part of the clinical interview. Structured or semistructured interviews can be used to systematically gather information about various childhood problems. Several options have demonstrated sensitivity and specificity in identifying relevant conditions and require varying levels of training and time to administer. Examples include the Diagnostic Interview Schedule for Children,[75] Children's Interview for Psychiatric Symptoms (ChIPS),[76,77] Diagnostic Interview for Children and Adolescents,[78] and the Washington University at St. Louis KSADS (WASH-U-KSADS),[79] which includes an expanded section on the diagnosis of manic symptoms. Variations of the KSADS, such as the WASH-U-KSADS, are most commonly used in research settings, but require

extensive time and specialized training for administration, which makes this instrument impractical for clinical use.[69] Symptoms of mania are often not thoroughly evaluated in developmentally appropriate terms in the briefer structured interviews; however the ChIPS shows the most promise for identifying manic symptoms in youth.[69]

Questionnaires

Diagnosis of mood disorders can never be made on the basis of questionnaires alone. However, questionnaires can be useful as screening instruments to guide a clinical interview or as another source of information to integrate with interview data. The Child Behavior Checklist (CBCL) is a norm-referenced and widely used instrument in clinical practice and research to assess a variety of behavior problems in children and adolescents.[80] The CBCL behavior scales are not specific enough to differentiate depressive from anxiety disorders; however, high scores on the internalizing scale signal that additional information should be gathered about specific mood and anxiety disorders. The Children's Depression Inventory[81] is a self-report measure specifically designed to assess the severity of depressive symptoms. This inventory has been shown to differentiate between psychiatric patients and control subjects, but it does not differentiate well among psychiatric diagnoses.[82]

Low scores on the externalizing scales of the CBCL are useful in ruling out bipolar disorder, but high scores are not specific enough to draw conclusions about the presence of bipolar disorder.[9] The General Behavior Inventory[83] is a questionnaire that is used specifically to assess manic symptoms. Parent and youth versions of this inventory have demonstrated excellent psychometric properties; however, the complexity of many items may make it difficult for individuals with limited education or reading abilities.[69] Data suggest that youth and teacher questionnaires do not add anything beyond parent questionnaire data in the prediction of bipolar disorder diagnosis.[9]

The Pediatric Symptom Checklist[84] has been developed specifically to screen for a variety of mental health problems in primary care settings. It is brief, has empirically derived cutoff scores, and has been validated with racially diverse populations and populations of low socioeconomic status.[1] In settings in which resources are available to score and interpret the CBCL, it may be administered before the clinician meets with the family and used to help guide the interview. When a mood disorder is suspected, the Children's Depression Inventory or General Behavior Inventory may be useful in the decision of whether to refer for a more thorough evaluation.

ASSOCIATED CONDITIONS

Comorbidity

Comorbidity is common among childhood diagnoses. Approximately 40% to 70% of children and adolescents with depression have at least one other psychiatric condition.[4] A meta-analysis by Angold and colleagues[85] found that depression is most closely associated with anxiety disorders (odds ratio, 8.2), followed closely by conduct disorders (odds ratio, 6.6) and ADHD (odds ratio, 5.5). Substance abuse disorders are also commonly comorbid with depression and tend to begin an average of 4.5 years after the onset of the depressive disorder.[4]

High rates of comorbidity have also been found with early-onset bipolar disorder, particularly with ADHD, behavior disorders, and anxiety disorders. Rates of comorbidity range from 66% to 75% for ADHD, 46% to 75% for oppositional defiant disorder, 5.6% to 37% for conduct disorder, 12.5% to 56% for anxiety disorders, and 11% for pervasive developmental disorders.[7,69] The rates of comorbid substance abuse disorders increase with age, with rates up to 40% in adolescents.[7]

Treatment of Comorbidity

In treating conditions comorbid with bipolar disorder, it is important to first stabilize the mood symptoms and then evaluate the need for psychosocial or pharmacological treatment of any comorbid conditions.[45] There are no clear guidelines for the treatment of comorbid conditions with depression. If the mood disorder appears to be secondary to another condition, such as social anxiety or post-traumatic stress disorder, it may be useful to treat the primary condition first or concurrently with the treatment for depression.

Suidical Ideation

Children with mood disorders are at increased risk for suicidal ideation, attempt, and completion. Suicidal ideation has been reported in more than 60% of depressed children and adolescents, and MDD is the most common diagnosis among suicide victims.[5,86] Children with bipolar disorder are also at high risk for suicide, particularly when depressed, during a mixed episode, or when psychotic.[8,55,87] Geller and colleagues[55] reported suicidal ideation in 25% of their 7- to 16-year old participants with bipolar disorder. Comorbidity between mood disorders and substance abuse or disruptive behavior disorders further increases the risk of suicide.[86] These data highlight the importance of assessing suicidality in youths with mood disorders. Data from a randomized controlled trial

indicate that assessing for suicidal ideation does not increase distress or suicidal ideation in adolescents.[88]

In assessing for suicide risk, several factors should be taken into account; these are outlined in the American Academy of Child and Adolescent Psychiatry's 2001 Practice Parameters regarding the assessment and treatment of adolescent suicidal behavior.[20] In addition to the presence of a mood and/or substance abuse disorder, individuals with previous suicide attempts, suicidal thoughts, plans for suicide, agitation, and psychosis are at greatest risk for suicide.[20] Other risk factors include family history of suicide; history of physical or sexual abuse; school problems; poor communication with parents; recent suicide of a peer; and gay, lesbian, or bisexual orientation.[86] Several questionnaires that have been developed to assess risk of suicide have high sensitivity but poor specificity because of the low base rates of suicide.[86] These questionnaires can best be used as screening tools in community samples. In children and adolescents at high risk for suicide, such as those with mood disorders, assessment should include direct interview with the child and parent.[20]

Psychosis

Psychosis is more common in child and adolescent mood disorders than in adult mood disorders. Approximately 33% to 50% of preadolescents with MDD and up to 31% of adolescents with MDD experience hallucinations, most commonly auditory hallucinations.[5] Estimates of the rates of psychosis in early-onset bipolar disorder range from 16% to 88%, depending on assessment strategy.[70] The most common type of psychotic symptom reported in early-onset bipolar disorder is mood-congruent grandiose delusions.[70]

TREATMENT

As evidenced by the prevalence, chronicity, and impairment associated with mood disorders described previously, effective intervention strategies are needed to manage these conditions. Treatment outcome studies for both biological and psychosocial therapies have helped informed treatment decisions for children with mood disorders. Considerable research on treatments for MDD has accumulated.[89,90] Much of the treatment research on childhood bipolar disorder, in contrast, is preliminary and is currently evolving.[45]

Depression

BIOLOGICAL INTERVENTIONS

Tricyclic antidepressants have not been found to be effective in the treatment of children and adolescents.[26] Only one SSRI, fluoxetine, has received approval from the U.S. Food and Drug Administration (FDA) to be marketed for children and adolescents.

Cheung and associates[91] reviewed the efficacy and safety of published and unpublished randomized controlled trials of antidepressants in children and adolescents. Throughout the studies reviewed, various outcome measures were used; however, a Clinical Global Impression Improvement (CGI-I) rating of 1 or 2 (*very much improved* or *much improved*) was the most frequent definition of response to treatment that produced significant results and these response rates are reported as follows: (1) Three large double-blind placebo-controlled trials of fluoxetine indicated significant differences in clinician-rated response and symptom level between fluoxetine and placebo across all three studies; response rates for fluoxetine ranged from 53% to 60%, in comparison with 33% to 37% rates for placebo.[90,92,93] (2) Of three double-blind, placebo-controlled studies of paroxetine, the one published study demonstrated superiority of paroxetine over placebo (66% response to paroxetine, 48% to placebo), whereas the other two adequately powered but unpublished studies failed to demonstrate significant results.[94] (3) Two studies of sertraline, combined a priori for analysis, were identified. Response rates were 69% for the sertraline recipients and 59% for the placebo recipients. The difference was statistically significant because of the large number of subjects; however, neither study produced significant results when analyzed separately.[95] (4) Two studies of citalopram were reviewed, one published and one unpublished, with an unusual pattern of results. Neither study revealed differences in CGI-I response rates; however, one did reveal group differences in depression symptom severity, as rated by the Children's Depression Rating Scale–Revised.[96] The meaning of this finding without CGI-I response differences is unclear. (5) Two studies of nefazodone were identified; one revealed a significant effect of the drug (65% response rate in comparison with 46% response rate with placebo), whereas the other study revealed no significant effect.[97] (6) In two studies of venlafaxine and two studies of mirtazapine, no differences were found between the drugs and placebo on any measure.[98] Additional details about the methods and results of all these studies were described by Cheung and associates.[91]

In October 2004, the FDA issued a black box warning requiring that antidepressant medications be accompanied by information indicating that antidepressant use is associated with increased risk of suicidality in children and adolescents. This warning was based on a review of 26 studies that demonstrated that the average risk of suicide-related events was 4% with antidepressants, in comparison with 2% with placebo.[99] No deaths by suicide were reported in any of the studies reviewed.[99] Examining the risk of sui-

cidal behavior associated with naturalistic antidepressant use in the United Kingdom, Jick and colleagues[100] found that risk was increased in the first month after initiation of antidepressant therapy and was highest in the first 1 to 9 days. Concerns have also been raised concerning children's and adolescents' risk of becoming agitated or switching to mania with antidepressant medications, which was found to occur in very small numbers of patients participating in randomized controlled trials.[91] The Society for Adolescent Medicine emphasizes the high risk of suicide associated with untreated depression, however, and supports the continued use of antidepressant medication in adolescents along with careful monitoring, particularly at the beginning of treatment and after dose changes.[99]

Herbal remedies are gaining popularity, and St. John's wort has been shown to have antidepressant effects superior to those of placebo in mild to moderate adult depression.[101] Open-label pilot studies in children and adolescents have indicated that St. John's wort is well tolerated and may be beneficial in treating MDD in youth.[101,102] Randomized clinical trials are needed to further evaluate the safety and efficacy of St. John's wort in children and adolescents.

Among adults who experience seasonal variation in mood symptoms, exposure to bright light or to dawn simulation has been found beneficial. Research extending these findings to pediatric samples has shown that light therapy is effective and superior to placebo in children and adolescents.[103]

Electroconvulsive therapy has been shown to be a very effective treatment for severe depression in adults, with remission rates of 70% to 90% in clinical trials.[104] Since 1990, several studies of the use of electroconvulsive therapy in adolescents with a variety of diagnoses have been published.[105] Response rates range from 50% to 100%, with higher response rates reported for mood disorders. In addition, high rates of satisfaction with the treatment have been reported among adolescents who received electroconvulsive therapy.[105] There are not enough data on the use of electroconvulsive therapy in preadolescents with which to draw conclusions about its efficacy. The American Academy of Child and Adolescent Psychiatry practice parameters advised that electroconvulsive therapy be considered for adolescents after previous interventions have been ineffective and if a second psychiatrist agrees to the appropriateness of the treatment.[105] Overall, electroconvulsive therapy is rarely used in adolescents despite the efficacy data and American Academy of Child and Adolescent Psychiatry guidelines.[106] Lack of both knowledge and experience with electroconvulsive therapy among child and adolescent psychiatrists and public controversy surrounding the treatment may contribute to the low rates of utilization.[105]

PSYCHOSOCIAL TREATMENT

The most extensively researched psychosocial treatment for depression in children and adolescents is cognitive-behavioral therapy (CBT). Compton and colleagues[89] reviewed 12 randomized controlled trials of CBT for depression in children and adolescents. Overall these studies showed that CBT is superior to no treatment. One study found that CBT was superior to an attentional control group;[107] however others have failed to find differences in comparison with nonfocused therapy, treatment as usual, or pill placebo.[90,108,109] In comparison with other specific treatment modalities, CBT has been found to be superior to relaxation training[110] and systemic behavior family therapy,[107] but no differences were found with interpersonal therapy.[111]

The cognitive-behavioral model is based on the idea that depression is maintained by cognitions and behavioral patterns that decrease effective interaction with the world.[89] Cognitive distortions are thought to bias the way an individual obtains and interprets information from the environment, leading to negative thoughts about one's self, the world, and the future and to attribution of negative events to stable, internal, and global factors. Deficits in social skills and problem solving also prevent successful interactions with the environment. Further, decreased participation in potentially enjoyable activities decreases opportunities for pleasure. Specific components of CBT include psychoeducation, goal setting, problem solving, and tailored interventions based on the individual's cognitive and behavioral patterns. As family conflict and disruption is quite common in child and adolescent depression, a parent or family component is often included in treatment. Two studies have specifically investigated the effect of adding a family component to individual therapy, and have failed to find group differences, however this may be due to insufficient power to detect incremental differences in treatment efficacy.[112,113]

Another psychosocial treatment that shows promise in the treatment of adolescents with depression is interpersonal psychotherapy (IPT). In randomized clinical trials, IPT has been shown to be more effective than control groups and has shown similar efficacy to CBT.[111,114,115] IPT focuses treatment on patterns of interpersonal interaction and communication. Specific targets of treatment include the problem areas of grief, interpersonal disputes, role transitions, interpersonal deficits, and single-parent families.[116]

COMBINATION BIOLOGICAL AND PSYCHOSOCIAL TREATMENT

The Treatment of Adolescents with Depression (TADS) study[90] is the first to systematically explore the relative efficacy of fluoxetine, CBT, and their combination in adolescent depression. Results suggest that the combination is most effective, followed by fluoxetine, which was superior to both CBT alone and placebo. The TADS study[90] showed that combination pharmacotherapy and CBT are more effective in decreasing both depressive symptoms and suicidal behavior than either intervention alone in adolescents with depression, highlighting the importance of a combination of interventions in the treatment of childhood-onset mood disorders.

Bipolar Disorders

BIOLOGICAL INTERVENTIONS

Pharmacological interventions are an essential component of comprehensive treatment for bipolar disorder.[116a] The only medication approved by the FDA for adolescent bipolar disorder is lithium. Only five randomized placebo-controlled studies to date have evaluated medications for use in child and adolescent bipolar disorder.[7] Lithium was shown to improve global functioning in adolescents with bipolar disorder and comorbid substance use disorders.[117] The only other study of lithium monotherapy, however, did not find continuing effects of lithium in a randomized discontinuation study.[118] Following mood stabilization with combination lithium and divalproex sodium, a comparison of the two medications indicated that they were equally effective in maintenance treatment.[119] DelBello and colleagues[120] found that the combination of quetiapine with divalproex sodium was more effective in treating adolescent mania than dovalproex sodium alone. In a study of children and adolescents with comorbid ADHD, the addition of Adderall following mood stabilization with divalproex sodium was found to be effective in treating the ADHD symptoms.[121] Much of the data used in determining treatment options for bipolar disorder in children and adolescents come from open trials, adult studies, and clinical experience.[45]

Kowatch and colleagues[45] developed treatment guidelines for children and adolescents with bipolar disorder based on the evidence currently available. For bipolar mania, with or without psychosis, various combinations of treatment with mood stabilizers and/or atypical antipsychotics were recommended. Following nonresponse to multiple medication trials, clozapine or electroconvulsive therapy was recommended. See Kowatch et al[45] for detailed treatment algorithms. No algorithm was developed for the treatment of bipolar depression, as the currently available data are too limited to draw conclusions about the treatment of depressive symptoms.

Despite the limited efficacy data for child and adolescent bipolar disorder treatments, mood stabilizers and antipsychotics are commonly used for the treatment of early onset bipolar disorder in clinical settings. American Academy of Child and Adolescent Psychiatry practice parameters recommend considering the evidence from child and adult studies, symptom presentation, phase of illness, medication safety profile, child's history of medication response, and family preference in choosing medication(s).[116a] The practice parameter also suggests that most youth with bipolar disorder will require ongoing medication treatment to prevent relapse.[116a]

PSYCHOSOCIAL TREATMENT

Medication is a critical component of treatment for bipolar disorder; however psychosocial interventions play an important role in promoting medication compliance and teaching skills to help decrease relapse.[7,116a] Outcome studies of medication treatment in children and adolescents are limited, as described above, however adult studies describe residual symptoms, poor outcomes for bipolar depression, and high medication nonadherence rates.[122] Additionally, while the cause of bipolar disorder in children appears to be strongly influenced by biological factors, the course can be shaped by psychosocial factors.[123] Adjunctive interventions are clearly needed to enhance treatment outcome and adult studies indicate family-based psychosocial interventions decrease relapse by 33%.[124,125]

The addition of psychotherapy to pharmacotherapy has been recommended as soon as the child's mood is stable enough to learn new skills.[45] Research to identify efficacious treatments for bipolar disorder is in the early stages of development and three research teams have developed and reported preliminary data on therapies for bipolar disorder. These therapies are all adjunctive, include family involvement, and are psychoeducationally focused.

Fristad and colleagues have conducted the only randomized controlled trials of a psychoeducational treatment for families of children with mood disorders to date. These studies included children age 8-11 with both depression and bipolar disorder. In a pilot study of 35 children, 46% of whom had bipolar disorder, Multi-Family Psychoeducation Groups (MFPG) were found to increase parental knowledge about mood disorders, increase positive family interactions, increase the parental support perceived by children, and increase utilization of appropriate services by families.[126] MFPG involves parents and children meeting separately in a group format to receive education, support, and learn skills to cope with symptoms and improve the child's functioning. Forming groups of children with both bipolar disorder and depressive disorder diagnoses had the benefits of

making it easier and faster to recruit an adequate number of families to start a group. Due to the significant portion of children initially diagnosed with MDD who later develop bipolar disorder, it was also considered important to provide information on the symptoms and management of bipolar disorder to families of children with both diagnoses. No difficulties were found in conducting these combined groups, but it was considered beneficial to include at least two children with each type of diagnosis in a group. In the pilot study, families of children with bipolar disorder had worse mood symptoms, a history of more treatment experiences, and greater knowledge about mood disorders at the beginning of treatment than the families of children with depressive disorders; however families of children with bipolar disorder and depressive disorders both benefited from treatment.[127] A larger randomized controlled trial of 165 children is currently underway to evaluate MFPG.

The content of MFPG has also been adapted for delivery in individual family sessions, which has been tested in a pilot study of 20 children with bipolar disorder. Results suggest treatment led to decreased severity of mood symptoms, with improvements continuing for 12 months following treatment, improved treatment utilization, more positive family climate, and high levels of satisfaction with treatment.[128] Further research with a larger sample size will be needed to more clearly evaluate the efficacy of individual family psychoeducation.[128]

Family-Focused Therapy (FFT) in adults with bipolar disorder has been shown to delay relapse, decrease hospitalization, decrease symptom severity, and improve medication adherence.[129-131] FFT involves patients and family members in education about bipolar disorder, communication training, and problem solving skills training. Miklowitz and colleagues[132] have adapted FFT for an adolescent population (FFT-A), and in open trials the combination of FFT-A and pharmacotherapy was associated with improvements in symptoms of mania and depression and reductions in problem behaviors. Pavuluri and colleagues[133] adapted the FFT model and combined it with cognitive behavioral principles to develop Child and Family-Focused Cognitive-Behavioral Therapy (CFF-CBT) for younger children. In open trials, CFF-CBT in addition to pharmacotherapy led to reductions in mood symptoms and improved global functioning.[133]

PREVENTION

Research has begun to address the prevention of depression in youth with subclinical symptoms. Group cognitive behavioral interventions for children and adolescents have shown promise in reducing symptoms and subsequent development of clinical depression; however data on the long term effects of these programs have been mixed.[134-136] Gilham and colleagues[134] found that benefits were sustained and the prevention effects grew over the course of two years, while Spence and colleagues[136] found that initial benefits were lost by one year follow up. Intervention programs in primary care have also targeted adolescents at risk for depression, and findings suggest that prevention programs can be successfully implemented in such settings with the consultation of mental health professionals or use of internet-based programs.[50,137]

Given the often chronic and relapsing course of mood disorders, the prevention of relapse in children who have had a prior mood episode is an important consideration. One study suggests that the continuation of fluoxetine treatment for depression may help reduce and delay relapse in children and adolescents over eight months.[138] Follow-up studies of CBT for depression have indicated that treatment gains are generally maintained or continue one to nine months following treatment, but over longer term follow-up (nine months to two years), lack of recovery and relapse are common.[89] Further research is needed to determine whether booster sessions of CBT may be helpful in maintaining treatment effects.[89] Research on pharmacological and psychosocial strategies for reducing and delaying relapse for children and adolescents with bipolar disorder is in the early stages and has not yet yielded any conclusive findings.[7]

CLINICAL IMPLICATIONS

Mood disorders in pediatric populations are associated with impairment at home, at school, and with peers. The experience of a mood disorder also increases risk for suicide and future mood problems. Identification of these disorders in children and adolescents is a crucial first step in reducing the associated impairment and risks. Developmental-behavioral pediatricians, as well as other health and educational professionals, play an important role in identifying mood disorders in this population and recommending appropriate treatments. A significant portion of mental health services are currently provided in primary care settings, with primary care visits accounting for nearly 40% of all mental health services among a small sample of privately insured children.[3] The availability of child and adolescent psychiatry services nationwide is far short of the need.[139] These data highlight the importance of all child and adolescent health care providers being educated about the symptoms and effective treatments for mood disorders. Further, only about half of children referred for services with a

mental health provider show up for their first appointment with that provider.[1] Families may be more likely to follow through with treatment when services are available in the primary care setting or there is significant collaboration among professionals.[1,2,50]

Models of collaboration among professionals to treat mental health problems in a primary care setting have been developed and show promise for providing cost-effective, beneficial services for children and adolescents. A stepped-care approach has been shown effective in treating adult mood disorders and has been adapted for the treatment of child mental health problems.[2,50,140] Campo and colleagues[2] described a program in which primary care physicians, advanced practice nurses, social workers, and pediatric psychiatrists work together to provide appropriate levels of care for children and adolescents. In their model, primary care physicians identify children with possible mental health issues and provide treatment for less complex cases. Advanced practice nurses with training in psychiatry complete on-site mental health assessments, make diagnoses, and provide patient education and support as needed. Social workers provide case management and on-site psychotherapy for cases of moderate to severe complexity. The pediatric psychiatrist manages more complex cases and provides consultation for the team. The team also met regularly to discuss ongoing cases. With this level of support, two-thirds of mental health cases were successfully managed by the primary care pediatrician and advanced practice nurse. Asarnow and colleagues[50] reported on a similar program testing the benefits of having a care manager with mental health training available in the primary care setting to coordinate and support the care of adolescents with depression. Adolescents who received the collaborative care reported fewer depressive symptoms, greater utilization of mental health services, and greater satisfaction with their treatment than those who received usual care. These models highlight the ways that mental health screening, in-house treatment options, and consultation among professionals can improve outcomes for children and adolescents.

RESEARCH IMPLICATIONS

Further research in childhood mood disorders is needed to improve prevention, identification, diagnosis, and treatment efforts. The existing research base is considerably stronger for depressive disorders than for bipolar disorders. There is a growing base of knowledge about the risk factors involved in mood disorders, including genetics, neurobiology, and environmental influences. Future molecular genetics research will improve our understanding and early identification of at-risk children. It will also be important for future research to examine the ways genetics, neurobiological factors, and environmental influences interact, which may lead to more targeted intervention strategies.[139] Research is necessary to establish a clear definition of bipolar disorder in children and determine its continuity with adult forms of the disorder. To accomplish this, developmentally appropriate criteria with high interrater reliability and validity will need to be developed.[139]

We now have a growing base of randomized controlled trials of treatments for depression to guide treatment decisions. Future research should expand on this knowledge by examining treatment options for treatment-resistant depression, identifying the active components of psychotherapy through dismantling studies, increasing attention to prevention strategies, and examining effectiveness in community-based studies.[139] There is currently very little research base for the treatment of bipolar disorder and the identification of effective pharmacological and psychosocial treatments will be very important in improving outcomes for the children and families who are coping with this chronic and relapsing condition.[139]

Changes are also needed in the way mental health services are provided to increase identification and appropriate treatment. Programs to increase knowledge about mood disorders among professionals who work directly with children, such as teachers and primary care physicians, should be developed and evaluated. Recent research has begun evaluating ways of incorporating mental health treatment into primary care.[2,50] Continued research and public policy changes to allow for more effective treatment will help improve access to appropriate services.[139]

REFERENCES

1. Simonian SJ: Screening and identification in pediatric primary care. Behav Modif 30:114-131, 2006.
2. Campo JV, Shaver S, Strohm J, et al: Pediatric behavioral health in primary care: A collaborative approach. J Am Psychiatr Nurses Assoc 11:276-282, 2005.
3. Ringel JS, Sturm R: National estimates of mental health utilization and expenditures for children in 1998. J Behav Health Res 28:319-333, 2001.
4. Birmaher B, Ryan ND, Williamson DE, et al: Childhood and adolescent depression: A review of the past 10 years: Part 1. J Am Acad Child Adolesc Psychiatry 35:1427-1439, 1996.
5. Hammen C, Rudolph KD: Childhood mood disorders. In Mash E, Barkley RA, eds: Child Psychopathology, 2nd ed. New York: Guilford, 2003, pp 233-278.
6. Kashani JH, Holcomb WR, Orvashel H: Depression and depressive symptoms in preschool children from the general population. Am J Psychiatry 143:1138-1143, 1996.
7. Pavuluri MN, Birmaher B, Naylor MW: Pediatric bipolar disorder: A review of the past 10 years. J Am Acad Child Adolesc Psychiatry 44:846-871, 2005.
8. Lewinsohn PM, Seeley JR, Klein DN: Bipolar disorder in a community sample of older adolescents: Prevalence, phenomenology, comorbidity and course. J Am Acad Child Adolesc Psychiatry 34:454-463, 1995.
9. Youngstrom EA, Findling RL, Calabrese JR, et al: Comparing the diagnostic accuracy of six potential screening instruments for bipolar disorder in youths aged 5 to 17. J Am Acad Child Adolesc Psychiatry 43:847-858, 2004.
10. Weissman MM, Wolk S, Goldstein RB, et al: Depressed adolescents grown up. JAMA 281:1707-1713, 1999.
11. Geller B, Tillman R, Craney JL, et al: Four-year prospective outcome and natural history of mania in children with a prepubertal and early adolescent bipolar disorder phenotype. Arch Gen Psychiatry 61:459-467, 2004.
12. U.S. Department of Education: FY 2004 Performance and Accountability Report. Washington, DC: U.S. Department of Education, 2004.
13. Office of Special Education Programs: 25th Annual (2003) Report to Congress on the Implementation of the Individuals with Disabilities Education Act, vol 1. Washington, DC: U.S. Department of Education, 2005.
14. Rudolph KD, Clark AG: Cognitions of relationships in children with depressive and aggressive symptoms: Social-cognitive distortion or reality? J Abnorm Child Psychol 29:41-56, 2001.
15. Puig-Antich J, Kaufman J, Ryan ND, et al: The psychosocial functioning and family environment of depressed adolescents. J Am Acad Child Adolesc Psychiatry 32:244-253, 1993.
16. Biederman J, Faraone SV, Wozniak J, et al: Further evidence of unique developmental phenotypic correlates of pediatric bipolar disorder: Findings from a large sample of clinically referred preadolescent children assessed over the last 7 years. J Affect Disord 82(Suppl 1):S45-S58, 2004.
17. Geller B, Craney JL, Bolhofner K, et al: Phenomenology and longitudinal course of children with a prepubertal and early adolescent bipolar disorder phenotype. In Geller B, DelBello MP, eds: Bipolar Disorder in Childhood and Early Adolescence. New York: Guilford, 2003, pp 7-24.
18. Hellander M, Sisson DP, Fristad MA: Internet support for parents of children with early-onset bipolar disorder. In Geller B, DelBello MP, eds: Bipolar Disorder in Childhood and Early Adolescence. New York: Guilford, 2003, pp 314-329.
19. World Health Organization: Mental health: New understanding, new hope. Geneva: World Health Organization, 2001.
20. American Academy of Child and Adolescent Psychiatry: Practice parameter for the assessment and treatment of children and adolescents with suicidal behavior. J Am Acad Child Adolesc Psychiatry 40:24S-50S, 2001.

21. Faraone SV, Glatt SJ, Tsuang MT: The genetics of pediatric-onset bipolar disorder. Biol Psychiatry 53:970-977, 2003.

22. Sullivan PF, Neale MC, Kendler KS: Genetic epidemiology of major depression: Review and meta-analysis. Am J Psychiatry 157:1552-1562, 2000.

23. Rice F, Harold G, Thapar A: The genetic aetiology of childhood depression: A review. J Child Psychol Psychiatry 43:65-79, 2002.

24. Lapalme M, Hodgins S, LaRoche C: Children of parents with bipolar disorder: A meta-analysis of risk for mental disorders. Can J Psychiatry 42:623-631, 1997.

25. Todd R, Neuman R, Geller B, et al: Genetic studies of affective disorders: Should we be starting with childhood onset probands? J Am Acad Child Adolesc Psychiatry 32:1164-1171, 1993.

26. Kaufman J, Martin A, King RA, et al: Are child-, adolescent-, and adult-onset depression one and the same disorder? Biol Psychiatry 49:980-1001, 2001.

27. Rao U: Sleep and other biological rhythms. *In* Geller B, DelBello MP, eds: Bipolar Disorder in Childhood and Early Adolescence. New York: Guilford, 2003, pp 215-246.

28. Nolan CL, Moore GJ, Madden R, et al: Prefrontal cortical volume in childhood-onset major depression. Arch Gen Psychiatry 59:173-179, 2002.

29. Byrum CE, Ahearn EP, Krishnan KR: A neuroanatomic model for depression. Prog Neuropsychopharmacol Biol Psychiatry 23:175-193, 1999.

30. Mirza Y, Tang J, Russell A, et al: Reduced anterior cingulate cortex glutamatergic concentrations in childhood major depression. J Am Acad Child Adolesc Psychiatry 43:341-348, 2004.

31. Rosenberg DR, Mirza Y, Russell A, et al: Reduced anterior cingulated glutamatergic concentrations in childhood OCD and major depression versus healthy controls. J Am Acad Child Adolesc Psychiatry 43:1146-1153, 2004.

32. Farchione TR, Moore GJ, Rosenberg DR: Proton magnetic resonance spectroscopic imaging in pediatric major depression. Biol Psychiatry 52:86-92, 2002.

33. Steingard RJ, Yurgelum-Todd DA, Hennen J, et al: Increased orbitofrontal cortex levels of choline in depressed adolescents as detected by in vivo proton magnetic resonance spectroscopy. Biol Psychiatry 48:1053-1061, 2000.

34. Ehilich S, Noam GG, Lyoo I, et al: White matter hyperintensities and their associations with suicidality in psychiatrically hospitalized children and adolescents. J Am Acad Child Adolesc Psychiatry 43:770-776, 2004.

35. Frazier JA, Ahn MS, DeJong S, et al: Magnetic resonance imaging studies in early-onset bipolar disorder: A critical review. Harv Rev Psychiatry 13:125-140, 2005.

36. Asarnow JR, Tompson M, Woo S, et al: Is expressed emotion a specific risk factor for depression or a nonspecific correlate of psychopathology? J Abnorm Child Psychol 29:573-583, 2001.

37. Kashani JH, Burgach DJ, Rosenberg TK: Perception of family conflict resolution and depressive symptomatology in adolescents. J Am Acad Child Adolesc Psychiatry 27:42-48, 1988.

38. Khaleque A, Rohner RP: Perceived parental acceptance-rejection and psychological adjustment: A meta-analysis of cross-cultural and intracultural studies. J Marriage Fam 64:54-64, 2002.

39. Puig-Antich J: Psychosocial functioning in prepubertal major depressive disorders: Interpersonal relationships during the depressive episode. Arch Gen Psychiatry 42:500-507, 1985.

40. Asarnow JR, Goldstein MJ, Tompson M, et al: One-year outcomes of depressive disorders in child psychiatric in-patients: Evaluation of the prognostic power of a brief measure of expressed emotion. J Child Psychol Psychiatry 34:129-137, 1993.

41. Hammen C, Burge D, Stansbury K: Relationship of mother and child variables to child outcomes in a high risk sample: A causal modeling analysis. Dev Psychol 26:24-30, 1990.

42. Hammen C, Brennan PA, Shih JH: Family discord and stress predictors of depression and other disorders in adolescents of depressed and nondepressed women. J Am Acad Child Adolesc Psychiatry 43:994-1002, 2004.

43. Geller B, Craney JL, Bolhofner K, et al: Two-year prospective follow-up of children with a prepubertal and early adolescent bipolar disorder phenotype. Am J Psychiatry 159:927-933, 2002.

44. Tillman R, Geller B, Nickelsburg MJ, et al: Life events in a prepubertal and early adolescent bipolar phenotype compared to attention-deficit hyperactive and normal controls. J Child Adolesc Psychopharmacol 13:243-251, 2003.

45. Kowatch RA, Fristad MA, Birmaher B, et al: Treatment guidelines for children and adolescents with bipolar disorder. J Am Acad Child Adolesc Psychiatry 44:213-239, 2005.

46. Carlson GA: The bottom line. J Child Adolesc Psychopharmacol 13:115-118, 2003.

47. Horwitz SM, Leaf PJ, Leventhal JM, et al: Identification and management of psychosocial and developmental problems in community-based, primary care pediatric practices. Am Acad Pediatrics 89:480-485, 1992.

48. Wildman BG, Kizibash AH, Smucker WD: Physicians' attention to parents' concerns about the psychosocial functioning of their children. Arch Fam Med 8:440-444, 1999.

49. Wren FJ, Scholle SH, Heo J, et al: Pediatric mood and anxiety syndromes in primary care: Who gets identified? Intl J Psychiatry Med 33:1-16, 2003.

50. Asarnow JR, Jaycox LH, Duan N, et al: Effectiveness of a quality improvement intervention for adolescent depression in primary care clinics: A randomized controlled trial. JAMA 293:311-319, 2005.

51. American Psychiatric Association: Diagnostic and Statistical Manual of Mental Disorders, 4th ed, text revision. Washington, DC: American Psychiatric Association, 2000.

52. Ryan ND, Puig-Antioch J, Ambrosini P, et al: The clinical picture of major depression in children and adolescents. Arch Gen Psychiatry 44:854-861, 1987.

53. Leibenluft E, Charney DS, Towbin KE, et al: Defining clinical phenotypes of juvenile mania. Am J Psychiatry 160:430-437, 2003.

54. Carlson GA, Kashani JH: Phenomenology of major depression from childhood through adulthood: Analysis of three studies. Am J Psychiatry 145:1222-1225, 1988.

55. Geller B, Zimerman G, Williams M, et al: DSM-IV mania symptoms in a prepubertal and early adolescent bipolar disorder phenotype compared to attention-deficit hyperactive and normal controls. J Child Adolesc Psychopharmacol 12:11-25, 2002.

56. Kagan J: Emotional development and psychiatry. Biol Psychiatry 49:973-979, 2001.

57. Geller B, Zimmerman B, Williams M, et al: Phenomenology of prepubertal and early adolescent bipolar disorder: Examples of elated mood, grandiose behaviors, decreased need for sleep, racing thoughts, and hypersexuality. J Child Adolesc Psychopharmacol 12:3-9, 2002.

58. Terwogt MM, Stegge H: The development of emotional intelligence. *In* Goodyear IM, ed: The Depressed Child and Adolescent. Cambridge, UK: Cambridge University Press, 2001, pp 24-45.

59. Baker JE, Sedney MA: How bereaved children cope with loss: An overview. *In* Corr CA, Corr DM, eds: Handbook of Childhood Death and Bereavement. New York: Springer, 1996, pp 109-129.

60. Fristad MA, Sisson DP: Sadness and depressive disorders. *In* Osborn LM, DeWitt TG, First LR, et al, eds: Pediatrics. Philadelphia: Elsevier, 2005, pp 1591-1595.

61. Dowdney L: Annotation: childhood bereavement following parental death. J Child Psychol Psychiat 41:819-830, 2000.

62. Cerel J, Fristad MA, Verducci J, et al: Childhood bereavement: Psychopathology in the two years postparental death. J Am Acad Child Adolesc Psychiatry 45:681-690, 2006.

63. Cerel J, Fristad, MA, Weller EB, et al: Suicide-bereaved children and adolescents: A controlled longitudinal examination. J Am Acad Child Adolesc Psychiatry 38:672-679, 1999.

64. Weller RA, Weller EB, Fristad MA, et al: Depression in recently bereaved prepubertal children. Am J Psychiatry 148:1536-1540, 1991.

65. Tillman R, Geller B, Craney JL, et al: Relationship of parent and child informant to prevalence of mania symptoms in children with a prepubertal and early adolescent bipolar disorder phenotype. Am J Psychiatry 161:1278-1284, 2004.

66. Ryan ND: Diagnosing pediatric depression. Biol Psychiatry 49:1050-1054, 2001.

67. Barkley RA: Attention-Deficit Hyperactivity Disorder: A Handbook for Diagnosis and Treatment, 2nd ed. New York: Guilford, 1998.

68. Mackinaw-Koons B, Fristad MA: Research in practice: Early-onset bipolar disorder: What every child clinician should know. Soc Clin Child Adolesc Psychol Newsl 17(4):6-7, 2004.

69. Youngstrom EA, Findling RL, Youngstrom JK, et al: Toward an evidence-based assessment of pediatric bipolar disorder. J Clin Child Adolesc Psychol 34:433-448, 2005.

70. Pavuluri MN, Herbener ES, Sweeney JA: Psychotic symptoms in pediatric bipolar disorder. J Affect Disord 80:19-28, 2004.

71. Poznanski EO, Mokros HB: Children's Depression Rating Scale, Revised Manual. Los Angeles: Western Psychological Services, 1996.

72. Fristad MA, Weller RA, Weller EB: The Mania Rating Scale (MRS): Further reliability and validity studies with children. Ann Clin Psychiatry 7:127-132, 1995.

73. Young RC, Biggs JT, Ziegler VE, et al: A rating scale for mania: Reliability, validity and sensitivity. Br J Psychiatry 133:429-435, 1978.

74. Axelson D, Birmaher BJ, Brent D, et al: A preliminary study of the Kiddie Schedule for Affective Disorders and Schizophrenia for School-Age Children mania rating scale for children and adolescents. J Child Adolesc Psychopharmacol 13:463-470, 2003.

75. Shaffer D, Fisher P, Lucas CP, et al: NIMH Diagnostic Interview Schedule for Children Version IV (NIMH DISC-IV): Description, differences from previous versions, and reliability of some common diagnoses. J Am Acad Child Adolesc Psychiatry 39:28-38, 2000.

76. Weller EB, Weller RA, Rooney MT, et al: Children's Interview for Psychiatric Syndromes (ChIPS). Washington, DC: American Psychiatric Press, 1999.

77. Weller EB, Weller RA, Rooney MT, et al: Children's Interview for Psychiatric Syndromes, Parent Version (P-ChIPS). Washington, DC: American Psychiatric Press, 1999.

78. Reich W: Diagnostic Interview for Children and Adolescents (DICA). J Am Acad Child Adolesc Psychiatry 39:59-66, 2000.

79. Geller B, Warner K, Williams M, et al: Prepubertal and young adolescent bipolarity versus ADHD: Assessment and validity using the WASH-U-KSADS, CBCL, and TRF. J Affect Disord 51:93-100, 1998.

80. Achenbach TM, Rescorla LA: Manual for the ASEBA School-Age Forms & Profiles. Burlington: University of Vermont, Department of Psychiatry, 2001.

81. Kovacs M: Children's Depression Inventory. North Tonawanda, NY: Multi-Health Systems, 1999.

82. Fristad MA, Weller RA, Weller EB, et al: Comparison of the parent and child versions of the Children's Depression Inventory. Ann Clin Psychiatry 3:341-346, 1991.

83. Depue RA, Slater JF, Wofstetter-Kaush H, et al: A behavioral paradigm for identifying persons at risk for bipolar depressive disorder: A conceptual framework and five validation studies. J Abnorm Child Psychol 90:381-437, 1981.

84. Jellinick M, Murphy JM: Screening for psychosocial disorder in pediatric practice. Am J Dis Child 109:371-378, 1988.

85. Angold A, Costello EJ, Erkanli A: Comorbidity. J Child Psychol Psychiatry 40:57-87, 1999.

86. Pfeffer CR: Diagnosis of childhood and adolescent suicidal behavior: Unmet needs for suicide prevention. Biol Psychiatry 49:1055-1061, 2001.

87. Dilsaver SC, Benazzi F, Rihmer Z, et al: Gender, suicidality and bipolar mixed states in adolescents. J Affect Disord 87:11-16, 2005.

88. Gould MS, Marrocco F, Kleinman M, et al: Evaluating iatrogenic risk of youth suicide screening programs: A randomized controlled trial. JAMA 293:1635-1643, 2005.

89. Compton SN, March JS, Brent D, et al: Cognitive-behavioral psychotherapy for anxiety and depressive disorders in children and adolescents: An evidence-based medicine review. J Am Acad Child Adolesc Psychiatry 43:930-959, 2004.

90. March J, Silva S, Petrycki S, et al: Fluoxetine, cognitive-behavioral therapy, and their combination for adolescents with depression: Treatment for Adolescents With Depression Study (TADS) randomized controlled trial. JAMA 297:807-820, 2004.

91. Cheung AH, Emslie GJ, Mayes TL: Review of the efficacy and safety of antidepressants in youth depression. J Child Psychol Psychiatry 46:735-754, 2005.

92. Emslie GJ, Heiligenstein JH, Wagner KD, et al: Fluoxetine for acute treatment of depression in children and adolescents: A placebo-controlled, randomized clinical trial. J Am Acad Child Adolesc Psychiatry 41:1205-1215, 2002.

93. Emslie GJ, Rush AJ, Weinberg WA, et al: Double-blind placebo controlled study of fluoxetine in depressed children and adolescents. Arch Gen Psychiatry 54:1031-1037, 1997.

94. Keller MB, Ryan ND, Strober M, et al: Efficacy of paroxetine in the treatment of adolescent major depression: A randomized, controlled trial. J Am Acad Child Adolesc Psychiatry 40:762-772, 2001.

95. Wagner KD, Ambrosini PJ, Rynn M, et al: Efficacy of sertraline in the treatment of children and adolescents with major depressive disorder. JAMA 290:1033-1041, 2003.

96. Wagner KD, Robb AS, Findling RL, et al: A randomized placebo-controlled trial of citalopram for the treatment of major depression in children and adolescents. Am J Psychiatry 161:1079-1083, 2004.

97. Emslie GJ, Findling RL, Rynn MA, et al: Efficacy and safety of nefazodone in the treatment of adolescents with major depressive disorder. J Child Adolesc Psychopharmacol 12:299, 2002.

98. Emslie GJ, Findling RL, Yeung PP, et al: Efficacy and safety of venlafaxine ER in children and adolescents with major depressive disorder. Presented at the annual meeting of the American Psychiatric Association, New York, May 2004.

99. Lock J, Walker LR, Rickert VI, et al: Suicidality in adolescents being treated with antidepressant medications and the black box label: Position paper of the Society for Adolescent Medicine. J Adolesc Health 36:92-93, 2005.

100. Jick H, Kaye JA, Jick SS: Antidepressants and the risk of suicidal behaviors. JAMA 292:338-343, 2004.

101. Simeon J, Nixon MK, Milin R, et al: Open-label pilot study of St. John's wort in adolescent depression. J Child Adolesc Psychopharmacol 15:293-301, 2005.

102. Findling RL, McNamara NK, O'Riordan MA, et al: An open-label pilot study of St. John's wort in juvenile depression. J Am Acad Child Adolesc Psychiatry 42:908-914, 2003.

103. Sweedo SE, Allen AJ, Glod CA, et al: A controlled trial of light therapy for the treatment of pediatric seasonal affective disorder. J Am Acad Child Adolesc Psychiatry 36:816-821, 1997.

104. Prudic J, Olfson M, Marcus SC, et al: Effectiveness of electroconvulsive therapy in community settings. Biol Psychiatry 55:3010-312, 2004.

105. American Academy of Child and Adolescent Psychiatry: Practice parameter for use of electroconvulsive therapy with adolescents. J Am Acad Child Adolesc Psychiatry 43:1521-1539, 2004.

106. Walter G, Rey JM: An epidemiological study of the use of ECT in adolescents. J Am Acad Child Adolesc Psychiatry 36:809-815, 1997.

107. Brent DA, Holder D, Kolko D, et al: A clinical psychotherapy trial for adolescent depression comparing cognitive, family, and supportive therapy. Arch Gen Psychiatry 54:877-885, 1997.

108. Clarke GN, Hornbrook M, Lynch F, et al: Group cognitive-behavioral treatment for depressed adolescent offspring of depressed parents in a health maintenance organization. J Am Acad Child Adolesc Psychiatry 41:305-313, 2002.

109. Vostanis P, Feehan C, Gratten E, et al: A randomized controlled outpatient trial of cognitive-behavioral treatment for children and adolescents with depression: A nine-month follow-up. J Affect Disord 40:105-116, 1996.

110. Wood A, Harrington R, Moore A: Controlled trial of a brief cognitive-behavioral intervention in adolescent patients with depressive disorders. J Child Psychol Psychiatry 37:737-746, 1996.

111. Rossello J, Bernal G: The efficacy of cognitive-behavioral and interpersonal treatments for depression in Puerto Rican adolescents. J Consult Clin Psychol 67:734-745, 1999.

112. Clarke GN, Rohde P, Lewinsohn PM, et al: Cognitive-behavioral treatment of adolescent depression: Efficacy of acute group treatment and booster sessions. J Am Acad Child Adolesc Psychiatry 38:272-279, 1999.

113. Lewinsohn PM, Clarke GN, Hops H, et al: Cognitive-behavioral treatment for depressed adolescents. Behav Ther 18:85-102, 1990.

114. Mufson L, Weissman MM, Moreau D, et al: Efficacy of interpersonal psychotherapy for depressed adolescents. Arch Gen Psychiatry 56:573-579, 1999.

115. Mufson L, Dorta KP, Wickramaratne P, et al: A randomized effectiveness trial of interpersonal psychotherapy for depressed adolescents. Arch Gen Psychiatry 61:577-584, 2004.

116. Mufson L, Dorta KP: Interpersonal psychotherapy for depressed adolescents. In Kazdin AE, Weisz JR, eds: Evidence-Based Psychotherapies for Children and Adolescents. New York: Guilford, 2003, pp 148-164.

116a. American Academy of Child and Adolescent Psychiatry: Practice parameters for the assessment and treatment of children and adolescents with bipolar disorder. J Am Acad Child Adolesc Psychiatry 46:107-125, 2007.

117. Geller B, Cooper TB, Sun K, et al: Double-blind and placebo-controlled study of lithium for adolescent bipolar disorders with secondary substance dependency. J Am Acad Child Adolesc Psychiatry 37:171-178, 1998.

118. Kafantaris V, Coletti DJ, Dicker R, et al: Lithium treatment of acute mania in adolescents: A placebo-controlled discontinuation study. J Am Acad Child Adolesc Psychiatry 43:984-993, 2004.

119. Findling RL, McNamara NK, Youngstrom EA, et al: Double-blind 18-month trial of lithium versus divalproex maintenance treatment in pediatric bipolar disorder. J Am Acad Child Adolesc Psychiatry 44:409-417, 2005.

120. DelBello MP, Schwiers ML, Rosenberg HL, et al: A double-blind, randomized, placebo-controlled study of quetiapine as adjunctive treatment for adolescent mania. J Am Acad Child Adolesc Psychiatry 41:1216-1223, 2002.

121. Scheffer RE, Kowatch RA, Carmody T, et al: Randomized, placebo-controlled trial of mixed amphetamine salts for symptoms of comorbid ADHD in pediatric bipolar disorder after mood stabilization with divalproex sodium. Am J Psychiatry 162:58-64, 2005.

122. Keck PE, McElroy SL: Pharmacological treatments for bipolar disorder. *In* Nathan PE, Gorman JM, eds: A Guide to Treatments That Work, 2nd ed. London: Oxford University Press, 2002, pp 277-299.

123. Lofthouse N, Fristad MA: Psychosocial interventions for children with early-onset bipolar spectrum disorder. Clin Child Fam Psychol Rev 7:71-88, 2004.

124. Colom F, Vieta E, Martínez-Arán A, et al: A randomized trial on the efficacy of group psychoeducation in the prophylaxis of recurrences in bipolar patients whose disease is in remission. Arch Gen Psychiatry 60:402-407, 2003.

125. Miklowitz DJ, Richards JA, George EL, et al: Integrated family and individual therapy for bipolar disorder: Results of a treatment development study. J Clin Psychiatry 64:182-191, 2003.

126. Fristad MA, Goldberg-Arnold JS, Gavazzi SM: Multifamily psychoeducation groups (MFPG) in the treatment of children with mood disorders. J Marital Fam Ther 29:491-504, 2003.

127. Fristad MA, Goldberg-Arnold JS, Gavazzi SM: Multifamily psychoeducation groups (MFPG) for families of children with bipolar disorder. Bipolar Disord 4:254-262, 2002.

128. Fristad MA: Psychoeducational treatment for school-aged children with bipolar disorder. Dev Psychopathol 18:1289-1306, 2006.

129. Miklowitz DJ, Simoneau TL, George EL, et al: Family-focused treatment of bipolar disorder: One-year effects of a psychoeducational program in conjunction with pharmacotherapy. Biol Psychiatry 48:582-592, 2000.

130. Miklowitz DJ, George EL, Richards JA, et al: A randomized study of family-focused psychoeducation and pharmacotherapy in the outpatient management of bipolar disorder. Arch Gen Psychiatry 60:904-912, 2003.

131. Rea MM, Tompson M, Miklowitz DJ, et al: Family focused treatment vs. individual treatment for bipolar disorder: Results of a randomized clinical trial. J Consult Clin Psychol 71:482-492, 2003.

132. Miklowitz DJ, George EL, Axelson DA, et al: Family-focused treatment for adolescents with bipolar disorder. J Affect Disord 82(Suppl 1):S113-S128, 2004.

133. Pavuluri MN, Graczyk,PA, Henry DB, et al: Child-and family-focused cognitive behavioral therapy for pediatric bipolar disorder: Development and preliminary results. J Am Acad Child Adolesc Psychiatry 43:528-537, 2004.

134. Gilham JE, Reivich KJ, Jaycox LH, et al: Prevention of depressive symptoms in schoolchildren: Two-year follow-up. Psychol Sci 6:343-351, 1995.

135. Clarke GN, Hawkins W, Murphy M, et al: Targeted prevention of uinpolar depressive disorder in an at-risk sample of high school adolescents: A randomized trial of group cognitive intervention. J Am Acad Child Adolesc Psychiatry 34:312-321, 1995.

136. Spence SH, Sheffield JK, Donovan CL: Long-term outcome of a school-based, universal approach to prevention of depression in adolescents. J Consult Clin Psychol 73:160-167, 2005.

137. Van Voorhees BW, Ellis J, Stuart S, et al: Pilot study of a primary care Internet-based depression prevention intervention for late adolescents. Can Child Adolesc Psychiatry Rev 14:40-43, 2005.

138. Emslie GJ, Heiligenstein JH, Hoog SL, et al: Fluoxetine treatment for prevention of relapse of depression in children and adolescents: A double-blind, placebo-controlled study. J Am Acad Child Adolesc Psychiatry 43:1397-1405, 2004.

139. Coyle JT, Pine DS, Charney DS, et al: Depression and bipolar alliance consensus statement on the unmet needs in diagnosis and treatment of mood disorders in children and adolescents. J Am Acad Child Adolesc Psychiatry 42:1494-1503, 2003.

140. Katon W, Von Korff M, Lin E, et al: Stepped collaborative care for primary care patients with persistent symptoms of depression: A randomized trial. Arch Gen Psychiatry 56:1109-1115, 1999.

18B.
Anxiety Disorders

KATHLEEN L. LEMANEK
KERI BROWN KIRSCHMAN

Anxiety is a multidimensional construct, involving three dimensions: subjective distress, physiological response, and avoidance or escape behaviors.[1] Clinical levels of anxiety and anxiety disorders are common in both referred and nonreferred children and adolescents. Pediatric anxiety disorders co-occur with other childhood disorders; persist over time; interfere with functioning at school, at home, and with peers; and may be predictive of dysfunction in later childhood, adolescence, and adulthood.[2,3] These conclusions are based on increased knowledge about the classification, etiology, assessment, and treatment of anxiety disorders in children and adolescents since the 1980s.[4] The two most recent editions of the *Diagnostic and Statistical Manual of Mental Disorders (DSM)*[5,6] detail the diagnostic criteria for 12 anxiety disorders that are applicable to children, adolescents, and adults: Panic Disorder with and without Agoraphobia, Agoraphobia without History of Panic Disorder, Specific Phobia, Social Phobia, Obsessive-Compulsive Disorder (OCD), Posttraumatic Stress Disorder (PTSD), Acute Stress Disorder, Generalized Anxiety Disorder (GAD), Anxiety Disorder Due to a General Medical Condition, Substance-Induced Anxiety Disorder, and Anxiety Disorder Not Otherwise Specified.

This chapter provides an overview of key terms in describing anxiety and fear in children and adolescents, along with prevalence rates of anxiety disorders in youths and their effect on functioning. Diagnostic considerations are presented with a description of the varied assessment methods and measures for pediatric and adolescent anxiety disorders. The diagnostic criteria and prevalence, causes, and unique assessment measures are delineated for seven specific disorders: GAD, separation anxiety disorder (SAD), panic disorder, PTSD, social anxiety, OCD, and phobias. The chapter concludes with general intervention and referral guidelines for primary care pediatrician and developmental-behavioral pediatricians, as well as conclusions to foster future research and clinical practice. Other chapters in this book address psychological and pharmacological treatments for childhood anxiety disorders.

OVERVIEW

Definition of Key Terms

Anxiety, worry, and fear are related and yet distinct concepts, and the terms should not be used interchangeably.[7,8] Simply stated, anxiety is a mood state characterized by worry or apprehension about future or anticipated situations.[9] The definition given by Barlow[10] is more elaborate: Anxiety is "a future-oriented emotion, characterized by perceptions of uncontrollability and unpredictability over potentially aversive events and a rapid shift in attention to the focus of potentially dangerous events or one's own affective response to these events" (p 104). It is represented by a tripartite response system, including verbal or cognitive components, motor or behavioral components, and somatic or physiological components.[11] The *cognitive component* pertains to thoughts, images, beliefs, and attributions about the situation and expected outcomes (e.g., "What if I have a heart attack because I cannot breathe?" "What if I fail this test and do not graduate?" "What if no one picks me up after school?"). The *behavioral component* consists of motor responses that involve escaping, avoiding, or taking action (e.g., trembling, running). The *physiological component* involves sensations of the flight-or-fight response or other somatic responses, such as muscle tension and increased heart rate.[12]

Worry involves thoughts and images that pertain to potentially threatening future events and is thus considered one of the cognitive components of anxiety.[13] Borkovec and colleagues[14] stated that "normal" worry manifests with minimal perceived or actual peripheral physiological activation and greater intrusions of negative thoughts in comparison with somatic aspects of anxiety. In addition, the content of worries differ from time to time and in response to changes in life circumstances. Silverman and Ollendick[15] indicated that both worry and avoidance reflect maladaptive coping efforts in response to aversive states that are pervasive, intense, or uncontrollable. As worry persists and becomes excessive, it is deemed a dysfunctional process according to the fourth edition of the *DSM (DSM-IV)*.[5]

Fear is an emotion that is related to the fight-or-flight system, which involves triggering the autonomic nervous system along with focusing attention on escaping the situation or fighting the potential threat.[16] Thus, fear is viewed as a physiological response and is linked to the biological alarm system.[8] Fear is essential in focusing attention to immediate danger, learning how to overcome dangerous situations, and learning how to differentiate threatening from harmless situations.[12] Two key differences between anxiety and fear are whether the interpretation of threat is immediate or future oriented and whether the physiological arousal is an alarm reaction or excessive apprehension.[9]

Complicating the conceptual distinction between anxiety and fear is the high correlation with depression. The construct of negative affectivity refers to the nonspecific component of generalized distress that is common to anxiety and depression.[15] Examples of symptoms that reflect negative affect include anxious or depressed mood, sleep difficulties, and irritability. An elaborate study implemented by Chorpita and colleagues[17] confirmed the distinction among anxiety, fear, and depression as separate constructs. Their data indicate that anxiety reflected general distress; fear was equated with heightened physiological arousal; and depression corresponded to low positive affect. Additional research is needed to further distinguish these constructs from others, such as attention-deficit/hyperactivity disorder (ADHD), and to describe their course of development.[12]

Function of Worry

Borkovec and colleagues[14,18] offered a detailed conceptualization of the formation and maintenance of worry, with implications for the development of anxiety disorders. According to these authors, worry represents the end result of an avoidance response to perceived threats. Behavioral inhibition is considered a temperamental category and appears related to the defensive reactions delineated by Barlow and colleagues.[10,16] It is defined in terms of reactions of withdrawal, wariness, avoidance, and shyness in novel situations.

Defensive reactions are started when a threatening stimulus (object, person, situation) is perceived by a person; these reactions include automatic activation and inhibition, behavioral avoidance and or inhibition, catastrophic images and thoughts. Worry as a cognitive process is considered an example of long-term cognitive avoidance of future catastrophes or negative events. Barlow and collagues[10,14] propose a suppression of physiological-affective processes as a direct outcome of such cognitive activity. They suggest that chronic worriers and nonanxious controls display activation of the frontal cortex during worrying, but chronic worriers display greater left than right frontal activation. Furthermore, worries about one topic tend to easily spread or generalize to related and unrelated topics. The results or consequences of such cognitive activity reportedly hinder new learning and maintain distressing emotional states.

Retrospective and prospective studies have linked certain early temperamental styles with anxiety and suggest that temperamental styles of high arousal, emotionality, and behavioral inhibition place youth at risk for developing later anxiety symptoms and disorders.[19] In addition, adverse life events, especially uncontrollable ones, place individuals at greater risk of developing an anxiety disorder. Finally, the difference between a vulnerability and a disorder is probably a function of symptom severity and interference with daily activities.

Worry may serve two purposes or functions.[20] One function is preparational, whereby worry at a moderate level may motivate a person to accomplish tasks. Within this function, worry supposedly suppresses somatic responses and decreases uncomfortable emotional reactions, thereby allowing the person to prepare for anticipated negative events.[14] A second function of worry is avoidance, with regard to distracting the person from other emotional events and situations. Worry involves efforts to prevent the occurrence of negative events or to cope if and, when these events occur, through problem-solving strategies. Theorists also propose that although worry may offer some advantages, such as initial reduction of somatic distress, it interferes with emotional processing of negative events. As such, efforts at problem solving are not often effective, and the anxiety response is maintained.[18,21]

Normative Data on Worry

Many studies document the relatively common occurrence of fears in children. Almost 70% of children report worrying. Girls report more fears than do boys; at some point during their development, children experience between 9 and 13 fears on average 2 or 3 days per week.[12,22] In studies on the frequency and content of children's worries, investigators have identified developmental, gender, and potentially ethnic differences.[8,23,24]

The frequency of fears decreases, and their focus changes with age. From birth through age 18 years, fears change: Among preschool-aged children, they concern separation from caregivers and imaginary or supernatural creatures; in children aged 5 to 6 years old, they concern threats to physical well-being; among older children, they concern personal and social performance.[24,25] In general, the worries of school-aged children (i.e., 7 to 14 years old) center on school performance, health, and personal harm. Young adolescents appear to worry more intensely about social issues, such as war, money, and disasters. Some studies (e.g., Vasey et al[24]) but not others (e.g., Silverman et al[8]) reveal age-related differences with regard to a greater number of worries in school-aged children than in younger children. Most experts in this area (e.g., Silverman et al[8]) suggest that the content of worries is associated with current social circumstances and media attention.

Girls are said to display more extreme symptoms and to report more worries than do boys in both clinical and community samples.[8,26] Children of African-American ethnicity reported more worries than did white or Hispanic children.[8]

Several studies have focused on the frequency, intensity, and content of worries of clinically referred children in comparison with community samples. Overall, it appears that the intensity but not the number of worries differs between these two samples.[27,28] The content of their worries—namely, school, health, disasters, and personal harm—are reflective of contemporary social challenges and concerns. The authors of these studies proposed that intensity more than specific content serves to differentiate children with anxiety syndromes or disorders from those without.

General Prevalence

The literature indicates that 18% of school-aged children are identified by their primary care clinicians as having a psychosocial problem.[29-31] Other studies (e.g., Wren et al[32]) have revealed that clinicians identify mood or anxiety syndromes on only 3.3% of visits. Differences in these rates appear related to how well the clinician knew the child, whether the visit was a well-child appointment rather than for acute care, and the presence of comorbid behavioral problems.[30,32] Prevalence rates of specific anxiety disorders in children and adolescents typically range from 2% to 7%,[3] whereas rates for clinical levels of anxiety among children range from 10% to 21%.[33] Some guidelines help distinguish "normal" fears and worries from those that are dysfunctional and suggest a true anxiety disorder[12]: First, the intensity of the worry/fear is out of proportion to the actual threat of the situation. Second, the frequency of the worry/fear increases despite reassurance. Third, the content of the worry/fear concerns a harmless object or situation that poses minimal harm. Fourth, the worry/fear seems spontaneous. Finally, escape or avoidance is often in reaction to the worry/fear.

Effect of Anxiety Disorders

Children and adolescents with anxiety syndromes or disorders are at risk for a variety of problems across domains of functioning. Longitudinal studies have demonstrated an association between anxiety disorders and educational underachievement and between these disorders and alcohol and other drug use.[3,34] The risk of other emotional problems is consistently documented in the literature[3,34]; the occurrence of anxiety disorders commonly precedes those of depressive disorders and substance abuse disorders.[35,36] Alcohol and other drugs may be used to self-medicate or to manage symptoms of anxiety.[37] Difficulties in social and peer relations that contribute to feelings of loneliness and low self-esteem also are related to anxiety disorders.[38]

The effect of anxiety disorders on health care utilization and health care costs is evident in the pediatric and adult literature. Studies on older adolescents and adults indicate high utilization of specialists and primary care physicians for symptoms of anxiety.[39,40] Increased utilization results from frequent visits to physicians and emergency rooms, extensive laboratory tests, medications, and prolonged hospitalizations.[40] Specialists most often seen include gastroenterologists for individuals with GAD, because of abdominal complaints; dermatologists and cardiologists for those with OCD, because of skin conditions and problems breathing; and neurologists and urologists for those with panic disorders, because of multiple physical symptoms. In one study, 54% of patients with irritable bowel syndrome had diagnoses of GAD, and 29% had diagnoses of panic disorder.[41]

Diagnostic Considerations

In a thorough review of the assessment literature on anxiety disorders, Silverman and Ollendick[15] indicated that anxiety disorder diagnoses co-occur most frequently with other anxiety disorders, next most frequently with depression, and third most frequently with externalizing disorders, such as ADHD or oppositional defiant disorder. Symptoms of anxiety and resultant diagnoses tend to persist over time, and the condition is often refractory to intervention.[42,43] Two constructs are critical in understanding the comorbidity patterns and course of anxiety disorders: (1) threshold for clinical significance and (2) sensitivity and specificity of assessment measures.

The term *threshold* pertains to the frequency and intensity of symptoms necessary to detect the presence of a disorder, along with level of impairment. The phrase "clinical level" is used in a case when all diagnostic criteria are met and impairment is severe.[29] The term *subthreshold*, refers to cases in which diagnostic criteria are met but impairment is mild to moderate. An optimal threshold for clinical significance is currently arbitrary, but low thresholds may help identify youth at risk for psychopathology, whereas higher thresholds help identify those requiring immediate treatment. Less stringent impairment thresholds may be preferred with regard to internalizing disorders, such as anxiety disorders, because the nature of the symptoms is less overt and disruptive than are symptoms.[29,44]

Silverman and Ollendick[15] also proposed that discriminating between anxiety and other constructs is related to the diagnostic accuracy of anxiety assessment measures. The diagnostic value of these measures pertains to their sensitivity and specificity. Silverman and Ollendick[15] defined *sensitivity* as the percentage of people who receive a diagnosis and who have been positively identified by rating scales, or true-positive cases. They defined *specificity* as the percentage of people who do not receive a diagnosis and who have not been identified by rating scales, or true-negative cases. Anxiety assessment measures are reviewed in the next section.

Research clearly indicates that anxiety disorders in youths share the same underlying constructs, display solid covariation with each other over time, seldom occur as singular conditions, and exhibit comparable familial constellations with adult anxiety and depressive disorders.[4,10,45] Clinicians within primary care settings are expressing the need for practical and validated screening measures for mood syndromes and disorders in children and adolescents.[32]

ASSESSMENT METHODS

Since the 1980s, attention has been directed toward developing reliable and valid assessment measures for anxiety disorders in children and adolescents for accurate diagnosis and for formulating treatment plans and monitoring treatment outcome.[4,46] Readers are referred to excellent reviews by Kearney and Wadiak,[46] Silverman and Ollendick,[15] and Velting and associates.[4] The following discussion outlines recommended assessment protocols from these reviews; measures specific to individual disorders are listed in subsequent sections.

A multimethod and a multisource assessment approach is recommended for examining biological, cognitive, and behavioral aspects of anxiety from a variety of sources, such as the child, the parents, and the teachers, through the use of diverse methods, including structured interviews, rating scales, and observations. Kendall and colleagues[47] also proposed a multistage sampling design in which a screening measure is administered first and followed by a more detailed diagnostic interview for persons identified from the initial screening. This process focuses on identifying the existence of an anxiety disorder and then determining the exact nature of the disorder. In general, self-report, parent, and teacher rating scales are frequently used for screening purposes. These rating scales also are administered to identify specific symptoms, to discriminate between anxiety and other constructs, and to examine treatment outcome. Semistructured and structured interviews are employed primarily to diagnose specific anxiety disorders, as well as to identify symptoms and to evaluate treatment effectiveness. Finally, rating scales, direct observations, and self-monitoring are used to identify specific aspects of anxiety that serve to maintain its occurrence and changes during treatment.

Various problems are evident with assessment methods and measures for anxiety disorders in youths. The predictive power of methods and measures requires further exploration. For example, a greater number of individuals may be identified as having anxiety symptoms or disorders at initial screening because of the higher false-positive values in comparison with true-positive values on self-report rating scales.[34] Many assessment methods are limited in terms of developmental differences, including age and gender.[46] Diagnostic interviews are difficult to administer, and self-report measures are less reliable with younger children.[48] Furthermore, self-monitoring and behavioral observations may be more reactive with older children and adolescents. Many assessment measures lack appropriate cultural variations, such as idioms of distress and interpretation of worry.[49]

A medical condition or substance use should be confirmed or ruled out when anxiety symptoms are assessed.[49] Therefore, a targeted medical examination should be completed before a final diagnosis is established, with the use of data from other methods. Individuals should be questioned about prescription medications; over-the-counter medications, especially those containing ephedrine and appetite suppressants; and caffeine intake, such as colas and chocolate. Othmer and Othmer[50] provide a detailed list of medication side effects related to mental health symptoms. Fong and Silien[49] describe a range of medical conditions associated with anxiety symptoms, such as specific neurological disorders (e.g., multiple sclerosis, temporal lobe epilepsy), endocrine disorders (e.g., hyperthyroidism, Cushing syndrome), immune and collagen disorders (e.g., lupus erythematosus), and cardiovascular disorders (e.g., anemia, mitral valve prolapse).

Semistructured and Structured Interviews

Semistructured and structured interviews offer the most reliable means of diagnosis because of the degree of information solicited from children and their parents.[51] However, the 2 to 3 hours needed to complete these interviews may be prohibitive in some settings.[4] The length appears related to the experience of the interviewer, the cooperation of the family, and the level of functional impairment of the youth. In addition, children report fewer symptoms than do their parents and may be less reliable in specifying symptom onset and duration.[52] Examples of common interviews for school-aged children and adolescents include the Schedule for Affective Disorders and Schizophrenia in School-Aged Children[53] and the Diagnostic Interview Schedule for Children.[54] The Anxiety Disorders Interview Schedule for Children[55] assesses for the presence and severity of anxiety, mood, and externalizing disorders, and it screens for learning and developmental disorders, substance abuse, eating disorders, psychotic symptoms, and somatoform disorders. This measure has strong psychometric properties and has been studied extensively in the literature on anxiety disorders.[15]

Self-Report Rating Scales

Self-report rating scales provide information from the youth's perspective about the frequency and intensity of cognitive, behavioral, and physiological aspects of anxiety. The majority of self-report scales for anxiety disorders require a second to third grade reading level but take only about 10 to 15 minutes to complete and can be manually scored easily.[4] Examples of self-report rating scales for general anxiety include the Revised Children's Manifest Anxiety Scale (RCMAS),[56] the State-Trait Anxiety Inventory for Children,[57] the Screen for Anxiety and Related Emotional Disorders (SCARED),[58] and the Children's Anxiety Sensitivity Index.[59] The Negative Affect Self-Statement Questionnaire[60] may be considered because of the relevance of negative affect and comorbidity between anxiety and depression. Finally, the Youth Self-Report[61] and the Behavior Assessment System for Children[62] may be given as general self-report measures of both internalizing problems and externalizing problems. The SCARED appears to be useful in clinical practice, whereas the RCMAS and the State-Trait Anxiety Inventory for Children are used often in research.[4,15] Appendix A provides a listing of resources for ordering specific self-report and parent and teacher rating scales. The specific websites should be consulted about restrictions of who may order and administer these measures. Measures not listed in Appendix A can be obtained by contacting the authors noted in the reference section.

Parent and Teacher Rating Scales

Data from multiple informants are crucial for accurate assessment because of the high parent-child discordance, especially with internalizing disorders such as anxiety and depression.[15] The perspective of parents and teachers should be solicited with regard to the range of symptoms shown by the youth, in order to place the anxiety symptoms within a context of other problems.[4] In addition, symptoms may be quantified and may be monitored over the course of treatment.[15] These rating scales are time and cost efficient and are fairly easy to administer and to score, with the use of hand-scoring templates or computer programs, but the problem of self-disclosure is considerable.[4,15] Examples of general, corresponding parent and teacher rating scales are the Child Behavior Checklist[63] and the Teacher Report Form,[64] the Conners' Parent and Teacher Rating Scales,[65] and a parent version of the SCARED. A measure of family environment, such as the Family Environment Scale,[66] or of

marital functioning, such as the Marital Adjustment Scale,[67] also may be administered to obtain additional data about family factors that affect the presence of anxiety symptoms.

Behavior Observations

Behavioral observations include such procedures as behavioral approach tests, observational ratings, and role-play tests. Behavioral approach tests usually consist of five 5-minute phases that are held in analogue settings (e.g., giving speech), under stimulated conditions (e.g., tape recordings of thunder or visual displays of spiders), or in a naturalistic setting (e.g., at school): adaptation, baseline, walking baseline, approach, and post-baseline to assess social anxiety, specific phobias, or generalized anxiety.[46] Observational ratings are provided by clinicians, parents, or teachers on diverse aspects of anxiety, including overt statements, trembling, and avoidance of the situation.[68] Direct observational procedures are most useful in specialty clinics or experimental settings because of their obtrusive nature and complexity of implementation.[15] An alternative approach may be to videotape at home and view the tape in the clinic setting.[4] Examples of direct observational measures include the Observer Rating Scale of Anxiety,[69] the Procedure Behavior Rating Scale,[70] and the Behavioral Assertiveness Test for Children.[71] An addition to these methods is to observe family interactions in order to examine the factors that may be maintaining anxiety symptoms, such as misinterpreting ambiguous situations and reinforcing avoidant behavioral styles.[15] These observations are categorized as the Family Behavioral Test.[17,72]

Self-Monitoring

Self-monitoring involves monitoring and recording components of anxiety, including physical sensations, related thoughts, and behavior, along with the situation in which these symptoms occur.[4] Self-monitoring is used to identify and quantify symptoms and controlling variables and to evaluate and monitor treatment outcomes.[73] Self-monitoring is of limited value because in many trials, only between 31% and 39% of children record requested information for a full 2-week period.[15] A brief description of symptoms, specific antecedents, and consequences of these symptoms can be recorded in a diary format. In addition, an anxiety rating (on a scale of 0 to 100) may be given to each description, as well as to an overall daily rating. Thought-listing and think-aloud procedures may be included within this method of assessment.[46] Thought listing consists of recording thoughts associated with the anxious reaction,[74] whereas think-aloud procedures involve audiotaping verbalizations of thoughts and placing these thoughts into categories.[75]

Physiological Assessment

Various physiological responses may be used as a measure of anxiety, although their reliability and validity have been mixed.[4,15] In addition, there are few normative data by which to compare baseline responses or changes after interventions. Examples of physiological measures include heart rate and blood pressure, to examine cardiovascular reactivity; respiration and skin temperature, to assess blood flow to extremities and physiological arousal; and electromyography, to measure electrical activity in tense muscles.[4,15]

SPECIFIC ANXIETY DISORDERS

According to the *DSM-IV*,[5] anxious apprehension is a critical process in all anxiety disorders; it is defined as the anticipation of future danger, accompanied by feelings of dysphoria or symptoms of tension. Multiple factors are judged to interact in the origin of anxiety disorders in children and adolescents, including biological predispositions, psychological vulnerabilities, environmental stressors, sociocultural demands, familial variables, and functional influences. Integrative models are currently emphasized, inasmuch as changes in cognitions and behaviors are assumed to effect neurobiological processes and genetic expression[76] (see Albano et al[12] for a review of integrative models of anxiety in children). Kearney and Wadiak[46] suggested that contemporary models belong to one of three categories: behavioral, cognitive, and physiological. A behavioral model highlights the learning principles of classical and operant conditioning within Mowrer's[77] two-factor theory or Delprato and McGlynn's[78] approach-withdrawal theory. In general, anxiety or avoidance is learned through classical conditioning and maintained by reinforcement of nonaversive reactions and situations. Cognitive models of fear and anxiety disorders include Beck and Emery's[79] schema theory and Reiss's[80] expectancy-anxiety sensitivity theory. In these models, normal physiological responses are misinterpreted as negative. Individuals avoid situations that cue these response because they expect negative consequences. Physiological models address genetic factors revealed through family and twin studies, along with a range of biological variables such as changes in the basal ganglia (OCD); mitral valve prolapse (panic disorder); and dysfunctions in neurochemical substances, including γ-amino butyric acid (GAD),

norepinephrine (panic disorder), and serotonin (OCD) (see Biederman et al,[81] for a detailed review of these physiological processes).

Generalized Anxiety Disorder

DIAGNOSTIC CRITERIA

The diagnostic criteria for GAD are outlined in Table 18B-1. Worry that is difficult to control is the most prominent clinical feature of GAD. Some authors[82] question the applicability of a GAD diagnosis in children because of differences in the occurrence of specific somatic complaints in children and adolescents. For example, headaches and stomachaches are the most common somatic complaints reported by children, but these complaints are not included in the symptoms of GAD in the fourth edition, text revision of the *DSM* (*DSM-IV-TR*).[6] In addition, although muscle tension is one physiological response that discriminates adults with a diagnosis of GAD from nonanxious controls,[83] muscle tension is least often reported by parents and children. On the other hand, reducing the number of symptoms required from criterion C in Table 18B-1 from three to one for children and adolescents may increase the diagnostic prediction of GAD.[84]

Finally, for a diagnosis of GAD, symptoms of anxiety cannot be caused by a substance, a medical condition, or other mental health disorder. The level of impairment in functioning required by all *DSM-IV-TR* diagnostic categories may prompt parents and teachers to seek referrals to health care or mental health care professionals.

COMORBIDITY

Additional findings reveal comorbidity with mood disorders; generalized anxiety most often occurs before depression.[36,85] Externalizing disorders, such as ADHD and oppositional defiant disorder, also appear to co-occur with GAD, but not more so than with any other anxiety disorder.[85,86]

PREVALENCE

The prevalence of GAD in children and adolescents is between 2% and 5%[87]; onset of the full syndrome generally occurs in later adolescence or early adulthood. The diagnosis is made twice as often in girls as in boys.[88] GAD is associated with a lower spontaneous recovery rate than are other anxiety disorders.[26]

CAUSES

The combined roles of biological factors, psychological factors, and environmental factors are consistently delineated in the literature on the causes of GAD.[19] Evidence is suggestive of a general predisposition toward anxiety rather than a specific heritability for GAD.[89] It appears that affected individuals possess an anxious vulnerability that is manifested as heightened sensitivity, greater emotionality, and enhanced physiological arousal in response to threat. This greater emotionality and physiological arousal foster a tendency to interpret situations as threatening and to develop an avoidant coping style. Avoidance of novel situations is rewarding by reducing distress and obtaining attention from others in the environment. Also, an anxious temperament allows the individual to solicit behaviors from others in the environment that support avoidant and other maladaptive coping styles. For example, parents' heightened attention to the youth's efforts to prevent or cope with anxiety may actually increase the youth's perception of the degree of threat, even though, if the threat were not real, minimal attention would be devoted to it. Modeling and verbal statements from the family, along with cultural and social influences, seem to transmit information about anxious behaviors to youths.

A multivariate twin analysis of more than 1000 pairs of twin girls[90] suggests that the genetic influences for anxiety disorders are accounted for by two factors: one for phobia, panic, and bulimia and the other for GAD and major depression. Studies also support a familial basis of anxiety in that parents exhibit a cognitive bias toward threats and reinforce an avoidant response in their children.[72]

The literature dictates that worry as the principal component of GAD reflects a style of cognitive avoidance.[19,23] Cognitive avoidance with regard to GAD is conceptualized as composed of cognitive activity or "verbal" content.[91,92] The verbal content of worry allows the person to avoid fearful images and to decrease arousal. Subsequently, the avoidance of fearful images and physiological arousal maintains worry, but at the cost of not dealing with the emotional aspect of the worries. In relation to worry, key features of GAD are intolerance of uncertainty and poor problem orientation.[93] This intolerance of uncertainty is defined as the way an individual perceives information in uncertain or ambiguous situations and responds to this information with a set of cognitive, emotional, and behavioral reactions.[94]

ASSESSMENT

In general, the range of assessment methods and measures outlined in this section are applicable for diagnosis, symptom identification, and treatment outcome in GAD. The SCARED is recommended by several investigators to detect GAD in children and adolescents because of sufficient sensitivity and specificity (e.g., Muris et al[95]). The RCMAS also is used in clinical practice to examine overall levels of anxiety.

Obsessive-Compulsive Disorder

DIAGNOSTIC CRITERIA

The diagnostic criteria for OCD are listed in Table 18B-1. The obsessions appear to be irrational, are difficult to remove, and usually pertain to perceived risk or harm.[96] The compulsions are performed in an effort to suppress, organize, or ignore the obsessive thoughts.[97] Common content of obsessions include contamination by dirt or germs, aggression, inanimate-interpersonal objects (e.g., locks, bolts), sex, and religion.[98] Compulsive behaviors often seen are hand washing, cleaning, checking, repetitive touching, counting, and ordering. These obsessions and compulsions generally take up more than an hour a day and cause distress or functional impairment in academics, with peers and family members, and with activities of daily living.[5]

Long-term follow-up studies of OCD in children and adolescents reveal a chronic, waxing-and-waning course, regardless of medication or behavior therapy treatment.[99,100] Symptoms persist but change over time; for example, checking rituals may become ordering compulsions, and contamination fears may

---

TABLE 18B-1 ■ Diagnostic Criteria for Generalized Anxiety Disorder (GAD) and Obsessive-Compulsive Disorder (OCD)

Diagnostic Criteria for GAD
A. Excessive anxiety/worry more days than not for at least 6 months, about a number of events or activities
B. Uncontrollability
C. One or more of the following:
  Restlessness/keyed up
  Easily fatigued
  Difficulty concentrating
  Irritability
  Muscle tension
  Sleep disturbance

Diagnostic Criteria for OCD
A. Either obsessions or compulsions and defined by:
  Intrusive thoughts, impulses, or images (i.e., obsessions)
  Not simply excessive worries about real-life problems
  Ignoring, suppressing, or neutralizing with other thoughts or actions
  Product of own mind
  Repetitive behaviors or mental acts the person feels driven to perform (i.e., compulsions)
  Behaviors or mental acts aimed at preventing or reducing distress
B. Obsessions or compulsions recognized as unreasonable
C. Causes distress and interferes with normal routine or functioning
D. Not caused by substance or medical condition

Data from American Psychiatric Association: Diagnostic and Statistical Manual of Mental Disorders, 4th ed, text revision. Washington, DC: American Psychiatric Association, 2000.

become counting rituals.[100] In two follow-up studies of OCD in children,[101,102] 43% to 68% of children continued to meet diagnostic criteria for OCD, and 28% to 57% did not have the disorder at follow-up. The literature provides minimal information on prognostic indicators other than that developmentally appropriate rituals are not predictive of obsessions or compulsions.[103,104]

Subtypes of OCD in adults appear applicable to youths with OCD. The first classification pertains to the presence or absence of a tic disorder; the second classification pertains to familial versus nonfamilial OCD.[105,106] Children without tics seem to have a higher incidence of contamination fears, washing, and repetitive requests for reassurance.[107] Children with nonfamilial OCD may have other disorders suggestive of a central nervous system dysfunction.[104] These subtypes may have implications for etiology and treatment response.[105,107]

There is some diagnostic confusion with regard to the phenomenological overlap between obsessions and worry and between pathological worry and covert compulsive behavior.[108] Although both worry and obsessions involve cognitive activity, worry may be more abstract and verbal in nature, whereas obsession is more imaginative in form.[109] Whether this distinction applies to children is not known, especially as it pertains to differential diagnosis between OCD and GAD.[109] Compulsive behavior in children with OCD and in children with GAD may be distinguished in terms of frequency, rigidity, quality, and function, but empirical verification of these differences is not available in the literature.[108]

COMORBIDITY

Coexisting symptoms and disorders are common in children and adolescents with diagnosed OCD; 62% to 84% exhibit co-occurrence[110] of SAD and GAD. Depressive symptoms and dysthymia[106] also co-occur frequently. Neurological conditions, particularly tics and Tourette syndrome, frequently co-occur in this group, especially in boys. Youths with OCD and Tourette syndrome tend to display more violent and aggressive obsessions and harm-avoidance compulsions.[111]

PREVALENCE

The average age at onset of OCD is between 7.5 years and 12.5 years,[112] and the prevalence is about 1% to 3%.[113] Another 1% to 19% of children may show "subthreshold" or problem levels of OCD.[114] It is diagnosed in twice as many boys as girls during childhood and adolescence, but this pattern reverses in adults with OCD.[115] Earlier age at onset seems related to a familial pattern of OCD.[116] Few differences appear in the frequency of specific obsessions or compulsions

across age groups,[100,117] although adolescent boys may report more religious/moral obsessions than do younger boys.[107]

CAUSES

Although the exact origin of OCD is not known, possible organic causes focus on focal brain lesions, specifically to the basal ganglia, and on immune-mediated sequelae of streptococcal infections.[104,116] Through neuroimaging techniques, the frontal-striatal-thalamic pathway is implicated in the pathophysiology of OCD, along with the neurotransmitters serotonin and ocytocin.[104,107]

The role of heredity was elucidated through one twin study and several family studies, in which the prevalence of OCD was higher among first-degree relatives of patients than among those of controls (11% to 25% vs. 2.7%).[118,119] Concordance for treated youths with OCD was 33% in monozygotic twins, in comparison with 7% in dizygotic twins.[120] A familial component is also suggested by a higher incidence of OCD diagnosed in relatives of youths who received diagnoses of OCD before the age of 17 years.[119] Even higher prevalence rates exist in parents considered to have subthreshold or problematic OCD (8.8% to 42%).

ASSESSMENT

A basic question that clinicians can ask youths is "Do you have thoughts that you cannot get out of your mind or have behaviors you do over and over?" The Leyton Obsessional Inventory–Child Version[121] is a 20-item self-report measure of obsessions and compulsions used for diagnostic screening. Several factors include general obsessive thoughts and rituals, dirt-contamination fears, lucky numbers, and school-related habits. This measure does not provide a rating of severity. Separate child and parent interviews are necessary to determine the extent and the nature of the obsessions and compulsions because of the covert aspect of these symptoms.[116] In addition, if parents have subthreshold or problematic obsessive and compulsive symptoms, they may either become involved in or accommodate the child's ritual.[116] The first choice for rating severity of OCD symptoms is the Children's Yale-Brown Obsessive-Compulsive Scale.[122] The basic 10-item scale is used to rate obsessions and compulsions in terms of degree of severity, interference, distress, resistance, and control. Normative data are available to assist with symptom identification and, subsequently, severity ratings.[116]

A neurological examination is recommended because of the high prevalence (33%) of soft signs and choreiform movements in youth with OCD,[123] reports of streptococcal pharyngeal infections triggering obsessive-compulsive symptoms,[124] and occurrence of obsessive-compulsive symptoms in various neurological disorders, including basal ganglia disorders, Huntington's chorea, and Tourette syndrome.[116] The presence of focal neurological signs may prompt a brain imaging study, such as computed tomography or magnetic resonance imaging study of the brain.[116]

Separation Anxiety Disorders

DIAGNOSTIC CRITERIA

Some difficulty separating from home or attachment figures is normal and expected for children aged 7 months to 6 years.[26] When this distress lingers beyond normal development or is abnormally intense, a child may meet *DSM-IV* criteria for SAD.[5] Furthermore, the *DSM-IV* specifies that the distress upon separation cannot be attributable primarily to pervasive developmental disorder or a psychotic disorder (e.g., schizophrenia) and, in adolescents, cannot be better accounted for by panic disorder with agoraphobia. Diagnostic criteria for SAD are provided in Table 18B-2.

Children with SAD may first come to the awareness of a physician because of refusal to go to school or physiological symptoms, such as recurrent abdominal pain. In a physician's office, these children may present as "clingy." Parents may complain about

---

TABLE 18B-2 ■ **Diagnostic Criteria for Separation Anxiety Disorder**

A. Excessive anxiety in separation from home, or from attachment figure(s), as evidenced by three of the following:
   1. Distress separating from home/attachment figure(s)
   2. Worry about loss of or harm to attachment figure(s)
   3. Worry that untoward event will lead to separation from attachment figure(s)
   4. Reluctance or refusal to go to school because of fear of separation
   5. Reluctance or fearful to be alone or without significant adults
   6. Reluctant/refusal to sleep alone or away from home
   7. Nightmares involving theme of separation
   8. Physical complaints when separation occurs or is anticipated
B. Disturbance of at least 4 weeks in duration
C. Onset before age 18 years
D. Distress/impairment in social, academic, or other area of functioning

Data from American Psychiatric Association: Diagnostic and Statistical Manual of Mental Disorders, 4th ed, text revision. Washington, DC: American Psychiatric Association, 2000.
Note: The *DSM-IV-TR* specifies that the distress on separation cannot be attributable primarily to pervasive developmental disorder or a psychotic disorder (e.g., schizophrenia) and, in adolescents, cannot be better accounted for by panic disorder with agoraphobia.

---

bedtime routines, nightmares, or a child's refusal to engage in normal peer relationships, such as spending time at a friend's house. SAD may initially manifest in situations in which the child is expected to separate from a caregiver (e.g., school), when the child becomes extraordinarily distressed and avoidant of separation situations. Careful observation of these symptoms may reveal a cyclical pattern in which symptoms are exaggerated during times when a child is anticipating or has separated from home or parent.[125] For example, if a child's symptoms may increase just before a parent leaves for work. Refusal to go to school may also be seen in other disorders, such as specific phobia, social phobia, and/or depression.

Symptom manifestation is related to developmental stage: Younger children with SAD tend to have more symptoms and focus on unrealistic worry about harm to a caregiver, whereas older children exhibit excessive distress during times of separation. In adolescence, SAD is typified by somatic complaints and refusal to go to school.[126]

PREVALENCE

The prevalence rate of SAD is approximately 4% among children and adolescents in community samples; the incidence of SAD is higher among girls and younger children.[87,127] The average age at first presentation is 7.5 years. In clinical samples, SAD accounts for approximately one third of anxiety referrals[128] and is the most frequently occurring anxiety disorder in preadolescents.[115] Although girls appear to show more symptoms of SAD than do boys in screening surveys, boys affirm separation anxiety more often in clinical samples, perhaps because these symptoms are less well accepted in boys. Therefore, SAD symptoms in boys may more likely result in a referral for treatment.[129]

CAUSES

Although the specific origin is largely unknown, SAD reportedly has an acute onset, with initial or subsequent occurrence often triggered by a major stressor, such as change of schools, death of a parent, or prolonged illness.[128] Familial patterns are noted for SAD; the risk is increased for children whose parents have panic disorder with features of agoraphobia.[130,131]

The course of SAD is generally favorable for most children. In a study of over 150 children and adolescents with SAD, 80% of cases were improved at an average of 18-month follow-up.[132] Individual and family factors related to a continued SAD diagnosis seem to include the presence of externalizing problems, such as oppositional defiant disorder or ADHD symptoms; parental psychopathology; and parental marital difficulties.[125] In addition, children with persistent SAD may be more likely to receive diagnoses of depressive disorder or another anxiety disorder at a later date.

ASSESSMENT

Parents' and children's reports of SAD symptoms differ; children report more symptoms than do parents, which highlights the importance of multi-informant assessment in diagnosis.[133] There is no parent or self-report questionnaire designed to assess solely diagnostic criteria for SAD. Several of the self-report measures of anxiety have separation anxiety subscales that can be used with children aged 8 years and older, including the SCARED,[58] the Multidimensional Anxiety Scale for Children[134] and the Spence Children's Anxiety Scale.[135] For the interested clinician, a full report regarding assessment of SAD can be found in Perwein and Bernstein.[133] Specific questions suggested for use in initial assessment of SAD include the following: "Are you afraid of something that might happen to your mom or dad?"; "Do you sometimes get nervous when you are alone?"; and "Do you worry about getting lost or kidnapped?" Questions to ask parents include "Does your child have difficulty falling asleep or sleeping alone?"; "Does your child cry or have temper tantrums when anticipating being left with others?"; "Does your child follow you from room to room?"; "Does your child's worries ever keep her or him from normal activities, including school or other fun activities away from home?"; and "Does your child complain of headaches, stomachaches, or body aches frequently on weekdays but not on weekends?"[136]

Post-traumatic Stress Disorder

DIAGNOSTIC CRITERIA

The types of trauma that children and adolescents may experience include motor vehicle collisions, house fires, natural disasters, child maltreatment, violence, and witnessing domestic abuse. These experiences make children vulnerable to PTSD. Table 18B-3 lists the *DSM-IV-TR* criteria for PTSD.[6]

If the child or adolescent's response to the extreme stressor does not meet full criteria for PTSD, or if the pattern of PTSD symptoms occurs for a situation that is not extreme (e.g., parental divorce), a diagnosis of Adjustment Disorder should be considered. Presence of avoidance, numbing, and increased arousal before the stressor are suggestive of another underlining pathological process, such as a different anxiety disorder or mood disorder. If the symptoms have occurred for less than 1 month, a diagnosis of Acute Stress Disorder is warranted initially. The types of PTSD to be specified are acute (less than 3 months), chronic

TABLE 18B-3 ■ Diagnostic Criteria for Posttraumatic Stress Disorder (PTSD)
A. Exposure to event(s) that involved actual or threatened death/injury or a threat to physical integrity. The response was intense fear, helplessness, horror, agitation, and/or disorganization.
B. The traumatic event is reexperienced in one or more of the following ways:
1. Distressing and intrusive recollections of the event or repetitive event-themed play
2. Distressing dreams; for children, frightening dreams with unrecognizable content
3. Acting or feeling as if the traumatic event were recurring; in young children, trauma-specific reenactment may occur
4. Intense psychological distress at exposure to event cues
5. Physiological reactivity on exposure to stimuli that resemble an aspect of the traumatic event
C. Avoidance of trauma reminders and numbing in responsiveness, indicated by at least 3 of the following:
1. Efforts to avoid thoughts, feelings, or conversations about the trauma
2. Avoidance of activities, places, or people that arouse recollections of the trauma
3. Disinterest in significant activities
4. Feelings of detachment or estrangement from others
5. Restricted range of affect
6. Sense of foreshortened future
D. Persistent symptoms of increased arousal, as indicated by 2 of the following:
1. Sleep difficulties
2. Irritability/anger
3. Difficulty concentrating
4. Hypervigilance
5. Exaggerated startle response
E. Duration of the disturbance more than 1 month
F. Significant impairment in social, academic, or other important areas of functioning

Data from American Psychiatric Association: Diagnostic and Statistical Manual of Mental Disorders, 4th ed, text revision. Washington, DC: American Psychiatric Association, 2000.

(longer than 3 months), or delayed onset (6 months after the most recent PTSD stressor).

Knowledge of developmental differences in the manifestation of PTSD is essential. Some scholars question the validity of the *DSM-IV-TR* criteria for very young children, because nearly half the criteria require verbal descriptions of thoughts and feelings that a young child is unlikely to articulate.[137] Young children may have trauma-specific nightmares initially but more generalized nightmares as time passes. Young children with PTSD symptoms may also exhibit fear of the dark, awake frequently at night, and report generalized fears such as "monsters."[138,139] All children may have difficulties separating from parents in the days or weeks after the trauma. Older children and adolescents may report difficulties concentrating on schoolwork or may attempt to self-medicate with drugs and alcohol to alleviate painful reminders of the event.[140] Adolescents may engage in risky behaviors to lesson emotional pain.[141] In addition, older children and adolescents may report extreme levels of guilt for surviving a traumatic experience, when others did not survive.

COMORBIDITY

Children who meet criteria for a diagnosis for PTSD may also meet criteria for other psychiatric conditions, especially mood disorders, such as major depressive disorder and dysthymic disorder.[142,143] The trauma experience, especially those involving maltreatment, may increase the susceptibility to a mood disorder[144] or dissociative disorder.[145] Comorbidity with externalizing disorders such as ADHD, oppositional defiant disorder, and conduct disorder suggests a need for a thorough psychological assessment.

PREVALENCE

The prevalence of PTSD in children and adolescents in the general population is largely unknown. In a clinical sample of children aged 6 to 18, just over 3% of youths in the juvenile justice system and 3% using mental health services met diagnosis for PTSD.[146] Children who were the victims of parental abuse were nearly twice as likely to show signs of PTSD as were those who witnessed domestic violence,[143] of whom 13% met criteria for PTSD.[147] After a category 4 hurricane, 30% of 568 students in third through fifth grades demonstrated severe or very severe PTSD symptoms 3 months later,[148] and 18% demonstrated severe or very severe symptoms 10 months after the hurricane.[149] In a British study, of children who experienced an automobile collision, 35% met diagnostic criteria for PTSD.[150] In general, girls tend to be more symptomatic than are boys.[150,151]

Children who are susceptible to anxiety conditions before a traumatic event are at greater risk for the development of PTSD after a stressor. For example, preexisting anxiety symptoms were predictive of a child's PTSD symptoms 3 and 7 months after Hurricane Andrew.[152] There is a strong association between PTSD and other anxiety conditions, such as GAD and SAD.[153,154]

CAUSES

Factors contributing to the development of PTSD include the severity of trauma, reactions of attachment figures to the trauma, and time since the trauma. Children and adolescents with a history of family psychopathology, violence, child behavior problems, and child maltreatment may be more susceptible to extreme stressors. Children's coping with traumatic stressors is often reflective of parental coping.[155]

ASSESSMENT

In order to make a diagnosis of PTSD, it is important to assess aspects of the child's earlier functioning, severity of the trauma and child's initial reaction, current symptoms, and their effect on the child's life. PTSD-specific assessment measures can help determine whether a child should be referred to a mental health provider for further assessment and treatment. The Traumatic Events Screening Inventory for Children[156] is a self-report checklist that assesses exposure and intensity of the child's response to the trauma and can be used for children as young as 8 years of age. The Children's Post-Traumatic Stress Reaction Index[157] is a 20-item instrument that assesses the severity of PTSD symptoms; however, not all *DSM-IV-TR* criteria are represented. This index can be read aloud to children as a semistructured interview as well.[158]

Because it is difficult for children to assess their reactions at the time of the trauma, an observer report is helpful. However, parents may have difficulty accurately reporting the intensity of their child's PTSD symptoms.[159] Parents' reports are necessary, but they should not be the sole informants. The Child Stress Disorders Checklist[160] is a 36-item observer report measure of PTSD and acute stress disorder. This measure assesses PTSD symptoms in five domains: reexperiencing, arousal, avoidance, numbing and dissociation, and impairment in functioning. Parent and teacher information is important for gaining a better understanding of pretrauma functioning, inasmuch as young children may not be able to reflect accurately on their previous thoughts and behaviors, because of their relative cognitive immaturity.[141]

In addition to self-report and observer report instruments, empirical evidence supports asking children directly about the exposure in order to assess symptoms of PTSD.[161] Initially, children should be given the opportunity to recall the event in their own words. Subsequently, prompts regarding specific aspects of the diagnosis are helpful: for example, "What did you think/feel/hear in your body when the trauma occurred?"[158]

Social Phobia

DIAGNOSTIC CRITERIA

The hallmark feature of social phobia, also known as social anxiety disorder, for children and adolescents is excessive fear of embarrassment in social or performance situations. These feelings of anxiety may advance into a panic attack,[162] and refusal to go to school is a common presenting problem. The diagnostic criteria for social phobia as it relates to children and adolescence is outlined in Table 18B-4.

TABLE 18B-4 ■ Diagnostic Criteria for Social Phobia, Specific Phobia, and Panic Disorder

Diagnostic Criteria for Social Phobia

A. Fear of social/performance situations; there must be evidence of capacity for age-appropriate social relationships, and anxiety must occur in peer settings

B. Exposure to feared stimulus evokes anxiety, and may result in panic attack

C. For children, recognition of fear as excessive not necessary

D. Feared social situation(s) are avoided or endured with intense anxiety

E. Fear interferes with routines, school, or social activities/relationships, or there is marked distress about having the phobia

Diagnostic Criteria for Specific Phobia

A. Excessive fear, cued by presence/anticipation of a specific object/situation

B. Exposure to the feared object/situation provokes an immediate anxiety response, often expressed by crying, tantrums, freezing, or clinging in children

C. The person recognizes the fear is excessive; in children, this feature may be absent

D. Avoidance of phobic situation; if it is not avoided, intense anxiety is present

E. Phobia interferes significantly with the routine, school, or social activities and relationships, or there is marked distress about having the phobia

Diagnostic Criteria for Panic Disorder (without Agoraphobia)

A. Unexpected panic attacks followed by at least 1 month of 1 or more of the following:
  1. Concern about additional attacks
  2. Worry about the implication/consequences of attacks
  3. Change in behavior related to the attacks

B. Absence of agoraphobia

Data from American Psychiatric Association: Diagnostic and Statistical Manual of Mental Disorders, 4th ed, text revision. Washington, DC: American Psychiatric Association, 2000.

Children and adolescents with social anxiety typically resist or avoid social activities or begin missing school because of the anxiety present in those social situations.[163] This fear or avoidance of social situations must not be accounted for directly by the effects of medication or substance use or by another mental disorder such as SAD or panic disorder. If another medical or psychological problem is present, the marked fear must be unrelated to it.

For the physician, children with social phobia may present for an office visit with a range of physiological problems, including stomachache and headache. Young children may have tantrums, freeze, or display selective mutism. Black and Uhde[164] reviewed selective mutism in children as it may relate to social phobia. Reports of performance anxiety, stage fright, and shyness are relatively normal in children and adolescents and should not be diagnosed as social phobia unless they interfere with the child's normal development or cause marked distress.[5]

PREVALENCE

Social phobia affects between 1% and 4% of children and adolescents.[87] Although age at onset varies substantially, children are most likely to present with social anxiety during adolescence[165,166] and, typically, approximately 3 years after the onset of symptoms.[167] At all ages, more girls than boys are affected.[168] Earlier onset is often related to greater impairment in functioning and a higher rate of coexisting disorders.[162]

CAUSES

Several studies represent compelling arguments to suggest a familial link to social anxiety. For example, of children whose parents meet criteria for an anxiety disorder, more than one third themselves met criteria for a diagnosis of social anxiety.[169] One tenth of children meet diagnosis criteria for social phobia when one parent has anxiety, whereas no children do when neither parent meets criteria. In addition, other psychopathological processes in parents may increase rates of social phobia in their children. For example, parental depression, panic disorder, and substance abuse increase the difficulties that children have in social situations.[170] Social isolation, rejection of the child, parental overprotectiveness, and frequent moves may contribute to the development of social anxiety in children and adolescents.[170,171]

Children with social phobia may perceive peers as being more negative, may misread cues, and may have trouble evaluating the nature of their peers' intentions. An information-processing framework has been used to describe the negative cognitions in which children with anxiety disorders perceive a neutral environment.[172]

ASSESSMENT

In comparison with other types of anxiety, the assessment of social phobia in children and adolescents is rather extensive. Morris and colleagues[173] conducted a full review of the measures and techniques used in the assessment of social anxiety. Among the most useful and psychometrically sound tools are self-report instrument for children aged 8 and older. The Social Anxiety Scale for Children[174] and the counterpart for adolescents, the Social Anxiety Scale for Adolescents,[175] are useful tools in assessing social anxiety in a self-report format. Both scales are 22-item measures on a 5-point Likert-type scale in which the individual's fear of negative evaluation, generalized social avoidance and distress, and social avoidance in situations with new or unfamiliar peers are evaluated.

The Social Phobia and Anxiety Inventory for Children[176,177] is a 26-item self-report measure designed to assess behavioral, cognitive, and physiological features of social phobia as it relates to the *DSM-IV* criteria.[5] This instrument can be used for children and adolescents 8 to 14 years of age and has five scales: assertiveness, general conversation, public performance, physical/cognitive symptoms, and behavioral avoidance. This measure has been noted to be particularly helpful in differentiating whether the anxiety is experienced with peers or adults, an important distinction in the diagnosis of social phobia in children and adolescence.[173]

Specific Phobias

DIAGNOSTIC CRITERIA

Mild fears (i.e., fears that do not interfere with a child's day-to-day functioning and are short-lived) are developmentally normal.[168] When fears exceed what would be typical of a particular developmental period and cause severe distress on the part of a child, a diagnosis of specific phobia should be considered.[178] Table 18B-4 provides the diagnostic criteria for Specific Phobia as it relates to children and adolescents.

The types of specific phobias include animal, natural environment (e.g., heights, storms), blood-injection-injury, or situational type (e.g., elevators, airplanes), or the phobia can be noted as "other." For accurate diagnosis, a clinician must differentiate between a specific phobia and an anxiety reaction caused by another anxiety disorders, such as avoidance of a situation because of PTSD, avoidance of school because of SAD or social phobia, or the uncued attacks of panic disorder.

PREVALENCE

Specific phobias are present in approximately 5% of children and adolescents, although reports from community samples vary from 2.4% in a sample of 11-year-olds in New Zealand[179] to 9.1% in a sample 7- to 11-year-olds in the United States.[180] Girls have higher prevalence rates for specific phobias than do boys.[178] Rates are similar among white, Hispanic,[181] and African American children.[182]

COMORBIDITY

Comorbidity patterns within the different types of specific phobias can be present in children, but rates are relatively low (5%).[178] Specific phobia and other types of anxiety disorders co-occur frequently, with separation anxiety disorder[25], social phobia, and obsessive compulsive disorder[178] among the most commonly cited. As with anxiety disorders in general, children and adolescents with specific phobias often have concurrent depression.

Fears and prevalence of phobia appear to be developmental in nature. Younger children report greater fears of animals and being alone in the dark, whereas older children and adolescents report fears associated with failure and criticism around social situations, illness, and bodily injury.[168] In short, fears tend to decline as a child grows older; the fear of death remains the top fear for all age groups.[183,184]

CAUSES

Specific phobias may develop quite early; animal phobias often emerge earliest. In reviews of the literature, Silverman and associates[8,15] noted the complexities among the factors that influence the development of phobias in children. That said, much literature supports the notion of Rachman's[185] proposal of three nonexclusive pathways through which a child or adolescent develops a phobia: experiencing a harmful event themselves through direct conditioning (e.g., snakebite); observing anxiety on behalf of caregivers through modeling; and hearing information from peers, family, or media. Among parents of 30 dog-phobic children, 27% attributed the fear to direct experience with an aversive event involving a dog, 53% believed the behavior was modeled, and 7% identified information as the source of their child's phobia.[186] Children's reported fears about a fictional, unknown doglike animal changed according to the type of information provided before exposure and generalized to similar animals.[187]

A Darwinian nonassociative viewpoint suggests that some individuals are primed to have fears associated with things that may have been a threat at one time and thus develop a fear at first exposure to the object or event.[188] With repeated and successful exposures, these fears decrease considerably for most children. In a study evaluating both associative and nonassociative development of fear of spiders, 46% of the children were noted to have always been afraid of spiders, and 41% of parents of these children attributed this phobia to a direct experience.[189]

Although parental modeling appears to play a role in the development of specific phobia, parental role in genetics should not be discounted. In a study of twins with specific phobias, monozygotic twins reported more similar types and intensities of fears than did dizygotic twin pairs.[190]

ASSESSMENT

Multi-informant (e.g., child, parent, teacher) and multimethod assessment is the "gold standard" in the assessment of specific phobias.[191] The Fear Survey Schedule for Children–Revised[22] is an 80-item scale and aids in the identification of specific fear-producing stimuli in children and adolescents aged 7 and older. There are five factors relating to specific fear types: failure and criticism, the unknown, injury and small animals, death and danger, and medical problems. Self-monitoring approaches are also helpful in gaining an understanding of the intensity of the fear. The Fear Thermometer[192] depicts a thermometer-like drawing and a scale from 1 to 10 for children to rate fears as they encounter potential stimuli throughout their day. Physiological measures, including heart rate, galvanic skin response, muscle tension, and blood pressure, are helpful in gauging the intensity of fear of the object.[191] For the trained clinician, presentation of feared objects while monitoring the child or adolescent physiological response may be helpful.

Panic Disorder

Since the 1990s, attention to panic disorder in children and adolescents has increased. Inherent within the definition of panic disorder is an intense concern regarding panic attacks. According to the *DSM-IV*,[5] a panic attack is a somatic event that contains four of the following physiological features in a 10-minute time frame: heart palpitations/tachycardia, hyperhidrosis, trembling, sensations of suffocation or shortness of breath, sensations of choking, chest pain or discomfort, abdominal distress/nausea, syncope episodes, derealization or depersonalization, fear of loss of control, fear of dying, paresthesias, and/ or chills or hot flashes. Furthermore, panic attacks can be defined as *uncued* and unexpected, *cued* and expected in certain situations, and *situationally predisposed*, whereby the panic attack is probably but not invariably going to happen. For a diagnosis of panic disorder, children and adolescents must experience panic attacks that are *uncued*.

DIAGNOSTIC CRITERIA

Further diagnostic criteria for Panic Disorder without Agoraphobia are listed in Table 18B-4. It is important to determine whether the panic attacks are drug-related or caused by a general medical condition such as hyperthyroidism. In addition, before a diagnosis of panic disorder is made, the clinician must explore potential triggers that may or may not be known to the child. For example, if panic attacks happen as a result of being away from home or from relatives, SAD should be considered. Similarly, if a child has panic attacks in response to school or other evaluative situations, a diagnosis of social phobia is warranted.[5]

COMORBIDITY

Up to 90% of patients with panic disorder have another anxiety disorder or mood disorder. Panic disorder also is associated with migraines and mitral valve prolapse.[5]

PREVALENCE

Children and adolescents were not traditionally thought to be susceptible to panic disorder; thus, there are only few reports regarding its prevalence. Prevalence rates in the community vary considerably; from 0.5% to 5% of children and adolescents have been reported to meet full diagnostic criteria for panic disorder.[193,194] Onset peaks in late adolescence. In adult retrospective studies, nearly 40% of affected individuals reported initial onset in adolescence or earlier.[193,194]

Although studies have documented an equal male-female distribution,[195] more severe panic attacks are reported by girls.[196] In one clinical study of 2000 high school students, the female : male ratio for lifetime history of panic disorder was 3 : 1. Panic attacks are not uncommon in adolescence; rates among adolescents are 10.2%, although clinician ratings may be lower than self-report ratings.[196] Of the adolescents who experience panic attacks, 75% report heart palpitations and racing heart as primary symptoms.[165]

CAUSES

Both environmental and genetic influences contribute to the development of panic disorder. Children and adolescents with more severe panic attacks report less social support and higher rates of family stressors.[197] Risk factors for panic disorder include a diagnosis of Major Depressive Disorder and family histories of depression and/or panic disorders.[196] High negative affectivity and fearful response to symptoms of anxiety contribute to having a panic attack in adolescence.[196]

ASSESSMENT

There exist few assessment measures that are specific to panic disorder. The Panic Attack Questionnaire[198] represents the only self-report instrument designed to assess specifically panic attacks in individuals older than 13. This measure helps assess the frequency, duration, intensity, and triggers of panic attacks. In addition to the diagnostic function of this instrument, it may be useful for self-monitoring. A parent and/or a child may document any triggers underlying panic attacks.

COLLABORATIVE CARE PRACTICES

A review of interventions for anxiety disorders in children and adolescents indicates that cognitive-behavioral therapy alone and cognitive-behavior therapy plus family anxiety management are considered probably efficacious.[2] The short-term (e.g., 3.5 years) and long-term (e.g., 6 years) treatment gains of cognitive-behavioral therapy have been supported by results of randomized clinical trials.[199,200] After a 16-week cognitive-behavioral treatment program for primary anxiety disorders (e.g., GAD, social phobias), 60% to 70% of youth demonstrated a positive response to treatment in terms of reduced anxiety, as well as decreased substance use–related problems.[201] Variables related to nonresponders, such as attrition and intensity of treatments, merit further exploration in the literature.[201]

Although promising interventions for pediatric anxiety disorders appear to exist, few youths are referred for, and fewer receive, such interventions. In general, only 16% to 20% of youths with identified psychosocial problems are referred for specialty treatment.[30,44] With regard to identified anxiety disorders, reports suggest that about 50% of such youths are not referred for treatment.[202] One report indicates that even among those who are referred, the majority (up to 72%) of children and adolescents with an anxiety disorder do not actually receive any treatment.[29]

These differential referral and treatment rates seem related to a variety of factors, with lower rates for children with mild problems and for those from ethnic minority backgrounds.[30,203] Patients in managed care plans, in comparison with those in fee-for-service plans, receive fewer referrals for specialty care and psychotherapy.[204] Such differing rates also may appear related to varying levels of treatment acceptability, stigma of mental health services, and early detection.[203] If pediatricians are the "de facto mental health service" for many children with psychosocial problems, knowledge about effective treatment options and referral sources is essential to ensure timely intervention.[44]

Methods to enhance the ability of pediatricians to identify and treat psychosocial problems include interdisciplinary training, training in specialties such as developmental-behavioral pediatrics, and anticipatory guidelines and prevention strategies offered through the American Academy of Pediatrics.[205] In addition, some strategies developed in tertiary care settings to identify and treat psychosocial problems could possibly be modified to make them feasible in primary care settings.[206] For example, a group of investigators outline a three-tiered approach to enhance the role of primary care in children with psychosocial problems.[207,208] The first level of care is more consistent identification and management by primary care and community professionals, such as home health care managers and case managers. The second tier is management by mental health specialists working in primary care settings. The third approach pertains to consultation-liaison, in which the mental health specialist supports management by the primary care physician but does not assume primary therapeutic responsibility. In an extension of this approach, pediatricians and psychologists work jointly within a practice team, to which developmental-behavioral pediatricians serve as consultants.[209]

A chronic disease management approach may be more applicable for youths with diagnoses of anxiety disorders, especially in view of the high frequency of somatic complaints observed in these children and adolescents. In one such approach, recommended by von Korff and colleagues,[210] the "patient" works with the health care provider to manage his or her disease by monitoring symptoms, adhering to medical regimens, and adopting more adaptive health habits and coping skills. This approach can be modified by including patients and parents in collaboration with their primary care and mental health care professionals in managing pediatric anxiety disorders. As in the study by von Korff and colleagues[210] on adult patients with GAD, children and adolescents with an anxiety disorder and their parents can be given written material on the characteristics and nature of GAD, pharmacological and psychological treatment options, and basic strategies for managing worry and anxiety. Allied health clinicians may then be available to provide more in-depth services and follow-up as needed. Parent involvement would be crucial in ensuring practice of skills outside of the clinic setting, supporting generalization of these skills, and offsetting modeling and reinforcement of anxious behaviors. Such involvement of the family is considered essential with regard to positive outcomes and maintenance of treatment gains.[2,201]

Within all these approaches, continuity of care is essential as continuity improves clinician recognition of psychosocial problems, receipt of preventive services, and patient satisfaction with care.[30,31] In addition, continuing medical education programs are needed for primary care physicians and other medical specialists to ensure optimal identification, diagnosis, and effective treatment options for mental health disorders, including anxiety disorders in youths.[39,210] Finally, strategies are needed to ensure effective collaboration between primary care pediatricians and mental health professionals, either working side by side or functioning as a consultants. The role of other consultants, such as developmental-behavioral pediatricians, also requires delineation in the management of youths with anxiety disorders.

Black and Nabors[211] outlined optimal strategies for psychologists for collaborating with pediatricians in primary care settings. These strategies also apply to collaboration with other consultants and subspecialists, such as developmental-behavioral pediatricians. One recommendation centers on novel strategies for screening and interventions. Prompt identification may be fostered by consistent use of behavior screening measures during primary care appointments. Changes in behaviors across visits could be monitored and referrals made as soon as the information indicates that these behaviors are outside normative values. Another recommendation pertains to training of both medical and mental health professionals with regard to knowledge about development and behavior, as well as factors that affect busy practices. For example, consistent use of the *DSM-PC*[212] may increase communication among professionals and agreement about when referrals need to be made to mental health professionals and other subspecialists. The type and range of stressful situations and problematic clusters could be used as an algorithm to determine referral patterns, especially challenges to primary support groups, emotions, and moods. Coordination of care also would be enhanced when referral procedures are efficient in terms of point of contact and appointment scheduling. Periodic meetings or telephone conference calls could be made between consultants to address referral difficulties and specific cases. A particularly relevant issue concerns performance and economic indicators necessary to demonstrate treatment effectiveness and "need" for services. The separation of health insurance plans into physical health and behavioral health segments has, unfortunately, reemphasized single-provider models of care that may be less effective although more fiscally viable.[211] The role of pediatricians and psychologists as professional educators, clinicians, and researchers is evident from these approaches to care and in continued attention to strategies to support collaboration.[209]

FUTURE DIRECTIONS

Research and clinical efforts since the 1980s have produced extensive information about all aspects of pediatric anxiety disorders. Further research is needed to facilitate early recognition, early identification, and intervention, as well as to develop clinical practice guidelines.

Two "normative-developmental" principles are relevant to accurate diagnosis and assessment. Normative data on anxiety, worry, and fears are necessary in order to examine quantitative and qualitative changes that occur with development and to compare behaviors across reference groups. Normative data on gender, race, culture, and socioeconomic status should be obtained. Such data will be critical in interpreting behaviors as "normal" or "excessive" and in tracking behavior change over time, with or without intervention.[15] Differences in cognitive, social, and emotional capacities of children and adolescents will assist in categorizing symptoms as either essential or associated features within each anxiety disorder. Comer and colleagues[108] are credited for this recommendation in terms of distinguishing worry and obsessions in youth diagnosed with GAD or OCD, but consider-

ation of developmental differences is applicable to all pediatric anxiety disorders.

Most researchers and clinicians emphasize the need for brief and valid screening instruments.[29,32] Development of an "integrated triage protocol" is encouraged for primary care settings, community settings, and specialty clinic settings. In addition, potential thresholds could be established for these settings through cross-validated factor analysis.[32] Along these lines, a structured, comprehensive, reliable measure of functional impairment to determine the level of impairment is needed because of its relevance to diagnosis.[29]

Longitudinal research is crucial for examining manifestations of pediatric anxiety disorders and treatment outcome and for answering a range of questions. For example, is the function of worry similar in children, adolescents, and adults?[18] Are the core features of worry and behavioral inhibition predictive of, or do they co-occur with, anxiety syndromes and/or disorders?[28] Family studies, investigations of neurotransmitters, and phenomenological observations would be helpful in more fully clarifying the role of genetics, neurobiology, and risk-protective factors in anxiety disorders.[116] Prospective studies are essential for delineating the pattern and course of specific symptoms to document disorder subtypes, along with the relationship between childhood-onset and adult-onset disorders.[116]

As researchers and clinicians explore these recommendations, there should be another surge of information regarding etiology, diagnosis, assessment, and treatment of pediatric anxiety disorders. Stephenson[213] raised the question of whether underfunded and overburdened health care and mental health care systems can serve the needs of an increasing number of identified youths with anxiety disorders. Specific factors that interfere with referral practices of physicians and follow-through by families include limited availability of specialists, cost and payor requirements, and scheduling delays.[31] In addition, impediments to mental health services involve social stigma, family beliefs and attitudes about such care, as well as socioeconomic factors in the family.[29] These barriers must be explored in more detail to ensure early identification, accurate assessment, and effective intervention for all children and adolescents with anxiety disorders.

REFERENCES

1. Beidel DC, Turner SM: Anxiety disorders. *In* Hersen M, Turner SM, eds: Adult Psychopathology and Diagnosis, 2nd ed. New York: Wiley, 1991, pp 226-278.
2. Ollendick TH, King NJ: Empirically supported treatments for children with phobic and anxiety disorders: Current status. J Clin Child Psychol 27:156-167, 1998.

3. Pine DS, Cohen P, Gurley D, et al: The risk for early-adulthood anxiety and depressive disorders in adolescents with anxiety and depressive disorders. Arch Gen Psychiatry 55:56-64, 1998.

4. Velting ON, Setzer NJ, Albano AM: Update on and advances in assessment and cognitive-behavioral treatment of anxiety disorders in children and adolescents. Prof Psychol Res Pract 35:42-54, 2004.

5. American Psychiatric Association: Diagnostic and Statistical Manual of Mental Disorders, 4th ed. Washington, DC: American Psychiatric Association, 1994.

6. American Psychiatric Association: Diagnostic and Statistical Manual of Mental Disorders, 4th ed., text revision. Washington, DC: American Psychiatric Association, 2000.

7. Muris P, Merckelbach H, Mayer B, et al: How serious are common childhood fears? Behav Res Ther 38:217-228, 2000.

8. Silverman WK, La Greca AM, Wasserstein S: What do children worry about? Worries and their relation to anxiety. Child Dev 66:671-686, 1995.

9. Albano A, Causey D, Carter B: Fear and Anxiety in Children, 3rd ed. New York: Wiley, 2001.

10. Barlow D: Anxiety and Its Disorders: The Nature and Treatment of Anxiety and Panic, 2nd ed. New York: Guilford, 2002.

11. Lang P: Fear reduction and fear behavior. *In* Schlein J, ed: Research in Psychotherapy. Washington, DC: American Psychological Association, 1968, pp 85-103.

12. Albano A, Chorpita B, Barlow D: Anxiety Disorders. New York: Guilford, 1996.

13. Barlow D: Anxiety and Its Disorders. New York: Guilford, 1988.

14. Borkovec T, Shadick R, Hopkins M: The nature of normal and pathological worry. *In* Rapee R, Barlow D, eds: Chronic Anxiety. General Anxiety Disorder and Mixed Anxiety-Depression. New York: Guilford, 1991, pp 29-51.

15. Silverman WK, Ollendick TH: Evidence-based assessment of anxiety and its disorders in children and adolescents. J Clin Child Adolesc Psychol 34:380-411, 2005.

16. Barlow DH, Chorpita BF, Turovsky J: Fear, panic, anxiety, and disorders of emotion. Nebr Symp Motiv 43:251-328, 1996.

17. Chorpita BF, Albano AM, Barlow DH: The structure of negative emotions in a clinical sample of children and adolescents. J Abnorm Psychol 107:74-85, 1998.

18. Borkovec T: The nature, functions, and origins of worry. *In* Davey G, Tallis F, eds: Worrying: Perspectives in Theory, Assessment and Treatment. London: Wiley, 1994, pp 5-33.

19. Hudson J, Rapee R: From anxious temperament to disorder. An etiological model. *In* Heimberg R, Turk C, Mennin D, eds: Generalized Anxiety Disorder: Advances in Research and Practice. New York: Guilford, 2004, pp 51-74.

20. Davey G, Hamptom J, Farrell J, et al: Some characteristics of worrying: Evidence for worrying and anxiety as separate constructs. Pers Individ Diff 13:133-147, 1992.

21. Mathews A: Why worry? The cognitive function of anxiety. Behav Res Ther 28:455-468, 1990.

22. Ollendick TH: Reliability and validity of the Revised Fear Surgery Schedule for Children (FSSC-R). Behav Res Ther 21:685-692, 1983.

23. Muris P, Meesters C, Merckelbach H, et al: Worry in normal children. J Am Acad Child Adolesc Psychiatry 37:703-710, 1998.

24. Vasey MW, Crnic KA, Carter WG: Worry in childhood: A developmental perspective. Cogn Ther Res 18:529-549, 1994.

25. Kashani JH, Orvaschel H: A community study of anxiety in children and adolescents. Am J Psychiatry 147:313-318, 1990.

26. Bernstein GA, Borchardt CM: Anxiety disorders of childhood and adolescence: A critical review. J Am Acad Child Adolesc Psychiatry 30:519-532, 1991.

27. Perrin S, Last CG: Worrisome thoughts in children clinically referred for anxiety disorder. J Clin Child Psychol 26:181-189, 1997.

28. Weems CF, Silverman WK, La Greca AM: What do youth referred for anxiety problems worry about? Worry and its relation to anxiety and anxiety disorders in children and adolescents. J Abnorm Child Psychol 28:63-72, 2000.

29. Chavira DA, Stein MB, Bailey K, et al: Child anxiety in primary care: Prevalent but untreated. Depress Anxiety 20:155-164, 2004.

30. Horwitz SM, Leaf PJ, Leventhal JM, et al: Identification and management of psychosocial and developmental problems in community-based, primary care pediatric practices. Pediatrics 89:480-485, 1992.

31. Kelleher KJ, Childs GE, Wasserman RC, et al: Insurance status and recognition of psychosocial problems. A report from the Pediatric Research in Office Settings and the Ambulatory Sentinel Practice Networks. Arch Pediatr Adolesc Med 151:1109-1115, 1997.

32. Wren FJ, Scholle SH, Heo J, et al: Pediatric mood and anxiety syndromes in primary care: Who gets identified? Int J Psychiatry Med 33:1-16, 2003.

33. Pine DS: Child-adult anxiety disorders. J Am Acad Child Adolesc Psychiatry 33:280-281, 1994.

34. Costello EJ, Angold A: Epidemiology in anxiety disorders in children and adolescents. *In* March JS, ed: Anxiety disorders in children and adolescnets. New York: Guilford, 1995, pp 109-124.

35. Abraham HD, Fava M: Order of onset of substance abuse and depression in a sample of depressed outpatients. Compr Psychiatry 40:44-50, 1999.

36. Brady EU, Kendall PC: Comorbidity of anxiety and depression in children and adolescents. Psychol Bull 111:244-255, 1992.

37. Manassis K, Monga S: A therapeutic approach to children and adolescents with anxiety disorders and associated comorbid conditions. J Am Acad Child Adolesc Psychiatry 40:115-117, 2001.

38. Chansky TE, Kendall PC: Social expectancies and self-perceptions in anxiety-disordered children. J Anxiety Disord 11:347-363, 1997.

39. Kennedy BL, Schwab JJ: Utilization of medical specialists by anxiety disorder patients. Psychosomatics 38:109-112, 1997.

40. Souetre E, Lozet H, Cimarosti I, et al: Cost of anxiety disorders: Impact of comorbidity. J Psychosom Res 38(Suppl 1):151-160, 1994.

41. Walker EA, Roy-Byrne PP, Katon WJ, et al: Psychiatric illness and irritable bowel syndrome: A comparison with inflammatory bowel disease. Am J Psychiatry 147:1656-1661, 1990.

42. Angold A, Costello EJ, Erkanli A: Comorbidity. J Child Psychol Psychiatry 40:57-87, 1999.

43. Seligman L, Ollendick T: Comorbidity of anxiety and depression in children and adolescents: An integrative review. Clin Child Fam Psychol Rev 1:125-144, 1998.

43a. American Academy of Pediatrics: The Classification of Child and Adolescent Mental Diagnoses in Primary Care: Diagnostic and Statistical Manual for Primary Care (DSM-PC) Child and Adolescent Version. Elk Grove, IL: American Academy of Pediatrics, 1996.

44. Costello EJ: Primary care pediatrics and child psychopathology: A review of diagnostic, treatment, and referral practices. Pediatrics 78:1044-1051, 1986.

45. Kendall P, Brady E: Comorbidity in the anxiety disorders of childhood. In Carig K, Dobson K, eds: Anxiety and Depression in Adults and Children. Newbury Park, CA: Sage Publications, 1995, pp 3-36.

46. Kearney C, Wadiak D: Anxiety disorders. In Netherton S, Holmes D, Walker C, eds: Child and Adolescent Psychological Disorders. A Comprehensive Textbook. New York: Oxford University Press, 1999, pp 282-303.

47. Kendall P, Cantwell D, Kazdin A: Depression in children and adolescents: Assessment issues and recommendations. Cogn Ther Res 13:109-146, 1989.

48. Ollendick TH, Vasey MW: Developmental theory and the practice of clinical child psychology. J Clin Child Psychol 28:457-466, 1999.

49. Fong M, Silien K: Assessment and diagnosis of DSM-IV anxiety disorders. J Couns Dev 77:209-217, 1999.

50. Othmer E, Othmer S: The Clinical Interview Using DSM-IV, Volume I: Fundamentals. Washington, DC: American Psychiatric Press, 1994.

51. March J, Albano A: Assessment of anxiety disorders in children and adolescents. In Riddle MA, ed: Annual Review of Psychiatry. Washington, DC: American Psychiatric Association, 1996, pp 405-427.

52. Silverman WK, Eisen AR: Age differences in the reliability of parent and child reports of child anxious symptomatology using a structured interview. J Am Acad Child Adolesc Psychiatry 31:117-124, 1992.

53. Puig-Antich J, Chambers W: The Schedule for Affective Disorders and Schizophrenia in School-Aged Children (Kiddie_SADS). New York: New York State Psychiatric Institute, 1978.

54. Costello EJ, Edelbrock CS, Costello AJ: Validity of the NIMH Diagnostic Interview Schedule for Children: A comparison between psychiatric and pediatric referrals. J Abnorm Child Psychol 13:579-595, 1985.

55. Silverman WK, Albano AM: Anxiety Disorder Interview Schedule for Children for DSM-IV (Child and Parent Version). San Antonio, TX: Psychological Corporation/Grayworld, 1996.

56. Reynolds CR, Paget KD: Factor analysis of the revised Children's Manifest Anxiety Scale for blacks, whites, males, and females with a national normative sample. J Consult Clin Psychol 49:352-359, 1981.

57. Spielberger C: Preliminary Manual for the State-Trait Anxiety Inventory for Children ("How I Feel Questionnaire"). Palo Alto, CA: Consulting Psychologists Press, 1973.

58. Birmaher B, Khetarpal S, Brent D, et al: The Screen for Child Anxiety Related Emotional Disorders (SCARED): Scale construction and psychometric characteristics. J Am Acad Child Adolesc Psychiatry 36:545-553, 1997.

59. Silverman W, Fleisig W, Rabian B, et al: Childhood anxiety sensitivity index. J Clin Child Psychol 20:162-168, 1991.

60. Ronan K, Kendall P, Rowe M: Negative affectivity in children: Development and validation of a self-statement questionnaire. Cogn Ther Res 18:509-528, 1994.

61. Achenbach T: Manual for the Youth Self-Report and 1991 Profile. Burlington: University of Vermont, Department of Psychiatry, 1991.

62. Reynolds C, Kamphus R: Behavioral Assessment Scale for Children. Circle Pines, MN: American Guidance Service, 1992.

63. Achenbach T: Manual for the Child Behavior Checklist/4-18 and 1991 Profile. Burlington: University of Vermont, Department of Psychiatry, 1991.

64. Achenbach T: Manual for the Teacher's Report Form and 1991 Profile. Burlington: University of Vermont, Department of Psychiatry, 1991.

65. Conners C: Conners' Rating Scales Manual. North Tonawanda, NY: Multi Health Systems, 1990.

66. Moos R, Moos B: Family Environment Scale Manual, 2nd ed. Palo Alto, CA: Consulting Psychologists Press, 1986.

67. Locke H, Wallace K: Short-term marital adjustment and prediction tests: Their reliability and validity. J Marriage Fam Living 21:251-255, 1959.

68. Kendall PC: Treating anxiety disorders in children: Results of a randomized clinical trial. J Consult Clin Psychol 62:100-110, 1994.

69. Melamed BG, Siegel LJ: Reduction of anxiety in children facing hospitalization and surgery by use of filmed modeling. J Consult Clin Psychol 43:511-521, 1975.

70. Jay SM, Elliott C: Behavioral observation scales for measuring children's distress: The effects of increased methodological rigor. J Consult Clin Psychol 52:1106-1107, 1984.

71. Bornstein MR, Bellack AS, Hersen M: Social-skills training for unassertive children: A multiple-baseline analysis. J Appl Behav Anal 10:183-195, 1977.

72. Barrett PM, Rapee RM, Dadds MM, et al: Family enhancement of cognitive style in anxious and aggressive children. J Abnorm Child Psychol 24:187-203, 1996.

73. Silverman WK, Kurtines WM: Anxiety and Phobic Disorders: A Pragmatic Approach. New York: Plenum Press, 1996.

74. Kendall P, Chansky TE: Considering cognition and anxiety-disordered children. J Anxiety Disord 5:167-185, 1991.

75. Houston B, Fox J, Forbes L: Trait anxiety and children's state anxiety, cognitive behaviors, and performance under stress. Cogn Ther Res 8:631-641, 1984.

76. Barlow D: Psychological interventions in the era of managed competition. Clin Psychol Sci Pract 1:109-122, 1994.

77. Mowrer O: Learning Theory and Behavior. New York: Wiley, 1960.

78. Delprato D, McGlynn F: Behavioral theories of anxiety disorders. In Turner SM, ed: Behavioral Treatment of Anxiety Disorders. New York: Plenum Press, 1984, pp 63-122.

79. Beck A, Emery G: Anxiety Disorders and Phobias: A Cognitive Perspective. New York: Basic Books, 1985.

80. Reiss S: Expectancy model of fear, anxiety, and panic. Clin Psychol Rev 11:141-153, 1991.

81. Biederman J, Rosenbaum J, Boldue-Murphy E, et al: Behavioral inhibition as a temperamental risk factor for anxiety disorders. Child Adolesc Psychiatr Clin North Am 2:667-684, 1993.

82. Last C: Somatic complaints in anxiety disordered children. J Anxiety Disord 5:125-138, 1991.

83. Hoehn-Saric R, McLeod DR, Zimmerli WD: Somatic manifestations in women with generalized anxiety disorder. Psychophysiological responses to psychological stress. Arch Gen Psychiatry 46:1113-1119, 1989.

84. Tracey SA, Chorpita BF, Douban J, et al: Empirical evaluation of DSM-IV Generalized Anxiety Disorder criteria in children and adolescents. J Clin Child Psychol 26:404-414, 1997.

85. Verduin TL, Kendall PC: Differential occurrence of comorbidity within childhood anxiety disorders. J Clin Child Psychol 32:290-295, 2003.

86. Kovacs M, Devlin B: Internalizing disorders in childhood. J Child Psychol Psychiatry 39:47-63, 1998.

87. Benjamin R, Costello E, Warren M: Anxiety disorders in a pediatric sample. J Anxiety Disord 4:293-316, 1990.

88. Gould R, Otto M: Cognitive-behavioral treatment of social phobias and generalized anxiety disorder. In Pollack M, Otto M, Rosenbaum J, eds: Challenges in Clinical Practice: Pharmacologic and Psychosocial Strategies. New York: Guilford, 1996, pp 171-200.

89. Brown G, Harris T: Etiology of anxiety and depressive disorders in an inner-city population: 1. Early adversity. Psychol Med 23:143-154, 1993.

90. Kendler KS, Walters EE, Neale MC, et al: The structure of the genetic and environmental risk factors for six major psychiatric disorders in women. Phobia, generalized anxiety disorder, panic disorder, bulimia, major depression, and alcoholism. Arch Gen Psychiatry 52:374-383, 1995.

91. Borkovec T, Lyonfields J: Worry: Thought suppression of emotional processing. In Krohne H, ed: Attention and Avoidance. Seattle: Hogrefe & Huber, 1993, pp 101-118.

92. Butler G, Wells A, Dewick H: Differential effects of worry and imagery after exposure to a stressful stimulus: A pilot study. Behav Cogn Psychother 23:45-56, 1995.

93. Dugas MJ, Gagnon F, Ladouceur R, et al: Generalized anxiety disorder: A preliminary test of a conceptual model. Behav Res Ther 36:215-226, 1998.

94. Ladouceur R, Talbot F, Dugas MJ: Behavioral expressions of intolerance of uncertainty in worry. Experimental findings. Behav Modif 21:355-371, 1997.

95. Muris P, Merckelbach H, Mayer B, et al: The Screen for Child Anxiety Related Emotional Disorders (SCARED) and traditional childhood anxiety measures. J Behav Ther Exp Psychiatry 29:327-339, 1998.

96. Scahill L: Contemporary approaches to pharmacotherapy in Tourette's syndrome and obsessive-compulsive disorder. J Child Adolesc Psychiatr Nurs 9(1):27-43, 1996.

97. March JS, Mulle K: Obsessive-compulsive disorder in children and adolescents: A review of the past 10 years. J Am Acad Child Adolesc Psychiatry 35:1265-1273, 1996.

98. Beidel DC: Anxiety disorders. In Hersen M, Turner S, eds: Diagnostic Interviewing, 2nd ed. New York: Plenum Press, 1994, pp 55-77.

99. Leonard HL, Lenane MC, Swedo SE, et al: Tics and Tourette's disorder: A 2- to 7-year follow-up of 54 obsessive-compulsive children. Am J Psychiatry 149:1244-1251, 1992.

100. Rettew DC, Swedo SE, Leonard HL, et al: Obsessions and compulsions across time in 79 children and adolescents with obsessive-compulsive disorder. J Am Acad Child Adolesc Psychiatry 31:1050-1056, 1992.

101. Bolton D, Luckie M, Steinberg D: Long-term course of obsessive-compulsive disorder treated in adolescence. J Am Acad Child Adolesc Psychiatry 34:1441-1450, 1995.

102. Flament MF, Koby E, Rapoport JL, et al: Childhood obsessive-compulsive disorder: A prospective follow-up study. J Child Psychol Psychiatry 31:363-380, 1990.

103. Leonard HL, Goldberger EL, Rapoport JL, et al: Childhood rituals: Normal development or obsessive-compulsive symptoms? J Am Acad Child Adolesc Psychiatry 29:17-23, 1990.

104. Riddle M: Obsessive-compulsive disorder in children and adolescents. Br J Psychiatry Suppl (35)173:91-96, 1998.

105. Leckman JF, Grice DE, Boardman J, et al: Symptoms of obsessive-compulsive disorder. Am J Psychiatry 154:911-917, 1997.

106. Riddle MA, Scahill L, King R, et al: Obsessive compulsive disorder in children and adolescents: Phenomenology and family history. J Am Acad Child Adolesc Psychiatry 29:766-772, 1990.

107. Scahill L, Kano Y, King RA, et al: Influence of age and tic disorders on obsessive-compulsive disorder in

a pediatric sample. J Child Adolesc Psychopharmacol 13(Suppl 1):S7-S17, 2003.

108. Comer JS, Kendall PC, Franklin ME, et al: Obsessing/worrying about the overlap between obsessive-compulsive disorder and generalized anxiety disorder in youth. Clin Psychol Rev 24:663-683, 2004.

109. Turner S, Beidel D, Stanley M: Are obsessional thoughts and worry different cognitive phenomena? Clin Psychol Rev 12:257-270, 1992.

110. Owens EB, Piacentini J: Case study: Behavioral treatment of obsessive-compulsive disorder in a boy with comorbid disruptive behavior problems. J Am Acad Child Adolesc Psychiatry 37:443-446, 1998.

111. Zolar AH, Pauls DL, Ratzoni G, et al: Obsessive-compulsive disorder with and without ties in an epidemiological sample of adolescents. Am J Psychiatry 154:274-276, 1997.

112. Geller D, Biederman J, Jones J, et al: Is juvenile obsessive-compulsive disorder a developmental subtype of the disorder? A review of the pediatric literature. J Am Acad Child Adolesc Psychiatry 37:420-427, 1998.

113. Leonard HL, Swedo SE, Lenane MC, et al: A 2- to 7-year follow-up study of 54 obsessive-compulsive children and adolescents. Arch Gen Psychiatry 50:429-439, 1993.

114. Zolar AH, Ratzoni G, Pauls DL, et al: An epidemiological study of obsessive-compulsive disorder and related disorders in Israeli adolescents. J Am Acad Child Adolesc Psychiatry 31:1057-1061, 1992.

115. Last CG, Perrin S, Hersen M, et al: DSM-III-R anxiety disorders in children: sociodemographic and clinical characteristics. J Am Acad Child Adolesc Psychiatry 31:1070-1076, 1992.

116. Grados M, Labuda M, Riddle M, et al: Obsessive-compulsive disorder in children and adolescents. Int Rev Psychiatry 9:1-20, 1997.

117. Scahill L, Riddle MA, McSwiggin-Hardin M, et al: Children's Yale-Brown Obsessive-Compulsive Scale: Reliability and validity. J Am Acad Child Adolesc Psychiatry 36:844-852, 1997.

118. Lenane MC, Swedo SE, Leonard H, et al: Psychiatric disorders in first degree relatives of children and adolescents with obsessive compulsive disorder. J Am Acad Child Adolesc Psychiatry 29:407-412, 1990.

119. Nestadt G, Samuels J, Riddle M, et al: A family study of obsessive-compulsive disorder. Arch Gen Psychiatry 57:358-363, 2000.

120. Carey G, Gottesman I: Twin and family studies of anxiety, phobic, and obsessive disorders. In Kein D, Rabkin J, eds: Anxiety: New Research and Changing Concepts. New York: Raven Press, 1981, pp 117-136.

121. Berg CJ, Rapoport JL, Flament M: The Leyton Obsessional Inventory–Child Version. J Am Acad Child Adolesc Psychiatry 25:84-91, 1986.

122. Goodman WK, Price L, Rasmussen S, et al: Children's Yale-Brown Obsessive-Compulsive Scale. New Haven, CT: Department of Psychiatry and Yale Child Study Center, 1991.

123. Denckla M: Neurological examination. In Rapoport J, ed: Obsessive-Compulsive Disorder in Children and Adolescents. Washington, DC: American Psychiatric Press, 1989, pp 107-118.

124. Swedo SE, Leonard HL, Mittleman BB, et al: Identification of children with pediatric autoimmune neuropsychiatric disorders associated with streptococcal infections by a marker associated with rheumatic fever. Am J Psychiatry 154:110-112, 1997.

125. Kearney CA, Sims KE, Pursell CR, et al: Separation anxiety disorder in young children: A longitudinal and family analysis. J Clin Child Adolesc Psychol 32:593-598, 2003.

126. Francis G, Last CG, Strauss CC. Expression of separation anxiety disorder: The roles of age and gender. Child Psychiatry Hum Dev 18(2):82-89, Winter 1987.

127. Lewinsohn PM, Hops H, Roberts RE, et al: Adolescent psychopathology: I. Prevalence and incidence of depression and other DSM-III-R disorders in high school students. J Abnorm Psychol 102:133-144, 1993.

128. Last CG, Strauss CC, Francis G: Comorbidity among childhood anxiety disorders. J Nerv Ment Dis 175:726-730, 1987.

129. Compton SN, Nelson AH, March JS: Social phobia and separation anxiety symptoms in community and clinical samples of children and adolescents. J Am Acad Child Adolesc Psychiatry 39:1040-1046, 2000.

130. Capps L, Sigman M, Sena R, et al: Fear, anxiety and perceived control in children of agoraphobic parents. J Child Psychol Psychiatry 37:445-452, 1996.

131. Weissman MM, Leckman JF, Merikangas KR, et al: Depression and anxiety disorders in parents and children. Results from the Yale family study. Arch Gen Psychiatry 41:845-852, 1984.

132. Foley DL, Pickles A, Maes HM, et al: Course and short-term outcomes of separation anxiety disorder in a community sample of twins. J Am Acad Child Adolesc Psychiatry 43:1107-1114, 2004.

133. Perwein A, Bernstein G: Separation anxiety disorder. In Ollendick T, March J, eds: Phobic and anxiety disorders in children and adolescents: A clinician's guide to effective psychosocial and pharmacological intervention. New York: Oxford University Press, 2004, pp 272-305.

134. March JS, Parker JD, Sullivan K, et al: The Multidimensional Anxiety Scale for Children (MASC): Factor structure, reliability, and validity. J Am Acad Child Adolesc Psychiatry 36:554-565, 1997.

135. Spence SH: Structure of anxiety symptoms among children: A confirmatory factor-analytic study. J Abnorm Psychol 106:280-297, 1997.

136. Adams T, Swank M, Masek B: Anxiety Disorders, 2nd ed. Philadelphia: Lippincott Williams & Wilkins, 2005.

137. Scheeringa MS, Zeanah CH, Drell MJ, et al: Two approaches to the diagnosis of posttraumatic stress disorder in infancy and early childhood. J Am Acad Child Adolesc Psychiatry 34:191-200, 1995.

138. Benedek E: Children and disaster: Emerging issues. Psychiatr Ann 15:168-172, 1985.

139. Drell M, Siegel C, Gaensbauer T: Post-traumatic stress disorder. *In* Zeanah C, ed: Handbook of Infant Mental Health. New York: Guilford, 1993.

140. Chilcoat HD, Breslau N: Posttraumatic stress disorder and drug disorders: Testing causal pathways. Arch Gen Psychiatry 55:913-917, 1998.

141. Cohen JA, Mannarino AP, Zhitova AC, et al: Treating child abuse–related posttraumatic stress and comorbid substance abuse in adolescents. Child Abuse Negl 27:1345-1365, 2003.

142. Brent DA, Perper JA, Moritz G, et al: Posttraumatic stress disorder in peers of adolescent suicide victims: Predisposing factors and phenomenology. J Am Acad Child Adolesc Psychiatry 34:209-215, 1995.

143. McCloskey LA, Walker M: Posttraumatic stress in children exposed to family violence and single-event trauma. J Am Acad Child Adolesc Psychiatry 39:108-115, 2000.

144. Pelcovitz D, Kaplan S, Goldenberg B, et al: Posttraumatic stress disorder in physically abused adolescents. J Am Acad Child Adolesc Psychiatry 33:305-312, 1994.

145. Famularo R, Fenton T, Augustyn M, et al: Persistence of pediatric post traumatic stress disorder after 2 years. Child Abuse Negl 20:1245-1248, 1996.

146. Garland AF, Hough RL, McCabe KM, et al: Prevalence of psychiatric disorders in youths across five sectors of care. J Am Acad Child Adolesc Psychiatry 40:409-418, 2001.

147. Graham-Berman S, Levendosky A: Traumatic stress symptoms in children of battered women. J Interpers Violence 13:111-128, 1998.

148. Vernberg EM, Silverman WK, La Greca AM, et al: Prediction of posttraumatic stress symptoms in children after Hurricane Andrew. J Abnorm Psychol 105:237-248, 1996.

149. La Greca A, Silverman WK, Vernberg EM, et al: Symptoms of posttraumatic stress in children after Hurricane Andrew: A prospective study. J Consult Clin Psychol 64:712-723, 1996.

150. Stallard P, Velleman R, Baldwin S: Prospective study of post-traumatic stress disorder in children involved in road traffic accidents. BMJ 317:1619-1623, 1998.

151. Shannon MP, Lonigan CJ, Finch AJ Jr, et al: Children exposed to disaster: I. Epidemiology of post-traumatic symptoms and symptom profiles. J Am Acad Child Adolesc Psychiatry 33:80-93, 1994.

152. La Greca AM, Silverman WK, Wasserstein SB: Children's predisaster functioning as a predictor of posttraumatic stress following Hurricane Andrew. J Consult Clin Psychol 66:883-892, 1998.

153. Clark DB, Bukstein OG, Smith MG, et al: Identifying anxiety disorders in adolescents hospitalized for alcohol abuse or dependence. Psychiatr Serv 46:618-620, 1995.

154. Yule W, Udwin O: Screening child survivors for post-traumatic stress disorders: Experiences from the "Jupiter" sinking. Br J Clin Psychol 30(Pt 2):131-138, 1991.

155. Sack WH, Clarke GN, Seeley J: Posttraumatic stress disorder across two generations of Cambodian refugees. J Am Acad Child Adolesc Psychiatry 34:1160-1166, 1995.

156. Ford JD, Racusin R, Daviss WB, et al: Trauma exposure among children with oppositional defiant disorder and attention deficit–hyperactivity disorder. J Consult Clin Psychol 67:786-789, 1999.

157. Frederick C: Selected foci in the spectrum of post traumatic stress disorders. *In* Murphy L, ed: Perspectives on Disaster Recovery. East Norwalk, CT: Appleton-Century-Crofts, 1985, pp 110-130.

158. Perrin S, Smith P, Yule W: The assessment and treatment of Post-traumatic Stress Disorder in children and adolescents. J Child Psychol Psychiatry 41:277-289, 2000.

159. Handford H, Mayes S, Mattison R, et al: Child and parent reaction to the Three Mile Island nuclear accident. J Am Acad Child Adolesc Psychiatry 25:346-356, 1986.

160. Saxe G, Chawla N, Stoddard F, et al: Child Stress Disorders Checklist: A measure of ASD and PTSD in children. J Am Acad Child Adolesc Psychiatry 42:972-978, 2003.

161. Wolfe DA, Sas L, Wekerle C: Factors associated with the development of posttraumatic stress disorder among child victims of sexual abuse. Child Abuse Negl 18:37-50, 1994.

162. Albano A, Chorpita B, Barlow D: Childhood Anxiety Disorders, In: Nash EJ, Barkley RA, eds. Child Psychopathology. 2nd ed. New York: Guilford Press; 2003;196-241.

163. Kearney CA: School Refusal Behavior in Youth: A Functional Approach to Assessment and Treatment. Washington, DC: American Psychological Association, 2001.

164. Black B, Uhde TW: Treatment of elective mutism with fluoxetine: A double-blind, placebo-controlled study. J Am Acad Child Adolesc Psychiatry 33:1000-1006, 1994.

165. Essau CA, Conradt J, Petermann F: Frequency of panic attacks and panic disorder in adolescents. Depress Anxiety 9:19-26, 1999.

166. Westenberg PM, Drewes MJ, Goedhart AW, et al: A developmental analysis of self-reported fears in late childhood through mid-adolescence: Social-evaluative fears on the rise? J Child Psychol Psychiatry 45:481-495, 2004.

167. Strauss C, Last C: Social and simple phobias in children. J Anxiety Disord 7:141-152, 1993.

168. Gullone E: The development of normal fear: A century of research. Clin Psychol Rev 20:429-451, 2000.

169. Merikangas KR, Avenevoli S, Dierker L, et al: Vulnerability factors among children at risk for anxiety disorders. Biol Psychiatry 46:1523-1535, 1999.

170. Bruch M, Heimberg R, Berger P, et al: Social phobia and perceptions of early parental and personal characteristics. Anxiety Res 2:143-154, 1989.

171. Arrindell WA, Kwee MG, Methorst GJ, et al: Perceived parental rearing styles of agoraphobic and

socially phobic in-patients. Br J Psychiatry 155:526-535, 1989.

172. Daleiden EL, Vasey MW: An information-processing perspective on childhood anxiety. Clin Psychol Rev 17:407-429, 1997.

173. Morris T, Hirshfeld-Becker D, Henin A, et al: Developmentally sensitive assessment of social anxiety. Cogn Behav Pract 11:12-28, 2004.

174. La Greca AM, Stone W: Social Anxiety Scale for Children–Revised: Factor structure and concurrent validity. J Clin Child Psychol 22:17-27, 1993.

175. LaGreca A, Lopez N: Social anxiety among adolescents: Linkages with peer relations and friendships. J Abnorm Child Psychol 26:83-94, 1998.

176. Beidel DC, Turner SM, Morris TL: A new inventory to assess childhood social anxiety and phobia: The Social Phobia and Anxiety Inventory for Children. Psychol Assess 7:73-79, 1995.

177. Beidel DC, Turner SM, Morris TL: Psychopathology of childhood social phobia. J Am Acad Child Adolesc Psychiatry 38:643-650, 1999.

178. Essau CA, Conradt J, Petermann F: Frequency, comorbidity, and psychosocial impairment of anxiety disorders in German adolescents. J Anxiety Disord 14:263-279, 2000.

179. Anderson JC, Williams S, McGee R, et al: DSM-III disorders in preadolescent children. Prevalence in a large sample from the general population. Arch Gen Psychiatry 44:69-76, 1987.

180. Costello EJ: Child psychiatric disorders and their correlates: A primary care pediatric sample. J Am Acad Child Adolesc Psychiatry 28:851-855, 1989.

181. Ginsburg G, Silverman W: Phobic and anxiety disorders in Hispanic and Caucasian youth. J Anxiety Disord 10:517-528, 1996.

182. Last CG, Perrin S: Anxiety disorders in African-American and white children. J Abnorm Child Psychol 21:153-164, 1993.

183. Burnhan J, Gullone E: The Fear Survey Schedule for Children–II: A psychometric investigation with American data. Behav Res Ther 35:165-173, 1997.

184. Spence SH, McCathie H: The stability of fears in children: A two-year prospective study: A research note. J Child Psychol Psychiatry 34:579-585, 1993.

185. Rachman S: The conditioning theory of fear-acquisition: A critical examination. Behav Res Ther 15:375-387, 1977.

186. King N, Ollendick T, Murphy G, et al: Animal phobias in children: Aetiology, assessment, and treatment. Clin Psychol Psychother 7:11-21, 2000.

187. Muris P, Bodden D, Merckelbach H, et al: Fear of the beast: A prospective study on the effects of negative information on childhood fear. Behav Res Ther 41:195-208, 2003.

188. Menzies RG, Clarke JC: A comparison of in vivo and vicarious exposure in the treatment of childhood water phobia. Behav Res Ther 31:9-15, 1993.

189. Merckelbach H, Muris P, Schouten E: Pathways to fear in spider phobic children. Behav Res Ther 34:935-938, 1996.

190. Torgersen S: Genetic factors in anxiety disorders. Arch Gen Psychiatry 40:1085-1089, 1979.

191. King N, Muris P, Ollendick T: Childhood fears and phobias: Assessment and treatment. Child Adolesc Ment Health 10:50-56, 2005.

192. Walk RD: Self ratings of fear in a fear-invoking situation. J Abnorm Psychol 52:171-178, 1956.

193. Moreau D, Follet C: Panic disorder in children and adolescents. Child Adolesc Psychiatr Clin North Am 2:581-602, 1993.

194. Von Korff MR, Eaton WW, Keyl PM: The epidemiology of panic attacks and panic disorder. Results of three community surveys. Am J Epidemiol 122:970-981, 1985.

195. King N, Ollendick TH, Mattis S, et al: Nonclinical panic attacks in adolescents: Prevalence, symptomatology, and associated features. Behav Change 13:171-183, 1997.

196. Hayward C, Varady S, Albano AM, et al: Cognitive-behavioral group therapy for social phobia in female adolescents: Results of a pilot study. J Am Acad Child Adolesc Psychiatry 39:721-726, 2000.

197. Costello EJ, Erkanli A, Fairbank JA, et al: The prevalence of potentially traumatic events in childhood and adolescence. J Trauma Stress 15:99-112, 2002.

198. Norton G, Dorward J, Cox B: Factors associated with panic attacks in nonclinical subjects. Behav Change 17:239-252, 1986.

199. Barrett PM, Duffy AL, Dadds MR, et al: Cognitive-behavioral treatment of anxiety disorders in children: Long-term (6-year) follow-up. J Consult Clin Psychol 69:135-141, 2001.

200. Silverman WK, Kurtines WM, Ginsburg GS, et al: Contingency management, self-control, and education support in the treatment of childhood phobic disorders: A randomized clinical trial. J Consult Clin Psychol 67:675-687, 1999.

201. Kendall PC, Safford S, Flannery-Schroeder E, et al: Child anxiety treatment: Outcomes in adolescence and impact on substance use and depression at 7.4-year follow-up. J Consult Clin Psychol 72:276-287, 2004.

202. Lavigne JV, Binns HJ, Christoffel KK, et al: Behavioral and emotional problems among preschool children in pediatric primary care: Prevalence and pediatricians' recognition. Pediatric Practice Research Group. Pediatrics 91:649-655, 1993.

203. Lavigne JV, Arend R, Rosenbaum D, et al: Mental health service use among young children receiving pediatric primary care. J Am Acad Child Adolesc Psychiatry 37:1175-1183, 1998.

204. Perneger TV, Allaz AF, Etter JF, et al: Mental health and choice between managed care and indemnity health insurance. Am J Psychiatry 152:1020-1025, 1995.

205. Schroeder CS: Commentary: A view from the past and a look to the future. J Pediatr Psychol 24:447-452, 1999.

206. Wren FJ, Scholle SH, Heo J, et al: How do primary care clinicians manage childhood mood and anxiety syndromes? Int J Psychiatry Med 35:1-12, 2005.

207. Bower P, Garralda E, Kramer T, et al: The treatment of child and adolescent mental health problems in primary care: A systematic review. Fam Pract 18:373-382, 2001.

208. Gask L, Sibbald B, Creed F: Evaluating models of working at the interface between mental health services and primary care. Br J Psychiatry 170:6-11, 1997.

209. Perrin EC: Commentary: collaboration in pediatric primary care: A pediatrician's view. J Pediatr Psychol 24:453-458, 1999.

210. Von Korff M, Gruman J, Schaefer J, et al: Collaborative management of chronic illness. Ann Intern Med 127:1097-1102, 1997.

211. Black M, Nabors L: Behavioral and developmental problems of children in primary care: Opportunities for psychologists. *In* Frans R, McDaniel S, Bray J, et al: eds: Primary Care Psychology. Washington, DC: American Psychological Association, 2004, pp 189-207.

212. Wolraich M, Felice M, Drotar D: The Classification of Child and Adolescent Mental Diagnosis in Primary Care. Elk Grove, IL: American Academy of Pediatrics, 1996.

213. Stephenson J: Children with mental problems not getting the care they need. JAMA 284:2043-2044, 2000.

The Effect of Substance Use Disorders on Children and Adolescents

HOOVER ADGER, JR. ■ HAROLYN M. E. BELCHER

Health professionals, including primary care pediatricians and developmental-behavioral pediatricians, encounter large numbers of children, adolescents, pregnant women, and other family members or adult caretakers who have or are affected by alcohol and other drug-related problems. Developmental-behavioral pediatricians and other health professionals are in an ideal position to identify substance use disorders and related problems in the children, adolescents, and families whom they care for and should be able to provide preventive guidance, education, and intervention. Although it is easiest to identify substance use disorders and related problems in children, adolescents, and families who are most severely affected, the bigger challenge is to identify affected individuals early in their involvement and to intervene quickly and effectively. The magnitude of the problem, the nature and effect of substance use disorders on individuals and families, and the role of the health care professional in the prevention, intervention, and treatment of substance use disorders must be appreciated.

INCIDENCE AND PREVALENCE

According to data from the 2004 National Survey of Drug Use and Health,[1] formerly called the National Household Survey, 121 million and 70.3 million U.S. citizens, aged 12 and older, are estimated to be current users of alcohol and tobacco, respectively. In 2004, about 10.8 million underage persons aged 12 to 20 (28.7%) reported drinking alcohol in the previous month. Past-month alcohol use rates ranged from 16.4% among Asians to 19.1% among black persons, 24.3% among Native Americans or Alaska Natives, 26.6% among Hispanic persons, and 32.6% among white persons. Nearly 7.4 million (19.6%) individuals in the age group were binge drinkers, and 2.4 million

(6.3%) were heavy drinkers. Among persons aged 12 to 20, binge drinking was reported by 22.8% of white persons, 19.0% of Native Americans or Alaska Natives, 19.3% of Hispanic persons, and 18.0% of persons reporting belonging to two or more races. However, binge drinking was reported by only 9.9% of black persons and 8.0% of Asians. Among youths aged 12 to 17 in 2004, an estimated 3.6 million (14.4%) had used a tobacco product in the previous month, and 3.0 million (11.9%) had used cigarettes. Current cigarette use increased with age up to the mid-20s and then declined. An estimated 2.8% of 12- or 13-year-olds, 10.9% of 14- or 15-year-olds, and 22.2% of 16- or 17-year-olds were current cigarette smokers in 2004.

Another 19.1 million United States citizens (7.9% of the population) aged 12 years or older currently use illicit drugs.[1] Among all youths aged 12 to 17 in 2004, 10.6% were current users of illicit drugs: 7.6% used marijuana, 3.6% used prescription-type drugs for nonmedical reasons, 1.2% used inhalants, 0.8% used hallucinogens, and 0.5% used cocaine.

The highest rate of illicit drug use, 19.4%, was reported among young adults aged 18 to 25 years. It is estimated that 22.5 million U.S. citizens met criteria for alcohol or drug dependence. The percentages of dependence were highest among Native Americans and persons of multiracial heritage: 20.2% and 12.2%, respectively. White and African American individuals had similar rates of dependence: 9.6% and 8.3%, respectively. Asian Americans had the lowest rates of dependence, 4.7%, whereas the rate for Hispanic Americans was 9.8%.[2]

Among pregnant women aged 15 to 44 years, 3.3%, representing slightly more than 130,000 births per year, reported using illicit drugs the month before interview; this rate was significantly lower than the rate among women who were not pregnant (10.3%).[1,3] Rates of drug use during pregnancy were highest among Native Americans/Alaska Natives (10.1%) and persons reporting a heritage of two or more races (11.4%). In 2002, marijuana was the most widely used illicit drug among pregnant women (2.9%).[3] Of all pregnant women in the United States, 1% used illicit drugs other than marijuana, including cocaine (or crack), heroin, hallucinogens, inhalants, or any prescription-type psychotherapeutic for nonmedical use of. Alcohol and tobacco remain significant preventable threats to favorable birth and neurodevelopmental outcomes. Among pregnant women, aged 15 to 25 years, 5% reported alcohol binge drinking (five or more drinks at the same time or within a couple of hours of each other) on at least one day within the month before the survey. Seventeen percent of pregnant women smoked cigarettes within the month before the survey.[1]

TOBACCO

Tobacco kills more individuals in the United States each year than do all other substances and firearms combined.[4] The average smoker starts smoking at age 12 years. Adolescent smokers are more likely to become nicotine dependent through smoking fewer cigarettes a day than are adult smokers.[5] Worldwide, the Global Youth Tobacco Survey[6] reports that 24% of youth surveyed began smoking before age 10, and younger women aged 13-15 years are as likely to use tobacco products as are young men. Adolescents see the positive aspects of smoking as helping with boredom, dealing with stress, staying thin, and appearing more mature, and they acknowledge negative aspects such as its making their teeth yellow, interfering with playing sports, being harder to quit, and causing bad breath.

Pharmacology

Human and animal studies confirm the addictive effects of nicotine, the primary active ingredient in cigarettes.[7,8] It produces a syndrome of dependence and withdrawal. Nicotine is absorbed by multiple sites in the body, including the lungs, skin, gastrointestinal tract, and buccal and nasal mucosa. The average nicotine content of one cigarette is 10 mg, and the average nicotine intake per cigarette ranges from 1.0 to 3 mg. Nicotine, as delivered in cigarette smoke, has a half-life of 10 to 20 minutes, with an elimination half-life of 2 to 3 hours. Nicotine's effect on the brain takes less than 20 seconds. The action of nicotine is mediated through nicotinic acetylcholine receptors. These receptors are located on noncholinergic presynaptic and postsynaptic sites in the brain. Cotinine is the major metabolite of nicotine via C-oxidation. It has a biological half-life of 19 to 24 hours and can be detected in urine, serum, and saliva.

Clinical Manifestations

Adverse health effects of smoking include chronic cough, increased mucus production, and wheezing. Smoking during pregnancy is associated with an average decrease in fetal weight of 200 g.[9] Smoking in combination with the use of estrogen-containing oral contraceptives is associated with an increased risk of myocardial infarction.[10] Tobacco smoke induces hepatic smooth endoplasmic reticulum and, as a result, may also influence metabolism of drugs and of endogenously produced hormones. Phenacetin, theophylline, and imipramine are examples of drugs affected in this manner.

Treatment

Consensus panels recommend the use of the "five As" (ask, advise, assess, assist, and arrange) and of nicotine replacement therapy in adults and adolescents, although evidence of efficacy in adolescents is limited. Nicotine patch studies to date in adolescents are suggestive of a positive effect on reducing withdrawal symptoms and that pharmacotherapy should be combined with behavioral therapy to reach higher cessation and lower relapse rates. Medications such as bupropion are not approved for use in anyone younger than 18 years; however, some pilot studies in adolescents report cessation efficacy. Clinical practice guidelines are available for practical office-based counseling strategies.[11] Health supervision and supportive counseling are necessary components of smoking cessation management in adolescents and older adults, because relapse is common (Table 19-1).

ALCOHOL

By 12th grade, close to three fourths of adolescents in high school report having used alcohol at some point, 25% having had their first drink before age 13 years.[12] The initiation of alcohol use at an early age is associated with an increased risk for alcohol-related problems. Although a legal drug, alcohol contributes to more deaths than do all the other illicit drugs combined. Among studies of adolescent trauma victims, alcohol is reported to be a factor in 32% to 45% of hospital admissions.[13] Motor vehicle crashes are the most frequent type of event associated with alcohol

TABLE 19-1 ■ **The Five As: Brief Strategies to Help Adolescents Quit Tobacco Use**	
Ask	Systematically identify all tobacco users, as well as tobacco experience at every visit. ■ Expand the current documentation of vital signs to include information regarding tobacco use.
Advise	Strongly urge all tobacco users to quit. When providing advice, be sure to offer a clear strong, and personalized message. ■ Clear—"I recommend you stop smoking, as it is harmful to your health." ■ Strong—"As our doctor, advising you to quit smoking is essential to protecting your health for the short and long term. We will work together in achieving this goal." ■ Personalized—Tie tobacco use to personal concerns of the patient, such as its impact on health or the high cost of addiction.
Assist	Assist the patient in the development of a quit plan, provide practical counseling, help the patient to identify social support, and recommend appropriate therapy. Preparation for a quit plan: ■ Set a quit date. ■ Involve friends, family members, or co-workers to offer support for the plan. Provide practical counseling: ■ Identify triggers, events, or events that may lead to relapse. ■ Identify and practice skills to cope. ■ Educate with basic facts. ■ Explain the addictive nature of tobacco-related products. Recommend appropriate therapy: ■ Provide information on the use of approved pharmacotherapies.
Arrange	Schedule follow-up and provide encouragement: ■ Establish a follow-up date soon after the quit date. ■ Praise success, and if relapse occurs, have the patient commit to quit again.
Anticipatory guidance	Discuss family and peer use, as well as health risks associated with short and long-term use of tobacco.

From Houston TP, Adger H, Bavishi M: The AFP Guide to Teen Tobacco Use Prevention and Treatment, Illinois Academy of Family Physicians, American Academy of Pediatrics and Illinois Department of Public Health, 2002.

use; the injuries reported span a wide variety, including self-inflicted wounds. Adolescents with alcohol-positive findings were also more likely to report a history of prior injury.[2] A study by the Institute of Medicine calls for U.S. society at large to address the underage drinking crisis responsible for costly traffic fatalities, violent crime, and other negative behaviors in youth.[14]

Pharmacology and Pathophysiology

Alcohol (ethyl alcohol or ethanol) is rapidly absorbed in the stomach and is transported to the liver and metabolized by two pathways. The primary pathway involves removal of two hydrogen atoms to form acetaldehyde, a reaction catalyzed by alcohol dehydrogenase through reduction of a cofactor nicotinamide-adenine dinucleotide. The removed hydrogen atoms supply energy (7.1 kcal/g of alcohol) and contribute to the excess synthesis of triglycerides, a phenomenon that is responsible for producing a fatty liver, even in persons who are well nourished. Engorgement of hepatocytes with fat causes necrosis, triggering an inflammatory process (alcoholic hepatitis), which is followed by fibrosis, the hallmark of cirrhosis. Early hepatic involvement may result in elevation in glutamyl transpeptidase and serum glutamic-pyruvic transaminase levels.

The second metabolic pathway, which is used at high serum alcohol levels, involves the microsomal system of the liver, in which the cofactor is reduced nicotinamide-adenine dinucleotide phosphate. The net effect of activation of this pathway is to decrease metabolism of drugs that share this system and to allow for their accumulation, enhanced effect, and possible toxicity (e.g., drinking alcohol and ingesting tranquilizers results in the potentiation of each).

Clinical Manifestations

Alcohol acts primarily as a central nervous system (CNS) depressant. It produces euphoria, grogginess, and talkativeness; impairs short-term memory; and increases the pain threshold. Alcohol's ability to produce vasodilation and hypothermia is also centrally mediated. At very high serum levels, respiratory depression occurs. Alcohol's inhibitory effect on pituitary antidiuretic hormone release is responsible for its diuretic effect. The gastrointestinal complications of alcohol use can occur as a result of a single large ingestion. The most common is acute erosive gastritis, which is manifested by epigastric pain, anorexia, vomiting, and guaiac-positive stools. Less commonly, vomiting and midabdominal pain may be caused by acute alcoholic pancreatitis; diagnosis is confirmed by the finding of elevated serum amylase and lipase activities.

In addition to the general risk factors noted for substance use, a positive family history of alcohol abuse is significant. The genetic influences for the predisposition to alcoholism are supported by family, twin, and adoption studies.[15-18] Children of alcoholic parents demonstrate a threefold to ninefold increased risk for alcoholism.

The alcohol overdose syndrome should be suspected in any teenager who appears disoriented, lethargic, or comatose. Although the distinctive aroma of alcohol may assist in diagnosis, confirmation by analysis of blood is recommended. There is a high correlation between results obtained by serum and breath analyses; therefore, the latter method may be reliable. At serum levels greater than 200 mg/dL, the adolescent is at risk of respiratory depression, and levels greater than 500 mg/dL (median lethal dose) are usually associated with a fatal outcome. When the level of depression appears excessive for the reported blood level, head trauma or ingestion of other drugs should be considered as possible confounding factors.

Treatment of Acute Alcohol Overdose Syndrome

The usual mechanism of death from the alcohol overdose syndrome is respiratory depression, and artificial ventilatory support must be provided until the liver can eliminate sufficient amounts of alcohol from the body. In a naive drinker, it generally takes about 20 hours to reduce the blood level of alcohol from 400 mg/dL to zero. Dialysis should be considered when the blood level is higher than 400 mg/dL. As a follow-up to acute management, patients can benefit from further assessment and referral for treatment of an identified alcohol use disorder. In emergency room settings, even brief interventions have shown some success in decreasing alcohol use and alcohol-related problems in adolescents.

INHALANTS

Young adolescents are attracted to these substances because of their rapid action, easy availability, and low cost. The inhalants most popular among adolescents are glue, gasoline, and volatile nitrites. "Huffing"—directly inhaling, or inhaling deeply from a paper bag containing a chemical-soaked cloth—is the common method used by teenagers.

Clinical Manifestations

The major effects of inhalants are psychoactive. Toluene, the main ingredient in airplane glue and some rubber cements, causes relaxation and hallucinations for up to 2 hours. Tolerance and physical dependence may occur. Gasoline, a substance popular among some adolescents, contains a complex mixture of organic solvents. Euphoria is followed by violent excitement, and coma may result from prolonged or rapid inhalation. Volatile nitrites, such as amyl nitrite, butyl nitrite, and related compounds marketed as room deodorizers, are used as euphoriants, enhancers of musical appreciation, and aphrodisiacs among older adolescents and young adults. Their use may result in headaches, syncope, and lightheadedness; profound hypotension and cutaneous flushing, followed by vasoconstriction and tachycardia; transiently inverted T waves and depressed ST segments on electrocardiography; methemoglobinemia; increased bronchial irritation; and increased intraocular pressure.

Complications

Toluene-based products such as airplane glue have been responsible for a wide range of complications related to chemical toxicity, to the method of administration (e.g., in plastic bags, with resultant suffocation), and to the often dangerous setting in which the inhalation occurs (e.g., inner-city roof tops). Gasoline toxicity is acute and chronic. Death in the acute phase may result from cerebral or pulmonary edema or myocardial involvement. Chronic use may cause pulmonary hypertension, restrictive lung defects or reduced diffusion capacity, peripheral neuropathy, acute rhabdomyolysis, hematuria, tubular acidosis, and possibly cerebral and cerebellar atrophy. Other behavioral disturbances such as inattentiveness, lack of coordination, and general disorientation have been linked to chronic solvent abuse.

Because of its brief effect, inhalant use is unlikely to be diagnosed unless there is a complication or death from use. Complete blood cell counts, coagulation studies, and hepatic and renal function studies may reveal the complications. In extreme intoxication, a user may manifest symptoms of restlessness, general muscle weakness, dysarthria, nystagmus, disruptive behavior, and occasionally hallucinations; thus, inhalant use is part of the differential diagnosis for acute intoxication of an adolescent. Toluene is excreted rapidly in the urine as hippuric acid, and the residual is detectable in the serum by gas chromatography.

Treatment of Acute Intoxication/Overdose

Treatment is generally supportive and directed toward control of arrhythmia and stabilization of respirations and circulation.

COCAINE

Cocaine, an alkaloid extracted from the leaves of the South American *Erythroxylon coca,* is supplied as the hydrochloride salt in crystalline form. It is rapidly absorbed from the nasal mucosa, detoxified by the liver, and excreted in the urine as benzoyl ecgonine. Its half-life is slightly more than 1 hour. The perceived effect of "snorting" cocaine may be influenced by some of the many diluents now being added to or actually substituted for the drug (heroin, amphetamines, phencyclidine, or fillers such as mannitol or quinine). Smoking the cocaine alkaloid ("freebasing") in pipes or cigarettes, mixed with tobacco, marijuana, or parsley, or as a paste, has become a popular method of use.

Accidental burns are potential complications of this practice. With crack cocaine, the smoker feels "high" almost immediately. The risk of addiction with this drug is higher, and the addiction more rapidly progressive, than from snorting cocaine. Tolerance develops, and the user must increase the dose or change the route of administration, or both, to achieve the same effect.

Clinical Manifestations

Cocaine produces euphoria, increased motor activity, decreased fatigability, and, occasionally, paranoid ideation. Its sympathomimetic properties are responsible for pupillary dilatation, tachycardia, hypertension, and hyperthermia. Binge patterns of use are common. Neurological effects such as dizziness, paresthesia, and seizures can occur. Use in group settings has been associated with sexual promiscuity and increased risks of acquiring sexually transmitted infections. Lethal effects are possible, especially when cocaine is used in combination with other drugs, such as heroin, in an injectable form known as a "speedball." Pregnant women who use cocaine place their fetus at risk for premature delivery, complications of low birth weight, and possibly congenital malformations and developmental disorders.

AMPHETAMINES

Stimulants, particularly amphetamines, are among the most frequently reported illicit drugs other than marijuana used by high school students. Methamphetamine, commonly known as "ice," accounts for more than 25% of stimulant use. Methamphetamine is particularly popular among adolescents and young adults because of its potency and ease of absorption. It can be ingested by snorting, by smoking, orally, or by absorption across mucous membranes, such as vaginal mucosa. Its use is especially common in the western and southwestern regions of the United States. Amphetamines have multiple CNS effects, among them the release of neurotransmitters and an indirect catecholamine agonist effect. In high doses, they may also affect serotonergic receptors.

Clinical Manifestations

The effects of amphetamines can be dose related. High doses produce slowing of cardiac conduction in the face of ventricular irritability. Hypertensive and hyperpyrexic episodes can occur, as can seizures. Binge effects result in the development of psychotic ideation with the potential for sudden violence. Cerebrovascular damage and psychosis can result from chronic use. There is a withdrawal syndrome associated with amphetamine use, with early, intermediate, and late phases. The early phase is characterized as a "crash" phase with depression, agitation, anergia, and desire for more of the drug. Loss of physical and mental energy, limited interest in the environment, and anhedonia characterize the intermediate phase. In the final phase, drug craving returns, often triggered by particular situations or objects.

Treatment of Acute Intoxication

Agitation and delusional behaviors can be treated with haloperidol or droperidol. Phenothiazines are contraindicated; they may cause a rapid drop in blood pressure or seizure activity. Other supportive treatment consists of a cooling blanket for hyperthermia and treatment of the hypertension and arrhythmias, which may respond to sedation with lorazepam (Ativan) or diazepam (Valium).

OPIATES

Heroin is hydrolyzed to morphine, which undergoes hepatic conjugation with glucuronic acid before excretion, usually within 24 hours of administration. The route of administration influences the timing of the onset of action. When the drug is inhaled ("snorted"), almost 30 minutes are required before the desired effect is achieved. Ingestion through the subcutaneous route ("skin-popping"), produces the effect within minutes; when the drug is injected intravenously, the effect is immediate. Tolerance develops with regard to the euphoric effect and only rarely to the inhibitory effect on smooth muscle, which causes both constipation and miosis.

Clinical Manifestations

The clinical manifestations are determined by the pharmacological effects of heroin or its adulterants, combined with the conditions and the route of administration. The cerebral effects include euphoria, diminution in pain sensation, and pinpoint pupils. An effect on the hypothalamus is suggested by the lowering of body temperature. Vasodilation is a major cardiovascular manifestation related to the method of administration of the drug. Respiratory depression is mediated centrally and is characterized by alveolar hypoventilation.

Pulmonary edema is common in death from the overdose syndrome, but it may also be an incidental radiological finding in an otherwise asymptomatic heroin abuser. The most common dermatological lesions are the "tracks," the hypertrophic linear scars that follow the course of large veins. Smaller, discrete peripheral scars, resembling healed insect bites, may be easily overlooked. Injection of heroin subcutaneously may lead to fat necrosis, lipodystrophy, and atrophy over portions of the extremities.

Attempts at concealment of these stigmata may include amateur tattoos in unusual sites. Abscesses secondary to unsterile techniques of drug administration are commonly found. A heroin user may resort to prostitution to support his or her habit, thus increasing the risk of acquiring sexually transmitted diseases (including human immunodeficiency virus infection), pregnancy, and other hazards.

Constipation results from decreased smooth muscle propulsive contractions and increased anal sphincter tone. Hepatic enzyme levels are frequently elevated in heroin users, and there may be serological evidence of viral infection with hepatitis B and/or C. The absence of sterile technique in injection may lead to cerebral microabscesses or endocarditis, usually caused by *Staphylococcus aureus*. Abnormal serological reactions, including false-positive Venereal Disease Research Laboratory and latex fixation test results, are also common.

Withdrawal Syndrome

After a period of 8 hours or more without heroin, the addicted individual undergoes, during a period of 24 to 36 hours, a series of physiological disturbances referred to collectively as *withdrawal* or the *abstinence syndrome*. The earliest sign is excessive yawning, followed by lacrimation, mydriasis, insomnia, "goose flesh," cramping of the voluntary musculature, hyperactive bowel sounds and diarrhea, tachycardia, and systolic hypertension. The administration of buprenorphine, an opiate agonist/antagonist is the most common method of detoxification. Another commonly used agent is methadone. This synthetic opiate is effective by the oral route and is pharmacologically similar to heroin, except for its lack of euphoric effect.

Overdose Syndrome

The overdose syndrome is an acute reaction after the administration of an opiate. It is the leading cause of death among drug users. The clinical signs include stupor or coma, seizures, miotic pupils (unless severe anoxia has occurred), respiratory depression, cyanosis, and pulmonary edema. The differential diagnosis includes CNS trauma, diabetic coma, and hepatic (and other) encephalopathy, as well as overdose of alcohol, barbiturates, phencyclidine, or methadone. Diagnosis of opiate toxicity is facilitated by intravenous administration of the opiate antagonist naloxone, 0.01 mg/kg (2 mg is a common initial dose for an adolescent or adult), which causes dilation of pupils constricted by the opiate. Diagnosis is confirmed by the finding of morphine in the serum. The treatment of acute overdose consists of maintaining adequate oxygenation and, when necessary, continued administration of naloxone every 5 minutes to improve and maintain adequate ventilation. Naloxone may have to be continued for 24 hours if methadone, rather than shorter-acting heroin, has been taken.

CLUB DRUGS

Flunitrazepam (Rohypnol), 3,4-methylenedioxymethamphetamine (MDMA), γ-hydroxybutyrate (GHB), and ketamine are among a group of drugs used by adolescents and young adults who are part of a nightclub, bar, rave, or trance scene; the drugs are often referred to as *club drugs*. Raves and trance events are generally night-long dances, often held in warehouses. Although many people who attend raves and trances do not use drugs, those who do may be attracted to their generally low cost and to the intoxicating highs that are said to deepen the rave or trance experience. Studies have shown changes to critical parts of the brain from use of these drugs.

MDMA

MDMA is a synthetic, psychoactive drug chemically similar to the stimulant methamphetamine and the hallucinogen mescaline. Street names for MDMA include "ecstasy," "XTC," and "hug drug." In high doses, MDMA can interfere with the body's ability to regulate temperature. This can lead to a sharp increase in body temperature (hyperthermia), resulting in liver, kidney, and cardiovascular system failure. Research in humans suggests that chronic MDMA use can lead to changes in brain function, affecting cognitive tasks and memory. MDMA can also lead to symptoms of depression several days after its use. These symptoms may occur because of MDMA's effects on serotonergic neurons. The serotonin system plays an important role in regulating mood, aggression, sexual activity, sleep, and sensitivity to pain. A study in nonhuman primates showed that exposure to MDMA for only 4 days caused damage of serotonin nerve terminals that was evident 6 to 7 years later.

Although similar neurotoxicity has not been definitively shown in humans, the wealth of animal research indicating MDMA's damaging properties suggests that MDMA is not a safe drug for human consumption.

γ-Hydroxybutyrate

Since about 1990, GHB has been abused in the United States for its euphoric, sedative, and anabolic (body building) effects. GHB is colorless, tasteless, and odorless and has been involved in poisonings, overdoses, date rapes, and deaths. It can be added to beverages and unknowingly ingested. It is a CNS depressant that was widely available over the counter in health food stores during the 1980s and until 1992. It was purchased largely by body builders to aid in fat reduction and muscle building. Street names include "liquid ecstasy," "soap," "easy lay," "vita-G," and "Georgia home boy." Coma and seizures can occur after abuse of GHB. Combining use with other drugs such as alcohol can result in nausea and breathing difficulties. GHB may also produce withdrawal effects, including insomnia, anxiety, tremors, and sweating.

Ketamine

Ketamine is an anesthetic that has been approved for both human and animal use in medical settings since 1970; about 90% of the ketamine legally sold is intended for veterinary use. It can be injected or snorted. Ketamine is also known as "special K" or "vitamin K." Certain doses of ketamine can cause dreamlike states and hallucinations. In high doses, ketamine can cause delirium, amnesia, impairment

of motor function, high blood pressure, depression, and potentially fatal respiratory problems.

Flunitrazepam (Rohypnol)

Flunitrazepam belongs to the benzodiazepine class of drugs. It can produce "anterograde amnesia," and may be lethal when mixed with alcohol and/or other depressants. It is not approved for use in the United States, and its importation is banned. Illicit use of flunitrazepam started appearing in the United States in the early 1990s, where it became known as "rophies," "roofies," "roach," and "rope."

Hallucinogens

Lysergic acid (LSD; also known as "acid," "big 'd,'" and "blotters") is one of the constituents found in rye fungus. Morning glory seeds contain lysergic acid derivatives, although the commercially packaged varieties have often been treated with toxic chemicals such as insecticides and fungicides. Although the specific mechanisms of action of LSD are still under study, it is proposed to alter neurotransmitters mediated by serotonin. LSD is a very potent hallucinogen; doses as low as 20 μg cause effects in some individuals. Its high potency allows effective doses to be applied to objects as small as postage stamps and paper blotters. It is rapidly absorbed from the gastrointestinal tract. The onset of action can occur in between 30 and 60 minutes, and its action peaks between 2 and 4 hours. By 10 to 12 hours, the user returns to the predrug state.

CLINICAL MANIFESTATIONS

The effects of LSD can be divided into three categories: somatic (physical effects), perceptual (altered changes in vision and hearing), and psychic effects (changes in sensorium). The common somatic symptoms are dizziness, dilated pupils, nausea, flushing, elevated temperature, and tachycardia. The sensation of synesthesia, such as "seeing" smells and "hearing" colors, has been reported with LSD use. Delusional ideation, body distortion, and suspiciousness to the point of toxic psychosis are the more serious of the psychic symptoms.

TREATMENT

An individual is considered to have a "bad trip" when the setting causes the user to become terrified or panicked. These episodes should be treated by removing the individual from the aggravating situation or setting and attempting to reestablish contact with reality through calm verbal interaction. Any physical complications such as hyperthermia, seizure, or hypertension should be treated supportively. "Flashbacks"—LSD-induced states that occur after the drug has worn off—and tolerance to the effects of the drug are additional complications of its use.

Phencyclidine

Phencyclidine (also known as "PCP," "angel dust," "hog," "peace pill," and "sheets") is an arylcyclohexalamine whose popularity is related, in part, to its ease of synthesis in home laboratories. One of the by-products of home synthesis causes cramps, diarrhea, and hematemesis. The drug is thought to potentiate adrenergic effects by inhibiting neuronal reuptake of catecholamines. Phencyclidine is available as a tablet, liquid, or powder, which may be used alone or sprinkled on cigarettes ("joints"). The powders and tablets generally contain 2 to 6 mg of phencyclidine, whereas joints contain an average of 1 mg for every 150 mg of tobacco leaves, or approximately 30 to 50 mg per joint.

CLINICAL MANIFESTATIONS

The clinical manifestations are dose related. Euphoria, nystagmus, ataxia, and emotional lability occur within 2 to 3 minutes after smoking 1 to 5 mg and last for hours. Hallucination may involve bizarre distortions of body image that often precipitate panic reactions. With doses of 5 to 15 mg, a toxic psychosis may occur, with disorientation, hypersalivation, and abusive language, lasting for more than 1 hour. Hypotension, generalized seizures, and cardiac arrhythmias commonly occur with plasma concentrations from 40 to 200 mg/dL. Death from hypertension, hypotension, hypothermia, seizures, and trauma has been reported during psychotic delirium. The coma caused by phencyclidine may be distinguished from that caused by the opiates by the absence of respiratory depression; the presence of muscle rigidity, hyperreflexia, and nystagmus; and lack of response to naloxone. Phencyclidine psychosis may be difficult to distinguish from schizophrenia. In the absence of history of use, analysis of urine must be depended on for diagnosis.

TREATMENT OF ACUTE INTOXICATION

Management of the phencyclidine-intoxicated patient includes placement in a darkened, quiet room on a floor pad, to provide safety from injury. Gastric absorption is poor; thus, for recent oral ingestion, induction of emesis or gastric lavage is useful. Diazepam, in a dose of 5 to 10 mg orally or 2 to 5 mg intravenously, may be helpful if the patient is agitated and not comatose. Rapid excretion of the drug is promoted by acidification of the urine. Supportive therapy for the comatose patient is indicated, with particular attention to hydration, which may be compromised by phencyclidine-induced diuresis.

Developmental and Behavioral Implications of Long Term Use of Drugs of Abuse

Although each of the drugs of abuse may have individual variation, they are similar in that they have a common pathway of biochemical interactions that are channeled through the reward system in the brain, and they all work by causing changes in brain chemistry. It is these changes in brain chemistry that lead to the experience of euphoria and secondarily to changes in behavior, and the changes in behavior are what often bring individuals to medical attention. Therefore, including drug use in the list of possible causes of unexplained behavior change, particularly in adolescents, is important. Moreover, early identification and intervention can play an important role in preventing many of the consequences that are associated with repeated and chronic use.

FAMILY EFFECTS OF ALCOHOL AND OTHER DRUG USE

Children of Parents Affected by Substance Use Disorders

The familial effects of substance use disorders, particularly for alcoholism, are well documented. Approximately one fourth of all children in the United States younger than 18 years are exposed to familial alcohol abuse or alcohol dependence.[19] Furthermore, it has been shown that children of an alcoholic parent are overrepresented in the mental health and general medical systems. They have higher rates of injury, poisoning, admissions for mental disorders and substance abuse, and general hospital admissions; longer lengths of stay; and higher total health care costs. Children of an alcoholic parent are at higher risk for learning disabilities. The effects of prenatal exposure to alcohol and the fetal alcohol syndrome (FAS)—the term generally applied to children who have been exposed and display a certain constellation of symptoms, such as growth retardation, CNS involvement to include behavioral and/or intellectual impairment, and characteristic facies (short palpebral fissures, thin upper lip, and elongated, flattened midface and philtrum)—are well known.

Some studies have demonstrated that parental alcoholism is associated with increased risk for attention-deficit/hyperactivity disorder (ADHD) in offspring, conduct disorder, or anxiety disorders.

These offspring have been shown to have more diagnosable psychiatric disorders (i.e., depression, ADHD, conduct disorder) and lower reading and math achievement scores.

Children of substance-abusing parents are at risk for neglect. These children appear to have more behavior disorders, anxiety disorders, poorer competency scores, and higher scores on both internalizing and externalizing subscales of the Child Behavior Checklist than do control groups of children.[20,21] Other investigators have questioned whether the increased psychiatric problems seen in these children are caused by the parental substance abuse or by the comorbid psychiatric disorders in these parents.[22] For example, there may be a link between both substance abuse and antisocial personality disorder (a frequent comorbid psychiatric disorder) in parents and conduct disorder in offspring or a link between both substance abuse and major depression in parents and conduct disorder in offspring.[23,24] Finally, the children of substance-abusing parents are at extreme risk to abuse substances themselves. This increased risk arises from two phenomena: First, there is a genetic predisposition for the development of substance use disorders; second, these children often receive inadequate parental supervision, which itself is a risk factor for the initiation of substance abuse.[25,26]

Core Competencies for Addressing Children and Adolescents in Families Affected by Substance Use Disorders

National leaders from pediatrics, family medicine, nursing, social work, and adolescent health have previously collaborated in the development of a set of core competencies (*Core Competencies for Involvement of Health Care Providers in the Care of Children and Adolescents in Families Affected by Substance Abuse*) that outline the core knowledge, attitudes, and skills that are essential for meeting the needs of children and youth affected by substance use disorders in the family.[27] These core competencies outline a model of practice and delineate the desired knowledge and skills of health professionals in this area. The model is an attempt to recognize and account for individual differences among health providers. Furthermore, it represents a recognition that although primary health and behavioral professionals may be responsible for identifying the problem, they should not be expected to manage it by themselves. Accordingly, three distinct levels of care are articulated that allow for flexibility of individuals to choose their role and degree or level of involvement (Table 19-2). A baseline or minimal level (level I) of competence is established, and all primary health care professionals should strive to achieve it. However, most developmental-behavioral pediatricians want and are expected to do more than is indicated in the level I competencies. For health professionals who desire competence at a higher level (levels II and III), a different and more advanced set of knowledge and skills is required.

EARLY IDENTIFICATION OF SUBSTANCE USE DISORDERS

In one study, 38% of Americans stated they had a family member with alcoholism.[28] Because of its high prevalence and lack of socioeconomic boundaries, developmental-behavioral pediatricians should expect to encounter families with alcoholism and other drug use disorders routinely. Several studies suggest strongly that children of women who are problem drinkers have an increased risk of experiencing serious, unintentional injuries and that children exposed to two parents with alcohol problems are at even greater risk.[29] Studies of the link between parental substance abuse and child maltreatment suggest that substance abuse is present in at least half of families known to the public child welfare system.[30]

If these families and children are identified early, some of the associated morbidity might be avoided. Developmental-behavioral pediatricians and other child and adolescent health care providers can have a tremendous influence on families of substance-abusing parents because of their understanding of family dynamics and their close long-standing relationship with the family. Information about family alcohol and other drug use should be obtained as part of routine history taking and when there are indications of family dysfunction, child behavioral or emotional problems, school difficulties, and recurring episodes of apparent accidental trauma and in the setting of recurrent or multiple vague somatic complaints by the child or adolescent. In many instances, family problems with alcohol or drug use are not blatant; rather, their identification requires a deliberate and skilled screening effort.

Another study indicated that fewer than half of pediatricians ask about problems with alcohol when taking a family history.[32] In contrast, Graham and colleagues[33] found that patients wanted their physicians to ask about family alcohol problems and believed that the physician could help them and/or the abusing family member deal with their problems. A family history of alcohol and other drug abuse is more likely than many other aspects of history to affect a child's immediate and future health. A thor-

TABLE 19-2 ■ Core Competencies for Involvement of Health Care Providers in the Care of Children and Adolescents in Families Affected by Substance Abuse

Level I

For all health professionals with clinical responsibility for the care of children and adolescents:
1. Be aware of the medical, psychiatric, and behavioral syndromes and symptoms with which children and adolescents in families with substance abuse present.
2. Be aware of the potential benefit to both the child and the family as a result of of timely and early intervention.
3. Be familiar with community resources available for children and adolescents in families with substance abuse.
4. As part of the general health assessment of children and adolescents, include appropriate screening for family history or current use of alcohol and other drugs.
5. On the basis of screening results, determine family resource needs and services currently being provided, so that an appropriate level of care and follow-up can be recommended.
6. Be able to communicate an appropriate level of concern, and offer information, support, and follow-up.

Level II

In addition to level I competencies, health care providers accepting responsibility for prevention, assessment, intervention, and coordination of care of children and adolescents in families with substance abuse should
1. Apprise the child and family of the nature of alcohol and other drug abuse and dependence and its effect on all family members and strategies for achieving optimal health and recovery.
2. Recognize and treat, or refer, all associated health problems.
3. Evaluate resources—physical health, economic, interpersonal, and social—to the degree necessary to formulate an initial management plan.
4. Determine the need for involving family members and significant other persons in the initial management plan.
5. Develop a long-term management plan in consideration of these standards and with the child's or adolescent's participation.

Level III

In addition to level I and level II competencies, the health care provider with additional training who accepts responsibility for long-term treatment of children and adolescents in families with substance abuse should
1. Acquire knowledge, by training and experience, in the medical and behavioral treatment of children in families affected by substance abuse.
2. Continually monitor the child's or adolescent's health needs.
3. Be knowledgeable about the proper use of consultations.
4. Throughout the course of health care treatment, continually monitor and treat, or refer for care, any psychiatric or behavioral disturbances.
5. Be available to the child or adolescent and the family, as needed, for ongoing care and support.

ough understanding of family members' use of alcohol or other drugs is as important as a history for hypertension, cancer, or diabetes mellitus. In addition, family problems with alcohol or other drugs can jeopardize a parent's ability to carry out necessary therapeutic regimens for their child.

The primary task of initial screening is to identify families with alcohol or other drug use problems that put their children and youths at risk for associated physical or mental health complications. Screening questions help identify individuals most likely to have a problem related to alcohol or other drug use. Information gathered should help the clinician decide whether there is a need for additional assessment by either the primary provider or a consultant. Screening is an important and time-efficient first step to identifying the probable existence of a problem, but it differs from assessment and establishing a final diagnosis. Assessment is a more lengthy and structured process designed to determine the extent of the problem, explore comorbid conditions, and assist in treatment planning for the entire family.

Screening can occur at three different levels. The first is screening the child or adolescent for physical or mental health problems that may be associated with alcohol- or drug use–related problems among other family members. As the child grows older, it becomes increasingly important to establish diagnostic concerns and related treatment plans that can be implemented with the child or adolescent directly. Many older children and adolescents can be assessed fully without need for referral.

A second screening concern relates to identifying family members at high risk for substance use problems. Family members who appear to be at high risk for substance use disorders probably need referral for more detailed assessment by substance abuse professionals. Screening for and intervening with other family members affected by the family situation are necessary endeavors to maximize the health of the child.

Third, as adolescents grows older, it is increasingly important to identify their own alcohol and other drug use problems, because children from homes or who have parents with substance use disorders are at higher risk for developing their own problems with alcohol and other drugs.

Although the ability to perform an in-depth assessment and make an actual diagnosis may be beyond the time limitations and skills of many practitioners, all developmental-behavioral pediatricians are responsible for screening and initial management or referral. The difficulty encountered sometimes in obtaining accurate social and psychological histories and behavioral self-reports related to alcohol or other drug use by family members should not deter the clinician from including such histories and interviews as part of routine office procedures.

INTERVIEWING CHILDREN, YOUTH, AND FAMILIES

Since the 1980s, there has been an increasing level of interest in, and appreciation for, the complexity of communication skills needed to establish effective physician-patient/family relationships. In efforts to organize concepts and knowledge about medical interviewing, investigators have established useful models for the medical interview.[34] In one particularly useful model for child and adolescent health care, the medical interview is viewed as having three central functions: (1) to collect information regarding a potential problem; (2) to respond to the patient and family's emotions; and (3) to educate the family and influence behavior.[35] These functions are highly germane to the identification and intervention of children living with substance-abusing parents, because all three functions may need to occur simultaneously and are necessary to promote the well-being of these children adequately.

Collecting Information

To collect information about potential parental substance use disorders, health care providers need to (1) screen for and identify the family alcohol or drug problem; (2) understand the child's response to his or her perceived situation; (3) monitor changes in the child's behavior or health condition; and (4) provide themselves with a knowledge base regarding the child and family that is sufficient for developing and implementing a treatment plan. Children should be encouraged to tell their story in their own words. The physician may be required to help create or facilitate the child's narration, to organize the flow of the interview, to use appropriate open- and closed-ended questions to clarify and summarize information, to show support and reassurance, and to monitor nonverbal cues.[34] Health care providers need to acquire the knowledge base of psychosocial and family issues that contribute to the child or adolescent's health condition. In addition, they may need to understand and respond to the child or adolescent patient and the family unit. Many children of substance-abusing parents display particular illness behaviors: that is, they develop a particular way of responding to their perceived overall situation. It is well established that children and youth, on the basis of individual and cultural differences, respond in different ways to similar biomedical and psychosocial conditions. Without an understanding of the psychological and social underpinnings of illness behavior, the clinician may fail to collect all the relevant information related to the child's health problems.

Establishing Rapport

The second function of the interview involves the communication of interest, respect, support, and empathy between the clinician and the parent and between the clinician and the child or adolescent, with the goal of forming a relationship with the family.[34,35] By recognizing and responding to the child and family's emotional responses, the provider can ensure the child or family's willingness to provide information and can ensure relief of the child's physical or psychological distress. Attending to a child's or family's emotions is essential for effective communication and treatment planning with any emotionally complex issue, particularly one as potentially controversial as parental substance abuse. The clinician needs to hear the child's (or the family's) story with all its associated emotional distress. The emotions may range from fear to sadness, anger, or shame. The ability of a child or family member to verbalize these feelings in the presence of someone who can tolerate them and not be frightened is, in itself, therapeutic. A nonusing but affected parent may be as confused and frightened about the problem as the child. The open communication of fear and anxiety has been found to be related to satisfaction and compliance.[36] The empathic clinician, by understanding the child's situation, can decrease the child's and family's anxiety, thereby increasing their trust, with associated willingness to offer more complete information and follow through with treatment recommendations.

Education and Behavior Change

Dealing with parental substance abuse requires education of the family and behavior change for the young patient but also for all family members. The third function of the medical encounter must build on the successes of the first two functions. Care must be taken to ensure the child's and family's understanding of the nature of addiction, its influence on family function and individual family members, and its role in undermining a child's health. The physician will probably need to negotiate additional assessment or treatment of family members, as well as a specific treatment plan for the child's physical and mental conditions. Emphasis may need to be placed on the child and family's coping styles and simple first-pass efforts at lifestyle change. This requires understanding and working with the social and psychological consequences of the parental substance use disorder.

These three functions often are interdependent. For example, an effective therapeutic relationship enables the child and family to share with the clinician important medical and personal information, thereby improving the chances of determining the nature of the problem correctly.

A DEVELOPMENTAL LIFESPAN PERSPECTIVE ON SCREENING

Anticipatory guidance throughout the lifespan of childhood and adolescence is a well-established principle of child health care. From the prenatal visit through each of the regularly scheduled health maintenance visits that occur from birth through adolescence, there are well-established tenets of health education, screening for health morbidities, and anticipatory guidance. These visits represent multiple opportunities for screening, early identification, and intervention for children living in families affected by substance abuse. Combining the principles of anticipatory guidance, screening, and early identification with the acknowledgment that families should be included in the process leads to a clear conclusion that screening for children affected by parental substance abuse must occur at all ages during infancy, childhood, and adolescence.

Developmental-behavioral pediatricians and other child health care providers are in a unique position to intervene in the early stages of parental substance abuse and are able to take advantage of the unique relationships they develop with most families. Discussions related to substance use disorders and related problems should begin with the prenatal visit by focusing on the responsibility of parents, parental lifestyle, and effects of parental use of alcohol and other drugs on the fetus, infant, child, and adolescent. Parents serve as important role models for their children. Attitudes and beliefs regarding alcohol, tobacco, and other drugs (ATOD) develop early in life. Parents need to be aware that their attitudes and beliefs can strongly influence and play a major role in shaping their child's behavior. Hence, it is important for the health care professional to explore the attitude of the family toward ATOD use and to provide basic education, screening, and early intervention services that are appropriate to the age and development of the child and the family situation. If inquiries about parental use of alcohol and other drugs are incorporated into the family history portion of a clinical interview, they may seem less out of place to all involved. If the clinician prefaces his or her questions with phrases such as, "Now I'm going to ask you about diseases that can run in families or have an effect on children's health," it may seem more natural and less intrusive to families.

Prenatal Visits

Although most developmental-behavioral pediatricians do not conduct prenatal visits, the earliest and perhaps the best time to bring up the subject of parental use of ATOD is at a prenatal visit, especially if both parents attend. Concern for the unborn child's health should be the focus. It may be less threatening to ask first whether there have been alcohol or other substance use problems in the parents' families. Questions about alcohol and other drugs can be coupled with questions about nutrition and smoking as part of a standard routine.

During pregnancy, parents are naturally concerned about the health of the fetus. Hence, it is worthwhile framing questions in two different contexts: the family history and the health of the fetus. The clinician may start questioning by addressing the use of over-the-counter medications, then prescription medications, then smoking, then alcohol use, and, finally, other drug use. An example of useful lead-ins is "Many parents seem to be confused about whether it is safe to drink alcohol during pregnancy. What is your understanding?" Questions also can be extended to the father.

Infancy and Early Childhood

During a child's infancy and early childhood, the target of screening efforts continues to be the parents. A good way to begin an interview with a parent may be by asking, "How are things going for you?" When verbal or nonverbal responses indicate depression, fatigue, unhappiness, or other emotional or interpersonal discomforts, it may be useful to pursue the underlying causes such as personal or spousal substance use. For example, "People handle stress in different ways. Some people exercise, some sleep, some people eat more, others smoke cigarettes or use alcohol or other drugs. How are you handling it?" The objective during infancy and early childhood is to reduce the amount and frequency of ATOD use occurring in the family and to which the young child is exposed. Child health care providers should learn about the alcohol and other drug use habits of all parents of infants and young children. This can be done in the context of a global family health assessment. Emphasis should be placed on how alcohol or drug use can affect parenting decisions, exacerbate stress and marital problems in the home, create a potentially unsafe home environment, and model drug use behaviors for children. The use of established screening tools such as the CAGE questionnaire (to be described) and the Alcohol Use Disorders Identification Test (AUDIT) may be helpful (Figs. 19-1 and 19-2).[37-40] If parents already have made a change in their alcohol or other drug use habits, this change should be reinforced. At a minimum, screening young adult parents for substance use disorders raises an important issue, gives feedback to the parents, and establishes the willingness of the provider to discuss the issue at a later time, if needed.

School Age

When children are asked from whom they learn most about health, the second most frequent response, after mothers, is their physician. Health care professionals can initiate or enhance the dialogue between children and their parents by asking whether alcohol and other drug use is being discussed in school and at home, inquiring about the specifics of what is being taught, and assessing whether the child understands the messages being delivered. It is important to ask whether alcohol or drug use is discussed among friends, whether alcohol or other drugs are present in the child's environment, about their perceptions of why some people use alcohol and other drugs, and

whether such use is harmful. This attention to common parenting and child behavior problems is valuable in preventing later problems.

Adolescence

Families continue to exert significant influence on adolescents and on the behaviors in which teenagers choose to engage. Early identification of families with alcohol- or drug-related problems is crucial for preventing substance abuse among adolescents themselves. Family issues to address include parent-child interactions and maladaptive family problem solving, which often involve avoidance of issues and conflict.[41,42] Families with marital discord, financial strains, social isolation, and disrupted family rituals (such as mealtimes, holidays, and vacations) also increase an adolescent's risk of problematic alcohol use.[43] Adolescents are particularly at risk if parents are either excessively permissive or punitive or if parents offer little praise or seem persistently neglectful of the adolescent.

Clear parent-defined conduct norms are an important protective factor.[42,44,45] Adolescents least likely to use alcohol or other drugs are emotionally close to their parents, receive advice and guidance from their parents, have siblings who are intolerant of drug use, and are expected to comply with clear and reasonable conduct rules. The parents of nonusers typically provide praise and encouragement, engender feelings of trust, and are sensitive to their children's emotional needs. Alcohol and/or other drug use should be included as a primary consideration in all behavioral, family, psychosocial, or related medical problems. The identification and assessment of high-risk behaviors and predisposing risk factors are key aspects in the early recognition of alcohol-related problems. As a routine part of the adolescent's visit, there should

---

CAGE Questionnaire

Have you ever felt you should *Cut* down on your drinking?
Have people *Annoyed* you by criticizing your drinking?
Have you ever felt bad or *Guilty* about your drinking?
Have you ever had an *Eye opener* or a drink in the morning to steady your nerves or to get rid of a hangover?

FIGURE 19-1 CAGE questionnaire.

Family CAGE

Have you ever felt that anyone in your family should *Cut* down on their drinking?
Has anyone in your family ever felt *Annoyed* by complaints about their drinking?
Has anyone in your family ever felt bad or *Guilty* about their drinking or something that has happened while drinking?
Eye opener: has anyone in your family ever had a drink first thing in the morning to steady their nerves or get rid of a hangover?

ALCOHOL USE DISORDERS IDENTIFICATION TEST (AUDIT)

Questions	0	1	2	3	4
1. How often do you have a drink containing alcohol?	Never	Monthly or less	2 to 4 times a month	2 to 3 times a week	4 or more times a week
2. How many drinks containing alcohol do you have on a typical day when you are drinking?	1 or 2	3 or 4	5 or 6	7 to 9	10 or more
3. How often do you have five or more drinks on one occasion?	Never	Less than monthly	Monthly	Weekly	Daily or almost daily
4. How often during the last year have you found that you were not able to stop drinking once you started?	Never	Less than monthly	Monthly	Weekly	Daily or almost daily
5. How often during the last year have you failed to do what was normally expected of you because of drinking?	Never	Less than monthly	Monthly	Weekly	Daily or almost daily
6. How often during the last year have you needed a first drink in the morning to get yourself going after a heavy drinking session?	Never	Less than monthly	Monthly	Weekly	Daily or almost daily
7. How often during the last year have you had a feeling of guilt or remorse after drinking?	Never	Less than monthly	Monthly	Weekly	Daily or almost daily
9. Have you or someone else been injured because of your drinking?	No		Yes, but not in the last year		Yes, during the last year
10. Has a relative, friend, doctor, or other health care worker been concerned about your drinking or suggested you cut down?	No		Yes, but not in the last year		Yes, during the last year
					Total

Note: This questionnaire is reprinted with permission from the World Health Organization. To reflect standard drink sizes in the United States, the number of drinks in question 3 was changed from 6 to 5. A free AUDIT manual with guidelines for use in primary care is available online at www.who.org.

FIGURE 19-2 Alcohol Use Disorders Identification Test (AUDIT). (From the World Health Organization. To reflect standard drink sizes in the United States, the number of drinks in question 3 was changed from 6 to 5. A free AUDIT manual with guidelines for use in primary care is available online at www.who.org.)

be an assessment of risk by reviewing risk factors and behaviors with youths and their parents.

APPROACHES TO SCREENING

Screening for alcohol and/or other drug use problems within families must begin with a careful and detailed psychosocial history. Information about the structure, function, and interpersonal problems of families, parents, children, and adolescents provides a necessary background from which the need for additional screening efforts can be determined. Evidence of child behavior problems, early school failure, parenting difficulties, family conflict, or changes in the home environment are commonly present in families affected by substance use disorders.

Screening for Alcohol- or Drug-Related Problems in the Family

In many instances, family problems related to alcohol and drug use are subtle and identifying them requires a deliberate and skilled screening effort. On the basis of the nature of a presenting medical problem or as a result of problem areas in the psychosocial history, screening may involve asking the child or adolescent patient questions directly, asking questions that are developmentally appropriate, and addressing their perceptions of problematic substance use in the family. The clinician can begin by asking a simple but important screening question: "Have you ever been concerned about someone in your family who is drinking alcohol or using other drugs?" This question sets the groundwork for possible later discussion. It also lets the family and the child or adolescent know that the clinician believes that use of alcohol and other drugs is a health concern and that the clinician is willing and able to assist the family. (The Web sites for the National Association for Children of Alcoholics [www.nacoa.org] and Contemporary Pediatrics [http://www.contemporarypediatrics.com/contpeds/article/articleDetail.jsp?id=141246] provide an extended discussion of strategies, tools, resources, and tips on organizing the office visit.)

Because of the high prevalence of unhealthy alcohol use, many authorities recommend that all adults be screened with a validated survey instrument such as the CAGE questionnaire (for which each letter in the acronym refers to one of the questions) or the AUDIT.[46] The CAGE questionnaire is brief but was designed primarily to detect dependence. The AUDIT is longer but detects a spectrum of unhealthy drinking (see Figs. 19-1 and 19-2).

The CAGE questionnaire is a four-item alcohol screening instrument with demonstrated relevance for primary care in clinical, educational, and research settings (see Fig. 19-1).[37-39] The questions concern whether the respondent has ever needed to *cut* down on their drinking, felt *annoyed* by complaints about his or her drinking, felt *guilty* about his or her drinking; or had an *eye*-opener—that is, a drink—first thing in the morning.

One technique for maximizing the usefulness of responses to screening questions is to apply them to all members of the household. The Family CAGE is a modified version of the commonly used CAGE questionnaire that simply broadens the standard CAGE items to include "anyone in your family" (see Fig. 19-1). The Family CAGE questions can be used to provide a proxy report regarding another individual, such as a parent or an older sibling. For example, if the patient is a 12-year-old who currently is not using alcohol or other drugs but is concerned about a parent's use of alcohol, the health care professional could screen for concerns about the parent's alcohol use by asking the child the CAGE questions in the following manner: "Do you think your mother needs to cut down on her alcohol use? Does your mother get annoyed at comments about her drinking? Does your mother ever act guilty about her drinking or something that happened while she was drinking? Does your mother ever have a drink early in the morning as an eye-opener?" One or more positive answers to the Family CAGE can be considered a positive screen result, and additional assessment is needed. The Family CAGE is intended to screen for alcohol problems in families, not to diagnose family alcoholism. A positive finding on the Family CAGE implies a greater relative risk for alcoholism in the family and should be followed by a more thorough diagnostic assessment. In one study, one positive response on the Family CAGE was more sensitive than a question about perceived family alcohol problems.[47] The specificity of the Family CAGE for family alcohol problems was 96%; the positive predictive value, 90%; the sensitivity, 39%; and the negative predictive value, 62%.[47] The Family CAGE results are also correlated with the degree of family stress, of family communication problems, and of marital dissatisfaction and with use of drugs other than alcohol. The ability to use the Family CAGE in this manner offers the potential for great flexibility for the pediatric encounter and provides a comfortable way of collecting pertinent screening information about or from children or adolescent patients and parents. By substituting the words *drug use* for *drinking*, the Family CAGE also can be used to screen for problematic use of drugs other than alcohol.[48]

Screening for the Effect of Family Substance Abuse

A longer written screening tool that may be useful is the Children of Alcoholics Screening Test.[49,50] This test was developed as an assessment tool that could identify older children, adolescents, and adult children of alcoholics. It is a 30-item self-report questionnaire designed to measure patients' attitudes, feelings, perceptions, and experiences related to their parents' drinking behavior, using a "yes"/"no" format. It may be useful when a written questionnaire is the preferred method with older children or adolescents.

The Family Drinking Survey also addresses how family members have been affected by a family member's alcoholism.[51] It is adapted from the Children of Alcoholics Screening Test, the Howard Family Questionnaire, and the Family Alcohol Quiz from Al-Anon and is suitable for use with adolescent patients or nonusing parents. It addresses the effects of family alcoholism on the patient's emotions, physical health, interpersonal relationships, and daily functioning. Many substance-abusing parents themselves are children of substance abusers. Inquiring about family histories of addiction while completing a three-generation genogram with parents can help them put their own substance abuse in an intergenerational context. This motivates some parents to seek treatment to prevent passing this self-destructive behavior on to their own children as their parents did to them. Acknowledging their own childhood experiences can also sensitize parents to the emotional devastation they are causing their children.

An important consideration of children, youths, and parents is the confidentiality of the information gathered. Although many family members are eager to facilitate help for the alcoholic family member, others are more reluctant. If the presenting child or adolescent patient or nonusing parent is reluctant to share his or her concerns, the physician can encourage individual counseling. Attendance at meetings of Al-Anon, Alateen, or Adult Children of Alcoholics groups is important for family members. Whether the family member affected does or does not obtain treatment, other family members may need to learn to care for themselves, and 12-step programs can be extremely supportive.

Screening Measures for Older Adolescents or Adult Family Members

The signs and symptoms of alcohol and other drug abuse in adolescents often are subtle. More telling than physical signs may be the indication of dysfunctional behaviors. A sudden lapse in school attendance, falling grades, or deterioration in other life areas may become more apparent as alcohol or other drug use escalates.[52] Often problems with interpersonal relationships, family, school, or the law become more evident as use increases. Depressive symptoms such as weight loss, change in sleep habits and energy level, depressed mood or mood swings, and suicidal thoughts or attempts may be presenting symptoms of alcohol or other drug use. A general psychosocial assessment of an adolescent's functioning is the most important component of a screening interview for alcohol misuse or abuse. It may be helpful to begin with a discussion of general topical areas, including home and family relationships, school performance and attendance, peer relationships, recreational and leisure activities, vocational aspirations and employment, self-perception, and legal difficulties. The information gathered helps determine whether alcohol or other drug use is a cause of behavioral dysfunction and the degree of patient impairment.

Although no single measure has been recommended for screening adolescents, the CRAFFT questionnaire (whose acronym is based on the questions) (Fig. 19-3), a brief screening tool that has been validated in adolescents, has been used by many clinicians and is easy to use.[53] Others find tools such as the AUDIT to be helpful because they incorporate questions about drinking quantity, frequency, and binge behavior, along with questions about consequences of drinking. A more detailed discussion of adolescent substance abuse screening and assessment is available in the Substance Abuse and Mental Health Services Treatment Improvement Protocol.[54]

EARLY INTERVENTION FOR SUBSTANCE USE DISORDERS

Developmental-behavioral pediatricians and others can have a major influence on families when there is an alcohol- or drug-related concern. Health providers can screen for problem use; offer interventions, support, information, and referrals; and provide guidance and direction for children at risk. Early intervention is a transitional component in the continuum of substance abuse care, between prevention and treatment, and can be distinguished in terms of target population and specific objectives.[55] A useful definition of early intervention would include services directed at (1) individuals or families whose use of ATOD places them or other family members at an unacceptably high level of risk for negative consequences, (2) individuals whose use of ATOD has resulted in clinically significant dysfunctions or consequences for themselves or family members, and (3) individuals or families who exhibit specific problem behaviors hypothesized to be precursors to ATOD problems. In the case of children of substance-abusing parents, an early intervention for the parent and family also should be viewed as prevention for the child. In addition, interventions by primary care pro-

---

CRAFFT: A New Brief Screen for Adolescent Substance Abuse

1. Have you ever ridden in a CAR driven by someone (including yourself) who was "high" or had been using AOD?
2. Do you ever use AOD to RELAX, feel better about yourself, or fit in?
3. Do you ever use AOD while you are by yourself, ALONE?
4. Do you ever FORGET things you did while using AOD?
5. Do your family or FRIENDS ever tell you that you should cut down on your drinking or drug use?
6. Have you ever gotten into TROUBLE while you were using AOD?

A CRAFFT score ≥2 had a sensitivity of 92.3% and specificity of 82.1% for AOD treatment need. The positive predictive value was 66.7% and the negative predictive value was 96.5%.

FIGURE 19-3 CRAFFT: a new brief screen for adolescent substance abuse. A CRAFFT score of 2 or more had a sensitivity of 92.3% and a specificity of 82.1% for alcohol and other drug (AOD) treatment need. The positive predictive value was 66.7%, and the negative predictive value was 96.5%.

viders, which lead to changes in the family's functioning and overall health, can be seen to affect the entire family.

Early intervention services can be distinguished from prevention in that early intervention services target specific individuals rather than the general population. Target populations have been defined on the basis of use patterns suggestive of abuse, the occurrence of use-related consequences for the family member or child, or the presence of risk factors within the family known to be associated with high risk for substance use disorders. Use in inappropriate settings, such as before driving, may be an indication for intervention, even before negative consequences have occurred. According to a consequence-based definition for problem drinking, patterns of use are not what determine the need for early intervention; rather, it is the appearance of negative consequences, which should include health risks or poor outcomes for anyone in the family of a substance abuser. Some substances, such as crack cocaine, heroin, or methamphetamines, are sufficiently dangerous that any use is, in fact, cause for intervention.

It is important for the physician to remember that a positive screen does not establish a diagnosis. A diagnosis that is reached too hastily and without a complete and thorough assessment may sever the physician-family relationship rather than strengthen it. To help the family members obtain the help that they may need, the physician must realize that the family has three issues to confront. The first is for family members to acknowledge their denial: that is, to recognize that a family member has a health problem and needs treatment. By collaborating with the family in the process of diagnosis, the physician not only gathers important and persuasive information about the patient but also helps the family members transcend their own denial. The second issue is for the family to understand the physical, psychological, social, and spiritual effects of the problem and that each member of the family may need help or treatment. If the non–substance-using but affected family member has presented to the physician with physical symptoms or has discussed family disruption, this information can indicate how the family is being affected by the disease. Often individual and family therapy is indicated. The third issue is for family members to realize that they did not cause the alcoholism or other drug use disorder but that their behavior can contribute to or help maintain it.

The physician should assist the family members in understanding their behaviors that keep the affected individual from facing the consequences of his or her use. By examining their enabling behaviors, the physician can help family members learn healthier actions

and, perhaps, motivate the substance-abusing person into treatment. Parents can be afforded the guidelines established by the National Institute on Alcohol Abuse and Alcoholism for nonrisky drinking: namely, (1) two drinks daily, and no more than four on a single occasion, for men and (2) no more than one drink daily and no more than three on a single occasion for nonpregnant women. One drink is defined as 12 oz of beer, 4 oz of wine, or 1.5 oz of liquor.

Even if the affected individual does not obtain treatment, the family can find relief from the stress or discomfort that is present. Often a 12-step program can be helpful. Al-Anon is recommended for spouses and other adults living with a chemically dependent person, and Alateen is recommended for older children and adolescents. Support groups also may be available through the child's school.

In addition to self-help groups, physicians can refer family members for therapy to counselors if the presenting problems warrant additional treatment. Because family members often do not recognize the extent to which they have been affected, it is important that the referral be made to a therapist who understands the effect of chemical substance use disorders on the family. School children and adolescents living with parents with a substance use disorder need to understand that the family's problems are not their fault, that their parents have a disease that is beyond their control and for which they need help, that many other young children feel the same way they do and have had the same experiences, and that help is available for them.

HEALTH AND NEURODEVELOPMENTAL OUTCOME STUDIES OF CHILDREN WITH INTRAUTERINE DRUG EXPOSURE

There are many factors that should be considered in reviewing the literature on neurodevelopmental outcome of children with intrauterine drug exposure. Drug dependence results from a complex, often multigenerational interplay among the individual, the drug, and the environment.

At the individual level, a parent with a history of drug dependence may impart genetic and environmental risk factors that contribute to poor neurobehavioral and neurodevelopmental outcomes in his or her children.[56-59] There is a higher incidence of childhood-onset ADHD and conduct disorder in individuals with alcohol and illicit drug dependence than in those without substance abuse disorders.[60,61] Women who become dependent on alcohol or drugs are shown to have had higher rates of depression, suicidal behavior, anxiety, and withdrawn behaviors during childhood.[57,62] In addition, women who abuse drugs are more likely to have experienced physical abuse and sexual abuse than their non–drug-dependent peers.[63]

Each drug has chemical properties that are associated with its addictive potential and neurophysiological effects on the individual, as well as on the fetus. Many infants of drug-dependent mothers are exposed to more than one potentially neurotoxic drug. The environment of the drug-dependent person may expose the child to risk factors that are associated with poor neurodevelopmental outcome. Lack of parental supervision, family chaos, increased duration of child self-care, community drug trafficking, and peer influences may all play pivotal roles in infant, child, and adolescent outcomes.

Fetal Alcohol Syndrome and Related Disorders

FAS is one of the leading identifiable and preventable causes of mental retardation and birth defects, occurring in 0.2 to 1.5 infants per 1000 live births in the United States.[64] Approximately 4 million infants each year are estimated to have been exposed to alcohol during gestation. It is estimated that 20% of pregnant women drink occasionally and fewer than 1% drink heavily. FAS occurs in 30% to 40% of pregnancies in which a women drinks heavily (more than one drink of 1.5 oz of distilled spirits, 5 oz of wine or 12 oz of beer per day). Although there is evidence of a dose response effect of alcohol on the developing fetus, no safe amount of alcohol consumption during pregnancy has been identified. Of importance is that FAS is 100% preventable; if a mother-to-be does not drink alcohol during pregnancy, her child will not have FAS.

FAS is associated with physical characteristics that include growth retardation, microcephaly, short palpebral fissures, flat midface, long philtrum, and thin upper lip.[65] A stepwise discriminant analysis of three facial features (ratio of reduced palpebral fissure length to inner canthal distance; smoothness of the philtrum; and thinness of the upper lip) identified children with FAS with 100% accuracy.[66] Sensitivity and specificity for identification of FAS by the three facial features were unaffected by race, age, and gender. CNS anomalies may include agenesis of the corpus callosum and cerebellar hypoplasia.[67]

Multiple studies have demonstrated alcohol's neurobehavioral teratogenic effects. Neuropsychological disorders associated with alcohol exposure include ADHD, depression, suicidal ideation, mental retardation, and learning disabilities.[68-71] Children with intrauterine alcohol exposure also are at risk for poor motor coordination, social functioning, and judgment that may place the child at further risk for poor school performance.[68]

In 1996, the Institute of Medicine proposed using the terms *alcohol-related neurodevelopmental disorder* and *alcohol-related birth defects* to describe the spectrum of clinical findings associated with alcohol exposure.[72] Furthermore, in 2004, the Centers for Disease Control and Prevention[73] released a report containing diagnostic criteria for FAS, including recommendations for prevention of alcohol exposure during pregnancy. There is currently general consensus that prenatal alcohol exposure results in a wide range of adverse effects that, as a whole, have been called *fetal alcohol spectrum disorders*. Birth defects associated with alcohol exposure affect multiple organ systems. The most common alcohol-related malformations include cardiac anomalies (e.g., atrial septal defects, ventricular septal defects, tetralogy of Fallot), skeletal anomalies (e.g., hypoplastic nails, shortened fifth digits, scoliosis, hemivertebrae, Klippel-Feil syndrome, radioulnar synostosis), renal anomalies (e.g., aplastic or dysplastic kidneys, horseshoe kidneys), ocular anomalies (e.g., strabismus, retinal vascular anomalies), and auditory impairments.

The annual U.S. cost of alcohol related disorders ranges from $75 million to $249.7 million.[74,74a]). Approximately 60% to 75% of the cost is attributable to care of individuals with FAS who have mental retardation. An estimated $75 million per annum is spent for supervised environments for individuals with IQs in the range of 70 to 85.[74a]

Early diagnosis of FAS and placement of the child in a safe, structured, nurturing environment is associated with improved outcomes. Behavioral and educational interventions to meet the child's individual needs may improve academic performance and peer relations. Nationally, support groups are available to provide information and resources for parents and caregivers of children with FAS or fetal alcohol exposure.

The Centers for Disease Control and Prevention has a Fetal Alcohol Syndrome Web site (*http://www.cdc.gov/ncbddd/fas/faqs.htm*) that answers frequently asked questions about FAS. Additional educational resources for caregivers and providers of services for children with fetal alcohol syndrome spectrum disorders include the Fetal Alcohol Syndrome Family Resource Institute (1-800-999-3429) http://*www.fetalalcholsyndrome.org*.

Tobacco

Nicotine, a colorless liquid alkaloid, is the active ingredient in tobacco. Ninety percent of nicotine is absorbed from inhalation, and the liver subsequently metabolizes 80% to 90% of the nicotine. The physiological effects of smoking one cigarette are similar to injecting 1 mg of nicotine intravenously.[75]). Nicotine is one the most toxic drugs known. It binds to the nicotinic acetylcholine receptors in the fetal brain, causing disruption of synaptic activity, cell loss, and neuronal damage. It has been determined that fetuses in the second and third trimesters are particularly susceptible to the negative effects of tobacco exposure, inasmuch as the number of nicotine receptor binding sites tends to increase significantly during these periods.[76]

Other biological studies indicate that carbon monoxide and nicotine lower maternal uterine blood flow by up to 38%.[9] This in turn reduces the concentration of oxygen in maternal tissues and fetal cord blood, thereby leading to fetal hypoxia and malnutrition. This chronic hypoxia may disrupt neuronal pathways and impair cognitive development.[77,78]

The teratogenic effects of smoking tobacco and passive transmission through environmental tobacco smoke are extensively documented in the literature. Children exposed to nicotine in utero have an increased risk for low birth weight, defined as birth weight of less than 2500 g.[79] This increased risk, resulting from intrauterine growth retardation, demonstrates a dose-response relationship at the rate of 5% weight reduction per pack of cigarettes smoked per day.[78] These infants weigh approximately 150 to 250 g less than non–tobacco-exposed infants and account for 20% to 30% of all infants with low birth weight.[9]

Inadequate fetal lung development and poor neonatal pulmonary functioning are associated with prenatal exposure to tobacco. Jaakkola and Gissler[79] tested the causal effect of maternal smoking during pregnancy on asthma development in childhood in a population-based cohort of Finnish singleton births ($N = 58,841$). These authors postulated that the direct effect of prenatal smoking on the risk for development of asthma in the first 7 years of life would be partially mediated by the presence of intrauterine growth retardation and preterm delivery. The results demonstrated that children whose mothers smoked more than 10 cigarettes per day during pregnancy had a 36% higher chance of developing asthma in the first 7 years of life. There appeared to be a small reduction in the direct effect when intrauterine growth retardation and preterm delivery were added to the model, which suggests that these mediating factors account for only a small proportion of the effect.

NEURODEVELOPMENTAL OUTCOME

Law and colleagues[9] examined the effects of smoking during pregnancy on neurobehavioral functioning in newborns. The NICU Network Neurobehavioral Scale[80] was completed for 56 neonates 48 hours after birth. Examiners were unaware of the prenatal smoking exposure status of the infants. Maternal smoking was measured through the Timeline Follow Back interview of smoking and alcohol use during pregnancy[81] and salivary cotinine bioassay. The results were suggestive of neurotoxic effects of in utero tobacco exposure on neurobehavior. Specifically, the exposed infants showed evidence of increased excitability, hypertonia, and stress/abstinence symptoms in the CNS, gastrointestinal system, and visual field. These findings were demonstrated at a dose rate (6 cigarettes per day) lower than the 10 cigarettes per day that is traditionally cited in the literature on the dose-response relationship. The authors noted that establishing these neuroteratogenic effects at birth may provide compelling evidence for the role of prenatal tobacco exposure, over and above postnatal contextual factors, on the development of long-term deficits such as lower IQ and ADHD.

Cornelius and associates[76] examined the longitudinal effects of prenatal smoking on neuropsychological functioning in a sample of 593 children. Participants were monitored prospectively from the fourth month of gestation to age 10 years. Neuropsychological tests were conducted at the 10-year follow-up to assess the effect of gestational smoking on learning, memory, problem solving, mental flexibility, attention, and eye-hand coordination. These longitudinal data demonstrated an adverse effect of gestational smoking on learning, memory, problem solving, and eye-hand coordination. These results remained statistically significant even when other prenatal and current maternal substance abuse, demographic, psychological, and environmental variables were accounted for. Fried and coworkers[82] found that prenatal cigarette exposure was negatively associated with overall intelligence in a sample of 145 adolescents aged 13 to 16 years old.

Prenatal nicotine exposure is also associated with deficits in language development.[78] Results from the Ottawa Prenatal Prospective Study[83] revealed that children prenatally exposed to cigarettes had decreased responsiveness on auditory items on the Bayley Scales of Infant Development (BSID) at 12 and 24 months of age. Delays in language development continued to exist at age 4 years. Cognitive deficits, specifically on measures of verbal intelligence, reading, and language, continued to persist into early adolescence, which constitutes further evidence of the dose-dependent response noted at earlier ages.[84]

The literature clearly demonstrates that prenatal tobacco exposure is a risk factor for development of behavior problems, specifically aggressive and antisocial behaviors.[85] This relationship also seems to follow a dose-response effect between the amount of prenatal exposure and the emergence of behavior problems.[78] Of importance is that although researchers have attempted to account for confounding factors when analyzing the statistical relationship between prenatal exposure and childhood conduct problems, the strength of the relationship relies primarily on correlational data. The effect of the relationship appears to be reduced when other known confounding factors are analyzed.

Silberg and colleagues[86] tested the causal relationship between prenatal tobacco exposure and childhood conduct disorder in a sample of 538 white male twins. General linear models were used to examine the direct effect of prenatal smoking on childhood conduct disorder. Mothers' conduct disorder symptoms in childhood were included as an operationalization of the latent variable "antisociality." The effects of prenatal smoking were significantly reduced when mothers' childhood conduct disorder symptoms and age were included in the model.

Further latent variable modeling indicated a significant relationship between the latent transmission variable and childhood conduct disorder. Excluding the direct path between prenatal smoking and child conduct disorder did not worsen the model fit; this suggests a stronger association between maternal conduct symptoms and child behavior than between tobacco exposure and child behavior.

Cocaine

Cocaine use during pregnancy is associated with adverse outcomes that include higher risk of sexually transmitted disease and of pregnancy-related complications such as premature rupture of membranes, abruption of the placenta, and fetal demise in comparison with women without a history of cocaine use.[87,88] In a case-control study of 400 maternal-infant dyads (200 with maternal cocaine use and 200 without drug use),[87] infants born to mothers with a history of cocaine use had a significantly higher risk of having respiratory distress syndrome, congenital syphilis, and prolonged hospital stay.

NEURODEVELOPMENTAL OUTCOME

Early case reports led to many premature conclusions about neurodevelopmental outcome of children with intrauterine cocaine exposure. One meta-analysis of 118 studies of children with intrauterine cocaine exposure demonstrated that 92% of the studies included children with exposure to multiple drugs, including alcohol, tobacco, marijuana, and opiates.[89] Over time, more sophisticated techniques were developed to identify and quantify cocaine and other drug use, and data collection and statistical analyses improved.

Impairment of brain growth in children with intrauterine cocaine/polydrug exposure (IUDE) is documented in multiple studies.[90-93] Disturbances of neuronal migration and differentiation have been reported in human infants exposed to cocaine during gestation.[94,95] The most common neurological anomaly found in children with cocaine/polydrug exposure is microcephaly.[96]

In a study of children with cocaine/polydrug exposure, mean birth head circumference for infants with only cocaine exposure was 1.71 standard deviations smaller than the mean, whereas head circumference was 1.0 and 1.52 standard deviations below the mean for infants exposed only to opiates and those exposed to cocaine and opiates, respectively.[92] Preliminary data from a small case-control magnetic resonance imaging study suggested smaller white matter volumes in the frontal lobes of children with cocaine or polydrug exposure than in those of children without drug exposure.[97] Midline prosencephalic developmental abnormalities, including agenesis of the corpus callosum, septo-optic dysplasia, and absence of the septum pellucidum, have been reported in case studies of children with intrauterine cocaine exposure.[98]

Cranial ultrasound data obtained during the neonatal period demonstrated that 35% of infants with intrauterine cocaine or polydrug exposure had one or more intracranial abnormalities.[99] Ultrasound findings were suggestive of degenerative changes or focal infarctions of the basal ganglia. In addition, schizencephaly and neuronal heterotopias have been documented in children born to cocaine-dependent mothers.[94,95,98]

Differences in attention, distractibility, and visual memory have been reported in infants with cocaine or polydrug exposure.[100-103] Studies of young school-aged children with IUDE have documented significantly higher externalizing (e.g., inattention, aggression, disruptive behavior) and internalizing behavior problems (e.g., withdrawn, anxious behaviors). Delaney-Black and associates[104] demonstrated gender and duration-specific effects of prenatal cocaine, finding that behavior of school-aged boys was more significantly and negatively affected by cocaine exposure than that of girls. In a study of 145 children (111 with IUDE and 34 nonexposed children) by Butz and coworkers,[105] parents and caretakers of children with intrauterine drug exposure reported significantly more overall behavior problems, especially anxious or depressed behaviors and deficits in attention in their children. In addition, stress levels were higher in caretakers of children with intrauterine drug exposure than in those of children without drug exposure.[102]

A longitudinal case-cohort study of 476 children (253 cocaine-exposed and 223 non–cocaine-exposed infants) documented performance deficiencies on measures of visual attention in 7-year-old children with intrauterine cocaine exposure, after adjusting for medical and sociodemographic variables and for alcohol, marijuana, and tobacco exposure.[100]

In a meta-analysis of 36 studies that met stringent criteria, including using only prospective controlled studies whose evaluators were unaware of drug of exposure and whose participants included children with cocaine exposure, without substantial opiate, amphetamine, or phencyclidine exposure, Frank and associates[106] concluded that if exposure to other drugs was controlled statistically or in the study design, prenatal cocaine exposure was not found to contribute to growth retardation. In addition, the majority of studies in which researchers controlled for other drug exposure did not reveal an association between intrauterine cocaine exposure and adverse cognitive and language outcomes. Three of the six studies analyzed demonstrated deficient motor skills in the first 7 months. Of most significance, findings did support a relationship between cocaine exposure and less affective expression during infancy and early childhood, as well as less optimal scoring on behavior rating scales and tests of sustained attention.

The Maternal Lifestyle Study is a prospective, longitudinal, multisite study (funded by the National Institute of Child Health and Human Development; the National Institute on Drug Abuse, the Administration on Children, Youth and Families; and the Center for Substance Abuse Treatment) to determine the association between cocaine and opiate exposure and developmental and behavioral outcome; a host of medical and psychosocial covariates are controlled.[89] Phase I, conducted between 1993 and 1995, included 11,811 mother-infant dyads. Meconium samples were collected from the infants for enzyme-multiplied immunoassay for cocaine, opiates, tetrahydrocannabinol, amphetamines, and phencyclidine, followed by gas chromatography/mass spectroscopy confirmation. In phase II, 1388 mother-infant dyads with and without drug exposure and matched for race, gender, and gestational age from the pool of 11,811 were studied. After adjustment for other drug exposure, results from the 1-month evaluation demonstrated subtle but consistent differences, including lower arousal, poorer quality of movement and self-regulation, increased hypertonia on the NICU Network Neurobehavioral Scale, and longer interpeak intervals I to III and shorter interpeak intervals III to V on auditory brain response testing. At 3 years of age, cocaine exposure was not associated with BSID–Second Edition Mental Developmental Index, Psychomotor Developmental Index, or Behavior Record Scale scores.[107]

In summary, although a direct causal effect of cocaine use that results in cognitive deficits was not apparent in this large prospective study, cocaine exposure was associated with factors such as low birth weight, disruptions in maternal care, low socioeconomic status, and low vocabulary scores, which themselves do place children at risk for lower cognitive functioning.

Marijuana

One large prospective study of more than 7000 pregnant women revealed no associations between marijuana use during pregnancy and low birth weight, preterm delivery, or abruptio placentae.[108] Another study of more than 700 infants revealed no increased incidence of pregnancy, labor, or delivery complications in association with marijuana use during pregnancy.[109] In addition, two large prospective studies—the Ottawa Prenatal Prospective Study (OPPS)[110] and the Maternal Health Practices and Child Development Projects (MHPCD)[109]—provide much of the knowledge about the effects of intrauterine marijuana exposure. Initiated in 1978, the OPPS is an ongoing longitudinal investigation of 190 children born to middle class, primarily college-educated women, of whom 140 had a history of marijuana use during pregnancy and 50 did not. The MHPCD recruited 763 primarily low-income women from Pittsburgh during the fourth month of pregnancy from 1983 to 1985 to monitor the developmental outcome of their children with and without exposure to marijuana and alcohol.[109]

These studies, along with others, revealed that marijuana use during pregnancy was not associated with fetal growth retardation.[109-111]

NEURODEVELOPMENTAL OUTCOME

Neonatal findings reported in infants with prenatal marijuana exposure include increased tremors and startles, abnormal sleep patterns characterized by decreased quiet sleep, and poorer habituation to light.[109,110]). Interestingly, in a prospective study of 24 Jamaican infants with marijuana exposure who were compared with nonexposed neonates, there were no differences between the groups on day 3, when the infants were assessed with the Brazelton Neonatal Assessment Scale, and at 1 month. Infants with heavy marijuana exposure demonstrated improved autonomic stability, quality of alertness, less irritability, and better self-regulation. Dreher's[112] study is important because the neonates in this study were generally exposed to higher potency marijuana and were less likely to be exposed to other drugs than were neonates in U.S. and Canadian studies.

Outcome evaluation of 12- and 24-month-old children with intrauterine marijuana exposure enrolled in the OPPS revealed no association between the BSID scores and marijuana exposure after home environment was controlled for. Marijuana exposure was negatively correlated with the home environment.[113]

Unadjusted hierarchical regression analyses of young elementary school–aged children with second trimester intrauterine marijuana exposure revealed that these children had more errors of commission on the Continuous Performance Test,[114] which was suggestive of increased impulsivity in marijuana-exposed children in comparison with children with no exposure.[115] At 10 years of age, children with heavy marijuana exposure during the first trimester had lower scores on the design memory and screening index of the Wide Range Assessment of Memory and Learning[116]; in addition, the finding of increased commission errors persisted.[117] The magnitude of the marijuana effects were small at this age, and on structural equation modeling, there were no significant associations between marijuana exposure and neuropsychological domains.[117] Functional magnetic resonance imaging studies of young adults, 18 to 21 years of age, with prenatal marijuana exposure demonstrated increased neural activity in bilateral prefrontal cortex and right premotor cortex and decreased cerebellar activation during response inhibition.[118] More commission errors continued to be present in young adults exposed to marijuana.[118]

In summary, intrauterine marijuana exposure appears to be associated with persistent deficits in prefrontal lobe functioning, as evidenced by both the longitudinal MHPCD and OPPS. As a result, children with intrauterine marijuana exposure have deficiencies in the stability of attention (e.g. the ability to maintain attention over time), as well as impulsivity.[115,119]

Opiates

The majority of studies suggest that infants with intrauterine opiate exposure weigh less and have smaller head circumferences than do their non–drug-exposed peers.[120-124] Infants with gestational opiate exposure have been reported to have a higher incidence of respiratory distress and infections and longer hospitalizations, attributable to withdrawal- and non–withdrawal-related morbidity.[121,122,124]

One of the major morbid conditions in infants with in utero opiate exposure is neonatal abstinence syndrome (NAS), or neonatal drug withdrawal. NAS is characterized by CNS and gastrointestinal symptoms, including irritability, tremors, disrupted sleep patterns, rigidity, seizures, poor suck, vomiting, diarrhea, dehydration, poor weight gain, temperature instability, and diaphoresis.[125-128]

The incidence of NAS varies in frequency and onset, depending of the dose and type of maternal opiate use.[120,122,129] Because of methadone's 15- to 57-hour half-life, neonatal withdrawal may not be observed until 72 hours after birth; however, the onset may be protracted and can occur up to 4 weeks after birth. In contrast, withdrawal from heroin is usually evident within 24 to 72 hours. Symptoms of NAS may be measured by a variety of instruments, including those developed by Finnegan[127] and Lipsitz[130] to determine whether pharmacological management is necessary.

Probably the most common pharmacological agents used to control the adverse effects of NAS are tincture of opium (10 mg morphine equivalent/mL), paregoric (containing anhydrous morphine, 0.4 mg/mL), methadone, and phenobarbital. Tincture of opium is preferred for treatment of NAS, because not only does tincture of opium substitute for the opiate that causes the withdrawal symptoms but it also contains fewer additives and less alcohol than does paregoric. Tincture of opium is usually diluted 25-fold (diluted tincture of opium) so that it has the same concentration of morphine equivalent as does paregoric. Initial diluted tincture of opium dose is 0.1 mL/kg (2 drops/kg) every 4 hours with feedings. This dosage may be increased by 2 drops/kg every 4 hours until NAS symptoms are controlled. The dosage is gradually tapered by decreasing the dose, not by increasing dosing interval.

Phenobarbital and diazepam have also been used to treat NAS. Phenobarbital reduces the irritability, tremulousness of NAS but does not control gastrointestinal signs. Poor feeding, weight gain, and feeding time was noted during phenobarbital therapy for NAS in comparison with paregoric. In addition, phenobarbital may cause CNS depression. In a study by Kaltenbach and Finnegan,[129] infants with NAS initially treated with phenobarbital were more likely to require a second drug to control NAS than were those treated with paregoric. A phenobarbital loading dose of 16 mg/kg in 24 hours controlled most narcotic symptoms, with maintenance doses of 2 to 8 mg/kg/day. Diazepam, 1 to 2 mg of every 8 hours, may result in rapid suppression of NAS signs; however, diazepam may cause CNS depression, poor suck, and late-onset seizures.

NEURODEVELOPMENTAL OUTCOME

A comparison of paregoric, phenobarbital (loading), phenobarbital (titration), diazepam, and no treatment (for infants with mild NAS symptoms) in infants with opiate exposure demonstrated no differences among the groups on the 6-month BSID Mental Developmental Index score.[129] In a longitudinal study of 39 infants (16 methadone-exposed infants and 23 non–drug-exposed infants) in which partial-order scalogram analyses were used to study the differences among the scores on the subtests of the Infant Behavior Rating, only motor coordination was different between the methadone-exposed and non–drug-exposed infants at 4 months, after family and medical risk factors were adjusted. By 12 months, the attention subtest distinguished between the two groups of infants.[131] Rosen and Johnson[123] studied 64 children, of whom 41 had been exposed to methadone and 23 had not been exposed, at ages 6, 12, and 18 months. At 12 and 18 months, significant differences, favoring the non–drug-exposed infants, were found in mean Mental Developmental Index and Psychomotor Developmental Index scores on the BSID. In the Maternal Lifestyle Study of children with cocaine and opiate exposure, 1227 infants (474 with cocaine exposure, 50 with opiate exposure, and 48 with cocaine and opiate exposure) were evaluated through 3 years of age.[107] Opiate exposure was not associated with overall Mental Developmental Index score at 2 or 3 years of age.

The unadjusted mean Psychomotor Developmental Index score was 3.9 points lower than in infants not exposed to opiates ($p = 0.003$). Once analysis models were adjusted for covariates (study site, infant age, infant birth weight, maternal care, Home Observation for Measurement of the Environment Inventory score, and ethnicity), opiate exposure was no longer associated with Psychomotor Developmental Index score at 3 years of age. No cocaine × opiate interactions were found in these analyses. In addition, there were no increases in clinically significant Behavior Rating Scale scores.

In summary, opiate exposure is associated with significant neonatal morbidity, including NAS, low birth growth parameters, and increased infections. Studies of infants with intrauterine opiate exposure now document potential maturation delays in midbrain development. However, the most recent longitudinal prospective data suggest no differences in Mental Developmental Index score, Psychomotor Developmental Index score, and evaluator ratings on behavior measures between 2- and 3-year-old children with opiate exposure and children without drug exposure.

PREVENTION AND TREATMENT

Research to date on children with intrauterine drug exposure has focused primarily on examining the developmental trajectory of children with IUDE. Studies have demonstrated that risk factors associated with prenatal substance exposure may be a potential contributor to negative neurodevelopmental outcomes. In view of this information, early intervention strategies are being developed to detect and prevent the onset of these problems and reduce their negative effects. Interventions geared toward treating the associated risk factors of IUDE may improve the quality of life for these children.

Home-based nursing intervention is one type of community-based educational intervention used for women who are drug dependent and for their children. By providing education, access to services, and enrichment experiences in the natural environment, home-based intervention are designed to promote the health and well-being of children and families at risk for poor developmental outcomes. Nurses are especially suited to provide intervention because of their expertise in the areas of women's and children's health, their capacity for handling complex clinical issues, and their ability to teach health awareness while improving access to medical care.[132]

Black and associates[133] examined the effect of a home intervention designed to support parenting and child development through the first 18 months post partum. Modest improvements were noted in recovery, emotional responsiveness of the mother, and attitudes toward parenting for the women in the intervention. There were no developmental differences between the intervention and control children at the 18-month follow-up. The findings revealed only modest changes on drug use and parenting behaviors as a result of the home intervention. In another randomized study of home-based nursing intervention for a cohort of 100 children with intrauterine drug exposure,[134] mothers perceived that children who received home-based nursing intervention had significantly fewer behavior problems.

Hofkosh and coworkers[135] found a similar pattern of results, noting that the developmental capabilities of the children in their home-based clinical intervention were age appropriate at 1 year. These authors noted that the ability of the mother to provide a developmentally supportive environment most significantly affected child development.

Schuler and associates[136] conducted a home-based nursing intervention for 131 women with active substance abuse problems up to 24 months after delivery. A preintervention-postintervention randomized control design was used with follow-up assessments at 6-month intervals through 24 months and yearly thereafter. The program was divided into two components. The parent component focused on teaching the parent to identify and to appropriately use family, community, and social systems for a range of services, including public assistance, domestic violence, and drug treatment. The child component focused on enhancing maternal-child relations by teaching parents how to play with their children in order to promote age-appropriate developmental skills. This home-based nursing intervention entailed a combination of the Infant Health and Development Program and the HELP at Home curriculum from the Hawaii Early Learning Program[137] that was modified to apply specifically to substance-abusing mothers and their children. Results indicate that children in the early intervention group demonstrated significant improvements in motor and mental development in comparison with children in the control group up to 18 months post partum. There were no differences between the groups on language development. Mothers receiving the intervention and mothers in the control group had similar rates of ongoing drug use: 43% and 36%, respectively.

There was no significant effect of the home-based intervention on maternal-child relations as operationalized by maternal competence and observed child responsiveness during mother-child interactions at the 18-month follow-up.[138] A sample of 108 cocaine-abusing mothers using the same home-based intervention[139] exhibited significant improvements in cognitive scores on the BSID after the home-based intervention. Ongoing maternal drug use was associated with poor infant cognitive developmental outcomes through 18 months post partum. These results suggest that ongoing maternal drug use is a critical environmental factor that appears to adversely affect the outcome of intervention trials in children exposed to IUDE.

Results of the home-based interventions yielded mixed outcomes. Overall, the findings suggest that these interventions result in some improvement of knowledge of parenting strategies, development of more positive attitudes toward parenting, and enhancement of the quality of maternal-child relationships. Studied interventions yield varied results on child development.

Other types of treatment approaches to improve maternal-child relations with drug-dependent mothers have focused on inclusion of multiple treatment methods within one model to provide a more comprehensive and holistic drug treatment approach. McComish and colleagues[140] evaluated the efficacy of a family-focused residential drug treatment program for drug-dependent women and their children. Significant improvements in the mother's parenting knowledge and treatment retention were noted. This study also demonstrated the importance of inclusion of children in early intervention with drug-dependent mothers. Although the children in the intervention did not initially show signs of developmental delay, longitudinal data revealed signs of motor and language delay for some of the children in the intervention group. Thus, early detection and, consequently, early treatment of developmental delays

occurred in the children as a result of their participation in this comprehensive residential program.

Although most studies have focused on adult mothers, substance abuse among mothers younger than 20 years is also an important public health concern. Studies show that young drug-abusing mothers are at increased risk for parenting problems because of a variety of factors, including lack of parenting experience, less education, and lack of financial resources. Furthermore, these mothers may have their own problems understanding and developing basic psychoemotional developmental skills such as developing trust, problem solving, and impulse control.[141] Field and coworkers[142] examined the effect of a multimodal intervention for adolescent mothers and their children with IUDE. The participants in this study attended a 4-month treatment program located within their vocational school. Mothers received drug and social rehabilitation, parenting and vocational courses, and relaxation therapy. Infants were placed in a nursery while their mothers attended high school or General Educational Development (GED) preparation classes. The mothers volunteered as teacher-aid trainees in the nursery and learned parenting skills while tending to their babies. At the 6-month follow-up, the mother-child interactions and child developmental outcomes of mothers and infants in the treatment group were similar to those of a non–drug-exposed control group.

The Mom Empowerment Too (ME2) program combined community-based nursing and drug treatment through a participatory action research model for a young adult population. Participatory action research allowed researchers to collect outcome data while modifying aspects of the intervention in response to the feedback of the participants.[143] Public health nurses used a variety of treatment modalities to provide case management services; access to drug treatment, medical care, and social services; educational and parenting classes; group therapy; and life skills training. The children (from birth to age 5 years) took part in developmental and health-promoting exercises while their parents attended their sessions. The investigators documented improvements in taking responsibility and learning to trust. Both areas of improvement are related to effective parenting.

In summary, intrauterine tobacco and illicit drug exposure are associated with adverse infant health outcomes. Studies suggest that infants exposed to these substances are at risk for attention and behavioral deficits during childhood. Data suggest that nicotine exposure places the child at risk for poorer cognitive outcome. Data concerning the causal associations between illicit drug exposure and cognitive outcome are less conclusive. More research is necessary to develop comprehensive prevention and intervention programs for this vulnerable population.

REFERENCES

1. Office of Applied Studies: The National Survey on Drug Use and Health Report: Pregnancy and Substance Abuse. Rockville, MD: Substance Abuse and Mental Health Services Administration, 2004.
2. Office of Applied Studies: *Results from the 2004 National Survey on Drug Use and Health: National Findings* (DHHS Publication No. SMA 05-4062, NSDUH Series H-28). Rockville, MD: Substance Abuse and Mental Health Services Administration, 2005. (Available at: *http://www.oas.samhsa.gov/p0000016.htm#2k4;* accessed 1/23/06.)
3. Office of Applied Studies: Illicit Drug Use in the Past Month among Females Aged 15 to 44, by Pregnancy Status and Demographic Characteristics: Percentages, 2002. Rockville, MD: Substance Abuse and Mental Health Services Administration, 2002.
4. U.S. Department of Health and Human Services: The Health Consequences of Smoking: A Report of the Surgeon General. Atlanta, GA: Centers for Disease Control and Prevention, National Center for Chronic Disease Prevention and Health Promotion, Office on Smoking and Health, 2004.
5. DiFranza JR, Savageau JA, Rigotti NA, et al: Development of symptoms of tobacco dependence in youths: 30 month follow up data from the DANDY study. Tobacco Control 11:228-235, 2002.
6. MMWR, Use of Cigarettes and Other Tobacco Products Among Students Aged 13-15 Years—Worldwide, 1999-2005, 55(20):553-556, May 26, 2006.
7. Henningfield J: Nicotine medications for smoking cessation. N Engl J Med 333(18):1196-1202, 1995.
8. Moolchan E, Ernst M, Henningfield J, et al: A review of tobacco smoking in adolescents: Treatment implications. J Am Acad Child Adolesc Psychiatry 39(6):682-693, 2000.
9. Law KL, Stroud LR, Lagasse LL, et al: Smoking during pregnancy and newborn neurobehavior. Pediatrics 111:1318-1323, 2003.
10. Acute myocardial infarction and combined oral contraceptives: Results of an international multicentre case-control study. WHO Collaborative Study of Cardiovascular Disease and Steroid Hormone Contraception. Lancet 349:1202-1209, 1997.
11. Fiore M, Bailey W, Cohen S, et al: A clinical practice guideline for treating tobacco use and dependence: A US Public Health Service Report. JAMA 283(24):3244-3254, 2000.
12. Johnston LD, O'Malley PM, Bachman JG, et al: Monitoring the Future National Results on Adolescent Drug Use: Overview of Key Findings, 2004 (NIH Publication No. 05-5726). Bethesda, MD: National Institute on Drug Abuse, 2005.
13. Smothers BA, Yahr HT, Ruhl CE: Detection of Alcohol Use Disorders in General Hospital Admissions in the United States. Arch Intern Med 164:749-756, 2004.
14. Bonnie RJ, O'Connell ME, eds: Committee on Developing a Strategy to Reduce and Prevent Underage Drinking, Board on Children, Youth, and Families, Division of Behavioral and Social Sciences and Education, National Research Council, Institute of Medicine: Reducing Underage Drinking, A Collective Responsibility. Washington, DC: National Academies Press, 2003.
15. Goodwin DW, Schulsinger F, Hermansen L, et al: Alcohol problems in adoptees raised apart from alcoholic biological parents. Arch Gen Psychiatry 28:238-243, 1973.
16. Goodwin DW, Schulsinger F, Knop J, et al: Alcoholism and depression in adopted-out daughters of alcoholics. Arch Gen Psychiatry 34:751-755, 1977.
17. Bohman M: Some genetic aspects of alcoholism and criminality: A population of adoptees. Arch Gen Psychiatry 35:269-276, 1978.
18. Cloninger CR, Bohman M, Sigvardsson S: Inheritance of alcohol abuse: Cross fostering analysis of adopted men. Arch Gen Psychiatry 38:861-868, 1981.
19. Grant BF: Estimates of US children exposed to alcohol abuse and dependence in the family. Am J Public Health 90:112-115, 2000.
20. Wilens TE, Biederman J, Kiely K, et al: Pilot study of behavioral and emotional disturbances in the high-risk children of parents with opioid dependence. J Am Acad Child Adolesc Psychiatry 34(6):779-785, 1995.
21. Stanger C, Higgins ST, Bickel WK, et al: Behavioral and emotional problems among children of cocaine- and opiate-dependent parents. J Am Acad Child Adolesc Psychiatry 38:421-428, 1999.
22. Clark DB, Pollock N, Bukstein OG, et al: Gender and comorbid psychopathology in adolescents with alcohol dependence. J Am Acad Child Adolesc Psychiatry 36:1195-1203, 1997.
23. Merikangas KR, Stolar M, Stevens DE, et al: Familial transmission of substance use disorders. Arch Gen Psychiatry 55:973-979, 1998.
24. Nunes EV, Weissman MM, Goldstein RB, et al: Psychopathology in children of parents with opiate dependence and/or major depression. J Am Acad Child Adolesc Psychiatry 37:1142-1151, 1998.
25. Chilcoat HD, Anthony JC: Impact of parent monitoring on initiation of drug use through late childhood. J Am Acad Child Adolesc Psychiatry 35:91-100, 1996.
26. Stronski SM, Ireland M, Michaud PA, et al: Protective correlates of stages in adolescent substance use: A Swiss national study. J Adolesc Health 26:420-427, 2000.
27. Adger H Jr, Macdonald DI, Wenger S: Core competencies for involvement of health care providers in the care of children and adolescents in families affected by substance abuse. Pediatrics 103(5, pt 2):1083-1084, 1999.
28. Harford TC: Family history of alcoholism in the United States: Prevalence and demographic characteristics. Br J Addict 87:931-935, 1992.
29. Bijur PE, Kurzon M, Overpeck MD, et al: Parental alcohol use, problem drinking, and children's injuries. JAMA 267:3166-3171, 1992.

30. Murphy JM, Jellinek M, Quinn QD, et al: Substance abuse and serious child maltreatment: Prevalence, risk, and outcome in a court sample. Child Abuse Negl 15:197-211, 1991.

31. Greer SW, Bauchner H, Zuckerman B: Pediatricians' knowledge and practices regarding parental use of alcohol. Am J Dis Child 144:1234-1237, 1990.

32. Duggan AK, Adger H, McDonald EM, et al: Detection of alcoholism in hospitalized children and their families. Am J Dis Child 145:613-617, 1991.

33. Graham AV, Zyzanski S, Reeb K, et al: Physician documentation of family alcohol problems. J Subst Abuse 6:95-103, 1994.

34. Lazare A, Putnam S, Lipkin M: Functions of the medical interview. *In* Lipkin M, Putnam S, Lazare A, eds: The Medical Interview: Clinical Care, Education, and Research. New York: Springer-Verlag, 1995, pp 3-19.

35. Cohen-Cole SA: The Medical Interview: The Three Function Approach. St Louis: Mosby–Year Book, 1991.

36. Hall JA, Roter DL, Rand CS: Communication of affect between patient and physician. J Health Soc Behav 22:18-30, 1981.

37. Ewing JE: Detecting alcoholism: The CAGE questionnaire. JAMA 252:1905-1907, 1984.

38. Bush B: Screening for alcohol abuse using the CAGE questionnaire. Am J Med 82:231-235, 1987.

39. King M: At risk drinking among general practice attenders: Validation of the CAGE questionnaire. Psychol Med 16:213-217, 1986.

40. Saunders JB, Aasland OG, Babor TF, et al: Development of the Alcohol Use Disorders Identification Test (AUDIT): WHO collaborative project on early detection of persons with harmful alcohol consumption. Addiction 88:791-804, 1993.

41. Hops H, Tildesley E, Lichtenstein E, et al: Parent-adolescent problem solving interactions and drug use. Am J Drug Alcohol Abuse 16:239-258, 1990.

42. Denoff MS: An integrated analysis of the contribution made by irrational beliefs and parental interaction to adolescent drug abuse. Int J Addict 23:655-669, 1988.

43. Wolin SJ, Bennett LA, Noonan DL, et al: Disrupted family rituals: A factor in the intergenerational transmission of alcoholism. Stud Alcohol 41:199-214, 1980.

44. Kandel DB, Andrews K: Processes of adolescent socialization by parents and peers. Int J Addict 22:319-342, 1987.

45. Cohn DA, Richardson J, LaBree L: Parenting behaviors and the onset of smoking and alcohol use: A longitudinal study. Pediatrics 94:368-375, 1994.

46. Saitz R: Clinical practice. Unhealthy alcohol use. N Engl J Med 352(6):596-607, 2005.

47. Frank SH, Graham AV, Zyzanski S, et al: Use of the Family CAGE in screening for alcohol problems in primary care. Arch Fam Med 1:209-216, 1992.

48. Brown RL, Rounds LA: Conjoint screening questionnaires for alcohol and other drug abuse: Criterion validity in a primary care practice. Wis Med J 94(3):135-140, 1995.

49. Jones J: Preliminary Test Manual: The Children of Alcoholics Screening Test. Chicago: Family Recovery Press, 1982.

50. Sheridan MJ: A psychometric assessment of the Children of Alcoholics Screening Test (CAST). J Stud Alcohol 56:156-160, 1995.

51. Whitfield C: Co-dependence. Healing the Human Condition. Deerfield Beach, FL: Health Communications, 1991.

52. Macdonald DI: Diagnosis and treatment of adolescent substance abuse. Curr Prob Pediatr 19:389-444, 1989.

53. Knight JR, Shrier LA, Bravender TD, et al: A new brief screen for adolescent substance abuse. Arch Pediatr Adolesc Med 153:591-596, 1999.

54. Winters KC: Screening and Assessing Adolescents for Substance Use Disorders. Treatment Improvement Protocol (TIP) Series 31, DHHS Publication No. (SMA) 99-3282. Rockville, MD: U.S. Department of Health and Human Services, Public Health Service, Substance Abuse and Mental Health Services Administration, Center for Substance Abuse Treatment, 1999. (Available at: *http://www.ncbi.nlm.nih.gov/books/bv. fcgi?rid=hstat5.chapter.54841;* accessed 1/23/07.)

55. Klitzner M, Fisher D, Stewart K, et al: Substance Abuse: Early Intervention for Adolescents. Princeton, NJ: Robert Wood Johnson Foundation, 1992.

56. Block J, Block JH, Keyes S: Longitudinally foretelling drug usage in adolescence: Early childhood personality and environmental precursors. Child Dev 59:336-355, 1988.

57. Luthar SS, Cushing G, Rounsaville BJ: Gender differences among opioid abusers: Pathways to disorder and profiles of psychopathology. Drug Alcohol Depend 43:179-189, 1996.

58. Conners NA, Bradley RH, Mansell LW, et al: Children of mothers with serious substance abuse problems: An accumulation of risks. Am J Drug Alcohol Abuse 30:85-100, 2004.

59. Wilens TE: Attention-deficit/hyperactivity disorder and the substance use disorders: the nature of the relationship, subtypes at risk, and treatment issues. Psychiatr Clin North Am 27:283-301, 2004.

60. Milin R, Halikas JA, Meller JE, et al: Psychopathology among substance abusing juvenile offenders. J Am Acad Child Adolesc Psychiatry 30:569-574, 1991.

61. Hovens JG, Cantwell DP, Kiriakos R: Psychiatric comorbidity in hospitalized adolescent substance abusers. J Am Acad Child Adolesc Psychiatry 33:476-483, 1994.

62. Wilsnack SC, Wilsnack RW, Kristjanson AF, et al: Alcohol use and suicidal behavior in women: Longitudinal patterns in a U.S. national sample. Alcohol Clin Exp Res 28:38S-47S, 2004.

63. Wilsnack SC, Vogeltanz ND, Klassen AD, et al: Childhood sexual abuse and women's substance abuse: National survey findings. J Stud Alcohol 58:264-271, 1997.

64. National Center for Birth Defects and Developmental Disabilities, Fetal Alcohol Spectrum Disorders, *http://www.cdc.gov/ncbddd/fas/fasask.htm#how*, 2007.

65. Bertrand J, Floyd RL, Weber MK: Guidelines for identifying and referring persons with fetal alcohol syndrome. MMWR Morb Mortal Wkly Rep 54:1-15, 2005.

66. Astley SJ, Clarren SK: A case definition and photographic screening tool for the facial phenotype of fetal alcohol syndrome. J Pediatr 129:33-41, 1996.

67. Riley EP, Mattson SN, Sowell ER, et al: Abnormalities of the corpus callosum in children prenatally exposed to alcohol. Alcohol Clin Exp Res 19:1198-1202, 1995.

68. Streissguth AP, Barr HM, Kogan J, et al: Understanding the Occurrence of Secondary Disabilities in Clients with Fetal Alcohol Syndrome (FAS) and Fetal Alcohol Effects (FAE) Final Report to the Centers for Disease Control and Prevention, Tech. Rep. No. 96-06. Seattle: University of Washington, Fetal Alcohol and Drug Unit, August 1996.

69. Jones KL, Smith DW, Ulleland CN, et al: Pattern of malformation in offspring of chronic alcoholic mothers. Lancet 1:1267-1271, 1973.

70. Clarren SK, Smith DW: The fetal alcohol syndrome. N Engl J Med 298:1063-1067, 1978.

71. Riley EP, Mattson SN, Li TK, et al: Neurobehavioral consequences of prenatal alcohol exposure: An international perspective. Alcohol Clin Exp Res 27:362-373, 2003.

72. National Academy of Sciences Committee of Fetal Alcohol Syndrome: Fetal Alcohol Syndrome: Diagnosis, Epidemiology, Prevention and Treatment. Washington, DC: National Academies Press, 1996.

73. Centers for Disease Control and Prevention, 2004; www.cdc.gov/ncbddd/fas/documents/FAS_guidelines_accessible.pdf.

74. Abel EL, Sokol RJ: A revised conservative estimate of the incidence of FAS and its economic impact. Alcohol Clin Exp Res 15:514-524, 1991.

74a. Abel EL, Sokol RJ: A revised estimate of the economic impact of fetal alcohol syndrome. Recent Dev Alcohol 9:117-125, 1991.

75. Ray O, Ksir C: Tobacco. In Ray O, Ksir C, eds: Drugs, Society, and Human Behavior, 7th ed. Boston: WCB/McGraw-Hill, 1996, pp. 266-290.

76. Cornelius MD, Ryan CM, Day NL, et al: Prenatal tobacco effects on neuropsychological outcomes among preadolescents. J Dev Behav Pediatr 22:217-225, 2001.

77. Albrecht SA, Maloni JA, Thomas KK, et al: Smoking cessation counseling for pregnant women who smoke: Scientific basis for practice for AWHONN's SUCCESS project. J Obstet Gynecol Neonatal Nurs 33:298-305, 2004.

78. DiFranza JR, Aligne CA, Weitzman M: Prenatal and postnatal environmental tobacco smoke exposure and children's health. Pediatrics 113:1007-1015, 2004.

79. Jaakkola JJ, Gissler M: Maternal smoking in pregnancy, fetal development, and childhood asthma. Am J Public Health 94:136-140, 2004.

80. Boukydis CF, Lester BM: The NICU Network Neurobehavioral Scale. Clinical use with drug exposed infants and their mothers. Clin Perinatol 26:213-230, 1999.

81. Brown RA, Burgess ES, Sales SD, et al: Reliability and validity of a smoking timeline follow-back interview. Psychol Addict Behav 12:101-112, 1998.

82. Fried PA, Watkinson B, Gray R: Differential effects on cognitive functioning in 13- to 16-year-olds prenatally exposed to cigarettes and marihuana. Neurotoxicol Teratol 25:427-436, 2003.

83. Fried PA: The Ottawa Prenatal Prospective Study (OPPS): Methodological issues and findings—It's easy to throw the baby out with the bath water. Life Sci 56:2159-2168, 1995.

84. Fried PA, Watkinson B, Siegel LS: Reading and language in 9- to 12-year olds prenatally exposed to cigarettes and marijuana. Neurotoxicol Teratol 19:171-183, 1997.

85. Maughan B, Taylor A, Caspi A, Moffitt TE: Prenatal smoking and early childhood conduct problems: testing genetic and environmental explanations of the association. Arch Gen Psychiatry 61:836-843, 2004.

86. Silberg JL, Parr T, Neale MC, et al: Maternal smoking during pregnancy and risk to boys' conduct disturbance: an examination of the causal hypothesis. Biol Psychiatry 53:130-135, 2003.

87. Ogunyemi D, Hernandez-Loera GE: The impact of antenatal cocaine use on maternal characteristics and neonatal outcomes. J Matern Fetal Neonatal Med 15:253-259, 2004.

88. Hladky K, Yankowitz J, Hansen WF: Placental abruption. Obstet Gynecol Surv 57:299-305, 2002.

89. Lester B: The Maternal Lifestyles Study. In Harvey JA, Kosofsky BE, eds: Cocaine: Effects on the Developing Brain. New York: New York Academy of Sciences, 1998, pp 296-305.

90. Azuma, 2001.

91. Chasnoff, 2002.

92. Butz AM, Kaufmann WE, Royal R, et al: Opiate and cocaine exposed newborns: Growth outcomes. J Child Adolesc Subst Abuse 8:1-16, 1999.

93. Hurt H, Brodsky NL, Braitman LE, et al: Natal status of infants of cocaine users and control subjects: a prospective comparison. J Perinatol 15:297-304, 1995.

94. Heier LA, Carpanzano CR, Mast J, et al: Maternal cocaine abuse: the spectrum of radiologic abnormalities in the neonatal CNS. AJNR Am J Neuroradiol 12:951-956, 1991.

95. Gomez-Anson B, Ramsey RG: Pachygyria in a neonate with prenatal cocaine exposure: MR features. J Comput Assist Tomogr 18:637-639, 1994.

96. Frank DA, Bauchner H, Parker S, et al: Neonatal body proportionality and body composition after in utero exposure to cocaine and marijuana. J Pediatr 117:622-626, 1990.

97. Belcher HME, Kraut MA, Slifer KJ, et al: Children with in-utero drug exposure: Preliminary MRI findings. Pediatr Res 2004.

98. Dominguez R, Aguirre Vila-Coro A, Slopis JM, et al: Brain and ocular abnormalities in infants with in utero exposure to cocaine and other street drugs. Am J Dis Child 145:688-695, 1991.

99. Dogra VS, Shyken JM, Menon PA, et al: Neurosonographic abnormalities associated with maternal

history of cocaine use in neonates of appropriate size for their gestational age. AJNR Am J Neuroradiol 15:697-702, 1994.

100. Bandstra ES, Morrow CE, Anthony JC, et al: Longitudinal investigation of task persistence and sustained attention in children with prenatal cocaine exposure. Neurotoxicol Teratol 23:545-559, 2001.

101. Pulsifer MB, Radonovich K, Belcher HM, et al: Intelligence and school readiness in preschool children with prenatal drug exposure. Child Neuropsychol 10(2):89-101, 2004.

102. Butz AM, Pulsifer MB, Leppert M, et al: Comparison of intelligence, school readiness skills, and attention in in-utero drug-exposed and nonexposed preschool children. Clin Pediatr (Phila) 42:727-739, 2003.

103 Struthers JM, Hansen RL: Visual recognition memory in drug-exposed infants. J Dev Behav Pediatr 13(2):108-111, 1992.

104. Delaney-Black V, Covington C, Nordstrom B, et al: Prenatal cocaine: Quantity of exposure and gender moderation. J Dev Behav Pediatr 25:254-263, 2004.

105. Butz, 2000.

106. Frank DA, Augustyn M, Knight WG, et al: Growth, development, and behavior in early childhood following prenatal cocaine exposure: A systematic review. JAMA 285:1613-1625, 2001.

107. Messinger DS, Bauer CR, Das A, et al: The Maternal Lifestyle Study: Cognitive, motor, and behavioral outcomes of cocaine-exposed and opiate-exposed infants through three years of age. Pediatrics 113:1677-1685, 2004.

108. Shiono PH, Klebanoff MA, Nugent RP, et al: The impact of cocaine and marijuana use on low birth weight and preterm birth: A multicenter study. Am J Obstet Gynecol 172:19-27, 1995.

109. Richardson GA, Day NL, McGauhey PJ: The impact of prenatal marijuana and cocaine use on the infant and child. Clin Obstet Gynecol 36:302-318, 1993.

110. Fried PA, Makin JE: Neonatal behavioural correlates of prenatal exposure to marihuana, cigarettes and alcohol in a low risk population. Neurotoxicol Teratol 9:1-7, 1987.

110a. Fried PA, O'Connell CM: A comparison of the effects of prenatal exposure to tobacco, alcohol, cannabis and caffeine on birth size and subsequent growth. Neurotoxicol Teratol 9:79-85, 1987.

110b. Fried PA, Watkinson B, Dillon RF, et al: Neonatal neurological status in a low-risk population after prenatal exposure to cigarettes, marijuana, and alcohol. J Dev Behav Pediatr 8:318-326, 1987.

111. Jacobson JL, Jacobson SW, Sokol RJ, et al: Effects of alcohol use, smoking, and illicit drug use on fetal growth in black infants. J Pediatr 124:757-764, 1994.

112. Dreher MC, Nugent K, Hudgins R: Prenatal marijuana exposure and neonatal outcomes in Jamaica: An ethnographic study. Pediatrics 93:254-260, 1994.

113. Fried PA, Watkinson B: 12- and 24-month neurobehavioural follow-up of children prenatally exposed to marihuana, cigarettes and alcohol. Neurotoxicol Teratol 10:305-313, 1988.

114. Lindgren S, Lyons D: Pediatric Assessment of Cognitive Efficiency (PACE). Iowa City: University of Iowa, Department of Pediatrics, 1984.

115. Leech SL, Richardson GA, Goldschmidt L, et al: Prenatal substance exposure: Effects on attention and impulsivity of 6-year-olds. Neurotoxicol Teratol 21:109-118, 1999.

116. Sheslow W, Adams W: Manual for the Wide Range Assessment of Memory and Learning. Wilmington, DE: Jastak Associates, 1990.

117. Richardson GA, Ryan C, Willford J, et al: Prenatal alcohol and marijuana exposure: Effects on neuropsychological outcomes at 10 years. Neurotoxicol Teratol 24:309-320, 2002.

118. Smith AM, Fried PA, Hogan MJ, et al: Effects of prenatal marijuana on response inhibition: An fMRI study of young adults. Neurotoxicol Teratol 26:533-542, 2004.

119. Fried PA, Watkinson B: Differential effects on facets of attention in adolescents prenatally exposed to cigarettes and marihuana. Neurotoxicol Teratol 23:421-430, 2001.

120. Fulroth R, Phillips B, Durand DJ: Perinatal outcome of infants exposed to cocaine and/or heroin in utero. Am J Dis Child 143:905-910, 1989.

121. Naeye RL, Blanc W, Leblanc W, et al: Fetal complications of maternal heroin addiction: Abnormal growth, infections, and episodes of stress. J Pediatr 83:1055-1061, 1973.

122. Kelly JJ, Davis PG, Henschke PN: The drug epidemic: Effects on newborn infants and health resource consumption at a tertiary perinatal centre. J Paediatr Child Health 36:262-264, 2000.

123. Rosen TS, Johnson HL: Children of methadone-maintained mothers: Follow-up to 18 months of age. J Pediatr 101:192-196, 1982.

124. Wilson GS, Desmond MM, Wait RB: Follow-up of methadone-treated and untreated narcotic-dependent women and their infants: Health, developmental, and social implications. J Pediatr 98:716-722, 1981.

125. Desmond MM, Wilson GS: Neonatal abstinence syndrome: Recognition and diagnosis. Addict Dis 2:113-121, 1975.

126. Kandall SR, Albin S, Gartner LM, et al: The narcotic-dependent mother: Fetal and neonatal consequences. Early Hum Dev 1:159-169, 1977.

127. Finnegan LP: Neonatal abstinence. *In* Nelson N, ed: Current Therapy in Neonatal-Perinatal Medicine. Hamilton, Ontario, Canada: BC Decker, 1984.

128. American Academy of Pediatrics, Committee on Drug Withdrawal: Neonatal drug withdrawal. Pediatrics 101:1079-1088, 1998.

129. Kaltenbach K, Finnegan LP: Neonatal abstinence syndrome, pharmacotherapy and developmental outcome. Neurobehav Toxicol Teratol 8:353-355, 1986.

130. Lipsitz PJ: A proposed narcotic withdrawal score for use with newborn infants: A pragmatic evaluation of efficacy. Clin Pediatr 14:592-594, 1975.

131. Marcus J, Hans SL, Jeremy RJ: A longitudinal study of offspring born to methadone-maintained women. III. Effects of multiple risk factors on development at

4, 8, and 12 months. Am J Drug Alcohol Abuse 10:195-207, 1984.

132. Olds DL: Prenatal and infancy home visiting by nurses: From randomized trials to community replication. Prev Sci 3:153-172, 2002.

133. Black MM, Nair P, Kight C, et al: Parenting and early development among children of drug-abusing women: effects of home intervention. Pediatrics 94:440-448, 1994.

134. Butz AM, Pulsifer M, Marano N, et al: Effectiveness of a home intervention for perceived child behavioral problems and parenting stress in children with in utero drug exposure. Arch Pediatr Adolesc Med 155:1029-1037, 2001.

135. Hofkosh D, Pringle JL, Wald HP, et al: Early interactions between drug-involved mothers and infants. Within-group differences. Arch Pediatr Adolesc Med 149:665-672, 1995.

136. Schuler ME, Nair P, Black MM, et al: Mother-infant interaction: Effects of a home intervention and ongoing maternal drug use. J Clin Child Psychol 29:424-431, 2000.

137. Furuno S, O'Reilly KA, Hosaka CM, et al: HELP at Home: Hawaii Early Learning Profile. Palo Alto, CA: VORT Corporation, 1991.

138. Schuler ME, Nair P, Black MM: Ongoing maternal drug use, parenting attitudes, and a home intervention: Effects on mother-child interaction at 18 months. J Dev Behav Pediatr 23:87-94, 2002.

139. Schuler ME, Nair P, Kettinger L: Drug-exposed infants and developmental outcome: Effects of a home intervention and ongoing maternal drug use. Arch Pediatr Adolesc Med 157:133-138, 2003.

140. McComish JF, Greenberg R, Ager J, et al: Family-focused substance abuse treatment: A program evaluation. J Psychoactive Drugs 35:321-331, 2003.

141. Baldwin JH, Rawlings A, Marshall ES, et al: Mom empowerment, too! (ME2): A program for young mothers involved in substance abuse. Public Health Nurs 16:376-383, 1999.

142. Field TM, Scafidi F, Pickens J, et al: Polydrug-using adolescent mothers and their infants receiving early intervention. Adolescence 33:117-143, 1998.

143. Rains JW, Ray DW: Participatory action research for community health promotion. Public Health Nurs 12:256-261, 1995.

BIBLIOGRAPHY

Azuma SD, Chasnoff IJ: Outcome of children prenatally exposed to cocaine and other drugs—A path-analysis of 3-year data. Pediatrics 92:396-402, 1993.

Barnard M, McKeganey N: The impact of parental problem drug use on children: What is the problem and what can be done to help? Addiction 99:552-559, 2004.

Bartecchi CE, MacKenzie TD, Schrier RW: Human costs of tobacco use. N Engl J Med 330:907-980, 1994.

Benowitz NL: Pharmacology of nicotine: Addiction and therapeutics. Annu Rev Pharmacol Toxicol 36:597-613, 1996.

Centers for Disease Control and Prevention: Trends in cigarette smoking among high school students—United States, 1991-1999. MMWR Morb Mortal Wkly Rep 49:755-758, 2000.

Chasnoff IJ: Cocaine, pregnancy, and the growing child. Curr Probl Pediatr 22:302-321, 1992.

Chilcoat HD, Dishion TJ, Anthony JC: Parent monitoring and the incidence of drug sampling in urban elementary school children. Am J Epidemiol 141:25-31, 1995.

Crum RM, Lillie-Blanton M, Anthony JC: Neighborhood environment and opportunity to use cocaine and other drugs in late childhood and early adolescence. Drug Alcohol Depend 43:155-161, 1996.

Crumb WJ Jr, Clarkson CW: Characterization of cocaine-induced block of cardiac sodium channels. Biophys J 57:589-599, 1990.

Finnegan LP, Mitros TF, Hopkins LE: Management of neonatal narcotic abstinence utilizing a phenobarbital loading dose method. NIDA Res Monogr 27:247-253, 1979.

Giros B, Jaber M, Jones SR, et al: Hyperlocomotion and indifference to cocaine and amphetamine in mice lacking the dopamine transporter. Nature 379:606-612, 1996.

Gold MS: Cocaine and (crack): Clinical aspects. *In* Lowinson JH, Ruiz PD, Millman RB, et al, eds: Substance Abuse: A Comprehensive Textbook, 2nd ed. Baltimore: Williams & Wilkins, 1992, pp 205-221.

Herzlinger RA, Kandall SR, Vaughan HG: Neonatal seizures associated with narcotic withdrawal. J Pediatr 91:638-641, 1971.

Jaffe JH: Opiates: Clinical aspects. *In* Lowinson JH, Ruiz PD, Millman RB, et al, eds: Substance Abuse: A Comprehensive Textbook, 2nd ed. Baltimore: Williams & Wilkins, 1992, pp 186-194.

Jarvik ME, Schneider NG: Nicotine. In Lowinson JH, Ruiz PD, Millman RB, et al, eds: Substance Abuse: A Comprehensive Textbook, 2nd ed. Baltimore: Williams & Wilkins, 1992, pp 334-356.

Jones LF, Tackett RL: Central mechanisms of action involved in cocaine-induced tachycardia. Life Sci 46:723-728, 1990.

Kandall SR, Gartner LM: Late presentation of drug withdrawal symptoms in newborns. Am J Dis Child 127:58-61, 1974.

Kandel DB, Simcha-Fagan O, Davies M: Risk factors for delinquency and illicit drug use from adolescence to young adulthood. J Drug Issues 16:67-90, 1986.

Karpen JW, Aoshima H, Abood LG, et al: Cocaine and phencyclidine inhibition of the acetylcholine receptor: Analysis of the mechanisms of action based on measurements of ion flux in the millisecond-to-minute time region. Proc Natl Acad Sci U S A 79:2509-2513, 1982.

Karpen JW, Hess GP: Cocaine, phencyclidine, and procaine inhibition of the acetylcholine receptor: Characterization of the binding site by stopped-flow measurements of receptor-controlled ion flux in membrane vesicles. Biochemistry 25:1777-1785, 1986.

Kaufmann WE: Developmental cortical abnormalities after prenatal exposure to cocaine. Soc Neurosci Abstracts 16:305, 1990.

Kron RE, Litt M, Eng D, et al: Neonatal narcotic abstinence: effects of pharmacotherapeutic agents and maternal drug usage on nutritive sucking behavior. J Pediatr 88:637-641, 1976.

Krumholtz A, Felix J, Goldstein P, McKenzie E: Maturation of the brain-stem evoked potential in preterm infants. Electroencephalogr Clin Neurophysiol 62:124-134, 1985.

Lester BM, Lagasse L, Seifer R, et al: The Maternal Lifestyle Study (MLS): Effects of prenatal cocaine and/or opiate exposure on auditory brain response at one month. J Pediatr 142:279-285, 2003.

Lester BM, Tronick EZ, Lagasse L, et al: The Maternal Lifestyle Study: Effects of substance exposure during pregnancy on neurodevelopmental outcome in 1-month-old infants. Pediatrics 110:1182-1192, 2002.

Luthar SS, Suchman NE: Relational Psychotherapy Mothers' Group: A developmentally informed intervention for at-risk mothers. Dev Psychopathol 12:235-253, 2000.

Macdonald DI, Blume SB: Children of alcoholics. Am J Dis Child 140:750-754, 1986.

McMurtrie C, Rosenberg KD, Kerker BD, et al: A unique drug treatment program for pregnant and postpartum substance-using women in New York City: Results of a pilot project, 1990-1995. Am J Drug Alcohol Abuse 25:701-713, 1999.

McPherson DL, Madden JD, Payne TF: Auditory brainstem-evoked potentials in term infants born to mothers addicted to opiates. J Perinatol 9:262-267, 1989.

Merriam AE, Medalia A, Levine B: Partial complex status epilepticus associated with cocaine abuse. Biol Psychiatry 23:515-518, 1988.

Milin R, Halikas JA, Meller JE, et al: Psychopathology among substance abusing juvenile offenders. J Am Acad Child Adolesc Psychiatry 30:569-574, 1991.

Murray AD: Newborn auditory brainstem evoked responses (ABRs): Prenatal and contemporary correlates. Child Dev 59:571-588, 1988.

National Institute on Drug Abuse: National Institute on Drug Abuse: Drug Use Among Racial/Ethnic Minorities 1995 (NIH Publication No. 95-3888). Rockville, MD: National Institute on Drug Abuse, 1995.

Ray O, Ksir C: Marijuana and hashish. In Ray O, Ksir C, eds: Drugs, Society, and Human Behavior. New York: McGraw-Hill, 1996a, pp 403-427.

Ray O, Ksir C: Opiates. In Ray O, Ksir C, eds: Drugs, Society, and Human Behavior, 7th ed. Boston: WCB/McGraw-Hill, 1996b, pp 336-367.

Ray O, Ksir C: Stimulants. In Ray O, Ksir C, eds: Drugs, Society, and Human Behavior, 7th ed. Boston: WCB/McGraw-Hill, 1996c, pp 134-163.

Richardson JL, Dwyer K, McGuigan K, et al: Substance use among eighth-grade students who take care of themselves after school. Pediatrics 84:556-566, 1989.

Streissguth AP, Aase JM, Clarren SK, et al: Fetal alcohol syndrome in adolescents and adults. JAMA 265:1961-1967, 1991.

Streissguth AP, Bookstein FL, Sampson PD, et al: Attention: Prenatal alcohol and continuities of vigilance and attentional problems from 4 through 14 years. Dev Psychopathol 7:419-446, 1995.

Substance Abuse and Mental Health Services Administration: Overview of Findings from the 2002 National Survey on Drug Use and Health (DHHS Publication No. SMA 03-3774). Rockville MD: Office of Applied Statistics, Substance Abuse and Mental Health Services Administration, 2003.

Sword W, Niccols A, Fan A: "New choices" for women with addictions: Perceptions of program participants. BMC Public Health 4:10, 2004.

Trammer RM, Aust G., Koser K, et al: Narcotic and nicotine effects on the neonatal auditory system. Acta Paediatrica 81:962-965, 1992.

Tunis SL, Webster DM, Izes JK, et al: Maternal drug use and the effectiveness of pharmacotherapy for neonatal abstinence. Pediatr Res 18:396, 1984.

U.S. Department of Health and Human Services: Healthy People 2010: Understanding and Improving Health, 2nd ed. Washington, DC: U.S. Government Printing Office, November 2000.

Xu Z, Seidler FJ, Ali SF, et al: Fetal and adolescent nicotine administration: Effects on CNS serotonergic systems. Brain Res 914:166-178, 2001.

Child Maltreatment: Developmental Consequences

EDWARD GOLDSON ▨ BARBARA L. BONNER

In the 21st century, child maltreatment continues to be a major medical, psychological, social, and public health issue that affects almost a million children every year in the United States. It is a problem that crosses all racial, ethnic, and socioeconomic boundaries and affects not only the victims but also their families and their communities.

Child maltreatment has been defined by the Federal Abuse Reporting Act of 1974 as "the physical or mental injury, sexual abuse or exploitation, negligent treatment, or maltreatment of a child by a person who is responsible for the child's welfare under circumstances which indicate harm or threaten harm to the child's health or welfare."[1] Helfer, a pediatrician who was one of the coauthors with Kempe and others of the seminal article on child abuse entitled, "The Battered Child,"[2] provided a definition that highlights the core elements of child maltreatment that are essential to the identification and appropriate treatment of these children. He defined child maltreatment as "any interaction or lack of interaction between family members which results in non-accidental harm to the individual's physical and/or developmental status."[3]

In considering maltreatment statistics, clinicians must keep certain issues in mind. The actual incidence and prevalence of child maltreatment is difficult to determine accurately for a number of reasons. No standard definitions of maltreatment are applied across professions and across state, federal, and tribal laws. Moreover, maltreatment can be defined differently, depending on the purpose of the definition (e.g., for investigation vs. treatment vs. research). Professionals from the fields of law enforcement, medicine, law, psychology, and social services may also have different interpretations of which acts constitute abuse and neglect because of differences in their professional training or roles. These definitional differences and interpretations can have

a profound effect on the substantiated rate of maltreatment.

There is currently no absolute checklist or set of symptoms or injuries by which clinicians can validly and reliably predict or verify that abuse or neglect has occurred to a child. There are certain physical findings that are known to be the result of inflicted injuries, such as spiral fractures of the femur in very young children, "bucket handle" fractures,[4] and immersion burns. In addition, professionals should be aware of situations that are frequently associated with valid abusive or neglectful incidents. These are situations in which professionals should consider that maltreatment may have occurred or that a child is at high risk for abuse or neglect.

Physical abuse should be considered when the history given by the caregiver or parent does not match the child's injury; when the child gives an unbelievable explanation for the injury; when the child reports an injury by a parent or caretaker; or when the child is fearful of going home or requests to stay at school, daycare, a clinic, or a hospital.

Sexual abuse should be considered when there is an injury to a child's genital area; when a child or adolescent has a sexually transmitted disease; when a young adolescent is pregnant; when a child reports inappropriate sexual behavior by a parent or caregiver; or when a child is engaged in highly inappropriate or aggressive sexual behavior.

Neglect should be considered when a child is significantly underweight for age for no apparent reason or when this could be the result of inadequate intake, excessive output, or a combination of both; when a child does not have necessary medical or dental care or has an untreated illness or injury; when a child has chronic poor hygiene, such as lice, body odor, or scaly skin; when a child reports no caregiver or adult in the home; when a child lacks a safe, sanitary shelter or appropriate clothing for the weather; or when a child is abandoned or left with inadequate supervision.

Psychological maltreatment should be considered when a child is rejected (there is no affection or acknowledgement of the child as a person), terrorized (the child is threatened with injury and/or lives in a climate of unpredictability), ignored (the parent or caretaker is psychologically unavailable), isolated (the child is prevented from having social relationships), or corrupted (the child is encouraged to engage in antisocial behavior).[5] These conditions can lead to the child's failure to thrive, being depressed and anxious, and not being responsive to his or her environment. These situations should be considered "red flags" for possible maltreatment, but, as mentioned earlier, some may also be children's responses to other stressful situations in their lives.

The methods and standards by which data are collected vary considerably. In 1993, the National Research Council reviewed the data-gathering process and made recommendations to improve the methods and reduce the disparity in the reports from the states. However, few changes have been made at the state or national levels to standardize the data-gathering process. Reporting or referral biases may skew the rate statistics of maltreatment in certain ethnic and socioeconomic groups. For example, African-American children[6] and children living in poverty[7] are more often reported and found to be maltreated than are children from other ethnic and socioeconomic groups.

Taking these caveats into consideration, we note that in 2003, about 3,353,000 reports of suspected child maltreatment were filed. About 31.7% of these reports, involving 906,000 children, were substantiated. The rate of victimization in 2003 was 12.4 per 1000 children; 61.9% of these children were neglected, 18.9% were physically abused, 9.9% were sexually abused, 2.3 % were medically neglected, and 16.9% met the "other" category, including abandonment, threats (psychological abuse), and congenital drug addiction. (These percentages add up to more than 100% because children who were victims of more than one kind of abuse were counted in each category.) Of the maltreated children, 48.3% were boys and 51.7% were girls. In addition, the rate of abuse by age was as follows: For every 1000 children aged 0 to 3 years, 16.4 were abused; for every 1000 aged 4 to 7 years, 13.8; and of children younger than 1 year, 9.8%. With regard to the variable of race, 53.6% of maltreated children were white, 25.5% were African-American, 11.5% were Hispanic, 1.7% were Native American or Alaskan, 0.6% were Asian, and 0.2% were Pacific Islanders. With regard to perpetrators, 83.8% of children were abused by either or both parents; 13.4%, by nonparental adults; and 2.8%, by unknown perpetrators. Finally, approximately 1500 children died in 2003 as a result of their maltreatment, of whom 78.7% were younger than 4 years.[8]

Children with disabilities are much more vulnerable to maltreatment.[9] In 2003, 6.5% of victims of maltreatment from the 34 states that reported this category had a disability, such as mental retardation, emotional disturbances, behavioral problems, physical disability, visual disturbances, and learning disabilities. Other studies suggest that children with disabilities are at least one to two times more likely to be abused than are typically developing children.[10] Goldson,[11] in a review of the literature on children with special health care needs, concluded that such children were at least three to four times more likely to be maltreated than were typically developing children.[12,13,14]

REPORTING, CLINICAL ASSESSMENT, AND TREATMENT OF THE MALTREATED CHILD

The clinical assessment and treatment of children who have been maltreated should be distinguished from forensic aspects (i.e., reporting and investigating allegations of abuse). However, an immediate concern for physicians and other medical staff who work with children is the legal requirement to report suspected child abuse and neglect. Every state in the United States has a mandatory child abuse and neglect reporting law, and physicians are typically mandated reporters: that is, they are required by law to report suspicions that a child is or has been physically or sexually abused, neglected, or emotionally maltreated. States implement these laws differently, and the requirements for reporting vary across the states. For example, some states require a report when there is only a suspicion of maltreatment, whereas others require a higher degree of certainty or knowledge that a child has been maltreated. If a mandated individual fails to report suspected abuse, he or she can be charged with a criminal offense, typically a misdemeanor punishable by a fine or civil liability. Laws in most states offer immunity from liability to individuals who report suspected abuse in good faith, even if the suspicion of maltreatment is not substantiated. Statues in some states permit the prosecution of individuals who intentionally make false allegations of child maltreatment. Physicians need to be familiar with the state laws and professional ethical standards and practices that require reporting suspected child maltreatment.

If a physician is the first professional to see a child and suspects maltreatment or is the person to whom a parent reports suspicions of abuse, he or she should document the history and perform a physical examination of the child. In addition, he or she must make a report to the appropriate state social services agency and/or the police. The investigation and substantiation of suspicions of abuse or neglect are the responsibility of the state or tribal child protection system or law enforcement, rather than the reporting individual. These agencies employ professionals who are trained to conduct investigations and are responsible for determining whether a child should be removed from the caregiver's custody. In many clinical programs, social workers are trained to conduct forensic interviews with suspected victims and to work closely with the child protection system and law enforcement during the investigation. Many larger communities have specialized children's advocacy centers with trained personnel to interview the child. Whenever child maltreatment is suspected, the physician must record accurate, complete documentation of the suspicion or allegations; how the suspicion of maltreatment occurred, such as an injury to the child or the child's statements; and the results of the examination and subsequent actions, such as contact with the child protection system, law enforcement, or other professionals. Careful documentation is important when a report of suspected abuse is made, during the investigation, and in any future legal or court involvement. Finally, physicians must avoid influencing the content of the child's report, being sure that the child speaks for himself or herself, both to maintain the child's credibility and also to best protect the child.

The approach to the clinical assessment and treatment should follow a developmental psychopathology model,[15] wherein the child's developmental functioning and abilities are taken into consideration. The goal of the clinical assessment is to determine the child and caregivers' overall functioning, adaptation, and level of symptoms. A thorough assessment of the family's strengths and problems should be conducted, including the types of problems that need to be addressed at the parental, child, family, and social systems levels.[16] The assessment may include interviews; paper-and-pencil measures; or structured observations with the child, siblings, and caregivers. In addition to the use of standard measures to assess cognitive functioning and general behavior, several specific measures have been developed and standardized to evaluate the child's symptoms associated with the abuse. These measures include general assessments of trauma symptoms, such as the Trauma Symptom Checklist for Children,[17] and a measurement of sexual behavior problems, such as the Child Sexual Behavior Inventory.[18] To assess psychological maltreatment, the Psychological Maltreatment Rating Scale[19] provides an observational structure for evaluating mother-child interactions. Bonner and colleagues[20] provided a complete review of assessment.

Evaluations of various treatment approaches for abused children and adolescents are increasing. Treatment interventions for abused children are conducted in therapeutic nurseries, day treatment programs, psychiatric or residential settings, and outpatient clinics. Clinicians must rely on techniques and approaches that are appropriate for the child's cognitive and developmental level of functioning and are effective in reducing the child's targeted symptoms. Reviews of the current treatment outcome literature indicate that abuse-specific cognitive-behavioral therapy is effective in reducing symptoms of posttraumatic stress disorder (PTSD).[21] The treatment components include anxiety management techniques, exposure, education, and cognitive therapy. Treatment for families in which physical abuse has occurred has typically focused on the abusive parents and, more recently, has addressed the symptoms in the child victims.[22-24] For some forms of neglect, research has yielded promising results for interventions that include home visitation as a primary approach.[25-27]

NEUROLOGICAL CONSEQUENCES OF NONACCIDENTAL TRAUMA

Although the focus of this chapter is on the cognitive and affective consequences of maltreatment, some of the physical consequences, particularly of injury to the central nervous system, are also considered. Ewing-Cobbs and associates[28] characterized the neuroimaging, physical, neurobehavioral, and developmental findings in 20 children aged 0 to 6 years old who had experienced traumatic brain injury (TBI) as a result of inflicted or nonaccidental trauma (NAT) and compared them with 20 children with accidental TBI 1.3 months after the injury. They found that in 45% of the children with NAT, there were signs of preexisting injuries, such as cerebral atrophy, subdural hygromas, and ventriculomegaly. There were no such findings among the children with accidental injuries. In addition, subdural hematomas and seizures were more common among the children with NAT, and none of the children with accidental injuries had retinal hemorrhages. Glasgow Coma Scale scores in the children with NAT were suggestive of a worse prognosis, and of these children, 45% had mental retardation, in comparison with 5% of the children with accidental TBI.

In a later paper, Ewing-Cobbs and associates[29] evaluated 28 children between the ages of 20 and 42 months, 1 and 3 months after their inflicted TBI, using the Bayley Scales of Infant Development–Second Edition. In comparing these children with those who had suffered accidental TBI, they found that the children with NAT had deficits in cognitive and motor functioning and that more than 50% showed persisting deficits in attention/arousal, emotional regulation, and motor coordination. As would be expected, the more severe the injury, as reflected in the lower Glasgow Coma Scale scores, the longer was the period of unconsciousness, and in the presence of cerebral edema and cerebral infarctions, the outcome was poorer. Perez-Arjona and coworkers,[30] in a review of the literature, found that children with cerebral NAT had worse clinical outcomes than did those with accidental TBI. The abused children were cognitively impaired and had more severe neurological consequences. Late findings on computed tomographic scans and magnetic resonance images provided evidence of cerebral atrophy in 100% and cerebral ischemia in 50% of the NAT group. Thus, the conclusions that can be drawn from these studies are that inflicted injuries to the central nervous system are significantly more harmful than accidental injuries and that the outcome for children sustaining NAT is quite poor.

EFFECTS OF CHILD MALTREATMENT

The short- and long-term effects of child maltreatment on children, adolescents, and adults have been well documented in the medical, psychological, and psychiatric literature since the 1960s. The effects range from mild, transitory symptoms to devastating disorders of behavior and affect. The symptoms may vary by the severity, intensity, and duration of the maltreatment and by the child's age and developmental stage. Symptoms such as low self-esteem, anxiety, or depression are frequently found in children who experience any form of abuse. Such symptoms are also associated with other stressful events in a child's life, such as a death in the family, parental separation or divorce, or living in a neighborhood with high levels of crime and/or violence. Other symptoms, such as highly sexualized behavior or sexual preoccupation, pregnancy in a young girl, or a sexually transmitted disease, are associated with a sexual abuse.

An issue of importance to developmental-behavioral pediatricians is the effect of child maltreatment on children with disabilities.[11] There has been a significant lack of research on the maltreatment of children with disabilities, and few state child welfare agencies document the presence or type of disability status of children entering the child protec-

tion system.[31] This issue was addressed by Sullivan and Knutson,[32] who studied a school-based population of more than 50,000 children to assess the prevalence of maltreatment among children identified with an existing disability; they related the type of disability to the type of abuse, and determined the effects of maltreatment on academic achievement and attendance rates for children with and without disabilities. They found a 31% prevalence rate of maltreatment of children with existing disabilities and a 9% rate among children without disabilities, which indicates that children with disabilities are 3.4 times more likely to be maltreated than are children who are not disabled. These authors further documented a significant relationship between maltreatment and disability that affected the child's school performance.

Three factors appear to contribute to the heightened effect of abuse on children with disabilities: (1) their state of dependency; (2) being in institutional care; and (3) communication problems.[33] Research has shown that physical disabilities that reduce a child's credibility, such as mental retardation, deafness, or blindness, increase children's risk for abuse,[34] which emphasizes the necessity of increased protective measures for such children.

Physical Abuse

Children who are physically abused experience different kinds of injuries, ranging from bruises to skull and other fractures and to death. Studies suggest that the severity of a child's physical injuries is related to young age,[35] and according to national statistics, child fatalities caused by maltreatment are substantially higher in infants and children younger than 4 years.[36] Earlier researchers explored the relationship between a child's early medical and health status and subsequent abuse. Their findings suggested that factors such as a physical disability, low IQ, or birth complications might increase a child's risk[37]; however, researchers did not find the factors to significantly increase a child's risk beyond parental characteristics.[38] Other studies have suggested that neonatal problems and failure to thrive were present in children who experienced physical abuse.[39]

Children's responses to physical abuse are related to their age, developmental status, the severity and duration of the abuse, and the physical and psychological effects on the child. Their responses range from becoming passive and withdrawn to having high levels of hostility and aggressive behavior. An extensive body of research documents the heightened levels of aggression and related externalizing behavior in physically abused children.[16] These problems include poor anger management[40]; increased rule violations, oppositional behavior, and delinquency[41];

drinking, smoking cigarettes, and drug use[42]; and property offenses and criminal arrests.[43] Other studies have reported a relationship between physical abuse and borderline personality disorder,[44] attention-deficit/hyperactivity disorder,[39] and high rates of depression and conduct disorders in adolescents.[45] Children who have been physically abused have also been found to have internalizing problems, such as depression and hopelessness[46]; Famularo and colleagues found that 30% of children and youth met criteria for PTSD, and 33% of the children with these criteria retained the full diagnosis 2 years later.[47,48]

Additional research has documented pervasive problems for victims of physical abuse in the areas of attachment, social competence, and interpersonal relationships. Studies report these children to have insecure attachments,[49] separation problems,[50] and difficulty making friends.[43] A control group study of adolescents revealed that a history of physical abuse was associated with greater deficits in social competence and increased coercive behavior in dating relationships.[51]

It is clear that physical abuse can result in long-term psychosocial problems in living skills and relationships. Well-designed, longitudinal studies have revealed that children with a history of physical abuse are at twice the risk of the general population for being arrested for a violent crime[52] and that they experience significant problems in adolescence and early adulthood, including suicidal ideation and attempts, depression, anxiety, and behavioral problems.[53,54]

Neglect

There are several forms of neglect that have varying effects on infants and children. These include (1) nutritional neglect (a lack of adequate food and nourishment); (2) educational neglect (failure to support attendance, achievement, and school activities, or allowing or encouraging truancy); (3) supervisory/protection neglect (leaving children unattended, not providing adequate supervision, or failing to protect children from maltreatment or dangerous situations); (4) physical/environmental neglect (failure to provide adequate, safe housing or appropriate clothing); (5) emotional neglect (failure to meet a child's needs for nurturance and interaction); and (6) neglect of medical or mental health conditions (failure to adhere to medical or therapeutic procedures recommended for serious diseases, injuries, or emotional and behavioral problems).[55]

In many cases, infants and children suffer from several forms of neglect that can have serious consequences on the child's development and behavior. Although physical and sexual abuses currently receive more public and professional attention, the majority of substantiated cases of maltreatment in the United States involve some form of neglect.[36]

Neglect can be chronic, such as long-standing lack of adequate nutrition, or a single episode, such as leaving children unattended for a period of time. For example, data demonstrate that children are most likely to die in fires when the fires are set by a child when appropriate adult supervision is lacking.[56] Other forms of fatal neglect occur when caregivers fail to provide necessary medical care[57] or fail to meet the nutritional and emotional needs of the child, which results in failure to thrive.[58]

The focus in research on neglected children has been mainly on physical and emotional neglect. In one of the first investigations to specifically study neglected children, Steele found learning problems, low self-esteem, and, as children grew older, a high rate of delinquency.[59] Subsequent research has revealed that neglected children are less interactive with their peers,[60] passive, tend toward helplessness in stressful situations, and display significant developmental delays.[49] They also have severe language delays and disorders[61] and experience a significant decline in school performance upon entering junior high school.[62] Longitudinal studies have shown the negative effects of physical neglect, particularly during preschool and primary grades, on the children's school behavior.[55] These problems continue into adolescence; these youth have low school achievement scores, heavy alcohol use, and school expulsions and dropouts. Clearly, physical neglect can have devastating effects on children's and adolescents' functioning and adjustment.

Since the 1990s, studies have focused on the neurobiological consequences of maltreatment, and results suggest that maltreatment leads to compromised central nervous system and brain development.[63] Studies have documented impairments in physiological functioning[64] and smaller intracranial and cerebral volumes in maltreated children with PTSD than in controls.[65,66] Perry[67] discussed the severe, long-term consequences for brain function if a child's needs for stable emotional attachments, physical touch from primary adult caregivers, and interactions with peers are not met. He suggested that if the necessary neuronal connections are lacking, the brain development for both caring behavior and cognitive capacities is damaged in a "lasting fashion."

Current research findings clearly demonstrate that neglect is a major social problem affecting thousands of children across the United States. The neglected children who survive have problems developing adequate confidence, concentration, and the social skills necessary to adapt successfully to school and interpersonal relationships.[55] In the absence of appropriate intervention in the family and for the child, the prognosis for these children is guarded.

Sexual Abuse

The short- and long-term effects of sexual abuse have the broadest research base of the four types of abuse. Since the 1980s, research findings have indicated that a variety of interpersonal and psychological problems are found more frequently in children with a history of sexual abuse than in nonabused children.[68] Although many of these studies were retrospective and involved clinical samples, a well-designed, prospective, longitudinal study of the general population revealed that sexual abuse was associated with subsequent depression and post-traumatic stress.[69] In evaluating the research in this area, investigators and clinicians agree that children who are sexually abused are at significant risk for problems in both the short term[70] and the long term.[33,71]

In reviews of the specific effects associated with sexual abuse, it has been noted that as a group, these children do not consistently report significant levels of emotional distress.[72] However, for many children, the experience can be frightening, confusing, and painful and can have significant negative effects on a child's developmental progress. Studies have revealed that sexually abused children have more symptoms of depression and anxiety and lower self-esteem than do nonabused peers.[73-75] Other research reports post-traumatic stress symptoms, including high levels of avoidance and reexperiencing of the event.[73] Several studies documented that more than one third of the abused children met criteria for PTSD.[76,77] Other documented symptoms include impaired cognitive functioning,[78] problems in social competency,[74,75] behavior problems,[79] and increased sexual behavior.[80]

Although most research has focused on the effects on younger children, several investigators have assessed the effects on adolescents. They have identified major problems in this age group, including substance abuse,[81] running away from home, bulimia,[82] having trouble with teachers,[83] and early pregnancy.[84] A 10-year review of the literature[33] revealed that a variety of psychiatric conditions—including major depression, somatization, substance abuse, borderline personality, PTSD, bulimia, and dissociative identity disorder—are later consequences of child sexual abuse. This comprehensive review identified three major problematic areas: psychiatric disorders; dysfunctional behaviors, particularly sexualized behaviors; and neurobiological dysregulation, including negative effects on the hypothalamic-pituitary-adrenal axis, the sympathetic nervous system, and, possibly, the immune system.

For some childhood victims, these symptoms continue into adulthood. Studies have revealed increased arrest rates for sex crimes and prostitution,[85] drug or alcohol dependence, and bulimia.[86-88] Another study documented increased rates of major depression, attempted suicide, conduct disorder, social anxiety, drug and nicotine dependence, rape after age 18, and divorce.[89] A meta-analysis of 37 studies revealed significant effects of child sexual abuse on later suicide, sexual promiscuity, and depression,[90] documenting a causal relationship between the later development of psychopathology and a history of child sexual abuse.[86]

Psychological Maltreatment

Because children are often victims of multiple forms of abuse, the effects of psychological maltreatment are often difficult to distinguish from other types of maltreatment. Many professionals consider psychological maltreatment to be a core component of all forms of child abuse and neglect.[91-94] Findings from longitudinal, cross-cultural, and comparison studies support this concept and document severe outcomes from chronic child neglect.

The Minnesota Parent-Child Project monitored a cohort of children from birth to adulthood whose mothers were at risk for parenting problems.[95-97] In comparison with children from the control group, the maltreated children exhibited serious consequences. Children whose mothers were hostile or verbally abusive demonstrated anxious attachments, lack of impulse control, distractibility, hyperactivity, angry and noncompliant behavior, difficulty in learning and problem solving, negative emotions, and lack of persistence and enthusiasm. Researchers noted the most devastating effects occurred when a mother was psychologically unavailable (i.e., denied emotional responsiveness to the child). The outcomes for such children included poor progress in competency from infancy through the preschool years, anxious-avoidant attachment, noncompliance, lack of impulse control, low self-esteem, high dependence, self-abusive behavior, and serious psychopathology. Other longitudinal studies have shown that parental rejection and lack of positive parent-child interactions are significant predictors of childhood aggression and delinquency.[98,99]

Psychological maltreatment includes both acts of commission (e.g., parental hostility and verbal aggression) and acts of omission (e.g., parental neglect and indifference or denial of emotional responsiveness). Anthropological studies have demonstrated that parental rejection has negative effects on children in many of the world's cultures.[100] Rejected children tend to be aggressive, to have poor self-esteem, to be emotionally unstable and unresponsive, and to have a negative world view.

Other researchers have compared the differential effects of psychological maltreatment with other forms of abuse. Claussen and Crittenden[92] found that psychological maltreatment was more accurately predictive of problematic developmental outcomes than was the severity of children's physical injury, which emphasizes the need for intervention in the psychological aspects of the child's environment. In comparing the effects of psychological maltreatment with those of physical and sexual abuse, investigators have found strong associations between psychological maltreatment and bulimia,[101] depression, and low self-esteem.[102,103] Although psychological harm is more difficult to observe and clearly document, research has established that it is a recognizable and serious condition that warrants increased attention to legal and child welfare policies and programs in order to intervene more effectively on behalf of children.[104]

EFFECTS ON ADULTS

Both retrospective and prospective studies have clearly documented long-term negative effects of childhood abuse or neglect on adults. These effects include poor psychosocial adjustment; delinquent and criminal behavior; engaging in frequent, indiscriminate sexual behavior and sexual assault; increased risk of human immunodeficiency virus infection, repeated victimization, depression and substance abuse, and intellectual and academic problems.[105-109] Researchers documented in adults the health-related consequences of maltreatment in childhood.[110] The authors found that the more severe the abuse during childhood was, the greater was the likelihood that victims would later smoke, be alcoholic, have chronic depression, have numerous sexual partners, and be involved in domestic violence, rape, and suicide.

In a retrospective study, McCord[111] studied 232 men identified in social service case records opened between 1939 and 1945. In 1957, these records were coded, and the parents in these families were divided into four groups: (1) rejecting parents, (2) neglectful parents, (3) abusive parents, and (4) loving parents. McCord found an increase in juvenile delinquency during adolescence in the maltreated children. Of the maltreated boys, 45% had an increased incidence of criminal records, alcoholism, mental illness, problems with control of aggression, and early death. Of men rejected by their parents, 53% were convicted of crimes, as opposed to 35% who were neglected or 39% who were physically abused. Only 23% of the men from loving families were convicted of crimes. Fifty-five percent of maltreated individuals appeared

to reach adulthood without significant social difficulties. The researches associated this positive outcome with a strong mother who was both educated and self-confident. Widom[112] also identified an increased incidence of criminal records, alcoholism, mental illness, problems with control of aggression, and early death, although an absence of crimes against children was also noted. Both studies raise the question of protective factors and interventions that might mitigate or ameliorate the later consequences of child maltreatment and enhance positive outcomes.

IMPLICATIONS FOR CHILDREN WITH DISABILITIES

Child maltreatment is a complex social, psychological, political, and cultural phenomenon. Knowledge of risk factors should enable clinicians to prevent, or at least diminish, its prevalence. Children living in poverty, those with atypical and disruptive behaviors, and those with disabilities are known to be at much higher risk for maltreatment.[11]

For example, Sobsey[113] and Verdugo and associates[114] invoked an ecological approach that involves changing attitudes that allow maltreatment of children with disabilities. The first task is to alter the way society views children with disabilities, leading to more positive perceptions of such children and a subsequent decrease in their risk of maltreatment. These authors suggested that relationships be established between families with children with special health needs and those with typical children, in an environment that positively acknowledges and celebrates the uniqueness of the disabled child and promotes education about children with special needs. Such settings may include daycare centers, schools, and hospitals. Because the most frequent perpetrators of abuse are family members, these authors also emphasize the need to support the children's caregivers.

Even when clinicians recognize risk factors and offer appropriate interventions, they do not prevent all maltreatment of children with special needs. Individuals who have contact with the child and family must alert the appropriate authorities when maltreatment is suspected. The observer does not need to make the diagnosis; to make such a report, he or she must only have reasonable cause to suspect that maltreatment is occurring.

Numerous professional organizations provide valuable information and support regarding child abuse and neglect for clinicians and institutions. Examples include the American Academy of Pediatrics (see www.aap.org for additional information), the National Association of Children's Hospitals and Related Institutions (NACHRI),[63] the American Professional

Society on the Abuse of Children (www.apsac.org), and the International Society on the Prevention of Child Abuse and Neglect (www.ISPCAN.org).

REFERENCES

1. Federal Child Abuse Prevention Treatment Act, 42 USC §5106g(4), 1974.
2. Kempe CH, Silverman FN, Steele BF, et al: The battered child syndrome. JAMA 181:17-24, 1962.
3. Helfer RE: The epidemiology of child abuse and neglect. Pediatr Ann 13:745-751, 1984.
4. Kleinman PK: Diagnostic Imaging of Child Abuse, 2nd ed. St. Louis: CV Mosby, 1998.
5. Garbarino J, Guttman E, Seeley JW: The Psychologically Battered Child. San Francisco: Jossey-Bass, 1986.
6. U.S. Department of Health and Human Services, Children's Bureau: Child Maltreatment 2001: Reports from the States to the National Child Abuse and Neglect System. Washington, DC: U.S. Government Printing Office, 2002.
7. ISCHHS, Children's Bureau, 2000.
8. U.S. Department of Health and Human Services, Children's Bureau. Child Maltreatment 2003: Reports from the States to the National Child Abuse and Neglect System. Washington, DC: U.S. Government Printing Office, 2005.
9. McPherson M, Arango P, Fox H, et al: A new definition of children with special health needs. Pediatrics 102:137-140, 1998.
10. Westat, Inc.: A Report on the Maltreatment of Children with Disabilities. Washington, DC: National Center on Child Abuse and Neglect, 1993.
11. Goldson E: Maltreatment among children with disabilities. Infants Young Child 13:44-54, 2001.
12. Ten Bensel RW, Rheinberger MM, Radbill SX: Children in a world of violence: The roots of child maltreatment. In Helfer ME, Kempe RS, Krugman RD, eds: The Battered Child, 5th ed. Chicago: University of Chicago Press, 1997, pp 3-18.
13. Zigler E, Hall NW: Physical child abuse in America: Past, present and, future. In Cicchetti D, Carlson V, eds: Child Maltreatment: Theory and Research on the Causes and Consequences of Child Abuse and Neglect. New York: Cambridge University Press, 1989, p 38.
14. Myers JEB: A History of Child Protection in America. Philadelphia: Xlibris, 2004.
15. Friedrich WN: An integrated model of psychotherapy for abused children. In Myers JEB, Berliner J, Briere J, et al, eds: The APSAC Handbook on Child Maltreatment, 2nd ed. Thousand Oaks, CA: Sage Publications, 2002, pp 141-158.
16. Kolko DJ: Child physical abuse. In Myers JEB, Berliner J, Briere J, et al, eds: The APSAC Handbook on Child Maltreatment, 2nd ed. Thousand Oaks, CA: Sage Publications, 2002, pp 21-54.
17. Briere J: Trauma Symptom Checklist for Children (TSCC) Professional Manual. Odessa, FL: Psychological Assessment Resources, 1996.
18. Friedrich WN: Child Sexual Behavior Inventory: Professional Manual. Odessa, FL: Psychological Assessment Resources, 1997.
19. Brassard MR, Hart SN, Hardy DB: The Psychological Maltreatment Rating Scale. Child Abuse Negl 17:715-729, 1993.
20. Bonner BL, Logue MS, Kaufman KL, et al: Child maltreatment. In Walker CE, Roberts MC, eds: Handbook of Clinical Child Psychology, 3rd ed. New York: Wiley, 2001, pp 989-1030.
21. Cohen JA, Berliner L, Mannarino AP: Treating traumatized children: A research review and synthesis. Trauma Violence Abuse 1:29-46, 2000.
22. Azar ST, Wolfe DA: Child physical abuse and neglect. In Mash EJ, Barkley RA, eds: Treatment of Childhood Disorders. New York: Guilford, 1998, pp 501-544.
23. Oats RK, Bross DC: What have we learned about treating physical abuse: A literature review of the last decade. Child Abuse Negl 19:463-473, 1995.
24. Wolfe D: Child Abuse: Implications for Child Development and Psychopathology, 2nd ed. Thousand Oaks, CA: Sage Publications, 1999.
25. Lutzker JR: Behavioral treatment of child neglect. Behav Modif 14:301-315, 1990.
26. Lutzker JR, Bigelow KM, Doctor RM, et al: An eco-behavioral model for the prevention and treatment of child abuse and neglect. In Lutzker JR, ed: Handbook for Child Abuse Research and Treatment. New York: Plenum Press, 1998, pp 239-266.
27. Olds DJ, Eckenrode J, Henderson CR, et al: Long-term effects of home visitation on maternal life course and child abuse and neglect. JAMA 278:637-643, 1997.
28. Ewing-Cobbs L, Kramer L, Prasad M, et al: Neuroimaging, physical and developmental findings after inflicted and noninflected traumatic brain injury in young children. Pediatrics 102:300-307, 1998.
29. Ewing-Cobbs L, Prasad M, Kramer L, et al: Inflicted traumatic brain injury: Relationship of developmental outcome to severity of injury. Pediatr Neurosurg 31:251-258, 1999.
30. Peerez-Arjona E, Dujovny M, Del Proposto Z, et al: Late outcome following central nervous system injury in child abuse. Child Nerv Syst 19:69-81, 2003.
31. Bonner BL, Crow SM, Hensley LD: State efforts to identify maltreated children with disabilities: A follow-up study. Child Maltreatment 2:56-60, 1997.
32. Sullivan PM, Knutson JF: Maltreatment and disabilities: A population-based epidemiological study. Child Abuse Neglect 24:1257-1273, 2000.
33. Putnam FW: Ten-year research update review: Child sexual abuse. J Am Acad Child Adolesc Psychiatry 42:269-278, 2003.
34. Westcott H, Jones D: Annotation: The abuse of disabled children. J Child Psychol Psychiatry 40:497-506, 1999.
35. Lung CT, Daro D: Current Trends in Child Abuse Reporting and Fatalities: The Results of the 1995 Annual Fifty State Survey. Chicago: National Committee to Prevent Child Abuse, 1996.

36. U.S. Department of Health and Human Services: Child Maltreatment 2003. Washington, DC: U.S. Government Printing Office, 2005.

37. Belsky J, Vondra J: Lessons from child abuse: The determinants of parenting. *In* Carlson CD, Carlson V, eds: Child maltreatment: Theory and Research on the Causes and Consequences of Child Abuse and Neglect. New York: Cambridge University Press, 1989, pp 153-202.

38. Ammerman RT: The role of the child in physical abuse: A reappraisal. Violence Victims 6(2):87-101, 1991.

39. Famularo R, Fenton T, Kinscherff RT: Medical and developmental histories of maltreated children. Clin Pediatr 31:536-541, 1992.

40. Beeghly M, Cicchetti D: Child maltreatment, attachment, and the self system: Emergence of an internal state lexicon in toddlers at high social risk. Dev Psychopathol 6:5-30, 1994.

41. Walker E, Downey G, Bergman A: The effects of parental psychopathology and maltreatment on child behavior: A test of the diathesis-stress model. Child Dev 60:15-24, 1989.

42. Kaplan S, Pelcovitz D, Salzinger S, et al: Adolescent physical abuse: Risk for adolescent psychiatric disorders. Am J Psychiatry 155:954-959, 1998.

43. Gelles RJ, Straus MA: The medical and psychological costs of family violence. *In* Straus MA, Gelles RJ, eds: Physical Violence in American Families: Risk Factors and Adaptations to Violence in 8,145 Families. New Brunswick, NJ: Transaction, 1990, pp 425-430.

44. Famularo R, Kinscherff R, Fenton T: Posttraumatic stress disorder among children clinically diagnosed as borderline personality disorder. J Nerv Ment Dis 179:428-431, 1991.

45. Pelcovitz D, Kaplan S, Goldenberg B, et al: Posttraumatic stress disorder in physically abused adolescents. J Am Acad Child Adolesc Psychiatry 33:305-312, 1994.

46. Allen DM, Tarnowski KG: Depressive characteristics of physically abused children. J Abnorm Child Psychol 17:1-11, 1989.

47. Famularo R, Fenton T, Kinscherff R, et al: Maternal and child posttraumatic stress disorder in cases of child maltreatment. Child Abuse Negl 18:27-36, 1994.

48. Famularo R, Fenton T, Augustyn M, et al: Persistence of pediatric post traumatic stress disorder after 2 years. Child Abuse Negl 20:1245-1248, 1996.

49. Crittenden PM, Ainsworth MDS: Child maltreatment and attachment theory. *In* Cicchetti D, Carlson V, eds: Child Maltreatment: Theory and Research on the Causes and Consequences of Child Abuse and Neglect. New York: Cambridge University Press, 1989, pp 432-463.

50. Lynch M, Cicchetti D: Patterns of relatedness in maltreated and non-maltreated children: Connections among multiple representational models. Dev Psychopathol 3:207-226, 1991.

51. Wolfe D, Werkele C, Reitzel-Jaffe D, et al: Factors associated with abusive relationships among mal-treated and non-maltreated youth. Dev Psychopathol 10:61-85, 1998.

52. Widom CS: Does violence beget violence? A critical examination of the literature. Psychol Bull 106:3-28, 1989.

53. Silverman AB, Reinherz HZ, Giaconia RM: The long-term sequelae of child and adolescent abuse: A longitudinal community study. Child Abuse Negl 8:709-723, 1996.

54. Brown J, Cohen P, Johnson JG, et al: Childhood abuse and neglect: Specificity of effects on adolescent and young adult depression and suicidality. J Am Acad Child Adolesc Psychiatry 38:1490-1505, 1999.

55. Erickson MF, Egeland B: Child neglect. *In* Myers JEB, Berliner L, Briere J, et al, eds: The APSAC Handbook on Child Maltreatment, 2nd ed. Thousand Oaks, CA: Sage Publications, 2002, pp 3-20.

56. Bonner BL, Crow SM, Logue MB: Fatal child neglect. *In* Dubowitz H, ed: Neglected Children. Thousand Oaks, CA: Sage Publications, 1999, pp 156-173.

57. Geffken G, Johnson SB, Silverstein J, et al: The death of a child with diabetes from neglect: A case study. Clin Pediatr 31:325-330, 1992.

58. Oates RK, Kempe RS: Growth failure in infants. *In* Helfer ME, Kempe RS, Krugman RD: eds: The Battered Child, 5th ed. Chicago: University of Chicago Press, 1997, pp 374-391.

59. Steele BF: Psychological Dimensions of Child Abuse. Presented at the meeting of the American Association for the Advancement of Science, Denver, February 1977.

60. Hoffman-Plotkin D, Twentyman CT: A multimodal assessment of behavioral and cognitive deficits in abused and neglected preschoolers. Child Dev 35:794-802, 1984.

61. Katz K: Communication problems in maltreated children: A tutorial. J Child Commun Dis 14:147-163, 1992.

62. Kendall-Tackett KA, Williams LM, Finklehor D: Impact of sexual abuse on children: A review and synthesis of recent empirical studies. Psychol Bull 113:164-180, 1993.

63. Perry BD: Incubated in terror: Neurodevelopmental factors in the "cycle of violence." *In* Osofsky JD, ed: Children in a Violent Society. New York: Guilford, 1997, pp 124-149.

64. Lewis DO: From abuse to violence: Psychophysiological consequences of maltreatment. J Am Acad Child Adolesc Psychiatry 31:383-391, 1992.

65. DeBellis MD, Baum AS, Birmaher B, et al: Developmental traumatology part I: Biological stress systems. Biol Psychiatry 45:1259-1270, 1999.

66. DeBellis MD, Keshavan MS, Clark DB, et al: Developmental traumatology part II: Brain development. Biol Psychiatry 45:1271-1284, 1999.

67. Perry BD: Childhood experience and the expression of genetic potential: What childhood neglect tells us about nature and nurture. Brain Mind 3:79-100, 2002.

68. Wolfe VV, Birt J: The psychological sequelae of child sexual abuse. Adv Clin Child Psychol 17:233-263, 1995.

69. Boney-McCoy S, Finklehor D: Psychosocial sequelae of violent victimization in a national youth sample. J Consult Clin Psychol 63:726-736, 1995.

70. Kendall-Tackett KA, Eckenrode J: The effects of neglect on academic achievement and disciplinary problems: A developmental perspective. Child Abuse Negl 20:161-169, 1996.

71. Fergusson DM, Horwood LJ, Lynseky MT: Childhood sexual abuse and psychiatric disorder in young adulthood: II. Psychiatric outcomes of childhood sexual abuse. Child Adolesc Psychiatry 34:1365-1374, 1996.

72. Berliner L, Elliott DM: Sexual abuse of children. *In* Myers JEB, Berliner L, Briere J, et al, eds: The APSAC Handbook on Child Maltreatment, 2nd ed. Thousand Oaks, CA: Sage Publications, 2002, pp 55-78.

73. McLeer SV, Dixon JF, Henry D, et al: Psychopathology in non-clinically referred sexually abused children. J Am Acad Child Adolesc Psychiatry 37:1326-1333, 1998.

74. Mannarino AP, Cohen JA: Abuse-related attributions and perceptions, general attributions, and locus of control in sexually abused girls. J Interpers Violence 11:162-180, 1996.

75. Mannarino AP, Cohen JA: A follow-up study of factors that mediate the development of psychological symptomatology in sexually abused girls. Child Maltreat 1:246-260, 1996.

76. Dubner AE, Motta RW: Sexually and physically abused foster care children and posttraumatic stress disorder. J Consult Clin Psychol 67:367-373, 1999.

77. Ruggiero KJ, McLeer SV, Dixon JF: Sexual abuse characteristics associated with survivor psychopathology. Child Abuse Negl 24:951-964, 2000.

78. Rust JO, Troupe PA: Relationships of treatment of child sexual abuse with school achievement and self-concept. J Early Adolesc 11:420-429, 1991.

79. Wind TW, Silvern LE: Type and extent of child abuse as predictors of adult functioning. J Fam Violence 7:261-281, 1992.

80. Friedrich WN, Dittner CA, Action R, et al: Child Sexual Behavior Inventory: Normative, psychiatric and sexual abuse comparisons. Child Maltreat 6:37-49, 2001.

81. Kilpatrick DG, Ruggiero KJ, Acierno RE, et al: Violence and risk of PTSD, major depression, substance abuse/dependence, and comorbidity: Results from the National Survey of Adolescents. J Consult Clin Psychol 71:692-700, 2003.

82. Hibbard RA, Ingersoll GM, Orr DP: Behavior risk, emotional risk, and child abuse among adolescents in a non-clinical setting. Pediatrics 86:896-901, 1990.

83. Boney-McCoy S, Finkelhor D: Is youth victimization related to trauma symptoms and depression after controlling for prior symptoms and family relationships? A longitudinal prospective study. J Consult Clin Psychol 64:1406-1416, 1996.

84. Herrenkohl E, Herrenkohl R, Egolf B, et al: The relationship between early maltreatment and teenage parenthood. J Adolesc 21:291-303, 1998.

85. Widom C, Ames M: Criminal consequences of childhood sexual victimization. Child Abuse Negl 18:303-318, 1994.

86. Kendler K, Bulik C, Silber J, et al: Childhood sexual abuse and adult psychiatric and substance abuse disorders in women. Arch Gen Psychiatry 57:953-959, 2000.

87. Schuck AM, Widom CS: Childhood victimization and alcohol symptoms in females: Causal inferences and hypothesized mediators. Child Abuse Negl 25:1069-1092, 2001.

88. Rich CL, Combs-Lane AM, Resnick HS, et al: Child sexual abuse and adult sexual revictimization. *In* Koenig LJ, Doll LS, O'Leary A, et al, eds: From Child Sexual Abuse to Adult Sexual Risk: Trauma, Revictimization, and Intervention. Washington, DC: American Psychological Association, 2004, pp 49-68.

89. Nelson EC, Heath AC, Madden PA, et al: Association between self-reported childhood sexual abuse and adverse psychosocial outcomes: Results from a twin study. Arch Gen Psychiatry 59:139-146, 2002.

90. Paolucci E, Genuis M, Violato C: A meta-analysis of the published research on the effects of child sexual abuse. J Psychol 135(1):17-36, 2001.

91. Binggeli NJ, Hart SN, Brassard MR: Psychological Maltreatment: A Study Guide. Thousand Oaks, CA: Sage Publications, 2001.

92. Claussen AH, Crittenden PM: Physical and psychological maltreatment: Relations among types of maltreatment. Child Abuse Negl 15:5-18, 1991.

93. Brassard MR, Germain R, Hart SN, eds: Psychological Maltreatment of Children and Youth. New York: Pergamon, 1987.

94. Garbarino J, Guttman E, Seeley J: The Psychologically Battered Child: Strategies for Identification, Assessment and Intervention. San Francisco: Jossey-Bass, 1986.

95. Egeland B: Mediators of the effects of child maltreatment on developmental adaptation in adolescence. *In* Cicchetti D, Toth SL, eds: Rochester Symposium on Developmental Psychopathology, Volume VIII: The Effects of Trauma on the Developmental Process. Rochester, NY: University of Rochester Press, 1997, pp 403-434.

96. Egeland B, Erickson M: Psychologically unavailable caregiving. *In* Brassard MR, Germain R, Hart SN, eds: Psychological Maltreatment of Children and Youth. New York: Pergamon, 1987, pp 110-120.

97. Erickson MF, Egeland B, Pianta R: The effects of maltreatment on the development of young children. *In* Cicchetti D, Carlson V, eds: Child Maltreatment: Theory and Research on the Causes and Consequences of Child Abuse and Neglect. New York: Cambridge University Press, 1989, pp 647-684.

98. Lefkowitz M, Eron L, Walder L, et al: Growing Up to Be Violent: A Longitudinal Study of the Development of Aggression. New York: Pergamon, 1977.

99. Loeber R, Stouthamer-Loeber M: Family factors as correlates and predictors of juvenile conduct problems and delinquency. *In* Tonry M, Morris N, eds: Crime and Justice, an Annual Review of the Research, 7th ed. Chicago: University of Chicago Press, 1986, pp 29-149.

100. Rohner RP, Rohner EC: Antecedents and consequences of parental rejection: A theory of emotional abuse. Child Abuse Negl 4:189-198, 1980.

101. Rorty M, Yager J, Rossotto E: Childhood sexual, physical, and psychological abuse in bulimia nervosa. Am J Psychiatry 151:1122-1126, 1994.

102. Briere J, Runtz M: Differential adult symptomatology associated with three types of child abuse histories. Child Abuse Negl 14:357-364, 1990.

103. Gross AB, Keller HR: Long-term consequences of childhood physical and psychological maltreatment. Aggress Behav 18:171-185, 1992.

104. Hart SN, Brassard MR, Binggeli NJ, et al: Psychological maltreatment. *In* Myers JEB, Berliner L, Briere J, et al, eds: The APSAC Handbook on Child Maltreatment, 2nd ed. Thousand Oaks, CA: Sage Publications, 2002, pp 79-103.

105. Koenig LJ, Clark H: Sexual abuse of girls and HIV infection among women: Are they related? *In* Koenig LJ, Doll LS, O'Leary A, et al, eds: From Child Sexual Abuse to Adult Sexual Risk: Trauma, Revictimization, and Intervention. Washington, DC: American Psychological Association, 2004, pp 69-92.

106. Perez CM, Widom CS: Childhood victimization and long-term intellectual and academic outcomes. Child Abuse Negl 18:617-633, 1994.

107. Putnam FW: Ten-year research update review: Child sexual abuse. J Am Acad Child Adolesc Psychiatry 42:269-278, 2003.

108. Rich CL, Combs-Lane AM, Resnick HS, et al: Child sexual abuse and adult sexual revictimization. *In* Koenig LJ, Doll LS, O'Leary A, et al, eds: From Child Sexual Abuse to Adult Sexual Risk: Trauma, Revictimization, and Intervention. Washington, DC: American Psychological Association, 2004, pp 49-68.

109. Schuck AM, Widom CS: Childhood victimization and alcohol symptoms in females: Causal inferences and hypothesized mediators. Child Abuse Negl 25:1069-1092, 2001.

110. Felitti VJ: The Relationship of Adverse Childhood Experiences to Adult Health Status: Turning Gold into Lead. Presented at the Snowbird Conference of the Child Trauma Network of the Intermountain West, Salt Lake City, UT, September 2003. (Available at: *www.acestudy.org;* accessed 1/29/07.)

111. McCord J: A forty year perspective on effects of child abuse and neglect. Child Abuse Negl 7:265, 1983.

112. Widom CS: Child abuse, neglect, and adult behavior: Research design and findings on criminality, violence and child abuse. Am J Orthopsychiatry 59:355-367, 1989.

113. Sobsey D: An integrated ecological model of abuse. *In* Violence and Abuse in the Lives of People with Disabilities: The End of Silent Acceptance? Baltimore: Paul H. Brookes, 1994, pp 145-174.

114. Verdugo MA, Bermejo BG, Fuentes J: The maltreatment of intellectually handicapped children and adolescents. Child Abuse Negl 19:205-215, 1995.

115. Dawes CG: Defining the Children's Hospital Role in Child Maltreatment. Alexandria, VA: National Association of Children's Hospitals and Related Institutions, 2005. (Available at: *www.childrenshospitals.net;* accessed 1/29/07.)

Pain and Somatoform Disorders

TONYA M. PALERMO ■ HEATHER KRELL ■ NORAH JANOSY
■ LONNIE K. ZELTZER

Pain complaints are common in children and adolescents seen in primary and subspecialty care. These complaints represent a broad spectrum of conditions, including acute medical pain, recurrent or chronic pain, pain related to chronic disease, and pain in the context of a somatoform disorder. Pain that persists can have a profound effect on many areas of child and family life and can lead to problems with pain in adulthood. Affected children often challenge the diagnostic and therapeutic acumen of physicians and mental health professionals who care for them. The goal of this chapter is to review the most common acute and chronic pediatric pain problems, as well as somatoform disorders. We examine the diagnostic criteria, the prevalence, functional effect, causes, and empirically supported methods of assessment and treatment of pain conditions and somatoform disorders. The chapter closes with a discussion and summary of implications for clinical care, training, and research on pain and somatoform disorders in children and adolescents.

DEFINITIONS OF PAIN AND SOMATOFORM DISORDERS

Some basic definitions are presented here to orient the reader to the problems of pediatric pain and somatoform disorders covered in this chapter. Pain is defined by the International Association for the Study of Pain as "an unpleasant sensory and emotional experience associated with actual or potential tissue damage, or described in terms of such damage."[1] Pain has a sensory and affective component. Neuroimaging studies[2,3] have demonstrated the differential pain perception areas of the cortex that are involved in affective pain perception and those involved in sensory pain perception. Pain can be categorized as acute or chronic, although there is no definite criteria

of how long pain must persist to become "chronic," other than an agreed-upon operational one (e.g., 3 months).

Acute Pain

Acute pain is usually a signal that there is some tissue injury, inflammation, or infection that may necessitate immediate attention. For example, a fall from a bicycle may produce a scraped and bruised knee. The knee is experienced as acutely painful because there is tissue injury, which activates local afferent nerve fibers through the local release of neural activators, such as prostanoids, substance P, and other local neurotransmitters. In turn, afferent nociceptive fibers provide messages to connector neurons in the spinal cord, with the release of other local neurotransmitters, and the ascending transmission of nociception up to pain perception areas in the brain is initiated. In acute pain, typically the descending neural inhibitory system is rapidly activated; then the pain process becomes diminished, and soon the pain goes away. Motor reflexes may also be activated, such as withdrawing a finger from a hot plate if the finger's sensation is experienced as too hot and painful. Phylogenetically, acute pain is protective and serves as a warning signal to take action. Acute pain is typically brief and usually ends shortly after the acute injury occurs; after it heals; after the inflammation has subsided; or when the stretch, contraction, or impingement on the body part has resolved. Examples include a broken arm, postsurgery pain, acute gastroenteritis, menstrual cramps, a sore throat, pain from an ear infection, or acute muscle cramps related to significant exercise. This type of pain can be mild to severe, but most acute pain conditions are readily diagnosable, which means that the source is fairly easily discovered. Although the source may be known (e.g., surgery), physical movement, emotions, beliefs, and environmental factors (e.g., what physicians, nurses, and parents do and say) can affect both the severity and duration of the pain, complicating the assessment and management of acute pain.

Chronic Pain

Chronic pain, on the other hand, may or may not be symptomatic of underlying, ongoing tissue damage or chronic disease. It can persist long after an initial injury has healed or another event has occurred (typically longer than 3 months) and no longer serves a useful warning function. Chronic or recurrent pain may be associated with ongoing underlying chronic or recurrent medical conditions, such as arthritis, cancer, nerve damage, Crohn disease, ulcerative colitis, chronic infection, or sickle cell disease. Cancer-related pain and pain associated with life-limiting and life-threatening medical conditions, as in end-stage diseases, are another form of serious chronic pain. Chronic and recurrent pain may be the problem itself, without an underlying clearly identifiable physical cause, as in pain associated with irritable bowel syndrome, headaches, musculoskeletal pain, or complex regional pain syndrome (CRPS). Chronic pain, whether the likely cause or contributory factors can be identified or not, can hinder the body's ability to heal itself and can affect quality of life, and so the pain itself becomes an additional or primary chronic problem.

With chronic pain, there are even greater opportunities over the longer time course for physical, emotional, behavioral, and social factors to affect the pain and the child's function, including sleep, school attendance, physical activities, and social and family engagement. For these reasons, even pain related to known causes, such as arthritis, can become more severe and continuous than would otherwise be expected if not adequately noted and well managed.

Somatoform Disorders

Somatoform disorders are a group of psychiatric disorders described in the *Diagnostic and Statistical Manual of Mental Disorders (DSM)*, 4th edition, Text Revision *(DSM-IV-TR)*[4] as the presence of physical symptoms suggestive of an underlying medical condition but for which the medical condition is neither found nor fully accounts for the level of functional impairment. In medicine, these conditions are classified as functional somatic syndromes.[5] *DSM-IV-TR* somatoform disorders include somatization disorder, conversion disorder, pain disorder, undifferentiated somatoform disorder, hypochondriasis, and body dysmorphic disorder. Except for body dysmorphic disorder, characterized by a preoccupation with an imagined or exaggerated defect in physical appearance, all the other somatoform disorders frequently have pain as part of the presenting complaint. Thus, the other somatoform disorders are included in this chapter, with the recognition of the limited research base in children and adolescents. However, because there may be precursors of adult somatoform disorders identifiable in children, we believe it is important to be inclusive of them in our review.

CLINICAL AND SCIENTIFIC SIGNIFICANCE OF PAIN AND SOMATOFORM DISORDERS

Prevalence of Pain and Somatoform Disorders

Pain among children and adolescents has been identified as an important public health problem. Acute pain is commonly encountered in hospitalized pediatric patients.[6] Chronic and recurrent pain is also commonly experienced. According to epidemiological study estimates, chronic and recurrent pain affects 15% to 25% of children and adolescents.[7,8] One population-based study revealed a pain prevalence of 54% in a large sample of youths aged 0 to 18 years; 25% of the respondents reported chronic pain lasting more than 3 months, and more than 25% of respondents reported a combination of multiple locations of pain.[8] The most commonly reported pain sites in epidemiological studies are the head, abdomen, and limbs.[7,8]

The prevalence of specific pain conditions has also been explored. Depending on the definitions of recurrent abdominal pain that are used, prevalence estimates range from 10% to 19% of children and adolescents.[9] Migraine is estimated to occur in 10% to 28% of children and adolescents.[10,11] Episodic tension-type headache has been estimated at a prevalence rate of 12.2% among school-aged children.[12] The prevalence of pediatric headache has apparently increased since the early 1980s. Musculoskeletal pain complaints have been reported as common in the general pediatric population; available prevalence estimates are 29% for back pain, 21% for neck pain, and 7.5% for widespread pain. Estimates of fibromyalgia syndrome in the general American adult population are 2%,[13] but specific estimates for the juvenile form are not available.

Pain also occurs in the context of chronic health conditions such as sickle cell disease, arthritis, and cancer. Recurrent and disabling pain symptoms have been reported to affect as many as 15% of patients with sickle cell disease.[14] On average, children with sickle cell disease experience pain episodes five to seven times per year and require hospitalization one or two times per year for pain.[15] For young and school-aged children, the majority of pain episodes occurs at home and are managed primarily by families.[15,16] Studies have shown that mild to moderate intensity pain is quite common in children with juvenile idiopathic arthritis[17] and occurs on a weekly basis for many such children. Epidemiological studies demonstrate that children with cancer experience frequent pain; an estimated 54% to 85% of pediatric hospitalized cancer patients report pain, and 26% to 35% of children in the outpatient setting report cancer-related pain.[18-20] Children with cancer may experience pain at the time of cancer diagnosis, during active treatment, and at the end of life.

Prevalence of Somatoform Disorders

Although there is little available information regarding the incidence and prevalence of specific somatoform disorders in the pediatric population, medically unexplained somatic symptoms, particularly pain, are common. The prevalence rates of recurrent somatic symptoms among children and adolescents generally range from 10% to 20%, the most common symptoms being recurrent head pain and abdominal pain.[7,8] Less common complaints include symptoms such as back and chest pain, low energy, fatigue, extremity numbness/tingling, and other gastrointestinal complaints.[21]

Somatoform disorders are common in adults seen in primary care; prevalence estimates are 10% to 15%.[22,23] Little information concerning the prevalence of specific somatoform disorders in children and adolescents is available. In an early survey conducted in pediatric primary care, the prevalence rate of psychosomatic diagnoses in children ranged between 5.7% and 10.8%.[24] However, in a community sample of 540 school-aged children, Garber and colleagues[25] found that only 1.1% of children met full diagnostic criteria for somatization disorder according to criteria of the third edition, revised, of the *DSM (DSM-III-R)*. There are multiple published case reports and case series documenting conversion disorder in children and adolescents, for example,[26] but no incidence data are available. Similarly, no incidence data for hypochondriasis, pain disorder, or undifferentiated somatoform disorder in children or adolescents are available. In general, diagnosed somatoform disorders are rarely documented in pediatric samples, probably because the diagnostic criteria were established for adults and it is controversial whether they are applicable to children. However, at present, an alternative, developmentally appropriate classification system is unavailable. In view of the profound effect of unexplained medical symptoms on children and adolescents, increasing the relevance of the diagnostic criteria for children will be a major advance in the classification system.

Consequences of Pediatric Pain and Somatoform Disorders

The functional consequences of pain and somatoform disorders on children and adolescents can be significant. In general, somatic symptoms are associated with increased risk for psychopathology, family conflict, parent-perceived ill health, school problems and absenteeism, and excessive use of health and mental health services.[27] Specifically, although many children with pain conditions cope very well, other children experiencing pain develop psychosocial difficulties, academic problems, disruptions in peer and family relationships, and anxiety and depression. Chronic pain, in particular, can have a major effect on the daily lives of children and adolescents. According to clinical descriptions of extreme chronic pain and disability in children,[28] some children who experience chronic pain develop significant impairments in their academic, social, and psychological functioning. These children frequently miss considerable amounts of school, may not participate in athletic and social activities, and may suffer anxiety or depression in response to uncontrolled pain.

There exists a continuum of functional consequences of pain on children and adolescents: At one end of the spectrum is the experience of pain symptoms but minimal day-to-day impairments; at the other end is the experience of pain symptoms accompanied by profound effects on most aspects of daily functioning and severely reduced quality of life. Health-related quality of life is a multidimensional construct that refers to an individual's perception of the effect of an illness, symptoms, and its consequent treatment on the person's physical, psychological, and social well-being.[29] Several examinations of health-related quality of life have been undertaken in children with chronic pain. Unexplained chronic pain in adolescents has been associated with poor quality of life in the adolescent, as well as in the family.[30] Children and adolescents with headaches suffer reductions in health-related quality of life in comparison with same-age peers without head pain.[31] Frequent pain in the context of chronic disease also impairs quality of life. Youth with sickle cell disease[32] and youth with cystic fibrosis[33] have been found to experience specific reductions in physical, psychological, and social functioning in relation to the experience of frequent pain.

Disability that results from chronic pain is a concept separate from pain itself and equally important to consider in assessment and management of pediatric pain patients.[34] *Disability* refers to the areas in an individual's life that are limited because of pain (i.e., the things that a person cannot do because of pain). For children, disability can be demonstrated in the home and school setting.[34,35] The domains of functioning that seem to be particularly affected by chronic pain and that are reviewed in the following sections include school and academics, participation in physical and social activities, sleep disturbance, and family disruption.

SCHOOL FUNCTIONING

In industrialized cultures, a child's sole responsibility is to attend school. Children with pain conditions often have difficulties accomplishing this important task. For example, children experiencing pain related to sickle cell disease,[16,36] widespread musculoskeletal pain,[37] and recurrent abdominal pain[38] have been found to have higher rates of school absenteeism than do controls. The number of missed school days is quite substantial. In one study, patients with sickle cell disease were absent from school on 21% of school days, or about 6 weeks.[16] Similarly, in a study of children with CRPS, affected children on average missed 40 school days.[39] Migraine headaches, which affect approximately 1 million children and adolescents, have been reported to lead to school absence rates of several hundred thousand missed days per month.[40] A high rate of absenteeism can have direct effects on academic performance and school success, as well as important effects on socialization and maintenance of peer relationships. Many children and adolescents with chronic pain experience extreme stress because of missing school and the subsequent difficulty in making up and keeping up with classwork. This can lead to a vicious cycle of missed school and increased stress that further compromises their ability to cope with the pain problem.

PHYSICAL AND SOCIAL ACTIVITIES

As with the effect on school attendance, recurrent and chronic pain affects children's participation in developmentally appropriate physical and social activities. Adolescents with headaches[41] and children with sickle cell disease[36] have reported a significant effect of pain on the amount of leisure time with peers in comparison with healthy controls. The majority of children with unexplained chronic pain suffer impairment in sports activities and social functioning.[42] Specific activities that are most often reported by children themselves as difficult to perform because of chronic pain are sports, running, gym class, schoolwork, going to school, and playing with friends.[43] In particular, when pediatric patients become severely disabled by chronic pain, their lives may become very isolated and restricted with few opportunities for enjoyment of friends and normative activities.

EMOTIONAL FUNCTIONING

Persistent pain can also have a substantial effect on the emotional status of children and adolescents. In general, children with recurrent pain experience more stress, feel less cheerful, and feel more depressed than do children without pain.[44] Higher levels of depressive symptoms are associated with higher levels of pain both in children with a chronic disease[45] and in children with chronic nonmalignant pain.[46] Moreover, increased depressive symptoms are associated with increased functional disability that children experience in relation to chronic pain.[46]

There have been only a few investigations to specifically report on the prevalence of psychiatric disorders in children and adolescents with chronic pain. Chronic pain does appear to be associated with psychiatric comorbidity, particularly anxiety and mood disorders. For example, in a sample of children seen in a primary care setting for recurrent abdominal pain, 79% of children met criteria for an anxiety disorder and 43% for a depressive disorder.[47] Further studies are needed to disentangle the temporal sequence of chronic pain and psychiatric disturbance. It is currently not clear whether psychiatric disturbance typically predates the pain problem or whether the psychiatric disturbance develops in reaction to living with unremitting or disabling pain.

SLEEP DISTURBANCE

Pain can also interfere with the quality and quantity of children's sleep, and sleep deprivation, in turn, can reduce children's ability to cope with pain and enhance pain sensitivity. More than half of children and adolescents with chronic pain report sleep difficulties.[7] Disturbed sleep has been identified in a number of specific chronic pain syndromes in children and adolescents, including juvenile rheumatoid arthritis, headache, CRPS, sickle cell disease, fibromyalgia, and recurrent abdominal pain. Researchers have begun to describe these sleep disturbances, finding that these children and adolescents experience difficulty falling asleep, frequent night and early morning awakening, and excessive daytime sleepiness. Inadequate sleep quantity and quality are linked to significant problems in several aspects of daily life for children and adolescents.[48] Daytime sleepiness resulting from both suboptimal sleep duration and sleep disturbance is associated with reduced academic performance, attentional difficulties, mood disturbance, and increased school absences.[48,49] For children and adolescents with chronic pain who may already be experiencing functional limitations in their daily lives, good quality sleep may be even more crucial than for their pain-free peers. The disruption in sleep in some children and adolescents may be a marker for problems with functional disability or may signal the progression into chronic pain syndromes. (Lewin and Dahl[50] reviewed the importance of sleep in the management of pediatric pain, highlighting the bidirectional effects between sleep and pain.) In adolescents with chronic pain, impaired sleep has been shown to reduce functioning in a broad range of physical and social activities and health-related quality of life.[51]

FAMILY AND SOCIETAL CONSEQUENCES

Childhood chronic pain is known to have negative effects on family life, including increased restrictions on parental social life and higher parental stress levels, in comparison with families whose children do not have chronic pain.[30,52] Parents are most often responsible for initiating a child's contact into the health care system and ultimately carry the burden of daily care for these children. In one study, parents' perception of more illness-related stress was the strongest predictor of health care use in children with sickle cell disease.[53]

Apart from the individual and family effects of chronic pain, there is also a potential societal effect of chronic pain that can be demonstrated in increased health care utilization and possible subsequent economic costs, whereby pain-related functional impairment prevents work.[34] The economic costs of adult chronic pain are well documented in terms of lost work productivity and costs of prescription pain medications.[54] The economic costs of childhood chronic pain have not yet been fully described. However, direct costs of pain treatment include medical costs such as hospitalization, doctor's visits, and medications. Indirect costs include parental time off work, transportation costs, child care, and incidental expenses. Children and adolescents with chronic pain may account for a disproportionate number of contacts with the health care system, contributing to millions of dollars spent annually on health care costs for chronic pain.[55] Prior studies have demonstrated that individuals living with chronic pain have increased usage of the health care system for routine medical visits, hospital overnight stays, and emergency room visits.[56,57] For example, in a population-based sample of 5424 children and adolescents, 25% reported chronic pain, and of these, 57% had consulted a physician for pain. In a similar epidemiological study, 53% of children and adolescents had used medication for pain, and 31% had consulted a general practitioner.[58]

RESEARCH ISSUES AND CONTROVERSIES

Pain and somatoform disorders can have a broad effect on children's daily functioning and well-being. As such, studies of children with pain conditions should include relevant outcome variables, including measures of pain and distress, function, quality of life, health care utilization, and economic factors. Although some progress has been made in describing specific areas of functioning that are affected by pain, very little is known about the effect of pain in other areas. For example, although adult chronic pain has been identified as among the most costly medical conditions in industrialized societies,[59] economic outcomes are only beginning to be measured in the pediatric population. In one study conducted in the United Kingdom,[60] a cost-of-illness analysis was completed with adolescents who received treatment for chronic pain; the mean cost was found to be £8027 per child per year, which is equivalent to approximately $14,000 in the United States, including direct service use costs, out-of-pocket expenses, and indirect costs (e.g., lost employment). The longer term costs of pediatric chronic pain are unknown because there are currently no data to indicate whether effective treatment results in reduced costs related to pain in adulthood. More longitudinal data on the outcome of adolescents with chronic pain are needed in order to estimate the true lifetime costs of pain.

CAUSES

Acute pain typically has a clear source and cause. In contrast, chronic pain often occurs without a clear cause. Somatoform disorders are assumed to result from psychological processes; however, the specific mechanisms by which this occurs are largely unknown. Various theories of acute and chronic pain in children have been presented over the years. Many of these theories focus on factors that explain the chronicity and impairment experienced from pain because there is no one-to-one correspondence between the severity of pain and the amount of disability or impairment. Some children may experience relatively severe pain but show surprisingly little impairment, whereas others with milder pain can have more problems in their day-to-day functioning. There may be different causes of pain and disability. For example, a child's pain may result from inflammatory bowel disease (IBD), but the child may not participate in school or recreational activities because the parent is overprotective and has reinforced a sick role. Illness and symptom-related factors are only one source of the variance in functional outcomes.[61]

Because considerable interindividual variability has been observed with regard to children's pain perception and extent of limitations in daily functioning, children's pain is understood in current models within a biopsychosocial framework. A number of models, including the biopsychosocial model of pain,[62] the fear and harm avoidance model,[63] and the self-efficacy model,[64] have this framework. Central to these models are interrelationships among physical, cognitive, affective, and social factors that influence pain and disability outcomes. The following sections summarize several etiological factors that arise from the biopsychosocial model, including developmental factors, sex, family factors, and physiological mechanisms. Although these models tend to include both pain and disability as outcomes with similar sets of contributing factors, we have divided the section below into two parts: (1) etiological factors that seem to play a larger role in the incidence of pain and somatoform disorders and (2) etiological factors that seem to determine the extent of children's pain-related disability.

Etiological Factors in the Incidence of Pain and Somatoform Disorders

In current conceptualizations of pain and somatoform disorders in children, the importance of age, sex, psychosocial stressors, and central nervous system mechanisms for understanding the etiology of pain problems is recognized. For example, the incidence of pain problems follows a clear developmental sequence. Headache increases dramatically with age. Before puberty, recurrent headache occurs at a low rate, and there is a slightly greater incidence of headache in boys.[65-68] With the onset of puberty, the incidence of both migraine and tension-type headaches increases dramatically, and the incidence of headache in girls is much higher, as is documented in adult studies.[67] Puberty plays an uncertain role in the development of chronic pain in children and youth.

In the pediatric population, somatoform disorders tend to follow with a developmental sequence, whereby younger children frequently present with a single somatic complaint, often as a consequence of affective stress, most frequently manifesting as abdominal pain and headaches. Teenagers are more likely to present with multiple complaints, and symptoms such as fatigue, extremity pain, aching muscles, and neurological symptoms increase with age.[69]

Sex differences have emerged in children's symptom reporting and development of endogenous pain and somatic complaints. In nonreferred samples, girls generally report higher pain intensity, longer lasting pain, and more frequent pain than do boys.[8] There is an increased prevalence of several pain problems in girls in comparison with boys, especially after puberty. For example, girls are more likely to be treated for CRPS, fibromyalgia, and migraine headaches. There appears to be a 2 : 1 ratio of girls to boys presenting with somatoform disorders across all age ranges.

Psychosocial stressors—including a parent with a physical illness, depression, anxiety, or somatization disorders; high levels of parental distress; and a history of physical or sexual abuse—are seen significantly more frequently in children in whom somatoform disorders are diagnosed.[69,70]

There are also various central nervous system pain mechanisms that may play a role in the persistence of pain. The neurophysiology of pain is an area of active research.[71,72] For example, in understanding functional bowel disorders, current theories suggest that the pain or symptoms are caused by abnormal brain-intestinal neural signaling that create intestinal or visceral hypersensitivity. Abdominal pain is thought to be brought on by visceral hyperalgesia, which may be caused by alterations in the sensory receptors of the gastrointestinal tract, abnormal modulation of sensory transmissions in the peripheral or central nervous system, or changes in the cortical perception of afferent signals.[73]

Etiological Factors in Pain-Related Disability

In considering etiological factors in children's pain-related disability, various factors have been conceptualized to play a role, including children's coping, anxiety and depressive symptoms, and family reinforcement of pain behavior.[34] Identification of factors that are predictive of disability related to pain is an active area of pediatric pain research,[74,75] particularly because many of these factors represent areas that can be directly targeted in behavioral interventions.

Investigations of children's coping responses to pain have revealed that certain coping strategies relate to better functional outcomes. Specifically, children who use more approach coping (i.e., direct attempts to deal with pain and the use of active methods to regulate feelings when in pain) report less pain-related disability.[61,74] Coping skills have been targeted in treatment studies to test the hypothesis that increasing children's use of adaptive coping responses would, in turn, decrease pain-related disability.[76,77]

Psychological distress, particularly anxiety and depressive symptoms, can be viewed as an outcome of a pain condition or as an etiological factor in the development of pain-related disability. Studies have demonstrated that increased depressive symptoms are associated with increased functional disability related to chronic pain.[46] Palermo[34] emphasized the importance of considering the relationship between emotional distress and children's functional status because emotional distress may affect many areas of functioning such as reduced participation in peer activities and sleep disturbances. For example, depressive symptoms were found to be predictive of reductions in health-related quality of life as a result of sleep disturbance in adolescents with chronic pain.[51] To date, there have been no investigations to specifically tease out the effects of psychological distress on specific aspects of children's pain-related disability.

A variety of familial factors have been identified as potentially important in the causes of pain-related disability, including parental responses to the child's pain, parental psychopathology, and parental history and modeling of chronic pain symptoms. A number of researchers have noted a family aggregation of pain complaints, finding that children with chronic pain often live in households in which other family members also have chronic pain.[78] Although preliminary twin studies indicate that there may be a genetic link, it is commonly thought that somatization is a learned behavior. Through the process of modeling, children may learn about pain perception and reaction to pain from others. Of importance is that in the context of chronic pain, parental modeling of avoidance behavior and poor coping skills may be particularly problematic, because they are at direct odds with the adaptive child behaviors that are needed to cope effectively with chronic pain.

Parental encouragement or reinforcement, sometimes referred to as *solicitous responses* (e.g., frequent attention to pain symptoms, granting permission to avoid regular activities), has been investigated in children with chronic pain.[79] The effect of parental responses on children's pain is presumed to occur because a parental solicitous response may be a reinforcing consequence of a pain behavior, thus serving to maintain or increase the likelihood that the behavior will occur. There is evidence that more solicitous or encouraging responses from parents toward their children's pain or illness behaviors do increase sick role behaviors in children with recurrent and chronic pain. Parental solicitous responses have been reported to be particularly problematic for children presenting with increased anxiety or depressive symptoms, who were the most disabled by pain when their parent demonstrated this response style.[80]

Natural History and Course of Pain

Despite any tendency of physicians to reassure parents that their child will "outgrow" recurrent pain complaints, the symptoms of many children with pain complaints persist. Although the overall base of knowledge of the natural history and course of pain is limited, the available data suggest that early exposure to pain may alter later pain response and that initial pain complaints often persist over time or may occur in another part of the body, or other somatic symptoms may develop in the child.

Investigators have examined whether early and prolonged exposure to pain alters later stress response, pain systems, and behavior and learning in childhood. There is some evidence that children who undergo pain or tissue damage as neonates may have increased pain sensitivity later in childhood.[81] This has important implications for the long-term care of these patients, because they may be more likely to develop problems with chronic pain in later life.

In short-term follow-up studies of children with chronic pain, a significant number of children are found to have continuing complaints of pain over 1- to 2-year follow-up periods. For example, in one study, children with recurrent benign pain were monitored over 2 years; 30% of the initial sample had continuing pain at the 2-year follow-up.[82] The children whose pain persisted over time were reported to have more emotional problems than did children without persisting pain complaints, and their mothers had poorer health than did the controls' mothers. Other studies have identified depressive symptoms as important in predicting generalization of pain from one localized site (i.e., neck pain) to widespread pain at the short-term follow-up.[83]

Long-term outcome studies suggest that children and adolescents who present with chronic abdominal or headache pain continue into adulthood with chronic pain, physical, and psychiatric complaints.[84-86] There is evidence that childhood history of recurrent abdominal pain may predispose children to irritable bowel syndrome in adulthood.[87] Children whose chronic pain limits their functioning may develop lifelong problems with pain and disability. It is unknown whether medical and psychological treatments alter these long-term outcomes for children with chronic pain.

RESEARCH ISSUES AND CONTROVERSIES

Potential areas of research focus within the causes and natural history of childhood pain may involve sociocultural studies, the developmental psychology of pediatric pain, and the relationship between pediatric and adult chronic pain. The available data on the etiology and natural history of childhood pain and somatoform disorders are insufficient to lead to effective prevention efforts. Longitudinal studies are needed to identify the course of pain and pain-related disability in different populations of children. Furthermore, longitudinal studies are needed to document the development of pain and somatoform disorders in at-risk groups. For example, retrospective studies have revealed an increased incidence of pain and physical comorbidity in girls with post-traumatic stress disorder,[88] but there have been no investigations to monitor children with this disorder over time to identify factors predictive of the development of pain conditions.

DIAGNOSIS/ASSESSMENT

We now briefly describe the most common types of pain problems in children and adolescents: acute pain; pain related to chronic disease, including sickle cell disease, IBD, juvenile arthritis, and cancer; headaches; CRPS; juvenile fibromyalgia syndrome; and functional bowel disorders. We also review the diagnostic category of somatoform disorders. We then describe assessment of pain symptoms, functional consequences, and specifically the clinical evaluation of the child with pain or a somatoform disorder.

Acute Pain

Acute, or nociceptive, pain arises from tissue inflammation or injury caused by a noxious event.[89] Examples of these processes include a broken arm, postsurgery pain, acute gastroenteritis, menstrual cramps, a sore throat, pain from an ear infection, or acute muscle cramps related to significant exercise. This type of pain can be mild to severe. Besides acute injuries and acute infections, the two most common types of acute pain include postoperative pain and medical procedure–induced pain. The majority of studies of medical procedure–induced pain have focused on pain related to intravenous insertions and phlebotomies[90-92] and to bone marrow aspirations and lumbar punctures in children with cancer.[93,94]

The child's experience of acute pain depends on relevant situational factors (e.g., understanding, predictability, and control) and emotional factors (e.g., fear, anger, and frustration), which are influenced by a child's sex, age, cognitive level, previous pain experience, learning, and culture.[89] Distress and anxiety are important factors to consider in acute pain because they can intensify the child's experience of pain and prolong recovery. Assessment of both pain and anxiety for postsurgical and medical procedure–related pain has received considerable research attention and, as detailed later in this chapter, there are many different tools and methods of measuring pain, including various self-report measures, observational measures of specific behaviors, and measures based on physiological monitoring.

Pain Related to Chronic Disease

SICKLE CELL DISEASE

Sickle cell disease is a genetic hematological disorder that affects the hemoglobin in red blood cells, causing the hemoglobin to form crystalloids that become less elastic than normal hemoglobin, resulting in long, misshapen red blood cells that have a "sickled" appearance. These abnormally shaped cells tend to aggregate rather than flow through blood vessels singly. This aggregation of red blood cells causes blockage in arteries, resulting in vaso-occlusive pain crises. Children with sickle cell disease are also vulnerable to infections (especially those caused by *Pneumococcus* organisms), organ damage related to episodes of ischemia, and, in some cases, early death.[95] Sickle cell disease is most prevalent among African-Americans and Hispanic-Americans; approximately 1 of every 500 African-American children and 1 of every 1400 Hispanic-American children are born with sickle cell disease.[96]

Ischemia causes pain through a buildup of certain nociceptive neurotransmitters, such as substance P and prostanoids, at afferent neural endings, and the ascending pain signal system is thus activated. Ischemic pain has been described by one of our clinic patients as "feeling like your arm is being squeezed by a blood pressure cuff that keeps getting tighter and tighter until your arm begins to ache and the pain may become unbearable." Pain may originate from many sources (e.g., musculoskeletal, visceral), and affected children may experience both acute and chronic pain (e.g., aseptic necrosis, bony infarction). For example, in children and adolescents with sickle cell disease, headaches[97] and low back pain can result from chronic muscle spasm and lack of oxygen in the spine; joint pain, especially in the hip, can result from aseptic necrosis of the femoral head; hip arthritis often causes a deep, aching "referred" pain in the lower thigh above the knee; and acute chest syndrome, with accompanying severe chest pain and shortness of breath, can develop, as can ischemia, which can affect almost any organ, causing visceral pain.

Children with sickle cell disease are also at risk for neurological sequelae and neuropsychological impairment.[98] It is estimated that 7% to 17% of children with sickle cell disease experience a clinical stroke before age 20,[99] and 10% to 20% of children may exhibit evidence of silent strokes, with associated cognitive deficits.[100] Learning impairment can increase school-related stress. Children with sickle cell disease often have short stature related to spinal infarcts and collapsed or narrowed vertebrae or renal disease; the short stature may add to social stress. In turn, stress can further exacerbate any pain.

Some children with sickle cell disease have frequent, repetitive bouts of pain, whereas others have a milder, intermittent form. The contributors to this variance may be related to aspects of the disease or to characteristics of the child and his or her environment.

INFLAMMATORY BOWEL DISEASE

IBD is a condition of ongoing or recurrent inflammation in the intestinal tract.[101] IBD is not to be confused with irritable bowel syndrome, which is a functional gastrointestinal disorder characterized by abdominal pain and altered bowel habits in the absence of specific and unique organic disease. There are several forms of IBD. The two most common are Crohn's disease and ulcerative colitis.[102] Crohn's disease is a condition that can affect the entire intestinal tract with patchy inflammation that can involve all the layers of the wall of the intestine. The early signs of Crohn's disease in children are often vague, making diagnosis difficult. Periumbilical pain or right-sided abdominal pain are the most common sites of pain and may appear long before significant diarrhea. Children with Crohn's disease may also have joint pain and fever before there are any changes in bowel patterns. Decreased appetite and weight loss are often symptoms misdiagnosed as anorexia nervosa, school anxiety, or other psychological problems.

Ulcerative colitis is an IBD that is limited to the large intestine. Early signs include left-sided abdominal pain that improves after bowel movements, joint pain, and progressive loosening of the stools, which are often bloody. Severe abdominal pain and bloody stools can create disabling symptoms for children when the disease is first diagnosed or during times of increased inflammation.

It is interesting that not all children with IBD have abdominal pain, even though there may be small areas of intestinal inflammation. Also, some children with IBD can also have irritable bowel syndrome, with far greater pain and other symptoms than the levels of inflammation would suggest. In addition, for some children who might be at risk for the development of chronic pain, such as those with an anxiety disorder, post-traumatic stress disorder, or other conditions associated with a hypersensitive neural system, severe bouts of inflammation-related abdominal pain or surgery can set off visceral hyperalgesia, or "phantom" intestinal pain. In this case, the brain-gut sensory system becomes dysregulated, and the intestinal tract becomes hypersensitive, with increased metabolic activity in pain perception areas of the brain. These central neuromodules create the same experience of pain as if there were active inflammation, even though the intestines may be normal after anti-inflammatory treatment. The sensation is called "phantom pain" because it can occur even if the colon has been removed. Extraintestinal symptoms, such as arthritis or arthralgias and skin rashes, may also occur in IBD. However, the hallmark of IBD is inflammation of the intestine and, typically, abdominal pain.

JUVENILE ARTHRITIS

Arthritis is an autoimmune disease, and juvenile arthritis is medically different from the adult form of rheumatoid arthritis or osteoarthritis. Juvenile arthritis can cause joint deformities and affect a child's skin, eyes, and visceral organs. More than 250,000 children in the United States have some form of arthritis.[103] It can start as early as infancy and lasts a lifetime. Arthritis is an inflammation in the joints that causes afferent neurons to transmit nociception to the spinal cord and to pain perception areas in the brain, resulting in joint pain. Juvenile rheumatoid arthritis is an autoimmune condition involving primarily pain and inflammation in the joints.[103] Sometimes involvement extends to only a single joint (monoarticular arthritis), sometimes to a few joints (pauciarticular arthritis), and sometimes to many joints (polyarticular arthritis). In some cases, other parts of the body are involved, such as the eyes, in which there may be inflammation of the uvea. There are other, less common causes of arthritis, besides juvenile rheumatoid arthritis, such as arthritis associated with IBD, infections of the joints, and other autoimmune diseases such as systemic lupus erythematosus. In contrast to affected adults, 30% to 50% of affected children go into remission after several years, depending on the arthritis subtype.[103]

CANCER

Medical-procedure pain is the most common acute pain associated with childhood cancer.[20] Common procedures include bone marrow aspiration and biopsy, lumbar puncture with or without the administration of intrathecal medication, intravenous insertion for chemotherapy administration (although most chemotherapy is now given through a central access catheter), and phlebotomy. Children who have vincristine chemotherapy may develop neuropathic pain associated with a peripheral neuropathy. Bone marrow transplantation is typically associated with a 7- to 10-day period of mucositis, with painful mouth, swallowing, urination, and defecation and pain in any areas involving mucosal surfaces (e.g., diarrhea associated with mucosal sloughing). Graft-versus-host disease may occur in some children after transplantation and can affect any organ, including skin. When solid tumors are increasing in size or if there is an acute hemorrhage within a tumor, the tumor can compress nearby or surrounding tissue, causing compression pain, capsular stretching pain, or hollow organ obstruction. Survivors of certain types of malignancies, such as bone tumors, other sarcomas, and Hodgkin disease, may continue to have pain long after treatment termination.

Headaches

Headache is a symptom that is almost universally experienced. Usually, headaches are considered a problem when they are severe, arise frequently, and start impeding sleep, eating, activities, or school performance. Headaches occur for a variety of reasons. Sometimes allergies or changes in barometric pressure can cause headaches in relation to fluid shifts in the sinus cavities. Caffeine, monosodium glutamate, and tannins in foods, as well as allergies to certain foods, also can trigger headaches. Other types of headaches include those occurring after head injury, those related to sensory "overload" (e.g., often in children with sensory integration problems, autism spectrum disorder, or Asperger syndrome), myofascial or tension headaches (often called "chronic daily headaches"), temporomandibular joint headaches (often called "facial pain" headaches), vision-related headaches, and migraine. It is not uncommon for children with occasional migraine headaches to develop chronic daily myofascial headaches. In a review of pediatric cases presenting to an emergency department with headache as the primary complaint, children's diagnoses included viral illness (39.2%), sinusitis (16%), migraine (15.6%), post-traumatic headache (6.6%), streptococcal pharyngitis (4.9%), and tension headache (4.5%).[104]

The International Headache Society classifies adulthood and childhood headaches as primary headaches (e.g., migraine and tension-type headaches), secondary headaches (e.g., headache attributed to infection or trauma), cranial neuralgias, facial pain, and other headaches. Pain in the head is a primary component of the diagnosis of primary headache disorders, although other symptoms such as nausea and vomiting may also accompany head pain. The reader is referred to the second edition of the International Classification of Headache Disorders[105] for a complete listing of the diagnostic criteria and classification of children's headaches.

Complex Regional Pain Syndrome (CRPS)

CRPS (formerly known as *reflex sympathetic dystrophy*) consists of a focal painful disorder in any part of the body, often one or both of the extremities.[106] Pain may occur after a minor injury or surgery but also may occur without an obvious prior event. The diagnostic criteria of this type of pain include severe pain; skin hypersensitivity, including allodynia (pain to light touch); and vasomotor instability. The first reported case of CRPS in children appeared in the literature in the 1970s, approximately 100 years after the first described adult case. The pain is often described as a burning, squeezing, or stabbing/shooting pain. The hallmark of CRPS is that the affected area is supersensitive to even light touch, has the type of pain just described, and often interferes with the use of the affected part (e.g., leg or arm). Sometimes there are swelling and color, skin, and hair changes from lack of touch to that body part, and there may be muscle atrophy and weakness from nonuse. There are many theories that exist to explain the pathophysiology of this syndrome; however, none fully explains the expression of this condition.

Juvenile Fibromyalgia

Fibromyalgia is a disease characterized by chronic widespread pain in the fibrous tissues of the muscles, ligaments, and tendons and often includes fatigue.[107] In children and adolescents, it is not well understood and often misdiagnosed. Many physicians continue to call this a "psychosomatic disease" and believe that it is psychological and not "real." In affected children, fibromyalgia is often mistakenly diagnosed as growing pains or psychological problems. Little is still known about juvenile fibromyalgia, even though research in adult fibromyalgia is increasing. In this condition, most rheumatological blood tests typically yield negative results, or the antinuclear antibody count may be mildly elevated. The diagnosis is based on a history of widespread pain and numerous tender points throughout the body.[108]

Fibromyalgia is characterized by an aroused and dysregulated central nervous system and is often accompanied by chronic fatigue, sleep disturbances, pain all over the body, and other neural imbalance problems such as irritable bowel syndrome and tension headaches. Sometimes, as with chronic fatigue syndrome, fibromyalgia symptoms can begin with a viral illness, but the flulike symptoms remain after the infection has cleared. When children are deprived of restorative, deep sleep, their neural systems become further dysregulated, and common neural and other bodily systems begin to unravel. For example, cognitive function can be impaired (sometimes called "fibro-fog"), physical and emotional exhaustion can develop, and depression can occur.

Functional Bowel Disorders

Functional bowel disorders are identified by abdominal pain with or without other gastrointestinal symptoms and are *not* associated with inflammatory, metabolic, or structural abnormality of the intestinal tract.[73,109] Recurrent abdominal pain was originally defined by Apley and Naish[110] as the child's experience of three episodes of abdominal pain within a 3-month period that affected his or her activities. Functional bowel disorders are currently classified according to the Rome criteria,[111] in which five types of functional gastrointestinal conditions associated with abdominal pain are characterized: functional abdominal pain (diffuse abdominal pain without any other gastrointestinal symptoms), functional dyspepsia (ulcer-like pain in one spot at the base of the sternum), irritable bowel syndrome (widespread abdominal pain with other gastrointestinal symptoms, such as nausea, vomiting, bloating, constipation, and/or diarrhea), abdominal migraines (which are rare), and aerophagia (abdominal distention due to intraluminal air). The pain or symptoms are caused by abnormal brain-intestinal neural signaling that create intestinal hypersensitivity and may thus result in increased pain. The pain relates to hypersensitivity rather than to intestinal contractility, although both may be linked. As mentioned, abdominal pain may be caused by alterations in the sensory receptors of the gastrointestinal tract, abnormal modulation of sensory transmissions in the peripheral or central nervous system, or changes in the cortical perception of afferent signals,[73] which may have been preceded by inflammation that has since resolved.

Description of Somatoform Disorders

By definition, somatoform disorders involve one or more symptoms that, after thorough medical evaluation, cannot be explained by any known pathophysiological process. Either the symptoms cannot be explained in their entirety or the patient's level of impairment grossly exceeds the level of impairment that would generally be expected with the patient's underlying medical condition. In order to meet the diagnostic criteria, these symptoms must also cause a significant decrease in the patient's level of functioning that is not better explained by another medical or psychological condition. Somatoform disorders are commonly referred to by more pejorative terms, including *nonorganic, functional,* or *psychosomatic disorders,* which leads many patients to believe that their symptoms are not real or are "all in their minds"; this constitutes disregard for the fact that psychological factors and physical symptoms often coexist and are intricately interrelated.

In the *DSM-IV-TR,*[4] Somatoform Disorders is defined as a broad diagnostic category to which a number of more specific diagnoses belong. Although the *DSM-IV-TR* diagnostic criteria were designed for adult patients,

at present they are also applied to the pediatric population, because, to date, no more age-specific, widely accepted, generalized classification system has been developed. Several of the disorders have a number of features in common with Axis II personality disorders involving character traits. Because character traits are viewed as evolving in childhood rather than firmly established, there is a reluctance to diagnose personality disorders in child psychiatric patients that also applies frequently to somatoform disorders.[69] Moreover, there has been much criticism in the psychiatry community in regard to this diagnostic category, and suggestions have been made for modification during the planning period for the fifth edition of the *DSM (DSM-V).*[112] Several specific criticisms of the somatoform disorder category include the unacceptability of the terminology to patients, the dualism splitting disease versus psychogenic causes, and incompatibility with other cultures. As outlined in the *DSM-IV-TR,* the broad category of somatoform disorders includes conversion disorder, pain disorder, body dysmorphic disorder, hypochondriasis, somatization disorder, and undifferentiated somatoform disorder. We describe each of these disorders briefly as follows, except for body dysmorphic disorder, which does not involve pain complaints.

SOMATIZATION DISORDER

Somatization disorder is a chronic condition consisting of multiple medically unexplained bodily complaints for which treatment has been sought over a prolonged period of time. The symptoms begin before 30 years of age, cause significant impairment in the patient's overall level of functioning, and are not feigned or intentionally produced. The patient presents with a specific constellation of symptoms, including four pain symptoms, two gastrointestinal symptoms, one sexual symptom, and one pseudoneurological symptom. The most common symptoms are pain in various parts of the body, dysphagia, nausea, bloating, constipation, palpitations, dizziness, and shortness of breath.[113] In pediatric populations, the full diagnostic criteria for somatization disorder are rarely met; however, many children do experience multiple medically unexplained symptoms.

CONVERSION DISORDER

Conversion disorder is characterized by medically unexplained deficits or alterations of voluntary motor or sensory function that is suggestive of a neurological or medical illness. These symptoms are judged to have either been initiated or perpetuated by psychological factors and are preceded by conflicts or other stressors. The symptom or deficit may not include pain, may be under voluntary control, may be intentionally produced or feigned, or may be a culturally sanctioned experience. The symptom or deficit cannot, after appropriate medical investigation, be entirely explained by a neurological or general medical condition or be substance induced. Documented conversion disorder is rare and is reported in fewer than 1% of individuals in community settings. Conversion disorder has been described in children and adolescents as involving a variety of motor and sensory symptoms.[114-116]

HYPOCHONDRIASIS

The term *hypochondriac* is commonly used colloquially; however, in order to fulfill the diagnosis of hypochondriasis, an individual must have a persistent preoccupation with fears of having a serious disease that is based on misinterpretation of bodily symptoms in spite of appropriate medical evaluation and reassurance.[117] This preoccupation must also cause significant distress or impairment in social, occupational, or other areas of functioning and must last at least 6 months. The condition cannot be better explained by an alternative psychiatric diagnosis, and may not be to the extent of a delusion. The prevalence is low in the adult population; fewer than 1% of community populations meet full diagnostic criteria.[118] There are no published descriptions of hypochondriasis in pediatric patients. The diagnosis would be complicated by the fact that parents are intricately involved in the seeking of health care for their children, as well as by the interpretation of children's medical symptoms.

PAIN DISORDER

The diagnosis of pain disorder is a relatively new classification, appearing first in the 4th edition of the *DSM (DSM-IV)*. Characteristics essential to the diagnosis include the patient's experience of pain with psychological factors judged to be a major factor in the pain's onset, severity, or duration. The pain must cause significant distress and/or functional impairment and cannot be feigned or accounted for by an alternative *DSM-IV-TR* diagnosis. This diagnosis can be difficult to make in the pediatric population because of the limited use of descriptive language and the effects of developmental stages on the ability to separate the psychological feelings associated with the pain from the pain sensation itself. To further complicate matters, it is essential to consider the effect that cultural issues often create differences in pain expression and behavior.

UNDIFFERENTIATED SOMATOFORM DISORDER

Undifferentiated somatoform disorder also first appeared in the *DSM-IV*. The diagnostic criteria include the experience of one or more physical complaints,

and the symptoms cannot be fully explained by a general medical condition, or when a medical condition is identified, the impairment is in excess of what would be expected by history, laboratory findings, or physical examination. Furthermore, the symptoms cause clinically significant distress or impairment and have been present for at least 6 months. This category has been particularly criticized because the criteria are overly broad; therefore, many individuals who have physical symptoms with associated disability would fulfill the criteria.[112]

Assessment of Pain in Children

In this section, we describe general principles in pain assessment in children, which are relevant to the assessment of acute or chronic pain or pain occurring as part of a somatoform disorder. Pain is both a sensory and emotional experience. Accurate assessment of children's pain should therefore include evaluation of the quality, duration, frequency, intensity, and location of the pain, as well as the environmental variables that may affect pain and the effect of pain on children's functional status and quality of life. When possible, the best way to learn about a child's pain is to ask the child directly. Finding out what makes it worse and what makes it better also provides clues to understanding the pain so that it can be optimally treated. There are times when self-report of pain is not feasible or becomes difficult for the clinician. The most obvious reasons are the age of the child (infant or toddler), severe developmental disability, or other communication difficulties (e.g., low-functioning autism, severe motor impairment as in cerebral palsy that affects understandable speech). Some children may not report pain because of fear, such as fear of talking to doctors, fear of disappointing or bothering others, fear of receiving an injection of medication, fear of finding out they are sick, or fear of returning to the hospital. For infants and nonverbal children, parents, pediatricians, nurses, and other caregivers must be called upon to interpret the child's distressed behaviors: that is, do the behaviors represent pain, fear, hunger, or a range of other perceptions or emotions? Therapeutic trials of comfort measures (cuddling, feeding) and analgesic medication, especially when the cause of the pain is likely known (e.g., postsurgical pain), can help to determine whether the behavioral distress represents pain behaviors.

Instruments measuring pain intensity, location, and affect are typically used to assess acute pain of relatively brief duration. Measurement of recurrent and chronic pain requires tools that also measure the frequency, duration, time course, and activity interference by pain. Examples of measures of these concepts are provided as follows.

PAIN-RELATED BEHAVIORS

Observing the child's behaviors can provide further clues about the location, extent, and severity of the pain. Clearly, behavioral manifestations of pain can be affected by many factors, including pain severity, child's age, fear and anxiety, past pain experiences, environmental factors (e.g., parent and peer presence), feelings of control, and other factors. For example, a 12-year-old boy who is injured on the soccer field may not demonstrate pain behaviors until he gets into the family car after the game. For these reasons, interpretation of meaning is involved in using behavior to assess pain. Acute pain and anxiety may be responded to behaviorally in a similar manner; these similarities result in debates about whether behaviors related to these two experiences can actually be separately identified or should be combined as "distress" behaviors.[119] In addition, with age, children learn how to mute some of their pain-related behaviors, as noted by LeBaron and Zeltzer.[120] Thus, for medical procedure–related pain behaviors, younger children may exhibit more crying and kicking, whereas adolescents may be more likely to clench their fists, grimace, and contract other muscles. This difference has affected the results of different behavioral scales used to assess acute pain across a wide age range of children and adolescents.

BEHAVIORAL AND PHYSIOLOGICAL SIGNS

Behavior and physiological signs are useful but can be misleading. A toddler may scream and grimace during an ear examination because of fear rather than from pain. Conversely, children with inadequately relieved persistent pain from cancer, sickle cell disease, trauma, or surgery may withdraw from their surroundings and appear very quiet, leading observers to conclude falsely that they are comfortable or sedated. In these situations, increasing dosages of analgesics may make the child become more, not less, interactive and alert. Similarly, neonates and young infants may close their eyes, furrow their brows, and clench their fists in response to pain. A child who is experiencing significant chronic pain may play "normally" as a way to distract attention from pain. This coping behavior is sometimes misinterpreted as evidence of the child "faking" pain when not distracted.

Investigators have devised a range of behavioral distress scales for infants and young children, mostly emphasizing the child's facial expressions, crying, and body movement. For example, the FLACC scale[121] is a 5-item scale that a rater uses to score each of five categories—face (F), legs (L), activity (A), cry (C), and consolability (C)—along a scale from 0 to 2. Facial expression measures appear most useful and specific in neonates and young infants. Autonomic signs can indicate pain but are nonspecific and may reflect other processes, including fever, hypoxemia, and cardiac or renal dysfunction.

SELF-REPORT OF PAIN

Children aged 3 years and older become increasingly articulate in describing intensity, location, and quality of pain. Scales involving drawings, pictures of faces, or graded color intensity have been validated, especially for children aged 5 years and older. For example, excellent psychometric properties have been reported with the Faces Pain Scale–Revised,[122] a revised version of a scale originally developed by Bieri and associates.[123] It consists of six gender-neutral line drawings of faces that are scored from 0 to 10.

Children's self-reports of pain can be obtained in the moment by asking about how much pain is currently present; in the past by using retrospective interview methods in which children or parents are asked to recall the frequency, intensity, and duration of pain over an identified time period such as 1 month; or in the future by using prospective monitoring of pain in daily diaries or logs. Because of the potential for children to have recall bias, prospective recording of recurrent or chronic pain complaints is recommended.[124] Novel methods have been emerging to enhance compliance in maintaining prospective records, including the use of electronic pain diaries with children.[125]

PAIN ASSESSMENT IN COGNITIVELY IMPAIRED CHILDREN

The measurement of pain in cognitively impaired children remains a challenge, and methods are being studied to determine ways of assessing pain in this population. There is increasing research on the development of pain assessment tools for understanding pain expression and experience in cognitively impaired children.[126-128] Cognitively impaired children may not have the language abilities to provide labels of quantity and quality to describe their pain. They also may not have the mathematical skills needed to rate their pain on the traditional rating scales. Their behavioral responses to pain may also lead to erroneous inferences about their pain. For example, children with Down's syndrome may express pain less precisely and more slowly than do children in the general population. Pain in individuals with autism spectrum disorders may be difficult to assess because these children may be both hyposensitive and hypersensitive to many different types of sensory stimuli, and they may have limited communication abilities. Readers are referred to the new editions of *Nelson Textbook of Pediatrics,* 18th edition,[129] and *Pain in Infants, Children, and Adolescents,* 3rd edition,[130] for detailed summaries of the different pain assessment tools currently available.

ASSESSMENT OF FUNCTIONAL CONSEQUENCES OF PAIN

Measurements of activity interference, functional disability, and quality of life are important for understanding the specific effects of pain on children. These functional consequences are considered important primary outcomes of pain treatment.[34] Validated measures have been developed to capture most of these domains.

There are general measures of disability and quality of life that may be useful for documenting the effect of pain on children's functioning and well-being. For example, the Functional Disability Inventory[35] and the Pediatric Quality of Life Inventory[131] have been the most widely used instruments to document disability and quality of life of children with chronic pain. Several more recently developed measures also show promise, including a new measure of pain-related activity interference in school age children and adolescents, the Child Activity Limitations Interview,[43] and a new composite measure of chronic pain in adolescents, the Bath Adolescent Pain Questionnaire.[132] Several measures of function and quality of life have been tailored to assess specific pain syndromes or chronic health conditions. For juvenile arthritis, for example, disease-specific measures of function and quality of life include the Childhood Health Assessment Questionnaire[133] and the Pediatric Quality of Life Inventory, Rheumatology Module.[134]

ASSESSMENT OF FAMILY FACTORS

The family has been described as an important context for understanding, assessing, and managing pediatric chronic pain,[135] and there is a growing body of research on family and parent factors and their relationship to pain and functional consequences. An integrative model of parent and family factors in pediatric chronic pain and associated disability has been proposed.[136] This model situates individual parenting variables (e.g., parenting style, parental reinforcement) within a broader context of dyadic variables (e.g., quality of parent-child interaction) and the more global familial environment (e.g., family functioning). A variety of instruments are available for assessing family variables at each level of assessment (e.g., the Illness Behavior Encouragement Scale[137]), although none have been widely used in pediatric pain research. Different family variables are important to consider, depending on developmental status of the child. For example, in adolescents with chronic pain, the level of autonomy and conflict in the parent-teenager rela-

tionship would represent developmentally relevant domains to consider in family assessment.

CLINICAL EVALUATION OF PAIN

Clinical evaluation of pain includes assessing pain and pain history, other physical symptoms, physical functioning, social functioning, academic functioning, family functioning, emotional and cognitive functioning, coping style and problem-solving capacity, perceived stressors, major life events, and pain consequences. For example, evaluating a child who presents with headaches includes assessment of all these factors and should not be aimed just at ruling out an organic pathological process.

Parents presenting with a child suffering from headaches want not only a diagnosis but also the clinician's help in reducing the pain and suffering of their child. Narratives are powerful tools with which to learn about a child's pain problem but also what the child and parents relate to the problem (e.g., the book by Arthur Frank, *The Wounded Storyteller,*[137a] provides detail on the narratives of patients and the relationship that develops between patient and health care provider through narrative). The use of pain narratives has been described in children[138] as a method of enhancing engagement between patient and provider on the basis of the experience of listening to the storyteller; that is, it is helpful to learn the child and parent's "stories" of the pain problem. After the child's and parent's pain narratives, further questions then can help elucidate the problem and help in planning for the treatment. For example, it would be important to learn what factors make pain worse and what helps, temporal qualities, location of the pain, and description of the pain experience. Through narratives, important differences in the perception of the nature, meaning, or consequences of pain may arise between the stories told by parents and those told by the children. Differences between parents and children in the reports of pain and pain-related disability have been found in several studies.[139] By elaborating parent and child interpretations of pain, the clinician may identify important areas for treatment, such as broader issues in parent-child communication.

It is also helpful to learn what has been tried and failed and what has helped, including medication and nonpharmacological treatment strategies. Invasive medical tests should not be the first approach unless the history and physical examination suggest an intracranial pathological process that can be visible on magnetic resonance imaging or computed tomography, such as a hemorrhage, tumor, or other lesion. For children with headaches or any type of chronic pain, it is important to assess for risk factors, such as past traumas, anxiety, learning disabilities, and other problems that affect pain.

With headaches, for example, the initial thinking by the clinician during the evaluation should be to rule out something structural in the brain (e.g., tumor, traumatic brain injury), chemical causes (e.g., monosodium glutamate reactions), or other identifiable "causes" that can be readily treated if diagnosed (e.g., sinus infection, poor vision). Clearly, observation and a history of unusual or sudden symptoms or signs—such as fever; morning vomiting; visual disturbances; seizures; paralysis; weakness; loss of sensation; shaking; or any sudden changes in alertness, speech, or thinking, especially after head trauma— would suggest the need for urgent evaluation with further diagnostic tools. However, most children presenting with chronic pain do not have easily identifiable single causes of the pain (e.g., sinus infection) and the longer pain has persisted, the more "baggage" the pain picks up along the way, such as secondary stressors of school absenteeism, muscle tension from restricting the painful body part, and pain-related anxiety. Although it is important to learn as much as possible about the pain, it is just as important to learn about pain-related functional disability; that is, inquiry can be directed to learn to what extent and in what ways the pain is interfering with the child's daily life, including sleep, appetite, school attendance and performance, social and physical activities, and family life.

The following questions can be asked of the child and parent to learn about the nature of the pain and how it is interfering with the child's daily life (adapted from Zeltzer and Schlank[140]).

- How long has your child (you) been bothered by the pain?
- Does the pain occur at any particular time of day (e.g., when your child [you] first awakens), week (e.g., school days only), or month (with menses, for girls)?
- How often do the pain episodes occur, and how long do they last?
- Do they come on suddenly or gradually?
- Is the pain preceded or followed by any other symptoms or unusual feelings?
- Where is the pain located, and what does it feel like (e.g., pounding, stabbing)?
- What makes it worse, and what helps it feel better?
- Did anything new or different, such as attending a new school, precede the pain? What do you think started the pain and what keeps it going?
- What medications (name, dose, how often and for how long) has your child taken for her pain and what is she still taking (and do they help)? What did not help? (For the child: What do you think helped most?)

- What herbs or nondrug therapies has your child tried for the pain (e.g., warm baths, ice packs, listening to music, physical therapy, massage, yoga, relaxation training, hypnotherapy, acupuncture, psychotherapy)? Did they help? Tell me more (why do you think [this therapy] helped?). (Ask same of child.)
- What does the pain stop your child (you) from doing (e.g., concentrating, doing homework, attending school, playing sports, attending social activities with friends, attending activities with family)?
- Does the pain interfere with falling asleep and/or staying asleep? Does your child (you) wake up feeling tired/not rested?
- Does the pain affect your child's (your) appetite? Has he or she (you) lost or gained weight because of the pain?
- What do you think is causing the pain?

PSYCHOSOCIAL ASSESSMENT

Some clinicians have recommended that psychosocial assessment begin as soon as noncoping occurs,[141] meaning that a child begins to miss school or curtail participation in regular activities because of the pain. Although the primary care physician should gather psychosocial information as part of the clinical evaluation of the pain problem, a referral to a psychologist or psychiatrist for a psychosocial assessment can greatly extend this inquiry. We believe the process of how the physician makes the referral for a psychosocial assessment is critical to the subsequent acceptance of psychological conceptualizations for symptoms and to management approaches and thus should be done with appropriate care. Patients and their families are more likely to accept a psychological referral and not feel abandoned by their physician if it is presented early and as a routine procedure in all cases of persistent pain causing disruption of normal activities. It is crucial that professionals avoid dichotomization between organic and psychogenic causes of pain[28] and to present the psychosocial assessment along with the physical investigation and follow-up. This procedure avoids the trap of waiting for psychosocial assessment as a last resort after all other physical attempts to understand the problem have failed.

Psychosocial assessment may consist of clinical interviews, record keeping, and observation of the interaction among family members. In detailed clinical interviewing, the clinician should assess developmental, behavioral, or psychiatric concerns in the patient's and family's history and should identify potential stressors and areas of maladaptive coping with regard to academic success, relationships, school absenteeism, and social activities. Observation and direct questioning concerning the roles of various family members toward pain and its management can uncover maladaptive patterns in how family members respond to the child's pain. Information concerning the parents' own emotional functioning, anxiety, and marital stress may also contribute to a more complete understanding of sources of stress within the child and family. Diaries and standardized self-report measures help provide information about the child's subjective experience of pain and may also provide information on the child's motivation and attitude toward pain treatment.

Standardized psychological measures may be administered to screen for mental health diagnoses, particularly anxiety and depressive symptoms, in order to assess coping behaviors, functional disability, and family functioning. No specific battery of psychological measures has been identified as particularly useful for assessment of all patients with pain. The choice of whether to administer such measures depends largely on the presenting concerns within the child and family. For patients with long-standing difficulties related to academic performance, referral for formal academic testing may be a useful adjunct for assessing whether children are functioning at grade level; undiagnosed learning disorders may hinder academic performance and contribute additional stress.

Because comorbid sleep disturbances are so prevalent in children with chronic pain, it is useful to obtain a detailed history of sleep patterns through clinical interview or a sleep diary. In particular, it is important to obtain description of any difficulties falling asleep or staying asleep. Children with chronic pain may develop extended problems with sleep because of arousal at bedtime, when negative thoughts and hypervigilance at bedtime are incompatible with settling to sleep. Many children meet diagnostic criteria for a clinically significant sleep disturbance, especially insomnia, that may require separate intervention.

It can be useful to conduct a psychosocial assessment with the child and parents separately to allow for greater understanding of each person's perception of the pain problem. Allowing the child (and parent) to describe a typical day can be an informative and nonthreatening way of getting specific detail about how pain interferes with the child's normal daily routine and accommodations that child and family have made because of the pain problem. It is also useful in this context to understand how much time the child spends in activity versus bed rest, because this may have important implications for the child's rehabilitation needs.

CLINICAL EVALUATION OF SOMATOFORM DISORDERS

In the assessment of a patient presenting with significant somatic symptoms, it is essential that a thorough workup be pursued in order to rule out pathophysiological processes that may have initiated or maintained these complaints. There are many pediatric illnesses, such as seizure disorders, multiple sclerosis, and Guillain-Barré syndrome, that can initially have vague, varied and even inconsistent findings. It is essential that these illnesses not be overlooked. A full history, including a detailed psychosocial history, a complete physical examination, and appropriate laboratory and imaging studies should be pursued.

It is crucial at this point to gather as much collateral information as possible, including medical records from all health care providers involved in the child's care, grandparents, teachers, the school nurse, and other caregivers such as babysitters or nannies. Many of the professional and laypeople involved in the care might be anxious or frustrated with these patients' difficult course. After the clinician reasonably concludes that a serious illness has not been missed, a multidisciplinary team should be initiated in order to complete a rounded biopsychosocial evaluation of the patient in his or her larger environs. The team members should then communicate that they are certain that a serious physical illness has not been missed. They should discuss the diagnostic impression of a somatoform disorder and thus lay the foundation for intervention, with assurance that regular reevaluation and reexamination of symptoms will continue. It is important to emphasize that many children may not reach diagnostic criteria for a somatoform disorder but do present with significant treatable symptoms that can be managed.

The diagnostic process for somatoform disorders involving pain complaints requires a quantification of the patient's pain, including how intense the pain is, when it occurs, its location, and its quality. Whenever possible, self-reports should be performed outside of the parents' presence, because children may hide or, alternatively, exaggerate pain in their parent's presence, and parental objectivity may be compromised. Pain disproportionate to the organic etiology does not alone establish the diagnosis. Positive evidence for the existence of psychological factors must be demonstrated to explain the patient's pain. Evidence that would support the diagnosis from a psychological point of view might include the onset of pain after a specific stress or trauma, disability that is disproportionate to the reported pain, and exacerbations that are predictably linked to stressful events or clear secondary gain. All of these factors should be independently assessed, as well as assessed with regard to the effect each factor has on the child's level of functional impairment or distress.

In their management model for pediatric somatization, Campo and Fritz[27] offered seven useful guidelines for assessment in the context of suspected somatization: (1) acknowledge patient suffering and family concerns; (2) explore prior assessments and treatment experiences; (3) investigate patient and family fears provoked by the symptoms; (4) remain alert to the possibility of unrecognized physical disease, and communicate an unwillingness to prejudge the origin of the symptom; (5) avoid excess and unnecessary tests and procedures; (6) avoid diagnosis by exclusion; and (7) explore symptom timing, context, and characteristics.

Standardized measures may provide useful information about children's specific somatic symptoms, as well as their level of functional disability. For example, the Children's Somatization Inventory[79] is a self-report instrument of somatic symptoms experienced by children and adolescents over a 2-week period. This may yield a quick and helpful overview of somatic symptoms. Functional disability can be assessed with the Functional Disability Inventory,[35] which provides information on the child's difficulty performing common physical and recreational activities.

RESEARCH ISSUES AND CONTROVERSIES

Diagnosis and assessment of pain conditions and somatoform disorders involves taking a comprehensive biopsychosocial perspective. Within the somatoform disorders, there remains controversy over nosology, and future research efforts focused on clarifying symptoms in children and adolescents will increase the relevance of this diagnostic category in pediatrics. There are some areas of pain assessment that are much further developed than others. For example, tremendous research attention has been devoted to devising developmentally appropriate rating scales for assessing pain intensity in children of various ages. However, much less attention has been devoted to validating measures of physical or emotional functioning in children with chronic pain. There has been movement in the pain field toward common assessment instruments to document patient response to treatment. The Initiative on Methods, Measurement, and Pain Assessment in Clinical Trials (IMMPACT) has accomplished this for adults, recommending a set of core domains to be considered in clinical trials of chronic pain in adults[142] and specific measures to assess each of these domains.[143] A similar effort is under way in pediatric pain (PedIMMPACT) with a current draft of a set of domains and recommended assessment tools to consider in all clinical

trials involving pediatric acute or chronic pain.[144] These efforts should greatly extend clinicians' ability to synthesize research findings and make treatment decisions.

TREATMENT STRATEGIES FOR PAIN AND SOMATOFORM DISORDERS

Pain, whether acute or chronic, is often thought of in the same way and not uncommonly treated in the same way. For many children with chronic pain, an acute pain treatment approach, in which pain is expected to be related to a single cause and resolve once treated, can lead to confusion and psychological attributions when the pain does not readily resolve. Also, inadequate treatment of acute pain or pain associated with medical procedures or injuries may actually worsen a preexisting chronic pain or may lead to the development of chronic pain. A variety of intervention strategies have been designed to reduce pain sensations, increase comfort, and/or reduce associated disability and dysfunction in children with pain conditions from infancy to adolescence. These intervention strategies may include pharmacological strategies, behavioral strategies, rehabilitation approaches, complementary and alternative treatments, or a combination of these.

The setting and providers involved in the care of children with pain conditions is variable. Most children and adolescents with chronic pain are not disabled by their pain and do not seek treatment. Of the children who seek treatment, most are seen in primary care. A minority of children with chronic pain are treated in a specialized pain clinic, which may involve outpatient multidisciplinary care or intensive inpatient rehabilitation.

In this section, we describe treatment strategies for pain conditions and somatoform disorders in childhood, with a focus on empirically supported treatment approaches. Within some areas of pediatric pain, the treatment research is fairly well developed, such as for pediatric migraine, whereas for many other chronic pain conditions, only a handful of treatment studies have been conducted. There have been no randomized controlled trials of treatments for somatoform disorders in children, and thus the empirical support for treatment of these conditions is much less robust.

This chapter is not intended to provide an exhaustive review of pediatric pain treatment strategies. More comprehensive reviews of treatments for specific pain conditions in children (disease-related pain,[145] migraine,[146] recurrent abdominal pain,[147] and chronic nonmalignant pain[148]) are available elsewhere. The reader is also referred to several published clinical practice guidelines available from the American Pain Society for the management of pain conditions in children, including for fibromyalgia pain,[108] sickle cell disease pain,[149] cancer pain,[150] and juvenile chronic arthritis.[103]

We have organized this section by reviewing treatment strategies for procedural pain; disease-related pain; recurrent pain conditions, including headache and recurrent abdominal pain; chronic nonmalignant pain; and somatoform disorders.

Management of Procedural Pain

A growing body of research has focused on the best ways to help children cope with and manage pain related to invasive procedures. In the 1980s, much of the treatment research was focused on children undergoing more extensive invasive procedures such as bone marrow biopsy and lumbar puncture. However, children now routinely undergo these procedures under sedation or general anesthesia,[151] with a corresponding reduction in the experience of pain and distress. Cutaneous procedures such as venipuncture for intravenous administration and intramuscular injections for immunizations are anxiety provoking for children and caregivers alike, and there are a variety of pharmacological agents, as well as psychological techniques, that have shown to be useful to assist children in coping with these necessary painful events.

Topical local anesthetics have been used to help prevent or alleviate skin pain associated with needle puncture and venous cannulation. A variety of local anesthetics have been studied, and although none have become the standard of care, there is a large body of evidence that different agents and methods of delivery can effectively decrease procedural pain (reviewed by Houck and Sethna[152]). Topical anesthetics such as lidocaine (ELA-Max), lidocaine-prilocaine (EMLA), liposomal lidocaine 4% cream, vapocoolant spray, iontophoresis, and amethocaine have all been evaluated. The application of topical anesthetic creams, such as EMLA, has been shown to help reduce pain that children experience but remains underused, primarily because of their slow analgesic onset (60 to 90 minutes for EMLA) and inconsistent effectiveness. Advances in transdermal delivery technology have led to the emergence of a number of new delivery approaches that accelerate the onset time to 20 minutes or less and provide more consistent and deeper sensory skin analgesia. Although still in the early stages of investigation, transdermal delivery of local anesthetics shows promise. The use of topical anesthetic techniques for cutaneous procedural pain in children continues to be an active area of research

as new agents and methods of delivery are developed. However, even with adequate analgesia from a topical anesthetic, it is still important for medical professionals to consider incorporating behavioral methods (such as coaching and distraction) to assist children who may still experience significant behavioral distress.

Psychological treatments to aid children in coping with invasive procedure pain have also been extensively reviewed.[94] Cognitive-behavioral techniques have been identified as a well-established treatment for procedure-related pain in children and adolescents.[153] Treatment includes various components such as breathing exercises, progressive muscle relaxation, positive mental imagery, filmed modeling, reinforcement/incentive, behavioral rehearsal, cognitive distraction, counterconditioning, and active coaching by a psychologist, parent, and/or medical staff member. Each of these techniques must be developmentally appropriate for the child. Techniques such as listening to music, watching videos, playing videogames, counting objects in the room, playing with toys or puppets, and reading books are a few of the many distraction modalities that have been shown to effectively decrease pain and distress in children undergoing injections, immunizations, and chemotherapy.[154] Discrimination training has been described as a useful treatment strategy for infants undergoing frequent invasive procedures. Visual and auditory signals can be used to let an infant know that an invasive procedure is about to occur and then immediately after the procedure the signal can be turned off to let the child discriminate "safe" times.[154]

There are a range of effective pharmacological and psychological modalities for procedure related pain in children. Developmentally appropriate psychological interventions help children cope with invasive procedures and side effects of the procedures and prepare for future similar procedures. Although many children undergo medical procedures without analgesics or behavioral intervention, there is a large body of evidence that procedural pain and distress can be significantly minimized for children.

Management of Disease-Related Pain

The management of pain related to a chronic health condition such as sickle cell disease, IBD, juvenile arthritis, and cancer involves largely medical management of the underlying condition. For example, treatment of IBD is aimed at reducing inflammation in the colon, usually by specific anti-inflammatory medication, which often reduces pain symptoms. Ongoing assessment, treatment, and, when possible, prevention of pain should be the rule for management of disease-related pain. Pain that persists beyond aggressive medical management may necessitate separate intervention. Moreover, the clinician should consider nonpharmacological strategies to improve coping and reduce pain (e.g., hypnotherapy, biofeedback). Several examples of treatment strategies for disease-related pain are offered in this section.

CANCER PAIN

Cancer pain in children is different from that experienced by adults because different types of cancer afflict children and adults and because the treatment protocols for their cancer are different. For example, children being treated for cancer commonly experience mucositis, stomatitis, and neuropathic pain from chemotherapy. The focus of pain treatment is twofold: (1) the pain caused by the neoplasm and (2) the pain caused by the treatment of the cancer. Both pharmacological and psychological treatment modalities have been investigated. Pharmacological pain management focuses mainly on analgesic drugs, such as ibuprofen, acetaminophen, and opioids; on tricyclic antidepressants; and on anticonvulsant medications. Although much research attention has been devoted to nonpharmacological management of procedural pain related to cancer treatment, only a handful of studies on nonpharmacological treatments for other types of cancer pain have been conducted to date. In a few case studies, researchers have investigated the use of hypnosis and imagery for management of cancer pain in children. However, there are currently no empirically validated psychological treatments for pediatric cancer–related pain.[145]

MUSCULOSKELETAL DISORDERS

Management of musculoskeletal disorders such as juvenile arthritis and hemophilic arthropathy has focused on anti-inflammatory drugs, as well as opioids and tricyclic antidepressants, with varying degrees of success. Treatments may differ, depending on the activity of the disease. In small trials of cognitive-behavioral therapy, children with arthritis were taught progressive muscle relaxation, guided imagery techniques with distraction, and methods of "blocking" transmission of pain messages.[155] Cognitive-behavioral interventions combined with antidepressant agents are currently being investigated in the treatment of juvenile fibromyalgia.

Physical therapy and maintaining a regular exercise program are important aspects of pain treatment in musculoskeletal disorders for several reasons. First, there is a tendency to avoid using painful parts of the body. In time, because of lack of use, these joints become stiff, with restricted range of motion. Also, muscles that are not used become weaker and atrophy. Treatment aimed at reducing inflammation, good pain management, and active physical therapy and exercise helps keep affected body parts healthy and functional.

A child with arthritis may experience pain during physical therapy, and the therapy-associated pain may create avoidance of physical therapy and anticipatory anxiety. Although the concept of "good pain" versus "bad pain" may seem paradoxical, children can learn the difference. Good pain is a sign that the child is working hard and doing more and more, resulting in greater range of motion of joints and greater physical abilities over time. Children can be taught that any new activity that involves the use of muscles that have not previously been used as strenuously may hurt. However, the pain typically lessens as the child becomes increasingly physically active. This type of pain is different from "bad pain," which continues long after the physical therapy sessions or exercise ends. Chronic pain is "bad pain"; it does not serve any purpose and should be treated. Iyengar yoga is an excellent self-help tool for children and adolescents who have arthritis, because it involves specified poses with the help of props and can build muscle mass, increase flexibility, and build confidence. As with any type of chronic pain, anxiety and other factors can magnify the pain, and reduced confidence about coping with the pain can contribute to pain-related disability. Psychological and complementary therapies can assist with coping, reduce pain, and help increase function.

SICKLE CELL DISEASE

Both acute and chronic pain treatment strategies are needed for children with sickle cell disease. For some children, vaso-occlusive pain episodes occur frequently and are difficult to manage. Ideally, management of a painful crisis begins with having a treatment plan, medication, and other strategies set up in advance of the pain. A number of barriers to successful treatment of pain have been identified in children with sickle cell disease, such as conflicting perceptions between patients, their families, and healthcare professionals about pain that is reported and analgesia that is required. Guidelines for the management of acute vaso-occlusive pain have been published.[149] Although there is considerable variability in the way sickle cell disease pain is managed, the standard treatment protocol for painful episodes has been rest, rehydration, and analgesia. There are a variety of analgesic agents to choose from, such as acetaminophen (paracetamol), oral or parenteral nonsteroidal anti-inflammatory drugs, and oral or parenteral opioids. Each of these options has advantages and disadvantages.[156] Continuous infusions of analgesics and patient-controlled analgesia have been shown to be effective and widely used in hospital settings to manage severe pain. However, the opioid dose required to achieve pain relief varies considerably during each painful episode, from one episode to another, and between individual patients. Patients with sickle cell disease pain may need higher doses of analgesics than do patients with other forms of pain.[149]

Physical, psychosocial, and complementary/alternative approaches may also be used to treat acute pain episodes, although there is currently limited published evidence for their effectiveness in reducing sickle cell disease pain. Physical and complementary therapies used in sickle cell disease consist of hydration, heat, massage, physical therapy, transcutaneous electrical stimulation, and acupuncture. Psychosocial interventions such as hypnosis, cognitive-behavioral therapy, and coping skills training have received some empirical support, particularly in providing children with sickle cell disease more adaptive pain management skills.[157]

The management of chronic pain associated with sickle cell disease is not as well documented. Like the management of other forms of chronic pain, a broad approach that integrates pharmacological, psychological, physical, and complementary therapies is expected to achieve the best results.

Management of Recurrent Pain Conditions

A fairly large body of treatment research is available on the management of pain related to recurrent headache and abdominal pain, probably because of the high prevalence rates of these conditions in children.

HEADACHE

Pediatric headache treatment research is focused mainly on pediatric migraine headache. There has been some interest in pediatric tension headache, with a few published studies; this section, however, focuses on published treatment studies of pediatric migraine headache. Hermann and colleagues[146] conducted a comprehensive review and meta-analysis of the treatment research with pharmacological and behavioral treatments for pediatric migraine headache. These authors reported that thermal biofeedback and the combination of biofeedback and progressive muscle relaxation produced the largest treatment effects. Thermal biofeedback involves teaching patients how to increase their peripheral temperature by using electronic instruments (a temperature probe on the finger) to measure temperature and a computer monitor to display reinforcing information back to the patient. These treatment modalities were more efficacious than other behavioral treatments,

psychological treatment, drug placebo, and prophylactic drug regimens. The use of thermal biofeedback and relaxation training in the treatment of pediatric migraine has continued to receive further support in more recent original treatment research. Pediatric migraine is one of the few pain conditions in childhood for which there is sufficient empirical support to recommend one specific treatment approach (biofeedback and/or relaxation).

RECURRENT ABDOMINAL PAIN OR FUNCTIONAL BOWEL DISORDERS

On the basis of the theory that functional bowel disorders results from dysfunction in the brain-intestine neural signaling, treatment consists of measures to reduce intestinal sensitivity and to re-regulate the neural signaling mechanism. This can be accomplished with specific medications (e.g., low-dose amitriptyline), adequate sleep and diet, and both physical interventions (e.g., Iyengar yoga) and psychological interventions (e.g., hypnotherapy). Certain medications are used in functional bowel disorders for constipation-predominant irritable bowel syndrome (e.g., tegaserod [Zelnorm]) and for diarrhea-predominant irritable bowel syndrome (e.g., low-dose amitriptyline [Elavil]). Constipation also can be treated with herbal remedies (apricot and linnem), sorbitol (candies for diabetics), polyethylene glycol (MiraLax), and stool softeners such as docusate sodium (Colace). Loperamide (Imodium) as a temporary measure can also ameliorate diarrhea. Finally, peppermint oil geltabs before meals have proved effective in reducing belly pain, and ginger taken in the form of ginger candy or dried sweetened ginger or tea brewed with pieces of fresh ginger can reduce nausea. However, a good treatment plan includes nondrug therapies, with or without medications.

In a review of randomized controlled trials for the treatment of recurrent abdominal pain in children, Weydert and associates[147] summarized available evidence of the effectiveness of pharmaceuticals, dietary changes, cognitive-behavioral therapy, and botanicals. These authors found evidence for treatment of recurrent abdominal pain through a number of different modalities. In the studies reviewed, there was evidence of successful treatment with the pharmaceuticals famotidine and pizotifen, cognitive-behavioral therapy, biofeedback, and peppermint oil enteric-coated capsules. Dietary changes such as the addition of fiber or the avoidance of lactose containing products were found to be less efficacious. It is difficult, however, to summarize these studies because of the differing definitions of recurrent abdominal pain that have been used. The Rome classification[111] should help with standardizing the definitions and samples of patients in future treatment studies of functional bowel disorders.

Numerous studies have focused on treatment of recurrent abdominal pain with cognitive-behavioral interventions. For example, in one study, cognitive-behavioral family intervention was compared to standard pediatric care for recurrent abdominal pain.[158] Children who received cognitive-behavioral family intervention participated in five 40-minute sessions and were trained in relaxation skills and positive self-talk; parents were taught to limit secondary gains from sick behavior. Children receiving the standard medical care group underwent usual and customary medical treatment, consisting of follow-up office visits, education, support, and medications as deemed appropriate by the treating physician. Children who received the cognitive-behavioral intervention reported significantly less pain after treatment and at the 1-year follow-up than did children receiving standard care; this outcome supports the use of cognitive-behavioral family interventions in children with abdominal pain.[158]

Other investigators examined the use of citalopram (Celexa) for the treatment of recurrent abdominal pain with comorbid anxiety and depressive disorders.[47] Citalopram is a selective serotonin reuptake inhibitor commonly used to treat both adult and pediatric anxiety and depression. Campo and coworkers conducted an open-label trial of citalopram in 25 patients aged 7 to 18 years in whom recurrent abdominal pain had been diagnosed. The children were enrolled in a 12-week protocol. At the end of the trial, children reported decreases in abdominal pain, anxiety, depression, somatic symptoms and functional impairment. The authors concluded that citalopram is a promising treatment for recurrent abdominal pain with comorbid anxiety or depression and that a double-blind randomized, controlled trial is needed to further assess the efficacy of this treatment.

Management of Chronic Nonmalignant Pain

In this section, we describe management strategies for chronic nonmalignant pain such as CRPS and amplified musculoskeletal pain. We begin with a general description of a multidisciplinary treatment approach that a child might receive in a specialized pediatric pain clinic for management of chronic nonmalignant pain.

MULTIDISCIPLINARY CARE OF CHILDREN WITH CHRONIC PAIN

Children with chronic nonmalignant pain may be referred for specialized pain care. Children who receive care in a multidisciplinary or interdisciplinary pediatric pain clinic are typically offered a rehabilitation approach to treatment. In this approach, pain is accepted as a symptom that might not be eradicated, and efforts are directed toward improvement of functioning. As functioning and coping skills are improved, pain often remits as well. Such treatment may involve pharmacological strategies, physical or occupational therapy, cognitive-behavioral therapy, family therapy, group therapy, and complementary and alternative approaches. The specific structure of each program differs; some programs emphasize intensive physical therapy and inpatient rehabilitation, whereas other programs treat children exclusively on an outpatient basis. Zeltzer and Schlank[140] listed pediatric pain and gastrointestinal pain programs in the United States, Canada, and elsewhere.

In general, there has been a paucity of treatment research on chronic nonmalignant pain in children. There are limited published trials of any one component of multidisciplinary treatment, although there is emerging support for psychological therapies and physical therapy. There are very few published data on pharmacological treatments for chronic pain in children, despite their widespread use. Eccleston and colleagues[148] reviewed about a dozen controlled trials of psychological therapy for children and adolescents with chronic pain (with meta-analysis of a subset for pain relief). These authors concluded that there is strong evidence that psychological therapies, principally relaxation and cognitive-behavioral therapy, are effective in reducing the severity and frequency of chronic pain in children and adolescents. The cognitive-behavioral therapy interventions primarily involved brief, standardized treatments in which children were taught specific coping skills (e.g., positive self-statements, relaxation).

There have been few descriptions of the outcomes of pediatric patients treated in multidisciplinary pain clinics. One was a treatment outcome study of the effectiveness of interdisciplinary cognitive-behavioral therapy.[159] In this study, 78 adolescents aged 11 to 18 years who had chronic nonmalignant pain and had suffered pain-associated disability for at least three months were enrolled in an intensive inpatient pain treatment program involving physiotherapy and psychological therapy. The treatment program included education regarding physiology and anatomy of pain, exercise and chronic pain, regular activity, and cognitive therapy. An adult family member was also involved in therapy with the adolescent patient. Conclusions after a 24-month assessment were that cognitive-behavioral therapy delivered in this interdisciplinary context is a promising treatment for adolescents suffering from chronic pain. The patients demonstrated improvement in physical performance and activity and in school attendance and a reduction in emotional distress after treatment.

COMPLEX REGIONAL PAIN SYNDROME

CRPS is an example of a condition that is often treated in a multidisciplinary pediatric pain clinic. Although many adult pain programs treat CRPS with epidural and other types of nerve blocks, most pediatricians who treat pain do not use these invasive methods, because there are no data to indicate their effectiveness over less invasive methods such as physical therapy, support of good sleep, medications aimed at neuropathic pain, and psychological interventions.

Treatment studies of CRPS in children, however, are scarce. Case studies report success in treating children with reflex sympathetic dystrophy and other neuropathic pain with gabapentin, a novel agent developed for the treatment of seizures.[160,161] However there have been no controlled studies of gabapentin in children with CRPS.

There have been several descriptions of intensive physical therapy and rehabilitation programs for the treatment of CRPS in children.[39,162] In one study, 103 children with a diagnosis of CRPS participated in intensive physical therapy–based exercise programs for 5 to 6 hours per day for a period of 6 to 8 weeks (either as inpatients or as outpatients). Findings demonstrated that symptoms resolved in 92% of the children and they were able to regain full function after the intensive exercise treatment protocol.[162] Similarly, the benefit of physical therapy and cognitive-behavioral treatment were demonstrated in a randomized controlled trial, which included 28 children with CRPS.[39] Each child was randomly assigned to receive physical therapy for 6 weeks either once a week or three times a week. Both groups received weekly cognitive-behavioral treatment. In general, all children showed reduced pain and improved function from physical therapy and cognitive-behavioral therapy. The frequency of the physical therapy did not alter outcome.

Treatment of Somatoform Disorders

Although functional pain symptoms are classified as psychiatric disorders, most children and adolescents with these symptoms are seen predominantly by primary care providers, with referrals to psychiatrists reserved for the most extreme or baffling cases. Furthermore, many physicians are loath to diagnose these disorders for fear that they are "missing something" or out of concern with alienating the patient and the parents by indirectly suggesting that the symptoms are "all in your head." In addition, both patient and parent may be resistant to the idea of

psychiatric treatment. These issues may contribute to the scant volume of evidence-based medicine, meta-analyses, or treatment research on somatoform disorders in children and adolescents. This paucity of research is further complicated by inconsistent terminology, widely differing study designs, and diagnostic criteria that are not specific to the child and adolescent population. The majority of empirical research on the treatment of somatoform disorders has focused on specific symptoms (e.g., abdominal pain, headaches) or the treatment of comorbid psychiatric disorders (e.g., panic disorder, depression).

Although there have been no controlled treatment outcome studies of somatoform disorder in children, various case reports and case series have described treatment of such problems as persistent somatoform pain disorder[163,164] and conversion reactions.[165,166] Treatments that have been successful in remedying symptoms and improving children's functioning include rehabilitation approaches,[167] behavioral techniques,[168] relaxation techniques, and family therapy.[163]

As with all illnesses, the treatment plan for somatoform disorders must be individualized to address the specific problems of the particular patient. All patients, but particularly those with pervasive, long-standing, or multiple symptoms, should be approached from a management point of view. First and foremost an alliance should be built between physician and patient, because resistance to the diagnosis of a somatoform disorder is generally the case. Patient, family, and professional roles should be clearly delineated with an emphasis on teamwork. The team should determine shared goals for all involved with a focus on functional improvement, rather than an unequivocal cure. The physician-patient relationship is also of the utmost importance in avoiding "doctor shopping," which often occurs when the patient or parent is dissatisfied by conservative management or when side effects or new symptoms arise when aggressive management is pursued. It could further be argued that when a physician antagonizes the patient, leading the patient to stop seeing the physician and "doctor shop," these patients often find physicians who are willing to prescribe "magic pills," providing a vast number of medications that include analgesics, tranquilizers, anxiolytics, and narcotics. A respect of the patient's need to express himself or herself with somatic language is necessary. Restraint is crucial with regard to direct confrontation of the psychological aspects of the patient's symptoms, because premature or pejorative confrontation can cause the patient to feel misunderstood or even angry enough to pursue treatment that is likely to cause more harm.

Therapeutic approaches should also include a switch from an emphasis on symptoms to an emphasis on increased level of functioning, and physician contact should not be contingent on escalating sick role behavior. Referral to a mental health professional, preferably a child psychiatrist with a strong background in pediatric medicine, is essential because the incidence of comorbid psychiatric disturbance is significant in the child or adolescent with a somatoform disorder. The incidence of anxiety, panic, and depressive disorders in adult patients with somatoform disorders has been shown to be treated effectively with psychotropic medications such as selective serotonin reuptake inhibitors; however, similar studies in the pediatric population are not available. Education is also of value in the treatment of somatoform disorders, with a focus on the clarification of when specific symptoms should be of concern, use of problem-solving coping techniques, and creation of a collaborative treatment plan. Cognitive-behavioral techniques, such as reinforcement of coping behavior, is effective as a method of reducing secondary gain related to the sick role, and they may increase compliance. Family therapy may significantly reduce pain and relapse rate in pediatric somatoform disorders. Individual and group therapies have also been demonstrated as useful in adult populations; however, data with regard to children and adolescents is, again, scant.[69] Guided imagery, biofeedback, hypnosis, and relaxation techniques have also been shown to be useful in the treatment of somatoform disorders. The patient should be encouraged to maintain regular sleep, hygiene, and mealtimes and to return to regular activities, including exercise, with the parents enlisted as cheerleaders.

THE REATTRIBUTION MODEL

One specific strategy for treatment of somatoform disorders that is gaining popularity is the reattribution model, as is the modified version, the extended reattribution and management model.[169-173] This mode of treatment was specifically designed to facilitate the general practitioner's identification and treatment of adult patients suffering from somatoform symptoms (summarized by Fink et al[172]). This model entails the use of the following stages: (1) feeling understood, (2) broadening the agenda, and (3) making the link, in order to facilitate the shift from the patient's acceptance of medical to the psychological standpoint. In several randomized controlled trials, investigators have compared general practitioner training in the reattribution model with standard practice.[173,174] These investigators found significant attitude changes after intervention, in that physicians felt more comfortable dealing with patients with somatic complaints.[174] The patients of practitioners trained in the reattribution model did evidence significant reductions in physical symptoms at the 6-month follow-up.[173] Although

developed for adult general practitioners, the reattribution model provides important education on the interrelationship between physical and psychological factors and on how they interact with each other, which would be equally relevant in working with pediatric patients.

SEQUENCE OF TREATMENT

In the initial stages of treatment, the development of a bond between physician and the patient and parents is essential, as is using a psychoeducational approach in a measured way to encourage the patient to understand the mind-body connection. A complete history should be pursued at this point, which in effect tells the patient that the physician is interested in the somatic symptoms, as well as the circumstances in which they arise. An intensive focus on psychosocial issues is crucial, because, as stated previously, somatic disorders frequently occur in a setting in which the parent is medically ill or has a somatization disorder. Other psychosocial issues that should be pursued as risk factors include a chaotic household; employment, legal, or financial difficulties in the home; low socioeconomic status; substance abuse; and physical or sexual abuse. Discussion should also focus on how certain psychiatric disorders include somatic symptoms as part of the illness: for example, that major depressive disorder causes anorexia, fatigue, and psychomotor retardation, or that panic disorder can produce the sensation of chest tightening, dizziness, and paresthesia. A complete physical examination with a focus on the patient's chief complaint is important at this stage to assure the patient that the physician takes the symptom seriously. Only appropriate laboratory testing should be done if necessary, on the basis of evidence from the history and physical examination.

In the second stage of treatment, assisting the patient in understanding the interrelatedness of mind and body in a more direct way may be necessary. This can be easily demonstrated in an office visit by merely showing how hyperventilating into a bag or spinning in a chair can cause panic attacks. The treating physician should then explain that symptoms tend to belong to three categories: (1) a verifiable physical disorder, (2) a demonstrable psychological symptom with a somatic manifestation, or (3) a combination of physical disease and psychological symptoms. Also during this stage, the patient is instructed to keep a diary of symptoms, which includes any possible environmental or social stressors, to check later for relationships. Finally, a family history should be documented to explore the role modeling of the sick person in his or her home, both when he or she was a child and in other family members who had medical illnesses or somatoform disorders. The patient's own complaints should be reframed in view of the identified patterns and stressors; this advances the patient's shift toward a more psychological perspective.

The final stage of treatment should involve solidifying the link between physical and psychological in a concrete manner. This may require additional explanations, particularly with the information the patient has provided about his or her own experience. Demonstrations may again need to be used, and printed literature and patient handouts can be useful in this stage. The patient must be given the opportunity to discuss the presenting complaints but encouraged to entertain the alternative explanations, all the while with the reassurance that the symptoms are real and not "all in your mind." Patience and persistence are required on the part of the physician, and the importance of building a rapport with the patient and his or her parents is essential for a collaborative relationship.

Regardless of the model used to address the symptoms of somatoform disorders, follow-up care should involve a multidisciplinary or interdisciplinary approach. A variety of treatments would follow this stage, including psychotherapy, focused on behavioral or cognitive techniques. This therapy often involves the use of relaxation techniques targeted to triggering situations identified in the mind-body diary and mindfulness training, with a focus on using the mind in order to distract or override the experiencing of the symptoms. Other therapies, including pharmacological agents (e.g., antidepressants), coping skills groups, group therapy, acupuncture, biofeedback, energy healing, and other complementary alternative medicine treatments may be considered to reduce somatic complaints, treat comorbid mental health disorders, or target behavioral changes in the patient's ability to cope with stress and/or physical symptoms. If the symptoms persist over time and treatment, a consultation with a specialist (e.g., a neurologist for a patient with neurological complaints) should be considered in order to assess for comorbid conditions or to examine remaining symptoms.[175]

During follow-up treatment, several issues, including patient and family fears provoked or increased by the symptoms, should be addressed. Anxiety can be pervasive in these disorders, affecting the patient, the family, and even the various medical professionals involved. This anxiety can exacerbate the symptoms and may even confound treatment. Separation fears in both the patient and the parents can be pervasive in the context of somatoform disorders, and people who care for and about these children frequently see them as "vulnerable." It is important to assuage these fears with frequent reminders of past successes over the course of treatment, particularly those that demonstrate an increase in level of functioning. The patient, parents, and other care providers should be reassured that the physician is continuing to explore the possibility of unrecognized disease. They should frequently be reminded that the physician is unwilling to prejudge the origin of the symptom and that a thorough exploration of the symptom will be pursued as warranted. As the patient's condition improves, care should be consolidated, with the primary medical provider arranging check-in appointments that the patient is expected to keep with or without a complaint. These visits serve to reassure the family that their concerns have not been dismissed. The physician involved may also be useful in dealing with the distress that this child has produced, either by frequent use of nurses or by absenteeism, and can act in a manner to repair the bond between patient, parents, and teachers. The primary physician by this point serves as an attachment figure within the family, further encouraging the individual to remain involved in a non–crisis-oriented way, such as with regular appointments, to avoid rejection sensitivity and abandonment issues, which often arise with these patents.

At this later stage in treatment, it is also helpful to redefine what constitutes medically legitimate excuses from school or other activities, as well as situations in which it is appropriate to contact the physician or present to an emergency room. A system should be worked out with the school whereby only one medical professional from the team be specified as the medical excuse writer, in order to decrease potential problems such as splitting within the team, as well as doctor shopping in outside institutions. The frequency of symptom monitoring should occur on a regular basis with a plan to taper it slightly with vast changes of symptoms. Although symptomatic relief is certainly desirable, functional improvement needs to be the focus of this patient's treatment. Some patients are loath to identify anything that has improved, saying everything is "the same as always"; thus, when specifics are asked about, such as school attendance, school performance, family and peer relationships, social functioning and health service use, the physician may observe improvements in a way that the patient cannot.

RESEARCH ISSUES AND CONTROVERSIES

Evidence-based treatment for pediatric pain and somatoform disorders is severely limited. Few overall studies have been conducted, and there are wide differences in populations and study designs. Currently there is insufficient available data to compare the effectiveness of treatment approaches for particular conditions or to indicate how treatment components work in concert. These are important areas for future research inquiry. In view of the small populations of patients at any one site, there is a particular need for multisite studies, which would be facilitated by the development of cooperative pediatric chronic pain research consortia.

SUMMARY AND IMPLICATIONS

Clinical Care: Role and Challenges for the Developmental-Behavioral Pediatrician

The developmental-behavioral pediatrician may play different roles in the provision of services to children with pain or somatoform disorders. In a primary care position, the developmental-behavioral pediatrician may be responsible for the initial diagnostic workup and management of the patient, as well as the coordination and follow-up of care. Alternatively, the developmental-behavioral pediatrician who has specific training and expertise in pain management may serve as a consultant and provide specific pain treatment to children with chronic pain, such as biofeedback, hypnosis, or relaxation training.

It is essential that a team approach be used in treating a child with chronic pain or a somatoform disorder. The developmental-behavioral pediatrician should consider enlisting a child or pediatric psychologist, child psychiatrist, and physical or occupational therapist to assist in both diagnosis and management of the pain or somatoform disorder. Communication among the team members should occur on a consistent basis, because providers may not be physically proximate. For example, locating service providers such as physical therapists or psychologists who have experience in managing chronic pain in children can be arduous, because these providers are not abundant and are often not present in small or rural communities. Many services are available only in major metropolitan areas, which may be geographically distant for families. Insurance barriers may also prevent children from accessing mental health services for which the physician wishes to refer the child, thereby compromising the optimal team approach.

In our experience, insurance constraints can often be surmounted on appeal. Clear statements concerning the management of chronic pain in children that can be provided to document the necessity of a team approach and the importance of psychological treatment are available (e.g., the Pediatric Chronic Pain position statement from the American Pain Society[175a]). If experts in chronic pain cannot be located, the developmental-behavioral pediatrician can assemble a team of knowledgeable professionals and serve as a coordinator to help educate the team about chronic pain treatment. Psychologists and rehabilitation therapists can play a useful role in treatment

even when they do not have expertise in pain management, if an overarching treatment plan is in place with specific assessments and interventions outlined.

Research

There are several areas of research inquiry that are needed in pediatric pain and somatoform disorders for diagnosis, treatment, and outcomes. With regard to diagnosis as highlighted in this chapter, pertinent research goals include describing specific areas of functioning that are affected by pain, conducting longitudinal studies to document the development of pain and somatoform disorders in at-risk groups, and validating measures of physical or emotional functioning in children with chronic pain. Furthermore, as noted, although medically unexplained physical symptoms such as chronic pain are common in children and adolescents seen in primary care,[176,177] there is little information available regarding the incidence and prevalence of specific somatoform disorders in children and adolescents. The nomenclature and diagnostic classification system for somatoform disorders in children may need to be revised in order for meaningful incidence data to be available. However, this represents a significant gap in the understanding of somatoform disorders.

A major area for which future research is needed is on treatment, particularly randomized controlled trials of pain treatment approaches. Various pharmacological, psychological, rehabilitation, and complementary approaches used in clinical practice have not yet been studied to document their effectiveness. Moreover, there has been limited comparisons of any treatment strategies, such as comparing medication to cognitive-behavioral therapy for chronic nonmalignant pain. As mentioned, the treatment of chronic pediatric pain would benefit from the development and support of cooperative pediatric chronic pain research consortia. There is a tremendous opportunity for pediatricians to contribute to the research base on evidence-based treatments for pediatric pain.

Finally, pediatricians are in a unique position to study the developmental trajectory of specific pain syndromes, risk factors that add to and hasten this trajectory, and the relevance of factors unique to childhood such as puberty and the development of socialized gender roles. Because sex differences emerge in many chronic pain conditions during adolescence, developmental-behavioral pediatricians should explore reasons for these sex differences, which might begin in infancy. Studies that determine salient risk factors along this developmental pathway can help define critical times during which specific intervention are likely to have the most effect not only in treating the pain but also, ideally, in preventing it.

Training

Pain management should be part of the educational curriculum of all health professionals who care for children. For example, assessment and management of pain in children should be a mandatory part of pediatric residency. Specifically, for the developmental-behavioral pediatrician, specialized training in pain and somatoform disorders in children is necessary to develop clinical and research competencies in this field. Curricula for professional education in pain are available from the International Association for the Study of Pain[178]; these are focused on general issues, assessment and psychology of pain, treatment of pain (pharmacology and other methods), and clinical states. Special consideration is given to pain in infants, children, and adolescents. Apart from formal curricula, there are opportunities for both didactic research and clinical training that would enhance the capacities of developmental-behavioral pediatricians. Links with anesthesiology programs, particularly with acute pain and sedation services, will provide important opportunities for the developmental-behavioral pediatrician to understand approaches to managing acute procedural and postsurgical pain. Multidisciplinary pediatric pain programs are a particularly valuable resource for training in pediatric chronic pain, and efforts should be made to arrange for time to be spent within such programs to observe the approach to treatment. Opportunities for didactic research training are present in many settings that reflect the diversity of specialists who conduct research on pain in children, such as anesthesiology, critical care, emergency medicine, pediatrics, psychology, nursing, and rehabilitation medicine. Last, education and training opportunities are available through professional organizations devoted to pain; for example, opportunities exist within the American Pain Society and the International Association for the Study of Pain, both of which have special interest groups on pain in children.

REFERENCES

1. Merskey H: Classification of chronic pain: Descriptions of chronic pain syndromes and definitions of pain terms. Pain Suppl 3:1-226, 1986.
2. Rainville P: Brain mechanisms of pain affect and pain modulation. Curr Opin Neurobiol 12:195-204, 2002.
3. Coghill RC, McHaffie JG, Yen YF: Neural correlates of interindividual differences in the subjective experience of pain. Proc Natl Acad Sci U S A 100:8538-8542, 2003.
4. American Psychiatric Association: Diagnostic and Statistical Manual of Mental Disorders, 4th ed, Text Revision. Washington, DC: American Psychiatric Association, 2000.
5. Wessely S, Nimnuan C, Sharpe M: Functional somatic syndromes: One or many? Lancet 354:936-939, 1999.
6. Cummings EA, Reid GJ, Finley GA, et al: Prevalence and source of pain in pediatric inpatients. Pain 68: 25-31, 1996.
7. Roth-Isigkeit A, Thyen U, Stoven H, et al: Pain among children and adolescents: Restrictions in daily living and triggering factors. Pediatrics 115(2):e152-e162, 2005.
8. Perquin CW, Hazebroek-Kampschreur AA, Hunfeld JA, et al: Pain in children and adolescents: A common experience. Pain 87:51-58, 2000.
9. Chitkara DK, Rawat DJ, Talley NJ: The epidemiology of childhood recurrent abdominal pain in Western countries: A systematic review. Am J Gastroenterol 100:1868-1875, 2005.
10. Abu-Arefeh I, Russell G: Prevalence of headache and migraine in schoolchildren. BMJ 309:765-769, 1994.
11. Split W, Neuman W: Epidemiology of migraine among students from randomly selected secondary schools in Lodz. Headache 39:494-501, 1999.
12. Anttila P, Metsahonkala L, Aromaa M, et al: Determinants of tension-type headache in children. Cephalalgia 22:401-408, 2002.
13. Wolfe F, Ross K, Anderson J, et al: Aspects of fibromyalgia in the general population: Sex, pain threshold, and fibromyalgia symptoms. J Rheumatol 22:151-156, 1995.
14. Hall H, Chiarucci K, Berman B: Self-regulation and assessment approaches for vaso-occlusive pain management for pediatric sickle cell anemia patients. Int J Psychosom 39(1-4):28-33, 1992.
15. Walco GA, Dampier CD: Pain in children and adolescents with sickle cell disease: A descriptive study. J Pediatr Psychol 15:643-658, 1990.
16. Shapiro BS, Dinges DF, Orne EC, et al: Home management of sickle cell-related pain in children and adolescents: Natural history and impact on school attendance. Pain 61:139-144, 1995.
17. Anthony KK, Schanberg LE: Pain in children with arthritis: A review of the current literature. Arthritis Rheum 49:272-279, 2003.
18. Collins JJ, Byrnes ME, Dunkel IJ, et al: The measurement of symptoms in children with cancer. J Pain Symptom Manage 19:363-377, 2000.
19. Ellis JA, McCarthy P, Hershon L, et al: Pain practices: A cross-Canada survey of pediatric oncology centers. J Pediatr Oncol Nurs 20:26-35, 2003.
20. Miser AW, Dothage JA, Wesley RA, et al: The prevalence of pain in a pediatric and young adult cancer population. Pain 29:73-83, 1987.
21. Albrecht S, Naugle AE: Psychological assessment and treatment of somatization: Adolescents with medi-

cally unexplained neurologic symptoms. Adolesc Med 13:625-641, 2002.

22. Kellner R: Functional somatic symptoms and hypochondriasis. A survey of empirical studies. Arch Gen Psychiatry 42:821-833, 1985.

23. Kroenke K, Spitzer RL, Williams JB, et al: Physical symptoms in primary care. Predictors of psychiatric disorders and functional impairment. Arch Fam Med 3:774-779, 1994.

24. Starfield B, Gross E, Wood M, et al: Psychosocial and psychosomatic diagnoses in primary care of children. Pediatrics 66:159-167, 1980.

25. Garber J, Walker LS, Zeman J: Somatization symptoms in a community sample of children and adolescents: Further validation of the Children's Somatization Inventory. Psychol Assess 3:588-595, 1991.

26. Gooch JL, Wolcott R, Speed J: Behavioral management of conversion disorder in children. Arch Phys Med Rehabil 78:264-268, 1997.

27. Campo JV, Fritz G: A management model for pediatric somatization. Psychosomatics 42:467-476, 2001.

28. Bursch B, Walco GA, Zeltzer L: Clinical assessment and management of chronic pain and pain-associated disability syndrome. J Dev Behav Pediatr 19:45-53, 1998.

29. Pal DK: Quality of life assessment in children: A review of conceptual and methodological issues in multidimensional health status measures. J Epidemiol Community Health 50:391-396, 1996.

30. Hunfeld JA, Perquin CW, Duivenvoorden HJ, et al: Chronic pain and its impact on quality of life in adolescents and their families. J Pediatr Psychol 26:145-153, 2001.

31. Nodari E, Battistella PA, Naccarella C, et al: Quality of life in young Italian patients with primary headache. Headache 42:268-274, 2002.

32. Palermo TM, Schwartz L, Drotar D, et al: Parental report of health-related quality of life in children with sickle cell disease. J Behav Med 25:269-283, 2002.

33. Palermo TM, Harrison D, Koh JL: Effect of disease-related pain on the health-related quality of life of children and adolescents with cystic fibrosis. Clin J Pain 22:532-537, 2006.

34. Palermo TM: Impact of recurrent and chronic pain on child and family daily functioning: A critical review of the literature. J Dev Behav Pediatr 21:58-69, 2000.

35. Walker LS, Greene JW: The functional disability inventory: Measuring a neglected dimension of child health status. J Pediatr Psychol 16:39-58, 1991.

36. Fuggle P, Shand PA, Gill LJ, et al: Pain, quality of life, and coping in sickle cell disease. Arch Dis Child 75:199-203, 1996.

37. Mikkelsson M, Salminen JJ, Kautiainen H: Nonspecific musculoskeletal pain in preadolescents. Prevalence and 1-year persistence. Pain 73:29-35, 1997.

38. Walker LS, Guite JW, Duke M, et al: Recurrent abdominal pain: A potential precursor of irritable bowel syndrome in adolescents and young adults. J Pediatr 132:1010-1015, 1998.

39. Lee BH, Scharff L, Sethna NF, et al: Physical therapy and cognitive-behavioral treatment for complex regional pain syndromes. J Pediatr 141:135-140, 2002.

40. Stang PE, Osterhaus JT: Impact of migraine in the United States: Data from the National Health Interview Survey. Headache 33:29-35, 1993.

41. Langeveld JH, Koot HM, Passchier J: Headache intensity and quality of life in adolescents. How are changes in headache intensity in adolescents related to changes in experienced quality of life? Headache 37:37-42, 1997.

42. Konijnenberg AY, Uiterwaal CS, Kimpen JL, et al: Children with unexplained chronic pain: Substantial impairment in everyday life. Arch Dis Child 90:680-686, 2005.

43. Palermo TM, Witherspoon D, Valenzuela D, et al: Development and validation of the Child Activity Limitations Interview: A measure of pain-related functional impairment in school-age children and adolescents. Pain 109:461-470, 2004.

44. Langeveld JH, Koot HM, Loonen MC, et al: A quality of life instrument for adolescents with chronic headache. Cephalalgia 16:183-196, 1996 [discussion, Cephalalgia 16:137, 1996].

45. Sandstrom MJ, Schanberg LE: Peer rejection, social behavior, and psychological adjustment in children with juvenile rheumatic disease. J Pediatr Psychol 29:29-34, 2004.

46. Kashikar-Zuck S, Goldschneider KR, Powers SW, et al: Depression and functional disability in chronic pediatric pain. Clin J Pain 17:341-349, 2001.

47. Campo JV, Perel J, Lucas A, et al: Citalopram treatment of pediatric recurrent abdominal pain and comorbid internalizing disorders: An exploratory study. J Am Acad Child Adolesc Psychiatry 43:1234-1242, 2004.

48. Wolfson AR, Carskadon MA: Sleep schedules and daytime functioning in adolescents. Child Dev 69:875-887, 1998.

49. Fallone G, Owens JA, Deane J: Sleepiness in children and adolescents: Clinical implications. Sleep Med Rev 6:287-306, 2002.

50. Lewin DS, Dahl RE: Importance of sleep in the management of pediatric pain. J Dev Behav Pediatr 20:244-252, 1999.

51. Palermo TM, Kiska R: Subjective sleep disturbances in adolescents with chronic pain: Relationship to daily functioning and quality of life. J Pain 6:201-207, 2005.

52. Walker LS, Greene JW: Children with recurrent abdominal pain and their parents: More somatic complaints, anxiety, and depression than other patient families? J Pediatr Psychol 14:231-243, 1989.

53. Logan DE, Radcliffe J, Smith-Whitley K: Parent factors and adolescent sickle cell disease: Associations with patterns of health service use. J Pediatr Psychol 27:475-484, 2002.

54. Rizzo JA, Abbott TA 3rd, Berger ML: The labor productivity effects of chronic backache in the United States. Med Care 36:1471-1488, 1998.

55. Latham J, Davis BD: The socioeconomic impact of chronic pain. Disabil Rehabil 16:39-44, 1994.

56. James FR, Large RG: Chronic pain and the use of health services. N Z Med J 105:196-198, 1992.

57. Perquin CW, Hazebroek-Kampschreur AA, Hunfeld JA, et al: Chronic pain among children and adolescents: physician consultation and medication use. Clin J Pain 16:229-235, 2000.

58. Perquin CW, Hunfeld JA, Hazebroek-Kampschreur AA, et al: Insights in the use of health care services in chronic benign pain in childhood and adolescence. Pain 94:205-213, 2001.

59. Maniadakis N, Gray A: The economic burden of back pain in the UK. Pain 84:95-103, 2000.

60. Sleed M, Eccleston C, Beecham J, et al: The economic impact of chronic pain in adolescence: Methodological considerations and a preliminary costs-of-illness study. Pain 119:183-190, 2005.

61. Reid GJ, Gilbert CA, McGrath PJ: The Pain Coping Questionnaire: Preliminary validation. Pain 76:83-96, 1998.

62. Turk DC, Flor H: Psychosocial factors in pain: Critical perspectives. In Gatchel RJ, Turk DC, eds: Chronic Pain: A Biobehavioral Perspective. New York: Guilford Press, 1999, pp 18-34.

63. Crombez G, Vlaeyen JW, Heuts PH, et al: Pain-related fear is more disabling than pain itself: Evidence on the role of pain-related fear in chronic back pain disability. Pain 80:329-339, 1999.

64. Cioffi D: Beyond attentional strategies: Cognitive-perceptual model of somatic interpretation. Psychol Bull 109:25-41, 1991.

65. Rhee H: Prevalence and predictors of headaches in US adolescents. Headache 40:528-538, 2000.

66. Sillanpaa M: Prevalence of migraine and other headache in Finnish children starting school. Headache 15:288-290, 1976.

67. Stewart WF, Lipton RB, Celentano DD, et al: Prevalence of migraine headache in the United States. Relation to age, income, race, and other sociodemographic factors. JAMA 267:64-69, 1992.

68. Unruh AM, Campbell MA: Gender variation in children's pain experience. In Finley G, McGrath P, eds: Chronic and Recurrent Pain in children and Adolescents. Seattle: IASP Press, 1999, pp 1999-1241.

69. Fritz GK, Fritsch S, Hagino O: Somatoform disorders in children and adolescents: A review of the past 10 years. J Am Acad Child Adolesc Psychiatry 36:1329-1338, 1997.

70. Silber TJ, Pao M: Somatization disorders in children and adolescents. Pediatr Rev 24:255-264, 2003.

71. Aguggia M: Neurophysiology of pain. Neurol Sci 24(Suppl 2):S57-S60, 2003.

72. Mayer EA, Gebhart GF: Basic and clinical aspects of visceral hyperalgesia. Gastroenterology 107:271-293, 1994.

73. Drossman DA: What does the future hold for irritable bowel syndrome and the functional gastrointestinal disorders? J Clin Gastroenterol 39(5, Suppl):S251-S256, 2005.

74. Eccleston C, Crombez G, Scotford A, et al: Adolescent chronic pain: Patterns and predictors of emotional distress in adolescents with chronic pain and their parents. Pain 108:221-229, 2004.

75. Logan DE, Scharff L: Relationships between family and parent characteristics and functional abilities in children with recurrent pain syndromes: An investigation of moderating effects on the pathway from pain to disability. J Pediatr Psychol 30:698-707, 2005.

76. Gil KM, Anthony KK, Carson JW, et al: Daily coping practice predicts treatment effects in children with sickle cell disease. J Pediatr Psychol 26:163-173, 2001.

77. Powers SW, Mitchell MJ, Graumlich SE, et al: Longitudinal assessment of pain, coping, and daily functioning in children with sickle cell disease receiving pain management skills training. J Clin Psychol Med Settings 9:109-119, 2002.

78. Goodman JE, McGrath PJ, Forward SP: Aggregation of pain complaints and pain-related disability and handicap in a community sample of families. In Jensen TS, Turner JA, Wiesenfeld-Hallin Z, eds: Proceedings of the 8th World Congress on Pain. Seattle: IASP Press, 1997.

79. Walker LS, Garber J, Greene JW: Psychosocial correlates of recurrent childhood pain: A comparison of pediatric patients with recurrent abdominal pain, organic illness, and psychiatric disorders. J Abnorm Psychol 102:248-258, 1993.

80. Peterson CC, Palermo TM: Parental reinforcement of recurrent pain: The moderating impact of child depression and anxiety on functional disability. J Pediatr Psychol 29:331-341, 2004.

81. Peters JW, Schouw R, Anand KJ, et al: Does neonatal surgery lead to increased pain sensitivity in later childhood? Pain 114:444-454, 2005.

82. Perquin CW, Hunfeld JA, Hazebroek-Kampschreur AA, et al: The natural course of chronic benign pain in childhood and adolescence: A two-year population-based follow-up study. Eur J Pain 7:551-559, 2003.

83. Mikkelsson M, Sourander A, Salminen JJ, et al: Widespread pain and neck pain in schoolchildren. A prospective one-year follow-up study. Acta Paediatr 88:1119-1124, 1999.

84. Campo JV, Di Lorenzo C, Chiappetta L, et al: Adult outcomes of pediatric recurrent abdominal pain: Do they just grow out of it? Pediatrics 108(1):E1, 2001.

85. Fearon P, Hotopf M: Relation between headache in childhood and physical and psychiatric symptoms in adulthood: national birth cohort study. BMJ 322:1145, 2001.

86. Hotopf M, Carr S, Mayou R, et al: Why do children have chronic abdominal pain, and what happens to them when they grow up? Population based cohort study. BMJ 316:1196-1200, 1998.

87. Howell S, Poulton R, Talley NJ: The natural history of childhood abdominal pain and its association with adult irritable bowel syndrome: Birth-cohort study. Am J Gastroenterol 100:2071-2078, 2005.

88. Seng JS, Graham-Bermann SA, Clark MK, et al: Posttraumatic stress disorder and physical comorbidity among female children and adolescents: Results from service-use data. Pediatrics 116:e767-e776, 2005.

89. McGrath PA: Pain in Children: Nature, Assessment, and Treatment. New York: Guilford Press, 1990.

90. Fowler-Kerry S, Lander J: Assessment of sex differences in children's and adolescents' self-reported pain from venipuncture. J Pediatr Psychol 16:783-793, 1991.

91. Goodenough B, Thomas W, Champion GD, et al: Unravelling age effects and sex differences in needle pain: ratings of sensory intensity and unpleasantness of venipuncture pain by children and their parents. Pain 80(1-2):179-190, 1999.

92. Koh JL, Harrison D, Myers R, et al: A randomized, double-blind comparison study of EMLA and ELA-Max for topical anesthesia in children undergoing intravenous insertion. Paediatr Anaesth 14:977-982, 2004.

93. Holdsworth MT, Raisch DW, Winter SS, et al: Pain and distress from bone marrow aspirations and lumbar punctures. Ann Pharmacother 37:17-22, 2003.

94. Kuppenheimer WG, Brown RT: Painful procedures in pediatric cancer. A comparison of interventions. Clin Psychol Rev 22:753-786, 2002.

95. Steinberg MH: Management of sickle cell disease. N Engl J Med 340:1021-1030, 1999.

96. National Heart Lung and Blood Institute: Sickle Cell Anemia (NIH Publication No. 96-4057). Washington, DC: U.S. Government Printing Office, 1996.

97. Palermo TM, Platt-Houston C, Kiska RE, et al: Headache symptoms in pediatric sickle cell patients. J Pediatr Hematol Oncol 27:420-424, 2005.

98. Bonner MJ, Gustafson KE, Schumacher E, et al: The impact of sickle cell disease on cognitive functioning and learning. School Psychol Rev 28:182-193, 1999.

99. Ohene-Frempong K, Weiner SJ, Sleeper LA, et al: Cerebrovascular accidents in sickle cell disease: rates and risk factors. Blood 91:288-294, 1998.

100. Schatz J, Brown RT, Pascual JM, et al: Poor school and cognitive functioning with silent cerebral infarcts and sickle cell disease. Neurology 56:1109-1111, 2001.

101. Hyams JS: Inflammatory bowel disease. Pediatr Rev 21:291-295, 2000.

102. Crohn's and Colitis Foundation of America: Inflammatory Bowel Diseases. (www.ccfa.org)

103. American Pain Society: Guideline for the Management of Pain in Osteoarthritis, Rheumatoid Arthritis, and Juvenile Chronic Arthritis (APS Clinical Practice Guidelines Series, No. 2). Glenview, IL: American Pain Society, 2002.

104. Burton LJ, Quinn B, Pratt-Cheney JL, et al: Headache etiology in a pediatric emergency department. Pediatr Emerg Care 13:1-4, 1997.

105. Headache Classification Subcommittee of the International Headache Society: The International Classification of Headache Disorders: 2nd edition. Cephalalgia 24(Suppl 1):9-160, 2004.

106. Burton AW, Bruehl S, Harden RN: Current diagnosis and therapy of complex regional pain syndrome: Refining diagnostic criteria and therapeutic options. Expert Rev Neurother 5:643-651, 2005.

107. Anthony KK, Schanberg LE: Juvenile primary fibromyalgia syndrome. Curr Rheumatol Rep 3:165-171, 2001.

108. Burckhardt C, Goldenberg D, Crofford L, et al: Guideline for the Management of Fibromyalgia Syndrome Pain in Adults and Children (APS Clinical Practice Guidelines Series, No. 4). Glenview, IL: American Pain Society, 2005.

109. Thompson WG, Longstreth GF, Drossman DA, et al: Functional bowel disorders and functional abdominal pain. Gut 45(Suppl 2):II43-II47, 1999.

110. Apley J, Naish N: Recurrent abdominal pains: A field survey of 1,000 school children. Arch Dis Child 33:165-170, 1958.

111. Walker LS, Lipani TA, Greene JW, et al: Recurrent abdominal pain: Symptom subtypes based on the Rome II criteria for pediatric functional gastrointestinal disorders. J Pediatr Gastroenterol Nutr 38:187-191, 2004.

112. Mayou R, Kirmayer LJ, Simon G, et al: Somatoform disorders: Time for a new approach in DSM-V. Am J Psychiatry 162:847-855, 2005.

113. Liu G, Clark MR, Eaton WW: Structural factor analyses for medically unexplained somatic symptoms of somatization disorder in the Epidemiologic Catchment Area study. Psychol Med 27:617-626, 1997.

114. Ikeda K, Osamura N, Hashimoto N, et al: Conversion disorder: Four case reports concerning motor disorder symptoms. J Orthop Sci 10:324-327, 2005.

115. Kumar S: Conversion disorder in childhood. J R Soc Med 97:98, 2004.

116. Pehlivanturk B, Unal F: Conversion disorder in children and adolescents: A 4-year follow-up study. J Psychosom Res 52:187-191, 2002.

117. Starcevic V, Lipsitt DR: Hypochondriasis: Modern Perspectives on an Ancient Malady. Oxford, UK: Oxford University Press, 2001.

118. Looper KJ, Kirmayer LJ: Hypochondriacal concerns in a community population. Psychol Med 31:577-584, 2001.

119. Katz ER, Sharp B, Kellerman J, et al: β-Endorphin immunoreactivity and acute behavioral distress in children with leukemia. J Nerv Ment Dis 170:72-77, 1982.

120. LeBaron S, Zeltzer L: Assessment of acute pain and anxiety in children and adolescents by self-reports, observer reports, and a behavior checklist. J Consult Clin Psychol 52:729-738, 1984.

121. Merkel SI, Voepel-Lewis T, Shayevitz JR, et al: The FLACC: A behavioral scale for scoring postoperative pain in young children. Pediatr Nurs 23:293-297, 1997.

122. Hicks CL, von Baeyer CL, Spafford PA, et al: The Faces Pain Scale–Revised: Toward a common metric in pediatric pain measurement. Pain 93:173-183, 2001.

123. Bieri D, Reeve RA, Champion GD, et al: The Faces Pain Scale for the self-assessment of the severity of

pain experienced by children: Development, initial validation, and preliminary investigation for ratio scale properties. Pain 41:139-150, 1990.

124. Palermo TM, Valenzuela D: Use of pain diaries to assess recurrent and chronic pain in children. Suffering Child 3:1-14, 2003.

125. Palermo TM, Valenzuela D, Stork PP: A randomized trial of electronic versus paper pain diaries in children: Impact on compliance, accuracy, and acceptability. Pain 107:213-219, 2004.

126. Fanurik D, Koh JL, Harrison RD, et al: Pain assessment in children with cognitive impairment. An exploration of self-report skills. Clin Nurs Res 7:103-119 [discussion, Clin Nurs Res 7:120-104, 1998].

127. McGrath PJ, Rosmus C, Canfield C, et al: Behaviours caregivers use to determine pain in non-verbal, cognitively impaired individuals. Dev Med Child Neurol 40:340-343, 1998.

128. Stallard P, Williams L, Velleman R, et al: The development and evaluation of the Pain Indicator for Communicatively Impaired Children (PICIC). Pain 98:145-149, 2002.

129. Kliegman R, Behrman RE, Jenson HB, et al: Nelson Textbook of Pediatrics, 18th ed. Philadelphia: Elsevier, in press.

130. Schechter N, Berde C, Yaster M: Pain in Infants, Children and Adolescents, 3rd ed. Philadelphia: Lippincott Williams & Wilkins, in press.

131. Varni JW, Seid M, Rode CA: The PedsQL: Measurement model for the pediatric quality of life inventory. Med Care 37:126-139, 1999.

132. Eccleston C, Jordan A, McCracken LM, et al: The Bath Adolescent Pain Questionnaire (BAPQ): Development and preliminary psychometric evaluation of an instrument to assess the impact of chronic pain on adolescents. Pain 118:263-270, 2005.

133. Singh G, Athreya BH, Fries JF, et al: Measurement of health status in children with juvenile rheumatoid arthritis. Arthritis Rheum 37:1761-1769, 1994.

134. Varni JW, Seid M, Smith Knight T, et al: The PedsQL in pediatric rheumatology: Reliability, validity, and responsiveness of the Pediatric Quality of Life Inventory Generic Core Scales and Rheumatology Module. Arthritis Rheum 46:714-725, 2002.

135. Chambers CT: The role of family factors in pediatric pain. In McGrath PJ, Finley GA, eds: Pediatric Pain: Biological and Social Context. Seattle: IASP Press, 2003, pp 99-130.

136. Palermo TM, Chambers CT: Parent and family factors in pediatric chronic pain and disability: An integrative approach. Pain 119:1-4, 2005.

137. Walker LS, Zeman JL: Parental response to child illness behavior. J Pediatr Psychol 17:49-71, 1992.

137a. Frank AW: The Wounded Storyteller: Body, Illness, and Ethics. Chicago: University of Chicago Press, 1997.

138. Carter B: Pain narratives and narrative practitioners: A way of working "in-relation" with children experiencing pain. J Nurs Manag 12:210-216, 2004.

139. Palermo TM, Zebracki K, Cox S, et al: Juvenile idiopathic arthritis: Parent-child discrepancy on reports of pain and disability. J Rheumatol 31:1840-1846, 2004.

140. Zeltzer L, Schlank C: Conquering Your Child's Chronic Pain: A Pediatrician's Guide for Reclaiming a Normal Childhood. New York: HarperCollins, 2005.

141. McGrath PJ, Unruh AM, Branson SM: Chronic nonmalignant pain with disability. In Tyler DC, Krane EJ, eds: Advances in Pain Research Therapy. New York: Raven Press, 1990, pp. 225-271.

142. Turk DC, Dworkin RH, Allen RR, et al: Core outcome domains for chronic pain clinical trials: IMMPACT recommendations. Pain 106:337-345, 2003.

143. Dworkin RH, Turk DC, Farrar JT, et al: Core outcome measures for chronic pain clinical trials: IMMPACT recommendations. Pain 113:9-19, 2005.

144. Initiative on Methods, Measurement and Pain Assessment in Clinical Trials, www.immpact.org.

145. Walco GA, Sterling CM, Conte PM, et al: Empirically supported treatments in pediatric psychology: Disease-related pain. J Pediatr Psychol 24:155-167, 1999 [discussion, J Pediatr Psychol 24:168-171, 1999].

146. Hermann C, Kim M, Blanchard EB: Behavioral and prophylactic pharmacological intervention studies of pediatric migraine: An exploratory meta-analysis. Pain 60:239-255, 1995.

147. Weydert JA, Ball TM, Davis MF: Systematic review of treatments for recurrent abdominal pain. Pediatrics 111(1):e1-e11, 2003.

148. Eccleston C, Morley S, Williams A, et al: Systematic review of randomised controlled trials of psychological therapy for chronic pain in children and adolescents, with a subset meta-analysis of pain relief. Pain 99:157-165, 2002.

149. Benjamin L, Dampier CD, Jacox AK, et al: Guideline for the Management of Acute and Chronic Pain in Sickle-Cell Disease (APS Clinical Practice Guidelines Series, No. 1). Glenview, IL: American Pain Society, 1999.

150. Miaskowski C, Cleary J, Burney R, et al: Guideline for the Management of Cancer Pain in Adults and Children. Glenview, IL: American Pain Society, 2005.

151. Evans D, Turnham L, Barbour K, et al: Intravenous ketamine sedation for painful oncology procedures. Paediatr Anaesth 15:131-138, 2005.

152. Houck CS, Sethna NF: Transdermal analgesia with local anesthetics in children: Review, update and future directions. Expert Rev Neurother 5:625-634, 2005.

153. Powers SW: Empirically supported treatments in pediatric psychology: Procedure-related pain. J Pediatr Psychol 24:131-145, 1999.

154. Slifer KJ, Tucker CL, Dahlquist LM: Helping children and caregivers cope with repeated invasive procedures: How are we doing? J Clin Psychol Med Settings 9:131-152, 2002.

155. Walco GA, Varni JW, Ilowite NT: Cognitive-behavioral pain management in children with juvenile rheumatoid arthritis. Pediatrics 89(6, Pt 1):1075-1079, 1992.

156. Stinson J, Naser B: Pain management in children with sickle cell disease. Paediatr Drugs 5:229-241, 2003.

157. Chen E, Cole SW, Kato PM: A review of empirically supported psychosocial interventions for pain and adherence outcomes in sickle cell disease. J Pediatr Psychol 29:197-209, 2004.

158. Robins PM, Smith SM, Glutting JJ, et al: A randomized controlled trial of a cognitive-behavioral family intervention for pediatric recurrent abdominal pain. J Pediatr Psychol 30:397-408, 2005.

159. Eccleston C, Malleson PN, Clinch J, et al: Chronic pain in adolescents: Evaluation of a programme of interdisciplinary cognitive behaviour therapy. Arch Dis Child 88:881-885, 2003.

160. McGraw T, Stacey BR: Gabapentin for treatment of neuropathic pain in a 12-year-old girl. Clin J Pain 14:354-356, 1998.

161. Mellick GA, Mellicy LB, Mellick LB: Gabapentin in the management of reflex sympathetic dystrophy. J Pain Symptom Manage 10:265-266, 1995.

162. Sherry DD, Wallace CA, Kelley C, et al: Short- and long-term outcomes of children with complex regional pain syndrome type I treated with exercise therapy. Clin J Pain 15:218-223, 1999.

163. Lock J, Giammona A: Severe somatoform disorder in adolescence: A case series using a rehabilitation model for intervention. Clin Child Psychol Psychiatry 4:341-351, 1999.

164. Palermo TM, Scher MS: Treatment of functional impairment in severe somatoform pain disorder: A case example. J Pediatr Psychol 26:429-434, 2001.

165. Donohue B, Thevenin DM, Runyon MK: Behavioral treatment of conversion disorder in adolescence. A case example of globus hystericus. Behav Modif 21:231-251, 1997.

166. Woodbury MM, DeMaso DR, Goldman SJ: An integrated medical and psychiatric approach to conversion symptoms in a four-year-old. J Am Acad Child Adolesc Psychiatry 31:1095-1097, 1992.

167. Brazier DK, Venning HE: Conversion disorders in adolescents: A practical approach to rehabilitation. Br J Rheumatol 36:594-598, 1997.

168. Campo JV, Negrini BJ: Case study: negative reinforcement and behavioral management of conversion disorder. J Am Acad Child Adolesc Psychiatry 39:787-790, 2000.

169. Goldberg D, Gask L, O'Dowd T: The treatment of somatization: Teaching techniques of reattribution. J Psychosom Res 33:689-695, 1989.

170. Rosendal M, Fink P, Bro F, et al: Somatization, heartsink patients, or functional somatic symptoms? Towards a clinical useful classification in primary health care. Scand J Prim Health Care 23:3-10, 2005.

171. Blankenstein AH, van der Horst HE, Schilte AF, et al: Development and feasibility of a modified reattribution model for somatising patients, applied by their own general practitioners. Patient Educ Couns 47:229-235, 2002.

172. Fink P, Rosendal M, Toft T: Assessment and treatment of functional disorders in general practice: The extended reattribution and management model—An advanced educational program for nonpsychiatric doctors. Psychosomatics 43:93-131, 2002.

173. Larisch A, Schweickhardt A, Wirsching M, et al: Psychosocial interventions for somatizing patients by the general practitioner: A randomized controlled trial. J Psychosom Res 57:507-514, 2004 [discussion, J Psychosom Res 57:515-516, 2004].

174. Rosendal M, Bro F, Sokolowski I, et al: A randomised controlled trial of brief training in assessment and treatment of somatisation: Effects on GPs' attitudes. Fam Pract 22:419-427, 2005.

175. Mathers NJ, Gask L: Surviving the "heartsink" experience. Fam Pract 12:176-183, 1995.

175a. American Pain Society: Pediatric Chronic Pain. (Available at: http://www.ampainsoc.org/advocacy/pediatric.htm; accessed 1/31/07.)

176. Garralda ME: A selective review of child psychiatric syndromes with a somatic presentation. Br J Psychiatry 161:759-773, 1992.

177. Campo JV, Fritsch SL: Somatization in children and adolescents. J Am Acad Child Adolesc Psychiatry 33:1223-1235, 1994.

178. Charlton JE: Core Curriculum for Professional Education in Pain. Seattle: IASP Press, 2005.

Sleep and Sleep Disorders in Children

JUDITH A. OWENS

NORMAL SLEEP IN INFANTS, CHILDREN, AND ADOLESCENTS

Although sleep in neonates and infants is quite different from that in adults, the structure of children's sleep and sleep-wake patterns begin to resemble those of adults as they mature.[1] In terms of sleep architecture, there is a dramatic decrease in the proportions of both rapid eye movement (REM) sleep and slow-wave sleep (delta or deep sleep) from birth through childhood to adulthood. Sleep cycles during the nocturnal sleep period (known as the *ultradian rhythm of sleep*) lengthen, which results in fewer spontaneous arousals. Several general trends in the maturation of sleep patterns over time have also been identified. First, there is a decrease in the 24-hour average total sleep duration from infancy through adolescence, with a less marked and more gradual continued decrease in nocturnal sleep amounts into late adolescence.[2] This decline includes a decrease in nocturnal sleep throughout childhood, as well as a significant decline in daytime sleep (scheduled napping) between 18 months and 5 years. There is also a gradual but marked circadian-mediated shift to a later bedtime and sleep onset time that begins in middle childhood and accelerates in early to middle adolescence. Finally, sleep-wake patterns on school nights and nonschool nights become increasingly irregular from middle childhood through adolescence. However, sleep patterns also reflect the complex combined influence of biological, environmental, and cultural factors and thus may differ substantially across different cultures and in different contexts.[3] The following section provides a more detailed description of normal sleep behaviors and patterns in different age groups.

Sleep in Newborns

Newborns sleep approximately 16 to 20 hours per day, generally in 1- to 4-hour periods asleep followed by 1- to 2-hour periods awake, and sleep amounts during the day are approximately equal to the amount of nighttime sleep. Sleep-wake cycles are largely dependent on hunger and satiety; for example, bottle-fed babies generally sleep for longer periods (3 to 5 hours) than do breastfed babies (2 to 3 hours). Newborns have two sleep state that are essentially analogous to adult REM and non-REM sleep: active ("REM-like," characterized by smiling, grimacing, sucking, and body movements; 50% of sleep) and quiet ("non–REM-like"), as well as a third "indeterminate" state. Unlike adults and older children, newborns and infants up to the age of approximately 6 months enter sleep through the active or REM-like state.[4]

Sleep in Infants (Aged 1 to 12 months)

Infants generally sleep about 14 to 15 hours per 24 hours at age 4 months and 13 to 14 hours total at age 6 months; however, there appears to be a very wide intraindividual variation in parent-reported 24-hour sleep duration in the first year of life.[2] Sleep periods last about 3 to 4 hours during the first 3 months and extend to 6 to 8 hours by the age of 4 to 6 months. Most infants between 6 and 12 months of age nap a total of 2 and 4 hours, divided into two naps, per day.[5]

Two important developmental "milestones" are normally achieved during the first 6 months of life; these are known as *sleep consolidation* and *sleep regulation*.[6] Sleep consolidation is generally described as an infant's ability to sleep for a continuous period of time that is concentrated during the nocturnal hours, augmented by shorter periods of daytime sleep (naps). Infants develop the ability to consolidate sleep between ages 6 weeks and 3 months, and approximately 70% to 80% of infants achieve sleep consolidation (i.e., "sleeping through the night") by age 9 months. Sleep regulation is the infant's ability to control internal states of arousal in order both to fall asleep at bedtime without parental intervention or assistance and to fall back asleep after normal brief arousals during the night. The capacity to self-soothe begins to develop in the first 12 weeks of life and is a reflection of both neurodevelopmental maturation and learning. However, the developmental goal of independent self-soothing in infants at bedtime and after night awakenings may not be shared by all families, and voluntary or lifestyle sharing of bed or room by infants and parents is a common and accepted practice in many cultures and ethnic groups. Sleep behavior in infancy, in particular, must also be understood in the context of the relationship and interaction between child and caregiver, which greatly affects the quality and quantity of sleep.[7,8]

Sleep in Toddlers (Aged 12 to 36 months)

Toddlers sleep about 12 hours per 24 hours. Napping patterns generally consist of $^1/_2$ to $3^1/_2$ hours per day, and most toddlers give up a second nap by age 18 months. During this stage, both developmental and environmental issues begin to have more of an effect on sleep; examples include the development of imagination, which may result in increased nighttime fears; an increase in separation anxiety, which may lead to bedtime resistance and problematic night awakenings; an increased understanding of the symbolic meaning of objects, which can lead to increased interest in and reliance on transitional objects to allay normal developmental and separation fears; and an increased drive for autonomy and independence, which may result in increased bedtime resistance. Sleep problems in toddlers are very common, occurring in 25% to 30% of this age group; bedtime resistance occurs in 10% to 15% of toddlers, and night awakenings occur in 15% to 20%.[9,10]

Sleep in Preschoolers (Aged 3 to 5 years)

Preschool-aged children typically sleep about 11 to 12 hours per 24 hours; most children give up napping by 5 years, although approximately 25% of children continue to nap at age 5, and there is some evidence that napping patterns and the preservation of daytime sleep periods into later childhood may be influenced by cultural differences.[11] Difficulties falling asleep and night awakenings (15% to 30%) are still common in this age group, in many cases coexisting in the same child.[12] Developmental issues affecting sleep include expanded language and cognitive skills, which may lead to increased bedtime resistance, as children become more articulate about their needs and may engage in more limit-testing behavior; a developing capacity to delay gratification and anticipate consequences, which enables preschoolers to respond to positive reinforcement for appropriate bedtime behavior; and increasing interest in developing literacy skills, which reinforces the importance of reading aloud at bedtime as an integral part of the bedtime routine. Bedtime routines and rituals, use of transitional objects, and sleep-wake schedules are all important sleep-related issues at this developmental stage.

Sleep in Middle Childhood (Aged 6 to 12 years)

Most children this age sleep between 10 and 11 hours a night. It is important to note that the presence of daytime sleepiness in an elementary school–aged child is likely to be indicative of significant sleep problems that cause insufficient or poor quality sleep, because of the high level of physiological alertness during the day that is characteristic of school-aged children. Middle childhood is also a critical time for the development of healthy sleep habits. Increasing independence from parental supervision and a shift in responsibility for health habits as children approach adolescence may result in less enforcement of appropriate bedtimes and inadequate sleep duration; parents may also be less aware of sleep problems if they do exist. Although sleep problems were previously believed to be rare in middle childhood, studies have revealed an overall prevalence of significant parent-reported sleep problems of 25% to 40%, ranging from bedtime resistance to significant sleep onset delay and anxiety at bedtime.[13,14]

Sleep in Adolescents (Aged 12 to 18 years)

Although a number of significant sleep changes occur in adolescence, adolescents' sleep needs do not differ dramatically from those of preadolescents, and optimal sleep amounts remain at about 9 to $9^1/_4$ hours per night. However, a number of studies across different environments and in different cultures have suggested that the average adolescent typically sleeps about 7 hours or less per night[15] and that this accumulating sleep debt may have a significant effect on functioning, performance, and quality of life. Biologically based pubertal changes also significantly affect sleep. In particular, around the time of onset of puberty, adolescents develop as much as a 2-hour sleep-wake "phase delay" (later sleep onset and waking times) in relation to sleep-wake cycles in middle childhood.[16] Environmental factors and lifestyle/social demands, such as homework, activities, and after-school jobs, also significantly affect sleep amounts in adolescents, and early start times of many high schools may contribute to insufficient sleep. There is significant weekday/weekend variability in sleep-wake patterns in adolescents, often accompanied by weekend oversleep in an attempt to address the chronic sleep debt accumulated during the week; this further contributes to decreased daytime alertness levels. All of these factors often combine to produce significant sleepiness in many adolescents and consequent impairment in mood, attention, memory, behavioral control, and academic performance.[17,18]

NEUROBEHAVIORAL AND NEUROCOGNITIVE EFFECT OF INADEQUATE AND DISRUPTED SLEEP IN CHILDREN

There is clear evidence from both experimental laboratory-based studies and clinical observations that insufficient and poor quality sleep result in daytime sleepiness and behavioral dysregulation and affect neurocognitive functions in children, especially the functions involving learning and memory consolidation and those associated with the prefrontal cortex (e.g., attention, working memory, and other executive functions).[19] Indeed, positron emission tomographic scans of sleep-deprived adults show decreased glucose metabolism in the prefrontal cortex, similar to the changes in neural function seen in attention-deficit/hyperactivity disorder (ADHD). Sleep loss and sleep fragmentation are known to directly affect mood (increased irritability, decreased positive mood, poor affect modulation). Behavioral manifestations of sleepiness in children are varied and range from those that are classically "sleepy," such as yawning, rubbing eyes, and/or resting the head on a desk, to externalizing behaviors, such as increased impulsivity, hyperactivity, and aggressiveness, to mood lability and inattentiveness.[20] Sleepiness may also result in observable neurocognitive performance deficits, including decreased cognitive flexibility and verbal creativity, poor abstract reasoning, impaired motor skills, decreased attention and vigilance, and impaired memory.[21,22]

Clinical experience, as well as empirical evidence from numerous studies and case reports, have demonstrated that childhood sleep disorders both arising from intrinsic processes, such as obstructive sleep apnea syndrome (OSAS), and those related to extrinsic or environmental factors, such as behavioral insomnia of childhood (sleep onset association type and limit-setting type) and insufficient sleep, may manifest primarily with daytime sleepiness and neurobehavioral symptoms. The pediatric sleep disorders that have been most frequently studied from this perspective include sleep-disordered breathing (SDB) (i.e., OSAS and snoring), and restless legs syndrome (RLS)/periodic limb movement disorder (PLMD). For example, a higher prevalence of parent-reported externalizing behavior problems, including impulsivity, decreased attention span, hyperactivity, aggression, and conduct problems has been frequently reported in studies of children with either polysomnographically diagnosed OSAS or symptoms suggestive of sleep-disordered breathing, such as frequent snoring.[23,24] Investigators who have compared neuropsychological functions in children with OSAS have found impairments on tasks involving reaction time and vigilance, attention, executive functions, motor skills, and memory. Although some studies have documented significant short-term improvement in daytime sleepiness, behavior, and academic performance[25] after treatment (usually adenotonsillectomy) for OSAS/SDB, other studies have suggested that young children with SDB may continue to be at high risk for poor academic performance several years after the symptoms have resolved.[26] Alternatively, the prevalence of SDB symptoms in children with identified behavioral and academic problems has also been examined in several studies; overall, these studies have revealed an increased prevalence of snoring in young children with behavioral and school concerns, which is suggestive of an approximately twofold increased risk of habitual snoring and SDB symptoms in children with high scores on behavior problem scales.[27]

Significant neurobehavioral consequences may also occur in relation to RLS/PLMD and, as described in several studies, may manifest with a symptom constellation similar to that of ADHD.[28,29] A number of studies have revealed an increased prevalence of periodic limb movements on polysomnography in children referred for ADHD; furthermore, treatment of these children with dopamine antagonists has been shown to result not only in improved sleep quality and quantity but also in improvement in "attention deficit/hyperactivity" behaviors previously resistant to treatment with psychostimulants.[30]

Other postulated health outcomes of inadequate sleep in children include potential deleterious effects on the cardiovascular, immune, and various metabolic systems, including glucose metabolism and endocrine function, and an increase in accidental injuries.[31] In addition, studies have documented secondary effects on parents (e.g., maternal depression), as well as on family functioning.[32]

COMMON SLEEP DISORDERS IN CHILDREN: ETIOLOGY, EPIDEMIOLOGY, PRESENTATION, EVALUATION, AND TREATMENT

It is helpful to the clinician to understand that four basic etiological mechanisms essentially account for most sleep disturbances in the pediatric population that result in excessive daytime sleepiness: Sleep either is *insufficient for individual physiological sleep needs* (e.g., "lifestyle" sleep restriction, sleep onset delay related to behavioral insomnia) or is adequate in amount but *fragmented or disrupted* by conditions that result in frequent or prolonged arousals (e.g., RLS, PLMD). *Primary disorders of excessive daytime sleepiness* (e.g., narcolepsy) are less common but important and underrecognized causes of sleep disturbance in children and adolescents. Finally, *circadian rhythm disorders,* in which sleep is usually normal in structure and duration but occurs at an undesired time (e.g., delayed sleep phase syndrome) may result in daytime sleepiness. For practical purposes, sleep disorders may also be defined as primarily behaviorally based, as opposed to organic or medically based, although, in reality, these two types of sleep disorders are often influenced by similar psychosocial and physical/environmental factors and frequently coexist.

Sleep-Disordered Breathing and Obstructive Sleep Apnea Syndrome

SDB in childhood includes a spectrum of disorders that vary in severity, ranging from OSAS to primary snoring (snoring without ventilatory abnormalities).[33-35] The prevalence is also variable, from 1% to 3% of children with OSAS to 10% of children with habitual snoring. The basic pathophysiological process of OSAS involves cessation of airflow through the nose and mouth during sleep (pathological duration of an apnea is determined by age-appropriate norms) despite respiratory effort and chest wall movement; this disrupts normal ventilation during sleep, resulting in hypoxemia and/or hypoventilation and a sleep pattern characterized by frequent arousals.[36] Common manifestations of SDB in childhood include loud, nightly snoring; choking/gasping arousals; and increased work of breathing characterized by noctur-

nal diaphoresis, paradoxical chest and abdominal wall movements, and restless sleep. However, as noted previously, SDB may manifest primarily with neurobehavioral symptoms, including inattention and poor academic functioning. Although repeated episodes of nocturnal hypoxia probably constitute an important etiological factor for neurobehavioral deficits in OSAS, sleep fragmentation resulting from frequent nocturnal arousals, which in turn leads to the daytime sleepiness, is also believed to play a key role.

Common risk factors for SDB are those contributing to a reduced upper airway patency and include the presence of obstructive features (e.g., adenotonsillar hypertrophy, allergies, reactive airway disease), reduced upper airway size (e.g., obesity, craniofacial syndromes, midfacial hypoplasia, or retrognathia/micrognathia), and/or reduced upper airway tone (e.g., neuromuscular disorders characterized by hypotonia, Down syndrome). Racial factors (e.g., African-American) and genetic factors (family history of SDB) may also play a role, as may environmental factors (e.g., exposure to secondary smoke).

Specific physical examination findings (growth abnormalities such as obesity or failure to thrive, nasal obstruction with hyponasal speech and "adenoidal facies" or mouth breathing, enlarged tonsils) may raise suspicion of OSAS. However, the presence of large tonsils and adenoids does not necessarily mean the patient has OSAS, and there is in fact no constellation of presenting symptoms and physical findings that have reliably been found to differentiate between OSAS and primary snoring in the ambulatory setting.[37] Overnight polysomnography remains the "gold standard" for evaluating pediatric SDB; it documents physiological variables during sleep, including sleep stages and arousals (electroencephalographic montage, eye movements, chin muscle tone), cardiorespiratory parameters (air flow, respiratory effort, oxygen saturation, transcutaneous or end-tidal CO_2, and heart rate), and limb movements and allows for both confirmation of the diagnosis and assessment of severity of OSAS.

Adenotonsillectomy is generally the first line of treatment for pediatric SDB, although adenoidectomy alone may not be curative when other risk factors such as obesity are present.[38] Adenoids may also "grow back" as the result of continued hypertrophy of residual adenoidal tissue after surgery. Reported cure rates after adenotonsillectomy range from 75% to 100% in normal healthy children. Nutrition and exercise counseling should be a routine part of treatment for SDB in obese children. Continuous Positive airway pressure, the most common treatment for OSAS in adults, can be an effective and reasonably well-tolerated treatment option for those children and adolescents for whom surgery is not an option or in children who continue to have OSAS despite surgery.[39,40] Little is known about the efficacy of other treatment modalities, such as oral appliances, palatal/pharyngeal surgery, or other noninvasive techniques such as external nasal dilators for OSAS in the pediatric population.

Parasomnias

Parasomnias are defined as episodic, often undesirable nocturnal behaviors that typically involve autonomic and skeletal muscle disturbances, as well as cognitive disorientation and mental confusion.[41] Parasomnias may be further categorized as occurring primarily during stage 4 slow-wave or deep (delta) sleep (partial arousal parasomnias), during REM sleep, or at the sleep-wake transition.

PARTIAL AROUSAL PARASOMNIAS

The *partial arousal parasomnias,* which include *sleepwalking and sleep terrors,* typically occur in the first third of the night at the transition out of slow-wave sleep and thus share clinical features of both the awake state (ambulation, vocalizations) and the sleeping state (high arousal threshold, unresponsiveness to the environment, amnesia for the event).[42] Sleep terrors are typically characterized by a very high level of autonomic arousal, whereas sleepwalking, by definition, usually involves displacement from bed. Both are more common in preschool- and school-aged children and generally disappear in adolescence, at least in part because of the relatively higher amount of slow-wave sleep in younger children. Sleep terrors are considerably less common (1% to 3% incidence) than sleepwalking (40% of the population have had at least one episode). Furthermore, any factors that are associated with an increase in the relative percentage of slow-wave sleep (certain medications, previous sleep deprivation, sleep fragmentation caused by an underlying sleep disorder such as OSAS) may increase the frequency of these events in a predisposed child.[43] Finally, there appears to be a genetic predisposition for both sleepwalking and night terrors, and it is not uncommon for individuals to have both types of episodes.

Atypical manifestations of partial arousal parasomnias are sometimes difficult to distinguish from nocturnal seizures; the index of suspicion for a seizure disorder should be higher in the presence of a history of seizures or risk factors for seizures, any unusual or stereotypic movements accompanying the episodes, or postictal phenomena.[44] Subsequent daytime sleepiness is also much more likely with nocturnal seizures. Home videotaping of the episodes may be helpful in making the diagnosis, but overnight polysomnography (with a full electroencephalographic seizure montage) may be necessary. The treatment of partial arousal parasomnias generally involves parental education and reassurance, avoidance of exacerbating factors such as sleep deprivation, and institution of safety precautions, particularly in the case of sleepwalking. Pharmacotherapy (with a slow-wave sleep–suppressing drug such as a benzodiazepine or tricyclic antidepressant) may be indicated in severe or chronic cases.

NIGHTMARES

In contrast, *nightmares,* the most common REM-associated parasomnia in childhood, are very common, occur primarily during the last third of the night when REM sleep is most prominent, generally include vivid recall of dream content, and are more likely to be triggered by anxiety or a stressful event. In general, nightmares are fairly easily managed with a combination of behavioral, cognitive, and relaxation strategies. However, frequent and persistent nightmares in a child warrant further investigation with regard to possible trauma, such as sexual abuse, and/or evaluation for a more global anxiety disorder.

RHYTHMIC MOVEMENT DISORDERS

Rhythmic movement disorders, including *body rocking, head rolling,* and *head banging,* are parasomnias that occur largely during sleep-wake transition and are characterized by repetitive, stereotypic movements involving large muscle groups. They are much more common in the first year of life and generally disappear by age 4 years, but in rare cases they persist into adulthood.[45] Although occasionally associated with developmental delay, most occur in normal children and do not result in physical injury to the child. Treatment is generally parental reassurance and, if appropriate, judicious padding of the sleeping surface.

BRUXISM

Bruxism, or repetitive nocturnal tooth grinding, occurs in as many as 50% of normal infants during eruption of primary dentition, and the incidence of at least occasional episodes approaches 20% in older children.[45] There is some speculation that the underlying pathophysiology may be linked to alterations in serotonergic and dopaminergic neurotransmission in the central nervous system. Treatment of symptomatic bruxism (e.g., temporomandibular joint pain, wearing of teeth surfaces) generally involves the use of occlusal splints, and behavioral treatment (e.g., biofeedback) may also be useful.

Restless Legs Syndrome and Periodic Limb Movement Disorder

RLS and PLMD are related sleep disorders that are frequently overlooked in both adult and pediatric clinical practice.[29] Although the prevalence of these disorders in the pediatric population is unknown, retrospective reports given by affected adults suggest that symptoms (such as restless sleep and discomfort in the lower extremities at rest) frequently first appear in childhood and can result in significant sleep disturbance. As in adults, RLS symptoms in children and adolescents are typically worse in the evening and are exacerbated by inactivity, leading to significant difficulty in falling asleep. Individuals with RLS describe uncomfortable, "creepy-crawly" sensations in the lower extremities rather than pain per se; however, these symptoms are often poorly articulated by the children themselves and may be expressed as "growing pains." Additional diagnostic clues may include iron deficiency anemia (specifically, a low ferritin level), exacerbation of symptoms by caffeine intake, and a positive family history of RLS/PLMD. Periodic limb movements, which often co-occur with RLS (as many as 80% of adults with RLS also have periodic limb movements), are characterized by brief, repetitive, rhythmic jerks primarily of the lower extremities during stages 1 and 2 of sleep; these may result in sleep fragmentation related to nocturnal arousals and awakenings. The underlying pathophysiology of both disorders probably involves alterations in dopaminergic neurotransmission, but whereas RLS is a clinical diagnosis, documentation of periodic limb movements associated with arousals requires an overnight sleep study. Pharmacological management with a variety of agents such as dopamine agonists, opioids, and anticonvulsants, as well as iron supplementation if appropriate, and avoidance of exacerbating factors are often quite helpful.[46]

Narcolepsy

Narcolepsy is a rare primary disorder of excessive daytime sleepiness that affects an estimated 125,00 to 200,000 Americans.[47,48] Narcolepsy is rarely diagnosed in prepubertal children, but retrospective surveys nonetheless suggest that in many cases it first manifests in late childhood and early adolescence. However, both pediatric and adult patients with narcolepsy often delay seeking medical attention and are frequently labeled as having mood disorders, learning problems, and academic failure before the underlying cause is identified, as long as several decades later.[49] In about 25% of cases, there is a family history of narcolepsy; secondary narcolepsy after brain injury or in association with other medical illnesses may also occur.

The cardinal and usual initial presenting feature of narcolepsy is repetitive episodes of profound sleepiness that may occur both at rest and during periods of activity (e.g., talking, eating). These "sleep attacks" may be very brief (3 seconds, or "microsleeps"), resulting primarily in lapses in attention. Other features of the so-called "narcoleptic tetrad" essentially represent "uncoupling" of REM phenomena or the intrusion of REM sleep features (muscle atonia, dream mentation) into wakefulness. In addition to daytime sleepiness, the tetrad includes cataplexy (sudden loss of total body or partial muscle tone, usually in response to an emotional stimulus); hypnagogic (at sleep onset) and/or hypnopompic (on waking) visual, auditory, or tactile hallucinations; and sleep paralysis (temporary loss of voluntary muscle control) at sleep onset or cessation. These symptoms of narcolepsy are also frequently misdiagnosed as part of a psychiatric or neurological disorder, such as psychosis or a conversion reaction. The pathophysiology of narcolepsy is thought to involve alterations in the hypocretin/orexin sleep neuroregulatory system. The "gold standard" of diagnosis is overnight polysomnography followed by a multiple sleep latency test. This test involves a series of opportunities to nap, during which patients with narcolepsy demonstrate a pathologically shortened sleep onset latency (<5 minutes), as well as periods of REM sleep occurring immediately after sleep onset. The treatment of narcolepsy generally involves a combination of medications to combat daytime sleepiness (stimulants) and REM sleep suppressants to prevent cataleptic attacks. Because appropriate and timely treatment of both the excessive daytime sleepiness and other symptoms can result in reversal or amelioration of at least some of the neurobehavioral consequences, early recognition of narcolepsy is an important goal for clinicians.

Delayed Sleep Phase Syndrome

Delayed sleep phase syndrome is a circadian rhythm disorder that involves a significant and persistent phase shift in sleep-wake schedule (later bed and wake time) that conflicts with the individual's school, work, and/or lifestyle demands.[50] Thus, it is the *timing* rather than the quality of sleep per se that is problematic; sleep *quantity* may be compromised if the individual is obligated to wake up in the morning before adequate sleep is obtained. Individuals with delayed sleep phase syndrome may complain primarily of sleep initiation insomnia; however, when allowed to sleep according to their preferred later bedtime and waking time (e.g., on school vacations), the sleep onset delays resolve. The typical sleep-wake pattern in delayed sleep phase syndrome is a consistently preferred bedtime/sleep onset time after midnight and a waking time after 10 a.m. on both weekdays and weekends. Adolescents with delayed sleep phase syndrome often complain of sleep-onset insomnia, extreme difficulty waking in the morning, and profound daytime sleepiness. Delayed sleep phase may be treated with a combination of the imposition of a strict sleep-wake schedule, exogenous melatonin, and bright light therapy to help reset the patient's inner clock.[51] Teenagers with a severely delayed sleep phase (more than 3 to 4 hours) may benefit from chronotherapy, in which bedtime ("lights out") and waking times are successively delayed (by 2 to 3 hours per day) over a period of days, until the sleep onset time coincides with the desired bedtime. If school avoidance or a mood disorder is part of the clinical picture, which is commonly the case, noncompliance with treatment is typical, and more intensive behavioral and pharmacological management strategies may be warranted.

Insomnia

BEHAVIORAL INSOMNIA OF CHILDHOOD

Insomnia should be viewed as a symptom and not a diagnosis. The causes of insomnia are varied, range from the medical (e.g., drug-related, pain-induced, associated with primary sleep disorders such as obstructive sleep apnea) to the behavioral (e.g., associated with poor sleep habits or negative sleep onset associa-tions), and are often the result of a combination of these factors. Insomnia in adults is generally defined as (1) difficulty initiating and/or maintaining sleep and/or (2) early morning awakening and/or nonrestorative sleep. However, the definition of insomnia or problematic sleep in children is much more challenging for a number of reasons. For example, parental concerns and opinions regarding their child's sleep patterns and behaviors, as well as the resulting stress on the family, must be considered in defining sleep disturbances in the clinical context. Parental recognition and reporting of sleep problems in children also vary across childhood; parents of infants and toddlers are more likely to be aware of sleep concerns than those of school-aged children and adolescents. In addition, culture-based values and beliefs regarding the meaning, importance, and role of sleep in daily life, as well as culture-based differences in sleep practices (e.g., sleeping space and environment, solitary sleep vs. cosleeping, use of transitional objects) have a profound effect not only on how a parent defines a sleep "problem" but

on the relative acceptability of various treatment strategies.

It is estimated that overall 20% to 30% of young children in cross-sectional studies are reported to have significant bedtime problems and/or night awakenings.[1] For didactic purposes, the subtypes of behavioral insomnia of childhood, sleep onset association and limit-setting subtypes, are defined as separate entities.[52] However, in reality, the two often coexist, and many children present with both bedtime delays and night awakenings.

Sleep Onset Association Subtype of Behavioral Insomnia

The presenting problem in the sleep onset association subtype of behavioral insomnia is generally one of prolonged night waking, which results in insufficient sleep. In this disorder, the infant learns to fall asleep only under certain conditions or in the presence of specific sleep associations, such as being rocked or fed, which are usually readily available at bedtime. During the night, when the child experiences the type of brief arousal that normally occurs at the end of each sleep cycle (every 60 to 90 minutes) or awakens for other reasons, he or she is not able to get back to sleep (self-soothe) unless the same conditions are available. The child then "signals" the caregiver by crying (or coming into the parents' bedroom if he or she is no longer in a crib) until the necessary associations are provided.

The Limit-Setting Sleep Subtype

The limit-setting sleep subtype is a disorder most common in preschool-aged and older children and is characterized by active resistance, verbal protests, and repeated demands at bedtime ("curtain calls") rather than night awakenings. If sufficiently prolonged, the sleep onset delay may result in inadequate sleep. This disorder most commonly develops from a caregiver's inability or unwillingness to set consistent bedtime rules and enforce a regular bedtime and is often exacerbated by the child's oppositional behavior. In some cases, however, the child's resistance at bedtime results from an underlying problem in falling asleep caused by other factors (e.g., medical conditions such as asthma or medication use, a sleep disorder such as RLS, or anxiety) or a mismatch between the child's intrinsic circadian preferences ("night owl" tendencies) and parental expectations.

A review of 52 treatment studies indicated that behavioral therapies produce reliable and durable changes for both bedtime resistance and night awakenings in young children.[53] Ninety-four percent of the studies reported that behavioral interventions were efficacious; more than 80% of children treated demonstrated clinically significant improvement, maintained for up to 3 to 6 months. In particular, results of controlled group studies strongly supported unmodified extinction, graduated extinction, and preventive parent education about sleep as efficacious behavioral treatment strategies. Extinction (or systematic ignoring) typically involves a program of withdrawal of parental assistance at sleep onset and during the night. Graduated extinction is a more gradual process of weaning the child from dependence on parental presence; in a common form, parents use periodic brief checks at successively longer time intervals during the sleep-wake transition. If the infant has become habituated to awaken for nighttime feedings ("learned hunger"), then these feedings should be slowly eliminated. In older children, the introduction of more appropriate sleep associations that are readily available to the child during the night (transitional objects such as a blanket or toy) in addition to positive reinforcement (e.g., stickers for remaining in bed) are often beneficial. Successful treatment of limit-setting sleep problems generally involves a combination of decreased parental attention for bedtime-delaying behavior, establishment of a consistent bedtime routine that does not include stimulating activities such as television viewing, "bedtime fading" (temporarily setting bedtime to the current sleep onset time and then gradually making bedtime earlier) and positive reinforcement (e.g., sticker charts) for appropriate behavior at bedtime. Older children may benefit from being taught self-relaxation techniques and cognitive-behavioral strategies to help themselves fall asleep more readily. For all of these behavioral strategies, parental consistency in applying behavioral programs is crucial to avoid inadvertent intermittent reinforcement of night awakenings; they should also be forewarned that protest behavior frequently temporarily escalates at the beginning of treatment ("postextinction burst").

Psychophysiological Insomnia

Psychophysiological insomnia (difficulty with sleep onset and/or sleep maintenance) occurs primarily in older children and adolescents. This type of insomnia is frequently the result of the presence of *predisposing* factors (such as genetic vulnerability, underlying medical or psychiatric conditions) combined with *precipitating* factors (such as acute stress) and *perpetuating* factors (e.g., poor sleep habits, caffeine use, maladaptive cognitions about sleep). In this disorder, the individual develops conditioned anxiety around difficulty falling or staying asleep, which leads to heightened physiological and emotional arousal and further compromises the ability to sleep.[54] Treatment usually involves educating the adolescent about principles of sleep hygiene, instructing him or her to use the bed for sleep only and to get out of bed if he or she is unable to fall asleep (stimulus control), restricting time in bed to the actual time asleep (sleep restriction), and teaching relaxation techniques to reduce anxiety.

SLEEP ISSUES IN SPECIAL POPULATIONS

Children with Neurodevelopmental Disorders

The high prevalence rates for sleep problems found in these populations of children, ranging from 13% to 85%, may be related to any number of factors, including intrinsic abnormalities in sleep regulation and circadian rhythms, sensory deficits, and medications used to treat associated symptoms.[55,56] It is estimated that significant sleep problems occur in 30% to 80% of children with severe mental retardation and in at least half of children with less severe cognitive impairment. Estimates of sleep problems in children with autism and/or pervasive developmental delay are similarly in the range of 50% to 70%. The types of sleep disorders that occur in these children are generally not unique to these populations; rather, they are more frequent and more severe than in the general population, and they typically reflect the child's developmental level rather than chronological age. Significant problems with initiation and maintenance of sleep, shortened sleep duration, irregular sleeping patterns, and early morning waking, for example, have been reported in a variety of different neurodevelopmental disorders, including Asperger syndrome, Angelman syndrome, Rett syndrome, Smith-Magenis syndrome, and Williams syndrome.[55]

Sleep problems, especially in children with special needs, are often chronic in nature and unlikely to resolve without aggressive treatment. In addition, sleep disturbances in these children often have a profound effect on the quality of life of the entire family. These children also frequently have multiple sleep disorders, which occur simultaneously or in succession. More severe degrees of cognitive impairment tend to be associated with more frequent and severe sleep problems. Psychiatric disorders, such as depression and anxiety in children and adolescents with developmental delays and autistic spectrum disorders, and medications used to treat these disorders (e.g., atypical antipsychotics) may further contribute to sleep problems.

Basic principles of sleep hygiene in children are particularly important to consider in preventing and treating sleep problems in children with developmental delays.[57] Ensuring the safety of these children, especially if night waking is a problem or there is a history of self-injurious behavior, also must be a key consideration in management. A range of behavioral management strategies used in normal children for night awakenings and bedtime resistance, such as graduated extinction procedures and positive reinforcement, may also be applied effectively in children with developmental delay. Collaboration with a behavioral therapist may be needed if there are complex, chronic, or multiple sleep problems or if initial behavioral strategies have failed. Finally, the use of pharmacological intervention in conjunction with behavioral techniques, including melatonin, has also been shown to be effective in selected cases.[58]

Children with Psychiatric Disorders

Sleep disturbances often have a significant effect on the clinical manifestations and symptom severity, as well as on the management, of psychiatric disorders in children and adolescents. Virtually all psychiatric disorders in children may be associated with sleep disruption.[59-61] Psychiatric disorders can also be associated with daytime sleepiness, fatigue, abnormal circadian sleep patterns, disturbing dreams and nightmares, and movement disorders during sleep. Studies of children with major depressive disorder, for example, have revealed a prevalence of insomnia of up to 75%, a prevalence of severe insomnia of 30%, and a prevalence of sleep onset delay in one third of depressed adolescents. Sleep complaints, especially bedtime resistance, refusal to sleep alone, increased nighttime fears, and nightmares, are also common in anxious children and in children who have experienced severely traumatic events (including physical and sexual abuse). Use of psychotropic medications that may have significant negative effects on sleep often complicates the issue. Conversely, growing evidence suggests that "primary" insomnia (i.e., insomnia with no concurrent psychiatric disorder) is a risk factor for later development of psychiatric conditions, particularly depressive and anxiety disorders.

Clinicians who evaluate and treat children with ADHD frequently report sleep disturbances, especially difficulty initiating sleep and restless and disturbed sleep.[62] Surveys of parents and children with ADHD consistently report an increased prevalence of sleep problems, including delayed sleep onset, poor sleep quality, restless sleep, frequent night awakenings, and shortened sleep duration, although more objective methods of examining sleep and sleep architecture (e.g., polysomnography, actigraphy) have overall disclosed minimal or inconsistent differences between children with ADHD and controls. Sleep problems in children with ADHD are likely to be multifactorial in nature, and potential causes range from psychostimulant-mediated sleep-onset delay in some children to bedtime resistance related to a

comorbid anxiety or oppositional defiant disorder in others. In some children, difficulties in settling down at bedtime may be related to deficits in sensory integration associated with ADHD, whereas in others, a circadian phase delay may be the primary etiological factor in bedtime resistance. Difficulty falling asleep related to psychostimulant use may respond to adjustments in the dosing schedule, inasmuch as in some children, the sleep onset delay results from a rebound effect of the medication's wearing off that coincides with bedtime, rather than a direct stimulatory effect of the medication itself. From a clinical standpoint, therefore, an important treatment goal in managing the individual child with ADHD should be evaluation of any comorbid sleep problems, followed by appropriate, diagnostically driven behavioral and/or pharmacological intervention.

Children with Chronic Medical Disorders

Relatively few data currently exist with regard to the effect on sleep problems of both acute and chronic health conditions such as asthma, diabetes, sickle cell disease, and juvenile rheumatoid arthritis in children.[63-66] However, particularly in chronic pain conditions, these interactions are likely to significantly affect morbidity and quality of life. A number of patient and environmental factors, such as the effects of repeated hospitalization, family dynamics, underlying disease processes, comorbid mood and anxiety disorders, and concurrent medications, are clearly important to consider in assessing the bidirectional relationship of insomnia and chronic illness in children. Specific medical conditions that may also increase risk of sleep problems include allergies and atopic dermatitis, migraine headaches, seizure disorders, other rheumatological conditions such as chronic fatigue syndrome and fibromyalgia, and chronic gastrointestinal disorders such as inflammatory bowel disease. For example, research indicates that one third of asthmatic children report at least one awakening per night,[1] and questionnaire-based studies have revealed that asthmatic children rate themselves as significantly more tired in the morning than do normal controls.[1] In pediatric populations, research has suggested that pain is positively correlated with sleep disturbances, and that children with juvenile rheumatoid arthritis report greater sleep anxiety, more awakenings per hour, and more daytime sleepiness than do normal controls.

In addition, many over-the-counter and prescription drugs have potentially significant effects on sleep and alertness in children, including direct pharmacological effects, disruption of sleep patterns (e.g., night awakenings), exacerbation of a primary sleep disorder (e.g., OSAS or RLS), withdrawal effects, and daytime sedation.[67] Drugs commonly used in children that may have effects on sleep include psychotropic drugs such as stimulants (amphetamines and methylphenidate may cause increased wakefulness and increased sleep onset latency) and antidepressants (selective serotonin reuptake inhibitors are often activating, and there are frequent reports of sleep disruption; tricyclic antidepressants suppress slow-wave sleep and may cause daytime sedation); antihistamines (first-generation drugs such as diphenhydramine, hydroxyzine, and chlorpheniramine cross the blood-brain barrier and promote sleep; they may also significantly reduce daytime alertness and impair performance); corticosteroids (which may be associated with insomnia and subjective increases in wakefulness); opioids (which may cause daytime sedation and disruption of sleep continuity and may worsen obstructive sleep apnea; their abrupt discontinuation may lead to insomnia and nightmares); and anticonvulsants (which may cause excessive daytime sedation). Also, caffeine, the most widely used drug in the world, has potent effects on sleep, resulting in difficulty initiating sleep and more frequent arousals.

A wide variety of medications have been prescribed or recommended by pediatric practitioners for sleep disturbances in children, including antihistamines, chloral hydrate, barbiturates, phenothiazines, tricyclic antidepressants, benzodiazepines, and α-adrenergic agonists.[68,69] In addition, over-the-counter medication such as diphenhydramine and melatonin and herbal preparations are frequently used by parents to treat sleep problems, with or without the recommendation of the primary care provider. The prescription of a wide array of medications for childhood sleep disturbances appears to be based largely on clinical experience, empirical data derived from studies on adults, or small case series of medication use, inasmuch as no medications are currently approved for use as hypnotics in children by the U.S. Food and Drug Administration. Although a combination of behavioral and pharmacological intervention may be appropriate in selected clinical situations and in specific populations (e.g., children with ADHD, autism spectrum disorders) to treat symptoms of insomnia in children and adolescents, most sleep disturbances in children are successfully managed with behavior therapy alone.

IMPLICATIONS FOR CLINICAL CARE AND RESEARCH

Every child who presents with mood, learning, or behavioral issues should be screened for sleep problems. Parents and the children themselves may not recognize the connection between behavioral and learning disorders and sleep problems and thus may fail to spontaneously volunteer such information. Furthermore, because parents of older children and adolescents, in particular, may not be aware of any existing sleep difficulties, it is also important to question the patient directly about sleep issues. A number of parent-report sleep surveys for use in primary care settings exist, as do several clinical screening tools. The latter category includes a simple tool known by its acronym, BEARS: Key areas of inquiry are: *b*edtime resistance/delayed sleep onset; *e*xcessive daytime sleepiness (e.g., difficulty in morning awakening, drowsiness); *a*wakenings during the night; *r*egularity, pattern, and duration of sleep; and *s*noring and other symptoms of sleep-disordered breathing.[70]

If a sleep problem is identified, a comprehensive evaluation includes assessment of current sleep patterns, usual sleep duration, and sleep-wake schedule, often best assessed with a sleep diary in which parents record daily sleep behaviors for an extended period (2 to 4 weeks). A review of sleep habits, such as bedtime routines, daily caffeine intake, and the sleeping environment (e.g., temperature, noise level) may reveal environmental factors that contribute to the sleep problems. Use of additional diagnostic tools such as polysomnographic evaluation are seldom warranted for routine evaluation but may be appropriate if organic sleep disorders such as OSAS or PLMD are suspected. Finally, referral to a sleep specialist for diagnosis and/or treatment should be considered in children or adolescents with persistent or severe bedtime issues that are not responsive to simple behavioral measures or that are extremely disruptive.[71]

Important treatment goals in managing children with sleep problems should include the implementation of appropriate *diagnostically driven* behavioral, educational, and/or pharmacological intervention targeted toward eventual improvement in daytime symptoms. In any discussion of the use of behavioral or pharmacological interventions in the treatment of pediatric insomnia, the clinician must acknowledge the importance of educating parents and children about normal sleep development and good sleep hygiene as a necessary component of every treatment package. *Sleep hygiene* refers to the basic environmental (e.g., temperature, noise level, ambient light), scheduling (e.g., regular sleep-wake schedule), sleep practice (e.g., bedtime routine), and physiological factors (e.g., exercise, timing of meals, caffeine use) that promote optimal sleep.

In view of the complexity of the relationship between sleep and mood, attention, learning, and behavior, further research is clearly needed. Key research areas include the neuroanatomical and neurophysiological basis for the relationship between the regulation of sleep and the regulation of mood, attention, and arousal; the relationship between primary sleep disorders, such as obstructive sleep apnea and RLS/PLMD, and symptoms of hyperactivity and inattention in children and adolescents, including identification of risk factors for irreversible central nervous system deficits; elucidation of the scope, magnitude, natural history, and effect on morbidity of sleep disturbances in children and adolescents with behavioral and developmental disorders in comparison with the general population; the efficacy of various treatment modalities for sleep problems in children, including behavioral interventions and pharmacotherapy, and the effect of treatment on the natural history of neurodevelopmental disorders into adulthood; and the potential utility of sleep problems in predicting the eventual emergence of psychiatric comorbid conditions (depression, anxiety, bipolar disorder). Further elucidation of these fundamental questions regarding the nature of the relationship between sleep and mood/learning/behavior will contribute significantly to the understanding of the relationship between specific brain functions, neuromodulator systems, sleep, and daytime behavior. The ultimate goal is to guide clinicians, parents, and patients in the identification of children with neurobehavioral and neurocognitive manifestations of primary sleep disorders, as well as in the management of sleep problems in children with developmental disorders and behavioral conditions.

REFERENCES

1. Mindell JA, Carskadon MA, Owens JA: Developmental features of sleep. Child Adolesc Psychiatr Clin North Am 8:695-725, 1999.
2. Iglowstein I, Jenni O, Molinari L, Largo R: Sleep duration from infancy to adolescence: Reference values and generational trends. Pediatrics 111:302-307, 2003.
3. Jenni O, O'Connor B: Children's sleep: An interplay between culture and biology. Pediatrics 115(1 Suppl): 204-216, 2005.
4. Sheldon S, Kryger MH, Ferber R, eds: Principles and Practices of Pediatric Sleep Medicine. Philadelphia: WB Saunders, 2005.
5. Mindell J, Owens J: A Clinical Guide to Pediatric Sleep: Diagnosis and Management of Sleep Problems in Children and Adolescents. Philadelphia: Lippincott Williams & Wilkins, 2003.
6. Goodlin-Jones B, Burnham M, Gaylor E, et al: Night-waking, sleep-wake organization, and self-soothing in the first year of life. J Dev Behav Ped 22:226-233, 2001.
7. Hiscock H, Wake M: Infant sleep problems and post natal depression: A community based study. Pediatrics 107:1317-1322, 2001.
8. Zuckerman B, Stevenson J, Bailey V: Sleep problems in early childhood: Continuities, predictive factors, and behavioural correlates. Pediatrics 80:664-671, 1987.
9. Kuhn B, Weidinger D: Interventions for infant and toddler sleep disturbance: A review. Child Fam Behav Ther 22(2):33-50, 2000.
10. Katari S, Swanson MS, Trevathan GE: Persistence of sleep disturbances in preschool children. J Pediatr 110:642-646, 1987.
11. LeBourgeois M, Giannotti F, Cortesi F, et al: The relationship between reported sleep quality and sleep hygiene in Italian and American adolescents. Pediatrics 115(1 Suppl):257-265, 2005.
12. Kerr S, Jowett S: Sleep problems in pre-school children: A review of the literature. Child Care Health Dev 20:379-391, 1994.
13. Blader JC, Koplewicz HS, Abikoff H, et al: Sleep problems of elementary school children. A community study. Arch Pediatr Adolesc Med 151:473-480, 1997.
14. Owens J, Spirito A, Mguinn M, et al: Sleep habits and sleep disturbance in school-aged children. J Dev Behav Pediatr 21:27-36, 2000.
15. Carskadon MA, Wolfson AR, Acebo C, et al: Adolescent sleep patterns, circadian timing, and sleepiness at a transition to early school days. Sleep 21:871-881, 1998.
16. Carskadon MA, Vieira C, Acebo C: Association between puberty and delayed phase preference. Sleep 16:258-262, 1993.
17. Wolfson AR, Carskadon MA: Sleep schedules and daytime functioning in adolescents. Child Dev 69:875-887, 1998.
18. Giannotti F, Cortesi F: Sleep patterns and daytime functions in adolescents: An epidemiological survey of Italian high-school student population. In Carskadon MA, ed: Adolescent Sleep Patterns: Biological, Social and Psychological Influences. New York: Cambridge University Press, 2002.
19. Fallone G, Owens J, Deane J: Sleepiness in children and adolescents: Clinical implications. Sleep Med Rev 6:287-306, 2002.
20. Smedje H, Broman JE, Hetta J: Associations between disturbed sleep and behavioural difficulties in 635 children aged six to eight years: A study based on parent's perceptions. Eur Child Adolesc Psychiatry 10:1-9, 2001.
21. Dahl RE: The regulation of sleep and arousal: Development and psychopathology. Dev Psychopathol 8:3-27, 1996.
22. Randazzo AC, Muehlbach MJ, Schweitzer PK, et al: Cognitive function following acute sleep restriction in children ages 10-14. Sleep 21:861-868, 1998.
23. Ali NJ, Pitson D, Stradlin JR: Natural history of snoring and related behaviour problems between the ages of 4 and 7 years. Arch Dis Child 71:74-76, 1994.
24. Gozal D: Sleep-disordered breathing and school performance in children. Pediatrics 102:616-620, 1998.
25. Ali NJ, Pitson D, Stradlin JR: Sleep disordered breathing; effects of adenotonsillectomy on behavior and psychological function. Eur J Pediatr 155:56-62, 1996.

26. Gozal D, Pope D: Snoring during early childhood and academic performance at ages thirteen to fourteen years. Pediatrics 107:1394-1399, 2001.

27. Chervin RD, Dillon JE, Bassetti C, et al: Symptoms of sleep disorders, inattention, and hyperactivity in children. Sleep 20:1185-1192, 1997.

28. Picchietti D: Periodic limb movement disorder and restless legs syndrome in children with attention-deficit hyperactivity disorder. J Child Neurol 13:588-594, 1988.

29. Picchietti D, Walters A: Restless legs syndrome and period limb movement disorders in children and adolescents. Child Adolesc Psychiatr Clin North Am 5:729-740, 1996.

30. Walters AS, Mandelbaum DE, Lewin DS, et al: Dopaminergic therapy in children with restless legs/periodic limb movements in sleep and ADHD. Dopaminergic Therapy Study Group. Pediatr Neurol 22:182-186, 2000.

31. Valent F, Brusaferro S, Barbone F: A case-crossover study of sleep and childhood injury. Pediatrics 107:E23, 2001.

32. Mindell JA, Durant VM: Treatment of childhood sleep disorders: Generalization across disorders and effects on family members. Special issue: Interventions in pediatric psychology. J Pediatr Psychol 18:731-750, 1993.

33. Marcus CL: Sleep-disordered breathing in children. Am J Respir Crit Care Med 164:16-30, 2001.

34. Schecter M; Section on Pediatric Pulmonology, Subcommittee on Obstructive Sleep Apnea Syndrome: AAP technical report: Diagnosis and management of childhood obstructive sleep apnea. Pediatrics 109(4):e69, 2002.

35. Section on Pediatric Pulmonology, Subcommittee on Obstructive Sleep Apnea Syndrome, American Academy of Pediatrics: Clinical practice guideline: Diagnosis and management of childhood obstructive sleep apnea. Pediatrics 109:704-712, 2002.

36. Lipton AJ, Gozal D: Treatment of obstructive sleep apnea in children: Do we really know how? Sleep Med Rev 7(1):61-80, 2003.

37. Guilleminault C, Palayo R, Leger D, et al: Recognition of sleep disordered breathing in children. Pediatrics 98:871-882, 1996.

38. Lalakea ML, Marquez-Biggs I, Messner AH: Safety of pediatric short-stay tonsillectomy. Arch Otolaryngol Head Neck Surg 125:749-752, 1999.

39. Waters KA, Everett FM, Bruderer JW, et al: Obstructive sleep apnea: The use of nasal CPAP in 80 children. Am J Respir Crit Care Med 152:780-785, 1995.

40. Marcus CL, Ward SL, Mallory GB, et al: Use of nasal continuous positive airway pressure as treatment of childhood obstructive sleep apnea. J Pediatr 137:88-94, 1995.

41. Mahowald MW: Arousal and sleep-wake transition parasomnias. In Lee-Chiong T, Sateia MJ, Carskadon MA, eds: Sleep Medicine. Philadelphia: Hanley & Belfus, 2002, Chapter 24.

42. Laberge L, Trembly RE, Vitaro F, et al: Development of parasomnias from early childhood to early adolescence. Pediatrics 106:67-74, 2000.

43. Rosen GM, Mahowald MW: Disorders of arousal in children. In Sheldon S, Kryger MH, Ferber R, eds: Principles and Practices of Pediatric Sleep Medicine. Philadelphia: WB Saunders, 2005, pp 293-304.

44. Sheldon SH, Glaze DG: Sleep in neurologic disorders. In Sheldon S, Kryger MH, Ferber R, eds: Principles and Practices of Pediatric Sleep Medicine. Philadelphia: WB Saunders, 2005, pp 269-292.

45. Sheldon SH: The parasomnias. In Sheldon S, Kryger MH, Ferber R, eds: Principles and Practices of Pediatric Sleep Medicine. Philadelphia: WB Saunders, 2005, pp 305-315.

46. Tabbal SD: Restless legs syndrome and periodic limb movement disorder. In Lee-Chiong T, Sateia MJ, Carskadon MA, eds: Sleep Medicine. Philadelphia: Hanley & Belfus, 2002, Chapter 26.

47. Wise MS: Childhood narcolepsy. Neurology 50 (Suppl 1):S37-S42, 1998.

48. Kotagal S, Hartse K, Walsh J: Characteristics of narcolepsy in pre-teenaged children. Pediatrics 82:205-209, 1990.

49. Dahl R, Holtum J, Trubnick L: A clinical picture of child and adolescent narcolepsy. J Am Acad Child Psychiatry 33:834-841, 1994.

50. Garcia J, Rosen G, Mahowald M: Circadian rhythms and circadian rhythm disturbances in children and adolescents. Semin Pediatr Neurol 8:229-240, 2001.

51. Sack RL, Lewy AJ, Highes RJ: Use of melatonin for sleep and circadian rhythm disorders. Ann Med 30:115-121, 1998.

52. The International Classification of Sleep Disorders: Diagnosis and Coding Manual (ICSD-2), 2nd ed. Westchester, IL: American Academy of Sleep Medicine, 2005.

53. Mindell J, Kuhn B, Lewin D, et al: Behavioral treatment of bedtime problems and night wakings in infants and young children. An American Academy of Sleep Medicine Review, Sleep 29:1263-1276, 2006 [erratum in Sleep 29:1380, 2006].

54. Hohagen F: Nonpharmacologic treatment of insomnia. Sleep 19:S50-S51, 1996.

55. Wiggs L: Sleep problems in children with developmental disorders. J Royal Soc Med 94:177-179, 2001.

56. Johnson C: Sleep problems in children with mental retardation and autism. Child Adolesc Psychiatr Clin North Am 5:673-681, 1996.

57. Didden R, Curfs LMG, van Driel S, et al: Sleep problems in children and young adults with developmental disabilities: Home-based functional assessment and treatment. J Behav Ther Exp Psychiatry 33:49-58, 2002.

58. Jan MMS: Melatonin for the treatment of handicapped children with severe sleep disorders. Pediatr Neurol 23:229-232, 2000.

59. Sadeh A, McGuire JP, Sachs H: Sleep and psychological characteristics of children on a psychiatric inpatient unit. J Am Acad of Child Adolesc Psychiatry 33:1303-1346, 1995.

60. Sachs H, McGuire J, Sadeh A, et al: Cognitive and behavioural correlates of mother reported sleep problems in psychiatrically hospitalized children. Sleep Res 23:207-213, 1994.

61. Dahl RE, Ryan ND, Matty MK, et al: Sleep onset abnormalities in depressed adolescents. Biol Psychiatry 39:400-410, 1996.

62. Owens J: The ADHD and sleep conundrum: A review. J Dev Behav Pediatr 26:312-322, 2005.

63. Rose M, Sanford A, Thomas C, et al: Factors altering the sleep of burned children. Sleep 24:45-51, 2001.

64. Lewin D, Dahl R: Importance of sleep in the management of pediatric pain. J Dev Behav Pediatr 20:244-252, 1999.

65. Bloom B, Owens J, McGuinn M, et al: Sleep and its relationship to pain, dysfunction and diseases activity in juvenile rheumatoid arthritis. J Rheumatol 29:169-173, 2002.

66. Sadeh A, Horowitz I, Wolach-Benodis L, et al: Sleep and pulmonary function in children with well-controlled stable asthma. Sleep 21:379-384, 1998.

67. Mindell J, Owens J: Sleep and medications. *In* A Clinical Guide to Pediatric Sleep: Diagnosis and Management of Sleep Problems. Philadelphia: Lippincott Williams & Wilkins, 2003, pp 169-182.

68. Owens J, Rosen C, Mindell J: Medication use in the treatment of pediatric insomnia: Results of a survey of community-based pediatricians. Pediatrics 111(5): e628-e635, 2003.

69. Owens J, Babcock D, Blumer J, et al: The use of pharmacotherapy in the treatment of pediatric insomnia in primary care: Rational approaches. A consensus meeting summary. J Clin Sleep Med 1:49-59, 2005.

70. Owens J, Dalzell V: Use of the "BEARS" sleep screening tool in a pediatric residents' continuity clinic: A pilot study. Sleep Med 6:63-69, 2005.

71. Kryger M: Differential diagnosis of pediatric sleep disorders. *In* Sheldon S, Kryger MH, Ferber R, eds: Principles and Practices of Pediatric Sleep Medicine. Philadelphia: WB Saunders, 2005, pp 17-25.

CHAPTER 23

Feeding and Eating Conditions

23A.
Introduction

JULIE C. LUMENG

Because eating is integral to survival, successful feeding of one's child forms the bedrock of a healthy and fulfilling parent-child relationship. Perturbations in eating and feeding frequently come to the attention of a developmental-behavioral pediatrician. These conditions require a conceptualization of child development from medical, social, and psychological perspectives. The biological brain-based relationships between feeding and stress, emotion, and affect regulation are only just beginning to be explored. Feeding and eating disorders highlight social injustices, health disparities based on race and socioeconomic status, and the unique pressures on girls and women in our society. Finally, feeding and eating are fluid processes that rely on interaction with others and the environment and respond differentially to various influences over the course of the child's development. They are, in summary, disorders particularly appropriate to the expertise of the developmental-behavioral pediatrician in the intersection of biology and behavior, parent-child relationships, the influence of societal issues on children's well-being, and, most fundamentally, the myriad ways in which children change, physically, cognitively, and emotionally, as they grow.

We begin this chapter by using disorders of feeding in infancy as a framework in which to discuss the emergence of the dyadic nature of feeding and the development of feeding in early childhood. Next, in the context of a discussion of failure to thrive (FTT) and undernutrition, we discuss more heavily the medical and biological contributors to poor weight gain, as well as social contributors to undernutrition in children. Finally, we conclude by discussing two seemingly disparate conditions, restrictive eating dis-

orders and obesity, and describe the paradoxical commonalities between them. Both problems emerge increasingly as children grow older. We discuss these disorders in tandem because they in particular highlight how affect, behavior, and weight intersect throughout the course of child and adolescent development. We review in this chapter how societal influences affect feeding and eating, as well as how mental health concerns, behavioral issues, and mental health diagnoses are intertwined with eating and feeding conditions. Perhaps most importantly, we highlight the limited evidence and data regarding the problems associated with feeding and eating and the urgent need for more research into mechanisms underlying these conditions, as well as their effective treatment. Developmental-behavioral pediatricians are in a key position to lead efforts in both advocacy and research that will improve children's well-being with regard to the development of healthy eating behaviors, a positive body self-image, emotional well-being, and a healthy weight status.

23B.
Infant Feeding Processes and Disorders

SHEILA GAHAGAN

FEEDING DEVELOPMENT

The Dyadic Nature of Feeding

THE NURSING PERIOD

The full-term human infant is first nourished by a reciprocal process between the newborn and the mother. Breastfeeding is the prototype of the dyadic maternal-infant feeding relationship during the nursing period (first 4 to 6 months after birth). The neonate is born with primitive reflexes, including sucking and rooting that allow suckling during the first hours after birth. Gagging, a competing primitive reflex, may initially interfere with infant feeding. However, the infant's suckling gradually increases in strength, frequency, and coordination over the first few days and, under normal circumstances, predominates over gagging. Colostrum, the first milk produced by the lactating breast, is produced in scant volume, which decreases the chance of choking, as well as regurgitation caused by overfilling of the stomach. The scant colostrum is gradually replaced with increasing volumes of transitional milk between the fourth and tenth postpartum day. By 14 days of age, the baby is usually an accomplished "nurser."

Maternal lactation is regulated by a positive feedback loop. When suckling occurs, oxytocin and prolactin are released by the maternal hypothalamus, controlling milk ejection. Oxytocin release occurs as a conditioned response in most women and can be induced by seeing the baby or hearing the cry even before the tactile stimulus of suckling.[1] Oxytocin and prolactin basal levels are elevated during the months of lactation and are higher 4 days post partum than during the third or fourth month of breastfeeding.[2] Oxytocin levels in the perinatal period are influenced by characteristics of the infant, such as the infant's birth weight. Levels are also influenced by exclusivity of breastfeeding over time, so that mothers who exclusively breastfeed have higher oxytocin and prolactin levels than do those who give supplementary feedings at 3 to 4 months. Prolactin and oxytocin have multiple influences on behaviors crucial to the survival of mammalian infants. Animal research demonstrates that oxytocin promotes maternal-infant bonding and prolactin inhibits sexual behaviors. Mammalian research contributes to the hypothesis that oxytocin and prolactin may contribute to maternal responsiveness during the attachment process. These neuroendocrine hormones may also contribute to decreased maternal interest in and responsiveness to outside stressors.

Both prolactin and oxytocin release are induced by suckling. Suckling-induced oxytocin release may be reduced by psychological stress, thereby reducing stimulation of milk flow (letdown).[3] Infant suckling (on demand or frequently), provides the primary impetus that determines the actual volume of milk produced. It is difficult to overfeed a breastfed infant, because the baby influences the volume of milk by his or her own appetite and satiety. The infant hypothalamus processes infant hunger and satiety signals and coordinates stimulation and inhibition of infant feeding. This positive feedback loop can be perturbed by infant impairment such as muscle weakness or fatigue. For example, the infant with a weak suck may provide inadequate stimulation to the breast to induce oxytocin release and maintain an adequate milk supply. The positive feedback loop can also be disrupted by maternal mammary-hypothalamic-pituitary-adrenal dysregulation related to maternal fatigue, distress, or medication.

Formula feeding during the nursing period follows a pattern similar to that of breastfeeding. However, the caretaker cognitively chooses how much milk to provide in response to the infant's cues. Theoretically, formula feeding is less fine-tuned to the infant's appetite-satiety system. More research is needed to understand how bottle-fed infants express satiety.

Social interaction takes place during feeding as well as during holding, rocking, stroking, and visual engagement. Social interaction develops with a burst in eye contact at 4 weeks of age.[4] The infant may become increasingly social during suckling with interruptions to engage, laugh, or look around. These behaviors may be erroneously interpreted as lack of interest in feeding or desire to discontinue feeding, but they more accurately reflect the infant's emerging capability of directing attention to other interests.

Feeding continues to be a social activity throughout childhood and into adulthood. As the infant's social capabilities increase, socialization during feeding diversifies, including involvement with other members of the family at mealtimes. Older infants, toddlers, and children should anticipate the social interactions associated with mealtimes with pleasure.

THE TRANSITIONAL FEEDING PERIOD

The transitional feeding period starts when the baby begins to ingest nonmilk food but continues to ingest a major portion of calories from milk. The timing and practices of the introduction of food to infants has varied historically and continues to vary widely across cultures. At about 1900, most infants in the United States were not fed solid food routinely until 12 months of age, but in the 1950s, mothers were encouraged to give 3-week old infants pureed or liquid food, such as pablum (rice cereal) and soft-cooked egg yolk. The American Academy of Pediatrics currently recommends gradual introduction of complementary foods containing iron at approximately 6 months of age.[5] These recommendations are based on the infant's neurodevelopmental ability to sit, hold the head erect, and turn the head when satiated, as well as scientific evidence that infants begin to need supplemental foods for calories and for iron in the second 6 months of life.

The dyadic nature of feeding does not diminish during the transitional feeding period. Infants lose some control over nutritional intake when supplemental foods are introduced, as they have less direct input into the timing, volume, and pace of feeding than during breastfeeding. However, if supplemental feeding begins beyond the neonatal and early infancy period (first 3 months), the infant's capability to communicate desires and dislikes can aide in the self-regulation of feeding. Infants have variable capacity to signal hunger and satiety. Most newborns cry when they are hungry, but their early cries are not easily differentiated from cries for other needs such as for sleep and physical comfort.[6] Therefore, these signals may be misinterpreted. As infants mature and develop relationships with caregivers, the human adult's perceptual and problem-solving capability for interpreting the infant cry improves.[6] It is quite likely that infants are sometimes fed when they are not hungry and that at times the amount may not match their desire.

During the first year of life, infants develop increasingly sophisticated communication skills. Expression of emotional states becomes more complex, including the ability to communicate displeasure without crying. The developing abilities to sit, to reach and grasp, and to turn the head all allow the infant to indicate desire or displeasure by motoric maneuvers. The infant has a great deal of power in his or her ability to turn away, throw food, or spit; however, these behaviors do not represent fine-tuned communication. The parent is left wondering whether the child is no longer hungry, does not like a particular food, or is having some other emotion or desire unrelated to food, such as a desire to get out of the chair.

ATTACHMENT THEORY

Feeding, beginning with the nursing period and continuing through the transitional feeding period and into the modified adult feeding period, is anchored in relationships. It is therefore important to consider attachment theory and how it relates to feeding development. Attachment is a behavioral system that conceivably operates in many infant behaviors, including normal feeding development. Furthermore, attachment theory can aid in the understanding of some feeding problems. In 1958, Bowlby hypothesized that human young must be equipped with a behavioral system that operates to promote sufficient proximity to the principal caregiver.[7] He argued that attachment was important for humans because of their long period of immaturity and vulnerability. This system facilitated parental protection and therefore infant survival. His theory was based on the Darwinian notion of adaptation for survival of the species. Specific behaviors that attract the caregiver include crying, suckling, calling, smiling, and seeking proximity. Attachment theory describes attachment behaviors as a behavioral system, which differs from the use of the word *attachment* to mean a bond. Bowlby emphasized the importance of the infant's confidence in the mother's accessibility and responsiveness.[8]

Bowlby described four phases of attachment.[9] The initial *preattachment* phase involves "orientation and signals without discrimination of figure." This phase comes to an end within a few weeks after birth, when the infant can discriminate the mother figure from others. During the second phase, *attachment in the making,* the system involves "orientation and signals toward one or more discriminated figures." The second phase lasts until the phase of *clear attachment,* which begins in the second half of the first year and involves the "maintenance of proximity to a discriminated figure by means of locomotion as well as signals." This stage of attachment has been studied empirically.[10] The final phase, *goal-corrected partnership,* which involves lessening of egocentricity and capability of seeing things from caretaker's point of view, does not begin for most children until age 3 or 4 years.

Attachment is clearly entwined with feeding, inasmuch as feeding behaviors are an intricate part of the system of behaviors during preattachment and attachment in the making. Feeding both facilitates attachment and can be disturbed by disorders of attachment throughout early childhood.[11] Feeding becomes a less important behavioral determinant of attachment during the phase of clear attachment as capabilities such as locomotion become operational.

The Context of Infant Feeding

CULTURE

Both within and outside of the United States, cultural norms strongly influence infant feeding practices. Breastfeeding initiation, frequency, and duration are influenced by cultural factors. Culture prescribes how the infant is held and for how long. Carrying and how the infant is carried (arms, sling, cradleboard, infant seat) is also culturally determined. Furthermore, where the infant sleeps, where the infant is placed when not held, and how the infant is clothed are all influenced by culture.[12] In return, these practices influence feeding.

Cultural practices dictate when solid foods are introduced and whether bottle supplementation is started early. Health care providers may be integral in some cultures and may influence other cultures by their recommendations. Many families choose to feed their infants solid food earlier than the range of 4 to 6 months recommended by the American Academy of Pediatrics.[5] Mothers are often encouraged to introduce solid food (before the time recommended by physicians) by grandmothers who believe that infants' sleep will improve if they have food in their stomachs at bedtime. Conversely, some groups choose to delay feeding until later than 6 months because of cultural beliefs (often related to a theory that longer exclusive breastfeeding is more natural and perhaps healthier for the baby). Similarly, toddler feeding may be accomplished in a high chair or by allowing the toddler to take food while moving from family member to family member. Parents may introduce food into their infant's mouth by hand or by various types of utensils. Many American Indian and African American mothers chew food for their infant and then introduce small amounts into the infant's mouth. This practice is seen in other contemporary and historical cultures. (Research on this practice as a risk for infectious diseases focuses on children exposed to this practice who present with infectious disease, and it suffers from lack of a denominator as well as control groups.)[12a]

In the United States, infants have typically been allowed to progress quickly from being spoon-fed by a caregiver to independent eating. They may achieve independence by eating "finger foods" or by learning to use utensils. It is not unusual for U.S. infants to self-feed early in the second year of life. Some families do not realize that many babies need some help during this period. This practice of early independence in eating differs radically from traditional practices in many cultures. For example, in China, it is not unusual for toddlers to be entirely spoon-fed by their caregivers until they are almost school age.

The choice of foods for infants is also highly influenced by culture. Culture evolves, and eating practices of many cultures have changed dramatically since the 1960s, with increasing consumption of prepared and processed foods, larger portion sizes, some meals taken while people watch television, and more meals consumed away from the family.

When pediatricians consider feeding milestones, they are formulating assessments about the family's childrearing practices and the infant's neurobehavioral adaptation to feeding. Within the context of society and the family, feeding milestones have cultural meaning. For example, the timing of initiating eating solid foods conveys information about the parental values and whether they conform or diverge from their cultural norms. Many cultures value the development of independence and therefore value an infant's ability to hold the bottle. Similarly, drinking from a cup signals a graduation of sorts from baby activities. In the toddler, emerging table manners conform to cultural norms. In most cultures (and in the pediatrician's office), the success of feeding is at least equally judged by the infant's physical growth.

The size of the baby may be equated with the success of parenting within many cultures.

FAMILY

Infant feeding is fraught with meaning for parents, especially mothers: "Successful feeding is inherently satisfying and a powerful affirmation of competence."[13] Conversely, mothers often interpret poor infant feeding as a sign that their mothering is defective. Some mothers generalize this belief and begin to feel that they themselves are defective because their babies do not eat. Clinical experience suggests that fathers also feel competent if their children eat well for them. However, fathers are less inclined to self-blame if their children have eating problems. The grandparents are often the repository of knowledge regarding childrearing and cultural practices. Therefore, grandparents view themselves as experts. This can be problematic if the parents do not choose to follow the feeding practices recommended by the grandparents. Conflicts between pediatric recommendations and grandparental recommendations about feeding are common. Some of these differences reflect changes that have taken place in pediatric knowledge and recommendations over a generation. Feeding problems can often cause stress for grandparents, who may wonder if they could do a better job than the parents. Grandparents do not always understand the complexity of feeding problems, which may stem from neurodevelopmental differences and parent-child relationship difficulties, often in a vicious cycle. Although parents need support from the grandparents, they also need consistent advice from all sources, including their family and doctors. Because infant/toddler feeding problems are poorly understood, the family is often confused by conflicting information and advice.

Normal Feeding Development

Full-term human infants are born with the ability to suck and swallow, to protect their airway, to perceive taste, and to regulate their appetite and satiety. Swallowing occurs as early as the 11th week of fetal life.[14] The coordination of sucking, swallowing, and breathing is related to neuromuscular coordination, which is a function of gestational maturity.[15] Although there is individual variation, most infants can adequately coordinate sucking, swallowing, and breathing by 35 weeks' gestational age. In preterm infants, nonnutritive sucking bursts are seen at 31 to 33 weeks' gestational age.[16] The duration of each sucking burst is about 4 seconds, and as the infants mature, the period of time between sucking bursts decreases. Nutritive sucking allows approximately one suck and swallow per second.

The infant's developing ability to take food off of a spoon and handle thicker foods depends on neuromuscular maturation, including loss of the extrusion reflex. Infants gradually develop the ability to keep their lips closed, thereby avoiding the loss of food from their mouth. Infants who are spoon-fed before 4 to 6 months of age are likely to use a sucking pattern to ingest pureed foods. By 9 months of age, most infants can chew by using a vertical jaw movement and can transfer food from the center of the mouth to the side. At this age, diagonal rotary jaw movements are emerging. By 12 months, most children can use a controlled, sustained bite for textured food, such as a soft cookie. Well-coordinated diagonal rotary and circular rotary jaw movements are attained by 18 and 24 months, respectively. Babies with neurodevelopmental disorders, including cerebral palsy, cleft lip and palate, and hypotonia syndromes, may present with feeding disorders or FTT. Extremes of oromotor tone—spasticity and hypotonia—often cause delay in feeding milestones. Sensory problems are discussed in the following section.

FEEDING CONCERNS, DISTURBANCES, AND DISORDERS

Deviations from normal development are described in the DSM-PC[16a] as *normal variations, problems,* and *disorders. Variations of normal feeding* may be accompanied by parental concerns, which are commonly handled by primary care pediatricians. They are included in this chapter because developmental-behavioral pediatricians are instrumental in training pediatric residents, and provide consultation about feeding problems to pediatric generalists and specialists. More serious *feeding problems,* as long as they do not impair growth, are called disturbances or perturbations in this chapter. *Feeding disorders* are more persistent than these problems and involve vomiting and/or poor growth. After these broad categories are discussed, more specific feeding disorders are described developmentally by presenting complaint.

Feeding Variations and Concerns

Parental concern about infant feeding problems is very common. At least 25% of parents of infants (in normative samples) express concern about their child's eating.[17-19] A longitudinal study of a normative sample of infants and toddlers in Sweden found that more than half of the mothers reported feeding concerns when their children were 10 months old and at the end of the second year. However, very few of

the children were experiencing highly problematic feeding at both ages. In these cases, both infant temperament and maternal sensitivity were believed to mediate the development and the maintenance of the problem.[20]

Although parental concern about feeding is common, it is distressing for the parent. We quote a letter written more than 50 years ago to Dr. Benjamin Spock by a mother of a boy in his practice:

"The one thing that I've found . . . to be the most irritating and long-lasting of the many problems having to do with child raising—that of eating. At just a little past a year of age my son, who had been eating everything and anything that would fit into his mouth, suddenly did a complete turnabout to the point where, today, his entire diet consists of little more than bacon, fruits and bread. . . . What is a mother to do? See that, above all, the baby's mealtime is happy and give him only those foods that he likes, or insist (through tears and tantrums) that he at least taste something new occasionally."

Dr. Spock comments, "I suspect this mother is quoting me—with a touch of irritation and sarcasm. . . . I agree that she is in no mood to create a happy mealtime when she's worried sick about a child's meager and lopsided diet. And it isn't just that she's anxious. She can't help being angry. She's bought and cooked and served good food and this tiny, opinionated whippersnapper turns it down day after day. . . . Her worry is not just over his . . . health . . . but what her husband, her mother, the doctor, and the neighbors will say about him as he grows thinner and thinner, and what they'll think about her. . . . The only thing she did, in the beginning, to bring this about was to be a conscientious mother. The guilt she feels for getting so mad, openly or inside, complicates the picture . . . as time goes on."[21]

Initial evaluation of feeding disorders is expected to take place in the primary care practice. Some physicians ask for developmental-behavioral pediatric consultation during the initial evaluation. When a parent expresses concern about a child's feeding behavior, the pediatrician's first task is to determine whether the child is growing adequately and then determine whether the feeding behavior is developmentally normal, problematic, or frankly disordered. Many parents are concerned about developmentally normal behavior, such as decreased intake at 1 year of age or throwing food at 9 months of age. When feeding behavior is normal, pediatric counseling can help parents avoid feeding battles. The development of frank feeding disorders may also be averted with appropriate anticipatory guidance, including pediatric counseling about age-appropriate feeding behaviors and normal growth parameters. The pediatrician can also explore parental strategies for feeding and support strategies that are helpful to the child. An example would include allowing the 12-month-old to do some finger feeding and limiting the mealtimes to 15 minutes in length (unless he is eating eagerly at 15 minutes). The pediatrician should listen for maladaptive strategies, such as force-feeding or punishing for not finishing food, and advise against such practices.

Feeding Disturbance

A feeding perturbation (intermittent problem) or disturbance (problem lasting more than one month) is diagnosed when an infant exhibits abnormal feeding with normal growth.[22] Although the infant maintains adequate growth, the abnormal behavior causes significant distress for the family. Furthermore, the feeding disturbance may put the child at risk for future eating problems. The following case from our practice is an example of a 10-month-old with a feeding disturbance:

> Larry was an 8-pound 10-oz, infant born at 41 weeks' gestational age to a primiparous 26-year-old mother and 30-year-old father. He was initially fed formula because his mother was taking medications for chronic back pain that precluded breastfeeding. The family history revealed a history of anxiety in the mother. Larry initially grew very rapidly, along the 95th percentile. When he was 3 months old, his mother attempted to return to her work as an occupational therapist, but Larry did not eat or sleep for the caretaker at the licensed day care home. Larry's mother decided that she should quit her job to stay home with him. He then developed vomiting, which was diagnosed as gastroesophageal reflux. His oral intake gradually decreased until at 10 months of age he took only 8 ounces of formula per day and a small amount of pureed foods. By this time the parents were force-feeding him and feeding him during sleep. His weight gain slowed, with his weight for age dropping from the 95th percentile for age to the 50th percentile for age. He then continued to grow along the 50th percentile. His triceps skin fold thickness continued to be between 1 and 2 standard deviations above the mean. He appeared very well nourished.

Feeding refusal sometimes begins in response to overfeeding or the infant's perception of being force-fed. In this case, maternal anxiety, and possibly depression, may have prevented the mother from interpreting her infant's satiety cues accurately. Furthermore, the infant may have been experiencing discomfort after feeding because of gastroesophageal reflux. The reflux may have been exacerbated by overfeeding. We hypothesize that between 5 and 12 months, the infant's appetite began to decrease in concert with a normally decreasing growth velocity combined with shifting linear growth. In other words, growth velocity in all babies slows between ages 5 and 12 months, but Larry's may have been more exaggerated for a combination of reasons, including his large size at birth. By 10 months of age, this child had developed an intense dislike of drinking milk and was willing to drink only enough to remain hydrated.

Growth velocity is very rapid during the first year. However, at 1 year of age, physical growth slows, and exploring, learning, and asserting individuality may take on greater importance than eating in the daily activity of many toddlers. The ravenous appetite of the first year must diminish in order for growth to slow. The decrease in appetite, followed by decreased intake, may be interpreted by the parents as feeding refusal. Vigorous attempts to improve the infant's intake may result in a feeding problem.

Initial evaluation for feeding problems may begin with the primary care physician. It is possible that simple interventions, such as education about normal feeding development and recommendations for adaptive parental feeding strategies appropriate for the developmental stage, will allow the family to ameliorate the child's feeding behavior. Parental coping, mental health, and attachment should be assessed in the case of an infant's feeding disorder. The primary care clinician may choose to refer the parent and the infant to developmental-behavioral pediatrics or mental health services. The pediatrician should remain involved to monitor the child's feeding and growth and to support the work of the mental health professional.

Feeding Disorder

A feeding disorder (in comparison with a normal variation or problem) is a dysfunctional behavior that persists across time and situations and involves abnormal growth or vomiting. It may necessitate more intensive intervention. A system of classification of feeding disorders currently used for research was developed by Chatoor (Table 23B-1).[23] These diagnostic categories were created on the basis of face validity (the extent to which the description of a category seems to accurately describe the characteristics of persons with a particular disorder).[24] Infantile anorexia is the one diagnosis that has been studied for descriptive validity (the extent to which the features of a disorder are unique in comparison with other mental disorders), and reliability (how reliably a condition can be identified, as judged by test-retest and interrater reliability). Although this diagnostic schema has some limitations for both research and clinical practice, it is the only system of classification for infant feeding disorders that has been studied empirically. The remainder of this chapter describes the developmental and symptom manifestations of infant feeding disorders.

TABLE 23B-1 ■ Infant Eating Disorders as Classified by Chatoor

Diagnosis	Presentation	Timing	Poor Weight Gain	Validity	Reliability Tested
State regulation	Difficulty maintaining calm, alert state for feeding	Start in neonatal period	+	Face	−
Caregiver-infant reciprocity	Lack of social responsivity during feeding Not caused solely by physical disorder or pervasive developmental disorder	Infancy	+	Face	−
Infantile anorexia	Refusal of adequate intake for at least 1 month No communication of hunger Not caused by traumatic event or underlying illness	Onset during transitional feeding period	+	Face Descriptive	Test-retest Interrater
Sensory food aversions	Refusal of specific tastes, textures, smells, or food appearances Nutritional deficiency or oromotor delay is present	Onset at introduction of new food type	+/−	Face	−
Associated with concurrent medical condition	Infant initiates feeding readily Infant shows distress and refusal during feeding Medical condition believed to cause distress Medical management improves but does not alleviate problem	Variable	+	Face	−
Post-traumatic feeding disorder	Refusal of bottle, spoon feeding, or other solid food feeding Infant may show distress when positioned for feeding, when approached with bottle, or if food is placed in mouth	Post-traumatic event or repeated insults to oropharynx or gastrointestinal tract	+/−	Face	−

TABLE 23B-2 ■ Feeding Problems during the Nursing Period That Are Related to Pathological Processes in the Infant

Infant Feeding Problem	Example
Developmental disorder	Prematurity
Neurological disorder	Cerebral palsy
Anatomical disorder	Cleft palate
Transient feeding difficulty	Poor latching on
Disordered alertness, vigor	Sedation, mild asphyxia
Oral-motor delays	Mild neurological disorder

SPECIFIC INFANT FEEDING DISORDERS

Feeding Problem—Nursing Period

Feeding problems involving a breastfed infant can be related to the infant, to the mother, or to the maternal-infant dyad. It is reasonable to expect that breastfeeding problems that begin as isolated infant or maternal problems will quickly progress to involve the maternal-infant dyad. Examples of breastfeeding problems include inability to adequately coordinate sucking, swallowing, and breathing or inability to stimulate adequate breast milk production (Table 23B-2). Feeding disorders in formula-fed infants during the first 6 months of life can also result from the same issues except for stimulating breast milk production.

A maternal problem with breastfeeding may relate to inadequate milk supply, often a function of maternal exhaustion or distress. Milk production may be delayed in mothers who had a precipitous delivery and who delivered by cesarean section. Some mothers misperceive their milk supply as inadequate and attempt to supplement feeding in an infant who does not need supplementation, thereby creating risk for an eating problem.

Eating disorders that take root in the maternal-infant dyad are common. A feeding disorder of caregiver-infant reciprocity (previously called *feeding disorder of attachment*) can manifest during the nursing period.[25] Both breastfed and formula-fed infants can develop feeding disorders when there is a disorder of caregiver-infant reciprocity. Criteria for this diagnosis include (1) onset between 2 and 8 months; (2) poor infant growth; (3) the presence of delays in cognitive, motor, or socioemotional development; (4) the presence of maternal psychopathological processes associated with lack of consistent care of the infant; and (5) poor parent-infant reciprocity during feeding. When feeding problems and poor growth are noted in the first 6 months of an infant's life, poor attachment should be included in the differential diagnosis. Along with many other causes of failure of attachment, the clinician can consider the "ghosts in the nursery" described by Selma Fraiberg, in which unconscious response to previous losses and painful experiences in the mother's life can distort interactions with the infant.[26] For example, a mother who experienced a significant loss, such as the death of a parent or spouse, may have difficulty forming attachment to her infant. Subconscious fear of the pain associated with loss prevents closeness with the baby. Her lack of attachment translates into behavior. For example, she may tune out the baby's crying or feed infrequently. Parents who have fewer unresolved losses are more available for knowing and responding to their child and interpreting the child's behavior.

Another psychological risk for infant eating disorder is projection of features of a problematic person onto the baby. For example, the baby "looks just like his father, who is in prison." The parent's mental representation of the infant often includes adult attributes. Some mothers attribute negative feelings and wishes to their infant. For example, crying may be seen as the infant's wish to disturb her. This can produce conflict in the desire to care for the infant and attachment may be impaired. The psychodynamic conflict appears as difficulty nurturing and feeding, which manifests to the pediatrician as poor growth.

Evaluation of the infant who is failing to thrive during breastfeeding includes history, physical examination, and observation. The detailed history focuses on possible associated medical conditions, as well as a mental health assessment of the family. It is important to screen for depression and psychosis in the mother and to refer for further evaluation if there are any concerns. Simultaneous evaluation of relationship factors and physiological factors is important for all cases of FTT, as discussed in detail later in this chapter. Observation of breastfeeding not only reveals mechanical problems related to latching on, positioning, and letdown but also assists with the assessment of attachment. Developmental-behavioral pediatricians may need to assess the volume of milk produced at a feeding. The evaluation of the formula-fed infant who is failing to thrive in the first 6 months of life differs little from that of the breastfed infant. A feeding observation focuses on the infant's ability to coordinate sucking, swallowing, and breathing, as well as on the infant-caregiver interaction. Milk volume is more easily assessed for the formula-fed infant.

Intervention for FTT and an infant's feeding disorder related to breastfeeding depends on the cause of the feeding disorder. Infant-initiated problems related to weakness or poor suck may be remedied by increasing the mother's milk supply through the use of an electric breast pump and a galactologue, such as metoclopramide. Most infants require bottle or nasogastric supplementation at least initially. Infants with neurodevelopmental disorders benefit from intervention by a skilled feeding therapist trained in occupational or speech therapy. Intervention for the formula-fed infant with a feeding disorder may also require a feeding therapist. Therapy focuses on the ability to make a good seal with the bottle nipple, to coordinate sucking and swallowing, and to avert feeding-avoidant behaviors. Feeding therapists are trained to address developmental delay in feeding and sensory aversion to feeding. Their intervention relies on excellent knowledge of development stages of feeding. They use behavior modification techniques and desensitization. Intervention in the case of a maternal mental health disorder requires treatment for the mother; ideally, an infant mental health professional assists. Attention to the mother-infant relationship provides the opportunity for the parents to receive supportive therapy.

Feeding Refusal (Birth to Age 6 Months)

Feeding refusal may be seen during the first 6 months of life. Most infants who refuse to eat during the nursing period have had medical problems such as prematurity, intubation, surgery, or conditions that cause anorexia. Many of these infants are nutritionally supported with gastrostomy or nasogastric feeding. Currently, feeding therapy is provided inconsistently to these infants, and there is little research addressing the utility of feeding therapy in the development of normal eating in infants who have required tube feeding. In our experience, most of these infants eventually eat if they have the neurological capability to do so. However, some feeding refusal persists well into school age.[27] A multidisciplinary approach to infant feeding refusal appears to be quite effective, albeit not empirically studied. An individualized combination of medical care, parental support, behavior modification, feeding practice, and desensitization for aversion is the current standard of care.

Feeding Refusal (Ages 6 to 18 Months)

Feeding problems during the transitional feeding period may be associated with an infant's problem, a caretaker's problem, or a disorder in the infant-

TABLE 23B-3 ■ Possible Causes for Infants' Feeding Refusal from 6 to 18 Months
Oral-motor delays
Self-feeding delays
Social feeding deficits
Eating rate extremes
Difficult temperament
Sensory deficit
Post-traumatic feeding disorder

caretaker dyad. Like feeding problems in the first 6 months of life, transitional feeding refusal associated with an infant's problem is often related to a developmental, neurological, or anatomical disorder. During this developmental phase, some infants develop transient feeding refusal related to illness or distress. Most feeding refusal associated with temporary problems resolves and does not progress to the stage of a disorder. Even when an infant experiences anorexia, most infants respond to thirst and drink enough to remain hydrated. Table 23B-3 lists some causes in infant for feeding refusal in the transitional feeding period.

Infants and toddlers may exhibit feeding refusal after trauma associated with the face or mouth or temporally with feeding. Post-traumatic feeding disorder has been well described in latency-age children after they experience choking, become preoccupied with a fear of eating, and refuse to eat.[28] The following criteria can be used to diagnose post-traumatic feeding disorders in infants: (1) The infant demonstrates food refusal after a traumatic event or repeated traumatic events to the oropharynx or esophagus (e.g., choking, severe gagging, vomiting, reflux, acute allergic reaction, insertion of nasogastric or endotracheal tubes, suctioning, force-feeding); (2) the event (or events) triggered intense distress in the infant; (3) the infant experiences distress when anticipating feedings (e.g., when positioned for feeding, when shown the bottle or feeding utensils, and/or when approached with food); and (4) the infant resists feedings and becomes increasingly distressed when force-fed. Conditioned dysphagia has also been described in children with congenital heart disease, tracheoesophageal fistula, and gastroesophageal reflux.[29-31] Research is needed to determine whether the pathophysiology of feeding problems associated with early oropharyngeal medical procedures or infantile illness is similar to that of post-traumatic feeding disorder in older children who have experienced choking.

Transition-stage feeding problems can relate to deficiencies in caretaker ability to assess the child's hunger, satiety, and feeding needs. Some caretakers are not good at reading the infant's hunger and satiety cues. The risk for cue insensitivity increases when the caretaker is inexperienced, exhausted, depressed, or hostile toward the infant. Some caretakers do not spontaneously interpret subtle signs, such as turning away, as infant communication. Furthermore, a developmentally inappropriate diet or feeding style can cause feeding refusal. Although some parents expect young infants to self-feed before they are capable, others continue to spoon-feed their infants long after the infant is capable of and desires self-feeding. Infants do not express hunger and satiety equally well. Refusal can result from a mismatch in the child's developmental ability and feeding opportunities provided by the caretaker. Infants eat optimally in a pleasant, social feeding environment. A distracting or unsupportive feeding environment may be problematic. At the other extreme, force-feeding is aversive conditioning, and feeding refusal can result. Feeding problems initiated by a caretaker's insensitivity or lack of knowledge can be best detected by a feeding observation. Standardized assessment tools are available for research.[32,33] Development of simple assessment tools for practice are needed.

Intervention for feeding refusal secondary to caretaker problems begins with education about developmentally appropriate feeding techniques. Close follow-up is essential to ensure that feeding strategies are changing and that the infant's symptoms are abating. Mental health services are usually needed to resolve caretaker ambivalence or hostility.

It is important to assess for individual infant-related and individual caretaker-related causes of feeding refusal; however, between 6 and 18 months of an infant's age, disorders are likely to occur in the caretaker-infant relationship. Feeding refusal during transition to solid feeding is not typically related to poor attachment. Early individuation or beginning to separate from the symbiotic phase of infancy is a developmental challenge during the second half of the first year.[34] Feeding problems may develop when caretakers are insensitive to the infant's new developmental needs. Chatoor[25,35] classifies feeding refusal during this developmental period as infantile anorexia with the following criteria: (1) refusal to eat adequate amounts of food for at least 1 month; (2) onset of the food refusal before 3 years of age, most commonly during the transition to spoon- and self-feeding, between 9 and 18 months of age; (3) lack of communication of hunger signals and lack of interest in food but interest in exploration and/or interaction with caregiver; (4) significant growth deficiency; (5) no preceding traumatic event; and (6) no underlying medical illness. Infantile anorexia is understood to stem from the infant's increasing need for autonomy, often beginning with a battle of wills over the infant's food intake. As the name *infantile anorexia* suggests, children with infantile anorexia characteristically lack appetite, beginning during infancy, seeming not to notice their own hunger. Although most infants with infantile anorexia have secure attachment to their mothers, they are somewhat more likely to have insecure mother-infant attachment than are picky eaters or normal controls. Furthermore, the likelihood of insecure attachment increases with worsening malnutrition.[36]

Selective Intake Disorder (Ages 6 to 18 Months)

Infants with a selective intake disorder are similar to "picky eaters"; however, their selectivity is severe. Typically, they eat only a small selection of foods. Some children with severe selective intake disorder restrict intake to carbohydrates such as rice and pasta. Other children restrict intake to one "safe food," such as a peanut butter sandwich. As these children get older, they may exhibit symptoms of anxiety, obsessive-compulsive disorder, or autism. In some children, severe selective intake disorder fits into the classification of sensory food aversion. This disorder can also be a less severe form of infantile anorexia or post-traumatic feeding disorder.

Evaluation of children with selective intake disorder includes a careful medical history, including attention to possible symptoms of food intolerance or allergies. It is not necessary to perform swallowing studies or allergy testing if the history supports food elimination or restriction in the diet. If the selective intake disorder persists, a mental health evaluation for the child is recommended.

Intervention for selective intake disorder includes parental support; strategies to reduce anxiety and distress at mealtimes; and mental health intervention for children who meet diagnostic criteria for anxiety or obsessive-compulsive disorders. Oromotor therapy is often beneficial for selective intake disorder. Habituation therapy can also be helpful. The child is asked to taste small pieces of a food that is not part of his or her usual repertoire. By tasting the same food every day, it may gradually become familiar and therefore acceptable. This type of therapy should be performed without emotion or forcing; however, a small reward or reinforcer (such as playing a short game with the parent) is frequently used. Children whose eating disorder has an oppositional component may not respond well to this type of intervention.

Eating Disorder Related to Deprivation

Eating disorders in children can be related to severe deprivation, such as that involved in institutionalization or abandonment. It is well accepted that depressed adults often experience disordered eating. Infants who have experienced severe trauma of abandonment have been described as withdrawn, apathetic, and uninterested. They often have sleep disorders in addition to disordered eating. These children urgently need placement in a nurturing home.

Rumination

Rumination is regurgitation of food, which is then partially or completely reswallowed or rechewed. Infants often initiate rumination by inserting a hand into the mouth. They may also bring up food by thrusting the tongue to the back of the mouth or by contracting their abdominal muscles. Rumination is poorly understood but believed to be self-stimulatory. It is often associated with child neglect. The differential diagnosis of rumination includes other causes of vomiting, such as gastroesophageal reflux. Some infants (usually premature or neurologically fragile) are observed to vomit in response to stimulation such as noise, human interaction, or movement. These infants may require behavioral strategies to decrease overstimulation. Vomiting is also seen in babies with chronic medical conditions (who may also experience the institutionalization of the hospital as nonintentional neglect caused by the medical environment). The diagnosis of rumination is made by observation. Intervention for children with rumination requires increased nurturing with attention to the infant-caretaker relationship.

SIGNIFICANCE AND IMPLICATIONS

Feeding disorders in infancy and early childhood present unique challenges to the child health professional, including the simultaneous assessment of the child's physical, developmental, and mental health; the parent's mental health; and the infant-caretaker relationship. Although the exact prevalence of eating disorders in infants and young children is not known, it is known that more than 25% of parents are concerned about their child's eating. Furthermore, poor growth is common in young children (5% to 10%). Eating disorders are commonly found in children with FTT when the evaluation includes systematic attention to eating behavior. The tools for this evaluation include a careful history of eating behavior; a feeding observation in the clinic, in the home, or by videotape; and a careful assessment of parental mental health and the parent-infant relationship. Feeding behavior in the infant and young child provides a window into the child's neurodevelopmental competence and developing independent psychological state and into the functionality of the caretaker-infant relationship.

REFERENCES

1. McNeilly AS, Robinson ICA, Houston MJ, et al: Release of oxytocin and prolactin in response to suckling. BMJ (Clin Res Ed) 286:257-259, 1983.
2. Uvnas-Moberg K, Widstrom AM, Werner S, et al: Oxytocin and prolactin levels in breast-feeding women. Correlation with milk yield and duration of breast-feeding. Acta Obstet Gynecol Scand 69:301-306, 1990.
3. Ueda T, Yokoyama Y, Irahara M, et al: Influence of psychological stress on suckling-induced pulsatile oxytocin release. Obstet Gynecol 84:259-262, 1994.
4. Wolff P: The Development of Behavioral States and the Expression of Emotions in Early Infancy: New Proposals for Investigation. Chicago: University of Chicago Press, 1987.
5. Gartner L, Morton J, Lawrence R, et al: Breastfeeding and the use of human milk. Pediatrics 115:496-506, 2005.
6. Barr RG, Hopkins B, Green JA, eds: Crying as a Sign, a Symptom, and a Signal. London: Mac Keith Press, 2000.
7. Bowlby J: The nature of a child's tie to his mother. Int J Psychoanal 39:350-373, 1958.
8. Bowlby J: Attachment and Loss, Volume 2: Separation. New York: Basic Books, 1973.
9. Bowlby J: Attachment and Loss, Volume 1: Attachment. New York: Basic Books, 1969.
10. Bretherton I, Waters E, eds: Growing points in attachment theory and research. Monogr Soc Res Child Dev 50(1-2, Serial No. 209), 1985.
11. Ward MJ, Kessler DB, Altman SC: Infant-mother attachment in children with failure to thrive. Infant Ment Health J 14:208-220, 1993.
12. Lawrence RA: Breastfeeding: A Guide for the Medical Profession. St. Louis: CV Mosby, 1989.
12a. Steinkuller JS, Chan K, Rinehouse SE. Prechewing of food by adults and streptococcal pharyngitis in infants. J Pediatr 120:563-564, 1992.
13. Kedesdy JH, Budd KS, eds: Childhood Feeding Disorders: Biobehavioral Assessment and Intervention. Baltimore: Paul H. Brookes, 1998.
14. Diamant NE: Development of esophageal function. Am Rev Respir Dis 131:S29-S32, 1985.
15. Bu'Lock F, Woolridge MW, Baum JD: Development of co-ordination of sucking, swallowing and breathing: Ultrasound study of term and preterm infants. Dev Med Child Neurol 32:669-678, 1990.
16. Hack M, Estabrook MM, Robertson SS: Development of sucking rhythm in preterm infants. Early Hum Dev 11:133-140, 1985.
16a. American Academy of Pediatrics: Diagnostic and Statistical Manual of Mental Disorders: Primary Care Version. Washington, DC: American Academy of Pediatrics, 1995.
17. Linscheid TR: Behavioral treatments for pediatric feeding disorders. Behav Modif 30:6-23, 2006.
18. McDonough S: Personal communication, 2007.
19. Gahagan S: Parental concern about eating behavior in early childhood. Submitted manuscript, 2007.
20. Hagekull B, Bohlin G, Rydell AM: Maternal sensitivity, infant temperament, and the development of early feeding problems. Infant Ment Health J 18:92-106, 1997.
21. Spock B: Dr. Spock Talks With Mothers—Growth and Guidance. Cambridge, MA: Riverside, 1961.
22. Anders TF: Clinical syndromes, relationship disturbances, and their assessment. In Sameroff AJ, Emde RN, eds: Relationship Disturbances in Early Childhood. New York: Basic Books, 1989, pp 125-144.
23. Chatoor I. Feeding disorders in infants and toddlers: diagnosis and treatment. Child and Adolescent Psychiatric Clinics of North America 11:163-183, 2002.
24. Spitzer RL, Williams JBW: Classification of mental disorders and DSM-III. In Kaplan H, Freedman AM, Sadock BJ, eds: Comprehensive Textbook of Psychiatry, vol 4. Baltimore: Williams & Wilkins, 1980, pp 1035-1072.
25. Chatoor I: Feeding disorders in infants and toddlers: Diagnosis and treatment. Child Adolesc Psychiatr Clin N Am 11:163-183, 2002.
26. Fraiberg S, ed: Clinical Studies in Infant Mental Health: The First Year of Life. New York: Basic Books, 1980.
27. Lumeng JC, Perez M, Gahagan S: Does Treatment of Undernutrition with Gastrostomy Tube Feeding Worsen Childhood Eating Disorders? PAS. May 1, 2001. Pediatric Research, 2001.
28. Chatoor I, Conley C, Dickson L: Food refusal after an incident of choking: A posttraumatic eating disorder. J Am Acad Child Adolesc Psychiatry 27:105-110, 1988.
29. Dellert SF, Hyams JS, Treem WR, et al: Feeding resistance and gastroesophageal reflux in infancy. J Pedatr Gastroenterol Nutr 17:66-71, 1993.
30. Di Scipio WS, Kaslon K: Conditioned dysphagia in cleft palate children after pharyngeal flap surgery. Psychosom Med 44:247-257, 1982.
31. Skuse D: Identification and management of problem eaters. Arch Dis Child 69:604-608, 1993.
32. Barnard K: Caregiver/Parent-Child Interaction Feeding Manual. Seattle: University of Washington School of Nursing, NCAST Publications, 1994.
33. Chatoor I, Getson P, Menville E, et al: A feeding scale for research and clinical practice to assess mother-infant interactions in the first three years of life. Infant Ment Health J 18:76-91, 1997.
34. Egan J, Chatoor I, Rosen G: Non-organic failure to thrive: Pathogenesis and classification. Clin Pro Child Hosp Nati Med Cent 36:173-182, 1980.
35. Chatoor I, Ganiban J, Surles J, et al: Physiological regulation and infantile anorexia: A pilot study. J Am Acad Child Adolesc Psychiatry 43:1019-1025, 2004.
36. Chatoor I, Ganiban J, Hirsch R, et al: Maternal characteristics and toddler temperament in infantile anorexia. J Am Acad Child Adolesc Psychiatry 39:743-751, 2000.

23C
Food Insecurity and Failure to Thrive

STEPHANIE BLENNER ■ MARYANN B. WILBUR ■ DEBORAH A. FRANK

EPIDEMIOLOGY AND CLINICAL SIGNIFICANCE

Food insecurity and nutritional growth failure, frequently termed *failure to thrive,* are common pediatric problems in the United States and even larger issues globally.[1,2] Although famine and malnutrition in the developing world are widely recognized, food insecurity in the United States remains relatively invisible. Food-insecure American children rarely resemble haunting images of hunger in the international media. However, many are not receiving adequate sustenance to support crucial development in early childhood. Insufficient nutrition, even without anthropometric changes, affects a child's behavior, learning, and social interactions.[3]

A startling number of American children are at risk for FTT. A U.S. Department of Agriculture study[4] revealed that in 2004, nearly 12% of U.S. households were "food insecure" (defined as being unable to obtain reliably sufficient nutritious food for an active, healthy life because of economic constraints). Food insecurity is even more prevalent among households with young children. Nearly 19% of American households with children younger than 6 years (the peak age for FTT) lacked consistent access to enough food for a healthy life in 2004.

Although not all children with FTT come from food-insecure families, poverty remains the most significant social risk factor for developing FTT. In some samples, as many as 10% of young, low-income American children meet criteria for FTT (see later "Diagnosis" section).[5] Developmental-behavioral clinicians usually do not become involved in a child's care until multiple cumulative experiences of food insecurity and associated medical and developmental risks manifest as FTT. As advocates for children, however, developmental-behavioral pediatricians should be aware that in low-income communities, children with FTT represent only part of a large problem. Many additional children experience food insecurity, which often acts as a precursor as well as a concomitant of FTT within a family, community, or population. FTT, in this regard, serves as a broad sentinel indicator of the health and well-being of children's communities.[6] The threshold at which per-

sistent developmental-behavioral risk emerges in young children on the continuum from household food insecurity without growth failure to FTT has not been established. Research findings from the Early Childhood Longitudinal Study[7] suggest that living in a food-insecure household during kindergarten is correlated with impaired social skills in girls and depressed third grade reading and math scores in both boys and girls, even after confound control.

Undernutrition in a young child, often in concert with other factors, is the key but not sole mechanism that disrupts cognitive and socioemotional development in children with FTT.[8] Studies of moderate to severe early malnutrition have shown detrimental effects on later cognitive measures,[9] increased rates of behavioral and mental health disorders,[10-13] and poorer school performance.[14-16] As noted, it is not only severely affected children with anthropometric deficits who are at risk. Children's physiology automatically conserves limited energy by decreasing social interaction and exploratory behavior.[17] This results in lost opportunities for language, cognitive, and social development. A meta-analysis revealed that even more mildly affected children with FTT managed in the outpatient setting had demonstrable decrements on later cognitive measures.[18] By virtue of their training, developmental-behavioral pediatricians are uniquely prepared to address the complex biopsychosocial factors, including proximal undernutrition, that contribute to FTT, with the goal of not only restoring growth but also ameliorating lasting developmental-behavioral sequelae.

ETIOLOGY

Too often, families of children with FTT are confronted with clinicians harboring the unstated assumption that the root cause of the child's difficulties is related to poor "mothering." This inaccurate perception springs from deep historical roots. The phrase *failure to thrive* was historically used by Spitz,[19,20] in his classic studies in the 1940s of "hospitalism," to describe children in orphanages suffering from "maternal deprivation." The concept was extended by Coleman and Provence[21] in the 1950s to describe two young children with feeding difficulties, growth retardation, and developmental delay living in college-educated families whose growth failure was, again, ascribed to "insufficient stimulation from the mother." The primary therapeutic intervention recommended for these home-reared children was "to modify the parents' attitude" or introduce a "mother substitute" via foster care.

Not until the groundbreaking work of Whitten and associates[22] in 1969 was the primary role of malnutrition in the development of FTT recognized. Since then, the field has advanced rapidly; the simplistic "maternal deprivation" model has been replaced by a more sophisticated understanding of the interplay of medical, nutritional, social, and developmental risks. However, historical stereotypes often persist, and many children are referred to developmental-behavioral pediatricians for the assessment of presumed primary and causal maternal incompetence, psychiatric disturbance, or culpability without systematic investigation of medical, nutritional, developmental, and social context.

Rather than accepting this presumption, the developmental-behavioral pediatric practitioner must draw on a spectrum of skills ranging from assessment of nutrition and feeding (as discussed in the earlier section on feeding disorders) to the diagnosis of acute and chronic medical illness and assessment of parent-child interaction, developmental risks, social stress, and family dynamics.

Moreover, developmental-behavioral pediatricians in their work with feeding disorders programs, neonatal follow-up clinics, and care of children with neurodevelopmental disabilities, autism, or other special health care needs may encounter children with complex cases of FTT. Thus, although diagnostically appealing, traditional dichotomous conceptualizations, such as organic versus nonorganic FTT, do not encompass the multifactorial causes of the disorder. Children with major medical conditions and FTT often have concomitant feeding or sensory issues. Families coping with a child's serious illness often lack adequate social and economic supports to buffer the stress of the child's condition. Conversely, apparently healthy children can have unidentified conditions like sleep-disordered breathing,[23] gastroesophageal reflux,[24] or subtle neurological dysfunction that contribute to their poor eating and growth. To be effective, the developmental-behavioral pediatrician must assess the child in the context of the entire family and, at a minimum, identify medical, nutritional, social, and developmental issues systematically and recommend further evaluation. In many settings, the developmental-behavioral pediatric practitioner must actually direct intensive diagnosis and treatment in these domains because effective management of affected children often exceeds the time available to primary care physicians. Rather than "ruling out" medical and nutritional conditions and then proceeding to address developmental and social issues, the successful practitioner, either alone or, ideally, with a multidisciplinary team, assesses and addresses these domains simultaneously, aware of how each affects the other. Current frameworks emphasize FTT as a "syndrome," a diagnosis of which is, for each child,

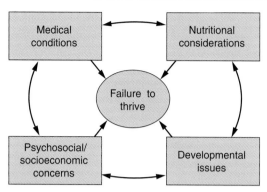

FIGURE 23C-1 A model for the development of failure to thrive.

identified through a complex network of contributions (Fig. 23C-1).

FTT, once established, often becomes self-perpetuating without clinical intervention. The behavioral effects of malnutrition contribute to the maintenance of FTT. Malnourished children, less likely to seek interaction and make demands to be fed, often do not elicit adequate nutrients or interpersonal stimulation from their caregivers. In addition, malnutrition depresses secretory immunoglobulin A levels, impairs cell-mediated immunity, and disrupts cytokine regulation.[25] Such compromised immune function manifests clinically as the frustrating malnutrition/infection cycle. As a result of functional immune compromise, children with FTT are more susceptible to illnesses such as gastroenteritis or otitis media. Caloric intake decreases, and utilization increases with each intercurrent illness, further inhibiting weight gain. From an ecological perspective, families struggle ineffectively to care for their ill and underweight child without adequate economic, physical, or social resources. The dynamic of a family dealing with a child's FTT parallels that of other chronic conditions during the time the child's growth is impaired. A complementary, multidisciplined approach—medical, nutritional, psychosocial, and developmental-behavioral—can validate caregivers' concerns and result in more thorough assessment and effective management.

DIAGNOSIS

Accurate diagnosis begins with careful anthropometric measurement, plotting of growth parameters, and consideration of growth trajectories over time. FTT is most commonly defined as a child's weight for age presenting at below the fifth percentile, a sustained decline in growth velocity, or a drop of more than two "major" percentiles after 18 months of age (e.g., a drop from the 50th to the 10th percentile). The child's height (or length under age 2 years) for age, weight for height (or body mass index in older children), and head circumference, in addition to weight for age, help determine the direction (or necessity) of diagnostic evaluation, as well as intervention.

Clinicians should use the most recent growth charts for sex and age published by the National Center for Health Statistics (NCHS), available online.[26] By international consensus, the NCHS growth charts serve currently as the references for evaluating growth in young children regardless of ethnic or racial background.[6] Despite their accepted use, these references include an unknown number of ill and deprived children and thus may be imprecise tools for identifying aberrant growth.[6] The World Health Organization[27] has developed standards for expected growth from a multiethnic, multinational sample restricted to healthy, initially breastfed children, which are publicly available.[6] To avoid a factitious diagnosis of FTT, it also is important to correct the following anthropometric measurements for prematurity: correct weight for age until 24 months chronological age, height for age until 42 months, and head circumference for age until 18 months.[28] Weight for length is not dependent on chronological or gestational age and does not require correction.

Frequently, scores on anthropometric measures of children with FTT fall below the lowest percentile shown on growth references, and growth failure must be classified more precisely than simply "less than the fifth percentile." Therefore, a standardized system for further ranking the severity of growth deficit, developed by Gomez and associates[29] and Waterlow,[30] defines anthropometric measurements as "percent standards" (percentage of the median). For example, a child's percent standard for weight for age is calculated by dividing his or her current weight by the median weight for chronological (or corrected) age and sex and multiplying by 100. This can be calculated for all four anthropometric measurements and allows identification of the degree of malnutrition. Table 23C-1 shows degrees of malnutrition based on percent standards for rapid clinical use. For research purposes, z-scores (standard deviation units) calculated from the NCHS growth grids are used, with parameters less than two standard deviations below the median (z-scores of −2 or lower) accepted as a threshold for identifying clinically serious malnutrition, even in developing countries.[2]

Consideration of all four anthropometric parameters is important because nutritional growth failure may manifest in several ways. Decreased weight for age may represent a composite indicator of either recent or past nutritional deprivation and can fluctuate acutely. Decreased height for age indicates more extended and chronic deprivation. It reflects slowed linear growth after weeks or months of inadequate

TABLE 23C-1 ■ Staging System for Malnutrition: Percent Standard as Indicator of Nutritional Deficit			
	Percent Standard		
Grade of Malnutrition	**Weight for Age**	**Height† for Age**	**Weight for Height†**
Normal	90-110	>95	>90
First degree (mild)*	75-89	90-94	80-89
Second degree (moderate)	60-74	85-89	70-79
Third degree (severe)	<60	<85	<70

*First-degree malnutrition is most common in the United States. "Mild" is a relative term; the consequences are clinically important, if not immediately life-threatening.
†Length is used under 2 years of age.

caloric intake. A depressed weight for length or height, along with a depressed height for age, may result from acute nutritional deprivation superimposed upon chronic deprivation. In chronic undernutrition, the child's weight for age typically "drops off," followed by a drop-off in height for age. This results in a child who appears proportionate, with a normal weight for height/length, or in older children, a normal body mass index, a pattern of growth impairment also seen with some genetic and endocrinological conditions. Although this child might look reasonably well nourished, he or she is actually "stunted." In acute malnutrition, a child's weight for age drops off while length/height for age remains in the normal range. This child appears emaciated, more like the images that the public and parents recognize as malnutrition. The ideal way to assess a child's growth is by looking at the child's growth trajectories over time. More sensitive than an isolated episodic measurement, this technique facilitates diagnosis by identifying the timing and sequence of anthropometric deficits.

ASSESSMENT

Assessment of the child who "fails to thrive" touches on core family dynamics: what it means to be a good parent able to nourish and provide for a child. Thorough assessment, even when performed skillfully, can cause caregivers to feel that their most fundamental abilities are being questioned. Initial clinical encounters should cultivate a supportive relationship and include overt acknowledgment of caregivers' desire to do the best for their child. Inviting families to partner with the clinical team lays a solid therapeutic foundation and empowers caregivers. At the same time, it is important to recognize the frustration many families feel when a child fails to thrive. Statements like "I can see you've tried several things to help Emily" and "We see many children with this problem" acknowledge the complementary perspectives of caregivers and clinicians, wherein one knows best the individual child and situation and the other has the benefit of broad experience and expertise. Because the origin of FTT is often multifactorial, a multidisciplinary assessment that includes medical, nutritional, psychosocial, and developmental parameters is important. Even in seemingly straightforward cases, thorough evaluation frequently identifies multiple causal contributors.

Medical History and Physical Examination

When participating in specialty evaluation or management of the child with FTT, the developmental-behavioral provider must first ensure that a thorough medical evaluation has been completed. The child's perinatal and postnatal medical history, as well as family history, should serve as starting points for evaluation. Caregiver report is crucial but should be supplemented by record review.

A history of low birth weight is associated with many developmental conditions and is a risk factor for later FTT.[31] Both prematurity and intrauterine growth restriction (IUGR) can result in low birth weight but can have different implications for postnatal growth. Although, as discussed previously, growth parameters for children born prematurely must be corrected for gestational age, growth rates should be comparable with (or greater than) those of full-term infants.[32] Formerly premature infants not growing at expected rates must be evaluated further. FTT in this population should not be attributed to "being born small." A history of prematurity is only a starting point that allows associated behavioral, oromotor, neurological, and other medical issues to be identified and addressed. Regardless of gestational age, infants with IUGR are at risk for postnatal FTT.[33] IUGR is conventionally defined as a birth weight less than the 10th percentile for gestational age. In this circumstance, it is important to determine the pattern of growth restriction. Symmetrical IUGR, with proportionate depression of weight, length, and head circumference at birth, carries a poorer prognosis for postnatal growth,[34] often portending long-term abnormalities of growth and development.[35] Asymmetrical growth restriction, which depresses weight to a greater degree than length or head circumference, has a better prognosis. This is because asymmetrical growth restriction is more likely to have had a maternal cause (such as preeclampsia) that is no longer present as an influence after birth. If provided optimal postnatal nutrition, infants with asymmetrical IUGR can often catch up in growth in the first years of life with subsequent normalization of growth trajectories.

TABLE 23C-2 ■ Common Medical Contributors to Failure to Thrive
Developmental conditions affecting intake and feeding (e.g., autism, cerebral palsy)
Syndromes (genetic, nongenetic)
Dental caries, adenoid-tonsillar hypertrophy
Allergies (food, environmental), eczema
Gastroesophageal reflux, celiac disease
Asthma, cystic fibrosis, congenital heart disease
Recurrent otitis media, enteric pathogens, HIV, hepatitis

HIV, human immunodeficiency virus.

Childhood conditions affecting growth are identified by a detailed history, review of systems, and physical examination. This should include information about chronic illnesses, consistency of medical care, hospitalizations or surgeries, medications, immunizations, allergies, and acquisition of developmental milestones. Family history should include both parents' attained heights[36] and both parents' ages at pubertal onset, if known, as well as medical, psychiatric, and developmental diagnoses. A thorough review of systems may identify previously undiagnosed contributing conditions. Clinicians should ask about symptoms that the caregiver may not recognize as related to poor growth, including diarrhea, vomiting, cough, gagging, snoring, fevers, rash, and painful teeth. The status and current management of previously diagnosed chronic conditions such as asthma or cerebral palsy, including effects on the child's daily appetite, energy demands, and dietary intake, as well as the effect on the quality of life of both child and caregivers, should be explored. Many medical conditions may contribute to the development of FTT. Although not an exhaustive summary, Table 23C-2 lists common medical contributors that can be identified by history, physical, and targeted laboratory assessment.

Laboratory Evaluation and Imaging

Historically it has been taught that laboratory evaluations identify very few occult causes of FTT. However, the data supporting this position date from the mid-1980s.[37] Despite the more recent emergence of new diagnostic assessments for food allergies, celiac disease, and subtle genetic and nongenetic syndromes, the current validity of this assumption has not been reevaluated. Nevertheless, it remains true that laboratory assessment should be guided primarily by meticulous history and physical examination. Basic laboratory evaluation includes complete blood cell count with differential, lead measurement, free erythrocyte protoporphyrins measurement, urinalysis/ urine culture, electrolyte measurements, blood urea nitrogen/creatinine measurements, and purified protein derivative skin test for tuberculosis; all of these are screens for common and treatable contributors to poor growth. Iron deficiency, with or without anemia, is seen at presentation in up to half of children with FTT, especially in low-income populations.[38] Iron deficiency directly impairs growth, development, and behavior. It also increases anorexia and enhances environmental lead absorption, raising the risk of lead toxicity.[39]

Additional laboratory work should be obtained only as indicated by history and physical examination findings. This may include human immunodeficiency virus testing, a sweat test for cystic fibrosis, or serum immunoglobulin A and anti-transglutaminase antibodies to screen for celiac disease.[40] Nutritional vitamin D deficiency can lead to rickets, especially in breastfed, dark-skinned infants in northern latitudes and should be sought in infants with suggestive physical findings or history.[41] Zinc deficiency impairs growth, taste perception, and functional activity level and may also be part of targeted screening.[42] Children with abdominal pain may benefit from testing for *Helicobacter pylori* infection.[43] If the child is a recent immigrant or traveler, is living in a shelter, is attending a childcare program, or has been camping and has diarrhea or abdominal discomfort, evaluation for enteric pathogens such as *Giardia lamblia* and *Cryptosporidium parvum* would be appropriate. Radioallergosorbent or skin testing for food allergies should be considered in children with atopic dermatitis, chronic rhinitis, or wheezing. Children with dysmorphic features and cardiac or other malformations should undergo careful assessment for genetic and nongenetic syndromes that may contribute to growth failure (see Chapter 10B). Since the advent of neonatal screening, previously undiagnosed inborn errors of metabolism (see Chapter 10C) and primary endocrine causes of FTT, such as hypothyroidism, are usually identified perinatally but must be considered in selected cases especially among children born overseas or in states without comprehensive neonatal screening programs.

For children whose weight is decreased in proportion to height and for whom underlying causes remain unclear, a bone age can be helpful in differentiating constitutional short stature from stunting resulting from undernutrition. Children with constitutional short stature have a bone age commensurate with chronological age; in nutritionally or hormonally stunted children, bone age is less than chronological age and similar to height age. When diagnosing constitutional short stature, clinicians should be aware of a study indicating that children with the diagnosis of idiopathic short stature often have more problematic (picky) eating behavior and reduced body mass index, which thus warrants an attempt at nutritional intervention.[44]

Nutritional Considerations

Comprehensive, longitudinal nutritional assessment is crucial. Current intake and feeding practices, along with historical information, must be elicited. As noted in the section on feeding disorders, particular attention should be paid to vulnerable nutritional transition points, such as weaning from breast or bottle or the introduction of solids, which are often associated with the onset of growth difficulties. The timing of growth failure, correlated with nutritional transitions, may suggest possible causes. For example, a clinician identifying FTT in a newly formula-fed infant is advised to consider whether there is incorrect preparation of formula or insufficient family resources to purchase adequate formula. FTT occurring after the introduction of cow's milk might suggest milk protein or lactose intolerance. Components of the nutritional assessment are summarized in Table 23C-3.

When assessing current feeding practices, the clinician should explore family mealtime routines in detail. It is very informative to inquire specifically who feeds the child and where and when the child is fed. Does the child sit at the table, in a high chair, or on an adult's lap? What happens if the child does not want to eat or wants to feed herself or himself? Are mealtimes stressful and, if so, in what way? A description of a typical meal, beginning with how the child signals hunger through to how meal termination is decided may be useful. Dietary recall from the preceding 24 hours and a 7-day food frequency are essential in determining the quality, quantity, and components of a child's diet. Once again, questions should be specific: for example, not only how many cups of juice, but how big is a "cup"? How many spoonfuls of cereal? Whole milk or 2% milk? When possible, observation of a feeding in the home or medical office can identify concerns not identified through caregiver report. This is especially true with difficult caregiver-child interactions or subtle neurological issues, which were discussed earlier in this chapter. Interactive difficulties are unlikely to be identified by history alone when the adult giving the history is a participant in the interaction.

Several feeding issues are frequent contributors to FTT in children and merit specific mention. In infants, poor weight gain often results from breastfeeding difficulties, formula preparation errors, dilution of formula to stretch limited resources,[45] and mixing large amounts of cereal into bottles. In toddlers and preschoolers, excessive consumption of juice,[46] water, soda, tea, sports drinks, or thin soups instead of solids or milk is a common contributor. "Grazing" (eating

TABLE 23C-3 ■ The Nutritional Assessment

Feeding History

Breast milk or formula
Age when solids were introduced
Age when switched to whole milk
Food allergy or intolerance
Vitamin or mineral supplementation
24-Hour dietary recall and 7-day food frequency

Current Feeding Behaviors

Difficulties with sucking, chewing, or swallowing
Frequency of feeding
Who feeds the child
Where the child is fed
Finickiness, negativism
Perceived appetite
Pica

Caretaker's Nutrition Knowledge

Language or literacy difficulties
Adequacy of developmentally appropriate nutrition
    information
Dietary beliefs (religious, fad diets, parental fears)

Adequacy of Financial Resources for Food Purchase

Food stamps
Nutrition program for Women, Infants, and Children (WIC)
Earned income
Recent change in income
Unemployment benefits
Transitional Assistance to Needy Families (TANF) (formerly
    "welfare")
Supplemental Social Security Income (SSI)
Family's budgeting abilities

Material Resources for Food Preparation and Storage

Refrigeration
Cooking facilities
Running water
Access to supermarkets

TABLE 23C-4 ■ Common Psychosocial Contributors to Failure to Thrive

Social

Resource constraint
Homelessness
Lack of access to food
Lack of access to food preparation (running water, stove,
    refrigeration)

Psychodynamic

Stressed home environment
Overcrowded, busy household
Overwhelmed or inexperienced caregiver
Caregiver depression
Family violence
Diffuse caregiving, chaotic schedules
Caregiver's cognitive limitations
Dysregulated parent-child interaction

Unusual Health Beliefs

Belief that adult diets benefit children
Low-fat, low-calorie diets
"Fad diets"
Belief that lots of water is good for children

frequently in very small amounts) suppresses appetite[47] and often leads to poor weight gain in young children.

Family Resources and Psychosocial Concerns

Inadequate resources and psychosocial stressors frequently play a role in families of children with FTT. It is important to inquire directly about family composition, income sources, housing, childcare, social supports, and availability of food throughout the month. Neither full-time work nor the receipt of public support ensures adequate food in the home. The Women, Infants, and Children (WIC) nutrition program and food stamps provide only a portion of a family's food expenses. These benefits are often tenuous, subject to time restrictions and maintenance of paperwork. Termination of benefits can tip the

scales in an at-risk household. Families whose welfare benefits are terminated or reduced have an almost 50% higher risk of being food insecure than do similar families whose benefits are intact.[48] Issues associated with poverty, including disconnected utilities and unreliable transportation, also negatively affect treatment success if not identified and addressed.

In all social strata, even the most privileged, the emotional functioning of family members is an important factor in children's growth. A wide range of psychosocial factors contributes to the development of FTT (Table 23C-4). Caregiver psychopathology (particularly depression), substance use, and interpersonal violence distort caregiver-child interactions and can lead to unresponsive parenting, erratic feeding schedules, and, at times, frank neglect. Stress caused by the child's condition may contribute additionally to caregiver depression. Sensitive interviewing helps identify these issues. Formal questionnaires also may be used to screen for caregiver depression.[49] One community study revealed that mothers of young children with FTT were more likely to report increased symptons on depression screening.[50] The quality of the home environment can be more difficult to ascertain without a home visit by a skilled clinician. Validated instruments such as the Home Observation for Measurement of the Environment scale are often used, particularly in research.[51]

In assessing these concerns, the clinician must determine whether a child's safety and well-being are at risk, and he or she must involve protective services when risk is indicated. In addition, although it is uncommon, school-aged children who present with the typical symptoms of hyperphagic short stature (formerly termed *psychosocial dwarfism*), including food scavenging, disrupted sleep, and encopresis or enuresis, often have a transient depression of growth hormone and are uniformly victims of serious and prolonged maltreatment. These children must be removed from the home or institution in which the maltreatment occurred.[52]

Developmental Issues

Developmental issues and temperamental characteristics of both caregiver and child must be considered. Specific caregiver concerns and how they are expressed may reveal inappropriate expectations. Particular attention should be paid to young or inexperienced caregivers and parents with cognitive limitations. A review of a caregiver's educational history, including learning problems, special education, and highest level of education completed, may identify caregiver challenges not obvious in casual conversation. Conversely, caregivers may not realize that the predictable developmental stages discussed earlier in this chapter are affecting a child's feeding behavior. Limited caregiver understanding of these stages may contribute to FTT.

Children with FTT are at higher risk for developmental delay and may have reductions in exploratory behaviors, both resulting from and contributing to their malnutrition. Less interactive children receive diminished environmental stimulation and reinforcement. Transactionally, this can exacerbate underlying developmental vulnerabilities and delays, which results in more significant morbidity.[53] The effects of early FTT on cognitive development are "dose" related: More severely affected children demonstrate a greater decrement on concurrent and later cognitive measures. In one analysis, pooled data from cases identified in primary care revealed FTT in infancy to have an effect size of −0.28 (−4.2 points) on later IQ testing.[18] Of importance is that because FTT often occurs in children with other risk factors affecting cognitive development, the decrement related to the FTT may be only one of several factors negatively affecting the child's development. Formal developmental assessment can identify delays and may lead to interventions that improve outcomes.

Children with underlying developmental conditions and specific difficulties contributing to FTT often benefit from additional evaluation. Examples include children with autism and food neophobia, oral aversion secondary to prolonged nasogastric feeding, poorly coordinated suck/swallow skills, and oromotor dysfunction.[54] Occupational or speech therapy evaluation, with swallow study when indicated, can be helpful for the child presenting with oromotor dyscoordination or maladaptive oral motor tone (discussed earlier in this chapter). Such a referral helps rule out tactile hypersensitivity, swallowing difficulties, and other contributing factors. It also informs subsequent development of an appropriate feeding plan for caregivers specifying how food, as well as what kinds of foods, should be offered.

MANAGEMENT

Effective management of the child who fails to thrive is directed by information gathered during the clinical assessment. Identified contributing factors unique to each child and family must be comprehensively addressed, as discussed later in this chapter. Frequent follow-up with practical, responsive interventions as the condition evolves are crucial for successful management. The importance of active caregiver involvement and a multidisciplinary approach cannot be overstated. Research shows improved outcome with management by a multidisciplinary team, which includes, for example, a physician, a nutritionist, a social worker, a mental health provider, and, potentially, a speech and/or an occupational therapist.[55]

Medical Treatment

The most immediate issue in managing a child with FTT, even in the context of developmental-behavioral subspecialty care, is ensuring the child's medical stability. Most children can be successfully managed as outpatients. Hospitalization is an added stress for families, disrupts mealtimes and feeding patterns, and increases risk for nosocomial infection. However, acute hospitalization is mandatory for a child classified as "severely malnourished" with third-degree malnutrition (see Table 23C-1) or for a child who fails to gain weight or continues to consistently lose weight despite aggressive outpatient management, as well as for children with serious, intercurrent infections or uncontrolled chronic illnesses.

After ensuring a child's acute stability, the physician must address issues uncovered during the assessment. Often, this involves intensified management of chronic conditions or additional specialty involvement for newly identified concerns. It is also crucial that the physician address the infection/malnutrition cycle with prompt identification and treatment of even low-grade infection. Children with FTT should receive all age-appropriate immunizations, including annual influenza vaccine after 6 months of age.

Nutritional Intervention

The initial objective of nutritional intervention is for the child to consume enough calories to enable catch-

TABLE 23C-5 ■ Recommended Daily Allowance (RDA) and Growth Rates for Children

Age	RDA (kcal/kg/day)	Median Weight Gain (grams/day)
0-3 months	108	26-31
3-6 months	108	17-18
6-9 months	98	12-13
9-12 months	98	9
1-3 years	102	7-9
4-6 years	90	6

From National Resource Council, Food and Nutrition Board: Recommended Daily Allowances. Washington, DC: National Academy of Sciences, 1989.

TABLE 23C-6 ■ Basic Nutritional Supplementation

Type	Calories Provided	How to Use
Fortified infant formulas	Variable	Increase caloric concentration
Polycose powder	23 kcal/tbsp	Add to formula or food
Instant breakfast mix	130 kcal/packet	Add to whole milk
PediaSure, Nutren, Boost, Bright Beginnings	30 kcal/oz	Ready to feed
Duocal	42 kcal/tbsp	Add to formula, milk, food

up growth. Adequate catch-up growth rates for children with FTT can be as much as two to three times average rates (available in Table 23C-5).[56] This is clearly a challenge because, by definition, these children are not maintaining even average rates of weight gain. Depending on severity of malnutrition at presentation, catch-up growth rates must be maintained for 4 to 9 months to restore a child's weight for height.[57]

Nutritional intervention begins with ensuring that caregivers are engaged and understand therapeutic goals. Success may necessitate involving all current caregivers of the child (for example, including a grandmother or childcare worker) or putting together nutritional plans for the preschool. Caregiver education about what constitutes a healthy diet and children's dietary needs at particular ages provides the basis for diet modification and additional intervention. Families receive nutritional misinformation from multiple sources including cultural traditions, well-meaning family and friends, television, and commercial advertising. Common misconceptions include the constipating effect of iron in infant formula, the nutritional value of fruit juice, perceived benefits of allowing an underweight child to graze and eat many sweets, and the appropriateness of adult low-fat diets for children.[58] In addition to correcting misconceptions, clinicians should not assume that caregivers are familiar with basic nutritional tenets. Important concepts must be explicit reviewed. Caregivers may need to be taught to offer solids before liquids, that young children require both morning and afternoon snacks, to decrease juice intake to 4 to 6 oz/day, and to limit snacks and drinks with low caloric density and nutritional value. The importance of structured family meals without television and the developmental basis for feeding behaviors and food choices often merit review with families.

Although caregiver education is crucial, it is equally important to present a concrete plan addressing a child's particular needs. Many caregivers respond positively to a formal feeding plan drawn up in collaboration with the clinician. A written schedule listing times for meals (three per day) and snacks (two to three per day), along with suggested meal choices based on a child's preferences, is helpful, especially for less experienced parents or multiple caregiver situations. Dietary modification and nutritional intervention should be based on a child's caloric needs. The caloric intake needed for catch-up growth can be estimated by dividing the average calorie requirement for age (as listed in Table 23C-5) by the child's weight as a percentage of median weight for age. For example, a 12-month-old (average requirement for age, 102 kcal/kg) who weighs 75% of the median weight for age would need 102/0.75, or 136 kcal/kg/day.[59] Depending on the severity of the initial malnutrition and the nutritional stresses of acute or chronic illness, a child may require as much as two times maintenance calories for adequate catch-up growth.

For some mildly affected children, target intake can be achieved by dietary manipulation: increasing caloric density without specialized supplementation. Many children, however, require a period of specialized oral supplementation, the options for which are presented in Table 23C-6 and depend on a child's age and needs. If available, consultation with a registered dietitian is recommended. It is rare for a child to be unable to consume adequate supplementation orally, but in such cases, nasogastric or gastrostomy tube feedings improve weight gain and must be implemented.[60] With these severely affected children, formal consultation with hospital-based nutrition support services is necessary. After a period of supplemental nutrition, a child should be monitored closely until the clinician ensures that the child can be weaned successfully to a regular diet administered orally and maintain normal rates of growth without supplementation.

Finally, the clinician must remember that a diet inadequate in calories and protein is frequently deficient in micronutrients as well. Catch-up growth rates increase micronutrient demand and may additionally deplete a child's micronutrient stores. For these reasons, all children with FTT should receive a daily multivitamin/multimineral preparation containing iron, calcium, and zinc. This ensures micronutrient intake, allowing caregivers to focus on increasing dietary calories rather than worrying about vitamin and micronutrient content. Children with frank anemia should receive therapeutic iron dosing until the anemia is corrected, and those with rickets should be treated with therapeutic doses of vitamin D.[41]

Psychosocial Support

Addressing the environmental context in which the child resides constitutes a crucial component of treatment. The goal must always be a thriving child in a thriving environment. After sensitively ascertaining what psychosocial needs are present, the clinician must address those needs practically. This may be as simple as supportive conversation and encouragement during the child's treatment. However, it often also involves mobilization of community resources. Social workers, while addressing mental health issues, may also link families to food pantries or cooperatives, food stamps, WIC, Supplemental Security Income, Temporary Assistance for Needy Families, housing subsidies, and energy programs to ensure a stable food supply, as well as utilities and means to cook and store food. The clinical approach must ensure that a family is capable of following through on clinical and nutritional recommendations. It is unfair and counterproductive to prescribe a diet and feeding regimen without confirming that the family has the means to follow recommendations.

In cases of caregiver psychopathology or disturbance of the parent-child relationship, it may be necessary to arrange formal counseling or psychiatric consultation for the child, caregiver, or family. If the clinic team does not include a mental health practitioner, clinicians should keep an active list of accessible mental health resources. If, after sufficient support has been provided, the family is unable to meet a child's nutritional and social needs, the clinical team must decide together whether this constitutes child neglect or maltreatment and mandates protective services involvement.

Addressing Developmental Needs

Finally, support for the child's developmental needs is crucial. Intervention begins with reframing typical developmental issues affecting feeding. Reflecting caregiver concerns or voicing observations of the parent-child interaction, in such ways as "Brandon is so active that he doesn't want to sit and eat" or "Katy really tries to feed herself, but it must be hard to deal with the mess," is often helpful in allowing parents to become thoughtful observers of their child's behavior. This is often the first step in addressing inappropriate expectations, decreasing power struggles, and cultivating more tolerant, nurturing interactions. Subsequent discussion of typical developmental struggles seen at particular ages helps put the child's behavior in a nonpathological perspective and helps caregivers appreciate their child's striving for independence and mastery.

Caregiver observation of formal developmental testing can invite discussion of a child's particular abilities and challenges. For children at risk for or found to have developmental delay, referral to early intervention programs (for children 36 months or younger) or to the public school system (for those older than 36 months) is imperative. Formal programs to enhance development result in improved outcomes for children with FTT,[61,62] particularly language and cognitive development in children younger than age 2 years.[63,64] Children with oromotor dysfunction secondary to neurological or developmental conditions often require specialized occupational therapy intervention with gradual introduction of foods and textures to develop age-appropriate competencies.[65]

Implications

Ironically, young children who are most vulnerable to the developmental effects of undernutrition are also most likely to experience it. Malnutrition uniquely affects the developing brain. In infants and young children, the growing brain accounts for up to 80% of the body's glucose usage.[66] This sensitive developmental period is characterized by biosynthetic capabilities and neural genesis that do not persist into later life.[54,67] When a young child experiences undernutrition, these processes are compromised. Depending on the timing, duration, and severity of malnutrition, the effect is potentially lifelong. Current deprivation and future life course are linked irrevocably.

Much remains to be learned about the long-term effects of food insecurity and FTT in childhood. Research findings suggest that the implications for later health may be broader than previously appreciated. Animal and human studies have identified catch-up growth in early childhood (rapid weight gain after a period of undernutrition) as a risk factor for obesity and adult-onset type 2 diabetes later in life.[68,69] In short, the same metabolic adaptations that work to minimize detrimental effects of undernutrition on brain growth during the perinatal period and early childhood period may paradoxically contribute to the development of obesity when nutrition is no longer compromised. Nevertheless, intact cognition and behavior are irreducible requirements for functioning successfully in the modern world, and they must be preserved.

Most pediatricians agree that hunger and malnutrition are unacceptable in the 21st century. In understanding the developmental implications, moral imperative becomes professional mandate. The relatively benign labels *food insecurity* and *failure to thrive* do not adequately convey the potential long-lasting implications for a child's development. Continued research into the processes of causation and prevention, as well as medical, psychosocial, and political interventions, are crucial for altering the potentially adverse trajectory for affected children.

REFERENCES

1. El-Ghannam A: The global problems of child malnutrition and mortality in different world regions. J Health Soc Policy 16(4):1-26, 2003.

2. deOnis M, Blossner M, Borghi E, et al: Estimates of global prevalence of childhood underweight in 1990 and 2015. JAMA 291:2600-2606, 2004.

3. Weinreb L: Hunger: Its impact on children's health and mental health. Pediatrics 110(4):e41, 2002.

4. Nord M, Andrews M, Carlson S: Household Food Security in the United States, 2003. Washington, DC: U.S. Department of Agriculture, Economic Research Service, 2004. (Available at: *http://www.ers.usda.gov/publications/err11/;* accessed 2/5/07.)

5. Frank D, Drotar D, Cook J, et al: Failure to thrive. *In* Reece R, Ludwig S, eds: Child Abuse: Medical Diagnosis and Management. Baltimore: Lippincott Williams & Wilkins, 2001, pp 307-338.

6. Garza C, deOnis M: Rationale for developing a new international growth reference. Food Nutr Bull 25(1): S5-S14, 2004.

7. Jyoti D, Frongillo E, Jones S: Food insecurity affects children's academic performance, weight gain, and social skills. J Nutr 135:2831-2839, 2005.

8. Galler JR, Barrett L: Children and famine: Long-term impact on development. Ambul Child Health 7(2):85-95, 2001.

9. Liu J, Raine A, Venables PH, et al: Malnutrition at age 3 years and lower cognitive ability at age 11 years. Arch Pediatr Adolesc Med 157:593-600, 2003.

10. Galler JR, Ramsey F: A follow-up study of the influence of early malnutrition on development: Behavior at home and at school. J Am Acad Child Adolesc Psychiatry 28:593-600, 1989.

11. St. Clair D, Xu M, Wang P, et al: Rates of adult schizophrenia following prenatal exposure to the Chinese famine of 1959-1961. JAMA 294:557-562, 2005.

12. Neugebauer R, Hoek H, Susser E: Prenatal exposure to wartime famine and development of antisocial personality disorder in early adulthood. JAMA 282:455-462, 1999.

13. Susser E, Neugebauer R, Hoek K, et al: Schizophrenia after prenatal famine: Further evidence. Arch Gen Psychiatry 53:25-31, 1996.

14. Galler JR, Famsey S, Solimano G: The influence of early malnutrition on subsequent behavioral development III: Learning disabilities as a sequel to malnutrition. Pediatr Res 18:309-313, 1984.

15. Kerr M, Black M, Krishnakumar A: Failure-to-thrive, maltreatment and the behavior and development of 6-year-old children from low-income, urban familes: A cumulative risk model. Child Abuse Negl 24:587-598, 2000.

16. Dykman R, Casey P, Ackerman P, et al: Behavioral and cognitive status in school-aged children with a history of failure to thrive during early childhood. Clin Pediatr 40:63-70, 2001.

17. Beaton G: Nutritional needs during the first year of life: Some concepts and perspectives. Pediatr Clin North Am 32:275-288, 1985.

18. Corbett S, Drewett R: To what extent is failure to thrive in infancy associated with poorer cognitive development? A review and metanalysis. J Child Psychol Psychiatry 45:641-654, 2004.

19. Spitz R: Hospitalism. Psychoanal Study Child 1:53, 1945.

20. Spitz R: Hospitalism: A following-up report. Psychoanal Study Child 2:113, 1946.

21. Coleman R, Provence S: Environmental retardation (hospitalism) in infants living in families. Pediatrics 19:285-292, 1957.

22. Whitten C, Pettit M, Fischhoff J: Evidence that growth failure from maternal deprivation is secondary to undereating. JAMA 209:1675-1682, 1969.

23. Bonuck K: Sleep-disordered breathing and failure to thrive: Research vs practice. Arch Pediatr Adolesc Med 159:299-300, 2005.

24. Hassall E: Decisions in diagnosing and managing chronic gastroesophageal reflux disease in children. J Pediatr 146:S3-S12, 2005.

25. Chevalier P, Sevilla R, Sejas R, et al: Immune recovery of malnourished children takes longer than nutritional recovery: Implication for treatment and discharge. J Trop Pediatr 44:304-307, 1998.

26. National Center for Health Statistics: 2000 CDC Growth Charts: United States. Hyattsville, MD: National Center for Health Statistics, 2000. (Available at: *www.cdc.gov/growthcharts;* accessed 2/5/07.)

27. World Health Organization: The WHO Child Growth Standards. Geneva, Switzerland: World Health Organization, undated. (Available at: *http://www.who.int/childgrowth/standards/en/;* accessed 2/5/07.)

28. Brandt I: Growth dynamics of low birthweight infants with emphasis on the perinatal period. *In* Falkner F, Tanner J, eds: Human Growth, Neurobiology and Nutrition. New York: Plenum Press, 1979, pp pp 415-475.

29. Gomez F, Galvan R, Frenk S, et al: Mortality in second and third degree malnutrition. J Trop Pediatr 2:77-83, 1956.

30. Waterlow J: Classification and definition of protein-calorie malnutrition. BMJ 3:566-569, 1972.

31. Dusick A, Poindexter B, Ehrenkranz R, et al: Growth failure in the preterm infant: Can we catch up? Semin Perinatol 27:302-310, 2003.

32. Casey P, Kraemer HC, Bernbaum J, et al: Growth status and growth rates of a varied sample of low birth weight, preterm infants: A longitudinal cohort from birth to three years of age. J Pediatr 119:599-605, 1991.

33. Hediger M, Overpeck MD, Maurer KR, et al: Growth of infants and young children born small or large for gestational age. Arch Pediatr Adolesc Med 152:1225-1231, 1998.

34. Luo Z, Albertsson-Wikland K, Karlberg J: Length and body mass index at birth and target height influences patterns of postnatal growth in children born small for gestational age. Pediatrics 102(6):E72, 1998.

35. Frisk V, Amsel R, Whyte H: The importance of head growth patterns in predicting the cognitive abilities and literacy skills of small-for-gestational-age children. Dev Neuropsychol 22:565-593, 2002.

36. Blair P, Drewett R, Emmett P, et al: Family, socioeconomic and prenatal factors associated with failure to thrive in the Avon Longitudinal Study of Parents and Children (ALSPAC). Int J Epidemiol 33:839-847, 2004.

37. Berwick DM, Levy JC, Kleinerman R: Failure to thrive: Diagnostic yield of hospitalization. Arch Dis Child 57:347-351, 1982.

38. Bithoney W, Ratbun J: Failure to thrive. *In* Levine M, Carey WB, Cracker AC, eds: Developmental-Behavioral. Pediatrics Philadelphia: WB Saunders 1983, pp 557-572.

39. Lozoff B, Jimenez E, Hagen J, et al: Poorer behavioral and developmental outcome more than 10 years after treatment for iron deficiency in infancy. Pediatrics 105(4):e51, 2001.

40. Catassi C, Farsano A: Celiac disease as a cause of growth retardation in childhood. Curr Opin Pediatr 16:445-449, 2004.

41. Gartner L, Greer F: Prevention of rickets and vitamin D deficiency: New guidelines for vitamin D intake. Pediatrics 111:908-910, 2003.

42. Black M: Zinc deficiency and child development. Am J Clin Nutr 68:464S-469S, 1998.

43. Yang Y, Sheu B, Lee S, et al: Children of *Helicobacter pylori*–infected mothers are predisposed to *H. pylori* acquisition with subsequent iron deficiency and growth retardation. Helicobacter 10:249-255, 2005.

44. Wudy S, Hagemann S, Dempfle A, et al: Children with idiopathic short stature are poor eaters and have decreased body mass index. Pediatrics 116(1):e52-e57, 2005.

45. Fein S, Falci C: Infant formula preparation, handling and related practices in the United States. J Am Diet Soc 99:1234-1240, 1999.

46. Dennison B: Fruit juice consumption by infants and children: A review. J Am Coll Nutr 15:4S-11S, 1996.

47. Haptinstall F, Puckering C, Skuse D, et al: Nutrition and meal-time behavior in families of growth retarded children. Hum Nutr Appl Nutr 41(A):390-402, 1987.

48. Cook J, Frank DA, Berkowitz C, et al: Welfare reform and the health of young children: A sentinel survey in 6 cities. Arch Pediatr Adolesc Med 156:678-684, 2005.

49. U.S. Preventive Services Task Force: Screening for Depression. Ann Intern Med 136:760, 2002.

50. O'Brien L, Heycock EG, Hanna M, et al: Postnatal depression and faltering growth: A community study. Pediatrics 113:1242-1247, 2004.

51. Caldwell C, Bradley R: Administration Manual: Home Observation for the Measurement of the Environment (HOME), rev ed. Little Rock: University of Arkansas, 1984.

52. Gilmore J, Skuse D: A case-comparison study of the characteristics of children with a short stature syndrome induced by stress (hyperphagic short stature) and a consecutive series of unaffected "stressed" children. J Child Psychol Psychiatr 40:969-978, 1999.

53. Sameroff D: Environmental context of child development. J Pediatr 109:192-200, 1986.

54. Skuse D, Pickles A, Wolke D, et al: Postnatal growth and mental development: Evidence for a "sensitive period." J Child Psychol Psychiatry 35:521-545, 1994.

55. Bithoney W, McJunkin J, Michalek J, et al: Prospective evaluation of weight gain in both nonorganic and organic failure-to-thrive children: An outpatient trial of multidisciplinary team intervention strategy. J Dev Behav Pediatrics 10:27-31, 1989.

56. Guo M, Roche A, Fomon S, et al: Reference data on gains in weight and length during the first two years of life. J Pediatr 119:355-362, 1991.

57. Casey P, Arnold W: Compensatory growth in infants with severe failure to thrive. South Med J 78:1057-1060, 1985.

58. Pugliese M, Weyman-Daum M, Moses N, et al: Parental health beliefs as a cause of nonorganic failure to thrive. Pediatrics 80:175-182, 1987.

59. Frank DA, Needleman R, Silva M: What to do when a child won't grow. Patient Care 15:107-135, 1994.

60. Shapiro B, Green P, Krick J, et al: Growth of severely impaired children: Neurological versus nutritional factors. Dev Med Child Neurol 28:729-733, 1986.

61. Black M: Nutrition and brain development. *In* Walker W, Duggan C, Watkins J, eds: Nutrition in Pediatrics. New York: BC Decker, 2003, pp 386-396.

62. Walker S, Grantham-McGregor S, Powell CA, et al: Effects of growth restriction in early childhood on growth, IQ, and cognition at age 11 to 12 and the benefits of nutritional supplementation and psychosocial stimulation. J Pediatr 137:36-41, 2000.

63. Black M, Dubowitz H, Hutcheson J, et al: A randomized clinical trial of home intervention for children with failure to thrive. Pediatrics 95:807-814, 1995.

64. Powell C, Baker-Henningham H, Walker S, et al: Feasibility of integrating early stimulation into primary care for undernourished Jamaican children: Cluster randomized controlled trial. BMJ 329:89, 2004.

65. Case-Smith J: Occupational Therapy for Children. St. Louis: Elsevier, 2005.

66. Sann L, Simonnet C: Recent data on cerebral circulation and metabolism of the brain in newborn infants. Presse Med 6:1465-1469, 1985.

67. Chugani H: A critical period of brain development: studies of cerebral glucose utilization with PET. Prev Med 27:184-188, 1998.

68. Ong K, Ahmed M, Emmett P, et al: Association between postnatal catch-up growth and obesity in childhood: prospective cohort study. BMJ 320:967-971, 2000.

69. Hales C, Ozanne S: The dangerous road of catch-up growth. J Physiol 547:5-10, 2003.

23D
Obesity and Restrictive Eating Disorders

JULIE C. LUMENG

As children mature and attain increasing autonomy over food choices and eating behaviors, developmental-behavioral goals for all children are (1) healthy dietary and physical activity habits, (2) maintenance of weight in a healthy range, and (3) the development of a positive and realistic self-concept and body image. Unfortunately, too many children struggle with each of these goals. Many children are unable to maintain a weight in a healthy range, becoming either underweight or overweight. Simultaneously, the media sends repeatedly conflicting messages that both encourage consumption of low-nutrition, high–caloric density foods and idealize an unattainable and unhealthy body type. In addition, the media promotes unhealthy methods of weight loss, including fad diets and dietary supplements that are expensive, time consuming, and often dangerous for children.

Both obesity and restrictive eating disorders have increased in frequency since the 1960s. Empirical data are more robust and the increases more dramatic for obesity. The causes of both restrictive eating disorders and obesity are complex and multifactorial, both disorders being the final common pathway resulting from the interaction of numerous biological and environmental risk factors. There is a substantial heritable contribution to both obesity risk and restrictive eating disorders.[1,2] However, the rapid shift in population prevalence is proof that these disorders are not caused by genetics alone but are at least in part a product of the changing environment.

Both restrictive eating disorders and obesity have implications for lifelong physical and emotional well-being, are difficult to treat, and have low rates of remission. Although treatment of both obesity and restrictive eating disorders focuses on healthy eating practices and a healthy body image, obesity prevention and treatment programs typically assume or promote dissatisfaction with body size. Current interventions encourage individuals to monitor and restrict intake and content of foods eaten.[3] Eating disorder prevention and treatment programs, on the other hand, promote self-acceptance regardless of weight, discourage self-consciousness about food consumption, and promote an overall goal of improved body self-image regardless of weight. Professionals and parents may be reluctant to address one condition (obesity or restrictive eating disorders) or the other for fear of inducing the opposite. Despite ample anecdotal reports, there have been no large trials to evaluate the risk that a prevention program for one condition will increase the risk for the other. Dieting behavior in general, however, appears to be a risk factor for the development of both conditions. Dieting behavior increases the risk of the development of an eating disorder during adolescence,[4] and self-reported dieting is associated with a greater likelihood of the development of obesity in 9- to 14-year-olds.[5] Many girls in fourth grade and younger self-report "being on a diet."[5]

This section compares and contrasts both disorders, which occur at opposite ends of the weight spectrum and have both convergent and divergent properties. A brief overview of each condition is provided first.

OBESITY

Childhood obesity is defined as a body mass index greater than or equal to the 95th percentile for age and gender, according to standardized growth charts. The prevalence of childhood obesity has increased from approximately 5% in the 1960s to a present rate of 15% of 6- to 11-year-olds.[6,7] The prevalence of obesity is increasing across racial/ethnic and socioeconomic groups; however, in both adults and children, the rate of increase is significantly greater in low-income and minority populations. In the 1980s, for example, the prevalence of obesity among upper-income white girls was approximately equal to that among lower-income black and Hispanic boys, both at about 7%. By the late 1990s, however, the prevalence in upper-income white girls had remained essentially unchanged, whereas the prevalence in low-income minority boys had nearly quadrupled to more than 27%.[8]

The genetic component of obesity is conceptualized primarily as rooted in differences in metabolism, although hard data to support such a view are limited. Perhaps the strongest evidence for genetically or metabolically mediated differences in the development of obesity is derived from the observation of early growth patterns. For example, maternal obesity during pregnancy contributes to increased obesity risk in the offspring in adulthood, as does a pattern of slow growth in utero followed by rapid growth in early childhood.[9] Early adiposity rebound has also been cited as a risk factor in several studies.[10,11] It remains unknown whether early adiposity rebound is simply a marker for a child with an underlying predisposition to obesity or is actually independently causative.

Most cases of childhood obesity are not associated with a specific identifiable genetic abnormality. There are five genetic syndromes that account for most "syndromic" obesity. Of note, all five syndromes are associated with short stature, whereas nonsyndromic obese children typically have advanced height for age. All five syndromes are also associated with hypogonadism. The most common is Prader-Willi syndrome, characterized by diminished fetal activity, obesity, muscular hypotonia, mental retardation, short stature, hypogonadotropic hypogonadism, and small hands and feet. It is caused by an abnormality on chromosome 15. The mechanism underlying the uncontrollable hyperphagia associated with Prader-Willi syndrome remains an active area of investigation but is presumably a different mechanism from that underlying obesity in the general population. The remaining four syndromes are Bardet-Biedl syndrome, Alström syndrome, Cohen syndrome, and Carpenter syndrome, all of which are significantly less common than Prader-Willi.

Hormonal aberrations must also be considered. Rare but serious neuroendocrine conditions such as hypothyroidism, Cushing syndrome, and generalized hypothalamic dysfunction can result in excessive weight gain and behavioral abnormalities. A medication review is also particularly important for children with coincident developmental or behavioral concerns, because many of the medications associated with excessive weight gain are anticonvulsants or psychopharmacological agents commonly used in this patient population. Medications that are associated with increased weight gain are listed in Table 23D-1.

TABLE 23D-1 ■ Medications Associated with Weight Gain
Glucocorticoids
Megestrol acetate (Megace)
Cyproheptadine
Phenothiazines and other antipsychotics
Atypical antipsychotics
Sedating tricyclic antidepressants
Antiepileptic medications (topiramate is an exception)
β-Adrenergic–blocking drugs
Insulin and drugs that stimulate insulin release
Selective serotonin reuptake inhibitors

The food environment is a primary contributor to obesity risk. The advertisement of calorie-dense, nutrient-poor foods has increased since the 1960s.[12] As fast food options for busy lifestyles expand, families eat meals prepared outside the home more today than ever before.[13] Portion sizes have also significantly increased since the 1960s, presumably providing added value for the customer but also, unfortunately, providing added calories (but not necessarily other important nutrients).[14]

The environment has also evolved since the 1980s to support lifestyles that include less physical activity. Fewer children walk to school than ever before,[15] and the layout of neighborhoods in many communities necessitates that families drive to schools and the nearest shopping area. The availability of safe and accessible neighborhood parks and playgrounds is an important contributor to the time that children spend outside, which affects directly the amount of physical activity they engage in.[16] Parental perception of the neighborhood as being unsafe is associated with increased obesity risk.[17] The growing perception, popularized by the media, is that violence and crime are increasing, although violence endangering children appears to be a localized rather than universal phenomenon.[18] Finally, the number of schools with mandatory physical education programs, and the frequency of physical activity in existing programs, have both decreased significantly since the 1980s.[19] Unfortunately, government mandates to improve academic achievement and test scores often remove funding and focus from physical education programs. All these areas are ripe for policy-level intervention.

Although the majority of obese children do not have behavioral or mental health concerns, the prevalence of these disorders is higher among obese children than among nonobese children. Thus, the underlying issue in the majority of overweight children is not one that requires individual or family therapy, and research studies have shown that for most overweight children, these types of interventions are not particularly effective.[20] Studies have shown, however, that school-aged children with significant externalizing or internalizing behavior problems are at higher risk for the development of obesity 2 years later.[21] Similarly, adolescents with significant depressive symptoms are at higher risk for the development of obesity 1 year later,[22,23] and children with depression are at greater risk of obesity in adulthood, regardless of a number of confounders.[24] In one study, chronic obesity in childhood was associated with oppositional defiant disorder in both genders, and depression in boys, although neither the onset of obesity nor the remission of obesity over childhood and adolescence was associated with psychiatric disorder.[25] There is less evidence to suggest that the presence of obesity portends the development of behavior problems in the future. In a study of 5-year-old children, obesity and behavior problems were concurrently associated in girls, but the presence of obesity was not predictive of the development of behavior problems in the future, which implies that obesity did not play a causative role in the development of future behavioral problems.[26] Many of the prior findings are particularly robust in girls but not boys; this observation requires further investigation.

About half of all children demonstrate declines in self-esteem through the preteen years. Obese children in this age range, however, demonstrate greater declines in self-esteem. In one study,[27] the declines in self-esteem associated with obesity were both race and gender dependent: Obese girls experienced a greater decline in self esteem than did obese boys, and obese white girls experienced a greater decline than did obese black girls. There are also developmental differences in the relationship between overweight and self-esteem or mental health concerns through childhood. In the same study,[27] there were no differences in self-esteem between obese and nonobese children at age 9 to 10 years or in younger children; these differences emerged during the early teen years. The self-esteem and mental health issues presumably associated with childhood obesity do not appear to emerge until the early teen years, which is consistent with the observation that the social stigmatization and marginalization of overweight children has been documented in adolescents but not clearly in younger children.[28] Nonetheless, poor self-esteem in overweight adolescents can contribute to a vicious cycle in which the poor self-esteem leads to more internalizing behaviors, fewer social activities, and more sedentary time at home eating and watching television, with the consequent increase in overweight. Intervening in this cycle is crucial.

Childhood obesity is very difficult to treat, and such children benefit from its prevention and early recognition. Weight loss during childhood tends to be more sustained than it is in adulthood; nearly one third of children maintain weight loss 10 years later.[29] Nonetheless, the most effective treatment programs for childhood obesity still result in relatively modest success rates. The older the age at which a child is obese in childhood, the greater is the likelihood that the child will remain obese into adulthood. A child who is obese at school age is at least 10 times more likely to be obese in adulthood than is a child who was not obese.[30] Table 23D-2 lists evidence-based clinical recommendations. Although these behaviors (if implemented) are associated with significantly reduced risk of overweight, healthier diets, and improved physical activity, there is no evidence that

TABLE 23D-2 ■ Evidence-Based Recommendations for Altering Childhood Overweight Risk That May Be Discussed in the Pediatric Office*
Encourage breastfeeding
Limit sweetened beverage consumption (juice, soda pop)
Reduce "screen time" (time spent watching television or at the computer)
Remove television from bedroom
Do not allow meals or snacks to be eaten during "screen time"
Spend more time outdoors (which leads to increased physical activity)
Increase intake of fruits, vegetables, and whole grains
Model healthy eating
Decrease intake of sweets, fats, and "empty-calorie" foods
Limit portion size
Limit visits to fast food restaurants or eating out
Do not use food as a reward for good behavior
Do not reward children for eating healthy foods (leads to decreased preference for these foods in the long term)
Encourage behavior change among all family members, particularly the mother
Present healthy foods repeatedly to increase liking

*Consider carefully financial limitations and barriers as well as cultural beliefs when making recommendations.

discussing these issues in the context of a clinic visit leads to significant behavior change.

Eating behavior is a key area for change, but change is also a formidable challenge for most parents. Therefore, it may be worth spending additional time discussing this topic in particular with families. Vegetables, which promote weight management and satiety because they are high in fiber and nutrients but low in fat and calories, are often one of the most difficult foods to persuade children to eat.[31] Children's vegetable consumption is related to parental consumption, and modeling of eating behavior can powerfully influence preference.[32] Therefore, encouraging changes in eating behavior in the entire family is important. In addition, the more times children are exposed to a vegetable, the greater is their preference for that vegetable[33]; thus, serving a wide variety of vegetables repeatedly may lead to increased preference over time.

Targeting reduction in sedentary behavior (such as television viewing) is an equally effective way to achieve weight loss in children, as is targeting increased physical activity; when children are prompted and positively reinforced for reducing sedentary behaviors such as watching television, they will replace the sedentary behavior with a more active behavior about one third of the time.[34] Thus, explaining to parents how to reinforce reduced television viewing is equally effective in achieving weight loss as is recommending that they institute a formal exercise program for the child. In addition, although all

TABLE 23D-3 ■ Behavioral Strategies Used Effectively for Treatment of Obesity in Adults, Adolescents, and Older Children

Strategy	Definition	Example
Reinforcement	Desired behavior is rewarded	Patient is given monetary reward for weight loss
Stimulus control	Identify and modify the environmental cues that are associated with overeating and inactivity	Eat only at the kitchen table without watching television; keep no snack foods in the house; and lay out exercise clothes the night before as a reminder to walk or jog in the morning
Stages of change	As people make a behavior change, they progress through a series of stages, including precontemplation, contemplation, preparation, action, and maintenance. Understanding where an individual is in terms of these stages is crucial for targeting interventions	An individual in the preparation stage may benefit from problem-solving and goal setting, whereas an individual in maintenance may benefit more from self-monitoring
Self-monitoring	The systematic observation and recording of target behaviors; the primary purpose is to become more aware of their behaviors and the factors that influence their behaviors in ways that are beneficial or detrimental	Keep a food diary and graph of physical activity per day; frequently check body weight
Problem solving and goal setting	Set an explicit short-term goal and a specific action plan for achieving it	Aim to exercise for a half hour each day next week; specify exactly what type of exercise and where and how it will be performed
Covert sensitization	By creating an association between an unwanted behavior such as overeating and an unpleasant consequence, the unwanted behavior is reduced	Learn to associate eating high-fat or unhealthy foods with not feeling well (e.g., nausea)

types of exercise studied reduce overweight, lifestyle exercise produces more sustained weight loss than does scheduled aerobic exercise.[29] Thus, incorporating activities such as walking to school or to the corner store, parking far from store entrances, and taking the stairs into the daily routine is generally more effective than a certain amount of running, walking, or other physical activity per day.

A number of resource-intensive, multilevel, community and school-based programs have been developed to prevent the development and progression of obesity in children. Unfortunately, most of these have had relatively limited success, despite invoking theory-based methods of behavior change and targeting both caloric intake and expenditure. Perhaps the most important barrier to effective treatment of overweight is family and/or child motivation (indeed, this is cited as the primary barrier perceived by pediatric providers). Understanding what motivates families to make changes toward healthier lifestyles is an active area of research. One study revealed that for mothers, the primary motivating factor for change with regard to childhood overweight was that the child's weight was adversely affecting his or her health.[35] Therefore, if there are clear health manifestations resulting from the child's weight, this may be a key point for discussion and a method of engaging the family's interest in pursuing treatment.

The developmental-behavioral pediatrician may play a role in recommending and implementing specific behavioral strategies to treat childhood obesity. The data in adults are robust, but there are unfortunately few studies of behavioral interventions in children. In a total of 36 randomized controlled trials involving nearly 3500 participants, researchers have evaluated the efficacy of a variety of "psychological" interventions for obesity in adults. Cognitive-behavioral therapies were the primary intervention tested and were found to result in significantly greater weight reductions than did placebo, both alone and in combination with diet and exercise. In addition, increasing intensity of the behavioral intervention resulted in greater weight loss.[36] Therapeutic techniques that have been studied are described in Table 23D-3.

The data in children are less robust. In 13 randomized controlled trials with nearly 750 participants, researchers have evaluated behavioral treatments of obesity in children. In most of these studies, there were fewer than 25 children in each treatment condition, and thus the studies lacked statistical power. In addition, most of these studies were conducted with homogeneous, motivated groups in tertiary care settings. It is therefore difficult to draw firm conclusions with the current data, and it is unclear how generalizeable the findings are. Nonetheless, in general, the

TABLE 23D-4 ■ *DSM-IV* Criteria for Anorexia Nervosa

Refusal to maintain body weight at or above a minimally normal weight for age and height (e.g., weight loss leading to maintenance of body weight at less than 85% of that expected or failure to make expected weight gain during period of growth, leading to body weight less of than 85% of that expected)

Intense fear of gaining weight or becoming fat, even though underweight

Disturbance in the way in which body weight or shape is experienced, undue influence of body weight or shape on self-evaluation, or denial of the seriousness of the current low body weight

In postmenarchal girls, amenorrhea (i.e., the absence of at least three consecutive menstrual cycles) (a woman is considered to have amenorrhea if her periods occur only after hormone treatment, e.g., estrogen administration)

Specify type:
Restricting type: During the current episode of anorexia nervosa, the person has not regularly engaged in binge-eating or purging behavior (i.e., self-induced vomiting or the misuse of laxatives, diuretics, or enemas)
Binge-eating/purging type: During the current episode of anorexia nervosa, the person has regularly engaged in binge-eating or purging behavior (i.e., self-induced vomiting or the misuse of laxatives, diuretics, or enemas)

DSM-IV, Diagnostic and Statistical Manual of Mental Disorders, 4th ed.[140a]

TABLE 23D-5 ■ *DSM-IV* Criteria for Bulimia Nervosa

Recurrent episodes of binge eating; an episode of binge eating is characterized by both of the following: (1) eating, in a discrete period of time (e.g., within any 2-hour period), an amount of food that is definitely larger than most people would eat during a similar period of time and under similar circumstances and (2) a sense of lack of control over eating during the episode (e.g., a feeling that one cannot stop eating or control what or how much one is eating)

Recurrent inappropriate compensatory behavior in order to prevent weight gain, such as self-induced vomiting; misuse of laxatives, diuretics, enemas, or other medications; fasting; or excessive exercise

Both the binge eating and inappropriate compensatory behaviors occur, on average, at least twice a week for 3 months

Self-evaluation is unduly influenced by body shape and weight

The disturbance does not occur exclusively during episodes of anorexia nervosa

Specify type:
Purging type: During the current episode of bulimia nervosa, the person has regularly engaged in self-induced vomiting or the misuse of laxatives, diuretics, or enemas
Nonpurging type: During the current episode of bulimia nervosa, the person has used inappropriate compensatory behaviors, such as fasting or excessive exercise, but has not regularly engaged in self-induced vomiting or the misuse of laxatives, diuretics, or enemas

DSM-IV, Diagnostic and Statistical Manual of Mental Disorders, 4th ed.[140a]

strategies described in Table 23D-3 have also been found to be effective in children and adolescents, although, obviously, the younger the child is, the more heavily the success of the intervention depends on parental implementation.

The role of parents in particular has also been studied. When parents received specific training in either problem-solving barriers or child management techniques, as well as when parents were targeted as the agents of change as opposed to the children, results of the standard behavioral interventions in Table 23D-3 were generally improved.[20] Clearly, the specific behavioral strategies and the role of the parent will differ according to individual characteristics of families and, in particular, the age of the child involved.

RESTRICTIVE EATING DISORDERS

A body image ideal of thinness is a primary risk factor for restrictive eating disorders, because it results in eating behaviors aimed at achieving a particular body weight or sense of control. Restrictive eating disorders include anorexia nervosa and bulimia nervosa, as well as eating disorder not otherwise specified. The *Diagnostic and Statistical Manual*, 4th edition,[37] criteria for anorexia nervosa and bulimia nervosa are provided in Tables 23D-4 and 23D-5.

The number of children and adolescents with restrictive eating disorders has increased since the 1950s. It is estimated that 0.5% of adolescent girls in the United States have anorexia nervosa and 1% to 5% have bulimia nervosa. In addition, however, 10% to 13% of adolescent girls and college-age women engage in eating-disordered practices,[38] and 45% of high school girls report that they are currently trying to lose weight.[39] Restrictive eating disorders are gradually extending from middle- to upper-income white girls to historically less affected groups: between 5% and 10% of diagnosed eating disorders occur in boys and men, and the prevalence of these disorders is increasing in younger and minority populations. White women still, however, account for 95% of diagnoses.

A genetic component of restrictive eating disorders is conceptualized as rooted in a predisposition to a particular behavioral style or risk for psychiatric illness. This genetic component is evidenced by the high coincidence of anorexia nervosa, bulimia nervosa, and anxiety disorders within families,[40] although the biological underpinnings of the disorders have yet to be fully determined. As yet, no clear genetic loci have been outlined as etiological for restrictive eating disorders. Other consistent, presumably biological, risk factors include a family history of obesity, affective illness, or alcoholism, and personality traits, including perfectionism.[2]

Low-self esteem has been associated with disordered eating behaviors and dieting, particularly in adolescence,[41] as well as with the occurrence of actual eating disorders.[42] Depression is a risk factor for the development of an eating disorder during adolescence,[4] and restrictive eating disorders are associated with high rates of depression, anxiety, alcoholism, substance abuse, and the development of other eating disorders.[40] In one study, about two thirds of individuals with eating disorders had received a diagnosis of an anxiety disorder at some prior point in their lives; the most common were obsessive-compulsive disorder (41%) and social phobia (20%). Most of these anxiety disorders began in childhood.[43] Nearly 25% of individuals with a diagnosis of a restrictive eating disorder also receive a diagnosis of alcohol abuse disorder at some point during their lives, and the onset of the restrictive eating disorder typically precedes the onset of the alcohol abuse.[44] Work with a therapist and psychiatrist is a critical component of the treatment of restrictive eating disorders.

The mortality rate for restrictive eating disorders is one of the highest for any disorder occurring in adolescence, at 5.6%. The longer these conditions are present and remain untreated, the poorer the recovery rate is. Long-term outcome of eating disorders is predicted by a number of factors. Patients with bulimia nervosa tend to have better outcomes than do patients with anorexia nervosa. Predictors of poorer outcomes include a lower body weight at the time of initial treatment, compulsion to exercise, premorbid asocial behavior, and disturbed family relationships. Early recognition and treatment are important because early treatment, as with most diseases, is predictive of improved outcomes.

The most effective treatment programs for eating disorders result in full recovery in fewer than 50% of patients.[45] There are relatively strong data in support of specific, manual-based cognitive-behavioral therapy for bulimia nervosa and other disorders associated with bingeing.[46] Despite the evidence for the efficacy of this intervention, however, bulimia remains very difficult to treat, with an estimated 50% response rate to therapy. In contrast to bulimia nervosa, no specific therapeutic strategy has emerged as clearly superior in the treatment of anorexia nervosa.[47] Family therapy is the generally accepted approach, but there have been few randomized controlled trials of its efficacy, and the samples have been small and results mixed.[48] Finally, there are growing efforts to enhance media literacy, improve body self-image, and promote healthy eating attitudes. Many prevention programs have effectively reduced risk factors for eating disorders or eating pathology, but there is currently insufficient evidence to indicate that any of these programs is efficacious in preventing the onset of actual eating disorders.[49] The prevention programs that do exist for eating disorders appear to be more effective when targeted at high-risk groups, girls, and adolescents older than 15 years.

TABLE 23D-6 ■ Commonalities and Differences in Restrictive Eating Disorders and Obesity		
Characteristic	Restrictive Eating Disorders	Obesity
Locus of control	Most commonly emerges in adolescence or late school age as children develop increasing control over their own eating	Control over eating rests primarily with parents in early childhood and gradually shifts to children; obesity may emerge at any time during childhood
Predictive value of early eating behaviors and feeding practices	Picky eating in early childhood is predictive of anorexia in later adolescence	Controlling or restricting children's eating is predictive of later overweight
Role of disordered eating (bingeing, purge, use of diet pills or laxatives)	Hallmarks of restrictive eating disorders	Most obese individuals do not binge or purge, although it is common in morbid obesity; obese adolescents commonly use diet pills or laxatives
Role of mental health disorders	Common comorbidity with restrictive eating disorders	Mental health disorders not present in most obese individuals but do increase risk of development of obesity
Self-esteem	Poor self-esteem commonly associated with restrictive eating disorders	Poor self-esteem associated with obesity only in adolescence and not earlier; poor self-esteem associated with obesity most strongly in white, middle-income girls
Academic achievement and attainment	No consistent difference detectable in studies to date	Academic achievement not associated with obesity in grade-school children, but lower academic attainment associated with obesity in adolescents
Media exposure	Linked to increased risk, presumably through the promotion of unrealistic, idealized body types	Linked to increased risk through increased sedentary activity and commercials promoting unhealthy foods

A DEVELOPMENTAL PERSPECTIVE

Comparing and contrasting obesity and restrictive eating disorders is useful, particularly in the context of reflecting on how these disorders unfold in the course of child development (Table 23D-6). We propose that the commonalities between the disorders begin to emerge primarily during school age and increase in adolescence.

Shifting Locus of Control around Eating Behavior

Obesity is prevalent in preschool- and young school-aged children, but disordered eating rooted in body image ideals or self-control is rare in this age range. Rather, the factors that contribute to obesity in all children, but perhaps less related to body-image and disordered eating than in older children, are components of the environment and parenting. The obesity–restrictive eating disorders dichotomy in older children may be conceptualized as a tension between the desire to eat and self-imposed restrictions. In younger children, there is no self-imposed restriction but, rather, generally a desire to eat that is molded by the parents and environment.

The role of the parents as an influence on child eating also changes throughout childhood. Parents exert nearly total control over the foods offered to very young children. In the early school years, schools begin to influence dietary preferences and intake. Thus, addressing obesity in early childhood requires supporting appropriate parenting behaviors concerning food and physical activity, as well as supporting policies that enable healthy food choices and daily activity through the schools and other locations that children frequent. Parents exert less (but certainly some) control over adolescents' eating behavior. Although peers always shape food preferences and eating, the role of peers in affecting weight-related self-esteem (and, through this, presumably eating behavior) appears to emerge in mid-childhood and strengthens during the adolescent years.

Early feeding behavior and maternal feeding practices have also been hypothesized to contribute to the risk of both restrictive eating disorders and obesity. A prospective study of 659 children monitored from 1 to 21 years of age revealed that picky eating in early childhood (defined by maternal report as not eating enough, being choosy about or uninterested in food, and eating unusually slowly) was predictive of symptoms of anorexia nervosa in later adolescence.[50] However, as reviewed extensively by other investigators, more than 30 different risk factors have been cited for adolescent eating disorders, and picky eating in early childhood does not consistently emerge as a major risk.[2] Conclusions about this association are currently difficult to draw, and further study is needed.

The potential relationship between early feeding practices and future overweight is equally difficult to disentangle. The studies conducted in an attempt to unravel the relationship have been primarily in middle-income white girls; therefore, it is unclear whether the findings can be applied to other gender, income, and ethnic groups. These studies have revealed that mothers who control or restrict their daughters' access to and consumption of certain foods are more likely to have children who are overweight several years later.[51] The underlying hypothesis is that by not allowing children to develop their own ability to respond to hunger or satiety, parents are inadvertently dysregulating eating behavior and causing increased obesity risk. Other researchers have studied whether maternal prompting to eat is associated with increased obesity risk in children, and results have been mixed. Some have found, however, that although obese mothers do not prompt their children to eat any more often than do nonobese mothers, the children of obese mothers are more compliant with maternal prompts to eat.[52] Research is needed in this area to determine what types of parental feeding practices may alter the risk of both restrictive eating disorders and obesity.

Another important point for comparison between the two conditions is the conceptualization of disordered eating. Disordered eating, such as bingeing and purging or the use of diet pills and laxatives, is a hallmark of restrictive eating disorders. In contrast, most obese individuals neither binge nor purge. Rather, obesity may be conceptualized as a normal response to an obesity-conducive environment. Disordered eating behaviors such as bingeing are frequently observed in morbid obesity, but most individuals with less severe obesity do not have these types of disordered eating behaviors.[53] Although dieting behavior is becoming more frequent at younger ages, disordered eating and dieting are not typically a characteristic of obese preadolescents. Obese adolescents, are, however, more likely than individuals of normal weight to engage in the types of disordered weight loss strategies associated with eating disorders, such as use of diet pills, self-induced vomiting, or use of laxatives.[39] Dieting behaviors or weight reduction efforts, paradoxically, are predictive of the later onset of obesity.[54]

Changing Association with Mental Health and Behavioral Concerns

Both restrictive eating disorders and obesity are strongly associated with mental health diagnoses, behavioral disorders, and poor self-esteem, but the time course varies. Although the majority of obese children do not have defined mental health disorders, the presence of mental health disorders does appear to increase the risk of obesity.[23] Distorted body image and poor self-esteem are often intertwined with both disorders. However, this once again highlights important developmental differences. For example, although poor self-esteem is strongly associated with the presence of restrictive eating disorders, poor self-esteem is associated with obesity only during adolescence, not at younger ages. The self-esteem issues associated with obesity appear to be race and gender dependent and are particularly prominent in white adolescent girls (the same group with the highest prevalence of restrictive eating disorders).

Associations with Intelligence and Academic Achievement

Relations of academic achievement with obesity and restrictive eating disorders also differ along a developmental trajectory and highlight the importance of understanding these conditions in a developmental context. Specifically, obesity is not independently associated with lower academic achievement in the primary grades,[55] although it does seem to be associated with lower academic achievement in adolescence and lower educational attainment into adulthood.[56] It seems likely that societal prejudice against obese adolescents, rather than actual decreased ability, explains the lower achievement. Although there is a clinical perception that young women with eating disorders are typically high-achieving, competitive, and successful, there are actually few to no data to support this impression. Understanding the potential relationship between academic attainment or achievement and these disorders is also difficult because of confounding by socioeconomic status. Data linking intellectual capacity (as measured by intelligence quotient) with either obesity or restrictive eating disorders in the general population are sparse; therefore, it is difficult to establish associations.[57]

Although no particular personality traits seem to be consistently associated with obesity, there do seem to be clusters of personality traits associated with restrictive eating disorders. Anorexia nervosa tends to be associated with personality traits such as introversion, conformity, perfectionism, rigidity, and obsessive-compulsive features, whereas bulimia nervosa tends to be associated with being extroverted, histrionic, and affectively unstable.[58] Certainly neither of these personality clusters consistently translates into differences in achievement, intelligence, or educational attainment in restrictive eating disorders that are supported by research data.

Changing Role of the Media

Children spend a significantly greater amount of time in front of the television and computers today than they did several decades ago.[59] Media exposure has been directly linked with increased risk for both obesity[60] and eating disorders.[61] The role of the media in influencing both eating disorders and childhood obesity also changes along the developmental trajectory of childhood.

During early childhood, media exposure increases overweight risk through its interference with physical activity, as well as through the content of advertising and television shows that promote the consumption of high–caloric density, unhealthy foods. Indeed, reduced television viewing is associated with a reduced prevalence of overweight in children.[62] Television does more than simply increase sedentary behavior. The relationship of restrictive eating disorders and obesity with media use is also related to the content of what is watched. Most advertising on television during children's programming is for unhealthy foods.[63] Such commercials can powerfully alter children's behavior with regard to the products they request from their parents, as well as their consumption. Children, especially preteenaged and younger, have very limited ability to critically appraise the messages in media and thus to restrict the effects that these messages may have on their behavior. One possible point for intervention is therefore to improve parents' and children's media literacy.[64] As children grow older into the preteen years and beyond, intervention can take the forms of both limiting media exposure and increasing their media literacy so that they can be critical consumers of the messages about nutrition and body image being portrayed. Media images of women have become increasingly thinner since the 1950s,[65] and a perceived ideal body shape that is very thin, along with body image dissatisfaction,[2] is a risk factor for eating disorders. The unrealistic portrayal of thinness in the media is believed to be one of the causative factors in the development of eating disorders, and a distorted body image or perceived body ideal is a hallmark of restrictive eating disorders. Promoting children's ability to accurately interpret the misleading nature of these messages may add to the benefits of supporting parents in generally limiting children's exposure to television, videogames, and the Internet.

SUMMARY

There are number of commonalities between childhood obesity and restrictive eating disorders that highlight the developmental components of each disorder, as well as how the environment and the media affect health. The growing disparities in obesity in the United States raise questions about health disparities in general, and how these relate to socioeconomic status in this country. The demographic distribution of eating disorders, on the other hand, raises questions about the particular pressures on the more privileged girls and women in this society. The treatment of obesity and restrictive eating disorders is complex and requires involvement of pediatricians, the public media, the advertising industry, multiple professional disciplines, communities, and policymakers. The developmental-behavioral pediatrician may play a key role in facilitating this type of care, as well as advocating for the necessary changes in the environment that can improve the well-being of all children.

REFERENCES

1. Hsu F, Lenchik L, Nicklas B, et al: Heritability of body composition measured by DXA in the Diabetes Heart Study. Obes Res 13:312-319, 2005.
2. Rome E, Ammerman S, Rosen D, et al: Children and adolescents with eating disorders: The state of the art. Pediatrics 111(1):e98-e108, 2003.
3. Irving L, Neumark-Sztainer D: Integrating the prevention of eating disorders and obesity: Feasible or futile? Prev Med 34:299-309, 2002.
4. Patton G, Selzer R, Coffey C, et al: Onset of eating disorders: Population based cohort over 3 years. BMJ 318:765-768, 1999.
5. Field A, Austin S, Taylor C: Relation between dieting and weight change among preadolescents and adolescents. Pediatrics 112:900-906, 2003.
6. Troiano R, Flegal K: Overweight children and adolescents: Description, epidemiology, and demographics. Pediatrics 101(Suppl 3):497-504, 1998.
7. Hedley A, Ogden C, Johnson C, et al: Prevalence of overweight and obesity among US children, adolescents, and adults, 1999-2002. JAMA 291:2847-2850, 2004.
8. Strauss R, Pollack H: Epidemic increase in childhood overweight. JAMA 286:2845-2848, 2001.
9. Parsons T, Power C, Manor O: Fetal and early life growth and body mass index from birth to early adulthood in a 1958 British cohort: longitudinal study. BMJ 323:1331-1335, 2001.
10. Owen C, Martin R, Whincup P, et al: Effect of infant feeding on the risk of obesity across the life course: A quantitative review of published evidence. Pediatrics 115:1367-1377, 2005.
11. Whitaker R, Pepe M, Wright J, et al: Early adiposity rebound and the risk of adult obesity. Pediatrics 101(3): e5, 1998.
12. Nestle M: Food politics: How the Food Industry Influences Nutrition and Health. Berkeley: University of California Press, 2002.
13. Lin B, Guthrie J, Frazao E: Quality of children's diets at and away from home: 1994-1996. Food Rev 22:2-10, 1999.
14. Nielsen S, Popkin B: Patterns and trends in food portion sizes, 1977-1998. JAMA 289:450-453, 2003.
15. Centers for Disease Control and Prevention: Barriers to children walking and bicycling to school—United States, 1999. MMWR Morb Mortal Wkly Rep 51:701-704, 2002.
16. Burdette H, Whitaker R, Daniels S: Parental report of outdoor playtime as a measure of physical activity in preschool-aged children. Arch Pediatr Adolesc Med 158:353-357, 2004.
17. Lumeng J, Appugliese D, Cabral H, et al: Neighborhood safety and overweight status in children. Arch Pediatr Adolesc Med 160:25-31, 2006.
18. Smith S, Steadman G, Minton T: Criminal Victimization and Perceptions of Community Safety in 12 Cities, 1998. Washington, DC: US Department of Justice, Bureau of Justice Statistics, Office of Community Oriented Policing Services, 1999.
19. Koplan J, Liverman C, Kraak V, eds: Preventing Childhood Obesity: Health in the Balance. Washington, DC: Institute of Medicine, National Academies Press, 2005.
20. Summerbell C, Ashton V, Campbell K, et al: Interventions for treating obesity in children. Cochrane Database Syst Rev (3):CD001872, 2003.
21. Lumeng J, Gannon K, Cabral H, et al: The association between clinically meaningful behavior problems and overweight in children. Pediatrics 112:1138-1145, 2003.
22. Richardson L, Davis R, Poulton R, et al: A longitudinal evaluation of adolescent depression and adult obesity. Arch Pediatr Adolesc Med 157:739-745, 2003.
23. Goodman E, Whitaker R: A prospective study of the role of depression in the development and persistence of adolescent obesity. Pediatrics 110:497-504, 2002.
24. Pine D, Goldstein R, Wolk S, et al: The association between childhood depression and adult body mass index. Pediatrics 107:1049-1056, 2001.
25. Mustillo S, Worthman C, Erkanli A, et al: Obesity and psychiatric disorder: Developmental trajectories. Pediatrics 111:851-859, 2003.
26. Datar A, Sturm R: Childhood overweight and parent- and teacher-reported behavior problems—Evidence from a prospective study of kindergarteners. Arch Pediatr Adolesc Med 158:804-810, 2004.
27. Strauss R: Childhood obesity and self-esteem. Pediatrics 105:e15, 2000.
28. Strauss R, Pollack H: Social marginalization of overweight children. Arch Pediatr Adolesc Med 157:746-752, 2003.
29. Epstein L, Myers M, Saelens B: Treatment of pediatric obesity. Pediatrics 101:554-570, 1998.

30. Whitaker R, Wright J, Pepe M, et al: Predicting obesity in young adulthood from childhood and parental obesity. N Engl J Med 337:869-873, 1997.

31. Falciglia G, Couch S, Gribble L, et al: Food neophobia in childhood affects dietary variety. J Am Diet Assoc 100:1474-1478, 2000.

32. Skinner J, Carruth B, Bounds W, et al: Children's food preferences: A longitudinal analysis. J Am Diet Assoc 102:1638-1647, 2002.

33. Birch L, Fisher J: Development of eating behaviors among children and adolescents. Pediatrics 101:539-549, 1998.

34. Epstein L, Paluch R, Gordy C, et al: Decreasing sedentary behaviors in treating pediatric obesity. Arch Pediatr Adolesc Med 154:220-226, 2000.

35. Rhee K, DeLago C, Arscott-Mills T, et al: Factors associated with parental readiness to make changes for overweight children. Pediatrics 116:e94-e101, 2005.

36. Shaw K, O'Rourke P, Del Mar C, et al: Psychological interventions for overweight or obesity. Cochrane Database Syst Rev (2):CD003818, 2005.

37. American Psychiatric Association: Diagnostic and Statistical Manual of Mental Disorders, 4th ed. Washington, DC: American Psychiatric Association, 1994.

38. Killen J, Taylor C, Telch M, et al: Self-induced vomiting and laxative and diuretic use among teenagers: Precursors of the binge-purge syndrome. JAMA 255:1447-1449, 1986.

39. Neumark-Sztainer D, Story M, Falkner N, et al: Sociodemographic and personal characteristics of adolescents engaged in weight loss and weight/muscle gain behaviors: Who is doing what? Prev Med 28:40-50, 1999.

40. Strober M, Freeman R, Lampert C, et al: Controlled family study of anorexia nervosa and bulimia nervosa: Evidence of shared liability and transmission of partial syndromes. Am J Psychiatry 157:393-401, 2000.

41. Neumark-Sztainer D, Hannan P: Weight-related behaviors among adolescent girls and boys: Results from a national survey. Arch Pediatr Adolesc Med 154:569-577, 2000.

42. Gaul P, Perez-Gaspar M, Martinez-Gonzalez M, et al: Self-esteem, personality, and eating disorders: Baseline assessment of a prospective population-based cohort. Int J Eat Disord 31:261-273, 2002.

43. Kaye W, Bulik C, Thornton L, et al: Comorbidity of anxiety disorders with anorexia and bulimia. Am J Psychiatry 161:2215-2221, 2004.

44. Franko D, Dorer D, Keel P, et al: How do eating disorders and alcohol use influence each other? Int J Eat Disord 38:200-207, 2005.

45. Johnson W, Tsoh J, Varnado P: Eating disorders: Efficacy of pharmacological and psychological interventions. Clin Psychol Rev 16:457-478, 1996.

46. Hay P, Bacaltchuk J, Stefano S: Psychotherapy for bulimia nervosa and binging. Cochrane Database Syst Rev (3):CD000562, 2006.

47. Hay P, Bacaltchuk J, Claudino A, et al: Individual psychotherapy in the outpatient treatment of adults with anorexia nervosa. Cochrane Database Syst Rev (4): CD003909, 2006.

48. Kolliakou A, Holliday J, Murphy R: Family therapy for anorexia nervosa (Protocol for Cochrane Review). Cochrane Database Syst Rev (3):CD004780, 2004.

49. Pratt B, Woolfenden S: Interventions for preventing eating disorders in children and adolescents. Cochrane Database Syst Rev (2):CD002891, 2006.

50. Marchi M, Cohen P: Early childhood eating behaviors and adolescent eating disorders. J Am Acad Child Adolesc Psychiatry 29:112-117, 1990.

51. Faith M, Scanlon K, Birch L, et al: Parent-child feeding strategies and their relationships to child eating and weight status. Obes Res 12:1711-1722, 2004.

52. Lumeng J, Burke L: Maternal prompts to eat, child compliance, and mother and child weight status. J Pediatr 149:330-335, 2006.

53. Wilson G: Behavioral treatment of childhood obesity: Theoretical and practical implications. Health Psychol 13:372-374, 1994.

54. Stice E, Cameron R, Killen J, et al: Naturalistic weight-reduction efforts prospectively predict growth in relative weight and onset of obesity among female adolescents. J Consult Clin Psychol 67:967-974, 1999.

55. Datar A, Sturm R, Magnabosco J: Childhood overweight and academic performance: National study of kindergarteners and first-graders. Obes Res 12:58-68, 2004.

56. Taras H, Potts-Datema W: Obesity and student performance at school. J School Health 75:291-295, 2005.

57. Blanz B, Detzner U, Lay B, et al: The intellectual functioning of adolescents with anorexia nervosa and bulimia nervosa. Eur Child Adolesc Pyschiatry 6:129-135, 1997.

58. Westen D, Harnden-Fischer J: Personality profiles in eating disorders: Rethinking the distinction between Axis I and Axis II. Am J Psychiatry 158:547-562, 2001.

59. Caroli M, Argentieri L, Cardone M, et al: Role of television in childhood obesity prevention. Int J Obes Relat Metab Disord 28:S104-S108, 2004.

60. Gortmaker S, Must A, Sobol A, et al: Television viewing as a cause of increasing obesity among children in the United States, 1986-1990. Arch Pediatr Adolesc Med 150:356-362, 1996.

61. Harrison K: The body electric: Thin-ideal media and eating disorders in adolescents. J Communication 50:119-143, 2000.

62. Robinson T: Reducing children's television viewing to prevent obesity: A randomized controlled trial. JAMA 282:1561-1567, 1999.

63. Harrison K, Marske A: Nutritional content of foods advertised during the television programs children watch most. Am J Public Health 95:1568-1574, 2005.

64. Steiner-Adair A, Purcell A: Resisting weightism: Media literacy for elementary-school children. *In* Piran N, Levine M, Steiner-Adair C, eds: Preventing Eating Disorders: A Handbook of Interventions and Special Challenges. Philadelphia: Brunner/Mazel, 1999.

65. Wiseman C, Gray J, Mosimann J, et al: Cultural expectations of thinness in women: An update. Int J Eat Disord 11:85-89, 1990.

Elimination Conditions

ALISON SCHONWALD ▉ LEONARD A. RAPPAPORT

TOILET TRAINING AS A DEVELOPMENTAL MILESTONE

Toilet training, like every developmental milestone, is the compilation of numerous neurobiological processes affected by social opportunities, cultural expectations, and temperamental tendencies. Infants develop object permanence, the basis for the toddler's fascination and fear of stool's disappearance down the toilet. As toddlers pass through the sensorimotor phase, they busily explore the world, entering the bathroom to investigate. The child younger than 2 years may have phases of separation difficulties and is eager to mimic. This creates opportunities to watch parents use the bathroom and imitate them by sitting on the potty chair at the same time. As the child enters the preoperational stage, language develops rapidly. Now the child can indicate when diapers are wet or when he or she needs to defecate. In this egocentric phase, the child is highly focused on himself or herself. Along with "It's mine" and "I do it," the child might interrupt anything and everything when the urge to defecate or urinate comes.

The toilet training period is a time of increased autonomy and initiative. Two- to 3-year-old children often want to pick their own clothes, feed a new baby, color the picture themselves, and explore every item in the room without parents' help. The developmental stage is set for toilet training, the ultimate skill of toddler independence. Toilet training requires the cognitive understanding of where stool and urine go, the motor skills to get there, and the desire to do it without help: skills that finally consolidate between 2 and 3 years of age in the typically developing child.

On the other hand, toilet training is like no other developmental milestone. Few childhood skills bring similar joy to parents when accomplished and frustration when delayed. Although stooling and urinating are universal bodily functions, they are nonetheless emotionally charged tasks. When a child uses the bathroom independently, parents are freed from the inconvenient and time-consuming task of regular diaper changes. The child who struggles with training can bring far more burden to the family than do children with other delayed milestones. For example, late talkers may communicate with pointing or word approximations; late walkers still can move from one place to another by crawling, cruising, or scooting. A child who is not toilet trained has no compensatory options. More so than those delayed in meeting other milestones, children who remain toilet untrained can be a source of enormous frustration and embarrassment to their families. Children with a persistent need for diapers or training pants (Pull-Ups®) can cause a significant financial, emotional, and time burden.

LOSS OF CONTINENCE CAN SIGNAL MEDICAL OR EMOTIONAL PATHOLOGY

Continence of stool is expected by 4 years of age, urine by 5. Loss of continence or failure to achieve continence carries a host of potential implications. Although incontinence is usually not indicative of major organic pathology, it does on rare occasions signal substantial concerns. Spinal cord abnormalities, tumors, and infections can manifest with incontinence; permanent morbidity may follow if identification of these causes is delayed. Although chronic incontinence rarely signals a serious psychiatric disorder, it can cause emotional distress and therefore necessitates attention and treatment. Children with stool or urine accidents are at increased risk for abuse; such substantial emotional traumas, although infrequent, must be considered in any child with incontinence.

TREATMENT OFTEN INCLUDES MEDICAL AND BEHAVIORAL INTERVENTION

Incontinence of urine and stool are treatable problems that can be managed in the primary care office. Once underlying neurological or other pathological disorders are ruled out by history and examination, treatment is mostly behavioral, with limited medical components. Behavior plans focus on reteaching the body to recognize signals to use the bathroom and to remain dry, as well as eliminating the stress that many children (and their families) are feeling about their incontinence. Medication is often aimed at softening stool so that defecation is not painful, and, at times, medication is used to stabilize bladder musculature so that bladder spasm decreases. Treatment must always include the consideration of the shame and blame that commonly develop around the incontinence, because that emotional component can become an obstacle interfering with every treatment plan.

TOILET TRAINING

Significance

TYPICAL AGE AT CONSOLIDATION AND TRENDS

Children in the United States typically become toilet trained between 2 and 3 years of age. At this stage, children are neurologically capable of sensing and containing stool and urine, and they have the language and motor skills to get to the toilet. Over the years, the completion of training has occurred at slightly older ages. Data from the late 1980s revealed that children completed toilet training at an average age of 24 to 27 months.[1] In contrast, in the 1990s, U.S. girls were found to complete toilet training at an average age of 35 months and boys at 39 months.[2]

Several explanations regarding the phenomenon of later toilet training are proposed. With cheaper, more effective, and larger-sized diapers and training pants, older and larger children can easily use them. Cultural norms and parenting styles have also changed. Years ago, parents were given direct parenting advice, specific instructions about when to put the child to bed, how much to give at each feeding, and when and how to toilet train. Beginning with Dr. Spock in the 1940s, parents have been increasingly encouraged to trust their own instincts when parenting a child, rather than to follow the same uniform directions for every child.[3] T. Berry Brazelton expanded this mindset specifically to toilet training.[4] Endorsing a child-centered approach, Brazelton allowed children to take the lead in the training process. Rather than forcing the child to adhere to an imposed schedule of when to train, parents were encouraged to read a child's signals that indicated readiness. When children express interest in toileting, have the developmental skills to accomplish the task, and have regularity in stooling and urinating, then parents step in to guide the process. Barton Schmitt later reincorporated specific parent responsibilities in the toilet training process, such as prompting practice runs, responding to successes, and responding to accidents.[5]

The parenting perspective may differ from one cultural group to another. For example, African American parents tend to start training their children at younger ages and are more likely than white parents to agree that it is important for a child to be trained before 24 months.[2] Not surprisingly, nonwhite children are more likely to be trained earlier than their white peers.[2]

Blum and colleagues studied a large cohort of children to identify factors associated with later toilet training.[6] More than 400 children, mostly Caucasian children at the top of the social strata, were monitored. The children who completed toilet training after age 3 years were compared with those who were trained before age 3. Later trainers started training later (at 22.3 vs. 20.6 months), were more likely to be constipated (41.7% vs. 13.2%), and exhibited more stool toileting refusal (56.7% vs. 17.9%) than peers who trained earlier. There were no differences between the two groups in parenting stress, birth order, or daycare participation.

TOILETING READINESS

Several developmental abilities are needed for a child to be toilet trained (Table 24-1). These are referred to as *readiness skills*. When parents ask when to train the child, it is helpful to provide a checklist of what the child needs to be able to do and an age range in which he or she is expected to do it.

The first step in training is the child's awareness of the sensation of a full bladder or rectum. As the rectum fills, stretch receptors send information to the brain that the stool is accumulating. For urine, a more complex interaction between the bladder and central nervous system is involved. Children often respond to these feelings with withholding behavior. This can be kneeling or freezing to hold in urine or "dancing" to hold in either urine or stool. Even infants have a sense of when they are about to stool, arching or crying in such a way that parents often recognize an imminent bowel movement. Before they are trained to use the toilet, some children hide in a corner or go to a specific room to stool privately. In these cases, the child can sense the urge to defecate.

To train, a child should be dry for 2 hours at a time. This indicates regularity and bladder capacity that are

TABLE 24-1 ■ Readiness Skills: Age at Acquisition

Readiness Skills	Age (Months) at Acquisition
Get to the toilet	12-16
Be aware of bladder/bowel sensation	15-24
Pull down pants and underpants	18-24
Sit on the toilet	26-31
Hold in urine/feces (dry for 2 hours)	26-35
Communicate the need to urinate/defecate	26-34
Use toilet without adaptive seat	31-36

adequate for using the toilet at reasonable intervals without interrupting daily activities. The child must communicate the need to go and his or her desire for access to the toilet. This can be accomplished with words, pointing, or signs. Families should be advised to pick toilet words that are socially acceptable and will be recognized in different settings, such as at school and at friends' homes. To be independent in toileting, a child must have the motor skills to get to the toilet and must be secure enough to sit comfortably on the toilet or potty chair. Children with neurological deficits may need special apparatus so that they are stable on the toilet. The ability to pull down underpants and pants, including fasteners, is an additional requisite motor skill.

A child cannot urinate or defecate on the toilet without relaxing; physiologically, the child has to relax the buttocks for the stool to be evacuated. The child must then push the stool out or relax the bladder's external sphincter, followed by wiping and flushing. Children should be taught to wipe from front to back to minimize spread of fecal bacteria.

In many cultures, infants are "trained" to defecate and urinate over the toilet.[7] This training is behavioral, accomplished by a parent very closely watching the child for signs of imminent voiding, such as a red face, a typical cry, or a typical posture. The parent removes diapers or underwear and holds the infant over a toilet. Infant training necessitates a great deal of consistency from parents and regularity in stooling and urinating patterns in infants. Interest in the US has resurged as "Elimination communication", considered an extension of parent-child connections and a step toward toilet training. Studies of the benefits, side effects, and long-term outcomes of infant toilet training are not available.

Current Practices

COMMON TOILETING STRATEGIES

In the United States, most children are trained easily and quickly through Brazelton's child-centered approach. Parents may first buy a potty chair, encouraging the child to pick it to boost excitement and investment. They can place the potty chair in the bathroom, and while parents use the big toilet, the child uses the small one, or pretends to do so. Parents may augment this experience with books and videos about toilet training. When the child is dry for at least 2 hours at a time, he or she may help choose new underwear, often decorated with superheroes or favorite cartoon characters. After stooling or urinating, the child can wear the special new underwear for an hour, successfully experiencing dryness. When parents see signs indicating that the child senses a full bladder or bowel, they can encourage the child to use the toilet. Often they can reward the child with a hug, sticker, or small treat. During the period that children are consolidating continence, they often make a transition from diapers to disposable training pants that can be pulled up and down like underwear.

Another common approach some parents use is to remove diapers or training pants altogether. Children who have the needed readiness skills and an easygoing temperament may do better with this method than do more developmentally impaired children or those with a less easygoing temperament. Parents prepare the child so that over a few days, the child learns to use the toilet. They often may chose a warm summer weekend for the house to become a "diaper-free" zone, when the child wears no diaper or training pant for much of the time. The child and parent stay home, waiting for the urine or stool to come so that the toilet can be used. Initially, they should expect accidents. Some parents increase output by having the child drink more than usual or even eat salty food to create more thirst. Although these techniques are an effective method in many instances, children at risk for physical abuse should not be trained this way, because of the high risk of accidents and often intense nature of this method.

Toilet sitting is another common technique that can be effective. Children are expected to sit on the toilet for 5 minutes at a time, at 2-hour intervals throughout the day and after each meal. Each time, the parent asks the child to try to urinate. When the child sits after meals, the natural gastrocolic reflex makes defecation more likely, and so the child is asked to stool. When bearing down, the child may place his or her hand on the lower abdomen to feel it push out. Parents usually give small rewards at first for trying and later for success. Reading books and singing songs can help make the sitting time pass pleasantly while the expectation is reinforced. Children who are toilet trained at preschool or daycare often learn through this method: they may be taken to the toilets at intervals, when they line up and wait their turns outside the bathroom. Peer activities can be an added incentive to motivate the children.

RELEVANT RESEARCH

There is little research support for a single best, evidence-based method of toilet training a child.[8] One review concluded that no randomized, controlled studies of preschoolers provide evidence for treating problems related to toilet training.[9] The largest body of evidence stems from Azrin and Foxx, whose intensive approach breaks training into individual steps and is effective for both developmentally abnormal and typically developing children.[10] Although Brazelton's child-oriented approach is currently perhaps the most commonly used,[11] no outcome data have been published since his original report.

Difficulty in Toilet Training

WHAT IS KNOWN ABOUT THIS PROBLEM?

Increasing data are available regarding children who are not able to toilet train or have more trouble than expected. Based on his extensive experience, Schmitt suggested that the most common cause of delayed toilet training is refusal or resistance but also emphasized that these children are often enmeshed in a power struggle with their parents.[12] Schonwald and associates furthered the understanding of difficulty in toilet training by demonstrating these children's significant tendency to have difficult temperamental traits outside of their toileting difficulties.[13] Children who were referred to a tertiary care center for failure to toilet train were less easygoing temperamentally and were more likely than easily trained children to have a negative attitude, be poorly adaptable, be less persistent, and be more hesitant in new situations. They were also substantially more constipated than were peers who trained easily. In comparisons of parents of such children with parents of typically trained children, no difference in parenting styles were found. Blum and colleagues confirmed that constipation in children with toilet training difficulty occurs before the toilet refusal[14]; theoretically, it hurts the child to stool, and so the temperamentally at-risk child then avoids stooling; this leads to more constipation and pain, and a vicious cycle ensues.

MANAGEMENT OF TOILET REFUSAL

Few interventions regarding late toilet training have been studied.[15] Successes associated with such interventions have been minimal. Taubman and coworkers demonstrated that (1) discouraging negative terms for feces and (2) praising children who defecate into diapers before training began (using a child-oriented approach) did not decrease the incidence of stool toilet refusal but did shorten its duration.[16]

Late toilet training interventions must account for the child's temperament, constipation status, and the parent-child dynamics that often develop around the toilet training power struggle. A group treatment approach has been one effective model that addresses these elements in a 6-week program.[17]

ENCOPRESIS

Significance

Encopresis is commonly defined as stool incontinence, typically of an involuntary nature as a result of overflow around constipated stool that dilates the distal rectum. The definition of the *Diagnostic and Statistical Manual of Mental Disorders,* 4th edition, however, identifies encopresis only as repeated passage of stool into inappropriate places by a child who is both chronologically and developmentally older than 4 years.[18] This definition can include both voluntary and involuntary situations but excludes those with stool incontinence resulting directly from physiological effects of a substance or caused by a general medical condition (except, of course, constipation). Because children typically are fully toilet trained by 3 years, those who are older than 4 years with stool that is evacuated anywhere other than into the toilet are considered abnormal. Their defecation must be considered medically and behaviorally; thus, those older than 4 years with ongoing symptoms are considered to have encopresis. In fact, most children with encopresis present before they are 7 years old.[19]

THE HIDDEN PROBLEM

Unfortunately, the private nature of toileting and the shame and disgust sometimes associated with defecation make encopresis a challenging disorder to identify. In the pediatric office, a child can demonstrate skills in walking, communicating, and socializing but is not expected to show the doctor his or her toileting skills! On occasion, providers find stool leakage in a child's underwear on examination, or a particularly stressed or worried parent asks for guidance. In general, the topic of encopresis must be explicitly queried by the provider to elicit the problem. Parents are often too embarrassed to bring up the subject on their own.

Unlike more obvious developmental and behavioral issues, encopresis is not easily discussed among parents. In contrast to children with sleep problems and tantrums, families of children with encopresis have rarely heard of another child with the same problem. Typically, families approach encopresis as a behavior problem, attributing willfulness as the cause. They may associate encopresis with filth, embarrassment, and serious psychiatric pathology, with no understanding of its underlying cause. Although

TABLE 24-2 ■ Incidence of Encopresis	
Age (Years)	Incidence
4	2.8%
5-6	4.1%
6	1.9%
10-11	1.6%
11-12	1.6%

Internet access creates unprecedented opportunities for research about medical conditions in the privacy of a parent's own home, few parents would know to search "encopresis."

INCIDENCE HARD TO CONFIRM

It is difficult to determine the true prevalence of encopresis because of its private nature and families' and children's reluctance to discuss it. Some authors report that 1% to 3% of children between ages 4 and 11 years suffer from encopresis[20] (Table 24-2); similarly, the prevalence of encopresis was 4.1% among 5- to 6-year-olds and 1.6% among 11- to 12-year-olds in a large, population-based study in The Netherlands, with an increased incidence among those with psychosocial problems.[21]

EMOTIONAL EFFECT RATHER THAN CAUSE

Traditionally, the perceived association between encopresis and serious emotional problems triggered mental health referrals for children presenting with stool leakage or larger accidents.[22] Children with stool accidents are at risk for physical and sexual abuse, perhaps because their accidents trigger anger in uninformed caregivers, although encopresis may also be a physical response to anal trauma.[23] Children who are traumatized can lose continence as a sign of regression, like all other fragile developmental skills that deteriorate in times of stress. Stool incontinence can also be a protection against abuse; a child may discover that stool in the underwear will keep an abuser away. In all cases of children presenting with encopresis, possible abuse must be explored, although it is rarely found.

Children with encopresis can develop emotional problems, which may be a consequence of being teased and embarrassed, leading to poor self-esteem, anxiety, reduced school performance, and impaired social success.[24] They may suffer when uneducated families exacerbate their sense of failure, expecting the child to stop the accidents despite his or her inability to control them. However, in most cases, encopresis is not symptomatic of a larger psychiatric problem.[25]

Cause

More than 90% of cases of encopresis result from constipation.[24] Anything that causes constipation can therefore cause encopresis. In rare cases, the cause is a neurological disorder, such as a tethered spinal cord. Children with tethered cords may have been continent and then regressed; as the child grows, the spinal cord stretches as a result of the abnormal tethering, causing neurological impairment. In addition to deterioration of continence, these children also may have gait changes, lower back pain, abnormal lower extremity reflexes, or lower back skin manifestations including lumbosacral dimples or hair tufts.

Another cause of encopresis without constipation is emotional trauma. Affected children may have been abused and, at times of stress, become disorganized and overwhelmed, which is manifested as stool accidents. Some children may purposely have accidents to keep an abuser away. Direct anal trauma may cause loss of sphincter control as well.

CONSTIPATION OF VARYING DEGREES

Most children with encopresis are constipated.[26] However, mild constipation can lead to overflow incontinence, whereas some severely constipated children have no encopresis. The critical variable seems to be the amount of rectal dilatation, not the absolute amount of stool in the bowel. Historical details elucidate the degree of impaction and dictate the intensity of intervention.

CAUSES OF CONSTIPATION

Constipation is common in U.S. children, affecting 5% of children aged 4 to 11 years.[27] In most children, there is no specific abnormality or disease that necessitates treatment. Again, history and physical examination identifies children in need of investigation for a pathological cause of constipation. The symptoms of slow growth, depression, and weight gain and a positive family history are indications for thyroid function testing to assess for hypothyroidism. A thorough physical examination should include an assessment for any signs of neuropathy or myopathy, which could manifest in the gastrointestinal tract with constipation. Conditions such as cerebral palsy or myelomeningocele are frequently associated with chronic constipation. It is also possible on physical examination to detect anatomical abnormalities, such as a very anterior ectopic anus or anal ring stenosis. Although inflammatory bowel disease more commonly manifests with loose stools, constipation is possible, and systemic symptoms, anal tags, weight loss, and a family history of autoimmune disorders may indicate the need for a workup for these conditions. Severe constipation is also possible in celiac disease.

Children with lifelong constipation symptoms may have Hirschsprung disease. They have had difficulty in evacuation from birth with recurrent abdominal distension. They may have frequent emesis and may suffer from failure to thrive and enterocolitis in infancy. Encopresis is rare in children with Hirschsprung disease and is found only in affected children with the rare short-segment form of Hirschsprung disease. In addition to historical information, a tight aganglionic rectum around the examining finger found during rectal examination should raise suspicion. Typically, children with encopresis have either normal rectal examination findings or decreased rectal tone and a palpable stool mass.

Many medications can cause constipation. Several psychoactive treatments can be constipating, such as selective serotonergic reuptake inhibitors, α-adrenergic agents (clonidine, guanfacine), and atypical neuroleptic agents. Anticholinergic medications, such as oxybutynin chloride (used for urinary incontinence), can be constipating as well.

IMPAIRED BOWEL SENSATION AND MUSCULAR STATUS

When encopresis is caused by constipation, impairment of bowel integrity is thought to be the cause. Stool is retained, dilating the rectum and sometimes the sigmoid colon. The bowel wall is stretched by the stool mass, and often the rectum becomes impacted with hard feces. Water is absorbed by the gut wall, and the feces becomes harder the longer they remain in the bowel. The stretched muscle layers lose ability to contract effectively against the large mass, and stool leakage around the stool mass develops.

BODY SIGNALS BECOME INCONSISTENT

When impacted stool blocks the rectum, stretch receptors are thought to lose the ability to sense when the rectal vault becomes filled, as the receptors remain stretched by the abnormally large fecal mass. Theoretically, no signal that the rectum is filling and the external sphincter should be contracted is sent to the brain. Softer stool formed proximally then leaks around or between hardened rocks of stool in the rectum, leaking into underwear without warning. This leakage is the main hallmark of encopresis. Leakage may be liquid or formed, daily or less frequent. Some children have more leakage just before evacuating, which indicates that the rectum has filled, has stretched, and cannot detect and respond to stool reaching the anus. For those children, they may have intact sensation when their rectum is not filled and thus frequently sense the need to defecate, voluntarily contract the external sphincter, and prevent accidents. However, as the impacted stool enlarges, sensation deteriorates, and accidents occur.

Diagnosis

HISTORY AND EXAMINATION REGARDING CONSTIPATION AND NEUROLOGICAL PATHOLOGY

The clinician should begin with a detailed history and physical examination, in order to diagnose encopresis and create a treatment plan. The history documentation should include questions about meconium passage after delivery and any early interventions needed for hard, painful stools. Very early symptoms are suggestive of Hirschsprung disease, which usually manifests with difficulty in evacuation from birth. It is helpful to identify any evidence of systemic diseases or medical causes of constipation from the medical and surgical history that indicate treatments other than laxatives and maintenance of stool regularity.

The current history should include the patient's urinary and bowel patterns, such as frequency of stool evacuation into the toilet, stool accidents, stool consistency, and the urge to defecate. More severe, prolonged constipation usually necessitates more aggressive treatment. A history of abuse or trauma suggests the possibility of an emotional basis for accidents and the need for further psychological assessment. Children may become incontinent in times of stress or as part of regressive behavior, even in the absence of specific sexual or physical abuse.

Abnormal urinary patterns and urine continence can be manifestations of neurological abnormalities underlying both stooling and voiding concerns. Constipation and encopresis also may be associated with urinary tract infections, especially in girls. Even without infection, enuresis can be caused by a dilated rectum pushing on and irritating the bladder, thus causing spasm. The history may reveal that increasing stool backup is associated with urine accidents. Families should be asked to chart defecation and urination into the toilet, accidents, and quality of stooling in order to clarify these temporal relationships.

As part of the developmental history, details of toilet training, when and which methods were used, and successes or failures can be helpful. Some children with stool accidents have never actually been toilet trained. They have never developed the skill to sense impending defecation, hold it in, and then evacuate on the toilet. These children require directed behavioral programming that focuses on identifying the body signal of a distended rectum, maintaining control over the body by contracting the external sphincter, and cooperating with using the toilet. Toilet refusal often leads to constipation as well, and thus treatment to improve bowel regularity and consistency is often needed.

The physical examination of the child with encopresis includes measurement of growth parameters, consideration of any signs of systemic disease, complete neurological examination, and inspection of the anal opening. Anal fissures cause chronic pain with repeated defecation, tags may indicate inflammatory bowel disease, and an absent anal wink or cremasteric reflex in boys raises concerns for a neurological abnormality. A child with an anteriorly placed anus requires referral to a surgeon. The rectal examination can aid in assessing for Hirschsprung disease and may offer information about the extent of rectal impaction to guide treatment. Rectal examination may divulge low anal pressure, which implies external and/or internal sphincter disease. The rectal examination, when performed with the child lying on his or her back in a modified lithotomy position, helps to minimize the patient's discomfort.

For children with a history of sexual abuse or who are struggling with the first public discussion of this private problem, a rectal examination may be deferred at the first visit, but visualization of the anal area is essential. A digital examination needs to be performed at least once to rule out organic causes of constipation, particularly in children who do not respond well to typical treatment in a timely manner.

RADIOLOGICAL EXAMINATIONS

For most children with encopresis, assessment can be limited to the history and physical examination alone. An abdominal radiograph is a useful adjunct when the history is vague, when the child is uncooperative with examination, or when the family and child would benefit from concrete evidence of constipation. The North American Society for Pediatric Gastroenterology and Nutrition recommends an abdominal film when the child's constipation history is in doubt, if the child or parent refuses a digital examination, or if the digital examination is to be avoided because of a history of trauma.[28] However, a review of 392 studies of the evaluation of children with constipation and encopresis revealed that the evidence of an association between the clinical symptoms of constipation and fecal load on radiographs was inconclusive.[29] Lumbosacral spine films or magnetic resonance imaging (MRI) is indicated when lower extremity neurological examination findings are abnormal or lumbosacral abnormalities are visualized. Children treated for encopresis for prolonged periods without expected improvement may also be considered for lumbosacral MRI in search of tethered cord with unusually silent neurological examination findings.

Treatment

BEHAVIORAL STRATEGIES

Encopresis treatment begins with demystification of the problem. Most children and their families have never met or heard of other people with this problem, and usually the child has been punished, blamed, or shamed. Explaining the underlying constipation that prevents the child from being able to control the stool accidents is an essential first intervention. Use of pictures or the child's own abdominal film can help the family understand the degree of impaction and need for stool evacuation.

From the start of treatment, patients and their families should learn that combined medication and behavioral interventions are vital for successful outcomes.[30] Because the bowel wall is stretched and cannot send the brain signals for defecation, a schedule for evacuation is necessary until normal feedback systems are restored. Even if the child does not feel the need to defecate, he or she should sit on the toilet and try to evacuate the bowel regularly. Sit-down times can take place 30 minutes after each meal, lasting for 10 minutes each. Most children do not want to sit during school, so the midday sit-down can take place on weekends only. Younger children may benefit from small rewards or treats for cooperating with the sit-down time and trying to defecate. Treats should be small and inexpensive, such as stickers, an extra story at bedtime, or use of a favorite toy. They also may find it helpful to blow up a balloon or place their hand on their lower abdomen and feel their abdomen push outward when bearing down.

Because children with stool accidents often hide dirty underwear and are frequently punished when the underwear is found, an important part of the intervention is to eliminate negative consequences and provide support for the child in coping with the accidents until symptoms resolve. Older children can be offered a bucket with water and bleach (out of the reach of small children) where dirty underwear can be placed discreetly.

MEDICATION FOR CONSTIPATION

In addition to the initial education and demystification, encopresis treatment starts with a bowel cleanout. More aggressive regimens tend to be associated with better results. Children aged 7 years and older usually can be treated with enemas. One effective treatment plan repeats a 3-day cycle consisting of an enema on day 1, a bisacodyl tablet on day 2, and a bisacodyl suppository on day 3; then the cycle is repeated three times, thereby running 12 to 15 days. Several cleanout schedules can be used regularly, including molasses enemas, polyethylene glycol with electrolyte cleanouts, and high doses of polyethylene glycol without electrolytes. No single cleanout method has been demonstrated to be most effective, but a major objective should be to avoid increasing the child's accident frequency during school hours.

After impacted stool has been evacuated, all treated children require maintenance management, and they usually require more than dietary changes alone. Recurrences of encopresis often develop after initial cleanouts when families and children fail to continue constipation treatment. Daily use of polyethylene glycol without electrolytes, mineral oil, lactulose, milk of magnesia, or methylcellulose (Citrucel®) is generally adequate. Some children need stimulants such as senna or bisacodyl on an intermittent basis as well. Daily toilet sitting after breakfast and dinner, combined with the medication regimen, is essential because by the time the child actually feels the need for a bowel movement, too much stool has reaccumulated in the previously dilated rectum.

RELEVANT RESEARCH OF EFFICACY

One review of 16 randomized or quasi-randomized trials of more than 800 children with encopresis revealed that behavioral intervention plus laxative therapy, rather than either alone, improved fecal continence in children with encopresis.[30] Most children treated for encopresis have meaningful improvement, although there are few data to guide prediction. Recovery rates have been reported as 30% to 50% after 1 year and 48% to 75% after 5 years.

ENURESIS

Primary Monosymptomatic Nocturnal Enuresis

Enuresis is defined as repeated voiding of urine into clothes during the day or into the bed during the night in a child who is chronologically and developmentally older than 5 years.[18] The accidents must occur at least twice per week for 3 months or cause significant distress or impairment. This broad category is divided into primary uncomplicated (monosymptomatic) nocturnal enuresis (no period longer than 6 months of being dry at night, no daytime symptoms), secondary or complicated nocturnal enuresis (nighttime wetness after a period of 6 months of being dry and/or the presence of daytime symptoms), and daytime incontinence. Monosymptomatic nocturnal enuresis rarely signifies an underlying organic abnormality, whereas presence of daytime symptoms is more likely to signify a disorder. Regardless of the type of enuresis, the workup and treatment needs to take into account both medical and psychological implications common to children with urine accidents.

SIGNIFICANCE

The achievement of nighttime continence results from a maturing of the urological and neurological systems. Sympathetic stimulation from nerves T11 to L2 induces detrusor muscle relaxation so the bladder can fill, while the internal sphincter muscle (bladder neck) contracts to contain the urine.[31] Infants have a small bladder that reflexively empties without voluntary control. To empty, parasympathetic fibers from nerves S2 to S4 activate the detrusor muscle to contract, increasing the intravesicular pressure and relaxing the bladder neck. Voluntary control comes from communication between the pontine micturition center and the sacral nerves, allowing voiding to be inhibited. Over the first 2 years of life, bladder capacity increases, along with central nervous system maturity, and thus the child develops greater awareness of bladder filling. Bladder capacity further increases between 2 and 4 years of age, when voluntary control during the day develops.

To maintain nighttime dryness, some children are aroused by a full bladder and wake to void. In most children, the amount of urine produced per hour decreases, and the functional bladder capacity to remain continent during sleep increases. When waking, children produce a large volume of concentrated urine. Nocturnal enuresis can therefore reflect a delay or defect in any of these elements.

INCIDENCE AND RESOLUTION RATE

Most children are continent at night within 2 years of completing daytime toilet training. However, by 7.5 years, 15.5% of children remain wet at night, although only 2.5% wet often enough to meet criteria for enuresis.[32] Each year, bed-wetting self-resolves in 15% of children,[33] so that 1% to 2% of 15-year-olds remain wet at night.[34] For unclear reasons, boys are twice as likely to suffer from this problem.[19] Bed-wetting seems to occur with similar prevalence across cultures, ethnicities, and socioeconomic classes.

EFFECT ON CHILDREN AND FAMILIES

Nocturnal enuresis is rarely associated with serious psychiatric disorders.[35] However, experiencing the frustration of persistent bed-wetting can affect the emotional well-being of affected children. At a minimum, affected children face barriers to activities involving an overnight stay, such as camp, sleepovers, and vacations. Furthermore, affected children have less competence socially, lower school success rates, and higher than expected levels of behavioral problems.[36] For example, 50 children with enuresis were compared with children suffering from asthma and heart problems with regard to their attitudes toward their conditions.[37] Children with bed-wetting had more negative feelings about their condition, more maladaptive coping strategies, and more negative adjustment to the stress bed-wetting causes, regardless of the frequency of nighttime accidents and history of treatment failures. Of importance is that positive attitude was correlated with improved response to treatment.

Nighttime bed-wetting typically is stressful to families of affected children, particularly when parents are uninformed about the accidental nature of the disorder. Parents of children who wet the bed report significant levels of withdrawn, anxious, and depressed symptoms in their children, which indicates the negative parental perception of these children.[35] Traditionally, children with enuresis have been considered at increased risk for child abuse; according to a study of 889 mothers in Turkey, child abuse was reported in 86% of children with enuresis.[38]

Other studies indicate that children with bed-wetting may have a higher incidence of attention-deficit/hyperactivity disorder (ADHD), a finding that matches common clinical experience. In one study of 120 children aged 6 to 12 years who were referred to an incontinence program, 37.5% met criteria for ADHD[39]; this percentage was far greater than the expected rate of 7.5%.[40] Similarly, children with ADHD seem to have more voiding dysfunction than do those without ADHD.[41] Furthermore, studies show significantly lower success rates of bed-wetting treatment by alarm or medication in children with ADHD than in those without ADHD, perhaps because of the greater difficulty with compliance by children with ADHD.[42]

CAUSES

The specific cause of enuresis is unknown, although it is thought to be multifactorial. Each affected child may have a single or multiple predisposing factors, which may indicate the most appropriate and successful treatment choice.

Genetics

It is unknown to most affected patients that nocturnal enuresis frequently runs in families. However, parents rarely reveal their own history of bed-wetting to a spouse or child, until specifically probed about the topic. In fact, most children with bed-wetting have an extended family history of the condition.[43] The child of one parent with a history of bed-wetting has a 44% risk of the same condition; if both parents wet their beds as children, their offspring have a 77% chance of also being affected.[44] Several studies have shown a strong genetic linkage on chromosomes 13q, 12q, 22q, and 8q, although heterogeneity exists.[45] Genetic testing is currently not useful in the diagnosis or treatment of enuresis.

Sleep

Some children with enuresis do not wake in response to the sensation of a full bladder. Parents have long claimed that their children with bed-wetting were heavy sleepers, a finding often attributed to a selection bias because their child with enuresis is the only child they awaken to urinate. However, studies have shown that children with bed-wetting have a higher threshold for arousal: for example, a stimulus that awakened 40% of controls awakened only 9% of enuretic patients in one sample of 33 boys.[46] Sleep studies of children with bed-wetting are not uniformly distinct from those of controls, and there is no specific time of the night or stage of sleep when enuresis is more likely to occur.[47]

Decreased Bladder Capacity

A mismatch between urine production and the amount of urine contained in the bladder at night seems to cause bed-wetting as well. In the normal circadian rhythm, the body produces less urine per hour at night than during the day; in some children nocturnal urine output may fail to decrease and therefore overwhelms the bladder's ability to prevent outflow. Other children may secrete insufficient amounts of antidiuretic hormone at night or may have resistance to antidiuretic hormone produced. This population may be helped by desmopressin (DDAVP), which decreases urine production and is further described in the section on medications. A final explanation for mismatch is decreased functional bladder capacity, which means the bladder empties before it is filled, although study findings are mixed.[48]

DIAGNOSIS

History

Obtaining a thorough history is vital in the diagnostic and therapeutic process for children with bed-wetting. The full medical and developmental histories may link bed-wetting to a systemic disorder or to global developmental problems. Details about urination and defecation clarify whether enuresis is primary or secondary and whether constipation is causal or comorbid. Constipation is a common cause of enuresis; a full bowel can interfere with bladder sensation, impede bladder emptying, and reduce bladder capacity. Information from the family history of nocturnal enuresis can help diagnostically, in view of the child's increased risk, and can relieve some of the child's isolation and shame instantly. Information from the social history should specifically include possible trauma, abuse, recent stressors, and emotional consequences of bed-wetting. The child and family should be asked how the bed-wetting has interfered with social opportunities and family function. Methods implemented to address the problem, such as alarms, incentives, punishments, and medications, must be reviewed in detail. Often, the parent may have used incentives without necessary strategies to address the cause of wetting (i.e., treat constipation), or they used alarms when the child was too young or they used them inappropriately.

Physical Examination

The physical examination first serves to rule out systemic organic disorders. Signs of constipation should also be noted. Because the innervations of the bladder and the sacral region and lower extremities are shared, special attention must be paid to these areas. Deep tendon reflexes of the patellae and Achilles tendons, as well as perianal and perineal sensation, and cremasteric reflexes in boys are important indicators of neurological status. The genitalia must be examined. The lower spine must be palpated and examined for defects such as hairy tufts and lumps, potential indicators of spinal cord abnormalities.

Testing

All children with nocturnal enuresis need to undergo urinalysis. This single, inexpensive, noninvasive test may suggest infection, concentrating defect, or diabetes as the cause. A urine culture is usually indicated in girls. In children with normal physical examination findings, unremarkable histories, and no daytime urinary symptoms, no further workup is indicated.

TREATMENT

The treatment of nocturnal enuresis begins with education and demystification. Because of the shame and blame common to families affected by bed-wetting, it is important to provide an explanation that the problem is not a voluntary behavior but rather physiological and often genetically mediated. In our clinical experience, this intervention can immediately help to change a family dynamic and a child's self-concept.

Alarms

Bed-wetting alarms, first described before 1900, are the mainstay of nocturnal enuresis treatment.[49] The alarm, which may sound or vibrate, is connected to the child's underwear and goes off when moisture is detected. The child must rouse or be aroused by parents, must urinate, must change his or her underwear and bed sheet, and re-place the alarm. Visualization should be practiced before going to sleep; the child imagines waking to the alarm, going to the bathroom, urinating, changing, fixing the bed and re-placing the alarm, and returning to sleep.[50] In addition, before bed, the child should complete a practice run, pretending to finish each of these steps. It is

helpful to recommend that parents reward their child in the morning; for the first week, children should receive a treat for waking with the help of a parent; for the second week, for waking independently; and after that, for waking up dry in the morning. Over the weeks, the urine mark will probably shrink in size, as the child wakes earlier in the void. For maximum success, after the child has been dry for 1 month, "over-treating" by having the child drink a glass of water before bed is effective.[51] Three to 4 months of alarm use is often required, and considerable motivation is necessary for both the child and parents. Alarms cost from $40 to $100 dollars and may or may not be covered by medical insurance. After use of the alarm, some children learn to wake to urinate, but most sleep through the night and remain dry. Alarms have been found to cure at least two thirds of affected children, with a low relapse rate.[52]

Medications

Medications also can be a useful component in enuresis treatment. DDAVP, an antidiuretic hormone analogue, is approved by the U.S. Food and Drug Administration for nocturnal enuresis. Given as a tablet or intranasal spray before bedtime, DDAVP decreases urine production for up to 7 hours.[53] On the basis of this mechanism of action, it seems that children with nocturnal polyuria are most likely to be responsive. DDAVP can be used on an as-needed basis, a method often preferred by families because of its high cost. DDAVP has few side effects, but drinking after taking DDAVP at night should be avoided in order to prevent water intoxication, which can rarely result in hyponatremic seizures. Imipramine, a tricyclic antidepressant, is also approved for bed-wetting, but its risk for cardiotoxicity and its narrow margin of safety limits its utility. The mechanism of imipramine is unknown, but it has an efficacy rate of 30% to 50%. When DDAVP or imipramine is discontinued, the relapse rate for both is 60%. Large meta-analyses confirm the greater success rates of alarms over these medications; a lower relapse rate and less toxicity are associated with alarm use.[54] Alternatively, DDAVP or imipramine can be used along with the alarm, in some cases leading to improved outcomes.[55]

Alternative treatments for nocturnal enuresis, although popular, currently lack conventional evidence to support their widespread use. Limited evidence-based data support the use of hypnosis, psychotherapy, and chiropractics in bed-wetting treatment[56]; however, a growing body of literature substantiates the role of acupuncture, long practiced in Chinese medicine and studied internationally in such countries as the United States, Italy, Japan, Korea, and Romania.[57]

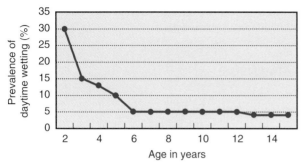

FIGURE 24-1 Prevalence of daytime wetting by age. (Adapted from Robson WL: Diurnal enuresis. Pediatr Rev 18:407-12, 1997.)

Daytime Incontinence

Children usually develop daytime continence between 2 and 4 years of age, with increasing bladder capacity, sensation of fullness, and voluntary control over the external sphincter. Children presenting with daytime incontinence caused by a physiological abnormality must be distinguished from those who have failed to toilet train in the context of developmental delays, because a stepwise approach with developmentally appropriate expectations is indicated for the latter population.

SIGNIFICANCE

Incidence

Daytime continence is achieved in 70% of children by age 3 years and in 90% by age 6 years (Fig. 24-1).[58] The exceptions raise suspicion for organic pathology, as do cases in which children were previously dry during the day and later suffer from accidents. Daytime incontinence is most commonly caused by treatable or benign conditions, but the rare and potentially serious origins must be investigated. Fortunately, a thorough history, physical examination, and urinalysis are generally adequate diagnostically to identify these conditions.

Causes

INCREASED OUTPUT

Several disorders of increased urine output can manifest with daytime or new-onset nighttime urine accidents. Urinalysis with glucose present helps identify patients who have diabetes mellitus, and urinalysis with a low specific gravity helps identify those with diabetes insipidus. A history of excessive water intake without an organic cause suggests a psychiatrically based condition. Children with sickle cell disease often have concentrating defects as well.

BLADDER INSTABILITY

Bladder instability is the most common cause for daytime accidents. The differential diagnosis should include, foremost, constipation, which should be con-

sidered as a trigger for bladder spasm. Constipation and encopresis occurred in 35% of children with daytime incontinence in one study of almost 1500 Swedish elementary school students[59]; this finding confirmed the clinical experience of this common copresentation. Dysuria also frequently signifies a urinary tract infection, diagnosed with a urine culture. In teenage girls, pregnancy must also be considered.

A number of dysfunctional voiding syndromes also underlie daytime accidents. Preschool- and elementary school–aged girls may have urge syndrome, caused by an uninhibited bladder that contracts at low volumes. This causes both urgency and frequency, and children may attempt to suppress detrusor contraction by squatting onto their heel. Symptoms generally improve or resolve with time, although anticholinergic agents can be helpful as well. Hinman syndrome, or nonneurogenic neurogenic bladder, may be an extreme form of urge syndrome. In addition to incontinence, affected children often have urinary tract infections, constipation, and encopresis. Urodynamic studies may be necessary, because of the complex nature of Hinman syndrome; they demonstrate poor coordination between the bladder and sphincter and may reveal a trabeculated bladder, postvoid residual, vesicoureteral reflux, a dilated upper urinary tract, and renal scarring. Urology referral and management are indicated.

Giggle incontinence generally affects school-aged girls whose entire bladders empty with laughter. This phenomenon may be familial and often resolves with age. When the condition persists, patients can be advised to void regularly to maintain an empty bladder and to sit when laughing to minimize incontinent symptoms. Others may have stress incontinence, when increased intra-abdominal pressure causes bladder contraction without contraction of the proximal urethra. Interventions are similar to those for giggle incontinence.

ABNORMAL SPHINCTER CONTROL

Spinal cord abnormalities rarely cause daytime incontinence, but because of their serious morbidity, they must be carefully considered in every patient with symptoms. Bladder function can be affected by a lesion at any level of the spine. A tethered cord manifests as a child grows. In contrast to the normally free-floating spinal cord within the canal, the tethered cord is abnormally attached to a local structure; with growth and movement, the cord and its blood supply stretch and are damaged. In addition to a change in bladder or bowel function, children with a tethered cord may have back pain, gait changes, scoliosis, and abnormal reflexes. External features include a sacral tuft or pit. Obtaining a sacral MRI is indicated, followed by a referral to a neurosurgeon if an abnormality is noted.

STRUCTURAL ABNORMALITIES

Structural defects complete the list of organic pathology that can manifest with incontinence. In vaginal reflux, urine does not clear the labia and drips out after voiding is complete. Girls with this condition experience wetness after leaving the bathroom, and they can treat the condition by pulling their underwear completely down when voiding and spreading their legs to open the labia; sometimes they may even need to sit backwards on the toilet to urinate. Other girls may have similar symptoms from labial fusion and can be treated with estrogen cream. In girls who have ectopic ureter with constant wetting, the urethral opening can be visualized adjacent to the urethral meatus or vagina, or it may be located on the cervix or uterus. The diagnosis is confirmed by intravenous pyelogram or computed tomography. Finally, urethral obstruction can be caused by valves, strictures, diverticula, and foreign bodies. Affected children may have an abnormal urine stream and may require increased intra-abdominal pressure to void. Voiding cystourethrography can be performed to assess for obstruction.

DIAGNOSIS

History

The diagnostic process begins with a detailed history. Routine documentation of medical history focuses on symptoms of systemic diseases or neurological dysfunction. The onset of incontinence must be reviewed, as must the presence or absence of associated symptoms. It is important to collect the details of the presenting symptoms, such as frequency, timing, and size of both voiding and accidents, in a diary completed by the family before the visit. The clinician needs to recognize comorbid constipation and/or encopresis. The social history must focus on any antecedent trauma, as well as emotional consequences of urine accidents.

Physical Examination

The physical examination is identical to that in the child with nighttime enuresis. It entails the close examination of the perineal, perianal, and sacral regions, as well as a detailed neurological assessment.

Testing

In any child with daytime urinary incontinence, an initial urinalysis is essential. Further investigation should be pursued on the basis of history and examination findings. In children who are unresponsive to the typical behavioral interventions to be described,

urodynamic studies, sacral MRI, and urological referral should be considered.

TREATMENT

Referrals

For children with suspected or confirmed structural defects, referral to a urologist for further assessment and surgery is often necessary. A neurosurgeon must be consulted for children with tethered spinal cord. However, most children with daytime incontinence can be managed in the primary care setting.

Behavioral

Like the treatment of primary nocturnal enuresis, behavioral interventions are the primary intervention for children with daytime accidents without surgical or medical treatment indications. First, the child and family should complete a log for several days. Data gathered includes time of void, urine accidents, amount voided, associated symptoms of pain, squatting, defecation, and stool accidents.

Expected functional bladder capacity in ounces is (age in years +2).[60] If the volume of urine voided is less than expected, the child has a small functional bladder capacity.

Again, education and demystification are the initial steps in the therapeutic process for children with incontinence. Reviewing the log together with the patient and parents provides the clinician with an opportunity to highlight successes and understand the cause of accidents. If constipation is present, it must be treated aggressively, before further efforts are made in addressing urinary symptoms. Children who squat can be taught about their inadvertent bladder muscle contractions and should be applauded for coming in to figure out a way to stop them. Children with giggle incontinence may be relieved to know that other children suffer from the same problem. Most children with daytime incontinence, regardless of the underlying cause, benefit from scheduled voids. A trip to the bathroom at 2-hour intervals gives the child a chance to void before involuntary contractions cause accidents. A watch that beeps every 2 hours can be helpful, or the child may participate in creating a schedule that does not interfere with school activities.

Children with small functional bladder capacity or involuntary bladder contractions may benefit from urge containment exercises. Once on or at the toilet to void, the child is asked to "hold it in," then void, then "hold it in again," and then fully void. The objectives are to strengthen both the child's sphincter and confidence.

Medication

Anticholinergics such as oxybutynin chloride and tolterodine tartrate may also be helpful in children with small bladder capacity caused by uninhibited detrusor contractions. Constipation is a common side effect and can be an obstacle to urinary continence.

SUMMARY OF CLINICAL CARE

Children with disorders of elimination commonly need a unique combination of both medical considerations and behavioral interventions. Acquisition of bowel and bladder continence requires developmentally obtained skills, neurological integrity, regularity of stooling and urination, and motivation and a favorable attitude on the part of the child. Unevenness in any of these realms can impede successful continence. Although limited, increasing evidence guides specific behavioral and medical interventions that can effectively improve the quality of life of most affected children and their families.

REFERENCES

1. Seim HC: Toilet training in first children. J Fam Pract 29:633-636, 1989.
2. Schum TR, McAuliffe TL, Simms MD, et al: Factors associated with toilet training in the 1990s. Ambul Pediatr 1:79-86, 2001.
3. Spock B: The Common Sense Book of Baby and Child Care. New York: Duell, Sloan & Pearce, 1946.
4. Brazelton TB: A child-oriented approach to toilet training. Pediatrics 29:121-128, 1962.
5. Schmitt BD: Toilet training: Getting it right the first time. Contemp Pediatr 21:105-122, 2004.
6. Blum NJ, Taubman B, Nemeth N: Why is toilet training occurring at older ages? A study of factors associated with later training. J Pediatr 145:107-112, 2004.
7. Sun M, Rugolotto S: Assisted infant toilet training in a Western family setting. J Dev Behav Pediatr 25:99-101, 2004.
8. Christophersen ER: The case for evidence-based toilet training. Arch Dis Pediatr Adolesc Med 157:1153-1154, 2003.
9. Brooks RC, Copen RM, Cox DJ, et al: Review of the treatment literature for encopresis, functional constipation, and stool-toileting refusal. Ann Behav Med 22:260-267.
10. Azrin NH, Foxx RM: Toilet Training in Less than a Day. New York: Simon & Schuster, 1974.
11. Brazelton TB, Sparrow JD: Toilet Training, The Brazelton Way. Cambridge, MA: De Capo Press, 2004.
12. Schmitt BD: Toilet training problems: Underachievers, refusers, and stool holders. Contemp Pediatr 21:71-82, 2004.
13. Schonwald A, Sherritt L, Stadtler A, et al: Factors associated with difficult toilet training. Pediatrics 113:1753-1757, 2004.
14. Blum NJ, Taubman B, Nemeth N: During toilet training, constipation occurs before stool toileting refusal. Pediatrics 113:e520-e522, 2004.
15. Shaikh N: Time to get on the potty: Are constipation and stool toileting refusal causing delayed toilet training? J Pediatr 145:12-13, 2004.
16. Taubman B, Blum NJ, Nemeth N: Stool toileting refusal: A prospective intervention targeting parental behavior. Arch Pediatr Adolesc Med 157:1193-1196, 2003.
17. Schonwald A, Huntington N, Lesser T, et al: Toilet School: A Promising Intervention for Difficult and Late Toilet Training. Poster presented at the Annual Meeting of the Pediatric Academic Societies, Washington, DC, May 2005.
18. American Psychiatric Association: Diagnostic and Statistical Manual of Mental Disorders, 4th edition, text revision. Washington, DC: American Psychiatric Press, 2000.
19. Schonwald A, Rappaport L: Consultation with the specialist: Encopresis: Assessment and management. Pediatr Rev 25:278-283, 2004.
20. Loening-Baucke V: Encopresis. Curr Opin Pediatr 14:570-575, 2002.
21. van der Wal MF, Benninga MA, Hirasing RA: The prevalence of encopresis in a multicultural population. J Pediatr Gastroenterol Nutr 40:345-348, 2005.
22. Foreman DM, Thambirajah M: Encopresis was associated with child sexual abuse. Child Abuse Negl 22:337, 1998.
23. Morrow J, Yeager CA, Lewis DO: Encopresis and sexual abuse in a sample of boys in residential treatment. Child Abuse Negl 21:11-18, 1997.
24. Benninga MA, Buller HA, Heymans HS, et al: Is encopresis always the result of constipation? Arch Dis Child 71:186-193, 1994.
25. Loening-Baucke V: Encopresis and soiling. Pediatr Clin North Am 43:279-298, 1996.
26. Voskuijl WP, Heijmans J, Heijmans HS, et al: Use of Rome II criteria in childhood defecation disorders: Applicability in clinical and research practice. J Pediatr 145:213-217, 2004.
27. Borowitz SM, Cox DJ, Tam A, et al: Precipitants of constipation during early childhood. J Am Board Fam Pract 16:213-218, 2003.
28. Baker SS, Liptak GS, Colletti RB, et al: Constipation in infants and children: Evaluation and treatment. A medical position statement of the North American Society for Pediatric Gastroenterology and Nutrition. J Pediatr Gastroenterol Nutr 29:612-626, 1999.
29. Reuchlin-Vroklage LM, Bierma-Zeinstra S, Benninga MA, et al: Diagnostic value of abdominal radiography in constipated children: A systematic review. Arch Pediatr Adolesc Med 159:671-678, 2005.
30. Brazzelli M, Griffiths P: Behavioural and cognitive interventions with or without other treatments for defaecation disorders in children. Cochrane Database

Syst Rev (4): CD002240, 2005 [update, Cochrane Database Syst Rev (2):CD002240, 2006].

31. Silverstein DM: Enuresis in children: Diagnosis and management. Clin Pediatr 43:217-221, 2004.

32. Butler RJ, Golding J, Northstone K, et al: Nocturnal enuresis at 7.5 years old: Prevalence and analysis of clinical signs. BJU Int 96:404, 2005.

33. Forsythe WI, Redmond A: Enuresis and spontaneous cure rate. Study of 1129 enuretics. Arch Dis Child 49:259-263, 1974.

34. Byrd RS, Weitzman M, Lanphear NE, et al: Bed-wetting in US children: Epidemiology and related behavior problems. Pediatrics 98:414-419, 1996.

35. Van Hoecke E, Hoebeke P, Braet C, et al: An assessment of internalizing problems in children with enuresis. J Urol 171:2580-2583, 2004.

36. Landgraf JM, Abidari J, Cilento BG Jr, et al: Coping, commitment, and attitude: Quantifying the everyday burden of enuresis on children and their families. Pediatrics 113:334-344, 2004.

37. Wolanczyk T, Banasikowska I, Zlotkowski P, et al: Attitudes of enuretic children towards their illness. Acta Paediatr 91:844-848, 2002.

38. Can G, Topbas M, Okten A: Child abuse as a result of enuresis. Pediatr Int 46:64-66, 2004.

39. Baeyens D, Roeyers H, Hoebeke P, et al: Attention deficit/hyperactivity disorder in children with nocturnal enuresis. J Urol 171:2576-2579, 2004.

40. Barbaresi W, Katusic S, Colligan R, et al: How common is attention-deficit/hyperactivity disorder? Towards resolution of the controversy: Results from a population-based study. Acta Paediatr Suppl 93:55-59, 2004.

41. Duel BP, Steinberg-Epstein R, Hill M, et al: A survey of voiding dysfunction in children with attention deficit–hyperactivity disorder. J Urol 170:1521-1523, 2003.

42. Crimmins CR, Rathbun SR, Husmann DA: Management of urinary incontinence and nocturnal enuresis in attention-deficit hyperactivity disorder. J Urol 170:1347-1350, 2003.

43. Elian M, Elian E, Kaushansky A: Nocturnal enuresis: A familial condition. J R Soc Med 77:529-530, 1984.

44. Bakwin H: The genetics of enuresis. *In* Kolvin I, MacKeith RC, Meadow SR, eds: Bladder Control and Enuresis. London: William Heinemann, 1973, p 73.

45. von Gontard, A, Schaumburg, H, Hollmann, E, et al: The genetics of enuresis: A review. J Urol 166:2438-2443, 2001.

46. Wolfish NM, Pivik RT, Busby KA: Elevated sleep arousal thresholds in enuretic boys: Clinical implications. Acta Paediatr 86:381-384, 1997.

47. Neveus T: The role of sleep and arousal in nocturnal enuresis. Acta Paediatr 92:1118-1123, 2003.

48. Korzeniecka-Kozerska A, Zoch-Zwierz W, Wasilewska A: Functional bladder capacity and urine osmolality in children with primary monosymptomatic nocturnal enuresis. Scand J Urol Nephrol 39:56-61, 2005.

49. Kristensen G, Jensen IN: Meta-analyses of results of alarm treatment for nocturnal enuresis—Reporting practice, criteria and frequency of bedwetting. Scand J Urol Nephrol 37:232-238, 2003.

50. Mellon MW, McGrath ML: Empirically supported treatments in pediatric psychology: Nocturnal enuresis. J Pediatr Psychol 25:193-214, 2000.

51. Wagner W, Johnson SB, Walker D, et al: A controlled comparison of two treatments for nocturnal enuresis. J Pediatr 101:302-307, 1982.

52. Fritz G, Rockney R, Bernet W, et al: Practice parameter for the assessment and treatment of children and adolescents with enuresis. J Am Acad Child Adolesc Psychiatry 43:1540-1550, 2004.

53. Glazener CMA, Evans JHC: Desmopressin for nocturnal enuresis in children. Cochrane Database Syst Rev (3):CD002112, 2002.

54. Glazener CM, Evans JH, Peto RE: Alarm interventions for nocturnal enuresis in children. Cochrane Database Syst Rev (2):CD002911, 2003.

55. Hjalmas K, Arnold T, Bower W, et al: Nocturnal enuresis: An international evidence based management strategy. J Urol 171:2545-2561, 2004.

56. Glazener CM, Evans JH, Cheuk DK: Complementary and miscellaneous interventions for nocturnal enuresis in children. Cochrane Database Syst Rev (2):CD005230, 2005.

57. Bower WF, Diao M, Tang JL, et al: Acupuncture for nocturnal enuresis in children: A systematic review and exploration of rationale. Neurourol Urodyn 24:267-272, 2005.

58. Robson WL: Diurnal enuresis. Pediatr Rev 18:407-412, 1997.

59. Soderstrom U, Hoelcke M, Alenius L, et al: Urinary and faecal incontinence: A population-based study. Acta Paediatr 93:386-389, 2004.

60. Casale AJ: Getting to the bottom of the issue. Contemp Pediatr 2:107-116, 2000.

Sexuality

25A.
Sexual Development and Sexual Behavior Problems

JANE F. SILOVSKY ■ LISA M. SWISHER

Sexual behavior problems (SBPs) are deviations from typical sexual development and are defined as child-initiated behaviors that involve sexual body parts (i.e., genitals, anus, buttocks, or breasts) and are developmentally inappropriate or potentially harmful to themselves or others.[1] Information about sexual development and guidelines for differentiating typical sexual behaviors from SBPs are rarely integrated in child development books or other types of parent educational materials. Thus, parents are often unsure how to determine whether sexual behaviors, such as interactions between children involving touching of genitals, are just "playing doctor" or something of concern. Parental guidance on sexual matters provided by developmental pediatricians facilitates caregiver's education and decision making. Sexual behaviors occur on a continuum ranging from typical to problematic; therefore, to accurately identify and manage problems related to sexual behavior of children and youth, a good foundation in sexual development is necessary. Research on childhood SBPs is relatively new, although significant progress has been made since the 1980s in distinguishing typical development from SBPs, as well as in understanding the origins, trajectory, and treatment of SBPs in youth.

This chapter provides an overview of typical sexual development, knowledge, and behavior of preschoolers, school-aged children, and adolescents. To facilitate understanding of the terms and concepts, definitions of key variables are provided. SBPs are defined with information on origins of the behavior,

developmental progression, assessment, and treatment outcome research for children and adolescents. Guidelines for distinguishing typical sexual behavior from SBPs are provided, as are references for parental education guidelines. Gender identity disorder is not discussed in this section; it is addressed in Chapters 25B and 25C.

We are not aware of another text designed specifically for developmental-behavioral pediatricians that covers both sexual development and the identification, assessment, treatment of, and response to SBPs across childhood and adolescence. A number of references provide pediatricians with information about typical sexual development and parental guidance suggestions, including provision of sex education.[2-6] In addition, Horner provided a pediatric-focused brief review of sexual development and SBPs in children, including two case studies.[7] The Association for the Treatment of Sexual Abusers (ATSA) Task Force on Children with Sexual Behavior Problems published a report on the identification, assessment, treatment, and public policies on children with SBPs, but this report does not address adolescence.[8] Older reviews include an excellent book on sexually aggressive youth by Araji[9]; a chapter that also includes information on children with SBPs, adolescent sexual offenders, and adult sexual offenders[10]; and practice parameters provided by the American Academy of Child and Adolescent Psychiatry.[11] Readers of these older reviews are advised to recognize that research published more recently updates previous assumptions, particularly regarding trajectory of the behaviors, long-term risk, and treatment outcome.

TERMINOLOGY

For this chapter, sex and gender are distinguished as follows: *Sex* is the classification by male or female reproductive organs,[12] whereas *gender* is the

TABLE 25A-1 ■ Terms Used in This Chapter, Their Definitions, and Areas of Knowledge

Term	Definition	Reference
Term Used in This Chapter		
Gender	Behavioral, cultural, or psychological traits typically associated with one sex	13
Sex	Classification by male or female reproductive organs	12
Genitals	The organs of the reproductive system; especially the external genital organs	13
Private parts or sexual body parts	Genitals, buttocks, anus, and breasts	
Sex role or gender role	The degree to which an individual acts out a stereotypical masculine or feminine role in everyday behavior	157
Sexual orientation	The inclination of an individual with regard to heterosexual, homosexual, and bisexual behavior	13
Sex preferences	Sex that children prefer to be like, to identify with, and to imitate in regard to sex role behavior	16
Childhood sexual behavior	Child-initiated behaviors involving sexual body parts (i.e., genitals, anus, buttocks, or breasts)	1
Sex play	Childhood sexual behavior that occurs spontaneously and intermittently, is mutual and non-coercive when it involves other children, and does not cause emotional distress	1
Sexual curiosity	Sexual behavior or questions about sexual matters motivated by inquisitive interest	
Sexual behavior problems in children and adolescents	Child and adolescents-initiated behaviors involving sexual body parts (i.e., genitals, anus, buttocks, or breasts) that are developmentally inappropriate or potentially harmful to themselves or others	1
Interpersonal or intrusive sexual behavior problems	Sexual behavior problems that involve two or more individuals and direct physical contact	146
Aggressive sexual behaviors	Sexual behavior problems that involve coercion, force, hostile intent, harm, or threatened harm	
Adolescent sexual offender	Adolescents between the ages of 13 and 17 years who commit illegal sexual behavior as defined by the sex crime statutes of the jurisdiction in which the offense occurred	121
Areas of Knowledge		
Labels of female genitalia	Terms for female genitalia, such as *vagina* or a slang term	18
Labels of male genitalia	Terms for male genitalia, such as *penis* or slang term	18
Physiological distinctions between sexes	Understanding of the basic genitalia differences between sexes (i.e., boys/men have penises and girls/women have vaginas) rather than basing sex differences on other physical, behavioral, or character differences, often related to cultural gender distinctions (e.g., for white American children, beliefs that boys/men have short hair and girls/women have long hair)	18
Pregnancy and birth	Knowledge related to conception, roles of both father and mother in conception, intrauterine growth, and birth process (i.e., cesarean or vaginal delivery)	18
Adult sexual behavior	Behavior of adults related to intimate interactions, arousal, and/or stimulation of genitals, including kissing, masturbation, and sexual intercourse; not limited to procreation	18
Knowledge of sexual abuse	Conceptualizations of sexual abuse, abusers, victims, and consequences of abuse	18

behavioral, cultural, or psychological traits typically associated with one sex.[13] *Genitals* refers specifically to external organs of the reproductive system, but references to "private parts" also include buttocks, anus, and breasts. Before specific information about how sexual knowledge and behavior evolve over the course of childhood and adolescents is provided, clarification in terminology would facilitate understanding of the research. In regard to knowledge about sexual matters, researchers have examined a wide range of children's understanding of sex and sexual matters. Table 25A-1 lists the terms used in this chapter with their definitions.

SEXUAL DEVELOPMENT

Early Childhood: Infants, Toddlers, and Preschoolers (Aged 0 to 6 years)

PHYSICAL DEVELOPMENT

Even as infants, children are capable of sexual arousal; newborn boys have penile erections, and baby girls are capable of vaginal lubrication.[14-16] Otherwise, until puberty, there is limited change in physical sexual development (including hormonal and gonad changes) during early childhood.[3]

SEXUAL KNOWLEDGE

Children as young as 3 years of age can identify their own sex and, soon after, identify the sex of others.[17,18] Initially distinctions between the sexes are based on visual factors found in the culture (such as hair), although by age 3 or 4 years, many children are aware of genital differences.[18,19] Both girls and boys have been found to be more likely to know labels of male than of female genitalia.[20-22]

Much of the research on sexual knowledge of preschool children was conducted before 1997.[19,20,23-26] Interestingly, the same pattern of results for toddlers and preschoolers have been found in a more recent study on knowledge of genital differences, pregnancy, birth, procreation, sexual activities, and sexual abuse.[18] Preschool children's understanding of pregnancy and birth tends to be vague until age 6, when most report knowledge of intrauterine growth, a third know about the concept of fertilization, and most know about birth by cesarean or vaginal delivery. Knowledge of adult sexual behavior was most often limited to behaviors such as kissing and cuddling; only 9% of 3-year-olds mention explicit sexual behaviors, increasing to 21% for the 6-year-olds, and another 8% of 6-year-olds can give detailed descriptions of the acts. The rate of this behavior is affected by abuse: Sexually abused 2- to 5-year-olds have been found to talk more about sex than do preschool-aged children in normative samples of (33% and 2%, respectively).[27]

SEXUAL BEHAVIOR

Preschool-aged children are curious in general and tend to actively learn about the world through listening, looking, touching, and imitating. Children as young as 7 months have been found to touch and play with their own genitalia; this behavior is found in both sexes but is more common in boys.[15,16] Infants' and young children's self-touch appear largely related to curiosity and pleasure seeking.[3] Children aged 2 to 5 years look at others when they are nude, intrude on others' physical boundaries (e.g., stand too close to others), touch their own genitalia even in public, and touch women's breasts (occurring in at least 25% of normative samples[27,28]). Preschool-aged children's general curiosity about the world manifests with questions and exploratory and imitative behaviors concerning sexual body parts.[3] Although gender role behavior is seen as early as age 1, dressing like the opposite sex is also not unusual throughout this developmental period (14% of boys and 10% of girls).[27,28] Boys demonstrate strong same-sex preferences early in the preschool years that increase in strength over time, whereas girls' same-sex preferences, strong in the preschool years, wanes in later years.[16]

Nonintrusive sexual play of showing sex parts to other children was found in 9% of preschoolers, and 4.5% were reported to have touched another child's sexual body parts (reported by mothers).[27] Sexual play is discussed in more details in the next section. Culture and social context affects the incidence of these typical behaviors, inasmuch as frequencies of these behaviors have been found to differ by the population and the situation studied.[29-32] Cultural effects are described in more detail later in this chapter.

Intrusive (putting finger or objects in another child's vagina or rectum), planned, and aggressive sexual acts were not reported by anyone in a normative sample of mothers of preschool children.[33] Other rare behaviors include putting objects in vagina/rectum, putting the mouth on sexual body parts, and pretending toys are having sex.[29,27,32]

School-Aged Children (Aged 7 to 12 Years)

PHYSICAL DEVELOPMENT

Pubertal development on average begins around 10 years of age, with girls starting earlier then boys, and can begin as early as 7 or 8 years of age. For girls, early puberty starts with a growth spurt in height, followed by a growth spurt in weight. Boys' growth spurts are often later than girls,[2] and occurs with acceleration of the growth of the testes and scrotum, enlargement of the larynx, and deepening of the voice.[16] There is wide variation, affected by a variety of factors (e.g., nutrition, heredity, race), in the onset and course of puberty, including a 4- to 5-year age range for the onset of puberty.[16] This variability can have significant effects on social adjustment of youth. Further information about puberty is provided later in the section on adolescent sexual development.

SEXUAL KNOWLEDGE

Knowledge of pregnancy, birth, and adult sexual activity increases during the school-age period. By age 10, most children have basic and more realistic understanding of puberty, reproductive processes, and birth.[3] Accuracy of knowledge depends in part on the child's exposure to correct informal and formal educational material.

SEXUAL BEHAVIOR

School-age children's behaviors become more guided by societal rules, which restrict the types of sexual behavior demonstrated in public. Sexual behavior continues to occur throughout the school-age period, but it is more concealed, and thus caregivers may not be directly aware of the behavior. In contrast to younger children, school-aged children are much less likely to touch their private parts in public or women's breasts.[27] However, they are more interested in media and are more likely to seek out television and pictures that include nudity.[27] Masturbatory behaviors occur, with an increase in frequency in boys during this developmental period.[16] Modesty emerges during this developmental period, particularly in girls, who become more shy and private about undressing and hygiene activities.[34]

During the early school years, children tend to seek out and interact with children of the same sex.[35] Interest in the opposite sex increases near the end of this developmental period with puberty, and interactive behaviors initiates with playful teasing of others. A small but substantial portion is involved in more explicit sexual activity, including sexual intercourse, at the end of this developmental period.[36]

SEXUAL PLAY

Sexual play is distinguished from problematic behaviors in that childhood sexual play involves behaviors that occur spontaneously and intermittently, are mutual and noncoercive when they involve other children, and do not cause emotional distress.[1,8] Sexual play typically occurs among children of similar age and ability who know and play with each other, rather than between strangers. Interpersonal sexual play often occurs between children of the same sex and can include siblings.[16,37,38] Experiencing sexual play at least once during childhood appears prevalent (reported by more than 66% to 80% of adults in retrospective research) and can occur in children as young as 2 or 3 years. Many incidents of sexual play in school-aged children may be unknown by caregivers, because the behaviors are more likely to be hidden with increased awareness of social norms.[37-39] Some degree of behavior focused on sexual body parts, curiosity about sexual behavior, and interest in sexual stimulation are a normal part of child development. This type of exploratory sexual play (periodic and without coercion or force and between children of similar age/abilities) has not been found to negatively affect long-term adjustment,[37,40-42] although inconsistent results have been found with sibling involvement.[43]

Childhood sexual play and exploration are not a preoccupation and usually do not involve advanced sexual behaviors such as intercourse or oral sex. Intrusive, planned, coerced, and aggressive sexual acts are not part of typical or normative sexual play of school-aged children; rather, they are perceived as problematic.[33] SBPs are discussed more extensively later in the chapter.

Adolescent Sexual Development (Ages 13 to 19 Years)

PHYSIOLOGICAL DEVELOPMENT

During adolescence, changes associated with puberty continue, including enlargement and maturation of the genitalia and secondary sex characteristics.[44] Most girls by age 16 have begun to menstruate; the average age at onset is 12 years.[3,45,46] Current research indicates that Caucasian girls enter puberty approximately 1 year earlier and African-American girls approximately 2 years earlier than previous studies have shown. The mean age for the beginning of breast development (sexual maturation rating stage 2) in African-American girls has been found to be 8.87 years, and that for white girls, 9.96 years.[47] By age 15, most boys are capable of ejaculation.[3] About 2 years after pubic hair growth begins, there is development of axillary and facial hair, as well as an acceleration of muscular strength. Hormonal changes that occur during puberty affect sexual interest, behavior, and fantasies.[48-50]

SEXUAL KNOWLEDGE AND BEHAVIOR

It is expected that adolescents have knowledge about sexual intercourse, contraception, and sexually transmitted diseases.[3] However, the quality of the knowledge they possess varies greatly across individuals. Evaluations of a variety of sex education programs (e.g., sex education, human immunodeficiency virus [HIV] education, teen pregnancy prevention) targeted at adolescents suggest that such programs do not lead to earlier onset of sex, more frequent sex, or more sexual partners. Many programs have been found to be associated with better outcomes for youths, including delay in the onset of sexual intercourse, increase in the use of contraceptives, and reduction in the number of sex partners. Programs more likely to affect teenagers' behavior contain several common characteristics, including having and reinforcing messages about abstinence and/or use of contraception, focusing on reducing at least one sexual behavior that leads to pregnancy or HIV infection and sexually transmitted diseases, and providing information about the risks of adolescent sexual activity.[51,52]

Many studies indicate that increases in sexual behavior during adolescence are not only influenced by hormones but are also affected by social factors, including parental supervision, peer influences, and community characteristics.[53-55] Several factors have been identified as being associated with the onset of sexual activity in adolescents: (1) less educated mothers; (2) having a boyfriend or girlfriend; (3) lower educational expectations (i.e., no intention of going to college); (4) authoritarian parenting; (5) poor communication with parents about sexuality; and (6) older siblings who are sexually active.[45]

The majority of teenagers engage in some form of sexual activity, whether masturbation or sexual intercourse. Studies have shown that 25% to 40% of adolescent girls and 45% to 90% of adolescent boys masturbate.[49,56] Sexual activity rates in adolescents have increased more than 79% since 1970.[57] In 2003, 47% of students in grades 9 to 12 reported that they had had sexual intercourse. Of these high school students, 14% reported having had sexual intercourse with four or more partners.[58] Research studies have revealed that 10% to 49% of adolescents have engaged in oral-genital contact, and the incidence is increasing.[59-61] Sexual experimentation and exploration is normative and may include behaviors with same-sex peers.

Risks associated with increased and early-onset sexual activity are notable, including sexually transmitted diseases, pregnancy, substance use, and exposure to and experiences of assault and unwanted sexual experiences. Although condom use has increased, it is not consistent, and approximately 25% of sexually active youths have been found to contract sexually transmitted diseases each year.[36] Furthermore, use of substances before sexual activity has increased.[62] Youths are at risk for experiences of sexual assault, force, coercion, and violence.[2] Other youths are often the offenders in these assaults, and information about management of adolescent sexual offenders is provided later in the chapter.

A summary of sexual development information by age group is provided in Table 25A-2.

TABLE 25A-2 ■ Sexual Development by Age

Development Description	Reference
Neonatal Period and Infancy	
Boys may have penile erections, and girls are capable of vaginal lubrication.	14, 15
Babies as young as 7 months touch their own genitalia.	15
Preschool Years (Ages 3-6 Years)	
Most 3-year-olds' knowledge of adult sexual behavior is limited to kissing and cuddling, and approximately 30% of 6-year-olds know about more explicit sexual acts.	18, 27
Children identify their own sex and sex of others, initially differentiating sexes by external characteristics (e.g., hair).	18
Children are aware of genital differences of the sexes by the end of this developmental period.	18, 19
Their understanding of pregnancy and birth tends to be vague.	18
They often have questions about, as well as exploratory and imitative behaviors concerning, sexual body parts.	3
They have a vague understanding of pregnancy and birth, with some knowledge of intrauterine growth and birth by cesarean or vaginal delivery by the end of this developmental period.	18
Nudity, looking at other people's bodies (particularly during hygiene activities), dressing like the opposite sex, and non intrusive sex play are not unusual.	27, 28
School Years (Ages 7-12 Years)	
Children tend to seek out and interact with same-sex children.	3
Girls become more shy and private about undressing and hygiene activities.	34
Children have a basic understanding of puberty, reproductive processes, and birth.	3
Pubertal development begins, with girls starting before boys.	2
Breast development begins in girls.	47
There is a wide variation in the onset and course of puberty.	16
Sexual behavior, including sexual play, occurs but is more likely to be concealed than during preschool years.	3
Sexual play typically occurs with children with whom they are interacting, including other children of the same sex and siblings.	16, 37, 38
Sexual play (periodic and without coercion or force and between children of similar age/abilities) has not been found to negatively affect long-term adjustment.	37, 41
Masturbatory behavior increases during this developmental period, particularly in boys.	16
Interest in the opposite sex increases with the onset of puberty.	35
Adolescence (Ages 13-17 Years)	
Enlargement and maturation of the genitalia and secondary sex characteristics occur.	44
Most boys by age 15 are capable of ejaculation.	3
Most girls by age 16 have begun to menstruate.	3, 45
Knowledge about sexual intercourse, contraception, and sexually transmitted diseases varies greatly across individuals.	3
Majority of adolescents engage in some form of sexual activity, whether masturbation, oral-genital contact, or sexual intercourse.	49, 56, 58-61
Experimentation and exploration of a range of sexual behaviors, including sexual behavior with the same and opposite sex, occurs.	2, 49

SPECIAL TOPICS ON SEXUAL DEVELOPMENT: CULTURAL FACTORS, SEXUAL ORIENTATION, DEVELOPMENTAL DISABILITIES, AND SEXUAL ABUSE

Cultural Factors Affecting Sexual Development and Behavior

Children's public and private sexual behavior, modesty, intimacy, and relationships are affected by their family's and communities' cultural values, beliefs, norms, religion, spirituality, socioeconomic, historical, and other factors. For example, social environments with norms in which nudity is acceptable, privacy is not reinforced, and exposure to sexualized material is common have been found to be related to higher frequencies of sexual behaviors in the children than are social environments that reinforce modesty and privacy.[28]

Parents' attitudes toward children's sexuality have been found to affect children's sexual knowledge and behavior.[19] Cultural beliefs may explain normative differences found in cross-cultural studies. For example, mothers of Dutch children report greater frequencies of sexual behaviors in their preschool-aged children than do mothers of American children, which may be related to a more permissive, positive attitude about sexuality and nudity in The Netherlands than in the United States.[30] Cultural differences in children's sexual knowledge (such as physiological distinctions between sexes, pregnancy, and birth) have also been found. For example, preschool-aged girls in the Western hemisphere have been found to perceive that babies were always in their mother's bellies, whereas Asian boys thought the baby was swallowed.[16]

Factors may interact, and differences in regard to norms between boys and girls are not uncommon. Implicit and explicit messages about sexual behavior are provided to children and youths through family, friends, neighbors, and the community, as well as a variety of media (including television, movies, music videos, music lyrics, video games, magazines, the Internet, and communications with cell phones). How children sort out the multiple and often conflicting messages about sex, sexuality, and relationships are not clearly understood. However, reduced risk-related behaviors have been found with attentive parenting with close supervision and good communication. Entertainment television can also have a positive effect on youth knowledge, particularly when paired with good communication with parents.[63] Ways in which culture may affect educational and intervention approaches are discussed later in the section on intervention.

Homosexuality

Homosexuality does not begin during adolescence. However, adolescence is the most likely time during childhood that concerns about sexuality, sexual orientation, and sexual behavior are presented to the developmental-behavioral pediatrician.

Many youths experiment with and explore a range of sexual behaviors, including sexual behavior with people of the same and opposite sex.[2,49] Sexual exploration and behavior are not synonymous with sexual orientation.[64] With whom youths have sexual behavior may be more strongly related to who is regularly in their social environment than with sexual orientation. Adolescents with homosexual experiences may identify themselves as having a heterosexual orientation. Furthermore, adolescents with no sexual experience or only heterosexual experiences may identify themselves as homosexual or bisexual.[49]

National data suggest that 2.3% of men and 1.3% of women in the United States are self-identified as homosexual.[60] In the same survey, 1.8% of men and 2.8% of women described themselves as bisexual.[60] Accurate prevalence rates are difficult to calculate because of the continuing stigmatization of homosexuality.[64] In a survey of junior and high school students from Minnesota, approximately 88% self-identified as heterosexual, 1.6% of boys and 0.9% of girls identified themselves as either primarily homosexual or bisexual, and more than 10% were "not sure" of their sexual orientation.[65] More information on homosexuality and development is available in Chapter 25C.

Children and Adolescents with Developmental Delays and Disabilities

Sexual development can be more variable when children and youth have developmental delays or disabilities or chronic medical conditions. Developmental disabilities and medical conditions may be associated with precocious or early-onset puberty (e.g., Down syndrome, traumatic brain injuries, and tumors, including hamartoma), delayed puberty (e.g., Prader-Willi syndrome), or disrupted sexual development (e.g., spinal cord injuries).[3,66,67] Historically, professionals and family members have inadequately understood, accepted, and responded to sexual development in individuals with disabilities.[3,67] However, as in all children, sexual arousal and sexual behaviors begins at or around birth, pubertal development with the associated sexual feelings typically occurs, and many adolescents with developmental disabilities date and are sexually active.[68] Unfortunately, many youths with developmental disabilities have not been provided developmentally appropriate sexual education.[67,69] Providing sex education for children with developmental delays is discussed in the section on recommendations concerning clinical care later in this chapter.

Effect of Sexual Abuse on Childhood Sexual Knowledge and Behavior

Sexual abuse affects children's sexual knowledge, as well as their sexual behavior. Furthermore, sexually abused children have been found to have greater frequencies of a wide range of sexual behaviors in comparison with normative samples and with children who were clinically referred with no known history of sexual abuse.[28,70,71] Sexually abused preschool-aged children are at greater risk for inappropriate sexual behaviors (35%) than are sexually abused school-aged children (6%).[70]

Although most sexually abused children do not demonstrate SBPs, the presence of SBPs raises concern about child sexual abuse and exposure to sexual material. Professionals need to be well aware of the child abuse reporting statutes in their jurisdiction, because reports of suspected sexual abuse may be necessary. Specific sexual behaviors (such as playing with dolls imitating explicit sexual acts and inserting objects in their own vaginas or rectums) are more likely to occur in children who have been sexually abused than in those who do not have a suspected history.[27,30,72] The presence of sexual behavior maybe enough to suspect sexual abuse and report to authorities for investigation; however, sexual behavior itself cannot be a sole determining factor for diagnosing sexual abuse.[8] Confirming sexual abuse in young children is quite complex, because often there is no physical evidence and no witnesses, and aspects of the abuse (e.g., threats by the perpetrator) hamper clear reporting by the child.[73] Additional information on identification and reporting of and response to suspected sexual abuse is provided in *The APSAC Handbook on Child Maltreatment* (2ed) by Myers JEB, Berliner L, Briere J et al, 2002.

SEXUAL BEHAVIOR PROBLEMS

Not all sexual behavior among youth is normative or appropriate. In the following discussion, SBPs in youth are defined, with information about the prevalence, origins, and trajectory of SBPs, as well as current findings on assessment, treatment, and management. Because of developmental and legal distinctions, children with SBPs are discussed separately from adolescents.

Problematic Sexual Behavior during Childhood (Ages 3 to 12 Years)

Sexual behavior in childhood occurs on a continuum from typical to concerning to problematic.[74] SBPs do not represent a medical/psychological syndrome or a specific diagnosable disorder; rather, they represent a set of behaviors that are well outside acceptable societal limits.[8] SBPs in this context are defined as child-initiated behaviors that involve sexual body parts (i.e., genitals, anus, buttocks, or breasts) and are developmentally inappropriate or potentially harmful to themselves or others.[1] SBPs may range from problematic self-stimulation (causing physical harm or damage) to nonintrusive behaviors (such as preoccupation with nudity, looking at others) to sexual interactions with other children that include behaviors more explicit than sexual play (such as intercourse) to coercive or aggressive sexual behaviors (of most concern, particularly when paired with large age differences between children).

Although the term *sexual* is used, the intentions and motivations for these behaviors may not be related to sexual gratification or sexual stimulation. Rather, the behaviors may be related to curiosity, anxiety, reenacting trauma, imitation, attention-seeking, self-calming, or other reasons.[1]

Children as young as 3 and 4 years of age with SBPs have been described in the literature.[75-78] Girls may be somewhat more likely than boys to be referred for services for SBPs during preschool years[78] and boys during the school years.[79,80] However, no population-based statistics on the incidence or prevalence of SBPs in children are available. By definition, most of the sexual behaviors involved are fairly rare.[28] Since the 1980s, there has been an increase in the number of children with SBPs who have been referred for child protective services, juvenile services, and treatment in both outpatient and inpatient settings.[81] The increase in referrals may represent an actual increase incidence of such behaviors, changing definitions of problematic sexual behavior, improved awareness and reporting of what has always existed, or some combination of these factors.[8]

The prevalence of sexual behavior for specific races, ethnic groups, religious groups, and socioeconomic groups is unknown. In groups in which there are extremely high rates of sexual abuse at a young age, the children are at higher risk for developing problematic sexual behaviors.

ORIGINS OF SEXUAL BEHAVIOR PROBLEMS IN CHILDREN

Social context, individual characteristics, disruptive experiences, and the interactions of these factors affect the course of sexual development.[9] Sexual abuse is one type of disruptive experience affecting sexual development. Children, particularly preschool age children,[70] who have been sexually abused are more likely to demonstrate SBPs than are children without such a history.[28] However, many children with SBPs have no known history of sexual abuse.[76,78,79,82] The development of SBPs appears to have multiple origins, including exposure to family violence, physical abuse, parenting practices, exposure to sexual material, absence of or disruption in attachments, heredity, and the development of other disruptive behavior problems.[33,83-85] For some children, SBPs may be one part of an overall pattern of disruptive behavior problems,[83,86,87] rather than an isolated or specialized behavioral disturbance.

RISKS AND COMORBIDITY OF SEXUAL BEHAVIOR PROBLEMS

Regardless of the causal pathway, a young child's demonstration of SBPs is associated with a variety of negative consequences in adjustment and development. Trauma histories and related trauma symptoms are common, particularly in young children with SBPs.[78,87] Children with SBPs often exhibit other behavior problems and disruptive behavior disorders.[78,79,84,87,88] Poor impulse-control skills, aggressive behaviors, and inaccurate perceptions of social stimuli hinder social relationships and cause problems at school.[9,79,88-90] Socialization difficulties and stigmatizing responses from peers and adults may impede developing self-concepts.[91] Poor boundaries and indiscriminate friendliness may increase risk of future victimization.[78,92] Furthermore, children with SBPs are at risk of separation from parents and of placement disruptions.[78,79,93,94]

CLASSIFICATION

There is much to be learned about subtypes of SBPs, because the research in this area is limited to a few studies. Youths with more frequent and more intrusive SBPs are more likely to have other behavior and emotional problems, to have caregivers with histories of trauma, and to have learning difficulties than are children with less frequent or nonintrusive sexual behaviors.[95,96] Typological examinations of comorbidity have suggested the differential effects of trauma and disruptive behavior, as well as gender's effect on rate of sexual behaviors.[87] Otherwise, how types of SBPs affect the functioning of the children demonstrating the behavior, the trajectory of SBPs and related concerns, and responsiveness to interventions are unknown.

EFFECT OF SEXUAL BEHAVIOR PROBLEMS ON OTHER CHILDREN

When children experience sexual behaviors initiated by other children, there can be a range of effects. The literature is scant but appears to suggest that sexual behaviors between children of similar age and ability that was of mutual agreement and without intrusive or aggressive behaviors is retrospectively viewed as neutral or positive. However, when the sexual behavior experienced is considered to be an SBP as previously defined, the experience can have potentially negative effects, perhaps similar to those of sexual abuse perpetrated by adolescents or adults. The research on the effect of child sexual abuse indicates that the level and severity of the effect are influenced by the duration; frequency; relationship with the initiator of the sexual acts; use of aggression, coercion, or force; the child's previous functioning; and the response and support by the caregivers.[97] Response can range from no or limited discernible symptoms to the development of trauma symptoms, other internalizing symptoms, behavior problems, sexual behaviors themselves, and/or social and peer problems.

ASSESSMENT OF SEXUAL BEHAVIOR PROBLEMS (AGES 3 TO 12 YEARS)

When caregivers report concern about the sexual behavior of children, an initial screening can facilitate the need for further clinical assessment. Gathering information about the type, frequency, duration, level of intrusiveness, harm, use of coercion, and course of behaviors can facilitate distinguishing typical from problematic sexual behaviors. The Child Sexual Behavior Inventory (CSBI)[27] is the only norm-based parental report measure of child sexual behavior with gender and age norms for ages 2 to 12 years. It is a 38-item measure used to assess boundary issues, showing of private parts, self-stimulation, sexual anxiety, sexual interest, sexual knowledge, interpersonal and intrusive sexual behavior, and looking at others' private parts. It is easy to administer and score; the Total Scale Score provides a T-score and a percentile that are based on age and gender norms. The published manual recommends that the CSBI be administered by mental health professionals with training in psychological assessments. It is important to note that this published version does not include any items concerning sexual aggression. Friedrich[33] evaluated four such items and found none of them to be endorsed by mothers in a normative sample. Friedrich also provided a checklist to assess exposure to sexualized material, supervision, and privacy, which facilitates developing a safety plan with the family.[33]

Assessment of the situations or circumstances under which SBPs seem to occur, the social ecology, exposure to sexualized materials, and success of attempts made to correct the behaviors can guide identifying points of intervention and treatment recommendations. The Child Sexual Behavior Checklist, 2nd revision, can help assess contributing factors and identify environmental intervention area, as it lists 150 behaviors related to sex and sexuality in children, asks about environmental issues that can increase problematic sexual behaviors in children, gathers details of children's sexual behaviors with other children, and lists 26 problematic characteristics of children's sexual behaviors.[98] However, the no norms have been published for the Child Sexual Behavior Checklist.

Comorbid disruptive behavior disorders, affective disorders, trauma-related symptoms, and learning deficits are not uncommon in children with SBPs.[78-80,84,87] Thus, a broad assessment is warranted and may include such measures as the Child Behavior Checklist (which includes items on sexual behavior),[99,100] or the Behavior Assessment System for Children.[101] To specifically assess trauma symptoms, the Trauma Symptom Checklist for Children (child report) and the Trauma Symptom Checklist for Young Children (caregiver report) are useful instruments that include subscales related to sexual concerns.[102,103] For preschool children, the Weekly Behavior Report[104] is useful in assessing a wide range of emotional and behavior problems, including SBPs, and in tracking progress over time.

A common misunderstanding is that if a child has SBPs, he or she must have a history of sexual victimization. Although a history of previous or ongoing sexual abuse increases the risk for developing SBPs,[70,72] there appear to be multiple pathways to the development of SBPs, and the presence of SBPs should not be presumed sufficient evidence of sexual abuse. However, when a child exhibits SBPs, it is appropriate for assessors to make direct inquiries into whether the child has been or is being sexually abused.[8] Suspected sexual abuse that had not been previously investigated by Child Protective Services necessitates responses consistent with state and regional child abuse reporting statutes. Additional information on management of suspected child sexual abuse is available in *The APSAC Handbook on Child Maltreatment* (2ed) by Myers JEB, Berliner L, Briere J, et al, 2002.

CASE EXAMPLE

A description of the application of these measures and assessment procedures to a case may facilitate application of the information. An example case of a young child follows:

Jill Doe is a 6-year-old girl who was referred by Child Protective Services after their investigation into possible sexual abuse. Their investigation was inconclusive. There were continued concerns regarding her sexual behaviors. Jill lives with her father and 3-year-old sister. She has sporadic visitations with her mother, who has a substance abuse problem. Jill's father provided the history of sexual behavior, in which he reported that Jill was found on top of a 4-year-old girl, kissing her and touching her genital area over the clothes. This behavior was followed by

observing her embracing and kissing two different young boys at a local park. A couple of months ago, she was found to be making her dolls "have sex," upon which her father responded by taking the dolls away. Around that time, she also found Jill visually examining her 3-year-old sister's vaginal area and touching their dog's private parts. All of these sexual behaviors have continued despite the father's efforts to stop the behaviors through distraction, removal of toys, and punishment (grounding). In addition to these sexual behaviors, Jill's father expressed concern about Jill's sleep problems, nightmares, moodiness, and temper tantrums.

Jill's father completed the CSBI and Child Behavior Checklist. On the CSBI, he endorsed items reflecting the sexual behaviors noted previously and the Total Standard Score of 23, which falls at the T-score of 108, in the clinical range. Thus, the sexual behaviors Jill has been exhibiting according to her father's report are much greater in frequency than those of the normative sample of girls her age. Problems were noted in regard to boundaries and interpersonal sexual behavior problems. The Safety Checklist suggested that Jill has been exposed to sexualized materials while in her mother's care. Furthermore, she often sleeps and bathes with her sister and, at times, her cousins. Jill was reported to have been exposed to violence and substance use. The Child Behavior Checklist scores were 68 for Total Problems, 67 for Externalizing Problems, and 65 for Internalizing Problems. The Weekly Behavior Report indicated that Jill is exhibiting sexual behavior problems a couple of times a week, as well is experiencing nightmares and temper tantrums four times a week. Services for sexual behavior problems and integrating strategies to address behavior problems, nightmares, and abuse prevention skills appear warranted. Work with the caregivers regarding privacy rules, boundaries, and protection from trauma and stress is also indicated. The Weekly Behavior Report measure is brief enough that frequent administration is not burdensome and can track treatment progress.

TREATMENT FOR SEXUAL BEHAVIOR PROBLEMS (AGES 3 TO 12 YEARS)

SBPs have been successfully treated with SBP-specific therapy services for school-age children and preschool children.[8,79,105,106] Further, Trauma-Focused Cognitive Behavior Therapy as a treatment for the effects child sexual abuse that includes SBP-specific elements effectively reduces SBPs in sexually abused preschool-aged children.[107-110] These treatments have been found to be more effective than time (wait periods), play therapy, and nondirective supportive treatment approaches. The types of SBPs found in the children involved in the studies have been wide ranging, with most children demonstrating interpersonal sexual behaviors, and include aggressive sexual behaviors.

One study provided results from a 10-year follow-up on children with SBPs who had been randomly assigned to receive group cognitive-behavioral treatment (CBT) or group play therapy. The study included a clinic comparison group of children with disruptive behavior problems but no SBPs.[105] Child welfare, juvenile justice, and criminal administrative data on all the children were collected and were aggregated. The CBT recipients were found to have had significantly fewer future sex offenses than the play therapy recipients (2% vs. 10%) and did not differ from the general clinic comparison (3%).[105] The overall rate of future sexual offenses not only was quite low with short-term outpatient CBT that involved families but also was indistinguishable from that of the comparison sample.

Common elements of the effective treatments are outpatient, short-term, cognitive-behavioral and educational approaches; caregiver direct involvement; teaching of rules about sexual behaviors and skills to facilitate maintaining these rules (such as feeling identification, impulse control, and problem-solving skills); sex education; and teaching caregivers efficacious behavior management strategies (such as praise, reinforcement, timeout, and logical consequences). This treatment should be distinguished from CBT approaches to treating adolescent and adult sexual offenders. Efficacious treatment for childhood SBPs have not included components more characteristic of treatment of adults, such as concepts of grooming, offense cycles, predation, or use of techniques such as confrontation or arousal reconditioning.[105] For children who have histories of sexual abuse and trauma-related symptoms, a trauma-focused CBT approach that includes SBP-specific strategies has been successful.[111-113]

For some children, the SBP may be part of a general pattern of disruptive and oppositional behaviors. Research on treatment for disruptive behaviors has consistently identified behavior management training as an effective modality.[114,115] Integrating SBP-specific treatment components with well-supported treatment models for early disruptive behavior disorders (such as Parent-Child Interaction Therapy,[114] The Incredible Years,[116] Barkley's Defiant Child protocol,[117] or the Triple P program[118]) might be considered; however, this approach has yet to be tested in regard to reducing SBPs.

The presence of attention-deficit-hyperactivity disorder is not uncommon in these youth,[106] and appropriate treatment is warranted to facilitate control of impulsive behaviors (see Chapter 16). In cases of neglectful, conflicted, or chaotic family environments, interventions focused on creating a safe, healthy, stable, and predictable environment may be the top priority.[119] For cases in which insecure attachment is a major concern, short-term interventions emphasizing parental sensitivity have been found to

be the most effective.[120] Family-based attachment-based treatment may be considered for complex cases involving significant family relationship concerns, as well as comorbid conditions,[86] although this approach has yet to be empirically validated.

Problematic Sexual Behavior during Adolescence

Adolescent sexual offenders are adolescents between the ages of 13 and 17 years who commit sexual behavior that is illegal as defined by the sex crime statutes of the jurisdiction in which the offense occurred.[121] In general, the legal system (i.e., family or juvenile court, probation officer, judge, district attorney) is involved when an adolescent commits a sexual crime, because of the adolescent's assumed culpability in committing the crime. The response of the legal system to an adolescent's sexual crime varies greatly by state and may include court-ordered treatment, probation, imprisonment in a juvenile or adult correctional facility, and/or inclusion in registrations and public notification systems. Approximately one third of sexual offenses against children are committed by adolescents. Sexual offenses against children younger than 12 years tend to be committed by boys aged 12 to 15 years.[122,123] The majority of adolescent sexual offenders are male, accounting for 93% of all juvenile arrests for sex offenses, excluding prostitution.[124]

ORIGINS OF SEXUAL BEHAVIOR PROBLEMS IN ADOLESCENTS

Adolescents with SBPs are a heterogeneous population.[125,126] Although it is commonly believed that adolescent sexual offenders were sexually abused themselves, most in fact were not childhood sexual abuse victims.[127,128] Some differences in maltreatment history between adolescent boys and girls with SBPs have been found. Adolescent girls with SBPs have been shown to have more severe physical and sexual abuse histories than have adolescent boys with SBPs. For adolescents with SBPs and who have been sexually abused, the girls tended to be sexually abused at younger ages and were more likely to have been abused by multiple perpetrators.[127-131] There appears to be multiple origins, including abuse history, family stability, and psychiatric disturbances in the development of SBPs in adolescence; however, for many adolescents, there is no known cause.[10]

RISKS, COMORBIDITY, AND TYPOLOGY

Although professionals have proposed subtypes of adolescent sexual offenders, these subtypes have not yet been confirmed in the literature. What is known is that adolescent sexual offenders are diverse. There are adolescent sexual offenders with few other behavioral or psychological problems and those with many nonsexual behavior problems or other (nonsexual) delinquent offenses. Some have psychiatric disorders. Some adolescent sexual offenders come from well-functioning families; others come from poorly functioning or abusive families.[10] Adolescents with SBPs tend to have poorer social skills, more behavior problems, learning disabilities, depression, and impulse control problems in comparison with nonoffending adolescents (see Becker[125] for a review). Some differences have been found between adolescents who rape peers and those whose sexual behavior is with younger children. Adolescents whose sexual behavior is with younger children have been found to be younger, to be less socially competent, to have less same-age sexual activity, to be more withdrawn, and to have fewer nonsexual behavior problems than do adolescents who rape peers.[132,133] Risk predictors that have been identified for sexual and nonsexual repeated offending, include antisocial tendencies, psychopathy, and larger numbers of victims.[134]

CONTRASTING ADOLESCENTS WITH SEXUAL BEHAVIOR PROBLEMS WITH ADULT SEXUAL OFFENDERS

Adolescents are different from adult sexual offenders in several important ways: (1) Adolescents are considered more responsive to treatment than are adults[135]; (2) of sexual offenders who receive treatment, adolescents have a lower sexual recidivism rate than do adults[136]; (3) adolescents have fewer victims and tend to engage in less aggressive behaviors than do adults[137]; and (4) most adolescents do not meet the criteria for pedophilia.[138] With regard to recidivism, adolescent sexual offenders are less likely to have sexual repeated offenses and are more likely to have nonsexual repeated offenses than are adults.[139]

ASSESSMENT OF ADOLESCENTS

There are no psychological tests available that can establish guilt or innocence of committing a sexual offense. However, there are some measures under development to assess the risk of future sexual offenses of adolescent sexual offenses. The National Center on Sexual Behavior of Youth *(www.ncsby.org)* provides more guidelines about assessment of adolescent sexual offenders.

For adolescents with histories (e.g., maltreatment, life stressors, behavior problems) that make it more likely that they will engage in high-risk sexual behaviors or have sexual concerns, it is important for clinicians to assess their sexual practices and concerns to guide intervention. The Adolescent Clinical Sexual Behavior Inventory (ACSBI) can be used as a screening tool with such adolescent clinical samples. The ACSBI has parent- and self-report versions (45 items

each), responses to which can provide information about adolescent's high-risk sexual behavior and help determine appropriate interventions. The ACSBI measures a range of sexual behaviors and yields five factors: sexual knowledge/interest, divergent sexual interest, sexual risk/misuse, fear/discomfort, and concerns about appearance.[140]

TREATMENT FOR ADOLESCENT SEXUAL OFFENDERS (AGED 13 TO 17 YEARS)

Rigorous research regarding treatment of adolescent sexual offenders is lacking. However, there is some evidence to support the use of sex offender–specific treatment for adolescent sexual offenders. Two randomized clinical trials with small sample sizes yielded results in support of the use of multisystemic therapy with adolescent sexual offenders. Multisystemic therapy is a home-based treatment intervention that targets the systems in which youth are embedded, as well as the factors that are associated with delinquency. Results from these studies indicated that youths who received multisystemic therapy had lower rates of sexual and nonsexual recidivism than did youths who received the usual services (e.g., individual or group treatment).[139,141,142] On the basis of what is known about juvenile sex offenders, state-of-the-art treatment recipients should include caregivers, so that relevant factors (e.g., parental monitoring and engagement) associated with delinquent behavior can be addressed.[139] Because of the low rates of pedophilia among adolescent sexual offenders, it is generally inappropriate to apply adult sexual reconditioning techniques to adolescent sexual offenders. The widely held belief that most adolescent sexual offenders will become adult sex offenders is not supported by research.[135]

RECOMMENDATIONS CONCERNING CLINICAL CARE

Parent Education and Clinical Management: Children (Aged 3 to 12 Years)

Concerns about sexual behavior of youth may manifest in a variety of ways in the medical office. During assessment of a wide range of behavior problems, concerns about respect of other's boundaries and sexual acts may arise. As sexual behavior, particularly in young children, often raises suspicion of sexual abuse, such children's caregivers may express concern about possible victimization of the child. Families and other professionals may seek advice for follow-up and management once SBPs have been identified.

Parents are generally interested in and expect pediatricians to discuss normal sexuality and sexual abuse prevention.[143] When there are concerns about SBPs, information provided depends on the results of the initial screening and, if warranted, further evaluation. In determining whether sexual behavior is inappropriate, it is important to consider whether the behavior is common or rare for the child's developmental stage and culture, the frequency of the behaviors, the extent to which sex and sexual behavior have become a preoccupation for the child, and whether the child responds to normal correction from adults or whether the behavior continues after normal corrective efforts.[119] In determining whether the behavior involves potential for harm, it is important to consider the age/developmental differences of the children involved; any use of force, intimidation, or coercion; the presence of any emotional distress in the children involved; whether the behavior appears to be interfering with the children's social development; and whether the behavior causes physical injury.[9,144,145]

Parent education may include information about typical sexual development and how to distinguish SBPs from sex play; specific instructions for reducing exposure to sexually stimulating media or situations in the home; instructions for monitoring interactions with other children; suggestions for how parents should respond to sexualized behaviors; and teaching children rules about privacy, sexual behavior, and boundaries.[119,146]

Parents and caregivers often are understandably concerned about the causes of the SBP. In some cases, there appears to be relatively clear sequence of events that explain the development of the SBP (such as young child's being sexually abused by an uncle, followed by the child's repeating the behavior with another child at daycare). However, such direct pathways are often not present, inasmuch as causes for human behavior can involve the interplay of multiple factors, and may not be fully knowable.[8] Parents can be reassured that children with SBPs can be treated successfully without clear evidence of the origins of the behavior, with the exception of situations of ongoing sexual abuse.

Ongoing sexual abuse is of serious concern, both for the child's welfare and for the success of intervention efforts. Indeed, subsequent sexual abuse appears to increase the likelihood of future SBPs.[105] In cases in which the Child Protective Services investigation of sexual abuse yields inconclusive results, interventions focused on educating children about sexual abuse, identifying whom children may tell if they were being abused, having significant adults support this message, and building support systems around the child have been recommended.[73] Repeated questioning and interviewing the child after thorough investigations are not recommended, because they may lead to inaccurate information and have potential deleterious effects on the child.[119]

Other parental concerns often relate to the misunderstanding about the meaning of childhood SBPs and likelihood of problematic adult sexual behavior, including pedophilia. The results of a 10-year prospective study of children with SBPs indicated low rates of future sexual offenses (2% to 10%, depending on treatment type).[105] A continuation of SBPs from childhood into adolescence and adulthood appears rare. Calm parental responses to these situations are advised.[147] Efficacious treatments have been outpatient and short-term and have involved helping the children while living in their natural environment and while attending school. Restricted environments and treatments should be reserved for children who pose immediate risk because of coercive, aggressive, harmful sexual behavior that has not been readily modifiable with appropriate parental interventions and treatment.[8]

Resources are available to professionals in their work with parents. Fact sheets addressing typical sexual development, SBPs, and common misconceptions about child with SBPs can be found on the Website of the National Center on the Sexual Behavior of Youth (www.ncsby.org). An information booklet on child sexual development and SBPs[145] is useful to supplement education for the caregivers (www.TCavJohn.com). Anticipatory guidelines on issues related to sexual development and behavior throughout childhood and adolescents with information on ways to approach issues of sexual development, sexuality, sexual behavior, and sexual abuse prevention designed for pediatric practice are available.[2,147] In addition, the report from the Task Force on Children with Sexual Behavior Problems of the Association of the Treatment of Sexual Abusers is a useful resource for professionals (www.atsa.org).[8] This report provides more a detailed review of the research and guidelines on the identification, clinical assessment, treatment, and policy issues relevant to children with SBPs.

Parent Education and Clinical Management: Adolescents (Aged 13 to 17 Years)

Caregivers and referring providers may need support in how to address sexual topics with youth. Furthermore, because of the sensitive and, at times, taboo nature of the topic, cultural considerations and sensitivity are necessary in approaching and educating about sexual matters. Guidelines for pediatricians and family practitioners on assessment and management sexual topics with adolescents and caregivers are available.[2,6,147] Caregivers often require education in addition to the youth. Helpful resources for caregivers can be found at *www.advocatesforyouth.org* and *www.talkingwithkids.org.*

When an adolescent is suspected of engaging in illegal sexual behavior, providers need to respond in a manner consistent with the reporting requirements for their state, including reporting suspected illegal sexual behavior with children as indicated. Developmental-behavioral pediatricians can help caregivers and adolescents by referring youths for clinical assessment and efficacious treatment when available.

Unfortunately, efficacious treatment is not available in all areas of the United States. If efficacious treatment is not available, then the developmental-behavioral pediatrician should look for cognitive-behavioral treatment programs that involve both adolescents and caregivers and do not use adult sex offender treatment interventions (e.g., penile plethysmograph, polygraph) that may be inappropriate for adolescents.

Typically, adolescent sexual offenders can be treated in the community in outpatient treatment programs. Most adolescent sexual offenders can remain in the community with appropriate supervision by caregivers and probation officers and can be treated on an outpatient basis.[135] In general, adolescent sexual offenders who are being treated in the community can attend school and engage in other activities, such as team sports and church. However, a small number of adolescent sexual offenders may need a higher level of care (i.e., residential or custodial placement).

Currently, there is no scientifically supported test to determine which adolescent sexual offenders are at high risk for recidivism. Usually, it is appropriate to treat an adolescent sexual offender as being at low risk for recidivism and in an outpatient setting, unless there is evidence that they are at higher risk. There are clinical guidelines to help identify youths at higher risk in order to help determine the level of care (outpatient vs. residential) that they may require. These factors are important in determining risk: (1) a history of multiple sexual offenses, particularly if sexual offenses continue despite appropriate treatment; (2) a history of multiple nonsexual juvenile offenses; (3) sexual attraction to children; (4) noncompliance with an adolescent sexual offender treatment program; (5) other "self-evident risk signs," including significant behavior problems and stated intent to commit repeated sexual offenses; and (6) caregivers' not providing the appropriate and recommended supervision and/or caregivers who are not compliant with treatment or probation.[121]

Collaboration with Family and Other Professionals and Agencies (Ages 3 to 17 Years)

As discussed in Chapter 8A, family-centered and collaborative approaches to service delivery are crucial for all children with developmental and behavioral needs. This is particularly true for children with SBPs and adolescent sexual offenders, for whom not only parents and caregivers but also other treatment providers, child welfare workers, schools, child care providers, juvenile justice staff, and court officials are involved in the care. The extent of collaboration and who may need to be included can be expected to vary considerably across cases. Main purposes of coordination and information sharing are to define service goals, articulate a clear plan and timetable of specific tasks needed to reach those goals, identify who on the team is responsible for each aspect of the plan, and evaluate plan implementation and goal attainment.[8]

OTHER RELEVANT TOPICS

Homosexuality

The sexual behavior of youth who identify themselves as gay, lesbian, or bisexual or who report homosexual or bisexual experiences are to be assessed with sensitivity and with nonjudgmental response and information. Education and intervention (e.g., information about relationships, decision making, self-care, reproduction, sexually transmitted diseases, protection) similar to that given to heterosexual youths often needs to be provided. In addition, the clinician should also be aware of the increased risk for other problems in homosexual or bisexual youths. These youths may feel extremely isolated from their peers and/or families and may have been the victims of violence and harassment.[148] Nonheterosexual youth are at higher risk for behavioral and emotional problems and risky behaviors, including drug use and abuse, self-harm, school problems, and suicide.[2,149] The American Academy of Pediatrics' Committee on Adolescence's clinical report on sexual orientation and adolescents provides useful information and guidelines for the care and support of youths.[64]

Children and Adolescents with Developmental Delays and Disabilities

In addition to the typical topics for sexual education, youths with disabilities may need focused information on ways to express physical affection, with whom, and under what circumstances, with an understanding of the youth's need for intimacy and affection.

Because of the increased risk of sexual abuse of such children, education should include sexual abuse prevention components. Self identity, developing relationships, and intimacy are important areas neglected in many sexual education programs for all youths. Caregivers and providers can be encouraged to provide guidance and education based on individual learning styles and disability-specific challenges, considering the use of visual supports (e.g., pictures, dolls), repeating information over time, and having the youth demonstrate or practice the information learned.[2,67] Issues of consent, marriage, and family planning are complicated and require collaborative care and an understanding of individuals' desires, choices, capabilities, supports, and needs. Curriculum on sex education for children and youths with disabilities are available[150] (see also the University of South Carolina Center for Disability Resource Library at *http://uscm. med.sc.edu/CDR/sexualeducation.htm*), as well as other useful information including one from the American Academy of Pediatrics.[67,151]

Cultural Factors Affecting Parental Education and Other Service Provision

Consideration of the child and family's cultural values, beliefs, and norms are of foremost importance in the provision of any mental health and social services. Race, ethnicity, religion, spirituality, socioeconomic factors, and other cultural factors can strongly affect individuals' and families' receptivity and response to treatment of child SBPs. Professionals are advised to account for the effect of the specific social ecology experience of the child. Significant variation among children exists, inasmuch as cultural and social context, as well as family attitudes and educational practices, affect children's knowledge and behavior.[18,19,30]

Because of the sensitive nature of the topic, clinicians must become knowledgeable about the family's and community's beliefs, values, traditions, and practices concerning sex, including the spoken and unspoken rules about public and private behavior, relationships, intimacy, and modesty. For example, discussions on sexual behavior with children may be considered appropriate for some individuals (e.g., aunts teaching nieces) but taboo for others (e.g., fathers talking with daughters). Provision of education in a manner consistent with the culture and family beliefs are recommended. African-American mothers have been found to integrate story telling in process of providing sex education.[152] Storytelling is also integral for American Indron Alaska Native, and Native Hawaiian families.[153] Beliefs about the appropriateness of children's touching their own private parts and about masturbation tend to be strong and

directly affect receptiveness to treatment. Understanding and respecting the cultural beliefs and values of families and providing services to enhance the family's ability to accept and receive the services is crucial not only for outcome but also for initiation and retention of families in services.

FUTURE DIRECTIONS

Although research on children and adolescent sexual knowledge began decades ago, research on children and adolescents with SBPs is a relatively new area of research. There remain many questions about knowledge and behavior of children and adolescents, particularly in the origins, typology, course, assessment, treatment, and long-term outcome for children and adolescents with SBPs. The following sections address some of the methodological challenges to research on the sexual knowledge and behavior of children and youth, as well as recommendations for future research.

Methodological Issues

Conducting research on the sexual knowledge and sexual behavior of children and youth has multiple challenges. Parents who allow their young children to participate in research on sexual knowledge may have distinct values and parenting practices from those who do not allow their children to participate. In one study, researchers noted that the majority of parents approached chose not to have their child participate; the concern about topic reported was the reason for declining.[18] The unknown effect of participation bias limits the generalizability of results.

Much of the research on children's sexual behavior has relied on caregivers' or teachers' reports. Self-reports of sexual behavior from adolescents suggest higher prevalence of sexual behaviors and sexual assaults than has been detected by administrative systems (such as child protective services, juvenile court system). Furthermore, retrospective research with adults suggests that caregivers are often unaware of sexual behavior that occurs among children. Retrospective research, although useful, relies on the memory of the adults, which is affected by a variety of factors. Administrative data sources track only the more severely maladaptive sexual behaviors and are also subjected to a variety of biases. The hidden nature of the sexual behavior of youths, particularly school-aged children and adolescents, challenges direct observations. Direct questioning of children and even adolescents about their sexual behavior is often restricted, particularly in the United States. Thus, reliable and valid information about children and adolescents sexual behavior is difficult to obtain, which further affects researchers' ability to track and examine factors that affect the trajectory of sexual behaviors.

Examination of treatment efficacy for SBPs of children and adolescent poses additional challenges. Because of the concerns about the ramifications of ongoing SBPs, randomized trials with no treatment or placebo control conditions are generally considered unethical. Quasi-experimental designs and preintervention/postintervention evaluations limit clinicians' ability to progress in understanding intervention efficacy. Randomly assigning children to receive one of two treatments when both interventions are believed to be efficacious requires a considerable sample size, perhaps multisite studies, to determine differences in effect sizes.

Recommendations for Future Research

Even basic information about SBPs in children and adolescents, such as prevalence and incidence data, is unavailable. National data on the incidence, prevalence, and frequency of types of sexual behaviors in children and youth would greatly enhance the literature. Clear, consistent definitions of types of sexual behaviors are necessary. Furthermore, because no single state or federal agency is designated as responsible for assessing and responding to sexual behavior of youths, the collection of incidence and prevalence data is challenged.

There is considerable research to be done in the area of clinical assessment of children and adolescents with SBPs. The CSBI[88] is the only norm-based measure of sexual behaviors of youth and is quite useful for clinical assessment, as well as monitoring treatment progress. The published version of the measure does not include items to assess aggressive or coercive sexual behaviors; however, Friedrich evaluated four such items after the published measure.[33] The published norms are based predominately on data from Caucasian and African-American children. Cross-cultural research with normative data from other populations is needed. No norms are available for the accompanying Safety Checklist.[33] The Child Sexual Behavior Checklist[98] includes items that assess broad issues such as environmental factors, in addition to specifics about the types and other details about SBPs. Although the measure is clinically useful, no norms have yet been published. Research is also needed in how to sensitively and culturally appropriately measure children's sexual thoughts and understanding of their sexual behaviors.

There is one measure of adolescent sexual behavior: the ACSBI.[140] This is a useful measure for clinically referred adolescents and can help guide treatment. However, there is no normative sample for this measure. The clinical sample used for development was primarily white and of middle to upper middle socioeconomic status. Research on normative sexual behavior of adolescents, including cross-cultural and economically diverse samples, is needed. One important assessment question is estimating the likelihood of sexual and nonsexual repeated offense. Although there are some adolescent sexual offender actuarial systems under development, this is still an area for continued research.

An untapped area of measurement concerns the caregivers' knowledge of, reaction to, and perception of their child and the sexual acts. Mothers' emotional reaction and support has been found to mediate treatment outcomes for preschool- and school-aged sexually abused children.[107,154,155] Clinically, caregivers' perceptions of their children who have demonstrated SBPs appear to strongly affect their willingness to support the child, engage in services, and respond to intervention. Psychometrically supported measures of caregiver's emotional reaction to, support of, and perceptions for this specific population would facilitate research in this area.

Origins, trajectory, risk factors, and treatment outcome probably vary for subgroups of children and adolescents with SBPs. Typologies have been proposed on the basis of the types of sexual behavior exhibited, as well as other factors (such as gender, comorbid conditions and nonsexual delinquent acts). No clear classification has yet emerged to advance understanding in this area.

Additional research on such service factors as group versus individual/family services, use of direct practice of skills with families in session, and need of specific components of treatment (such as acknowledging past SBPs) would advance the field. Because of the low base rates of subsequent sexual offenses in children,[105] it is unlikely that refined services would significantly lower this rate any further. However, researchers could examine improvements of less severe sexual behaviors, receptivity of services by families, reduced treatment burden, treatment attrition, comorbid symptom relief, and gains in coping skills and resiliency factors.

Research on services in more restrictive settings (i.e., inpatient and residential interventions) for children and adolescents with persistent, aggressive SBPs is limited to clinical descriptions and quasi-experimental designs. These youths are also more likely to have histories of severe trauma, comorbid conditions, and problematic family histories and situations (e.g., mental illness, substance abuse, maltreatment, community and domestic violence).

Many youths with SBPs have comorbid conditions of post-traumatic stress disorder, separation anxiety, and/or disruptive behavior disorders (including oppositional defiant disorder, attention-deficit/hyperactivity disorder, and conduct disorder). Although evidence-based treatments exist for each of these conditions, research on the most efficacious and efficient manner to integrate these services for children with comorbid conditions, in such a way that it is also palatable for families, is needed.

In many ways, the treatment outcome research on children with SBPs is more advanced than the research literature on adolescent and adult sex offender treatment outcomes. Only investigations of multisystemic therapy have amassed any controlled trial data with adolescents. Thus, many treatment questions remain. Comparisons of community-based treatments with residential treatment are particularly important, in view of the possible iatrogenic effects of residential placement.

The results of the prospective studies on children and adolescents with SBPs are encouraging but limited to a few studies focusing on administrative data sources. Longitudinal research integrating administrative data with self- and caregiver-disclosed rates of SBPs, other delinquent acts, victimization, and trauma experiences is warranted. Preschool-aged children with SBPs have been found to have much more frequent SBPs, more severe comorbid conditions, and greater rates of placement disruptions than do school-aged children with SBPs.[78] Trajectories of nonsexual disruptive behaviors (particularly physical aggression) have been found to be distinct, depending in part on age at onset, wherein a younger onset is related to more severe and pervasive problems (e.g., Broidy et al[156]). Longitudinal research with preschool- as well as school-age onset of SBPs would facilitate the examination of whether SBPs have a pattern similar to that of other disruptive behaviors.

In summary, initial results in this relatively new area of research are encouraging, but further research is warranted for prevalence and incidence data, assessment, typology, treatment mediators and outcome, and longitudinal trajectories.

SUMMARY

Children are sexual beings from birth, capable of sexual arousal and behavior even as infants. Sexual knowledge and behavior are affected not only by physiology but also by family, culture, and societal factors. Curiosity and exploratory play are typical in early childhood. Sexual activity and risky sexual behaviors increase throughout childhood, particularly with the onset of puberty. Sensitivity in provision of care is recommended, particularly for populations who have experienced disparities in

health care, including nonheterosexual youths, individuals with disabilities, and individuals from non-dominant cultures.

SBPs are, by definition, deviations from the normal course of sexual development and have been found in children as young as 3 years of age. Sexual abuse is a significant risk factor for the development of SBPs, but multiple factors appear to contribute to the onset and maintenance of SBPs, including exposure to family violence, physical abuse, parenting practices, exposure to sexual material, absence of or disruption in attachments, heredity, and comorbidity (including disruptive behavior disorders and trauma-related symptoms). Most children and youth with SBPs can be successfully treated in their community with outpatient services. Collaborative care is crucial for the success of interventions.

REFERENCES

1. Silovsky JF, Bonner BL: Sexual behavior problems. *In* Ollendick TH, Schroeder CS, eds: Encyclopedia of Clinical Child and Pediatric Psychology. New York: Kluwer Press, 2003, pp 589-591.
2. Duncan P, Dixon R, Carlson J: Childhood and adolescent sexuality. Pediatr Clin North Am 50:765-780, 2003.
3. Gordon BN, Schroder C: Sexuality: A Developmental Approach to Problems. New York: Plenum Press, 1995.
4. Lipsius SH: Normal sexual development of children: Physician roles in bridging gaps in parent-child communication. Md Med J 41:401-405, 1992.
5. Smith M: Pediatric Sexuality: Promoting normal sexual development in children. Nurse Pract 18:37-44, 1993.
6. Thornton AC, Collins JD: Teaching parents to talk to their children about sexual topics. Clin Fam Pract 6:801-819, 2004.
7. Horner G: Sexual behavior in children: Normal or not? Pediatrics 18:57-64, 2004.
8. Chaffin M, Berliner L, Block R, et al: Report of the ATSA Task Force on Children with Sexual Behavior Problems. Beaverton, OR: Association for the Treatment of Sexual Abusers, 2006.
9. Araji SK: Sexually aggressive children: Coming to understand them. Thousand Oaks, CA: Sage Publications, 1997.
10. Chaffin M, Letourneau E, Silovsky JF: Adults, adolescents and children who sexually abuse children. *In* Berliner L, Myers J, Briere J, et al, eds: The APSAC Handbook on Child Maltreatment. Thousand Oaks, CA: Sage Publications, 2002.
11. American Academy of Child and Adolescent Psychiatry: Practice parameters for the assessment and treatment of children and adolescents who are sexually abusive of others. J Am Acad Child Adolesc Psychiatry 38(12):55-76, 1999.

12. ten Bensel RW: Integrated glossary of normal child sexuality and child sexual abuse terms for juvenile justice professionals. Reno, NV: National Council of Juvenile and Family Court Judges, 1987.

13. National Institutes of Health, National Institutes of Health: Medline Plus Medical Dictionary, 2006. (Available at: *www.nlm.nih.gov/medlineplus/mplusdictionary.html;* accessed 2/16/07).

14. Masters WH, Johnson VE, Kolodny RC: Human Sexuality. Toronto, Ontario: Little, Brown, 1982.

15. Martinson FM: Eroticism in infancy and childhood. *In* Constantine LL, Martinson FM, eds: Children and Sex: New Findings, New Perspectives. Boston: Little, Brown, 1981, pp 23-35.

16. Rutter M: Normal psychosexual development. J Child Psychol Psychiatry 11:259-283, 1971.

17. Gessell A: The First Five Years of Life. London: Methuen, 1940.

18. Volbert R: Sexual knowledge of preschool children. J Psychol Hum Sex 12:5-26, 2000.

19. Gordon BN, Schoeder CS, Abrams M: Age and social-class differences in children's knowledge of sexuality. J Clin Child Psychol 19:33-43, 1990.

20. Bem SL: Genital Knowledge and gender constancy in preschool children. Child Dev 60:649-662, 1989.

21. Fraley MC, Nelson EC, Wolf AW, et al: Early genital naming. Dev Behav Pediatr 12:301-305, 1991.

22. Moore JE, Kendall DC: Children's concepts of reproduction. J Sex Res 7:42-61, 1971.

23. Cohen B, Parker S: Sex information among nursery-school children. *In* Oremland EK, Ormland JD, eds: The Sexual Gender Development of Young Children: The Role of the Educator. Cambridge, MA: Ballinger, 1977.

24. Goldman R, Goldman J: Children's Sexual Thinking. London: Rutledge & Kegan Paul, 1982.

25. Goldman R, Goldman J: Children's perceptions of sex differences in babies and adolescents: A cross-national study. Arch Sex Behav 12:277-294, 1983.

26. Kreitler H, Krietler S: Children's concepts of sexuality and birth. Child Dev 37:363-378, 1996.

27. Friedrich WN: Child Sexual Behavior Inventory: Professional Manual. Odessa, FL: Psychological Assessment Resources, 1997.

28. Friedrich WN, Fisher J, Dittner C, et al: Child Sexual Behavior Inventory: Normative, psychiatric, and sexual abuse comparisons. Child Maltreat 6:37-49, 2001.

29. Davies SL, Glaser D, Kossoff R: Children's sexual play and behavior in pre-school settings: Staff's perceptions, reports, and response. Child Abuse Negl 24:1329-1343, 2000.

30. Friedrich WN, Sandfort TG, M., Oostveen J, et al: Cultural differences in sexual behavior: 2-6 Year old Dutch and American Children. J Psychol Hum Sex 12:117-129, 2000.

31. Larsson I, Svedin CG, Friedrich WN: Differences and similarities in sexual behaviour among pre-schoolers in Sweden and USA. Nord J Psychiatry 54:251-257, 2000.

32. Larsson I, Svedin CG: Sexual behaviour in Swedish preschool children, as observed by their parents. Acta Paediatr 90:436-333, 2001.

33. Friedrich WN: Psychological Assessment of Sexually Abused Children and Their Families. Thousand Oaks, CA: Sage Publications, 2002.

34. Gordon B: Sexual development. *In* Ollendick TH, Schroeder CS, eds: Encyclopedia of Clinical Child and Pediatric Psychology. New York: Kluwer Academic/Plenum, 2003, pp 591-594.

35. Schroeder CS, Gordon BN: Assessment and Treatment of Childhood Problems. New York: Guilford, 1991.

36. Centers for Disease Control and Prevention: Trends in sexual risk behaviors among high school students—United States: 1991-2001. MMWR Morb Mortal Wkly Rep 51:856-861, 2002.

37. Lamb S, Coakley M: "Normal" childhood play and games: Differentiating play from abuse. Child Abuse Negl 17:515-526, 1993.

38. Larsson I: Children and Sexuality: "Normal" Sexual Behavior and Experiences in Childhood. Linköping, Sweden: Linköping University, Department of Health and Environment, Division of Child and Adolescent Psychiatry, 2001.

39. Reynolds M, Herbenick D, Bancroft J: The nature of childhood sexual experiences: Two studies 50 years apart. *In* Bancroft J, ed: Sexual development. Bloomington: Indiana University Press, 2003, pp 134-155.

40. Friedrich WN, Whiteside SP, Talley NJ: Noncoercive sexual contact with similarly aged individuals: What is the impact? J Interpers Violence 19:1075-1084, 2004.

41. Greenwald E, Leitenberg H: Long-term effects of sexual experiences with siblings and non-siblings during childhood. Arch Sex Behav 18:389-399, 1989.

42. Okami P, Olmstead R, Abramson PR: Sexual experiences in early childhood: 18-Year longitudinal data from the UCLA Family Lifestyles Project. J Sex Res 34:339-347, 1997.

43. Finkelhor D: Sex among siblings: A survey of prevalence, variety, and effects. Arch Sex Behav 9:171-194, 1980.

44. Tanner JM: Puberty. *In* McLaren A, ed: Advances in Reproductive Physiology, vol 2. New York: Academic Press, 1967, pp 311-347.

45. Ollendick TH, Schroeder CS: Encyclopedia of Clinical Child and Pediatric Psychology. New York: Kluwer Academic/Plenum, 2003.

46. Kinsey AC, Pomeroy WB, Martin CE: Sexual Behavior in the Human Male. Oxford, UK: WB Saunders, 1948.

47. Herman-Gidden M, Slora E, Wasserman R, et al: Secondary sexual characteristics and menses in young girls seen in office practice: A study from the Pediatric Research in Office Settings Network. Pediatrics 99:505-512, 1997.

48. Halpern CT, Udry JR, Suchindran C: Testosterone predicts initiation of coitus in adolescent females. Psychosom Med 59:161-171, 1997.

49. Blythe MJ, Rosenthal SL: Female adolescent sexuality: Promoting healthy sexual development. Obstet Gynecol Clin North Am 27:125-141, 2000.

50. DeLatmter J, Friedrich W: Human sexual development. J Sex Res 39:10-14, 2002.

51. Kirby D: Emerging Answers: Research Findings on Programs to Reduce Teen Pregnancy (Summary). Washington, DC: National Campaign to Prevent Teen Pregnancy, 2001.

52. Alford S: Science and Success: Sex Education and Other Programs That Work to Prevent Teen Pregnancy, HIV, and Sexually Transmitted Infections. Washington: Advocates for Youth, 2003.

53. Miller BC: Families Matter: A Research Synthesis of Family Influences on Adolescent Pregnancy. Washington, DC: National Campaign to Prevent Teen Pregnancy, 1998.

54. Kinsman SB, Romer D, Furstenberg FF, et al: Early sexual initiation: The role of peer norms. Pediatrics 102:1185-1192, 1998.

55. Santelli JS, DiClemente RJ, Miller KS, et al: Sexually transmitted diseases, unintended pregnancy, and adolescent health promotion. Adolesc Med 10:87-108, 1999.

56. Neinstein LS: Adolescent sexuality. *In* Neinstein LS, ed: Adolescent Health Care: A Practical Guide. Baltimore: Williams & Wilkins, 1996, pp 628-629.

57. Maynard R: Kids Having Kids: A Robin Hood Foundation Special Report on the Costs of Adolescent Childbearing. New York: Robin Hood Foundation, 1996.

58. Grunbaum JA, Kann L, Kinchen S, et al: Youth risk behavior surveillance—United States, 2003. MMWR Surveill Summ 53(2):1-96, 2004.

59. Gates G, Sonenstein FL: Heterosexual genital sexual activity among adolescent males: 1988 and 1995. Fam Plann Perspect 32:295-297, 2000.

60. Mosher WD, Chandra A, Jones J: Sexual behavior and selected health measures: Men and women 15-44 years of age, United States, 2002. Adv Data (362):1-55, 2005.

61. Prinstein MJ, Meade CS, Cohen GL: Adolescent oral sex, peer popularity, and perceptions of best friends' sexual behavior. J Pediatr Psychol 28:243-249, 2003.

62. Terry E, Manlove J: Trends in Sexual Activity and Contraceptive Use among Teens. Washington: Child Trends, 2000.

63. Collins RL, Elliott MN, Berry SH, et al: Entertainment television as a healthy sex educator: The impact of condom-efficacy information in an episode of *Friends.* Pediatrics 112:1115-1121, 2003.

64. Frankowski BL, American Academy of Pediatrics, Committee on Adolescence: Sexual orientation and adolescents. Pediatrics 113:1827-1832, 2004.

65. Remafedi G, Resnick M, Blum R, et al: Demography of sexual orientation in adolescents. Pediatrics 89:714-721, 1992.

66. Siddiqi S, Van Dyke DC, Donohoue P, et al: Premature sexual development in individuals with neurodevelopmental disabilities. Dev Med Child Neurol 41:392-395, 1999.

67. Woodward LJ: Sexuality and disability. Clin Fam Pract 6:941-954, 2004.

68. Gordon BN, Schroder C: Sexuality: A Developmental Approach to Problems. New York: Plenum Press, 1995.

69. Berman H, Harris D, Enright R, et al: Sexuality and the adolescent with a physical disability: Understandings and misunderstandings. Issues Comprehens Pediatr Nurs 22:183-196, 1999.

70. Kendall-Tackett K, Williams LM, Finkelhor D: Impact of sexual abuse on children: A review and synthesis of recent empirical studies. Psychol Bull 113:164-180, 1993.

71. White S, Haplin BM, Strom GA, et al: Behavioral comparisons of young sexually abused, neglected, and nonreferred children. J Clin Child Psychol 17:53-61, 1988.

72. Friedrich WN: Sexual victimization and sexual behavior in children: A review of recent literature. Child Abuse Negl 17:59-66, 1993.

73. Hewitt SK: Assessing allegation of sexual abuse in preschool children: Understanding small voices. Interpersonal Violence: The Practice Series. Thousand Oaks, CA: Sage Publications, 1999.

74. Johnson TC: Children who act out sexually. *In* McNamara J, McNamara BH, eds: Adoption and the Sexually Abused Children. Portland: University of Maine, 1990, pp 63-73.

75. Friedrich WN: Behavior problems in sexually abused children: An adaptational perspective. *In* Wyatt GE, Powell GJ, eds: Lasting Effects of Child Sexual Abuse. Newbury Park, CA: Sage Publications, 1988, pp 171-191.

76. Johnson TC: Child perpetrators—Children who molest other children: Preliminary findings. Child Abuse Negl 12:219-229, 1988.

77. Johnson TC: Female child perpetrators: Children who molest other children. Child Abuse Negl 13:571-585, 1989.

78. Silovsky JF, Niec L: Characteristics of young children with sexual behavior problems: A pilot study. Child Maltreat 7:187-197, 2002.

79. Bonner BL, Walker CE, Berliner L: Children with Sexual Behavior Problems: Assessment and Treatment (Final Report, Grant No. 90-CA-1469). Washington, DC: Administration of Children, Youth, and Families, U.S. Department of Health and Human Services, 1999.

80. Gray A, Busconi A, Houchens P, et al: Children with sexual behavior problems and their caregivers: Demographics, functioning, and clinical patterns. Sex Abuse 9:267-290, 1997.

81. Vermont Social and Rehabilitation Services: Vermont Child Abuse and Neglect. Waterbury, VT: Social and Rehabilitative Services, July 1996.

82. Bonner BL, Fahey WE: Children with aggressive sexual behavior. *In* Singh NN, Winton ASW, eds: Comprehensive Clinical Psychology Special Population. Oxford, UK: Elsevier Science, 1998, pp 453-466.

83. Friedrich WN, Davies W, Fehrer E, et al: Sexual behavior problems in preteen children: Developmental, ecological, and behavioral correlates. Ann N Y Acad Sci 989:95-104, 2003.

84. Gray A, Pithers WD, Busconi A, et al: Developmental and etiological characteristics of children with sexual behavior problems: Treatment implications. Child Abuse Negl 23:601-621, 1999.

85. Langstrom N, Grann M, Lichtenstein P: Genetic and environmental influences on problematic masturbatory behavior in children: A study of same-sex twins. Arch Sex Behav 31:343-350, 2002.

86. Friedrich WN: Children with Sexual Behavior Problems: Family-Based, Attachment-Focused Therapy. New York: WW Norton, in press.

87. Pithers WD, Gray A, Busconi A, et al: Children with sexual behavior problems: Identification of five distinct child types and related treatment considerations. Child Maltreat 3:384-406, 1998.

88. Friedrich WN, Luecke W, Beilke RL, et al: Psychotherapy outcome with sexually abused boys: An agency study. J Interpers Violence 7:396-409, 1998.

89. Gil E, Johnson TC: Sexualized children: Assessment and treatment of sexualized children and children who molest. Rockville, MD: Launch Press, 1993.

90. Horton CB: Children who molest other children: The school psychologist's response to the sexually aggressive child. School Psychol Rev 25:540-557, 1996.

91. Heiman M: Helping parents address their child's sexual behavior problems. J Child Sex Abuse 10:35-37, 2001.

92. Pearce J: Intervention Strategies with Preadolescent Children with Sexual Behavior Problems. Presented at the 11th Oklahoma Conference on Child Abuse and Neglect and Healthy Families, Norman, OK, September 17-19, 2003.

93. Baker AJL, Schneiderman M, Parker R: A survey of problematic sexualized behaviors in the New York City child welfare system: Estimates of problem, impact on services, and need for training. J Child Sex Abuse 10:67-80, 2002.

94. McKenzie W, English D, Henderson J: Family centered case management with sexually aggressive youth: Final report of the Sexually Aggressive Youth Project. Olympia: Washington State Department of Social and Health Services, Division of Children, Youth and Family Services, 1987.

95. Bonner BL, Walker CE, Berliner L, et al: Cluster Analyses of Children with Sexual Behavior Problems. Manuscript in preparation.

96. Hall DK, Mathews F, Pearce J: Sexual behavior problems in sexually abused children: A preliminary typology. Child Abuse Negl 26:389-312, 2002.

97. Berliner L, Elliott D: Sexual abuse of children. *In* Berliner L, Meyers JE, Briere J, et al, eds: The APSAC Handbook on Child Maltreatment. Thousand Oaks, CA: Sage Publishing, 2002, pp 55-78.

98. Johnson TC, Friend C: Assessing young children's sexual behaviors in the context of child sexual abuse evaluations. *In* Ney T, ed: True and False Allegations of Child Sexual Abuse: Assessment and Case Management. Philadelphia: Brunner/Mazel, 1995, pp 49-72.

99. Achenbach TM, Rescorla LA: Manual for ASEBA Preschool Forms & Profiles. Burlington: University of Vermont, Research Center for Children, Youth, and Families, 2000.

100. Achenbach TM, Rescorla LA: Manual for ASEBA School-Age Forms & Profiles. Burlington: University of Vermont, Research Center for Children, Youth & Families, 2001.

101. Reynolds C, Kamphaus R: Behavior Assessment System for Children Manual. Circle Pines, MN: American Guidance Service, 1992.

102. Briere J: Trauma Symptom Checklist for Children: Professional Manual. Odessa, FL: Psychological Assessment Resources, 1996.

103. Briere J, Johnson K, Bissada A, et al: The Trauma Symptom Checklist for Young Children (TSCYC): Reliability and association with abuse exposure in a multisite study. Child Abuse Negl 25:1001-1014, 2001.

104. Cohen JA, Mannarino AP: The weekly behavior report: A parent-report instrument for sexually abused preschoolers. Child Maltreat 1:353-360, 1996.

105. Carpentier M, Silovsky JF, Chaffin M: Randomized trial of treatment for children with sexual behavior problems: Ten year follow-up. J Consult Clin Psychol 74:482-488, 2006.

106. Pithers WD, Gray A, Busconi A, et al: Children with sexual behavior problems: Identification of five distinct child types and related treatment considerations. Child Maltreat 3:384-406, 1999.

107. Cohen JA, Mannarino AP: A treatment outcome study for sexually abused preschool children: Initial findings. J Am Acad Child Adolesc Psychiatry 35:42-50, 1996.

108. Cohen JA, Mannarino AP: A treatment study for sexually abused preschool children: Outcome during one-year follow-up. J Am Acad Child Adolesc Psychiatry 36:1228-1235, 1997.

109. Hall-Marley SE, Damon L: Impact of structured group therapy on young victims of sexual abuse. J Child Adolesc Group Ther 3:41-48, 1993.

110. Stauffer LB, Deblinger E: Cognitive behavioral groups for nonoffending mothers and their young sexually abused children: A preliminary treatment outcome study. Child Maltreat 1:65-76, 1996.

111. Cohen JA, Mannarino AP: A treatment model for sexually abused preschoolers. J Interpers Violence 8:115-131, 1993.

112. Cohen JA, Mannarino AP, Deblinger E: Treatment Trauma and Traumatic Grief in Children and Adolescents. New York: Guilford, 2006.

113. Deblinger E, Heflin AH: Treating sexually abused children and their nonoffending parents: A cognitive behavioral approach. Thousand Oaks, CA: Sage Publications, 1996.

114. Brestan EV, Eyberg SM: Effective psychosocial treatments of conduct-disordered children and adolescents: 29 Years, 82 studies, and 5,272 kids. J Clin Child Psychol 27:180-189, 1998.

115. Nixon R: Treatment of behavior problems in preschoolers: A review of parent training programs. Clin Psychol Rev 22:525-546, 2002.

116. Webster-Stratton C: The Incredible Years: A training series for the prevention and treatment of conduct

problems in young children. *In* Hibbs ED, Jensen PS, eds: Psychosocial Treatments for Child and Adolescent Disorders: Empirically Based Strategies for Clinical Practice. Washington, DC: American Psychological Association, 2005, pp 507-555.

117. Barkley R, Benton C: Your Defiant Child: Eight Steps to Better Behavior. New York: Guilford, 1998.

118. Sanders MR, Cann W, Markie-Dadds C: The Triple P—Positive parenting programme: A universal population-level approach to the prevention of child abuse. Child Abuse Rev 12:155-171, 2003.

119. Chaffin M, Berliner L, Block R, et al: Draft Report of the ATSA Task Force on Children with Sexual Behavior Problems. Beaverton, OR: Association for the Treatment of Sexual Abusers, 2005.

120. Bakersman-Kranenburg MJ, Van IJzendoorn MH, Juffer F: Less is more: Meta-analyses of sensitivity and attachment interventions in early childhood. Psychol Bull 129:195-215, 2003.

121. Chaffin M, Bonner B, Pierce K: What Research Shows about Adolescent Sexual Offenders. Fact Sheet Oklahoma City. National Center on the Sexual Behavior of Youth, 2003.

122. Synder HN, Sickmund M: Juvenile Offenders and Victims: 1999 National Report. Washington, DC: U.S. Department of Justice, Office of Juvenile Justice and Delinquency Prevention, 1999.

123. Davis GE, Leitenberg H: Adolescent sexual offenders. Psychol Bull 101:417-427, 1987.

124. Snyder H: Juvenile Arrests 2000 (Cooperative Agreement No. 1999-JN-FX-K002). *In* OJJDP Juvenile Justice Bulletin. Washington, DC: U.S. Department of Justice, Office of Juvenile Justice and Delinquency Prevention, 1-12, 2002.

125. Becker JV: What we know about the characteristics and treatment of adolescents who have committed sexual offenses. Child Maltreat 3:317-329, 1998.

126. Knight RA, Prentky RA: Exploring characteristics for classifying juvenile sex offenders. *In* Barbaree HE, Marshall WL, Hudson SM, eds: The Juvenile Sex Offender. New York: Guilford, 1993, pp 45-83.

127. Hanson RK, Slater S: Sexual victimization in the history of sexual abusers: A review. Ann Sex Res 1:485-499, 1988.

128. Widom CS: Victims of Childhood Sexual Abuse—Later Criminal Consequences. Washington, DC: U.S. Department of Justice, Office of Justice Programs, National Institute of Justice, 1995.

129. Mathews R, Hunter JA, Vuz J: Juvenile female sexual offenders: Clinical characteristics and treatment issues. Sex Abuse 9:187-199, 1997.

130. Bumby KM, Bumby NH: Adolescent female sex offenders. *In* Schwartz BK, Cellini HR, eds: The Sex Offender: Corrections, Treatment and Legal Practice. Kingston, NJ: Civic Research Institute, 1997, pp 10.1-10.16.

131. Hunter JA, Lexier LJ, Goodwin DW, et al: Psychosexual attitudinal, and developmental characteristics of juvenile female sexual perpetrators in a residential treatment setting. J Child Fam Stud 2:317-326, 1993.

132. Krauth A A: A comparative study of male juvenile sex offenders. Diss Abstr Int B Sci Eng 58:4455, 1998.

133. Carpenter DR, Peed SF, Eastman B: Personality characteristics of adolescent sexual offenders: A pilot study. Sex Abuse 7:195-203, 1995.

134. Prentky RA, Harrris B, Frizell K, et al: An actuarial procedure for assessing risk with juvenile sex offenders. Sex Abuse 12:71-93, 2000.

135. Association for the Treatment of Sexual Abusers: The Effective Legal Management of Juvenile Sex Offenders. Beaverton, OR: Association for the Treatment of Sexual Abusers, 2000. (Available at: *http://www.atsa.com/ppjuvenile.html;* accessed 2/16/07.)

136. Alexander MA: Sexual offender treatment efficacy revisited. Sex Abuse 11:101-116, 1999.

137. Miranda AO, Corcoran CL: Comparison of perpetration characteristics between male juvenile and adult sexual offenders: Preliminary results. Sex Abuse 12: 179-188, 2000.

138. American Psychiatric Association: Diagnostic and Statistical Manual of Mental Disorders, 4th ed. Washington: American Psychiatric Press, 1994.

139. Letourneau EJ, Miner MH: Juvenile sex offenders: A case against the legal and clinical status quo. Sex Abuse 17:293-312, 2005.

140. Friedrich WN, Lysne M, Sim L, et al: Assessing sexual behavior in high-risk adolescents with the Adolescent Clinical Sexual Behavior Inventory (ACSBI). Child Maltreat 9:239-250, 2004.

141. Borduin CM, Henggeler SW, Blaske DM, et al: Multisystemic treatment of adolescent sexual offenders. Int J Offender Ther Comp Criminol 34:105-113, 1990.

142. Borduin CM, Schaeffer CM: Multisystemic treatment of juvenile sex offenders: A progress report. J Psychol Hum Sex 13:25-42, 2002.

143. Thomas D, Flahery E, Binns H: Parent expectations and comfort with discussion of normal childhood sexuality and sexual abuse prevention during office visits. Ambul Pediatr 4:232-236, 2004.

144. Hall DK, Mathews F, Pearce J: Factors associated with sexual behavior problems in young sexually abused children. Child Abuse Negl 22:1045-1063, 1998.

145. Johnson TC: Helping Children with Sexual Behavior Problems—A Guidebook for Parents and Substitute Caregivers, 2nd ed. South Pasadena, CA: Toni Cavanagh Johnson, 2004.

146. Silovsky JF, Niec L, Bard D, et al: Treatment for Preschool Children with Sexual Behavior Problems: Pilot study. Journal of Clinical Child and Adolescent Psychology, in press.

147. Grant L: Sex and the Adolescent. *In* Zwellerman B, Parker S, ed: Behavioral and Developmental Pediatrics. Boston: Little, Brown, 1995, pp 269-277.

148. Russell ST, Franz BT, Driscoll AK: Same-sex romantic attraction and experiences of violence in adolescence. Am J Public Health 91:903-906, 2001.

149. Russell ST, Driscoll AK, Truong N: Adolescent same-sex romantic attractions and relationships: Implications for substance use and abuse. Am J Public Health 92:198-202, 2002.

150. Kupper L: Comprehensive sexuality education for children and youth with disabilities. SIECUS Rep 23:3-8, 1995.

151. American Academy of Pediatrics, Committee on Children with Disabilities: Sexuality education of children and adolescents with developmental disabilities. Pediatrics 97:275-278, 2000.

152. Nwoga IA: African American mothers use stories for family sexuality education. MCN Am J Matern Child Nurs 25:31-36, 2000.

153. Bigfoot DS, Dunlap M: Storytelling as a healing tool for American Indians. *In* Witko TM, ed: Mental Health Care for Urban Indians—Clinical Insights from Native Practitioners. Washington, DC: American Psychological Association, 2006.

154. Cohen JA, Mannarino AP: Factors that mediate treatment outcome of sexually abused preschool children: Six and twelve month follow up. J Am Acad Child Adolesc Psychiatry 37:44-51, 1998.

155. Cohen JA, Mannarino AP: Predictors of treatment outcome in sexually abused children. Child Abuse Negl 24:983-994, 2000.

156. Broidy L, Cauffman E, Espelage DL, et al: Sex differences in empathy and its relation to juvenile offending. Violence Victims 18:503-516, 2003.

157. Sex role [definition]. *In* Online Medical Dictionary. Newcastle upon Tyne, UK: University of Newcastle upon Tyne, Centre for Cancer Education, 2000. (Available at: http://cancerweb.ncl.ac.uk/cgi-bin/omd?sex+role ; accessed 2/16/07.)

25B.
Gender Identity

KENNETH J. ZUCKER

This chapter focuses on children and adolescents with sex-typed behavioral patterns that correspond to the diagnosis of Gender Identity Disorder (GID), as defined in the fourth edition, text revision, of the *Diagnostic and Statistical Manual of Mental Disorders (DSM-IV-TR)*.[1] Most children who meet *DSM-IV-TR* criteria for GID do not show any gross clinical signs of an abnormal or atypical physical sex differentiation (e.g., the sex chromosomes, the prenatal hormonal milieu); however, some children with physical intersex conditions (disorders of sex differentiation) do exhibit problems in their gender development; accordingly, some consideration is also given to this population.

Numerous television series have had story lines on the topic, and several critically acclaimed films, such as *Ma Vie en Rose (My Life in Pink)* in 1997, *Boys Don't Cry* in 1999, and *Transamerica* in 2005, have also focused an artistic gaze on the subject. The print media has also given attention to GID, including articles in *Time*[2] and *Saturday Night.*[3] On May 12, 2004, the *Oprah Winfrey Show,* with over 20 million viewers in the United States alone, featured several prepubertal "transgendered" children and their families, and on March 12, 2006, *60 Minutes,* with about 14 million viewers, provided a snapshot of 9-year-old fraternal twin boys markedly discordant for gender behavior: one boy was conventionally masculine, and the other boy was conventionally feminine and expressed the desire to be a girl. Thus, it is timely to provide an updated review on children and youth who experience discomfort about their gender identity.

CLINICAL AND SCIENTIFIC SIGNIFICANCE

Parents commonly rely on health professionals to help them sort out whether the behavior of their child warrants clinical attention. This is as true for gender and sexuality issues as it is for any other behavioral developmental matter. Thus, pediatricians are at the forefront in helping parents appraise their child's development. Moreover, primary care pediatricians can consult with pediatricians with expertise in developmental and behavioral issues in helping them differentiate between behavioral or emotional difficulties that are transient and those that are more pervasive.[4]

Issues surrounding gender and sexual development often cause intense anxiety for parents. Are the behaviors in question "only a phase" that the child will grow out of, or are the behaviors in question prognostic of longer term developmental issues? Regarding gender development, parents often want to know whether the behaviors of their young child are prognostic of a later homosexual sexual orientation or of transsexualism, the desire to receive contrasex hormonal treatment and physical sex change (e.g., in men, penectomy/castration and the surgical creation of a neovagina; in women, mastectomy and the surgical creation of a neophallus). Parents also often worry about the stigma that their child's pervasive cross-gender behavior might elicit within the peer group and in society at large. Similarly, when an adolescent engages in atypical sexual behavior (e.g., the use of women's undergarments for the purpose of sexual arousal), parents wonder what the behavior means. Is it only an experimental phase of sexual exploration and curiosity, or does it signify something else that might cause problems and complications in their adolescent's intimate life?

These kinds of questions require a familiarity with normative gender and sexual development, which allows the developmental-behavioral pediatrician to make decisions about differential diagnosis and to consider therapeutic options. This requires a good understanding of what is known about the basic mechanisms that underlie typical gender and sexual development.

TERMINOLOGY

Table 25B-1 provides a brief description of several terms that are used throughout this chapter.[5-15]

PREVALENCE

The prevalence of GID in children has not been formally studied by epidemiological methods. Prevalence estimates of GID in adults suggest an occurrence of 1 per 11,000 to 37,000 men and 1 per 30,400 to 150,000 women.[1,16]

Among children, some information can be derived from the widely used Child Behavior Checklist (CBCL),[18-19] a parent-report behavior problem questionnaire. The CBCL includes 2 items (of 118) that pertain to cross-gender identification: "behaves like opposite sex" and "wishes to be of opposite sex." On the CBCL, ratings are made on a 3-point scale (0 = *not true,* 1 = *somewhat or sometimes true,* and 2 = *very true or often true*). In the standardization study, answering both items affirmatively was more common for girls than for boys, regardless of age and clinical status (referred vs. nonreferred).[20]

Among nonreferred boys (aged 4 to 11 years), 3.8% received a rating of 1 and 1.0% received a rating of 2 for the item "behaves like opposite sex," but only 1.0% received a rating of 1 and 0.0% received a rating of 2 for the item "wishes to be of opposite sex." The comparable percentages among nonreferred girls were 8.3%, 2.3%, 2.5%, and 1.0%, respectively. Comparable findings have been reported in an epidemiological sample of twins.[21] Collectively, these data suggest that there is a sex difference in the occurrence of mild displays of cross-gender behavior but not with regard to more extreme cross-gender behavior. The main problem with such data, however, is that they do not identify adequately patterns of cross-gender behavior that would be of use in determining caseness. Thus, such data may be best viewed as screening devices for more intensive evaluation.

SEX DIFFERENCES IN REFERRAL RATES

Among children between the ages of 3 to 12, boys are referred clinically more often than girls for concerns regarding gender identity. In my own clinic, Cohen-Kettenis and colleagues reported a boy-to-girl ratio of 5.75 : 1 ($N = 358$) on the basis of consecutive referrals from 1975 to 2000.[22] In this study, comparative data were available from children evaluated at the sole gender identity clinic for children in Utrecht, The Netherlands. Although the sex ratio was significantly smaller at 2.93 : 1 ($N = 130$), it still reflected referral of more boys than girls. Among adolescents between the ages of 13 to 20, however, the sex ratio in my clinic narrowed considerably, at 1.32 : 1 ($N = 72$).[23]

TABLE 25B-1 ■ Terminology		
Term	**Brief Definition**	**References**
Sex	Attributes that collectively, and usually harmoniously, characterize biological maleness and femaleness (e.g., the sex-determining genes, the sex chromosomes, the H-Y antigen, the gonads, sex hormones, the internal reproductive structures, and the external genitalia)	5, 6
Gender	Psychological or behavioral characteristics associated with boys/men and girls/women	7
Gender identity	Basic sense of self as a boy/man or a girl/woman	8, 9
Gender role	Behaviors, attitudes, and personality traits that a society, in a given culture and historical period, designates as masculine or feminine: that is, more "appropriate" to or typical of the male or female social role	7
Sexual orientation	A person's relative responsiveness to sexual stimuli (erotic preference); the most salient dimension of sexual orientation is probably the sex of the person to whom one is attracted sexually, as in heterosexual, bisexual, or homosexual	10-12
Sexual identity	Self-labeling of one's sexual orientation	13
Paraphilias	A sexual orientation or erotic preference that is considered abnormal or atypical, as in transvestic fetishism or pedophilia	14, 15, 17

TABLE 25B-2 ■ *DSM-IV-TR* Diagnostic Criteria for Gender Identity Disorder

A. A strong and persistent cross-gender identification (not merely a desire for any perceived cultural advantages of being the other sex).

In children, the disturbance is manifested by at least four (or more) of the following:

1. Repeatedly stated desire to be, or insistence that he or she is, the other sex
2. In boys, preference for cross-dressing or simulating female attire; in girls, insistence on wearing only stereotypical masculine clothing
3. Strong and persistent preferences for cross-sex roles in make-believe play or persistent fantasies of being the other sex
4. Intense desire to participate in the stereotypical games and pastimes of the other sex
5. Strong preference for playmates of the other sex

In adolescents . . . the disturbance is manifested by symptoms such as a stated desire to be the other sex, frequent passing as the other sex, desire to live or be treated as the other sex, or the conviction that he or she has the typical feelings and reactions of the other sex.

B. Persistent discomfort with his or her sex or sense of inappropriateness in the gender role of that sex.

In children, the disturbance is manifested by any of the following: in boys, assertion that his penis or testes are disgusting or will disappear or assertion that it would be better not to have a penis, or aversion toward rough-and-tumble play and rejection of male stereotypical toys, games, and activities; in girls, rejection of urinating in a sitting position, assertion that she has or will grow a penis, or assertion that she does not want to grow breasts or menstruate, or marked aversion toward normative feminine clothing.

In adolescents . . . the disturbance is manifested by symptoms of such as preoccupation with getting rid of primary and secondary sex characteristics (e.g., request for hormones, surgery, or other procedures to physically alter sexual characteristics to simulate the other sex) or belief that he or she was born the wrong sex.

C. The disturbance is not concurrent with a physical intersex condition.

D. The disturbance causes clinically significant distress or impairment in social, occupational, or other important areas of functioning.

Specify if (for sexually mature individuals):

Sexually Attracted to Males
Sexually Attracted to Females
Sexually Attracted to Both
Sexually Attracted to Neither

From the American Psychiatric Association: Diagnostic and Statistical Manual of Mental Disorders, 4th ed, text revision [*DSM-IV-TR*]. Washington, DC: American Psychiatric Press, 2000.

This ratio was remarkably similar to the 1.20 : 1 (*N* = 133) boy-to-girl ratio reported by Cohen-Kettenis and Pfäfflin[24] in the Netherlands. Thus, across both clinics, there was a sex-related skew in referrals during childhood, but this lessened considerably during adolescence.

DIAGNOSIS AND ASSESSMENT

Reliability and Validity

In the clinical research literature, very little attention has been paid to reliability of diagnosis for GID. One study demonstrated that clinicians can reliably make the diagnosis in children[25] but, to my knowledge, no investigators have evaluated the reliability of the diagnosis for adolescents.[26]

It is relatively uncommon, at least in specialized child and adolescent gender identity clinics, to encounter an adolescent who has only very mild gender dysphoria. Thus, it is important to keep in mind that the indicators of GID are meant to capture a "strong and persistent cross-gender identification" and a "persistent discomfort" with one's gender, not transient feelings.[27-28]

The *DSM-IV-TR* criterion with regard to the "preoccupation" with primary and secondary sex characteristics (Point B-2) reflects well the adolescent expression of gender dysphoria as it pertains to discomfort with somatic sex, inasmuch as the distress over physical sex markers is so pervasive (Table 25B-2).

As noted previously, there is only one clinician-based reliability study of GID in children; however, there is a much more extensive literature in which its discriminant validity has been examined. Since the early 1970s, a variety of measurement approaches have been developed to assess the sex-typed behavior in children referred clinically for GID, including observation of sex-typed behavior in free play tasks, on semiprojective or projective tasks, and on a structured Gender Identity Interview schedule. In addition, several parent-report questionnaires pertaining to various aspects of sex-typed behavior have been developed. In this line of research, several comparison groups have typically been used: siblings of children with GID, clinical controls, and nonreferred (or "normal") controls.[29-31]

The results of these studies have demonstrated strong evidence for the discriminant validity of the various measures, with large effect sizes.[29] In addition, several studies have shown that gender-referred children can be distinguished as a function of whether they met the complete *DSM-IV-TR* criteria for GID (i.e., threshold vs. subthreshold cases).[31-35]

Two self-report and one parent report instruments are described. All three of these measures have practical utility in an office-based practice and can complement a detailed clinical interview. The first is the Gender Identity Interview for Children, which contains 11 items. Each item is coded on a 3-point response scale. On the basis of factor analysis, Zucker and associates[32] identified two factors, which were labeled *affective gender confusion* (seven items) and *cognitive gender confusion* (four items) and accounted for 38.2% and 9.8% of the variance, respectively. An item example from the first factor is "In your mind, do you ever think that you would like to be a girl (boy)?" and an item example from the second factor is "Are you a boy or a girl?" Both mean factor scores significantly differentiated gender-referred probands ($n = 85$) from controls ($n = 98$). Cutoff scores of either three or four deviant responses yielded high specificity rates (88.8% and 93.9%, respectively), but lower sensitivity rates (54.1% and 65.8%, respectively).

The second instrument is the Gender Identity Questionnaire for Children, a parent-report questionnaire.[33-34] This questionnaire consists of 16 items pertaining to various aspects of sex-typed behavior that are reflected in the GID diagnostic criteria, each rated on a 5-point response scale. A factor analysis based on 325 gender-referred children and 504 controls (siblings, clinic-referred, and nonreferred), with a mean age of 7.6 years, identified a one-factor solution containing 14 items, accounting for 43.7% of the variance. The gender-referred children had a significantly more total deviant score than did the controls, with a large effect size of 3.70, established by Cohen's *d*. With a specificity rate set at 95% for the controls, the sensitivity rate for the probands was 86.8%.

The third instrument is the Gender Identity/Gender Dysphoria Questionnaire for Adolescents and Adults (GIDQ-AA), another self-report questionnaire.[36] The GIDQ-AA consists of 27 items pertaining to various aspects of gender dysphoria, each rated on a 5-point response scale and with the past 12 months used as a time frame. In the female version, for example, items included: "In the past 12 months, have you felt more like a man than like a woman?" and "In the past 12 months, have you wished to have an operation to change your body into a man's (e.g., to have your breasts removed or to have a penis made)?" A factor analysis based on 389 university students (heterosexual and nonheterosexual) and 73 clinic-referred patients with GID identified a one-factor solution containing all 27 items, which accounted for 61.3% of the variance. The GIDQ-AA strongly distinguished the GID patients from both the heterosexual and non-heterosexual controls. With a cutpoint of 3.00, sensitivity was 90.4% for the patients with GID, and specificity was 99.7% for the controls.

Associated Behavior Problems

A considerable amount of evidence suggests that in the presence of GID symptoms, it is important to assess for the presence of behavior problems. The most systematic information on general behavior problems in children with GID comes from parent-report data on the CBCL. On the CBCL, clinic-referred boys and girls with GID display, on average, significantly more general behavior problems than do their siblings and nonreferred children[22,31] and levels comparable to those of demographically matched clinical controls[31]; moreover, CBCL-identified behavior problems are significantly more prevalent among adolescents with GID than among their GID child counterparts.[23,26]

According to the CBCL responses, boys with GID have a predominance of internalizing behavioral difficulties, whereas girls with GID do not.[31] Two studies have shown that boys with GID demonstrate high rates of separation anxiety traits.[37,38] Several studies have shown that increasing age was significantly associated with degree of behavior problems in boys with GID, which is probably mediated by peer ostracism,[20,22,31] and another study has shown that a composite index of maternal psychopathology was also a strong predictor of behavior problems.[39]

DEVELOPMENTAL TRAJECTORIES

Adolescents and adults with GID, particularly those who have a homosexual orientation (i.e., sexual attraction to members of one's birth sex), invariably recall a pattern of cross-sex–typed behavior during childhood that corresponds to the *DSM-IV-TR* criteria for GID.[36] Another line of research showed that adults with a homosexual sexual orientation, unselected for gender identity, were also more likely, on average, to recall patterns of childhood cross-sex–typed behavior in comparison with their heterosexual counterparts.[40] According to these retrospective studies, therefore, children with GID (which is at the extreme end of a continuum of cross-gender identification) monitored prospectively may be disproportionately likely to have persistent GID and/or a homosexual sexual orientation.

Follow-up Studies of Boys

Green's study[41] constitutes the most comprehensive long-term follow-up of behaviorally feminine boys, the majority of whom would likely have met *DSM-IV-TR* criteria for GID. His study contained 66 feminine and 56 control boys (unselected for gender identity) assessed initially at a mean age of 7.1 years (range, 4 to 12). Forty-four feminine boys and 30 control boys were available for follow-up at a mean age of 18.9 years (range, 14 to 24). The majority of the boys were not in therapy between assessment and follow-up. Sexual orientation in fantasy and behavior was assessed by means of a semistructured interview. Kinsey ratings were made on a 7-point continuum, ranging from exclusive heterosexuality (a Kinsey rating of 0) to exclusive homosexuality (a Kinsey rating of 6).[42] Depending on the measure (fantasy or behavior), 75% to 80% of the previously feminine boys were either bisexual or homosexual (Kinsey ratings between 2 and 6) at follow-up, in contrast to 0% to 4% of the control boys. Green also reported on the gender identity status of the 44 previously feminine boys. He found that only one youth, at the age of 18 years, was gender-dysphoric to the extent of considering sex-reassignment surgery.

Data from six other follow-up reports on 55 boys with GID were summarized by Zucker and Bradley.[31] In these studies, the percentage of boys who exhibited persistent GID was higher than that reported by Green (11.9% vs. 2.2%, respectively), but the percentage who were homosexual (62.1%) was somewhat lower.

Zucker and Bradley[31] reported preliminary follow-up data on a sample of 40 boys first observed in childhood (mean age at assessment, 8.2 years; range, 3 to 12). At follow-up, these boys were, on average, 16.5 years old (range, 14 to 23). Gender identity was assessed by means of a semistructured clinical interview and by questionnaire. Sexual orientation (for a 12-month period before the time of evaluation) was assessed for fantasy and behavior with the Kinsey scale in a manner identical to Green's study.[41]

Of the 40 boys, 8 (20%) were classified as gender-dysphoric at follow-up. With regard to sexual orientation in fantasy, 20 (50%) were classified as heterosexual, 17 (42.5%) were classified as bisexual/homosexual, and 3 (7.5%) were classified as "asexual" (i.e., they did not report any sexual fantasies). Regarding sexual orientation in behavior, 9 (22.5%) were classified as heterosexual, 11 (27.5%) were classified as bisexual/homosexual, and 20 (50.0%) were classified as "asexual" (i.e., they did not report any interpersonal sexual experiences).

Cohen-Kettenis[43] reported preliminary data on a sample of 56 boys first observed in childhood (mean age at assessment, 9 years; range, 6 to 12) and who had now reached adolescence. Of these, 9 (16.1%) requested sex-reassignment, and all 9 had a homosexual sexual orientation (P. T. Cohen-Kettenis, per-

sonal communication, February 1, 2003). Thus, the rate of GID persistence, at least into adolescence, was higher than that reported by Green[41] and comparable to the rate obtained by Zucker and Bradley,[31] as noted previously.

Follow-up Studies of Girls

To date, the most systematic follow-up of girls with GID was conducted by Drummond[44] of patients seen in my clinic. A total of 25 girls, originally assessed at a mean age of 8.8 years (range, 3 to 12), were interviewed at follow-up at a mean age of 23.2 years (range, 15 to 36). Of these 25 girls, 3 (12%) had persistent GID (at follow-up ages of 17, 21, and 23 years), of whom 2 had a homosexual sexual orientation and 1 was "asexual" (i.e., did not report any sexual orientation). The remaining 22 girls (88%) had a "normal" gender identity.

With regard to sexual orientation in fantasy (Kinsey ratings) for the 12 months preceding the follow-up assessment, 15 (60%) girls were classified as exclusively heterosexual, 8 (32%) were classified as bisexual/homosexual, and 2 (8%) were classified as "asexual" (i.e., did not report any sexual fantasies). Regarding sexual orientation in behavior, 11 (44%) girls were classified as exclusively heterosexual, 6 (24%) were classified as bisexual/homosexual, and 8 (32%) were classified as "asexual" (i.e., they did not report any interpersonal sexual experiences).

In another study, Cohen-Kettenis[43] reported preliminary data from a sample of 18 girls first seen in childhood (mean age at assessment, 9 years; range, 6 to 12) and who had now reached adolescence. Of these, 8 (44.4%) requested sex reassignment, and all had a homosexual orientation (P. T. Cohen-Kettenis, personal communication, February 1, 2003). Thus, the rate of GID persistence, at least into adolescence, was high (and much higher than the rate of persistence for the boys with GID).

Summary

In taking stock of these outcome data, Green's[41] study clearly showed that boys with GID were disproportionately, and substantially, more likely than the control boys to differentiate a bisexual/homosexual orientation. The other follow-up studies yielded somewhat lower estimates of a bisexual/homosexual orientation. In this regard, at least one caveat is in order. In Zucker and Bradley's[31] follow-up, for example, the boys were somewhat younger than were the boys in Green's follow-up; thus, their lower rate of a bisexual/homosexual orientation outcome should be interpreted cautiously, inasmuch as, if anything, these youth would be expected to underreport an atypical sexual orientation because of social desirability considerations. But even these lower rates of a bisexual/homosexual orientation are substantially higher than the currently acknowledged base rate of about 2% to 3% of men with a homosexual orientation that has been identified in epidemiological studies.[13] A similar conclusion can be drawn with regard to girls with GID. Using prevalence estimates of bisexuality/homosexuality in fantasy among biological females (anywhere between 2% and 5%), Drummond[44] reported that the odds of reporting bisexuality/homosexuality in fantasy was 8.9 to 23.1 times higher than in the general population. The odds of reporting bisexuality/homosexuality in behavior was 6.7 to 15.5 times higher than in the general population.

A more substantive difference between Green's[41] study and the other follow-up reports of boys pertains to the persistence of gender dysphoria. Both Zucker and Bradley[31] and Cohen-Kettenis,[43] for example, found higher rates of persistence than did Green. At present, the reasons for this are unclear. One possible explanation pertains to sampling differences. Green's study was carried out in the context of an advertised research study, whereas Zucker and Bradley's and Cohen-Kettenis's samples were clinic-referred. Thus, it is conceivable that their samples may have included more extreme cases of childhood GID than did the sample ascertained by Green.

With regard to girls with GID, the odds of persistent gender dysphoria in Drummond's[44] sample was 4084 times the odds of gender dysphoria in the general population.[16]

DISJUNCTIONS BETWEEN RETROSPECTIVE AND PROSPECTIVE DATA

A key challenge for developmental theories of psychosexual differentiation is to account for the disjunction between retrospective and prospective data with regard to GID persistence: It is clear that only a minority of children monitored prospectively show a persistence of GID into adolescence and young adulthood.

One explanation concerns referral bias. Green[45] argued that children with GID who are referred for clinical assessment (and then, in some cases, therapy) may come from families in which there is more concern than is the case for adolescents and adults, the majority of whom did not receive a clinical evaluation and treatment during childhood. Thus, a clinical evaluation and subsequent therapeutic intervention during childhood may alter the natural history of GID. Another possibility is that the diagnostic criteria for GID, at least as they are currently formulated,

simply are not sharp enough to distinguish children who are more likely to show a persistence in the disorder from those who are not.

An additional clue comes from consideration of the concepts of developmental malleability and plasticity. It is possible, for example, that gender identity shows relative malleability during childhood, with a gradual narrowing of plasticity as the gender-related sense of self consolidates as a child approaches adolescence. Some support for this idea comes from follow-up studies of adolescents with GID, who appear to show a much higher rate of GID persistence as they are monitored into young adulthood.[46,47]

ETIOLOGY

The cause of GID has been examined with regard to both biological and psychosocial mechanisms. Research on etiology is controversial because it is embedded in complex "political" matters, and the developmental-behavioral pediatrician needs to be aware of this social context. Parents, for example, hold all kinds of biases and beliefs regarding causality. Some parents adhere to a biological explanation for their child's cross-gender behavior ("He must have been born that way"), whereas others adhere to a psychosocial explanation ("His father was never around"). In many respects, parental perspectives mirror the general scientific debate on the relative roles of nature and nurture with regard to psychosexual differentiation. Regardless of their accuracy, parental perspectives on etiology are important because they may be correlated with their views on their child more generally, what they want from the clinician, and their attitudes and goals about therapeutics.

Biological Mechanisms

Contemporary biological research on human psychosexual differentiation includes investigations of molecular genetics, behavioral genetics, prenatal sex hormones, prenatal maternal stress, maternal immunization, neurodevelopmental processes, pheromones, temperament, anthropometrics, and neuroanatomical substrates. Some of these parameters have been studied with regard to both children and adults with GID, some have been investigated in relation to sexual orientation, and others have been examined in nonclinic populations (e.g., twin studies).

Experimental studies—from mice to monkeys—have shown quite clearly how manipulation of the prenatal hormonal milieu can affect postnatal sex-dimorphic behavior.[48] In humans, the effects of the prenatal hormonal environment have been examined in various physical intersex conditions. Consider, for example, studies of congenital adrenal hyperplasia (CAH), the most common physical intersex condition that affects genetically female humans. CAH is an autosomal recessive disorder associated with enzyme defects that result in abnormal adrenal steroid biosynthesis. Indeed, for affected genetically female fetuses, testosterone assayed from amniotic fluid during midgestation shows values in the range of unaffected genetically male fetuses. Because of this high level of androgen production during fetal development, masculinization of the external genitalia is common. On the basis of data from lower animals and on theory, it has been presumed that some masculinization of the fetal brain may also have occurred.

There is very clear evidence that the gender role behavior of girls with CAH is more masculine and/or less feminine than that of unaffected control girls.[29,49] Moreover, adult follow-up studies of girls with CAH indicate that they have higher rates of bisexuality and homosexuality (particularly in fantasy) than do controls. Thus, for both gender role behavior and sexual orientation, there is a shift away from the female-typical pattern and toward the male-typical pattern. The evidence that CAH results in an altered gender identity is much less convincing. Although the percentage of genetically female girls with CAH—about 5%—who develop gender dysphoria or change gender from female to male is higher than that of girls in the general population, most girls and women with CAH appear to have an uncomplicated female gender identity.[50] Together, these findings suggest that the prenatal hormonal milieu may have a greater effect on gender role and sexual orientation than it does on gender identity in girls and women with CAH.

As applied to GID (in both children and adults), classical prenatal hormone theory has, at least in its simple form, been challenged because there is no compelling evidence that the prenatal hormonal milieu is grossly abnormal because the differentiation of the external genitalia is normal. Thus, at least in terms of gross markers of biological sex, it appears that most individuals with GID are somatically normal.[51] This has led some researchers to consider alternative biological pathways that might affect psychosexual differentiation or to reconsider prenatal hormone theory in terms of behavioral-genital dissociations: that is, hormonal effects on the brain but not the genitals. Such researchers have has examined behavior genetics (the liability for cross-gender behavior),[21,52] altered ratio of the length of the second digit to that of the fourth digit,[53] handedness,[54,55] sibling sex ratio and birth order,[56-58] and neuroanatomical substrates.[59,60] This line of research reviewed has begun to identify some characteristics of children and adults with GID that may well have a biological basis. In some respects, however, it has been easier to rule out candidate biological explanations, such as the influence of gross anomalies in prenatal hormonal exposure.[61-62] Nonetheless, the study of new potential biological markers of variation in psychosexual differentiation has opened up avenues for novel empirical inquiry that will probably be pursued in the years to come.

Psychosocial Mechanisms

Psychosocial factors, to truly merit causal status, must be shown to influence the emergence of marked cross-gender behavior in the first few years of life. Otherwise, such factors are better conceptualized as perpetuating rather than predisposing. A few of the more prominent hypotheses and relevant data are discussed as follows.

PRENATAL GENDER PREFERENCE

It is common for parents to express a gender preference before a child is born. Other things being equal, parents have a child of the nonpreferred sex about 50% of the time. Are parents of children with GID more likely than control parents to report having had a desire for a child of the opposite sex? The simple answer appears to be no, at least with regard to the mothers of boys with GID.[63] We did find, however, that the maternal wish for a girl was significantly associated with the sex composition and birth order of the sibship. In families of affected boys with only older brothers, the percentage of mothers who recalled a desire for a daughter was significantly higher than among the families of probands with other sibship combinations; however, the same pattern was observed in a control group.[63] It was, noted, however, that among mothers of boys with GID who had desired daughters, a small subgroup appeared to experience what might be termed *pathological gender mourning*.[31] The wish for a daughter was acted out (e.g., by crossdressing the boy) or expressed in other ways. These mothers often had severe depression, which was lifted only when the boy began to act in a certain feminine manner. This clinical observation, however, must be examined in much greater detail, including understanding how the wish for a girl, when it occurs, is resolved in most cases.

SOCIAL REINFORCEMENT

Understanding the role of parent socialization in the genesis and/or perpetuation of GID (e.g., through reinforcement principles or modeling) has been influenced by the normative developmental literature on sex-dimorphic sex-typed behavior.[7] It has also been influenced by the seminal but controversial observations of Money and colleagues[61] that the rearing environment was the predominant determinant of gender identity in children with physical intersex conditions.

Clinicians of diverse theoretical persuasions have consistently reported that the parental response to early cross-gender behavior in children with GID is typically neutral (tolerance) or even encouraging.[31] Regarding boys with GID, Green[45] concluded that "what comes closest so far to being a *necessary* variable is that, as any feminine behavior begins to emerge, there is *no* discouragement of that behavior by the child's principal caretaker" (p 238; italics in original). An example of this is illustrated in the following email correspondence from a mother, who was considering an assessment of her 5-year-old son, who strongly desired to be a girl:

> *We adore Darryl just the way he is and wouldn't want to change a thing about him. We indulge him in Barbies, My Little Ponies, and princess dress-up clothing . . . whatever he wants, he gets.*

In my clinic, Mitchell,[64] in a structured interview study, found that mothers of GID boys were more likely to tolerate/encourage feminine behaviors and less likely to encourage masculine behaviors than were the mothers of both clinical patients and normal control boys. The reasons for such tolerance appear to be quite variable, including parental values and goals regarding psychosexual development; feedback from professionals that the behavior is within normal limits and "only a phase"; parental conflicts about issues of masculinity and femininity; and parental psychopathology and discord, which leave the parents relatively preoccupied and thus unresponsive to their child's behavior. Such underlying motivations can be examined only in a thorough clinical evaluation.

TRANSACTIONAL PROCESSES

Many scholars adhere to a transactional model of gender differentiation.[7] A child's gender identity is constructed gradually over time: even if a biological predisposition does affect the likelihood of a child engaging in varying degrees of sex-typical versus sex-atypical behavior, many other factors probably either accentuate or attenuate its expression. Parental responses, as noted earlier, may be one such factor. Children themselves contribute to this process as they develop complex cognitive constructions of what it means to be a boy or a girl.[65] The child's behavior may be both affected by and influence the quality of the relationship with his or her parents. A child's gender identity will affect emerging peer relationships, and the peer group may play a role in further gender differentiation.[7]

As another example of the direction-of-effect conundrum, consider the literature on parent-child relationships. In clinical studies of boys with GID, Stoller[66] described a situation in which the relationship between mother and son was overly close and that between father and son was distant and peripheral. Stoller claimed that such qualities were of etiological relevance: "The more mother and the less father, the more femininity" (p 25). He argued that GID in boys was a "developmental arrest . . . in which an excessively close and gratifying mother-infant symbiosis, undisturbed by father's presence, prevents a boy from adequately separating himself from his mother's female body and feminine behavior" (p 25). Green[41] assessed quantitatively the amount of shared time between fathers of feminine boys and control boys during the first 5 years of life. The fathers of feminine boys reported spending less time with their sons from the second to fifth year than did the fathers of the controls.

The picture that emerges for GID boys, then, is one in which they feel closer to their mothers than to their fathers.[41] From a causal perspective, however, the direction-of-effect question can be raised: Do GID boys feel this way because their own behavior influences the quality of parent-child relations, or are there predisposing parental characteristics that are influential? Or are both factors involved, resulting in a complex transactional chain?

SUMMARY

The research reviewed here has identified several psychosocial mechanisms thought to be involved in the genesis and perpetuation of GID. Some specific, relatively simple hypotheses have been shown to be incorrect. Others, such as parental response to cross-gender behavior when it first emerges, appear to have greater clinical and empirical support. The emphasis here, however, has also been to highlight the complex psychosocial chain and the difficulties in identifying direction-of-effect processes. On this point, considerably more research attention is clearly warranted.

THERAPEUTICS

Ethical Considerations

Consider the following clinical scenarios:

1. A mother of a 4-year-old boy called a well-known clinic that specializes in sexuality throughout the lifespan. She described behaviors consistent with the *DSM-IV-TR* diagnosis of GID. The clinician tells the mother, "Well, we don't consider 'it' to be a

problem." This mother then sent me an email, asking, "What should I do?"

2. A mother of a 4-year-old boy called a well-known clinic that specializes in gender identity problems. She described behaviors consistent with the *DSM-IV-TR* diagnosis of GID. She said that she would like her child treated so that he does not grow up to be gay. She also worried that her child would be ostracized within the peer group because of his pervasive cross-gender behavior. What should the clinician say to this mother?

3. The parents of a 6-year-old boy (somatically male) concluded that their son is really a girl, so they sought the help of an attorney to institute a legal name change (from Zachary to Aurora) and informed the school principal that their son would attend school as a girl. The local child protection agency was notified, and the child was removed from his parent's care.[2] If a clinician were asked to evaluate the situation, what would be in the best interest of the child and family?

4. A 15-year-old adolescent girl with GID asked to be seen for treatment. She wanted cross-sex hormones and a mastectomy immediately. The patient said that if refused, she would kill herself. What should the clinician do?

5. A 16-year-old adolescent boy with GID asked for sex-reassignment surgery. He stated that he is sexually attracted to biological boys and wants a sex-change because that would make his sexual feelings for boys "normal." He stated that homosexuality is against his religious beliefs and is taboo in his culture of origin. What should the clinician do?

Any contemporary pediatric clinician responsible for the therapeutic care of children and adolescents with GID is quickly introduced to complex social and ethical issues pertaining to the politics of sex and gender in post-modern Western culture and will have to think them through carefully. The scenarios just described, as well as many others, require the clinician to think long and hard about theoretical, ethical, and treatment issues.

Treatment of Children

Elsewhere, I have identified five rationales for intervention in the treatment literature on children with GID: (1) reduction in social ostracism, (2) treatment of underlying psychopathology, (3) treatment of the underlying distress, (4) prevention of transsexualism in adulthood, and (5) prevention of homosexuality in adulthood.[67]

In my view, the first four rationales are clinically defensible, but the fifth is not. Therefore, on this last point, further explication is warranted. Some critics have argued that clinicians consciously or unconsciously accept the prevention of homosexuality as a legitimate therapeutic goal.[68] Others have asserted, albeit without empirical documentation, that treatment of GID results in harm to children who are "homosexual" or "prehomosexual."[69]

The various issues regarding the relation between GID and homosexuality are complex, both clinically and ethically. Three points, although brief, can be made. First, until it has been shown that any form of treatment for GID during childhood affects later sexual orientation, Green's[41] discussion of whether parents have the right to seek treatment to maximize the likelihood of their child becoming heterosexual is moot. From an ethical standpoint, however, the treating clinician has an obligation to inform parents about the state of the empirical database. Second, I have argued elsewhere that some critics incorrectly conflate gender identity and sexual orientation, regarding them as isomorphic phenomena, as do some parents.[70] In psychoeducational work with parents, clinicians can review the various explanatory models regarding the statistical linkage between gender identity and sexual orientation[71] but also discuss their distinctness as psychological constructs. Third, many contemporary pediatric clinicians emphasize that the primary goal of treatment with children with GID is to resolve the conflicts that are associated with the disorder, regardless of the child's eventual sexual orientation.

If the clinician is to provide treatment for a child with GID, it is important to bear in mind that there has been no single randomized controlled treatment trial. The practitioner must rely largely on the "clinical wisdom" that has accumulated in the case report literature and the conceptual underpinnings that inform the various approaches to intervention.

Behavior Therapy

The literature contains 13 single-case reports in which investigators employed a behavior therapy approach to the treatment of GID in children.[67,71] The classical behavioral approach is to assume that children learn sex-typed behaviors much as they learn any other behaviors and that sex-typed behaviors can be shaped, at least initially, by encouraging some and discouraging others. Accordingly, behavior therapy for GID systematically arranges to have rewards follow gender-typical behaviors and to have no rewards (or perhaps punishments) follow cross-gender behaviors.

One type of intervention employed has been termed *differential social attention* or *social reinforcement*. This type of intervention has been applied in clinic settings, particularly to sex-typed play behaviors. The therapist first establishes with baseline measures that the child prefers playing with cross-sex toys or dress-up apparel rather than same-sex toys or dress-up apparel. A parent or stranger is then introduced into the playroom and instructed to attend to the child's same-sex play (e.g., by looking, smiling, and verbal praise) and to ignore the child's cross-sex play (e.g., by looking away and pretending to read). Such adult responses seem to elicit rather sharp changes in play behavior.

The field of behavior therapy has produced no new case reports since the 1980s, although its principles are often used in broader treatment approaches that involve the parents. This publication gap is odd, because more contemporary behavioral approaches, such as cognitive-behavior therapy, are now used so widely with other disorders.

Behavior therapy with an emphasis on the child's cognitive structures regarding gender could be an interesting and novel approach to treatment. There is now a fairly large literature on the development of cognitive gender schemas in nonreferred children.[65] It is possible that children with GID have more elaborately developed cross-gender schemas than same-gender schemas and that more positive affective appraisals are differentiated for the latter than for the former (e.g., in boys, "Girls get to wear prettier clothes" vs. "Boys are too rough"). A cognitive approach to treatment might help children with GID to develop more flexible and realistic notions about gender-related traits (e.g., "Boys can wear pretty cool clothes, too" or "There are lots of boys who don't like to be rough"), which may result in more positive gender feelings about being a boy or being a girl.

Psychotherapy

There is a large case report literature on the treatment of children with GID through psychoanalysis, psychoanalytic psychotherapy, or psychotherapy, some reports of which are quite detailed and rich in content.[67,71] The psychoanalytic treatment literature is more diverse than the behavior therapy literature, including varied theoretical approaches to understanding the putative cause of GID (e.g., classical, object relations, and self psychology); nevertheless, a number of recurring themes can be gleaned from this case report literature.

Psychoanalytic clinicians generally emphasize that the cross-gender behavior emerges during the "pre-oedipal" years;[66] accordingly, they stress the importance of understanding how the GID relates to other developmental phenomena salient during these years (e.g., attachment relations and the emergence of the autonomous self). Oedipal issues are also deemed important, but these are understood within the context of prior developmental interferences and conflicts. Psychoanalytic clinicians also place great weight on the child's overall adaptive functioning, which they view as critical in determining the therapeutic approach to the specific referral problem.

Apart from the general developmental perspective inherent to a psychoanalytic understanding of psychopathology, there is also a gender-specific perspective on development.[7] Many developmental psychologists, for example, note that the first signs of normative gender development appear during the toddler years, including the ability to correctly self-label as a boy or a girl. Thus, early gender identity formation intersects quite neatly with analytical views on the early development of the sense of self in more global terms. It is likely, therefore, that the putative pathogenic mechanisms identified in the development of GID are likely to have a greater effect only if they occur during the alleged sensitive period for gender identity formation.[61]

An overall examination of the available case reports suggests that psychotherapy, like behavior therapy, does have some beneficial influence on the sex-typed behavior of children with GID. However, the effectiveness of psychoanalytic psychotherapy, like that of behavior therapy, has never been demonstrated in an outcome study comparing children randomly assigned to treated and untreated conditions. Moreover, many of the cases cited previously did not consist solely of psychoanalytic treatment of the child. The parents were often also in therapy, and, in some of the cases, the child was an inpatient and thus exposed to other interventions. It is impossible to disentangle these other potential therapeutic influences from the effect of the psychotherapy alone.

Treatment for the Parents

Two rationales have been offered for parental involvement in treatment. The first emphasizes the hypothesized role of parental dynamics and psychopathology in the genesis or maintenance of the disorder. According to this perspective, individual therapy with the child probably proceeds more smoothly and quickly if the parents are able to gain some insight into their own contribution to their child's difficulties. Many clinicians who have worked extensively with gender-disturbed children subscribe to this rationale.[72,73,74] Assessment of psychopathology and the marital relationship in the parents of children with GID reveals great variability in adaptive functioning, which may well prove to be a prognostic factor.[31,39]

In addition, parents benefit from regular, formalized contact with the therapist to discuss day-to-day management issues that arise in carrying out the overall therapeutic plan. Work with parents can focus on the setting of limits with regard to cross-gender behavior, such as cross-dressing, cross-gender role and fantasy play, and cross-gender toy play and, at the same time, attempting to provide alternative activities (e.g., encouragement of same-sex peer relations and involvement in more gender-typical and neutral activities). In addition, parents can work on conveying to their child that they are trying to help him or her feel better about being a boy or a girl and that they want their child to be happier in this regard. Some parents, especially the well-functioning and intellectually sophisticated ones, are able to carry out these recommendations relatively easily and without ambivalence. Many parents, however, require ongoing support in implementing the recommendations, perhaps because of their own ambivalence and reservations about gender identity issues.[71]

Supportive Treatments

Clinicians critical of conceptualizing marked cross-gender behavior in children as a disorder have provided a dissenting perspective to the treatment approaches described so far.[75-77] These clinicians conceptualize GID or pervasive gender-variant behavior from an essentialist perspective—that it is fully constitutional or congenital in origin—and are skeptical about the role of psychosocial or psychodynamic factors. As an example of this perspective, Bockting and Ehrbar[78] argued that "instead of attempts to change the child's gender identity or role, treatment should assist the family to accept the child's authentic gender identity and affirm a gender role expression that is most comfortable for that child" (p 128). Along similar lines, Menvielle and Tuerk[75] noted that although it might be helpful to set limits on pervasive cross-gender behaviors that may contribute to social ostracism, their primary treatment goal (offered in the context of a parent support group) was "not at changing the children's behavior, but at helping parents to be supportive and to maximize opportunities for the children's adjustment" (p 1010). Menvielle and associates[76] took a somewhat stronger position, by arguing that "Therapists who advocate changing gender-variant behaviors should be avoided" (p 45).

Because comparative treatment approaches are not available, it is not possible to say whether this supportive or "cross-gender affirming" approach will result in both short-term and long-term outcomes any different from the more traditional approaches to treatment. The supportive approach does, however, highlight a variety of theoretical and clinical disagreements, which will be resolved only by more systematic research on therapeutics.

Adolescents

In adolescents with GID, there are three broad clinical issues that require evaluation: (1) the phenomena pertaining to the GID itself, (2) sexual orientation, and (3) psychiatric comorbidity. Gender-dysphoric adolescents with a childhood onset of cross-gender behavior typically have a homosexual orientation (i.e., they are attracted to members of their own "birth sex"). Some such adolescents may not report any sexual feelings, but follow-up typically reveals the emergence of same-sex attractions. Thus, the clinician must evaluate simultaneously two dimensions of the patient's psychosexual development: current gender identity and current sexual orientation.

The psychotherapy treatment literature on adolescents with GID has been very poorly developed and is confined to a few case reports.[31,67,71] In general, the prognosis for adolescents in resolving the GID is more guarded than it is for children. This state of affairs is similar to that of other child psychiatric disorders: The longer a disorder persists, the less is the likelihood that it will remit, with or without treatment. From a clinical management point of view, two key issues need to be considered: (1) Some adolescents with GID are not particularly good candidates for psychotherapy because of comorbid disorders and general life circumstances, and (2) some adolescents with GID have little interest in psychologically oriented treatment and are quite adamant about proceeding with hormonal and surgical sex reassignment.

Before recommending hormonal and surgical interventions, many clinicians encourage adolescents with GID to consider alternatives to this invasive and expensive treatment. One area of inquiry can, therefore, explore the meaning behind the adolescent's desire for sex reassignment and whether there are viable alternative lifestyle adaptations. The most common area of exploration in this regard pertains to the patient's sexual orientation. Some adolescents with GID recall that they always felt uncomfortable growing up as boys or as girls but that the idea of "sex change" did not occur until they became aware of homoerotic attractions. For some of these youngsters, the idea that they might be gay or homosexual is abhorrent (internalized homophobia).

For some such adolescents, psychoeducational work can explore their attitudes and feelings about homosexuality. Youth support groups or group therapy may provide an opportunity for youngsters to meet gay adolescents and can be a useful intervention. In some cases, the gender dysphoria may resolve, and a homosexual adaptation ensues.

For adolescents with persistent gender dysphoria, there is considerable evidence that it often interferes with general social adaptation, including general psychiatric impairment, conflicted family relations, and dropping out of school. For these youngsters, therefore, the treating clinician can consider two main options: (1) supportive management until the adolescent turns 18 and can be referred to an adult gender identity clinic or (2) "early" institution of contrasex hormonal treatment.

An option for treatment of gender-dysphoric adolescents is to prescribe puberty-blocking luteinizing hormone–release agonists (e.g., depot leuprolide or depot triptorelin) that facilitate more successful passing as the opposite sex.[79] Such medication can suppress the development of secondary sex characteristics, such as facial hair growth and voice deepening in adolescent boys, which make it more difficult to pass in the female social role. Cohen-Kettenis and van Goozen[46] reported that early cross-sex hormone treatment for adolescents younger than 18 years facilitated the complex psychosexual and psychosocial transition to living as a member of the opposite sex and resulted in a lessening of the gender dysphoria (see also Smith et al[47]). Although such early hormonal treatment remains controversial,[80] it may be the treatment of choice once the clinician is confident that other options have been exhausted.[26,81]

Summary

The treatment literature on GID in children and adolescents has many gaps. As reviewed previously, the literature for children has been confined to a lot of case reports from varying theoretical perspectives, with little in the way of comparative evaluation. Clinicians have varied perspectives on what to treat, and thus the developmental-behavioral pediatrician needs to be aware of the complex ideological, political, and theoretical perspectives that underlie the different positions. For adolescents, there is an emerging consensus by clinicians who work with gender-dysphoric adolescents that cross-sex hormone treatment may well be a reasonable early therapeutic intervention once it becomes clear that psychosocial approaches have not resulted in a reduction of the gender dysphoria.[82] For both children and adolescents, it is advisable, in my view, that referrals be made to clinicians with a strong background in child and adolescent developmental psychopathology and, when feasible, to therapists with at least some familiarity with the literature on both normative and applied gender development.

FUTURE DIRECTIONS

Although gender development and its disorders has been studied by a relatively small number of trained clinicians and researchers, considerable progress has been made in a number of areas since the introduction of the GID diagnosis to the third edition of the *Diagnostic and Statistical Manual of Mental Disorders* in 1980. This has included careful description of phenomena, the development of valid assessment techniques, some studies on causes, and follow-up studies on natural history.

Nonetheless, various issues require further attention. These include consideration of refinements to the *DSM-IV-TR* criteria for GID, a better understanding of body image development in children with GID, more research on causes, and continued study of long-term outcome. Of most importance, perhaps, is what is lacking in the literature: well-designed treatment studies, particularly for children. In an era in which increasing emphasis is placed on best-practice and evidence-based treatment, it is important to fill this gap in order to resolve the contemporary debates regarding how to most effectively provide clinical care for children and adolescents who experience tremendous distress and conflict about their gender identity.

REFERENCES

1. American Psychiatric Association: Diagnostic and Statistical Manual of Mental Disorders, 4th ed, Text Revision. Washington, DC: American Psychiatric Association, 2000.
2. Cloud J: His name is Aurora. Time (September 25):90-91, 2000. (Available at: *http://www.time.com/time/magazine/article/0,9171,998007,00.html*; accessed 2/18/07.)
3. Bauer G: Gender bender. Saturday Night 117(6):60-62, 64, 2002.
4. Sroufe LA: Considering normal and abnormal together: The essence of developmental psychopathology. Dev Psychopathol 2:335-347, 1990.
5. Grumbach MM, Hughes IA, Conte FA: Disorders of sex differentiation. *In* Larsen PR, Kronenberg HM, Melmed S, et al, eds: Williams Textbook of Endocrinology, 10th ed. Philadelphia: WB Saunders, 2003, pp 842-1002.
6. Vilain E: Genetics of sexual development. Annu Rev Sex Res 11:1-25, 2000.
7. Ruble DN, Martin CL, Berenbaum SA: Gender development. *In* Eisenberg N, ed: Handbook of Child Psychology, Volume 3: Social, Emotional, and Personality Development, 6th ed (Damon W, Lerner RM, series eds). New York: Wiley, 2006, pp 858-932.
8. Kohlberg L: A cognitive-developmental analysis of children's sex-role concepts and attitudes. *In* Maccoby EE, ed: The Development of Sex Differences. Stanford, CA: Stanford University Press, 1966, pp 82-173.
9. Stoller RJ: The hermaphroditic identity of hermaphrodites. J Nerv Ment Dis 139:453-457, 1964.
10. Chivers ML, Rieger G, Latty E, et al: A sex difference in the specificity of sexual arousal. Psychol Sci 15:736-744, 2004.
11. Rosen RC, Beck JG: Patterns of Sexual Arousal: Psychophysiological Processes and Clinical Applications. New York: Guilford, 1988.

12. Schrimshaw EW, Rosario M, Meyer-Bahlburg HFL, et al: Test-retest reliability of self-reported sexual behavior, sexual orientation, and psychosexual milestones among gay, lesbian, and bisexual youths. Arch Sex Behav 35:225-234, 2006.

13. Laumann EO, Gagnon JH, Michael RT, et al: The Social Organization of Sexuality: Sexual Practices in the United States. Chicago: University of Chicago Press, 1994.

14. Freund K, Watson R, Rienzo D: Heterosexuality, homosexuality, and erotic age preference. J Sex Res 26:107-117, 1989.

15. Zucker KJ, Blanchard R: Transvestic fetishism: Psychopathology and theory. In Laws DR, O'Donohue W, eds: Sexual Deviance: Theory, Assessment, and Treatment. New York: Guilford, 1997, pp 253-279.

16. Bakker A, van Kesteren PJM, Gooren LJG, et al: The prevalence of transsexualism in The Netherlands. Acta Psychiatr Scand 87:237-238, 1993.

17. Långström N, Zucker KJ: Transvestic fetishism in the general population: Prevalence and correlates. J Sex Marital Ther 31:87-95, 2005.

18. Zucker KJ: Cross-gender-identified children. In Steiner BW, ed: Gender Dysphoria: Development, Research, Management. New York: Plenum Press, 1985, pp 75-174.

19. Achenbach TM, Edelbrock C: Manual for the Child Behavior Checklist and Revised Child Behavior Profile. Burlington: University of Vermont, Department of Psychiatry, 1983.

20. Zucker KJ, Bradley SJ, Sanikhani M: Sex differences in referral rates of children with gender identity disorder: Some hypotheses. J Abnorm Child Psychol 25:217-227, 1997.

21. Beijsterveldt CEM, Hudziak JJ, Boomsma, DI: Genetic and environmental influences on cross-gender behavior and relation to behavior problems: A study of Dutch twins at ages 7 and 10 years. Arch Sex Behav 35:647-658, 2006.

22. Cohen-Kettenis PT, Owen A, Kaijser VG, et al: Demographic characteristics, social competence, and behavior problems in children with gender identity disorder: A cross-national, cross-clinic comparative analysis. J Abnorm Child Psychol 31:41-53, 2003.

23. Zucker KJ, Owen A, Bradley SJ, et al: Gender-dysphoric children and adolescents: A comparative analysis of demographic characteristics and behavioral problems. Clin Child Psychol Psychiatry 7:398-411, 2002.

24. Cohen-Kettenis PT, Pfäfflin F: Transgenderism and Intersexuality in Childhood and Adolescence: Making Choices. Thousand Oaks, CA: Sage Publications, 2003.

25. Zucker KJ, Finegan JK, Doering RW, et al: Two subgroups of gender-problem children. Arch Sex Behav 13:27-39, 1984.

26. Zucker KJ: Gender identity disorder. In Wolfe DA, Mash EJ, eds: Behavioral and Emotional Disorders in Adolescents: Nature, Assessment, and Treatment. New York: Guilford, 2006, pp 535-562.

27. Lee T: Trans(re)lations: Lesbian and female to male transsexual accounts of identity. Womens Stud Int Forum 24:347-357, 2001.

28. McCarthy L: Off That Spectrum Entirely: A Study of Female-Bodied Transgender-Identified Individuals. Unpublished doctoral dissertation, University of Massachusetts, Amherst, 2003.

29. Zucker KJ: Measurement of psychosexual differentiation. Arch Sex Behav 34:375-388, 2005.

30. Zucker KJ: Gender identity disorder. In Hooper SR, Hynd GW, Mattison RE, eds: Child Psychopathology: Diagnostic Criteria and Clinical Assessment. Hillsdale, NJ: Erlbaum, 1992, pp 305-342.

31. Zucker KJ, Bradley SJ: Gender Identity Disorder and Psychosexual Problems in Children and Adolescents. New York: Guilford, 1995.

32. Zucker KJ, Bradley SJ, Lowry Sullivan CB, et al: A gender identity interview for children. J Pers Assess 61:443-456, 1993.

33. Johnson LL, Bradley SJ, Birkenfeld-Adams AS, et al: A parent-report Gender Identity Questionnaire for Children. Arch Sex Behav 33:105-116, 2004.

34. Cohen-Kettenis PT, Wallien M, Johnson LL, et al: A parent-report Gender Identity Questionnaire for Children: A cross-national, cross-clinic comparative analysis. Clin Child Psychol Psychiatry 11:397-405, 2006.

35. Fridell SR, Owen-Anderson A, Johnson LL, et al: The Playmate and Play Style Preferences Structured Interview: A comparison of children with gender identity disorder and controls. Arch Sex Behav 35:729-737, 2006.

36. Deogracias JJ, Johnson LL, Meyer-Bahlburg HFL, et al: The Gender Identity/Gender Dysphoria Questionnaire for Adolescents and Adults. J Sex Res, in press.

37. Coates S, Person ES: Extreme boyhood femininity: Isolated behavior or pervasive disorder? J Am Acad Child Psychiatry 24:702-709, 1985.

38. Zucker KJ, Bradley SJ, Lowry Sullivan CB: Traits of separation anxiety in boys with gender identity disorder. J Am Acad Child Adolesc Psychiatry 35:791-798, 1996.

39. Zucker KJ: Predictors of Psychopathology in Boys with Gender Identity Disorder. Presented in the Institute on Gender Identity Disorder in Children and Adolescents (Bradley SJ, Chair), American Academy of Child and Adolescent Psychiatry and Canadian Academy of Child Psychiatry, Toronto, October 2005.

40. Bailey JM, Zucker KJ: Childhood sex-typed behavior and sexual orientation: A conceptual analysis and quantitative review. Dev Psychol 31:43-55, 1995.

41. Green R: The "Sissy Boy Syndrome" and the Development of Homosexuality. New Haven, CT: Yale University Press, 1987.

42. Kinsey AC, Pomeroy WB, Martin CE: Sexual Behavior in the Human Male. Philadelphia: WB Saunders, 1948.

43. Cohen-Kettenis PT: Gender identity disorder in DSM? [Letter]. J Am Acad Child Adolesc Psychiatry 40:391, 2001.

44. Drummond KD: A follow-up study of girls with gender identity disorder. Unpublished master's thesis, Ontario Institute for Studies in Education of the University of Toronto, 2006.

45. Green R: Sexual Identity Conflict in Children and Adults. New York: Penguin, 1974.

46. Cohen-Kettenis PT, van Goozen SHM: Sex reassignment of adolescent transsexuals: A follow-up study. J Am Acad Child Adolesc Psychiatry 36:263-271, 1997.

47. Smith YLS, van Goozen SHM, Cohen-Kettenis PT: Adolescents with gender identity disorder who were accepted or rejected for sex reassignment surgery: A prospective follow-up study. J Am Acad Child Adolesc Psychiatry 40:472-481, 2001.

48. Wallen K, Baum MJ: Masculinization and defeminization in altricial and precocial mammals: Comparative aspects of steroid hormone action. Horm Brain Behav 4:385-423, 2002.

49. Cohen-Bendahan CCC, van de Beek C, Berenbaum SA: Prenatal sex hormone effects on child and adult sex-typed behavior: Methods and findings. Neurosci Biobehav Rev 29:353-284, 2005.

50. Dessens AB, Slijper FME, Drop SLS: Gender dysphoria and gender change in chromosomal females with congenital adrenal hyperplasia. Arch Sex Behav 34:389-397, 2005.

51. Meyer-Bahlburg HFL: Introduction: Gender dysphoria and gender change in persons with intersexuality. Arch Sex Behav 34:371-373, 2005.

52. Coolidge FL, Thede LL, Young SE: The heritability of gender identity disorder in a child and adolescent twin sample. Behav Genet 32:251-257, 2002.

53. Schneider HJ, Pickel J, Stalla GK: Typical female 2nd-4th finger length (2D : 4D) ratios in male-to-female transsexuals—Possible implications for prenatal androgen exposure. Psychoneuroendocrinology 31:265-269, 2006.

54. Zucker KJ, Beaulieu N, Bradley SJ, et al: Handedness in boys with gender identity disorder. J Child Psychol Psychiatry 42:767-776, 2001.

55. Green R, Young R: Hand preference, sexual preference, and transsexualism. Arch Sex Behav 30:565-574, 2001.

56. Blanchard R, Zucker KJ, Bradley SJ, et al: Birth order and sibling sex ratio in homosexual male adolescents and probably prehomosexual feminine boys. Dev Psychol 31:22-30, 1995.

57. Zucker KJ, Green R, Coates S, et al: Sibling sex ratio of boys with gender identity disorder. J Child Psychol Psychiatry 38:543-551, 1997.

58. Green R: Birth order and ratio of brothers to sisters in transsexuals. Psychol Med 30:789-795, 2000.

59. Zhou J-N, Hofman MA, Gooren LJ, et al: A sex difference in the human brain and its relation to transsexuality. Nature 378:68-70, 1995.

60. Kruiver FPM, Zhou J-N, Pool CW, et al: Male-to-female transsexuals have female neuron numbers in a limbic nucleus. J Clin Endocrinol Metab 85:2034-2041, 2000.

61. Money J, Hampson J, Hampson J: Imprinting and the establishment of gender role. Arch Neurol Psychiatry 77:333-336, 1957.

62. Meyer-Bahlburg HFL, Gruen RS, New MI: Gender change from female to male in classical congenital adrenal hyperplasia. Horm Behav 30:319-332, 1996.

63. Zucker KJ, Green R, Garofano C, et al: Prenatal gender preference of mothers of feminine and masculine boys: Relation to sibling sex composition and birth order. J Abnorm Child Psychol 22:1-13, 1994.

64. Mitchell JN: Maternal Influences on Gender Identity Disorder in Boys: Searching for Specificity. Unpublished doctoral dissertation, York University, Downsview, Ontario, 1991.

65. Martin CL, Ruble DN, Szkrybalo J: Cognitive theories of early gender development. Psychol Bull 128:903-933, 2002.

66. Stoller RJ: Presentations of Gender. New Haven, CT: Yale University Press, 1985.

67. Zucker KJ: Gender identity disorder in children, adolescents, and adults. In Gabbard GO, ed: Gabbard's Treatments of Psychiatric Disorders, 4th ed. Washington, DC: American Psychiatric Press, in press.

68. Pleak RR: Ethical issues in diagnosing and treating gender-dysphoric children and adolescents. In Rottnek M, ed: Sissies & Tomboys: Gender Nonconformity & Homosexual Childhood. New York: New York University Press, 1999, pp 44-51.

69. Isay RA: Remove Gender Identity Disorder in DSM. Psychiatric News 32(Nov 21):9, 13, 1997.

70. Zucker KJ: Gender Identity Disorder in the DSM-IV [Letter]. J Sex Marital Ther 25:5-9, 1999.

71. Zucker KJ: Gender identity disorder in children and adolescents. In Gabbard GO, ed: Treatments of Psychiatric Disorders, 3rd ed, vol 2. Washington, DC: American Psychiatric Press, 2001, pp 2069-2094.

72. Coates S, Wolfe S: Gender identity disorder in boys: The interface of constitution and early experience. Psychoanal Inq 15:6-38, 1995.

73. Newman LE: Treatment for the parents of feminine boys. Am J Psychiatry 133:683-687, 1976.

74. Zucker KJ, Bradley SJ, Doering RW, et al: Sex-typed behavior in cross-gender–identified children: Stability and change at a one-year follow-up. J Am Acad Child Psychiatry 24:710-719, 1985.

75. Menvielle EJ, Tuerk C: A support group for parents of gender non-conforming boys. J Am Acad Child Adolesc Psychiatry 41:1010-1013, 2002.

76. Menvielle EJ, Tuerk C, Perrin EC: To the beat of a different drummer: The gender-variant child. Contemp Pediatr 22(2):38-39, 41, 43, 45-46, 2005.

77. Lev AI: Transgender Emergence: Therapeutic Guidelines for Working with Gender-Variant People and Their Families. New York: Haworth, 2004.

78. Bockting WO, Ehrbar RD: Commentary: Gender variance, dissonance, or identity disorder? J Psychol Hum Sex 17(3/4):125-134, 2005.

79. Gooren L, Delemarre-van de Waal H: The feasibility of endocrine interventions in juvenile transsexuals. J Psychol Hum Sex 8(4):69-84, 1996.

80. Beh H, Diamond M: Ethical concerns related to treating gender nonconformity in childhood and adolescence: Lessons from the Family Court of Australia. Health Matrix Clevel 15:239-283, 2005.

81. Cohen-Kettenis PT: Gender identity disorders. *In* Gillberg C, Harrington R, Steinhausen H-C, eds: A Clinician's Handbook of Child and Adolescent Psychiatry. Cambridge, UK: Cambridge University Press, 2005, pp 695-725.

82. Meyer W, Bockting WO, Cohen-Kettenis P, et al: The Harry Benjamin International Gender Dysphoria Association's Standards of Care for Gender Identity Disorders, Sixth version. J Psychol Hum Sex 13(1):1-30, 2001.

25C.
Variations in Sexual Orientation and Sexual Expression

ELLEN C. PERRIN

The majority of adults are content with gender definitions that are consistent with their anatomical sex and are physically and emotionally attracted to adults of different sex. An increasingly visible minority of adults are convinced that their social and emotional gender is discordant with their biological sex (i.e., they are transgendered) or are attracted to people of the same sex (i.e., they are homosexual). Teenagers and occasionally even preteenagers may find themselves believing that or questioning whether they are in either of these categories. Because both homosexuality and transgenderism are severely stigmatized in society, this process of a person's wondering and coming to believe that he or she is gay, lesbian, bisexual, or transgender is frequently associated with considerable distress for these young people and their families. Family and social support may provide protection against some of the disastrous effects of stigmatization. Pediatricians in primary care, adolescent medicine, and developmental-behavioral pediatrics, and their professional colleagues, have an important role to play in providing and bolstering this support.

This section of the chapter on sexuality is in four sections: (1) current theories about the genesis of variations in sexual orientations; (2) the development of a gay, lesbian, or trangender identity; (3) the well-being of children whose parents are gay or lesbian; and (4) opportunities for pediatric interventions.

Only a few general reviews have covered this particular assortment of topics since the 1990s. Summaries of the trajectory of gay and lesbian development, concerns about these adolescents, and resources for improvement are included in several recent reviews[1,2,4] and form the basis of the American Academy of Pediatrics' revised Clinical Statement on Homosexuality.[3]

Two reviews of the well-being of children who were raised by lesbian or gay parents have been published.[5,6] In addition, these data are summarized in support of marriage as a potential benefit for these children.[7]

EXPLANATIONS FOR VARIATIONS IN SEXUAL ORIENTATION

The complex interplay among biological and environmental factors in the determination of sexual orientation remains an enigma. Psychoanalytic, social learning, and social constructionist theories have postulated various mechanisms explaining the development of sexual orientation, although few differences have been found in the family and social environments of homosexual and heterosexual individuals. There is no evidence that the development of a homosexual orientation is related to traumatic experiences in childhood or adolescence such as sexual abuse.[8]

The futility of the typical polarization between "biological" and "social" influences on sexual orientation is described by one author as follows:

> It is impossible to separate biological and psychological contributions. . . . The public debate about the ontogeny of sexual orientation seems especially misguided because there is profound agreement between scientists who favor psychosocial theories and those who favor biological theories that sexual orientation is determined very early in life and is not a matter of individual choice.
> —S. M. Breedlove[9]

Neuroanatomical Phenomena

Some morphological differences have been found between heterosexual and homosexual men. Two of the four interstitial nuclei of the anterior hypothalamus have been found to be larger in men than in women; one of these has been found to be much larger in heterosexual men than in homosexual men.[10] Increased cell number and volume have been reported in the suprachiasmatic nucleus of homosexual men,[11] but environmental and psychological factors appear to play some part in this.[12] There may be a link between cerebral lateralization and sexual orientation,[13] and there appears to be less pronounced hemispheric asymmetry in homosexual men than in heterosexual men.[14,15] The significance of these findings in explaining the origins of homosexuality is unclear.

Psychoendocrine Factors

No differences have been found in the sex steroid levels of heterosexual and homosexual adults,[16-19] but in many mammalian species, prenatal sex hormones appear to be associated with structural differences in the brain and with sex-linked behaviors.[20,21]

Some support for the contribution of prenatal estrogen to the development of homosexuality comes from the finding of a modest association of prenatal diethylstilbestrol (DES) exposure with increased incidence of homosexuality in women.[22] Prenatal androgen exposure (e.g., resulting from congenital adrenal hyperplasia) also may be associated with a greater propensity for "tomboyish" behaviors.[23,24]

On the basis of animal studies, there is considerable controversy about whether homosexual men might have a positive estrogen feedback mechanism to regulate the secretion of luteinizing hormone; such a mechanism is usually present only in women.[25-28] More recent investigations of these relationships posit complex relationships between prenatal stress, genetic factors, and psychoendocrine changes in the development of a homosexual orientation.[29,30]

Genetic Studies

Early suggestions of a genetic component to the determination of sexual orientation stemmed from observations of family genograms. According to the first reports, more than one third of male homosexual patients had homosexual relatives, and there was concordance for homosexuality in six of seven pairs of identical twins. A tabulation of several earlier reports concluded that some families seemed to have an aggregation of homosexual members that exceeded the numbers expected by chance.[31] Several studies have reported concordances of between 52% and 66% among monozygotic male twins as and of between 22% and 30% among dizygotic male twins.[32,33] Concordance rates have been somewhat lower for women: 48% among monozygotic twins and 16% among dizygotic twins.[34] Although a high degree of concordance is found repeatedly in studies of twins,[35-37] all reports also include some identical twins whose sexual orientations were unquestionably different. Of course, twins share more than genes: their family and social environments are also far more similar than those of nontwin siblings. To address this concern, a few sets of twins who have been raised separately have been studied, and they also are reported to show greater than expected concordance in sexual orientation.[33,38]

Some investigations have suggested a chromosomal marker of sexual orientation. Of 40 pairs of gay brothers, 33 were found to have the same alleles at five adjacent marker sites at the Xq28 region of the X chromosome.[39,40] Unfortunately, no similar study has been done with lesbians, and this initial finding has not been replicated.

How genes exert their influence and in combination with what environmental factors remains unclear. It is possible that genes influence the development of particular areas of the brain, which then leads to the neuroanatomical and endocrine variations referred to previously. The interaction of genetic markers with familial and social patterns may result in predictable patterns of behaviors.[41,42] What seems increasingly clear is that whatever combination of biological and environmental factors influences sexual orientation seems to act very early in life and seems to be rather tenacious. A delightful summary of the complexity involved in understanding the biological origins of sexual orientations can be found in an essay by Money[43] titled "Sin, Sickness, or Status?"

The complexity of these processes should not be minimized. One neuroanatomist and psychiatrist summarizes the "state of the art" thus:

> While all mental phenomena must have an ultimate biological substrate, the precise contribution of biological factors to the development of sexual orientation remains to be elucidated. Does biology merely provide the slate of neural circuitry upon which sexual orientation is inscribed by experience? Do biological factors directly wire the brain so that it will support a particular orientation? Or do biological factors influence sexual orientation only indirectly, perhaps by influencing personality variables that in turn influence how one interacts with and shapes the environment as it contributes to the social relationships and experiences that shape sexual orientation as it emerges developmentally?
>
> —W. Byne[44]

Family and Social Factors

Psychoanalytic, social learning, and social constructionist theories have postulated mechanisms explaining the development of sexual orientation.

PSYCHOANALYTIC THEORY

Psychoanalytic theorists believe that relationships with parents early in childhood are central to the development of gender identity, gender roles, and sexual orientation. According to traditional psychoanalytic theory, gender development is rooted in the phallic stage of psychosexual development. The development of a lesbian or gay sexual orientation is viewed as a negative outcome resulting from the unsuccessful resolution of the oedipal conflict. This outcome is predicted for boys in the presence of a domineering mother and a weak father; a lesbian orientation is thought to result from a hostile and fearful relationship of a girl with her mother.[45]

Empirical studies have not supported this theory. Studies of gay men have found no evidence that they were overindulged by or more strongly attached to their mothers than were heterosexual men.[46,47] Research on the early family relationships of lesbian women has suggested that their mothers tended to be dominant and their fathers weaker,[46,48] contrary to theoretical predictions.

SOCIAL LEARNING THEORY

According to social learning theory, the family interpersonal environment and parental expectations are determining factors in the development of sexual orientation.[49] Important processes are thought to be *modeling* and *differential reinforcement.* Parents are known to treat their sons and daughters differently as early as infancy and to encourage different activities for older boys and girls.[50-53] Some theorists suggest that children develop culturally typical patterns of behavior and gender roles as a result of parental modeling and/or reinforcement.[54]

Some social learning theorists suggest that fathers may be more important to children's gender-role development than are mothers.[55] Fathers have been observed to make greater distinctions between sons and daughters and to interact with boys and girls in ways that are far more differentiated than do mothers. From this observation comes the prediction that fathers' behavior promotes typically gender-typed behavior in both boys and girls more strongly than does mothers' behavior. Fathers are said to be more likely to encourage their sons to take on an instrumental, independent style of behavior, whereas they encourage their daughters to seek help and be more dependent.[56,57]

SOCIAL CONSTRUCTIONIST THEORY

Social constructionist theories emphasize individuals' active role, guided by the culture, in creating their sexual identity.[58-60] According to these theorists, individuals first become aware of cultural norms for sexual encounters and then develop internal fantasies and interpersonal scripts associated with sexual arousal. Many children may experience attraction to peers of the same gender, but social sanctions force them to reject these attractions.[61]

DEVELOPMENT OF A GAY OR LESBIAN IDENTITY

In many ways, gay and lesbian youths share the experiences of all other adolescents regardless of sexual orientation[62]; in other ways, lesbian and gay youths share important elements of a developmental process in common with other lesbian and gay youths. Many factors intersect to affect the expression of an individual's sexual orientation. Several patterns expressed in the process of development of mature homosexuality have been described. Most often cited are the theoretical pathways outlined by Cass[63] and by Troiden (see Tables 25C-2 and 25C-3).[64,65]

Early Evidence of Gender Variance

Many gay adolescent boys remember a vague but distinct sense of being different from other boys as early as preschool and the early school years. They report a sense of "not fitting in" and were aware of not having the same interests as other boys. Some have intense, pervasive, and persistent interests and behaviors characterized as typical of the other gender, including play and sport activities, toys and hobbies, clothing and external appearance, identification with role models, preference for other-gender playmates, and a desire to be the other sex. Young boys with gender variance (or Gender Identity Disorder; see Table 25B-2) may have an intense interest in Snow White, or may want nothing for their birthday except a new Barbie doll. Their interests tend to be restricted to typically feminine ones, they generally are uncomfortable with typically masculine pursuits, and they avoid rough-and-tumble play. Similarly, young girls with marked gender variance typically show distinct discomfort with activities that are typically associated with girls, refuse to wear skirts and dresses, and often insist that they want to be a boy.

Although gender variance exists in children of both sexes, fewer girls than boys are seen by developmental-behavioral pediatricians and mental health clinicians. This pattern may reflect a true difference in prevalence, but it is also affected by the fact that the range of behavior that is considered acceptable in most modern societies is far broader for girls than for boys.[2]

The only available longitudinal data suggest that the majority of boys with marked gender variance during the preschool period later identified themselves as gay.[66] About 6% identified themselves as transgender,[67] and about 25% as heterosexual.[68] It is not possible to predict which outcome will occur for which boys. Very little research has been done on girls.

Children referred for so-called gender identity disorder are reported by their parents to have both internalizing and externalizing symptoms in greater number than do their peers, most consistently after 6 years of age.[68] Their distress is likely to emanate from a complex combination of forces in the family and social climate. There is no intrinsic disadvantage caused to a boy by wearing dresses and makeup or to a girl with short hair who competes in contact sports. However, girls and boys with atypical play and playmate preferences confront stigma from peers and adults; they are isolated and teased. Their parents, too, face stigmatization and may feel embarrassed, conflicted, and insecure, which in turn may lead them to respond to their children critically and punitively. Emotional and behavioral symptoms are likely to be a reflection of this distress.

When parents express concerns about their child's gender-variant behaviors, pediatricians generally have offered reassurance, hoping that these behaviors are evidence of the child's greater-than-average flexibility. This approach may not be in the best interest of the child and the family. It is important to acknowledge the considerable challenge of parenting a gender-variant child.[69] Siblings, grandparents, aunts, and uncles also may need information, support, and guidance to come to a new understanding and acceptance of the gender-variant child. Overlooking or minimizing the child's differences deprives families of the opportunity to be actively affirming in preparation for the possibility that the child is gay. The serious risks that gay, lesbian, and transgender adolescents typically face may be partly averted if children have the clear knowledge early in childhood that they are known, loved, and accepted just as they are. Their parents and professional advisers have an opportunity to provide active support for diversity in sexual orientation and sexual expression from early childhood onward (Table 25C-1).

Adolescent Development

Sexual experimentation typically begins during early or middle adolescence and frequently includes sexual activity with both opposite-sex and same-sex partners. The timing and process of consolidation of an individual's sexual identity depends on many factors, including access to reliable information, the avail-

---

TABLE 25C-1 ■ Tips for Parents of Children with Gender-variant Behavior

Remember that your child's sexual orientation is not your responsibility: You are not responsible for your child's gender variance or sexual orientation any more than you are responsible for a child's being left-handed. The child's sexual orientation is uncertain and will remain so until the time that the child is fully conscious of his or her sexual attractions, able to label his or her sexual orientation appropriately, and willing to disclose it to others.

Create a safe space: Your home may be your child's only place of safety. Allowing the child to be "who he or she is" in your home can make a big difference to the child's self-esteem. Preschoolers may need your help to recognize social situations in which people might react negatively. Older children learn to make decisions on their own about how to express themselves and what interests to pursue in public.

Encourage activities appropriate for your child: Encourage the child to find activities that fit with his or her interests and talents. "Prescribing" activities to change the child is always a failure. Children overly focused on very few interests should be introduced to alternative activities, given adequate time with each parent to support these new activities, and praised for just trying. Protect a regular time commitment for the child to spend with the parent or another adult of his or her gender. Avoid emotional withdrawal just because your child's interests are very different from yours.

Encourage communication: Listen to the child's concerns and wishes without criticizing, so that the child feels understood and remains open with you. Talk with the child matter-of-factly and in positive terms about his or her being different. Model tolerance and acceptance of various kinds of diversity for your children. Include siblings in these discussions.

Avoid stereotyping: Avoid using statements such as "Only girls play with dolls" and "Boys love to play ball but girls do not." Instead, tell your child that there are many kinds of boys and girls. Become vigilant about the language you use, avoiding assumptions about boyfriends, girlfriends, and marriage. Keep in mind that gay men and lesbians form long-term committed relationships that often include children. Express affirming opinions towards homosexuality (e.g., through family discussions of news events, books and movies).

Help the child with bullying: Look for resources to guide you on how to teach the child to handle bullying. Do not blame the child if he or she is bullied. Ask the child to tell you about any bullying that occurs. Be alert to possible warning signs that indicate that the child may be in trouble, such as refusal to attend school, pains and aches, or crying excessively.

Advocate with schools: Insist that your local schools adopt a zero tolerance policy toward bullying. Teachers are more likely to actively intervene if parents explain the issues and anticipate potential problems. Request that children's books on diversity, including sexual orientation and gender identity, be available in the library.

Advocate with extended family and friends: You might need to educate grandparents, aunts and uncles, other relatives, and neighbors. They may also benefit from some of the materials suggested as resources. Use all opportunities to educate children and adults about the value of respecting people who are unique or in some way different.

ability of supportive peers and adult role models, and the breadth of individual experience and sophistication. Adolescents may recognize and identify themselves as gay or lesbian during early, middle, or late adolescence; some (especially women) do not come to understand their sexual orientation until their 20s or even later. The age at self-identification as gay or lesbian appears to be decreasing[70,71]; some children as young as 10 to 12 feel certain of their homosexual orientation and disclose it to their parents.[72,73] One report documented that the majority of youths who had identified themselves as gay, lesbian, or bisexual maintained their self-identification over time. Adolescent girls were somewhat less likely to change their identities than were adolescent boys.[74] Both teenaged boys and girls typically discuss emerging questions about their sexual orientation first with same-sex friends, especially if any have self-identified as lesbian or gay. Teachers, coaches, physicians, and nurses can also provide advice and support as teenagers prepare to disclose their sexual orientation to family members and other friends.

Little is known about variations in the prevalence of homosexuality associated with differences in ethnic, religious, and racial affiliations and among people of lower socioeconomic status. There is considerable evidence that the prevalence of homosexual orientations varies little among cultures and ethnic groups, although attitudes about it vary greatly. Population-based data suggest that the prevalence of exclusive homosexuality among young men is between 1% and 4% and among women is 1% to 2%.[75-77]

GAY MALE DEVELOPMENT

Among the best-articulated models of the trajectory of development of a gay male identity during adolescence is that described by Troiden[65,78] and Cass[63] (Tables 25C-2 and 25C-3). Troiden described four discrete stages but conceptualized the process of homosexual identity formation as analogous to a horizontal spiral and said that "progress through the stages occurs in back-and-forth, up-and-down ways; the characteristics of stages overlap and recur in somewhat different ways for different people. In many cases, stages are encountered in consecutive order, but in some instances they are merged, glossed over, bypassed, or realized simultaneously."[79]

Many factors influence the process of sexual identity development in any individual. Religious, racial, and ethnic affiliation results in differences in the timing and the process of sexual identity development, disclosure to family members, and sexual behavior.[80,81] Meanings, values, and attitudes about sexuality and gender differ across different ethnic and cultural communities.[82-85] Lesbian and gay youth from certain ethnic/racial subcultures have to manage more than one stigmatized identity, often without family support, which creates additional stress and isolation. Relatively low rates of disclosure to families have therefore been reported among Asian, African-American, and Latino gay men and lesbians.[86,87]

The four stages that Troiden described are sensitization, identity confusion, identity assumption, and commitment. *Sensitization* occurs before puberty and

---

TABLE 25C-2 ■ Stages in the Formation of a Homosexual Identity[65]

Sensitization

Gender-neutral or cross-gender interests; feelings of marginality and difference from same-sex peers

Identity Confusion

Same-sex arousal and/or sexual activity; absence of heterosexual arousal; inner turmoil and confusion
Problematic responses: Denial or seeking change of homosexual feelings; inhibiting homosexually-oriented interests, activities; avoiding situations that precipitate or confirm homosexual desires; becoming socially isolated to avoid being "discovered"; redefining homosexual attractions as temporary, situational, or a "special case"; becoming immersed in heterosexuality, often including antihomosexual attitudes and actions

Identity Assumption

Self-definition as homosexual; acceptance of same-sex contacts and activities; exploration of homosexual subculture and sexual activity
Problematic responses: Same-sex activity kept secret, avoided, or criticized; stereotyped "homosexual" behavior paraded

Commitment

Homosexual identity accepted and disclosed to heterosexual family and peers; same-sex intimacy; involvement with homosexual community
Problematic responses: Homosexual identity kept secret and resulting in social isolation; escape through alcohol and other drug use; depression and diminished self-esteem through internalized homophobia

Troiden RR: Homosexual identity development. J Adolesc Health Care 9:105-113, 1988.

TABLE 25C-3 ■ Stages in Lesbian and Gay Identity Formation[63]

I. Identity Confusion

Recognition that "there is something about me/my behavior/thoughts/feelings that could be called homosexual"

II. Identity Comparison

Feelings of estrangement and alienation are felt as the possibility of membership in a stigmatized minority group is entertained; feelings of rejection and grief are common

III. Identity Tolerance

Management of difference between self and members of the heterosexual majority; careful disclosure of identity to selected others

IV. Identity Acceptance

Understanding of oneself as a member of a minority but valued group; increasing sense of peace and fulfillment with inclusion in the category of homosexuals; increasing disclosure to others

V. Identity Pride

Recognition of clash between dominant heterosexual population and personal acceptance of self as nonheterosexual; devaluing of heterosexuality and strong sense of group solidarity with homosexual community

VI. Identity Synthesis

Interactions with others at increasingly public level; sense of belonging to a broadly diverse world community; heightened self-esteem and empowerment

Cass VC: Homosexual identity formation: A theoretical model. J Homosex 4(3):219-235, 1979.

is not seen as related to sexuality. Many gay men report having felt "different" from their peers and unable to share interests or activities with them.[88]

During early adolescence, lesbians and gay men come to understand that their feelings, behaviors, or both might be identified as homosexual. This realization that they might be lesbian or gay is often surprising and is dissonant with previously held self-images, thus resulting in what Troiden[64,65] labeled *identity confusion*. In the context of a heterosexist social environment, considerable distress may accompany this new recognition, about which there is often ambiguity and ambivalence. These adolescents are no longer comfortable with their previously assumed heterosexual identities, but they have not yet developed a self-perception of themselves as homosexual. The social stigma and perceived need for secrecy discourages adolescents from discussing their emerging desires and activities with family members or friends, which results in increasing social isolation.

The age at which this early stage of recognition occurs has decreased since the 1980s. Gay men were formerly said to begin to suspect that they might be

homosexual at an average age of 17 years and lesbians at an average age of 18 years.[89] Data collected more recently suggest much earlier onset of this questioning. In a Massachusetts study, for example, college-age men and women who identified themselves as gay or lesbian were asked when they remembered being sure of their sexual orientation. Of these students, 13% of men and 7% of women believed themselves to be homosexual before 12 years of age, and 71% of the women were sure they were lesbian and 48% of the men identified themselves as gay by the age of 19.[90]

Adolescents may respond to identity confusion in various ways, such as with denial, repair, avoidance, redefinition, and/or acceptance. Which of these strategies they choose may determine in part the level and types of risk they encounter in the process of their development through adolescence.

■ *Denial* reflects simply ignoring the homosexual feelings, fantasies, or activities. Many young adolescents continue to act as if they are heterosexual, struggling with ambivalence and feelings of inauthenticity as they participate in typical adolescent social and romantic activities. For some, this may include promiscuous heterosexual activity, which carries the risk of pregnancy. Others actively limit their interactions with same- and opposite-sex peers in order to avoid the challenges inherent in them and, in so doing, increase their isolation.

■ *Repair* involves attempts to eradicate homosexual feelings and behaviors, often by soliciting the help of religious or conservative "therapies." There is no evidence that these attempts to "cure" homosexuality do anything but increase confusion and guilt.[91] Some reports suggest that these methods can lead to lasting damage to adolescents' self-esteem and mental health.[92]

■ Attempts at *avoidance* result from the belief that homosexual fantasies and behaviors are unacceptable. Some adolescents actively avoid learning about homosexuality, fearing that the information they obtain might confirm their suspected homosexuality. Others attack and ridicule homosexual persons and homosexuality as a way to fend off their worry about their own sexual orientation. Still others avoid their conflicts by abusing various chemical substances, thus temporarily relieving their identity confusion.

■ *Redefining* their homosexual feelings and behaviors refers to viewing them as a "special case," evidence of bisexuality, or as a temporary phenomenon. Homosexual feelings may be viewed as one-time occurrences or as a stage or phase of development that will pass in time rather than reflecting a new emerging identity.

■ Adolescents are increasingly resolving identity confusion successfully and finding *acceptance*. With acceptance, men and women acknowledge that their behavior, feelings, and fantasies may be homosexual and seek out additional sources of information to learn more about their sexual feelings. Their gradual recognition that they are homosexual and that there is a community of people with somewhat similar histories and feelings may diminish their sense of isolation and provide them with a reassuring label for the "differentness" that many of them have felt for several years.[62,93]

The stigma surrounding homosexuality contributes to this identity confusion by discouraging adolescents from discussing their emerging feelings and activities with either peers or their families. The notion that they might be homosexual often creates considerable consternation, guilt, and secrecy. Lack of available information and accurate knowledge about homosexuality and a paucity of recognizable role models also contribute to identity confusion. This stage at which gay and lesbian adolescents, and those who are questioning their sexual orientation, are particularly vulnerable is also one when they are often particularly open to approaches by supportive adults (e.g., teachers, school nurses, physicians) who can support and advise them.

Adolescents who accept the possibility or the recognition that they are homosexual are poised to enter successfully into the next stage of identity development, *commitment*. This stage is characterized by tolerance and acceptance of this new identity, initial tentative associations with other homosexual persons, and (usually) sexual experimentation. When teenagers have come to accept their homosexual identity and present themselves in this way to other homosexual peers, the lengthy and complex process of identity *disclosure* begins. As they come to understand that they belong to a group that includes others with similar histories and concerns, the pain caused by stigma and discrimination lessens. It is helpful for adolescents during this stage to find and nurture meaningful contacts with homosexual mentors, so that they can obtain accurate information, learn about social organizations for homosexual youth, and discover a social group to which they can belong. This process diminishes feelings of solitude and alienation and gives adolescents role models from whom they can learn strategies for stigma management, the range of social opportunities available to them, and the norms governing homosexual conduct.

During all phases of this developmental progression, support of family, friends, and professional advisers facilitates homosexual identity formation. Individuals feel more capable of acting on their sexual feelings and recognizing their meaning when they believe that those close to them will accept them as they are. Fears of rejection by family and friends and stigmatization in educational and employment settings interfere with healthy identity formation. Fears about discrimination in educational or employment opportunities may force homosexual adolescents and young adults to "hide in the closet"—a destructive pattern of coping. Many factors such as legal and economic constraints, racial and ethnic group membership, geographic area, family situation, and the availability of support systems determine the extent to which disclosure is possible. Ideally pediatricians and other professional colleagues can help teenagers as they assess and carry out the complex process of disclosure.

Adolescents who do not successfully navigate this stage may maintain an internalized stigmatizing view of homosexuality, experience self-hatred and despair, and avoid homosexual activity. Others may express their homosexuality in an exaggerated and stereotyped manner. Most commonly, they simply "pass" as heterosexual, concealing their sexual orientation and behaviors from heterosexual family, friends, and colleagues in order to avoid stigmatization. "Passing," or "staying in the closet," results in segregating their social worlds into peers who are heterosexual and peers who are homosexual, in continuing fear, and in the constantly draining efforts of maintaining secrecy: "careful, even torturous, control of information."[94]

Ideally, acceptance and comfort with self-identification as homosexual are achieved and homosexuality is accepted as a way of life. At this point, adolescents can develop same-sex intimate relationships, a widening circle of homosexual contacts, and increasing desire to disclose their homosexual identity to heterosexual friends and family. When Bell and Weinberg[95] asked homosexual adults whether they would remain homosexual even if a magic pill would enable them to become heterosexual, 95% of the lesbians and 86% of the gay males responded that they would not take the magic pill. With increasing societal understanding and acceptance of homosexuality since the 1980s, it is likely that these levels of acceptance are even stronger.

VARIATIONS AMONG WOMEN

There has been less systematic investigation and analysis of the process of lesbian identity development. Some parallels are clear; many women experience a linear and orderly progression from feelings of marginality to feelings of self-acceptance and pride in a new minority identity.[63,65,96] It has become clear that there are other, more idiosyncratic pathways and wide variability in the timing, sequence, and outcome of developmental stages among these women.[97,98] A historical analysis suggested that the typical age at which women became aware of their homosexuality, disclosed it, and initiated sexual involvement has decreased incrementally since the 1970s[98] and emphasizes wide geographic, socioeconomic, and individual variability. Some women appear to recognize their homosexual attractions and identity much later than others, as late as their 30s.[97] Inconsistencies among women's prior and current behavior, ideation, and attractions have been documented extensively.[99-101] The development of bisexuality appears to take an even more variable course.[102,103] Race and ethnicity also affect the timing and process of disclosure of a lesbian identity.[81,104]

Furthermore, neither feelings of "differentness" nor childhood gender atypicality are correlated as strongly with homosexual orientations among women as they are among men. For example, one study revealed that only 60% of adult lesbians reported any childhood indicators of homosexuality, and even among those who did, there was considerable variation in their experience.[97] Women may experience their first same-sex attractions and begin questioning their sexual identities at later ages than men do. Whereas a substantial proportion of young gay men report experiencing same-sex attractions, engaging in same-sex activity, and identifying themselves as gay before graduating from high school, many women do not consider the possibility of a same-sex relationship until entering college or later.[97] Some women first experience a same-sex relationship before any questioning of their heterosexual orientation, and the progression from entering a same-sex relationship, self-identifying as lesbian, and "coming out" may take place in a far shorter time period than has been described for gay men.[105]

In association with this later development of a stable sexual orientation, higher rates of prior heterosexual activity are reported by adult lesbians than by homosexual men. Nearly 40% of participants in one study reported having undergone changes in their sexual attractions over time that they did not attribute to changes in awareness.[97] It is important to recognize that both men and women experience this process of sexual identity development in idiosyncratic ways[96] and that cultural and religious affiliations affect individual challenges in many ways.[106]

Medical and Psychosocial Risks

Despite greater societal acceptance of homosexuality, gay and lesbian teenagers continue to be stigmatized, isolated, and harassed. Table 25C-4 enumerates some of the special risks faced by gay and lesbian adoles-

TABLE 25C-4 ■ Potential Risks to Homosexual Adolescents	
Traumatic Conditions	**AIDS and Its Complications**
Anal fissures	Viral, bacterial, fungal, and
Rectosigmoid tears	parasitic infections
Hemorrhoids	Neoplasms
Penile edema	Autoimmune reactions
Urethritis	**Unanticipated Pregnancy**
Gonorrhea	
Chlamydia infection	
Anogenital Conditions	**Oropharyngeal Conditions**
Pediculosis pubis	Gonorrhea
Scabies	Syphilitic chancres
Tinea cruris	Herpes simplex
Condylomata acuminata	Condylomata acuminata
Syphilis	*Chlamydia* infection
Herpes simplex	Candidiasis
Psychosocial Difficulties	**Gastrointestinal Conditions**
Family conflict	Proctitis
Social isolation	Gonorrhea
School failure	*Chlamydia* infection
Truancy	Herpes simplex
Prostitution	Syphilis
Homelessness	Human papillomavirus
Substance abuse	Colitis
Violence	*Shigella* infection
Depression, anxiety	*Salmonella* infection
Suicide	*Campylobacter* infection
	Yersinia infection
	Entamoeba histolytica infection
	Enteritis
	Giardia lamblia infection
	Opportunistic gastrointestinal infections associated with human immunodeficiency virus infection
	Hepatitis
	Types A, B, and C
	Cytomegalovirus

AIDS, acquired immunodeficiency syndrome.

cents. They are exposed repeatedly to reminders of homophobia and heterosexism.[114] During adolescence, when the approbation of peers is critical, the rejection and both verbal and physical abuse that they face can be particularly devastating.[115,116] In addition to societal homophobia, many homosexual youth incorporate these negative attitudes about homosexuality into a negative self-image. This internalized homophobia is manifested by self-doubts and sometimes overtly self-destructive and self-abusive behavior.[117,118] Internalized homophobia may result in depression, anxiety,[119] tolerance of discriminatory and abusive treatment by others, and abandonment or reduction of educational and vocational goals. Stigma, prejudice, and discrimination create a hostile and stressful social environment that leads to increased risk for mental health problems of various types.[119,120] Health professionals involved with gay and lesbian youth can play an important role in recognizing and intervening to limit self-defeating behavior before it becomes self-destructive.[2,21]

SCHOOL PROBLEMS

Academic underachievement, truancy, and dropout are common among homosexual youth.[122,123] Schools can be especially humiliating and dangerous environments for students who are perceived to be not typical.[124] Fear of discovery of their sexual orientation and the difficulties of maintaining secrecy in an unsympathetic environment may prove too much to bear. When the slang expression "that's so gay" continues in common use; the worst insult that boys and young men call each other is "fag;" and the worst insults for young women are "lesbi" or "dyke," emotional distress and multiple problem behaviors should come as no surprise. More than 75% of gay and lesbian high school students reported experiencing at least one homosexuality-related stressful event during the previous 3 months; 50% of them reported being ridiculed because they were gay.[125] In addition to these stressors, gay adolescents reported up to five times more stress unrelated to homosexuality than did heterosexual peers, such as arguments with parents and problems at school.[126]

Schools are traditionally not welcoming to gay and lesbian students. In one study, two thirds of school counselors and 8 of 10 prospective teachers had negative attitudes about gay and lesbian youth, while 14% to 42% ignored students' jokes about their gay peers.[127] In surveys of adolescents' experiences in high school, fewer than one in five lesbian and gay adolescents could identify *anyone* who had been supportive in school.[128] One 19-year-old is quoted as saying, "If someone would have been 'out' at my school, if the teachers wouldn't have been afraid to stop the 'fag' and 'dyke' jokes, if my human sexuality class had even mentioned homosexuality (especially in a positive light), if the school counselors would have been open to discussion of gay and lesbian issues, perhaps I wouldn't have grown up hating what I was, and perhaps I wouldn't have attempted suicide."[129]

HOMELESSNESS

Homosexual adolescents are at risk of rejection by their families when they disclose their sexual orientation, especially if this disclosure is done without support and advice and, as done too often, in anger.[130] Some investigators have reported that up to half of gay adolescents have run away from home at least once as a result of family conflicts related to their sexual orientation.[130] Although it is impossible to know precisely, social service agencies have estimated

that 25% to 35% of homeless youth in large urban centers are gay or lesbian.[131] Clearly, homeless youth have multiple health and social needs and are exposed to drugs, sexual abuse, and illegal activities, such as prostitution, drug-dealing, and theft. Homeless youth are at high risk for HIV infection, and prostitution and "survival sex" result in high rates of sexually transmitted diseases. Alcohol and drug abuse are pervasive and further increase the risk for trauma and sexually transmitted diseases.[129] Homeless youths are among the groups at highest risk for suicide as well.[132] Among homeless youths, those who identified themselves as gay, lesbian, bisexual, or transgender were found to be at increased risk for victimization, substance abuse, and mental health disorders.[133]

VIOLENCE

Youths who report same-sex attractions and/or sexual activity are at particularly high risk for violence.[134-136] Data from the National Longitudinal Study of Adolescent Health document increased odds of perpetrating, witnessing, and being the victim of violence among youths who report attraction to people of the same sex[77] (Table 25C-5). Up to 80% of homosexual youth

TABLE 25C-5 ■ Odds of Fighting, Victimization, and Witnessing Violence by Romantic Attraction

Experience of Violence	n	OR*	95% CI
Physical Fight (N = 10,582)			
Romantic attraction to same sex	108	0.88	0.52-1.48
Romantic attraction to both sexes	524	1.11	0.90-1.38
Medical Treatment Needed (N = 10,582)			
Romantic attraction to same sex	108	1.93	1.13-3.29
Romantic attraction to both sexes	524	1.57	1.16-2.12
Threat of Violence (N = 10,584)			
Romantic attraction to same sex	108	1.17	0.63-2.18
Romantic attraction to both sexes	523	1.08	0.77-1.51
Jumped (N = 10,582)			
Romantic attraction to same sex	108	1.14	0.60-2.16
Romantic attraction to both sexes	524	1.37	1.01-1.84
Violent Attack (N = 10,587)			
Romantic attraction to same sex	108	1.86	0.86-4.01
Romantic attraction to both sexes	524	1.43	1.01-2.01
Witnessing Violence (N = 10,579)			
Romantic attraction to same sex	108	1.89	1.09-3.28
Romantic attraction to both sexes	523	1.48	1.06-2.06

Data from the National Longitudinal Study of Adolescent Health.
*Adjusted for race/ethnicity, parental education, poverty status, intact family status, age, urban/rural context, and neighborhood drug problems.
CI, confidence interval; OR, odds ratio.

have reported receiving verbal abuse; 43%, being physically assaulted; and 10%, being assaulted with a weapon.[137] In a study conducted in nine cities and three states, one third to half of lesbian and gay junior and senior high school students reported victimization.[138]

Antigay verbal and physical abuse has been common on college campuses as well.[139,140] More than half of gay and lesbian college students have expressed worries about their future safety. In one study, 55% to 72% of lesbian and gay college students reported being the victim of violence; 64% of the perpetrators were peers and 23% were faculty or staff.[132]

The threat of violence increases anxiety among youths who are questioning their sexual orientation and among lesbian and gay youths who have not yet disclosed their homosexuality. This threat reinforces their sense of vulnerability and isolation, discourages them from "coming out," and may restrict their educational and career aspirations.[141] Anxiety, depression, sleep disorders, substance abuse, and frank post-traumatic stress disorder may follow the experience or witnessing of antigay violence. Lesbian and gay youth may blame themselves for the violence, further exacerbating the destructive effects of internalized homophobia.[142,143]

Responses to victimization may be moderated, depending on the support of the family and the individual's level of self-acceptance. Teenagers who are involved with an organized youth support group or other supportive network and who have "come out" and feel accepted by their families are better able to resist the challenges of antigay hostility and violence.[86]

SUBSTANCE ABUSE

Substance use is prevalent among all adolescents in the United States; therefore, it is somewhat difficult to discern particular risks for gay and lesbian youths. Depending on the source of data, up to 80% of high school seniors report having used alcohol, and 35 to 45% have used marijuana.[129,144,145]

Historically, one of the few social meeting places for gay men and lesbians was in bars, fostering substance use and abuse. Fortunately, other venues for socialization and supportive community networks have become available to teenagers and adults. Nevertheless, the incidence of overall drug and alcohol use has been reported to be double among gay and bisexual adolescents.[146,147] Similar findings concern cigarette smoking among gay and bisexual men.[148] A national survey of lesbian women showed that rates of drug and alcohol use were higher among young lesbians than among heterosexual women. One in three smoked cigarettes daily; 13% were concerned about their overuse of alcohol, 5.9% about marijuana

use, and 2.4% about cocaine use.[149] These findings were replicated in a more recent study.[150]

Among 12- to 17-year-olds in the northeastern United States, boys and girls who identified themselves as "mostly heterosexual" were more likely to smoke than students who identified themselves as "clearly heterosexual." In addition, female students who identified themselves as lesbian were almost 10 times more likely to acknowledge that they smoke cigarettes than were heterosexual girls, but no parallel differences were observed between gay and heterosexual boys.[151] Separate analyses of other data from the same study demonstrated similar findings for alcohol use: Both girls and boys who identified themselves as "mostly heterosexual" acknowledged significantly greater use of alcohol than their "clearly heterosexual" counterparts. Lesbian and bisexual girls reported greater alcohol use behaviors than did their heterosexual peers but gay boys did not.[152]

Among 772 college students at a Southeastern metropolitan campus, the 21 lesbian students were 4.9 times as likely to smoke, 10.7 times as likely to drink, and 4.9 times as likely to use marijuana as were heterosexual women. There were no differences in reported substance use between the 20 gay men and the heterosexual men.[153]

The vulnerability of gay and lesbian youth to substance abuse is a part of the complex process of coping with stigmatization, shame, and discrimination. This risk is compounded by the dearth of emotional and practical support and information available to gay and lesbian youth. Abuse of substances is a part of the process of managing stigma. It represents one way of escaping from the conflict engendered by same-sex attractions. Intervention programs should include youth in their design and implementation and should be integrated with support and guidance to help youth counteract stigma and isolation.[154]

EATING DISORDERS

Suggestive evidence points to an increased risk for restrictive eating disorders among gay men and adolescents.[155-157] Gay men have reported greater body dissatisfaction than have heterosexual men, whereas lesbian adolescents reported better body image than did heterosexual girls.[158] One study revealed that clinical eating disorders could be diagnosed in 17% of gay men, 14% of heterosexual women, 4.2% of lesbians, and 3.4% of heterosexual men.[159,160]

Among 10,583 adolescents in a 1999 study, "mostly heterosexual" boys and girls had greater concerns with their weight and appearance and were less happy with their bodies than were students who identified themselves as "clearly heterosexual." In addition, the "mostly heterosexual" girls were twice as likely to use laxatives and to binge-eat than were their heterosexual peers. Boys who identified themselves as gay were 15 times more likely to report binge-eating than were their heterosexual counterparts.[161]

Lesbians are at greater risk for being overweight or obese than are heterosexual women, but the reasons for this increased risk are not clear.[162,163]

DEPRESSION AND ANXIETY

Evidence from numerous surveys documents a high prevalence of anxiety and mood disorders among homosexual adults.[164-166] The prevalence of psychological distress may be even higher among minority ethnic and racial groups.[167]

Lesbian and gay youth also often experience depression and anxiety as they come to recognize their homosexuality and its implications.[168,169] Considerations of how and when to "come out" to family members and friends create heightened anxiety. With appropriate guidance and support, many gay teenagers eventually note improved self-esteem and mood after they have accepted and disclosed their identity.[170] Assessment of adolescents' emotional states, degree of isolation or support, and risk for suicide are important functions for all health care professionals who help care for teenagers.

SUICIDE

The increased rates of suicide among homosexual youth have been reported repeatedly. As in other areas of research with homosexual youths, studies have been hampered by nonprobability sampling and difficulties in identification of sexual orientation. Despite daunting difficulties in documenting the association between struggles with issues of sexual orientation and suicidal tendencies in adolescence, there is convincing evidence is that at least 50% of gay youth have seriously contemplated suicide and that at least 25% have attempted suicide one or more times before the age of 21.[171-174] Lesbian and bisexual girls did not differ significantly from the generally high rates of suicidal tendencies among young women in general.[172] The 2004 Minnesota Student Survey of 9th and 12th grade students revealed (once again) that more than half of gay, lesbian, and bisexual students had thought about suicide and that 37.4% reported a suicide attempt.[174a] Of more interest is that gay lesbian and bisexual students report significantly lower levels of four protective factors than did their heterosexual peers. Teenagers' reports of family connectedness, adult caring, and school safety were protective against suicidal ideation and attempts.[175]

A population-based survey demonstrated that high school youth who had had same-sex experiences (including but not limited to lesbian, gay, and bisexual youth) were four times more likely than their heterosexual peers to have attempted suicide during the previous year.[122] A study of male twin pairs, in each of which one was gay and the other not, revealed a substantially increased risk of suicidal tendency in homosexual men that was not associated with substance use or other psychiatric conditions.[176] Thus, convincing data have accumulated to establish that an increased risk of suicidal tendency does indeed accompany homosexuality in adolescence and young adulthood.[164,171,177-179] The reasons for this increased risk are multifactorial.[180]

SEXUALLY TRANSMITTED DISEASES

The medical needs of gay and lesbian teenagers are, for the most part, similar to those of heterosexual teenagers. All adolescents are at risk for sexually transmitted diseases, and this risk is increased with unprotected sexual behaviors. Because sexual experimentation is common in adolescence, an individual's sexual behavior often does not necessarily reflect sexual orientation. Homosexual adolescents may engage in heterosexual sex or may not be sexually active at all. Similarly, heterosexual adolescents may experiment with sexual activity with a person of the same sex. It is the adolescent's sexual *activity* that is associated with particular risks, not her or his sexual *orientation*.

High-risk sexual behavior among gay teenagers has remained quite common, despite the threat of HIV infection.[181,182] In addition, many teenagers engage in sexual activity with partners with whom they are not well acquainted and communicate poorly about protection against HIV infection and sexually transmitted diseases, as well as about pregnancy prevention. Young gay teenagers report using sexual experience as a way to learn about being gay. Unfortunately, unprotected intercourse puts them at high risk for HIV infection and other sexually transmitted diseases, such as urethritis, anogenital conditions, oropharyngeal conditions, gastrointestinal disease, hepatitis, and herpes (see Table 25C-3).[183-185]

HIV/AIDS

The age at which infection with HIV occurs has been declining; at least 25% of new infections occur in people younger than 21 years.[186] Among adolescents, sexual activity between boys has been implicated in 50% to 75% of the reported cases of acquired immunodeficiency syndrome (AIDS).[187-190a] Sexual minority adolescents report behavior with higher HIV risk, especially in association with sexual victimization.[135]

The current status of the HIV epidemic among gay adolescent boys and young men is of great concern. Most young adults who develop AIDS were infected during their teens. Adolescents of racial and ethnic minorities and homeless youth are at particularly high risk for HIV. The American Academy of Pediatrics recommends that all providers who work with teenagers include AIDS prevention education as part of *routine* care.[3]

A large number of adolescents engage in same-sex activity, even though they do not later identify themselves as gay. Thus, the extent of the risk for HIV transmission is even higher than would be expected from prevalence figures alone. For example, among those with a positive test results for HIV at an adolescent AIDS clinic, 9 of 10 patients reported same-sex intercourse, but only half (54%) identified themselves as gay.[191] More negative attitudes toward homosexuality, more substance abuse symptoms, and fewer intentions to use safer sex practices have been found to be predictive of greater sexual risk behaviors.[118]

PREGNANCY

Heterosexual activity is common among lesbian and gay adolescents. Four of every five lesbian adolescents and more than 50% of gay male adolescents reported a history of heterosexual intercourse.[192] Among high school students in Massachusetts, 30% of those who were classified as gay, lesbian, or bisexual acknowledged that they had "been or gotten someone pregnant," as compared with 11% of heterosexual students.[75] Unintended pregnancy is clearly a risk for these teenagers that might be reduced with appropriate counseling and education.

Community and Social Support Building Efforts

A serendipitous byproduct of the epidemic of HIV and AIDS since the early 1980s has been greater recognition of the diversity of sexual orientation and sexual behavior, as well as expansion of social discourse about sexuality in general and homosexuality in particular. Since the mid-1990s, sex education has been presented in the public media and in schools at all levels, and gay issues have been discussed frequently in mainstream newspapers and television programs. Many magazines and books are available to inform teenagers and adults about the range of responsible sexuality and its risks, and youth groups in many schools and communities create a network of peer support and role models for all students. In contrast to the earlier secrecy and the dearth of information available about homosexuality, many websites, listserves, hotlines, national organizations with local branches, and independent community youth groups are available for gay and lesbian teenagers and their friends. A growing volume of excellent fiction published since the 1990s helps all teenagers understand and appreciate the struggles of teenagers who may not be heterosexual.[193]

Stigma is painful. It marginalizes and dehumanizes people. It leads people to feel vulnerable and devalued. But when people gather together and recognize their power to confront stigma, they may be motivated to mobilize resources they did not formerly recognize they had. Some gay and lesbian youth, along with their adult counterparts, have empowered themselves and begun to confront the isolation and discrimination that has marginalized them.

High schools and colleges have developed "gay-straight alliances" that seek to support one another and to educate the community about the diversity of sexual orientation. The Gay, Lesbian, and Straight Education Network (GLSEN) helps students start such groups. Some evidence suggests that implementation of school-based programs for gay, lesbian, bisexual, and transgender students has been difficult for many school districts.[194] Many community-based support groups also combine health, mental health, and social services provided by trained professionals, as well as peer counselors and extensive outreach.

These local community youth support networks generate resilience and strength among adolescents and their adult mentors, work to counteract discrimination against gay and lesbian youth, and provide a safe community to nurture their development. They provide a resource for recreation and socialization. Opportunities for public speaking and political advocacy have empowered gay and lesbian youth to reject "homonegative" attitudes and heterosexism and to take pride in their own personal and group identity. The Internet and national telephone hotlines similarly counteract the isolation created by stigma and discrimination.

Criticism of community and school-based support groups for gay and lesbian students comes from various sources. They have become a rallying point for individuals and groups opposed to homosexuality on religious or ethical grounds. They have also highlighted questions about whether, and how explicitly, sex education should be taught in schools. In addition, there has been uneasiness about whether such groups encourage teenagers to experiment sexually beyond their emotional maturity. Many concerns have been raised about whether the increased visibility and social acceptability of homosexuality might encourage high school students to identify themselves as gay or lesbian when they have not yet fully sorted out their sexuality. Ideally, the leader of these groups is a trusted and admired faculty member or a responsible community leader; he or she will foster discussions that encourage explorations of social, emotional and sexual development and encourage individuality in the process of sorting out the place and orientation of sexuality in each student's emerging identity.

The high profile and relentless media coverage of political efforts to provide equal opportunities for gay and lesbian adults have been both beneficial and challenging for children and teenagers who are potentially affected by these decisions. Open discussions about diversity in sexual orientation and family constellation, and increasingly broad definitions of equal opportunity policies provide tangible evidence of social acceptance. The expansion of opportunities (e.g., adoption, civil union, marriage) and the slow erosion of institutional evidence of discrimination (e.g., Equal Employment Opportunity Commission policies that include sexual orientation, domestic partner benefits) provide hope and strength for gay and lesbian adolescents and their parents. On the other hand, it has been difficult for them to hear the public opposition to these efforts, which have been fueled by blatant homophobia and moral condemnation of homosexuality on ethical, religious, and personal grounds.

Disclosure of Sexual Orientation

Self-esteem and positive adolescent adjustment are enhanced for most adolescents after "coming out," especially if the process is managed with sensitivity and understanding of its likely effect. Fear of rejection and disapproval may restrain some teenagers, especially if they have not yet developed a supportive network of peers and adults. An important contribution health care providers can make is to encourage teenagers to "come out" to their parents and siblings and to help them plan an appropriate time and process to do so.

The process of "coming out" is rarely smooth. Teenagers typically begin to disclose their questions about their sexual orientation to close friends, preferably first to a gay or lesbian friend if they know of any who has already "come out." Adult role models (e.g., a nurse, a teacher) who are known to be homosexual may be among the first adults with whom a teenager feels sufficiently safe to disclose her or his concerns. Siblings and parents are rarely the first to hear about a teenager's emerging homosexual orientation, because the fear of rejection and approbation is great and the stakes are high. It is helpful if adolescents are already involved in a supportive community at school to buffer difficult experiences of disclosure and "information management" of their sexual orientation.

Unfortunately, many teenagers do experience rejection and loss of heterosexual friendships after they disclose their homosexual identity; they may also experience stigmatization and both verbal and physical violence. Professional mentors (teachers, nurses, physicians) who have made an effort to be available and accepting can help in making the "coming-out" process as affirming as possible. The ongoing dilemma of "information management" faces these teenagers repeatedly, if heterosexuality is assumed.

All too often, disclosure of homosexuality occurs in a manner that is hurtful to everyone involved and not conducive to the nurturance and support that the teenager most needs at this time of intense stress. If the teenager has been worried about her or his emerging sexual identity but has kept these concerns secret from family members and friends, the information may be disclosed prematurely, unwittingly, or in the course of an argument. An important role for pediatricians and their professional colleagues is to help these teenagers plan how they will tell their parents, siblings, and friends about their sexual identity in a manner that maximizes success for all concerned.[129]

After a teenager "comes out," parents may experience considerable guilt and shame and may benefit also from advocacy and support from health care professionals. Parents have been described as advancing through a series of stages in the awareness and acceptance of their child's homosexuality.[195] These stages are described as (1) *subliminal awareness,* when the child's gay identity is suspected (2) *impact,* when the gayness is discovered or disclosed; (3) *adjustment,* when the family denies the homosexuality or attempts to keep it a secret; (4) *resolution,* when the family mourns the loss of the anticipated heterosexual identity; and (5) *integration,* when new relationships are established on the basis of new understanding.

Siblings, grandparents, and other family members sometimes experience a similar process in recognizing and adjusting to a teenagers' homosexuality, although it is typically less strongly influenced by guilt and self-criticism. No research has focused on the possibly protective roles that siblings, grandparents, aunts, uncles and others might play in helping adolescents to disclose their homosexuality to their parents.

Families of a gay or lesbian adolescent may anticipate and/or experience the isolation and disapproval of "second-hand stigma" or "stigma by association."[196] They should be encouraged to avoid keeping their teenager's sexual orientation a secret from other family members, neighbors, and colleagues. Most crucial for a teenager who is struggling with a minority sexual orientation is that his or her family is unconditionally supportive of his or her emerging identity and further development.

A growing number of publications, websites, and community support networks may make families' transition to full acceptance easier. Most parents report improved relationships with the adolescent after disclosure.[197,198] For families who have greater difficulty accepting their adolescent's homosexuality, a colleague trained in family therapy may be able to facilitate a more constructive dialogue.

"Treating" Homosexuality

Before homosexuality was recognized as a normal variation of human sexual experience, various "therapeutic" methods were used to change people's attractions from homosexual to heterosexual. The various forms of "reparative" therapies are based on the outdated belief that homosexuality is intrinsically pathological rather than on the more current view that it is the force of social stigma that creates distress for people of homosexual orientation.

Although some such efforts continue,[199] they are generally considered ineffective and may be associated with significant negative outcomes.[91,92] The American Academy of Pediatrics[200] has stated that "therapy directed specifically at changing sexual orientation is contraindicated, since it can provoke guilt and anxiety while having little or no potential for achieving changes in sexual orientation." The American Psychiatric Association[201] concurs, stating that "there is no evidence that any treatment can change a homosexual person's deep-seated sexual feelings for others of the same sex."

Many professional organizations have stated explicitly that the change necessary is in societal attitudes and behaviors, not in individuals' sexual orientation. They have called, for example, for "the enactment of civil rights legislation at local, state, and national levels that would offer homosexual citizens the same protections now guaranteed to others"[201]; for "the repeal of all discriminatory legislation singling out homosexual acts by consenting adults in private"[202]; and for "the elimination and prevention of discriminatory statutes, policies, and actions that diminish the quality of life for lesbian and gay people and that force many to live their lives in the closet."[203]

TRANSGENDER YOUTH

Transgender persons maintain a strong and persistent cross-gender identification; that is, they feel themselves to be fundamentally mismatched with their anatomic and genetic sex. As difficult as it may be for gay and lesbian youths to acknowledge their sexual orientation in a society in which so-called gay bashing is all too common, transgender teenagers are confronted by an even greater lack of public understanding and acceptance. The current classification of transgender individuals is Gender Identity Disorder[107] and includes gender dysphoria (discomfort and distress with one's anatomical gender) and cross-gender identification.

Transgender individuals are severely stigmatized. In one study, approximately 60% reported harassment and violence and 37% various forms of economic discrimination.[108] Drug and alcohol abuse complicate social isolation and underachievement in education and employment.[109] Most of the psychosocial problems described above for gay and lesbian youth are even more challenging for transgender youth. Analyses have revealed an extremely high rate of human immunodeficiency virus (HIV) infection—up to 35%—among male-to-female transgender persons. In addition, 55% to 62% of transgender adults were found to be clinically depressed, and 32% had attempted suicide.[110]

It is more acceptable for women to dress in masculine clothing, whereas men wearing typically feminine attire are more noticeable. Of importance is that transgenderism signifies gender identity, not sexual orientation. In their chosen gender identity, they have the same propensity as anyone else to be heterosexual, homosexual, or bisexual.[111]

The rare transgender, middle or high school, student who decides to attend school with a new name and attire presents a special challenge for the school community. Administrators, nurses, and teachers encounter many issues ranging from avoidance of harassment to gym assignment and bathroom use. Many transgender students wait until they move into an entirely new environment (e.g., college) before expressing themselves in their chosen gender.

Transgender people face significant discrimination in employment, housing, and access to health care. Child health professionals can assist adolescents who consider themselves transgender by ensuring a safe environment, providing information about community and national resources, and enforcing policies regarding confidentiality and nondiscrimination.[112,113] Consultation with an endocrinologist familiar with gender-related concerns is appropriate if a teenager considers the option of hormonal and/or surgical interventions.

CHILDREN WHOSE PARENTS ARE GAY OR LESBIAN

Most children who have one or two gay or lesbian parents were born in the context of a heterosexual relationship. That relationship may still exist or may have been dissolved; if the latter, either or both partners may have found new partners of the same or different gender (Table 25C-6 contains examples of family constellations) Increasing numbers of gay and lesbian adults are bringing children into long-term

TABLE 25C-6 ■ Examples of Family Structures in Which Children May Grow Up

Child born to or adopted by heterosexual parents; one or both parents subsequently "come out" as gay/lesbian
    Parents decide to stay together.
    Couple divorce. Mother may remain single, have a male partner, or have a female partner. Father may remain single, have a male partner, or have a female partner. Custody/visitation decisions are complex.
Child born to or adopted by a gay or lesbian couple (or a single gay man or a single lesbian)
    Variable level of information is available to child about donor, surrogate, birth parents.
    Variable level of involvement is available from donor or surrogate with child.
    Anonymous donor, surrogate
    Information/contact at 18
    Three or four parent families
    Family friend
    "More than an uncle, less than a dad"
Issues to consider
    Do children have a *right* to know who their parents are?
    The effects of secrets
    Role models of both sexes

partnerships through adoption, alternative insemination, and surrogacy. Donors and surrogates may be anonymous or involved with the child and family to a variable degree.

Parenting Attitudes and Behavior, Personality, and Adjustment of Parents

Many questions have been posed about possible ways that lesbian mothers and gay fathers are similar to or different from heterosexual parents and how any differences might affect their children's well-being. However, few differences have been found in research since the 1970s in which lesbian and heterosexual mothers' self-esteem, psychological adjustment, and attitudes toward childrearing have been compared.[204-211] Lesbian mothers are within the range of normal psychological functioning according to interviews and psychological assessments, and report scores on standardized measures of self-esteem, anxiety, depression, and parenting stress are indistinguishable from those reported by heterosexual mothers.[208,212]

Lesbian mothers strongly endorse child-centered attitudes and commitment to their maternal roles[209,213,214] and have been shown to be at least as concerned with providing male role models for their children as are divorced heterosexual mothers.[215] Lesbian and heterosexual mothers describe themselves similarly in marital and maternal interests, current lifestyles, and childrearing practices.[209,211] They report similar role conflicts, social support networks, and coping strategies.[216] Descriptive studies of lesbian parents and their children are summarized in Table 25C-7.

Gay fathers demonstrate substantial evidence of nurturance and investment in their paternal role and show no differences from heterosexual fathers in providing appropriate recreation or encouraging autonomy.[217,218] Gay fathers have been described to adhere to strict disciplinary guidelines, to place greater emphasis than do heterosexual fathers on guidance and the development of cognitive skills, and to be involved in their children's activities.[219,220] Overall, there are more similarities than differences in the parenting styles and attitudes of gay and nongay fathers.[221-223]

Children's Emotional and Social Development

A great deal of investigation into the well-being of children who were raised by gay or lesbian parents can be divided historically and for clarification into three "waves" of research. In the first wave, children who were in the custody of their lesbian mothers after divorce were compared with children who were in the custody of their heterosexual mothers after divorce. In the second wave, children who were born or adopted by an already-existing lesbian couple were studied. The third wave is still small and consists of community-based or random sampling techniques to assess children whose parents are lesbian. These three waves of research are summarized in Table 25C-8.

CHILDREN AFTER DIVORCE

Because many biological parents who are gay or lesbian have been divorced, their children's subsequent psychological development in relation to the divorce has to be understood in that context. Whether they are subsequently raised by one or two separated parents and whether a stepparent has joined either of the biological parents are important factors for children that have rarely been addressed in research assessing psychological outcomes for these children. Similarly missing is an analysis of the role of the divorced noncustodial parent in the child's life.

The considerable research literature that has accumulated addressing this issue has generally revealed that children of divorced lesbian mothers grow up in ways that are very similar to children of divorced heterosexual mothers. Several studies in which children who had a lesbian mother were compared with children who had a heterosexual mother have failed to document any differences between the groups on personality measures, measures of peer group rela-

TABLE 25C-7 ■ Qualitative Investigations of Gay and Lesbian Parents and Their Children		
Author	**Sample**	**Outcome of Interest**
Green (1978)[264]	37 Children 21 Lesbian mothers 16 Transsexual parents	Sexual orientation
Miller (1979)[265]	14 Children with a gay father 40 Gay fathers	Sexual orientation Father-child relationship
Turner et al (1990)[266]	Children with a gay or lesbian parent	Early play preferences Sexual orientation
Osterweil (1991)[267]	30 Lesbian couples and their children	Relationship satisfaction Children's behavior Children's self-concept
Koepke et al (1992)[215]	47 Lesbian couples	Relationship satisfaction
Bailey et al (1994)[268]	82 Adult sons with gay fathers	Sexual orientation
Hare (1994)[216]	51 Children with lesbian mothers	Family relationships Parents' concerns
Patterson (1994)[232] (Bay Area Families Study)	37 Children with lesbian mother(s)	Contact with extended family Children's behavior Children's self-concept Children's sex-role preference Relationship satisfaction
Patterson (1995)[240]	26 Lesbian couples	Division of labor Parental relationship Mothers' mental health
Gartrell et al (1996, 2000, 2005, 1999)[213,235,239,269] (National Lesbian Family Study)	154 Lesbian mothers (84 families)	Parental relationship Social supports Coping strategies Division of labor Relationships with family-of-origin Children's experiences of homophobia
Mitchell (1996)[270]	32 Lesbian couples	Division of labor
Sullivan (1996)[271]	34 Lesbian couples	Division of labor
Barrett and Tasker (2001)[221]	101 Gay fathers	Difficulty of parenting experience Child's responses to gay parent

tionships, self-esteem, behavioral difficulties, academic success, or warmth and quality of family relationships.[209,224-230] Children's self-esteem has been shown to be higher among adolescents whose mothers (of any sexual orientation) were in a new partnered relationship after divorce than among those whose mothers remained single, and higher among those who found out at a younger age that their parent was homosexual than among those who found out when they were older.

Concern has been raised that social stigmatization might lead to teasing and embarrassment of children about their parent's sexual orientation or their family constellation, and restrict their ability to form and maintain friendships. Adult children of divorced lesbian mothers have indeed recalled more teasing by peers during childhood than have adult children of divorced heterosexual parents.[226,231] In general, children whose parents are gay or lesbian have been found to have normal relationships with childhood peers and to maintain social relationships appropriate for their developmental levels.[230]

CHILDREN BORN TO OR ADOPTED BY LESBIAN WOMEN

Children born to and reared by lesbian couples seem to develop very much like children reared by heterosexual parents. Ratings by their mothers and teachers have demonstrated these children to have normal social competence and the same prevalence of behavioral difficulties as population norms.[213,232-235] In fact, growing up with parents who are lesbian or gay may confer some advantages to children. Although the sample sizes have been small, there have been suggestions that these children may be more tolerant of diversity and more nurturing toward younger children than are children whose parents are heterosexual.[236-238]

TABLE 25C-8 ■ Studies Comparing Children Whose Parents Are Gay versus Not Gay

Author	Sample	Comparison Group	Ages of Children (Years)	Findings
Hoeffer (1981)[224]	20 Children of lesbian mothers	20 Children of divorced heterosexual mothers	6-9	Children with lesbian mothers were more androgynous
Kirkpatrick et al (1981)[225]	10 Children of divorced lesbian mothers	10 Children of divorced heterosexual mothers	5-12	No difference in prevalence of psychiatric disorders
Golombok et al (1983)[226]	37 Children of 27 divorced lesbian mothers	38 Children of 27 divorced heterosexual mothers	5-17	No differences in psychiatric disorders, children's behavior, gender identity, sex-role behavior, peer relationships Children of lesbian mothers had more contact with fathers
Green et al (1986)[209]	56 Children of 50 divorced lesbian mothers	48 Children of 40 divorced heterosexual mothers	3-11	No differences in parental stress or in children's intelligence, sexual orientation, gender-role preference, interpersonal relationships, or adjustment Lesbians more likely to have a partner after divorce
Steckel (1987)[237]	11 Children born to lesbian couples	11 Children born to heterosexual couples	1-5	No difference in separation-individuation or independence Children of lesbians were rated less aggressive, more affectionate
Gottman (1989)[227]	35 Children of divorced lesbian mothers	70 Children of divorced heterosexual mothers	Adults	No differences in gender identity, social adjustment, sexual orientation
Huggins (1989)[228]	18 Adolescents with a lesbian mother	18 Adolescents with a heterosexual divorced mother	13-19	No difference in self-esteem
Bigner and Jacobsen (1989b)[218]	33 Children of gay fathers	33 Children of heterosexual fathers	3-24	No differences in father's level of involvement, intimacy; gay fathers more concerned about limit-setting, guidance
Javaid (1993)[229]	26 Children of 13 lesbian mothers	15 Children of divorced heterosexual mothers	6-18	No difference in attitudes toward marriage and procreation
Golombok and Tasker (1994)[230]	25 Young adults raised by lesbian mothers	21 Young adults raised by single heterosexual mothers	17-35	No differences in psychiatric problems, family relationships, sexual orientation, children's adjustment (anxiety, depression), family well-being Children of lesbians had more gay/lesbian friends; more likely to consider same-sex sexual relationship; recall more stigma regarding own sexuality

Cont'd

TABLE 25C-8 ■ Studies Comparing Children Whose Parents Are Gay versus Not Gay—cont'd

Author	Sample	Comparison Group	Ages of Children (Years)	Findings
Flaks et al (1995)[272]	Children of 15 lesbian couples	Children of 15 heterosexual couples	3-9	No differences in cognitive functioning, behavioral adjustment, parents' relationship Lesbians more knowledgeable about parenting skills
Brewaeys et al. (1997)[273] (European Study of Assisted Reproduction)	30 Children with lesbian mothers (children conceived by donor insemination)	38 Children with heterosexual parents (children conceived by donor insemination) 30 Children with heterosexual parents (conceived naturally)	4-8	No difference in parent-child relationships, children's behavior Girls conceived by donor insemination in heterosexual families had more emotional problems Lesbian coparents had more "developmental" orientation Lesbian parents shared child care more equally
Golombok et al (1997)[231] (British Longitudinal Study)	15 Children with a single lesbian mother 15 Children with lesbian couple mothers	42 Children of single heterosexual mothers 41 Children of heterosexual couples	3-9	No differences in parenting stress, maternal anxiety, maternal depression, children's emotional adjustment, children's peer relationships Mother-child relationship better when father was absent (no difference by sexual orientation) Children's self-esteem better when father present (no difference by sexual orientation)
Chan et al (1998)[274] (Contemporary Families Study)	34 Children with lesbian couple mothers 21 Children with a single lesbian mother	16 Children of heterosexual couples 9 Children of heterosexual single mothers	5-11	No differences in children's adjustment by sexual orientation, but better when parental relationship was better No differences in parental adjustment, stress, depression, self-esteem, relationship satisfaction
Chan et al (1998)[241]	30 Children with lesbian couple mothers	16 Children of heterosexual couples	5-11	No differences in parental satisfaction with child care Children's adjustment (parent report and teacher report) better when child care shared Lesbian parents preferred equal distribution of child care responsibilities
Golombok et al (2003)[243]	39 Children with lesbian mothers (19 in a couple; 20 single/divorced)	134 Children with heterosexual mothers (74 married; 60 single/divorced)	7-8	No differences in mother-child relationships, self-esteem, peer relationships, behavior or emotional symptoms, gender-typical behavior Lesbian mothers reported more imaginative play

TABLE 25C-8 ■ Studies Comparing Children Whose Parents Are Gay versus Not Gay—cont'd				
Author	Sample	Comparison Group	Ages of Children (Years)	Findings
				Fathers reported more conflicts and hitting than did co-mothers
				Single parents reported more stress, more conflict, more hitting
				Teachers reported more behavior problems in children with single parents
Wainright et al (2004)[244]	44 Students with female couple parents	44 Students with male-female parents	12-18	Both groups similar with regard to psychosocial adjustment, school outcomes, romantic attractions, relationships with parents
Wainright et al (2006)[275]	44 Students with female couple parents	44 Students with male-female parents	12-18	No differences in frequency of delinquent behavior, substance abuse, experience of victimization

In one study, children of heterosexual parents saw themselves as being somewhat more aggressive than did children of lesbian parents, and they were seen by parents and teachers as more bossy, negative, and domineering. Children of lesbian parents saw themselves as more lovable and were seen by parents and teachers as more affectionate, responsive, and protective of younger children than were children of heterosexual parents.

The adjustment of children who have two mothers seems to be related to their parents' satisfaction with their relationship and specifically with the division of responsibility they have worked out with regard to child care and household chores.[234,235,240] Children with lesbian parents who reported greater relationship satisfaction, more egalitarian division of household and paid labor,[241] and more regular contact with grandparents and other relatives[242] were rated by parents and teachers to be better adjusted and to have fewer behavioral problems. These findings are consistent with general knowledge among students of child development: namely, that greater stability and nurturance within a family system are predictive of greater security and fewer behavioral problems among children. In a longitudinal study of children born to lesbian women using alternative insemination, 40% of children reported experiences of stigmatization by the time they were 10 years.[239]

COMMUNITY-BASED SAMPLES

Early studies in which researchers attempted to evaluate the well-being of children whose parents were gay or lesbian encountered predictable challenges in sample selection, sample size, investigator bias, and measurement. More recently, investigators have attempted to overcome some of these challenges and to clarify some factors that promote optimal well-being of this growing population of children.

The importance of these studies is that the research was planned and carried out by people who had no particular interest or investment in research regarding same-gender parents. In both cases, the investigations regarding lesbian parents and their children were post hoc analyses; thus, neither the sample nor the methods were influenced by a bias in support of gay parents.

The first of these community-based studies is based on data from a cohort study of 14,000 mothers of children born within a particular county in England during 1 year. The study examined the quality of parent-child relationships and the socioemotional and gender development of a community sample of 7-year-old children with lesbian mothers. Thirty-nine families headed by lesbian mothers were compared with 74 families with two heterosexual parents and 60 families headed by single heterosexual mothers.[243] No differences were found in maternal warmth, emotional involvement, enjoyment of motherhood, frequency of conflicts, supervision of the child, abnormal behaviors reported by parents or teachers in the child, children's self-esteem, or psychiatric disorders.

In the same study, parents who raised children alone reported greater stress; increased severity of parent-child conflicts; and less warmth, enjoyment of parenting, and imaginative play than did parents in a couple relationship, whether lesbian or heterosexual. Teachers reported more behavioral problems among children in single-parent families than among children who had two parents in the home, regardless of the parents' sexual orientation.

In the second study, researchers used data from the National Longitudinal Study of Adolescent Health, a randomly selected, nationally representative sample of 12,105 U.S. adolescents in grades 7 through 12. The authors demonstrated that 12- to 18-year-olds living with two women in a "marriage-like" family arrangement ($n = 44$) were similar to peers whose parents were heterosexual in measures of self-esteem, depression, anxiety, school "connectedness," and school success. Overall, these adolescents reported positive family relationships, including parental warmth, care from others, personal autonomy, and neighborhood integration, and there were no systematic differences between the families with same-sex and opposite-sex parents.[244]

Research on the diversity of parental relationships among gay and lesbian partners is just beginning. The legalization of same-sex marriage in Massachusetts in 2004 offers the first true opportunity to study how same-sex marriage affects family life and child development. In addition to the findings just discussed, current research on same-sex couples who have been able to jointly adopt and establish legal ties between children and both parents suggests that legal recognition of same-sex marriage may strengthen ties between partners, with their children, and with their extended families. Civil marriage among same-sex partners might be expected to be beneficial to children as a result of increased financial stability, as well as the permanence, stability, and social recognition that define marriage in general.[7,245] Another benefit of civil marriage is the protection provided by divorce laws, which exist in large part as a way to guarantee that the best interests of children are considered in case of dissolution of the parental relationship.

Children's Gender Identity and Sexual Orientation

There has been considerable interest in the psychosexual development of children who were raised by lesbians or gay men. Some researchers postulate that family influences might affect children's gender role development and sexual orientation. For children who were conceived by a lesbian woman and/or for whom a gay man served as the sperm donor, the possible genetic influences on the determination of sexual orientation might be expected to result in somewhat increased likelihood of gay or lesbian sexual orientation. Although of some academic interest, this question typically has its source in an assumption that an adolescent's self-identification as gay or a lesbian would be evidence of harm caused by being raised by parents who were not heterosexual.

There are few longitudinal data from which to determine whether there is an association between family constellation and eventual sexual orientation. The gender identity of preadolescent children raised by lesbian mothers has been found consistently to be in line with their biological sex. None of more than 500 children studied has shown evidence of gender identity confusion, wished to be the other sex, or consistently engaged in cross-gender behavior. No differences have been found between the toy, game, activity, dress, or friendship preferences of boys or girls who had lesbian mothers and those of children who had heterosexual mothers.[232,243,246]

In the only long-term longitudinal study, young men and women who had a divorced lesbian mother were slightly more likely than those who had a divorced heterosexual mother to consider the possibility of having a same-sex partner,[230] but in each group, similar proportions of adult men and women identified themselves as homosexual. A more recent study revealed no significant differences in gender development for either boys or girls according to the mother's sexual orientation.[243] According to data from a national sample of adolescents, there was no difference according to whether the parents were the same or different sexes in the proportion of adolescents who reported having had sexual intercourse or in the number who reported having a "romantic relationship" within the previous 18 months. So few adolescents in either group reported same-sex attractions or same-sex romantic relationships that a statistical comparison was not possible.[244] A long-term follow-up of adolescents raised by single lesbian mothers after divorce revealed similarly that their gender role orientation (level of masculinity or femininity) was similar to that of those who were raised by a single heterosexual mother after divorce or by a heterosexual couple. Boys from families headed by single heterosexual mothers and those from families headed by lesbian mothers scored higher on the scale of femininity, but they did not differ on the score of masculinity.[247] Data about the gender identity of adult children of gay fathers are scant. In the most extensive study available, 9% of sons of gay fathers identified themselves as bisexual or homosexual in orientation.[248]

OPPORTUNITIES AND RESPONSIBILITIES OF HEALTH CARE PROVIDERS

Early Gender Variance

Parents and clinicians concerned about a child with gender variant behaviors are legitimately obligated to

(1) help children feel more secure about their gender identity as boys or girls, perhaps preventing adult transgenderism; (2) diminish as much as possible peer ostracism and social isolation; and (3) treat evidence of associated behavioral/emotional distress. Attempts to alter a possible developmental pathway toward a homosexual orientation are neither ethical nor likely to be effective.

The best advice for parents is the same as for all children: to support their children, to foster their strengths, and to model desired behavior. The positive and nurturing qualities of both parents, and their contentment with their own gender roles, should be made evident to their children. Families can help children learn techniques of recognizing and combating the damaging effects of stigma. For example, they can explain that particular behaviors are not typical of boys or girls of the child's age, acknowledge that he or she may be unfairly criticized, and provide strategies and language to help children resist teasing and criticism.

Discussion with a developmental-behavioral pediatrician about their young child with gender-variant behavior can help parents to consider how they might feel if their child were to be gay or lesbian. Most families can come to accept a homosexual son or daughter, especially if given adequate time, information, and support. Parent-to-parent support may be invaluable, either locally or through electronic technology.[69,249] Table 25C-9 provides some suggestions for parents who are faced with the challenge of supporting a gender-variant child.

Most children respond positively to their parents' acceptance and encouragement. Referral for further mental health services is appropriate if the child is anxious, depressed, or angry; exhibits self-destructive behavior; or experiences significant social isolation; and if these problems do not improve with short-term counseling. Therapists should be selected carefully, as those who are competent in dealing with other childhood issues are not necessarily appropriately prepared to deal with gender variance.

Adolescents and Their Families

In its first policy statement about homosexuality among adolescents, the American Academy of Pediatrics[200] stated that "the physician's responsibility is to provide comprehensive health care and guidance to all adolescents, including gay and lesbian adolescents and those young people struggling with issues of sexual orientation. Pediatricians who care for teenagers need to understand the unique medical and psychosocial issues facing homosexually oriented youths." The most recently revised policy statement[250]

reiterates and expands further on pediatricians' responsibilities to gay and lesbian youth and their families. It continues to be difficult for gay and lesbian patients to communicate comfortably with their physicians.[251,252]

Meetings with teenagers without parents present, explicit reassurance and explanations of the limits of confidentiality, and care in recording private information in charts and in letters of referral will facilitate adolescents' sense of safety with their health care provider. First and foremost, providers must learn new ways to ask questions about sexual behavior and sexual orientation that do not assume heterosexuality (Table 25C-10), must ask the same questions of all adolescents, and must refrain from making assumptions about an adolescent's behavior or sexual orientation on the basis of appearances or social stereotypes.

Pediatricians report an interest in supporting gay, lesbian, bisexual, and transgender youths and their families, but they also report lack of comfort and skills regarding how to approach such discussions and lack of awareness of resources available.[253-256]

All adolescents—gay or not—worry about and may experience disapproval and stigmatization in medical settings. Assurance and repeated reminders of policies regarding confidentiality, and visible indications of acceptance and knowledge about homosexuality help them confide in clinicians about the whole range of their concerns and health care needs. A great deal of information about community networks of support, books, and Internet contacts can be provided as a resource for these adolescents and their families. Visible displays of information directed at gay and lesbian teenagers make these teenagers feel more welcome. For example, the American Academy of Pediatrics has a brochure titled *Gay, Lesbian, and Bisexual Teens: Facts for Teens and Their Parents.*[257] The routine use of previsit questionnaires to be completed by teenagers provides an opportunity for sensitive information to be communicated more readily. There is good evidence that adolescents are more likely to identify concerns about sensitive topics (e.g., sexual orientation and behavior, substance abuse) when completing a paper-and-pencil questionnaire than if asked directly by their pediatrician.

Parents who are having difficulty understanding or coming to terms with their adolescent's sexual orientation may appreciate guidance or counseling from the pediatrician. On a community level, pediatricians also have an opportunity to guide and advise schools about an appropriate curriculum about sexuality from kindergarten through high school and to advise libraries about purchasing books about sexual orientation and family diversity.[2]

TABLE 25C-9 ■ Suggestions for Parents of Gender-Variant Children

Create an atmosphere of acceptance so that your child feels safe within your family to express his or her interests

Identify and praise your child's talents

Encourage your child to develop activities that help him or her to "fit in" socially but still respect his or her interests and talents

Strengthen your child's relationship with an adult role model of the same sex (e.g., a parent, aunt or uncle, close friend)

Help your child learn specific language and strategies to counteract criticism and stigma

Use gender-neutral language in discussing romantic attachments

Watch together television programs and movies that include gay and lesbian adults and families

Read books about gay and lesbian heroes in history and in fiction

Discuss news stories about gay and lesbian issues with compassion and explicit acceptance

Highlight personal experiences and news stories of discrimination and negative stereotyping as inappropriate

Describe particular activities and interests concretely rather than labeling them as "girlish" or "boyish"

Educate others in your child's life; be sure to let your child's siblings, your parents and siblings, neighbors, and friends know that you love and support your child unconditionally

Facilitate classroom discussions about diversity and tolerance

Ensure that school and community libraries have, for all age groups, reading materials (both fiction and nonfiction) that include evidence of the diversity of sexual orientations

Ask your primary care physician to provide reading materials and contact information for organizations of other parents and children with similar questions

If it is indicated, arrange a referral to a psychotherapist with expertise in issues related to gender identity and sexual orientation

Recommended Resources

Books for Parents

Fanta-Shyer M, Shyer C: Not Like Other Boys. Boston: Houghton-Mifflin, 1996.

Cantwell MA: Homosexuality: The Secret a Child Dare Not Tell. Chicago: Rafael Press, 1998.

Rottnek M, ed: Sissies and Tomboys: Gender Non-conformity and Homosexual Childhood. New York: New York University Press, 1999.

Richardson J, Schuster MA: Everything You Never Wanted Your Kids to Know about Sex (But Were Afraid They'd Ask). New York: Random House, 2003.

If You Are Concerned about Your Child's Gender Behaviors. (Available at: *www.Dcchildrens.com/gendervariance;* accessed 2/11/07.) Printed copies can be ordered by writing to *pgroup@cnmc.org.* The Website also provides information on how to access a discussion group for families of gender-variant children.

Movies/Videos

Ma Vie en Rose (My Life in Pink) (Video), A film by Alain Berliner. Sony Picture Classics.

For Older Children and Adults

The Dress Code (video/DVD), a film by Shirley MacLaine. MGM/UA Studios (PG 13).

Oliver Button Is a Star (Video), directed by John Scagliotti and Dan Hunt, with Tomie de Paola and others. (Available at: *http://www.oliverbuttonisastar.com;* accessed 2/11/07.)

Books for Children

de Paola T: Oliver Button is a Sissy. Philadelphia: Voyager Books, Harcourt Brace, 1979. (For children at reading levels 4-8.)

Fierstein H, Cole H (Illustrator): The Sissy Duckling. New York: Simon & Schuster, 2002. (For children at reading levels 4-8.)

Harris R: It's Perfectly Normal. Cambridge, MA: Candlewick Press, 1994. (For children aged 10 and older.)

Bell R: Changing Bodies, Changing Lives. New York: Random House, 1998. (For teenagers.)

Transgender Youth

Transgender individuals may seek gender reassignment treatments. The process of gender reassignment is long and involves psychiatric, endocrinological, and surgical components. Hormone therapy precedes any surgical procedures and may itself be associated with various medical risks.[258]

The development of the typical secondary sexual characteristics of their anatomical sex in transgender teenagers may result in profound depression and recurrent self-mutilation and even suicidal gestures or attempts. Some consideration is currently focused on giving carefully evaluated adolescents an opportunity to suppress pubertal manifestations through the administration of gonadotrophin-inhibiting gonadotrophin-releasing hormone analogues.[259,260] Pubertal maturation is thus delayed without creating permanent physical changes. Upon reaching legal age, these teenagers can then authorize treatment with the hormones of choice to induce desired changes in the larynx, hair follicles, or breasts. At the age of 18, they may be considered candidates for irreversible surgery on breasts and genitals.

Treatment of the teenager experiencing gender dysphoria should include an assessment by a mental

TABLE 25C-10 ■ Asking Gender-Neutral Questions

It is helpful to reassure *all* adolescents that questions about sexuality are a routine part of the health supervision visit. Questions such as these can be included in a written health history form or be part of an office interview. Adolescents should be assured that these questions are asked routinely and that responses are confidential.

Examples of appropriate questions include the following:
  Do you have a boyfriend or a girlfriend?
  Some of my patients your age date—some boys, some girls, some both. Are you interested in dating?
  Have you ever dated or gone out with someone?
  Have you ever been attracted to any boys or girls?
  Are you especially attracted to any boys or girls?
  There are many ways of being sexual with another person: petting, kissing, hugging, as well as having sexual intercourse. Have you had any kinds of sexual experiences with boys or girls or both?
  Are you currently involved in a steady relationship with a boy or a girl?
  How do you protect yourself and your partner against sexually transmitted diseases and pregnancy?
  Do you have any concerns about your sexual feelings or the sexual things you have been doing?
  Have you discussed these concerns with your parents or any other adults? Any of your friends?
  Do you consider yourself to be gay/lesbian, bisexual, or heterosexual ("straight")?

health clinician experienced with the condition, as well as an endocrinologist. A decision to intervene hormonally requires approval by the parent or guardian unless the patient is an emancipated minor.

The Harry Benjamin International Gender Dysphoria Association, a multidisciplinary society dedicated to disseminating knowledge and preventing exploitation of transgender individuals, has established a set of "standards of care." For example, a patient has to have lived in the desired gender for at least a year before undergoing surgery.

Children Whose Parents Are Gay or Lesbian

Health care providers have important roles to play in supporting families headed by gay or lesbian parents.[2,7] First, they must (of course) ensure that the direct clinical care they provide is supportive, nonjudgmental, and affirming. Second, they can work within their offices and hospital contexts to support equal access and to eliminate practices that result in discomfort or exclusion. In addition, pediatricians who are motivated can find many opportunities for local and regional political advocacy to break down barriers and stigma and to support these nontraditional families and their children.

In general, pediatricians and their staff (including nurses, receptionists) must be aware of and sensitive to the history of stigma and discrimination of people who are not heterosexual and of the damaging personal and social effects of this stereotyping. As a result, policies ensuring privacy and confidentiality must be even more than usually explicitly displayed and discussed, and strict policies forbidding homophobic comments and jokes must be in place. Explicit evidence of knowledge and acceptance of parents who are gay or lesbian should be evident in the waiting room and office: for example, lists on the bulletin board of local and national resources for gay and lesbian parents and their children, books about gay and lesbian parents on the office bookshelf, posters or photographs displaying families that include two mothers or two fathers, and brochures about children whose parents are gay or lesbian (e.g., the American Academy of Pediatrics' *Gay, Lesbian, or Bisexual Parents: Information for Children and Parents*[261]) in the general brochure rack.

Office literature and forms should be revised so they do not assume heterosexuality—for example, asking for names of parent #1 and parent #2 rather than mother and father—and describe a variety of family constellations rather than uniformly mothers and fathers. There are now many children's books that can be displayed in the waiting room and examination rooms that describe the many forms of diversity that represent children's families. Similarly, hospital policies and admitting forms should be inclusive of a wide variety of family forms (e.g., policies that allow only legal parents to visit may exclude a child's true parent).

Pediatricians and nurses must make an effort to ask about and know the constellation of children's families: for example, whether the parents are divorced, whether there is a blended family, and whether the parents are of the same sex. Parents who are gay or lesbian generally appreciate honest discussions about their families and the acceptance that such discussion communicates. Honest and direct discussions with the children are also appreciated, with appropriate acknowledgment of who their parents are.

Some of the typically troubling transitions of childhood may be more challenging for parents who are gay or lesbian, and they provide opportunities for pediatricians to offer advice and guidance. For example,

1. Preschool children's normal curiosity about "where did I come from" may be more difficult for a lesbian couple who used an anonymous sperm donor.
2. The entry to school is a challenge for many parents, but parents who are gay or lesbian have the addi-

tional worry about whether their family will be acknowledged and accepted by the broader community of the school (teachers, other parents) and whether their child will be subjected to teasing, ostracism, and stigma on account of their sexual orientation or family constellation.

3. Children in early adolescence (aged 12 to 14) typically are curious about their roots and personal identity. This is a challenging period, for example, for children who were adopted and for children whose parents are divorced and estranged. For adolescents with gay or lesbian parents, this period of exploration may present special challenges, depending on their own particular family history.

4. Children in later adolescence begin exploring their own sexuality. For those whose parents are gay or lesbian, the known range of possible sexual orientations may be broader, but open discussions about sexual behavior are difficult for all types of families. Pediatricians can be helpful to parents by recommending appropriate books and by encouraging honest discussions about sexuality.

Pediatricians and other health care clinicians are important community opinion leaders. Their advocacy and involvement in community-based activities provides considerable support to gay and lesbian parents and their children. For example, they may provide advice to schools about inclusion of information describing family diversity in the curricula from kindergarten through high school. They may advise school and community libraries about the large number of available books for children and for adults that describe and discuss children whose parents are gay or lesbian and the consequences of stigma and discrimination. Pediatricians can also serve as advisers to local groups of gay and lesbian parents (e.g. Family Pride) and/or of their children (e.g., Children of Lesbians and Gays Everywhere [COLAGE]). Professionals who have developed a stronger passion for advocacy in this realm may choose to engage in political work or in continuing education for various professional groups about the strengths and challenges of these nontraditional families.

A great deal more research is needed to understand the strengths and vulnerabilities of the new family constellations that are being created by committed gay and lesbian parents. For example, little is known of the well-being of children raised by gay male couples, because most research has concerned lesbian parents. The appropriate role of a sperm donor, egg donor, and/or surrogate parent in the life of a child is unclear. Mechanisms for including in the child's life a role model of the opposite sex from single-sex parents is unknown. Some families are being created with two lesbian parents and a gay male couple all

having quasi-parental roles with the child.[262] Others are growing up with a sperm donor (often a relative of one mother) involved with and known to the child as "more than an uncle; less than a dad."

SUMMARY

Almost all experts in human sexuality view heterosexuality and homosexuality as the extremes of a theoretical continuum rather than as discrete identities. People are seen as occupying various points along this continuum in their sexual behaviors and responsiveness from exclusive heterosexuality to exclusive homosexuality. To whatever degree sexual orientations are established before birth, grow out of gender-role preferences established early in childhood, and/or are organized on the basis of family and social experiences, people construct their sexual orientation over time by making sense of their sexual feelings in the context of the wider culture.

In nearly all models of homosexual identity formation, development is viewed as taking place against a backdrop of stigma, which affects the processes of formation and expression of sexual identity. Although stigma still surrounds all sexual minorities, there is evidence that exposure (e.g., through college) erodes negative stereotypes.[263] It seems increasingly implausible to consider that genes, hormones, neuroanatomical differences, and different social environments either would have *no* part in the process or would act *alone* to result in anything so complex as human sexual behavior and orientation. Rather, biological, temperamental, and personality traits probably interact with the familial and social milieu in which a child is nurtured as her or his sexuality emerges.

Ample evidence about lesbian mothers and their children provides reassurance that these families support their children in much the same ways that parents in other family structures do. The evidence is clear that children thrive with the nurturance, security, and care provided by the parents, largely independently of their gender and sexual orientation. Research is just beginning about the families created by gay fathers. We have a great deal more to learn about the particular strengths gay and lesbian parents bring to their children that allow them to counteract stigma and maintain normal development and psychosocial adjustment.

REFERENCES

1. Perrin EC, ed: Gay and lesbian issues in pediatric health care. Curr Probl Pediatr Adolesc Health Care 34:355-398, 2004.

2. Perrin EC: Sexual Orientation in Child and Adolescent Health Care. New York: Kluwer-Plenum, 2002.

3. Frankowski BL, Committee on Adolescence: Sexual Orientation and Adolescents. Pediatrics, 113:1827-1832, 2004.

4. Remafedi G: Health disparities for homosexual youth. *In* Wolitski R, Valdiserri, R, eds: Unequal Opportunity: Health Disparities among Gay and Bisexual Men in the United States. New York: Oxford University Press, in press.

5. Tasker F: Lesbian mothers, gay fathers, and their children: A review. J Dev Behav Pediatr, 26:224-240, 2005.

6. Schorzman CM, Gold M: Gay and lesbian parenting. Curr Probl Pediatr Adolesc Health Care 34:375-383, 2004.

7. Pawelski JG, Perrin EC, Foy JM, et al: The effects of marriage, civil union, and domestic partnership laws on the health and well-being of children. Pediatrics 118:349-364, 2006.

8. Remafedi G: Fundamental issues in the care of homosexual youth. Med Clin North Am, 74:1169-1179, 1990.

9. Breedlove SM: Sexual differentiation of the human nervous system. Annu Rev Psychol 45:389-418, 1994.

10. LeVay S: A difference in hypothalamic structure between heterosexual and homosexual men. Science 253:1034-1037, 1991.

11. Swaab DF, Hofman MA: An enlarged suprachiasmatic nucleus in homosexual men. Brain Res 537:141-148, 1990.

12. Swaab DF, Hofman MA: Sexual differentiation of the human hypothalamus in relation to gender and sexual orientation. Trends Neurosci 18:264-270, 1995.

13. Geschwind N, Galaburda AM: Cerebral lateralization. Biological mechanisms, associations, and pathology: I. A hypothesis and a program for research. Arch Neurol 42:428-459, 1985.

14. Alexander JE, Sufka KJ: Cerebral lateralization in homosexual males: A preliminary EEG investigation. Int J Psychophysiol 15:269-274, 1993.

15. Reite M, Sheeder J, Richardson D, et al: Cerebral laterality in homosexual males: Preliminary communication using magnetoencephalography. Arch Sex Behav 24:585-593, 1995.

16. Downey J, Ehrhardt AA, Schiffman M, et al: Sex hormones and lesbian and heterosexual women. Horm Behav 21:347-357, 1987.

17. Gartrell NK: Hormones and homosexuality. *In* Paul E, Weinrich JD, Gonsiorek JC, et al, eds: Homosexuality: Social, Psychological and Biological Issues. Beverly Hills, CA: Sage Publications, 1982, pp 169-182.

18. Meyer-Bahlburg HFL: Psychoendocrine research on sexual orientation. Current status and future options. Progr Brain Res 61:375-398, 1984.

19. Meyer-Bahlburg HFL: Psychobiologic research on homosexuality. Child Adolesc Psychiatr Clin North Am 2:489-500, 1993.

20. Gerall AA, Moltz H, Ward IL, eds: Handbook of Behavioral Neurobiology, Volume 11: Sexual Differentiation. New York: Plenum Press, 1992.

21. Tallal P, McEwen BS, guest eds: Neuroendocrine effects on brain development and cognition [special issue]. Psychoneuroendocrinology 16(1-3):3-6, 1991.

22. Meyer-Bahlburg HFL, Ehrhardt AA, Rosen LR, et al: Prenatal estrogens and the development of homosexual orientation. Dev Psychol 31:12-21, 1995.

23. Friedman RC, Downey J: Neurobiology and sexual orientation: Current relationships. J Neuropsychiatry Clin Neurosci 5:131-153, 1993.

24. Ehrhardt AA, Meyer-Bahlburg HFL: Effects of prenatal sex hormones on gender-related behavior. Science 211:1312-1318, 1981.

25. Doerner G: Neuroendocrine response to estrogen and brain differentiation in heterosexuals, homosexuals, and transsexuals. Arch Sex Behav 17:57-75, 1988.

26. Gladue BA, Green R, Hellman RE: Neuroendocrine response to estrogen and sexual orientation. Science 225:1496-1499, 1984.

27. Gooren L: The neuroendocrine response of luteinizing hormone to estrogen administration in heterosexual, homosexual, and transsexual subjects. J Clin Endocrinol Metab 63:583-588, 1986.

28. Gooren L: The neuroendocrine response of luteinizing hormone to estrogen administration in the human is not sex specific but dependent on the hormonal environment. J Clin Endocrinol Metab 63:589-593, 1986.

29. Doerner G: Hormone-dependent brain development and neuro-endocrine prophylaxis. Exp Clin Endocrinol 94:4-22, 1989.

30. Doerner G, Poppe I, Stahl, F, et al: Gene- and environment-dependent neuroendocrine etiogenesis of homosexuality and transsexualism. Exp Clin Endocrinol 98:141-150, 1991.

31. Pillard RC, Poumadere J, Carretta RA: Is homosexuality familial? A review, some data, and a suggestion. Arch Sex Behav 10:465-475, 1981.

32. Bailey JM, Pillard RC: A genetic study of male sexual orientation. Arch Gen Psychiatry 48:1089-1096, 1991.

33. Whitam FL, Diamond M, Martin J: Homosexual orientation in twins: A report on 61 pairs and three triplet sets. Arch Sex Behav 22:187-206, 1993.

34. Bailey JM, Pillard RC, Neale MC, et al: Heritable factors influence sexual orientation in women. Arch Gen Psychiatry 50:217-223, 1993.

35. Kendler KS, Thornton LM, Gilman SE, et al: Sexual orientation in a U.S. national sample of twin and nontwin sibling pairs. Am J Psychiatry 157:1843-1846, 2000.

36. King M, McDonald E: Homosexuals who are twins: A study of 46 probands. Br J Psychiatry 160:407-409, 1992.

37. Pillard RC, Poumadere J, Carretta RA: A family study of sexual orientation. Arch Sex Behav 11:511-520, 1982.

38. Eckert ED, Bouchard TJ, Bohlen J, et al: Homosexuality in monozygotic twins reared apart. Br J Psychiatry 148:421-425, 1986.

39. Hamer DH, Hu S, Magnuson VL, et al: A linkage between DNA markers on the X chromosome and male sexual orientation. Science 261:321-327, 1993.

40. Turner WJ: Homosexuality, type 1: An Xq28 phenomenon. Arch Sex Behav 24:109-134, 1995.

41. Bailey JM, Dunne MP, Martin NG: Genetic and environmental influences on sexual orientation and its correlates in an Australian twin sample. J Pers Soc Psychol, 78:524-536, 2000.

42. Dawood K, Pillard RC, Horvath C, et al: Familial aspects of male homosexuallity. Arch Sex Behav 29:155-163, 2000.

43. Money J: Sin, sickness, or status? Homosexual gender identity and psychoneuroendocrinology. In Garnets LD, Kimmel DC, eds: Psychological Perspectives on Lesbian and Gay Male Experiences. New York: Columbia University Press, 1993, pp 130-167.

44. Byne W: Why we cannot conclude that sexual orientation is primarily a biological phenomenon. J Homosex 34(1):73-80, 1997.

45. Bieber I, Dain H, Dince P, et al: Homosexuality: A Psychoanalytic Study. New York: Basic Books, 1962.

46. Bene E: On the genesis of male homosexuality: An attempt at clarifying the role of parents. Br J Psychiatry 111:803-813, 1965a.

47. Siegleman M: Parental background of male homosexuals and heterosexuals. Arch Sex Behav 6:89-96, 1974.

48. Newcombe M: The role of perceived relative parent personality in the development of heterosexuals, homosexuals, and transvestites. Arch Sex Behav 14:147-164, 1985.

49. Mischel W: A social-learning view of sex differences in behavior. In Maccoby EE, ed: The Development of Sex Differences. Stanford, CA: Stanford University Press, 1966, pp 56-81.

50. Fagot BI: Sex differences in toddlers' behavior and parental reaction. Dev Psychol 10:554-558, 1974.

51. Fagot BI: Sex differences in toddlers' behavior and parental reactions. Developmental Psychology, 10: 554-558, 1974.

52. Rheingold HL, Cook KV: The contents of boys' and girls' rooms as an index of parent behavior. Child Dev 46:459-463, 1975.

53. Shakin M, Shakin D, Sternglanz SH: Infant clothing: Sex labeling for strangers. Sex Roles 12:955-963, 1985.

54. Bussey K, Bandura A: Social cognitive theory of gender development and differentiation. Psychol Rev 106:676-713, 1999.

55. Block JH: Issues, problems, and pitfalls in assessing sex differences: A critical review of "The Psychology of Sex Differences." Merrill Palmer Q 22:283-308, 1976.

56. Johnson MM: Sex role learning in the nuclear family. Child Dev 34:315-333, 1963.

57. Johnson MM: Fathers, mothers, and sex typing. Sociol Inq 45:15-26, 1975.

58. Kitzinger C: The Social Construction of Lesbianism. London: Sage Publications, 1987.

59. Simon W, Gagnon JH: A sexual scripts approach. In Geer JH, O'Donohue WT, eds: Theories of Human Sexuality. London: Plenum Press, 1987, pp 363-383.

60. Tiefer L: Social constructionism and the study of human sexuality. In Shaver P, Hendrick C, eds: Sex and Gender: Review of Personality and Social Psychology, vol 7. London: Sage Publications, 1987, pp 70-94.

61. Plummer K: Sexual Stigma: An Interactionist Account. London: Routledge & Kegan Paul, 1975.

62. Eccles TA, Sayegh MA, Fortenberry JD, et al: More normal than not: A qualitative assessment of the developmental experiences of gay male youth. J Adolesc Health 35:425.e11-425.e18, 2004.

63. Cass VC: Homosexual identity formation: A theoretical model. J Homosex 4(3):219-235, 1979.

64. Troiden RR: Becoming homosexual: A model of gay identity acquisition. Psychiatry 42:362-373, 1979.

65. Troiden RR: Homosexual identity development. J Adolesc Health Care 9:105-113, 1988.

66. Green R: The "Sissy Boy Syndrome" and the Development of Homosexuality. New Haven, CT: Yale University Press, 1987.

67. Pickstone-Taylor S: Children with gender non-conformity. J Am Acad Child Adolesc Psychiatry 42:266, 2003.

68. Zucker KJ, Bradley SJ: Gender Identity Disorder and Psychosexual Problems in Children and Adolescents. New York: Guilford, 1995.

69. Menvielle EJ, Tuerck C, Perrin EC: To the beat of a different drummer: The gender-variant child. Contemp Pediatr 22, 2005.

70. Savin-Williams RC: . . . And Then I Became Gay. New York: Routledge, 1998.

71. Floyd FJ, Bakeman R: Coming out across the life course: Implications of age and historical context. Arch Sex Behav 35:287-296, 2006.

72. Wildman S: Coming out early. Advocate (October 10):39, 2000.

73. Smith SD, Dermer SB, Astromovich RL: Working with nonheterosexual youth to understand sexual identity development, at-risk behaviors, and implications for health care professionals. Psychol Rep 96:651-654, 2005.

74. Rosario M, Scrimshaw EW, Hunter J, et al: Sexual Identity development among gay, lesbian, and bisexual youths: consistency and change over time. J Sex Res 43:46-58, 2006.

75. Blake SM, Ledsky R, Lehman T, et al: Preventing sexual risk behaviors among gay, lesbian, and bisexual adolescents: The benefits of gay-sensitive HIV instruction in schools. Am J Public Health 91:940-946, 2001.

76. Gilman SE, Cochran SD, Mays VM, et al: Risk of psychiatric disorders among individuals reporting same-sex sexual partners in the National Comorbidity Survey. Am J Public Health 91:933-9, 2001.

77. Russell ST, Franz BT, Driscoll AK: Same-sex romantic attraction and experiences of violence in adolescence. Am J Public Health 91:903-906, 2001.

78. Troiden RR: The formation of homosexual identities. J Homosex 17(1-2):43-73, 1989.

79. Troiden RR: The formation of homosexual identities. *In* Garnets LD, Kimmel DC, eds: Psychological Perspectives on Lesbian & Gay Male Experiences. New York: Columbia University Press, 1993, pp 191-217.

80. Dube EM, Savin-Williams RC: Sexual identity development among ethnic sexual-minority male youths. Dev Psychol 35:1389-1398, 1999.

81. Rosario M, Schrimshaw EW, Hunter J: Ethnic/racial differences in the coming-out process of lesbian, gay, and bisexual youths: A comparison of sexual identity development over time. Cultur Divers Ethnic Minor Psychol 10:215-28, 2004.

82. Greene B: Ethnic minority lesbians and gay men: Mental health treatment issues. J Consult Clin Psychol 62:243, 1994a.

83. Greene B: Lesbian women of color: Triple jeopardy. *In* Comas-Diaz L, Greene B, eds: Women of Color: Integrating Ethnic and Gender Identities in Psychotherapy. New York: Guilford Press, 1994.

84. Chan CS: Issues of identity development among Asian-American lesbians and gay men. J Counsel Dev 68:16, 1989.

85. Icard L: Black gay men and conflicting social identities: Sexual orientation versus racial identity. J Soc Work Hum Sex 4:83, 1986.

86. Loiacano D: Gay identity issues among black Americans: Racism, homophobia, and the need for Validation. *In* Garnets & Kimmel, pp 364-375.

86a. Chan, Connie S: Issues of identity development among Asian-American lesbians and gay men. *In* Garnets & Kimmel as cited above, pp 376-387.

87. Tremble B, Schneider M, Appathurai C: Growing up gay or lesbian in a multicultural context. J Homosex 17(3-4):253-267, 1989.

88. Bell AP, Weinberg MS, Hammersmith SK: Sexual Preference: Its Development in Men and Women. Bloomington: Indiana University Press, 1981.

89. Schafer S: Sexual and social problems among lesbians. J Sex Res 12:50-69, 1976.

90. Campbell L, Perrin EC: Social Support among Gay and Lesbian Adolescents. Presented at the annual meeting of the Pediatric Academic Societies, Washington, DC, May 4, 1997.

91. Stein TS: A critique of approaches to changing sexual orientation. *In* Cabaj RP, Stein TS, eds: Textbook of Homosexuality and Mental Health. Washington, DC: American Psychiatric Press, 1996, pp 525-537.

92. Haldeman DC: Sexual orientation conversion therapy: A scientific examination. *In* Gonsiorek JC, Weinrich JD, eds: Homosexuality: Research Implications for Public Policy. Newbury Park, CA: Sage Publications, 1991, pp 149-160.

93. Halpin SA, Allen MW: Changes in psychosocial well-being during stages of gay identity development. J Homosex 47(2):109-126, 2004.

94. Humphries L: Being odd against all odds. *In* Federico RC, ed: Sociology, 2nd ed. Reading, MA: Addison-Wesley, 1979, pp 238-242.

95. Bell AP, Weinberg MS, Hammersmith SK: Sexual Preference: Its Development in men and women. Bloomington Indiana: University of Indiana Press, 1981.

96. Cass VC: Homosexual identity formation: Testing a theoretical model. J Sex Res 20:143-167, 1984.

97. Diamond LM: Development of sexual orientation among adolescent and young adult women. Dev Psychol 34:1085-1095, 1998.

98. Parks CA: Lesbian identity development: An examination of differences across generations. Am J Orthopsychiatry 69:347-363, 1999.

99. Golden C: What's in a name? Sexual self-identification among women. *In* Savin-Williams RC, Cohen KM, eds: The Lives of Lesbians, Gays, and Bisexuals: Children to Adults. Fort Worth, TX: Harcourt Brace, 1996, pp 229-249.

100. Kitzinger C, Wilkinson S: Transitions from heterosexuality to lesbianism: The discursive production of lesbian identities. Dev Psychol 31:95-104, 1995.

101. Rust P: The politics of sexual identity: Sexual attraction and behavior among lesbian and bisexual women. Soc Prob 39:366-386, 1992.

102. Savin-Williams RC: Lesbian, gay male, and bisexual adolescents. *In* D'Augelli AR, Patterson CJ, eds: Lesbian, Gay, and Bisexual Identities over the Lifespan. New York: Oxford University Press, 1995, pp 165-189.

103. Weinberg MS, Williams CJ, Pryor DW: Dual Attraction: Understanding Bisexuality. New York: Oxford University Press, 1994.

104. Parks CA, Hughes TL, Matthews AK: Race/Ethnicity and sexual orientation: Intersecting identities. Cultur Divers Ethnic Minor Psychol 10:241-54, 2004.

105. Levine H: A further exploration of the lesbian identity development process and its measurement. J Homosex 34(2):67-78, 1997.

106. Espin OM: Issues of identity in the psychology of Latina lesbians. *In* Garnets L, Kimmel D, eds: Psychological Perspectives on Lesbian and Gay Male Experiences. New York: Columbia University Press, 1993, pp 348-363.

107. American Psychiatric Association: Diagnostic and Statistical Manual of Mental Disorders, 4th ed. Washington, DC: American Psychiatric Press, 1994.

108. Lombardi EL, Wilchins RA, Priesing D, et al: Gender violence: Transgender experiences with violence and discrimination. J Homosex 42(1):89-101, 2001.

109. HIV Prevention and Health Service Needs of the Transgender Community in San Francisco: Results from Eleven Focus Groups. San Francisco: San Francisco Department of Public Health, AIDS Office, 1997.

110. Clements-Nolle K, Marx R, Guzman R, et al: HIV prevalence, risk behaviors, health care use, and mental health status of transgender persons: Implications for public health intervention. Am J Public Health 91:915-921, 2001.

111. Cohen-Kettenis PT, Gooren LJG: Transsexualism: A review of etiology, diagnosis and treatment. J Psychosom Res 46:315, 1999.

112. Lombardi EL: Integration within a transgender social network and its effect on members' social and political activity. J Homosex 37(1):109-126, 1999.

113. Lombardi EL: Enhancing transgender health care. Am J Public Health 91:869-872, 2001.

114. Burn SM, Kadlec K, Rexer R: Effects of subtle heterosexism on gays, lesbians, bisexuals. J Homosex 49(2):23-38, 2005.

115. Garofalo R, Harper GW: Not all adolescents are the same: Addressing the unique needs of gay and bisexual male youth. Adolesc Med 14:595-611, 2003.

116. Harper GW, Schneider M: Oppression and discrimination among lesbian, gay, bisexual, and transgendered people and communities: A challenge for community psychology. Am J Community Psychol 31:243-252, 2003.

117. Rosario M, Schrimshaw EW, Hunter J, et al: Gay-related stress and emotional distress among gay, lesbian, and bisexual youths: A longitudinal examination. J Consult Clin Psychol 70:967-975, 2002.

118. Rosario M, Schrimshaw EW, Hunter J: A model of sexual risk behaviors among young gay and bisexual men: Longitudinal associations of mental health, substance abuse, sexual abuse and the coming-out process. AIDS Educ Prev 18:444-460, 2006.

119. Igartua KJ, Gill K, Montoro R: Internalized homophobia: A factor in depression, anxiety, and suicide in the gay and lesbian population. Can J Commun Ment Health 22:15-30, 2003.

120. Meyer IH: Prejudice, social stress, and mental health in lesbian gay and bisexual populations: conceptual issues and research evidence. Psychol Bull 129:674-697, 2003.

121. King M, Nazareth I: The health of people classified as gay, lesbian, and bisexual attending family practitioners in London. BMC Public Health 6:127-130, 2006.

122. Garofalo R, Wolf CR, Kessel S, et al: The association between health risk behaviors and sexual orientation among a school-based sample of adolescents. Pediatrics 101:895-902, 1998.

123. Bontempo DE, D'Augelli AR: Effects of at-school victimization and sexual orientation on lesbian, gay, or bisexual youths' health risk behavior. J Adolesc Health 30:364-374, 2002.

124. Kosciw JG, Diaz EM: The 2005 National School Climate Survey: The Experiences of Lesbian, Gay, Bisexual and Transgender Youth in Our Nation's Schools. New York: Gay, Lesbian, and Straight Education Network, 2006.

125. Rosario M, Rotheram-Borus MJ, Reid H: Gay-related stress and its correlates among gay and bisexual male adolescents of predominantly bBlack and Hispanic background. J Community Psychol 24:136-159, 1996.

126. Rotheram-Borus MJ: Suicidal behavior and gay-related stress among gay and bisexual male adolescents. J Adolesc Res 9:498, 1994.

127. Sears J: Educators, homosexuality, and homosexual students: Are personal feelings related to professional beliefs? J Homosex 22(3-4):29-79, 1991.

128. Telljohann SK, Price JH: A qualitative examination of adolescent homosexuals' life experience. J Homosex 26(1):41-56, 1993.

129. Ryan C, Futterman D: Lesbian and gay youth: Care and counseling. Adolesc Med 8:2, 1997.

130. Remafedi G: Adolescent homosexuality: Psychosocial and medical implications. Pediatrics 79:331, 1987.

131. Kruks G: Gay and lesbian homeless/street youth: Special issues and concerns. J Adolesc Health 12:515, 1991.

132. Savin-Williams RC: Verbal and physical abuse as stressors in the lives of lesbian, gay male and bisexual youths: Associations with school problems, running away, substance abuse, prostitution and suicide. J Consult Clin Psychol 62:261, 1994.

133. Cochran BN, Stewart AJ, Ginzler JA, et al: Challenges faced by homeless sexual minorities: Comparison of gay lesbian, bisexual, and transgender homeless adolescents with their heterosexual counterparts. Am J Public Health 92:773-777, 2002.

134. Hunter J: Violence against lesbian and gay male youths. In Herek GM, Berrill KT, eds: Hate Crimes: Confronting Violence against Lesbians and Gay Men. Newbury Park, CA: Sage Publications, 1992.

135. Saewyc EM, Skay CL, Pettingell SL, et al: Hazards of stigma: The sexual and physical abuse of gay, lesbian, ad bisexual adolescents in the United States and Canada. Child Welfare 85:195-213, 2006.

136. Williams T, Connoly J, Pepler D, et al: Questioning and sexual minority adolescents: High school experiences of bullying, sexual harassment and physical abuse. Can J Community Ment Health, 22:47-58, 2003.

137. D'Augelli AR, Hershberger SL: Lesbian, gay and bisexual youth in community settings: Personal challenges and mental health problems. Am J Community Psychol 21:421-448, 1993.

138. Pilkington NW, D'Augelli AR: Victimization of lesbian, gay, and bisexual youth in community settings. Am J Community Psychol 23:34, 1995.

139. D'Augelli AR: Lesbians' and gay men's experiences of discrimination and harassment in a university community. Am J Community Psychol 17:317-321, 1989.

140. Herek GM: Documenting prejudice against lesbians and gay men on campus: The Yale Sexual Orientation Survey. J Homosex 25(4):15-30, 1993.

141. Woods J: The Corporate Closet: The Professional Lives of Gay Men in America. New York: Free Press, 1993.

142. Hamilton JA: Emotional consequences of victimization and discrimination in "special populations" of women. Psychiatr Clin North Am 12:35, 1989.

143. Hershberger SL, D'Augelli AR: The impact of victimization on the mental health and suicidality of lesbian, gay and bisexual youths. Dev Psychol 31:65, 1995.

144. Youth risk behavior surveillance-United States, 2005. Morbidity and Mortality Weekly Report 55:1-108, 2006.

145. Farrow JA: Adolescent chemical dependency. Med Clin North Am 74:1265, 1990.

146. Bickelhaupt EE: Alcoholism and drug abuse in gay and lesbian persons: A review of incidence studies. J Gay Lesbian Soc Serv 2:5, 1995.

147. McKirnan DJ, Peterson PL: Alcohol and drug use among homosexual men and women: Epidemiology and population characteristics. Addict Behav 14:545, 1989.

148. Stall RD, Greenwood GL, Acree M, et al: Cigarette smoking among gay and bisexual men. Am J Public Health 89:1875-1878, 1999.

149. Bradford J, Ryan C, Rothblum ED: National lesbian health care survey: Implications for mental health care. J Consult Clin Psychol 62:228, 1994.

150. Gruskin EP, Hart S, Gordon N, et al: Patterns of cigarette smoking and alcohol use among lesbians and bisexual women enrolled in a large health maintenance organization. Am J Public Health 91:976-979, 2001.

151. Austin SB, Ziyadeh N, Fisher LB, et al: Sexual orientation and tobacco use in a cohort study of US adolescent girls and boys. Arch Pediatr Adolesc Med 158:317-322, 2004.

152. Ziyadeh NJ, Prokop LA, Fisher LB, et al: Sexual orientation, gender, and alcohol use in a cohort study of U.S. adolescent girls and boys. Drug Alcohol Depend 87:119-130, 2007.

153. Ridner SL, Frost K, Lajoie AS: Health information and risk behaviors among lesbian, gay, and bisexual college students. J Am Acad Nurse Pract, 18:374-378, 2006.

154. Remafedi G, Carol H: Preventing tobacco use among lesbian, gay, bisexual, and transgender youths. Nicotine Tob Res 7:249-56, 2005.

155. French SA, Story M, Remafedi G, et al: Sexual orientation and prevalence of body dissatisfaction and eating disordered behavior in a population-based study of adolescents. Int J Eat Disord 19:119, 1996.

156. Heffernan K: Sexual orientation as a factor in risk for binge eating and bulimia nervosa: A review. Int J Eat Disord 16:335, 1994.

157. Herzog DB, Norman DK, Gordon C, et al: Sexual conflict and eating disorders in 27 males. Am J Psychiatry 141:989, 1984.

158. Brand PA, Rothblum ED, Solomon LJ: A comparison of lesbians, gay men and heterosexuals on weight and restrained eating. Int J Eat Disord 11:253, 1992.

159. Heffernan K: Eating disorders and weight concerns among lesbians. Int J Eat Disord 19:127, 1996.

160. Siever MD: Sexual orientation and gender as factors in socioculturally acquired vulnerability to body dissatisfaction and eating disorders. J Consult Clin Psychol 62:252, 1994.

161. Austin SB, Ziyadeh N, Kahn JA, et al: Sexual orientation, weight concerns, and eating-disordered behaviors in adolescent girls and boys. J Am Acad Child Adolesc Psychiatry 43:1115-1123, 2004.

162. Yancey AK, Cochran SD, Corliss HL, et al: Correlates of overweight and obesity among lesbian and bisexual women. Prev Med 36:676-683, 2003.

163. Mravcak SA: Primary care for lesbians and bisexual women. Am Fam Physician 74:279-286, 2006.

164. Cochran SD, Mays VM: Lifetime prevalence of suicidal symptoms and affective disorders among men reporting same-sex sexual partners: Results from NHANES III. Am J Public Health 90:573-578, 2000.

165. Cochran SD, Mays VM: Relation between psychiatric syndromes and behaviorally defined sexual orientation in a sample of the US population. Am J Epidemiol 151:516-523, 2000.

166. Standfort TG, Graaf R, Bijl RV, et al: Same-sex sexual behavior and psychiatric disorders. Arch Gen Psychiatry 58:85-91, 2001.

167. Diaz RM, Ayala G, Bein E, et al: The impact of homophobia, poverty, and racism on the mental health of gay and bisexual Latino men: Findings from 3 US cities. Am J Public Health 91:927-932, 2001.

168. Fergusson DM, Horwood LJ, Beautrais AL: Is sexual orientation related to mental health problems and suicidality in young people? Arch Gen Psychiatry 56:876-880, 1999.

169. Lock J, Steiner H: Gay, lesbian, and bisexual youth risks for emotional, physical, and social problems: Results from a community-based survey. J Am Acad Child Adolesc Psychiatry 38:297-304, 1999.

170. Herdt G, Boxer, A: Children of Horizons: How Lesbian and Gay Teens Are Leading a New Way Out of the Closet, 2nd ed. Boston: Beacon Press, 1996.

171. Remafedi G: Death by Denial: Studies of Suicide in Gay and Lesbian Teenagers. Boston: Alyson Publishing, 1994.

172. Remafedi G, French S, Story M, et al: The relationship between suicide risk and sexual orientation: Results of a population-based study. Am J Public Health 88:57, 1998.

173. Rotheram-Borus MJ, Rosario M, Meyer-Bahlburg H, et al: Sexual and substance use acts of gay and bisexual male adolescents in New York City. J Sex Res 31:47, 1994.

174. D'Augelli AR, Grossman AH, Salter NP, et al: Predicting the suicide attempts of lesbian, gay and bisexual youth. Suicide Life Threat Behav 35:646-660, 2005.

174a. Eisenberg ME, Resnick MD: Suicidality among gay, lesbian and bisexual youth: the role of protective factors. J Adolesc Health 39(5):662-668, 2006.

175. Eisenberg ME, Resnick MD: Suicidality among gay lesbian and bisexual youth: The role of protective factors. J Adolesc Health 39:662-668, 2006.

176. Herrell R, Goldberg J, True WR, et al: Sexual orientation an suicidality: A co-twin control study in adult men. Arch Gen Psychiatry 56:867-874, 1999.

177. Remafedi G, Farrow JA, Deisher RW: Risk factors for attempted suicide in gay and bisexual youth. Pediatrics 87:869, 1991.

178. Rich CL, Fowler RC, Young D, et al: San Diego suicide study: Comparison of gay to straight males. Suicide Life Threat Behav 16:448, 1986.

179. van Heeringen C, Vincke J: Suicidal acts and ideation in homosexual and bisexual young people: A study of prevalence and risk factors. Soc Psychiatry Psychiatr Epidemiol 35:494-499, 2000.

180. Kitts RL: Gay adolescents and suicide: Understanding the association. Adolescence 40:621-628, 2005.

181. Remafedi G: Predictors of unprotected intercourse among gay and heterosexual youth: Knowledge, beliefs, and behavior. Pediatrics 94:163-168, 1994.

182. Rosario M, Meyer-Bahlburg HF, Hunter J, et al: Sexual risk behaviors of gay, lesbian, and bisexual youths in New York City: Prevalence and correlates. AIDS Educ Prev 11:476-496, 1999.

183. Osmond DH, Charlebois E, Haynes WS, et al: Comparison of risk factors for hepatitis C and hepatitis B virus infection in homosexual men. J Infect Dis 167:66, 1993.

184. Paroski PA: Health care delivery and the concerns of gay and lesbian adolescents. J Adolesc Health Care 8:188, 1987.

185. Remafedi G: Sexually transmitted diseases in homosexual youth. Adolesc Med 1:565-581, 1990.

186. Gourevitch MN: The epidemiology of HIV and AIDS. Med Clin North Am 80:1223, 1996.

187. Abadalian SE, Remafedi, G: Sexually transmitted diseases in young homosexual men. Semin Pediatr Infect Dis 4:122, 1993.

188. Povinelli M, Remafedi G, Tao G: Trend and predictors of human immunodeficiency virus antibody testing by homosexual and bisexual adolescent males. Arch Ped Adolesc Med 150(1):33-38, 1996.

189. Rosenberg PS: Back calculation models of age-specific HIV incidence rates. Stat Med 13:1975-1990, 1994.

190. Rosenberg PS, Biggar RJ, Goedert JJ: Declining age at HIV infection in the United States. N Eng J Med 330(11):789-790, 1994. No abstract available.

190a. Biggar RJ, Rosenberg PS: HIV infection/AIDS in the United States during the 1990s. Clin Infect Dis 1: S219-S223, 1993.

191. Futterman D, Hein K, Ruben N, et al: HIV-infected adolescents: The first 50 patients in a New York City program. Pediatrics 91:730, 1993.

192. Rosario M, Meyer-Bahlburg HFL, Hunter J, et al: Psychosexual Development of Lesbian, Gay, and Bisexual Youths: Sexual Activities, Sexual Orientation, and Sexual Identity. Presented at the Second International Conference on the Biopsychosocial Aspects of HIV Infection, Brighton, UK, 1996.

193. Day FA: Lesbian and Gay Voices: An Annotated Bibliography and Guide to Literature for Children and Young Adults. Westport, CT: Greenwood, 2000.

194. Rienzo BA, Button JW, Sheu JJ, et al: The politics of sexual orientation issues in American schools. J Sch Health 76:93-97, 2006.

195. Strommen EF: Family reactions to the disclosure of homosexuality. In Garnets LD, Kimmel DC, eds: Psychology Perspectives on Lesbian and Gay Male Experiences. New York: Columbia University Press, 1993, pp 248-266.

196. Goffman E: Stigma: Notes on the Management of a Spoiled Identity. New York: Simon & Schuster, 1963.

197. Borhek MV: Helping gay and lesbian adolescents and their families: A mother's perspective. J Adolesc Health Care 9:123-128, 1988.

198. Boxer AM, Cook JA, Herdt, G: Double jeopardy: Identity transitions and parent-child relations among gay and lesbian youth. In Pillemer K, McCartney K, eds: Parent-Child Relations throughout Life. Hillsdale, NJ: Erlbaum, 1991.

199. Nicolosi J, Byrd AD, Potts RW: Retrospective self-reports of changes in homosexual orientation: A consumer survey of conversion therapy clients. Psychol Rep 86:1071-1088, 2000.

200. American Academy of Pediatrics: Homosexuality and adolescence. Pediatrics 92:631, 1993.

201. American Psychiatric Association: Gay and Lesbian Issues Fact Sheet. Washington, DC: American Psychiatric Association, 1994.

202. American Psychological Association: Policy Statement on Discrimination against Homosexuals. Washington, DC: American Psychological Association, 1991.

203. National Association of Social Workers: Position Statement Regarding "Reparative" or "Conversion" Therapies for Lesbians and Gay Men. Washington, DC: National Association of Social Workers, 1992.

204. McNeill KF, Rienzi BM, Kposowa A: Families and parenting: A comparison of lesbian and heterosexual mothers. Psychol Rep 82:59-62, 1998.

205. Miller J, Jacobsen R, Bigner J: The child's home environment for lesbian vs. heterosexual mothers: A neglected area of research. J Homosex 7(1):49-56, 1981.

206. Pagelow M: Heterosexual and lesbian single mothers: A comparison of problems, coping, and solutions. J Homosex 5(3):189-204, 1980.

207. Parks CA: Lesbian parenthood: A review of the literature. Am J Orthopsychiatry 68:376-389, 1998.

208. Rand C, Graham DLR, Rawlings EI: Psychological health in lesbian mother trials. J Homosex 8(1):27-39, 1982.

209. Green R, Mandel J, Hotvedt M, et al: Lesbian mothers and their children: A comparison with solo parent homosexual mothers and their children. Arch Sex Behav 15, 1986.

210. Harris MB, Turner PH: Gay and lesbian parents. J Homosex 12(2):101-113, 1986.

211. Kweskin SL, Cook AS: Heterosexual and homosexual mothers' self-described sex-role behavior and ideal sex-role behavior in children. Sex Roles 8:967-975, 1982.

212. Golombok S, Cook R, Bish A, et al: Families created by the new reproductive technologies: Quality of parenting and social and emotional development of the children. Child Dev 66:285-298, 1995.

213. Gartrell N, Hamilton J, Banks A, et al: The National Lesbian Family Study: 1. Interviews with prospective mothers. Am J Orthopsychiatry 66:272-281, 1996.

214. Benkov L: Reinventing the Family. New York, Crown Publishers, 1994.

215. Koepke L, Hare J, Moran M: Relationship quality in a sample of lesbian couples with children and child-free lesbian couples. Fam Relat 41:224-229, 1992.

216. Hare J: Concerns and issues faced by families headed by a lesbian couple. Fam Society 75(1):27-35, 1994.

217. Bigner J, Jacobsen R: The value of children to gay and heterosexual fathers. J Homosex 18(1-2):163-172, 1989.

218. Bigner J, Jacobsen R: Parenting behaviors of homosexual and heterosexual fathers. J Homosex 18(1-2):173-186, 1989.

219. Bigner J, Jacobsen R: Adult responses to child behavior and attitudes toward fathering: Gay and nongay fathers. J Homosex 23(3):99-112, 1992.

220. Bigner JJ, Bozett FW: Parenting by gay fathers. In Bozett FW, Sussman MB, eds: Homosexuality and Family Relations. New York: Harrington Park Press, 1990, pp 155-157.

221. Barrett H, Tasker F: Growing up with a gay parent: Views of 101 gay fathers on their sons' and daughters' experiences. Educ Child Psychol 18:62-75, 2001.

222. Bozett FW: Gay men as fathers. In Hanson SMH, Bozett FW, eds: Dimensions in Fatherhood. Beverly Hills, CA: Sage Publications, 1985.

223. Bozett FW: Gay fathers: A review of the literature. J Homosex 18(1-2):137-162, 1989.

224. Hoeffer B: Children's acquisition of sex-role behavior in lesbian-mother families. Am J Orthopsychiatry 51:536-544, 1981.

225. Kirkpatrick M, Smith C, Roy R: Lesbian mothers and their children: A comparative survey. Am J Orthopsychiatry 51:545-551, 1981.

226. Golombok S, Spencer A, Rutter M: Children in lesbian and single parent households: Psychosexual and psychiatric appraisal. J Child Psychol Psychiatry 24:551-572, 1983.

227. Gottman J: Children of gay and lesbian parents. Marriage Fam Rev 14:177-196, 1989.

228. Huggins SL: A comparative study of self-esteem of adolescent children of divorced lesbian mothers and divorced heterosexual mothers. In Bozett FW, ed: Homosexuality and the Family. New York: Harrington Park Press, 1989, pp 123-135.

229. Javaid G: The children of homosexual and heterosexual single mothers. Child Psychiatry Hum Dev 234:235-248, 1993.

230. Golombok S, Tasker F: Children in lesbian and gay families: Theories and evidence. Annu Rev Sex Res 5:73-100, 1994.

231. Golombok S, Tasker F, Murray C: Children raised in fatherless families from infancy: Family relationships and the socioemotional development of children of lesbian and single heterosexual mothers. J Child Psychol Psychiatry 38:783-791, 1997.

232. Patterson CJ: Children of the lesbian baby boom: Behavioral adjustment, self-concepts, and sex-role identity. In Greene B, Herek G, eds: Contemporary Perspectives on Lesbian and Gay Psychology: Theory, Research, and Application. Beverly Hills, CA: Sage Publications, 1994, pp 156-175.

233. Patterson CJ: Lesbian mothers and their children: Findings from the Bay Area Families Study. In Laird J, Green RJ, eds: Lesbians and Gays in Couples and Families: A Handbook for Therapists. San Francisco: Jossey-Bass, 1996, pp 420-438.

234. Patterson C: Children of lesbian and gay parents. Clin Child Psychol 19:235-281, 1997.

235. Gartrell N, Banks A, Reed N, et al: The National Lesbian Family Study: 3. Interviews with mothers of five-year-olds. Am J Orthopsychiatry 70:542-548, 2000.

236. McCandlish B: Against all odds: Lesbian mother family dynamics. In Bozett FW, ed: Gay and Lesbian Parents. New York: Praeger, 1987.

237. Steckel A: Psychosocial development of children of lesbian mothers. In Bozett FW, ed: Gay and Lesbian Parents. New York: Praeger, 1987, pp 75-85.

238. Stacey J, Biblarz TJ: (How) Does the sexual orientation of parents matter? Am Sociol Rev 66:159-183, 2001.

239. Gartrell N, Deck A, Rodas C, et al: The National Lesbian Family Study: 4. Interviews with the 10-year-old children. Am J Orthopsychiatry 75:518-524, 2005.

240. Patterson CJ: Families of the lesbian baby boom: Parents' division of labor and children's adjustment. Dev Psychol 31:115-123, 1995.

241. Chan R, Raboy B, Patterson C: Psychosocial adjustment among children conceived via donor insemination by lesbian and heterosexual mothers. Child Dev 69:443-457, 1998.

242. Patterson C, Hurt S, Mason CD: Families of the lesbian baby boom: Children's contact with grandparents and other adults. Am J Orthopsychiatry 68:390-399, 1998.

243. Golombok S, Perry B, Burston A, et al: Children with lesbian parents: A community study. Dev Psychol 39:20-33, 2003.

244. Wainright J, Russell S, Patterson C: Psychosocial adjustment, school outcomes, and romantic relationships of adolescents with same-sex parents. Child Dev 75:1886-1898, 2004.

245. Meezan W, Rauch J: Gay marriage, same-sex parenting, and America's children. Future Child 15:97-115, 2005.

246. Weisner TS, Wilson-Mitchell JE: Nonconventional family lifestyles and sex typing in six year olds. Child Dev 61:1915-1933, 1990.

247. MacCallum F, Golombok S: Children raised in fatherless families from infancy: A follow-up of children of lesbian and single heterosexual mothers at early adolescence. J Child Psychol Psychiatry 45:1407-1419, 2004.

248. Bailey JM, Bobrow D, Wolfe M, et al: Sexual orientation of adult sons of gay fathers. Dev Psychol 31:124-129, 1995.

249. Rosenberg M: Children with gender identity issues and their parents. J Am Acad Child Adolesc Psychiatry 41:619-621, 2002.

250. Frankowski BL, American Academy of Pediatrics Committee on Adolescence: Sexual orientation and adolescents. Pediatrics 113:1827-1832, 2004.

251. Klitzman RL, Greenberg JD: Patterns of communication between gay and lesbian patients and their health care providers. J Homosex 42(4):65-75, 2002.

252. Meckler GD, Elliott MN, Kanouse DE, et al: Nondisclosure of sexual orientation to a physician among a sample of gay, lesbian and bisexual youth. Arch Pediatr Adolesc Med 160:1248-1254, 2006.

253. Perrin EC: Pediatricians' Caring for Complex Psychosocial Issues. Presented at the annual meeting of the Society for Research in Child Development, Atlanta GA, April 1997.

254. Perrin EC: Attitudes of Pediatricians about Psychosocial Issues. Presented at the annual meeting of the Ambulatory Pediatric Association, Washington DC, May 1997.

255. Lena SM, Wiebe T, Ingram S, et al: Pediatricians' knowledge, perceptions, and attitudes towards providing health care for lesbian, gay, and bisexual adolescents. Ann R Coll Physicians Surg Can 35:406-410, 2002.

256. Lena SM, Wiebe T, Ingram S, et al: Pediatric residents' knowledge, perceptions, and attitudes towards homosexually oriented youth. Ann R Coll Physicians Surg Can 35:401-405, 2002.

257. American Academy of Pediatrics: Gay, Lesbian, and Bisexual Teens: Facts for Teens and Their Parents.

258. Futterweit W: Endocrine therapy of transsexualism and potential complications of long-term treatment. Arch Sex Behav 27:209-226, 1998.

259. Cohen-Kettenis PT, van Goozen SHM: Pubertal delay as an aid in diagnosis and treatment of a transsexual adolescent. Eur Child Adolesc Psychiatry 7:246, 1998.

260. Gooren L, Delemarre-van de Waal H: The feasibility of endocrine interventions in juvenile transsexuals. J Psychol Hum Sex 8:69-74, 1996.

261. American Academy of Pediatrics: Gay, Lesbian, or Bisexual Parents: Information for Children and Parents.

262. Bowe J: Gay donor or gay dad? N Y Times Mag (November):1966, 2006.

263. Lambert EG, Ventura LA, Hall DE, et al: College students' views on gay and lesbian issues: does education make a difference. J Homosex 50(4):1-30, 2006.

264. Green R: Sexual identity of 37 children raised by homosexual or transsexual parents. American Journal of Psychiatry 135:692-697, 1978.

265. Miller B: Gay fathers and their children. The Family Coordinator 28:544-552, 1979.

266. Turner PN, Scadden L, Harris MB: Parenting in gay and lesbian families. Journal of Gay and Lesbian Psychotherapy 1:55-66, 1990.

267. Osterweil DA: Correlates of relationship satisfaction in lesbian couples who are parenting their first child together (Unpublished doctoral dissertation, California School of Professional Psychology, Berkeley, 1991.)

268. Bailey JM, Bobrow D, Wolfe M, et al: Sexual orientation of adult sons of gay fathers. Developmental Psychology 31(1):124-129, 1995.

269. Gartrell N, Banks A, Hamilton J, et al: The National Lesbian Family Study: 2. Interviews with mothers of toddlers. American Journal of Orthopsychiatry 69(3):362-369, 1999.

270. Mitchell V: Two moms: Contribution of the planned lesbian family to the deconstruction of gendered parenting. *In* Laird J, Green RJ, eds: Lesbians and gays in couples and families: A handbook for therapists (pp 343-357). San Francisco: Jossey-Bass, 1996.

271. Sullivan J: "Rosie and Harriet?": Gender and family patterns of lesbian co-parents. Gender and Society 10:747-767, 1996.

272. Flaks D, Ficher I, Masterpasqua F, et al: Lesbians choosing motherhood: A comparative study of lesbian and heterosexual parents and their children. Developmental Psychology 31(1):105-114, 1995.

273. Brewaeys A, Ponjaert I, van Hall EV, et al: Donor insemination: Child development and family functioning in lesbian mother families. Human Reproduction 12(6):1349-1359, 1997.

274. Chan R, Raboy B, Patterson C, et al: Psychosocial adjustment among children conceived via donor insemination by lesbian and heterosexual mothers. Child Development 69(2):443-457, 1998.

275. Wainright J, Russell S, Patterson C, et al: Psychosocial adjustment, school outcomes, and romantic relationships of adolescents with same-sex parents. Child Dev 75:1886-1898, 2004.

Atypical Behavior: Self-Injury and Pica

ROWLAND P. BARRETT

Atypical behavior, in the form of self-injury and pica, are among the most perplexing forms of psychopathology in children and adolescents. Both are highly conspicuous behavioral phenomena that, despite many years of clinical interest and dedicated research, are not well understood. A variety of theories have been offered to explain the motivational and biological bases underlying these behaviors. However, the true reason why children and adolescents engage in such activities remains a mystery. The purpose of this chapter is to review the definition, taxonomy, and prevalence of self-injury and pica in children and adolescents. In addition, the chapter contains a review of advances made toward understanding the motivational and biological bases for engaging in these behaviors, a discussion of the indications for intervention, and a review of the latest empirically based treatment approaches.

SELF-INJURIOUS BEHAVIOR

Self-injurious behavior is defined as the deliberate infliction of harm to one's own body.[1] Self-injury in children and adolescents may take various forms, ranging from severe and suicidal behavior to relatively mild and socially acceptable tattooing, piercing, and branding. This chapter, however, focuses on the two subtypes of self-injurious behavior with which patients most commonly present for treatment: stereotyped self-injury and impulsive self-injury. *Stereotyped self-injury* is repetitive in nature and are observed mostly in children and adolescents with autism spectrum disorders, mental retardation, and developmental disabilities.[2] *Impulsive self-injury* takes the form of a habitual behavior frequently encountered in adolescents and associated with serious personality disorder.[3]

Common forms of stereotyped self-injury in children and adolescents with developmental disabilities include self-biting, self-punching, self-scratching, self-pinching, and repetitive banging of the head and limbs against solid, unyielding surfaces such as walls, tables, and floors. Less common forms of stereotyped self-injury include repeatedly dislocating and relocating joints (especially the fingers and jaw); repetitive eye pressing and gouging; pulling out one's own hair, teeth, or fingernails; and twisting or tearing of the ears and genitals. Deliberate and forceful striking of the knee to the face and head is a unique and potentially lethal form of stereotyped self-injury that may result in detached retinas, serious damage to soft tissue, and fracture of the mandible and periorbital area. In rare cases, death results. Fortunately, most children with developmental disabilities who engage in stereotyped self-injury respond favorably to treatment. Behavior therapy with positive reinforcement strategies,[4] medication,[5] and various combinations of behavior therapy and medication[6] are frequently reported as successful in virtually eliminating the disorder. However, a significant minority of children with special needs are unresponsive to treatment. Stereotyped self-injury in this refractory group is at high risk of escalating to life-threatening proportions, and as a result, affected children must use highly restrictive protective equipment, such as helmets, padded mitts, and arm and leg restraints, among other individually tailored pieces of protective clothing.[7]

The principal forms of impulsive self-injury, sometimes referred to as *self-mutilation*, include skin cutting and skin burning.[8] However, episodic self-hitting, self-rubbing, self-scratching, and needle-sticking also may be observed. Skin cutting may be performed with a sharp conventional instrument, such as a razor blade, scissors, or a paring knife, or with a relatively blunt mechanism, such as a table knife. Skin cutting also may be accomplished with unconventional but nonetheless sharp objects, such as a wood splinter, a nail or screw, a bottle cap, a glass shard, and paper. Skin burning is frequently accomplished with lighted cigarettes and matches. However, the use of heated metal is not uncommon, and the use of a heated light bulb is an overlooked source. The typical profile associated with impulsive self-injury involves a mid- to late adolescent child of average or above average intelligence with comorbid borderline personality disorder and/or depression.[9] Impulsive self-injurious acts are typically superficial in nature, with a low risk of lethality. Approximately two thirds of adolescents who have engaged in impulsive self-injury have reported experiencing some form of a sense of relief after an episode.[10] Psychosocial approaches to the treatment of impulsive self-injury tend to focus on the underlying personality disorder or affective illness and include behavior modification, cognitive-behavioral therapy (specifically, cognitive restructuring), and dialectical behavior therapy (DBT).[11] Similarly, pharmacotherapy for impulsive self-injury follows loosely established guidelines for treatment of personality disorder and affective disorder; selective serotonin reuptake inhibitors (SSRIs) and low-dose atypical antipsychotic medications are first- and second-line drug treatments, respectively.[12]

Prevalence

Stereotyped self-injurious behavior affects approximately 16% of the child and adolescent population with pervasive developmental disorder (autism, Rett syndrome, Asperger syndrome, pervasive developmental disorder not otherwise specified), and mental retardation.[13] Prevalence rates vary in accordance with the level of severity of developmental disability. Self-injury is rare (1%) in children with mild mental retardation. Prevalence rates of self-injury are 9% among children with moderate mental retardation, whereas they are 16% and 27% among children with severe and profound mental retardation, respectively. There is a slightly higher relative prevalence among boys (53%).

Impulsive self-injury affects approximately 1.5% to 3% of the adolescent population.[14] Rates of 40% to 61% have been reported for samples of adolescent psychiatric inpatients.[15] Prevalence rates of impulsive self-injury as high as 80% have been reported among adolescents and young adults with borderline personality disorder. Intermittent explosive disorder (75%), post-traumatic stress disorder (60%), substance abuse disorder (50%), and eating disorder (48%) are additional psychiatric conditions with elevated prevalence rates of self-injury.[16] Conduct problems, anxiety disorders, obsessive-compulsive disorder, affective disorder, eating disorder, substance abuse, family violence, family alcohol abuse, sexual abuse, and physical abuse are also frequently present in the developmental histories of adolescents with impulsive self-injury.[17]

Cause

The mechanisms by which self-injurious behavior is developed and maintained are not well understood. For the most part, children and adolescents who engage in either stereotyped or impulsive self-injury are a heterogeneous and ill-defined group. Despite the fact that they may be grouped into two broad categories (i.e., developmental disabilities and personality disorder) on the basis of diagnoses, the reasons why a particular child or adolescent engages in self-injury may be entirely different from those for another child or adolescent who engages in self-injury, even if the diagnoses of the two children are the same and the self-injurious behavior in question takes the same form. In this regard, researchers[18-20] have delineated a number of motivational and biological hypotheses fundamental for children and adolescents who engage in self-injurious behavior. Of importance is that none of the proposed hypotheses are viewed as excluding each other. It is highly likely—and, in fact, expected—that one hypothesis overlaps with and complements one or more of the other hypotheses.

LEARNING THEORY

Learning theory encapsulates two differing rationales to account for self-injurious behavior, regardless of whether the nature of the behavior is stereotyped or impulsive. These include (1) the *positive reinforcement hypothesis,* whereby self-injurious acts are performed to gain access to a preferred goal state, and (2) the *negative reinforcement hypothesis,* whereby self-injurious acts are engaged in order to escape an aversive condition. According to learning theory, a child or adolescent may engage in self-injurious behavior, such as stereotyped head banging or impulsive skin cutting, either to gain access to something that they experience as pleasant, such as social attention, which is contingent on performance of the self-injurious act (positive reinforcement), or to escape from something that they experience as unpleasant, such as social demands, suspension of which is contingent on performance of the self-injurious act (negative reinforcement). In either case, when self-injury results in access to a pleasant condition or facilitates escape from an unpleasant circumstance, the result is a strengthening (reinforcement) of the self-injurious behavior.

Self-injury in children and adolescents is a dramatic event that draws immediate attention and concern from adults. Parents, siblings, teachers, and friends, acting in good faith, may intuitively seek to provide comforting measures or modify and suspend limits or demands on a child or adolescent because it has the effect of stopping the self-injury, at least for the time being. In this regard, learning theory provides a useful insight as to how self-injury may be inadvertently reinforced and maintained by caretakers. Under certain circumstances, comforting measures intended to stop self-injury may result, paradoxically, in an increased frequency of the child's self-injurious behavior because the child receives attention and caring after engaging in self-injury.[20a] Similarly, modifying or eliminating expectations in response to a child's self-injury also runs the risk of inadvertently teaching the child that self-injury is an effective way to communicate protest and to escape from nonpreferred tasks or stressful situations. The immediate effects of providing either comforting measures or "giving in" to the child's protests quite often results in the temporary interruption of self-injurious behavior. In the long run, however, these approaches are likely to have the unintentional effect of promoting and strengthening self-injurious behavior and worsening the child's problem.

SELF-REGULATORY (HOMEOSTATIC) THEORY

According to homeostatic theory, both stereotyped and impulsive self-injurious behaviors are considered self-stimulatory in nature and take the form of either arousal-inducing or arousal-reducing behaviors. In this perspective, when the optimal level of psychological stimulation is not available to a child, the child engages in compensatory activity, including self-injury, in an attempt to generate a more favorable or comfortable level of stimulation. Thus, the child is seen as self-regulating sensory stimulation by altering his or her level of arousal in relation to perceived changes in psychological stimuli. Underlying self-regulatory theory is the belief that children and adolescents (as well as adults) strive inherently to maintain a balanced level of central nervous system activation. That a certain degree of sensory stimulation is not only optimal, but also necessary, is a central tenet of the self-regulatory (homeostatic) hypothesis. Environmental sources of sensory stimulation, in the form of auditory, visual, tactile, vestibular, and kinesthetic modalities must be balanced and maintained at sufficient levels in order to avoid an internal sensation of discomfort. The same is true for cognitive and affective sources of sensory stimulation. According to self-regulatory theory, when the existing source of psychological stimulation does not fulfill the needs of the child, the underaroused child engages in self-injurious acts in an attempt to reach a balanced and sufficient level of sensory stimulation. Conversely, self-injurious acts also may function as self-stimulatory behaviors that regulate central nervous system activity when a child is overaroused. Engaging in proximal and monotonous self-injury is viewed as a means of effectively blocking potentially overwhelming psychological stimulation and achieving a lower and balanced arousal level.

The increased level of stereotyped self-injurious behavior displayed by children with autism spectrum disorder and mental retardation is hypothesized to be the result of striving to achieve this balance within a central nervous system that may be less reactive to distal environmental stimuli and more reactive to proximal stimulus conditions, because of the underlying nature of a developmental disability typified by cognitive deficit. This same self-regulatory hypothesis may be applied to adolescents with impulsive self-injury, who may experience underarousal or overarousal as a function of personality disorder or an affective illness, such as major depression, dysthymia, or bipolar disorder. When the adolescent's internal balance of cognitive and/or affective sources of sensory stimulation is disrupted and he or she becomes either overaroused because of a perceived abundance of psychological stimulation or underaroused because of a perceived lack of stimulation, self-injurious behavior may serve a compensatory function and act to restore homeostasis.

DEVELOPMENTAL THEORY

According to developmental theory, self-injury is a unique subset of behaviors emerging from the larger category of repetitive behaviors commonly observed in infancy.[21] In this regard, repetitive behavior is seen as occurring during the normal progression of early developmental stages and reflective of the child's maturational process. Piaget[22] viewed repetitive motor movements as reflecting the earliest stages of intellectual growth (i.e., sensorimotor period of development). For the infant, engaging in repetitive acts, or "circular reactions," as Piaget termed them, emerges from an innate propensity for repetition, which allows infants to learn about their bodies. During the first year of life, the extent to which infants continue to engage in repetitive activity affects their ability to develop adaptive environment manipulation, which ultimately, helps them understand the world. Repetitive behavior would then decrease across the normal developmental trajectory as the child learns more adaptive and mature behavior, such as communication, to interact with the environment.

For children not progressing in accordance with the normal developmental trajectory, engaging in repetitive behavior was said to have become "fixated" at levels of primary and secondary circular reactions. Repetitive motor mannerisms directed toward the self were said to represent primary circular reactions, whereas repetitive motor mannerisms directed toward the environment were said to represent secondary circular reactions. Fixation, in this regard, was representative of not only a slower development but also a deceleration and termination of progress in the latter stages of the developmental period, in which continuing cognitive growth was anticipated. In sum, fixation was thought to occur when the course of normal development was disrupted as a result of inadequate learning experience, lack of appropriate stimuli, absence of critical role models, or physical and/or cognitive impairment.

Accordingly, self-injurious behavior is viewed as resulting from the stalling of an otherwise normal and transient stage of development. Repetitive self-injurious behavior has been observed in 5% of normally developing infants and toddlers before the age of 36 months,[23] usually in the form of head banging in the crib and usually with the clear communicative intent to be picked up, fed, burped, changed, or comforted because of sickness. The advent of language in the normally developing child results in no further self-injury. For children with autism spectrum disorder and mental retardation who fail to acquire language, repetitive self-injurious behavior becomes stereotypic in nature because of a "fixed primary circular reaction" based in earlier learning, in which it proved to be an efficacious means of communicating protest and discomfort and/or gaining access to care and comforting measures. It may be argued that this same line of reasoning, which overlaps extensively with the positive and negative reinforcement hypotheses of learning theory, may be applied to adolescents with impulsive self-injurious behavior and borderline personality disorder, in which a constant demand for attention is characteristic of the disorder, or those with affective disorder, in which the need to communicate distress and access safety and comforting measures may be paramount.

ORGANIC THEORY

According to organic theory, self-injurious behavior may be the product either of a genetic disorder or a nongenetic health condition. Smith-Magenis syndrome,[24] Lesch-Nyhan syndrome,[25] Prader-Willi syndrome,[26] Cornelia de Lange syndrome,[27] and Rett syndrome[28] are examples of mental retardation syndromes in which chronic self-injury is characteristic of the developmental disorder. A complex motor tic, such as self-slapping or skin picking, associated with Tourette syndrome[29] also is an example of a genetic disorder that may involve stereotyped self-injury. However, organic theory also allows for self-injurious behavior to occur as an artifact of a nongenetic health condition, such as epilepsy,[30] otitis media,[31] headache, toothache and constipation,[32] menstrual pain,[33] gastroesophageal reflux disease,[34] and sleep difficulties.[35] Children with autism spectrum disorders and mental retardation who are nonverbal and lack an effective means for communicating distress and illness may

resort to self-injury in the form of repeatedly pressing or hitting an affected area possibly to achieve an anesthetic effect, or they may merely attack the affected area out of frustration over the discomfort it creates. Adolescents with personality disorder and/or affective illness also may experience an increased risk of impulsive self-injury as the result of an unrecognized health condition that produces pain, elevates discomfort, increases anxiety and agitation, or depresses mood. In this regard, they, too, may engage in self-injurious behavior in order to gain access to the "sense of relief" commonly reported to follow an episode of impulsive self-injury.

NEUROBIOLOGICAL THEORY

Research on the neurobiological mechanisms that underlie self-injurious behavior is an outgrowth of studies aimed at understanding why children with developmental disabilities engage in the larger class of stereotypic responding and, similarly, why adolescents with borderline personality disorder and comorbid affective disorder may experience an impulse to engage in self-injury. In this regard, the neurobiological perspective views dopaminergic, serotoninergic, and opioid mechanisms as playing a major role in the advent and maintenance of self-injurious behavior.

The dopamine hypothesis[36] is pursued largely because of the known association of alterations in basal ganglia dopamine with repetitive behaviors and the behavioral comparability of seemingly driven repetitive behavior with stereotypical and impulsive forms of self-injury. According to the dopamine hypothesis, self-injurious behavior results from a deficiency of dopamine that causes receptor sites to develop "supersensitivity" to the neurotransmitter, so that low levels of dopamine across the transmission sites create exaggerated excitability and result in basal ganglia dysfunction. Support for a dopamine hypothesis is derived from positron emission tomographic studies that demonstrate dopaminergic deficits associated with Lesch-Nyhan syndrome, a disorder characterized by stereotyped self-injury in the form of repetitive lip and finger biting. Additional support may be observed in studies of children with autism in which bromocriptine, a dopamine agonist, produced marked improvement in a variety of repetitive behavior disorders, as well as studies of so-called atypical antipsychotics, which block D_2 dopamine receptors and have been observed to be moderately effective in decreasing self-injury in children with developmental disabilities.

According to the serotoninergic hypothesis,[37] self-injurious behavior is caused by alterations in serotoninergic functioning that result in pathologically altered mood and, ultimately, failure of impulse control. Approximately 50% of adolescents with personality disorder and/or affective disorder admit to thinking about engaging in self-injury less than 1 hour before acting to cut or burn themselves. The serotonin hypothesis also gains support from findings that serotonin uptake inhibitors, such as clomipramine, have been demonstrated as a moderately effective treatment of self-injurious behavior. Additional support for a serotoninergic hypothesis is derived from studies that have shown increased self-injury after depletion or administration of selected precursors that act on serotoninergic neurotransmission.

The role of endogenous opiates[38] in self-injurious behavior is sought to explain both stereotyped and impulsive responding. In this regard, it has been hypothesized that for some children and adolescents, specifically, those with a demonstrated insensitivity to pain, self-injury may occur in response to a state of sensory depression brought about by chronic elevation of endogenous opiates. A second and more widely postulated theory suggests that some children with autism spectrum disorder and mental retardation may engage in stereotyped self-injurious behavior in order to gain access to endogenous opiates and, more specifically, to the favorable sensory consequence associated with its narcotic effect. This same line of reasoning may be applied to adolescents with borderline personality disorder or affective illness. Thus, gaining access to endogenous opiates through self-injury may, ironically, result in an improved sense of well-being. It is further speculated that the same children and adolescents may continue to hurt themselves, day after day, because they become addicted to the rewarding sensory consequence of the endorphins.

PSYCHODYNAMIC THEORY

Psychodynamic theory was formulated primarily as an attempt to explain impulsive self-injury in adolescent (and adult) populations with comorbid personality and affective disorders.[39] It is based on the self-disclosures of individuals with a history of self-injurious behavior and, to a greater extent, on the interpretation of these self-reports by professionals charged with providing treatment. Consequently, several hypotheses generated by psychodynamic theory cannot be empirically validated. However, many of the proposed causal mechanisms very clearly and extensively overlap with much of what has been previously reviewed with regard to learning, self-regulatory, developmental, organic, and neurobiological theories. In this regard, psychodynamic theory purports that children and adolescents engage in self-injury for a variety of reasons,[40] including (1) to gain access to care and comforting; (2) to distract themselves from emotional pain by causing physical pain;

(3) to act as a compromise between life and death drives; (4) to punish themselves; (5) to relieve tension; (6) to feel "real" by feeling pain or seeing evidence of injury; (7) to end a dissociative episode; (8) to feel numb, "zoned out," calm, or at peace; (9) to experience euphoric feelings; (10) to communicate their pain, anger, or other emotions to others; and (11) to nurture themselves through the process of the self-care of their wounds.

Diagnosis and Assessment Issues

Although most stereotyped and impulsive self-injurious responders are children with developmental disabilities and adolescents with serious personality disorders and/or affective illness, respectively, not every child or adolescent with these diagnoses engages in self-injurious behavior. Therefore, the assessment of self-injury must go beyond merely identifying neurodevelopmental characteristics and comorbid psychiatric features. It also must advance beyond listing the topography of the self-injury and establishing its magnitude or severity. The assessment of self-injury must be comprehensive and designed to identify the reason why the child or adolescent engages in the behavior. Seeking to establish the role of self-injury in the behavioral repertoire of a child or adolescent is an approach known as the *functional assessment of behavior*.[41] Conducting a functional assessment of self-injurious behavior is crucial in determining which of the previously mentioned motivational and/or biological hypotheses (and combinations thereof) may be operational for any specific child.

A functional behavioral assessment of self-injury includes analyzing both the antecedent and consequent conditions that surround the self-injurious act: that is, assessing the conditions that immediately preceded the self-injurious response, as well as what resulted for the child or adolescent after he or she engaged in the self-injurious behavior. The goal of the functional assessment is to delineate causal circumstances—the events that prompted or cued the child or adolescent to engage in self-injury—as well as to identify the function or role served by the self-injurious behavior. Did the self-injury result in social attention? Did it facilitate escape from a nonpreferred or unpleasant situation? Was it a response to isolation or boredom? Did it appear to have a communicative intent, such as protest? Was the child sick (fever, headache, toothache, stomachache)? Does the child have a history of complex motor tic disorder? Does the child have a genetic disorder (mental retardation syndrome) or a chronic medical condition (epilepsy) or psychiatric condition (affective disorder)? Did the injury appear (ironically) to provide relief from discomfort? These and similar questions, including the developmental history of the behavior, must be addressed through a careful analysis of conditions surrounding the self-injurious event in order to determine the function or role played by self-injury and, consequently, how best it may be treated.

A variety of structured interviews, such as the Functional Assessment Interview,[42] the Functional Assessment Checklist for Teachers and Staff,[43] and the Student Guided Functional Assessment Interview,[44] as well as standardized questionnaires, such as the Questions About Behavioral Function Scale,[45] the Motivation Assessment Scale,[46] the Stereotypy Analysis Scale,[47] and the Detailed Behavior Report,[48] may be used to gather information about the antecedent and consequent stimuli that may be acting to maintain stereotyped self-injurious behavior in children and adolescents with developmental disabilities. Similarly, a functional approach to the assessment of self-harm in adolescents who engage in impulsive, superficial forms of self-injury may use a variety of structured interview techniques and questionnaires, including the Functional Assessment of Self-Mutilation Scale,[49] the Self-Harm Behavior Questionnaire,[50] and the Self-Harm Inventory.[51] The Scale Points for Lethality Assessment[52] also may prove useful in helping the clinician determine the potential risk of harm inherent to the patient's impulsive self-injurious acts.

Treatment

STEREOTYPED SELF-INJURY

More than $20 billion has been spent in the care and treatment of children with autism spectrum disorders and mental retardation who have engaged in stereotyped self-injurious behavior since 2000. Most children with stereotyped self-injury respond favorably to behavior modification approaches in which positive reinforcement strategies are used. The majority of these approaches are complicated multimodal treatments that include careful functional behavioral analysis, differential reinforcement procedures, and intensive communication skills training. However, a few simple and straightforward learning-based approaches also have proved to be effective.

Behavior Modification

Studies in which learning-based behavior modification strategies are used[53] account for the majority of the applied research on children with special needs who engage in stereotyped self-injurious behavior. Behavior modification aims to decrease the magnitude (frequency, duration, intensity) of a child's self-injury by directly manipulating the causal antecedents and consequences surrounding the behavior.

ENVIRONMENTAL MODIFICATION

Environmental modification is the simplest example of a behavior modification strategy. This approach targets reliably occurring environmental antecedents of self-injury and facilitates making changes in the environment that will lead to a reduction in the behavior. Environmental analysis can provide a means for assessing the conditions likely to promote stereotyped self-injurious behavior and provide indications for structural rearrangements. For example, stereotyped self-injurious behavior is well known to vary with situational factors, such as room size, the number of people present in a room, and noise level. Stereotyped self-injurious behavior also may vary in accordance with the availability of a preferred activity within a particular setting. For example, a classroom or home setting that includes a smaller room with fewer people and less noise, is highly structured with a predictable routine, and is well managed, in that it facilitates access to preferred activities, often is the foundation for observations of decreased self-injurious responding.

DIFFERENTIAL USE OF POSITIVE REINFORCEMENT

The differential use of positive reinforcement is another behavior modification strategy frequently used to reduce a child's stereotyped self-injurious behavior. This approach is considered labor intensive. It requires a great deal of time and energy in terms of close observation of the child across designated time periods, maintenance of a careful timing procedure, and delivering rewards in an accurate and timely manner. Attention to procedural detail is crucial for success. The most successful differential positive reinforcement strategy involves training adaptive behavior that is incompatible with engaging in self-injury, such as teaching children with autism and mental retardation to play with a variety of toys, followed by rewards in the form of edibles, tickles, or music or rewarding the omission of self-injury for progressively longer periods of time with tokens that may be "cashed in" for access to preferred activities.

COMMUNICATION SKILLS TRAINING

The development of functional communication skills is an additional form of learning-based training and an effective means of intervention, regardless of whether the self-injurious behavior is attention seeking or escape motivated. In this regard, a child who is nonverbal may be taught to attract social attention or request to leave an uncomfortable, distressing, or simply nonpreferred situation in a more adaptive manner by using an alternative form of communication, such as sign language, a picture communication board, and gestures. The use of differential reinforcement strategies, in combination with alternative forms of communication, is also a commonly employed and successful strategy for decreasing self-injurious behavior in children with developmental disabilities.

EXTINCTION (PLANNED IGNORING) AND INTERRUPTION-EXTINCTION (RESPONSE PREVENTION)

Self-injurious behavior that is escape driven and maintained by negative reinforcement may be an indication for the use of *extinction* as a viable treatment. Extinction occurs when a previously rewarded behavior is no longer rewarded. In other words, self-injurious behavior, rewarded because it resulted in the avoidance or escape from an unpleasant circumstance, diminishes and is eventually extinguished if it no longer results in a reward. If, for example, a child engages in self-injurious behavior to avoid classroom tasks, ignoring the self-injury results in its extinction. By not being allowed to avoid the tasks, the child learns that engaging in self-injurious behavior does not result in a discontinuation of (or escape from) the activity. Of course, use of the extinction model is often compromised by the reality that the child cannot be left to engage in self-injury as a means of learning that it will no longer be rewarded. In situations in which an extinction approach is indicated but, realistically, cannot be employed, a modified strategy known as *interruption-extinction* may prove to be effective. In this approach, the self-injurious behavior is prevented from occurring by blocking the intended response. If, for example, a child slaps his or her face in an attempt to escape a classroom task, placement of a teacher's aid whose job is to interrupt all attempts at face slapping and keep the child working on the task at hand will, across time, result in the child's abandoning the self-injurious behavior because it no longer results in the desired escape from the activity.

Pharmacotherapy

Approximately 65% of children and adolescents with developmental disabilities respond favorably to treatment of their self-injury with behavior modification. An additional 30% of children with developmental disabilities respond favorably to the use of behavior modification in combination with various medications.[5,6] Neuroleptic drugs have a long history of being used to combat self-injury by children and adolescents with autism spectrum disorders and mental retardation, with mixed results.[54] Both low and high doses of thioridazine have been found equally effective in reducing the rate of stereotyped behavior, including self-injury. Several additional studies with D_2 antagonists, such as haloperidol, have demonstrated decreased stereotyped responding, as well as decreased social withdrawal, hyperactivity, angry affect, and negative attitude. However, the presence of significant adverse effects associated with the use of neuroleptic agents, such as dystonia and tardive dyskinesia, has prompted the increased exploration of newer, alternative medications such as the so-called atypical antipsychotic drugs (e.g., risperidone, olanzapine) as treatment of self-injury.[55] These medications block D_2 dopamine receptors, as well as 5-HT_2 receptors, and have been reported as effecting decreases in stereotyped self-injury in adolescents and young adults with mental retardation. Unfortunately, few controlled studies have been performed. Nevertheless, there is a promise of efficacy associated with these new medications that rests in the relative absence of any negative effect on cognition, as well as fewer other adverse effects typically associated with the use of older neuroleptic medications.[56] SSRIs also represent a newer class of drugs that have been investigated as treatment for stereotyped self-injury, in part because of the similarity of seemingly driven stereotyped self-injury with compulsive behavior and also because of the fewer side effects associated with these medications. Fluoxetine is one such SSRI that has been studied in several open clinical trials and has been found to decrease perseverative, compulsive, and stereotyped behavior,[57] as well as inappropriate speech, mood lability, and lethargy.

An opiate antagonist, naltrexone, is also used clinically. Preliminary data support the notion that self-injurious responding in some children and adolescents with developmental disabilities may be linked to defects in the pro-opiomelanocortin (POMC) system.[38] If a child demonstrates hyposensitivity to pain, naltrexone may upregulate receptors and improve nociception. Consequently, self-injury may decrease if it is experienced by the child as an aversive event. For children who may engage in repetitive self-injury in order to gain access to the narcotic effect of endogenous opiates, naltrexone acts to block opiate receptors and, consequently, eliminates the favorable sensory consequence serving to reward and maintain the behavior.[58] In the absence of a favorable sensory consequence, the self-injurious behavior should be extinguished.

Despite the potential benefits that may be derived from pharmacotherapy in any particular case involving self-injurious behavior, parents and professionals continue to express concern regarding the use of medication, particularly with children who have special needs. Direct care staff members responsible for the day-to-day management of children with developmental disabilities considered behavior modification to be a viable alternative to drug treatment for stereotyped self-injury.[59] Similarly, mothers seeking behavior management training for their children with mild to moderate mental retardation preferred positive reinforcement procedures over medication.[60] Although the opinions of parents and paraprofessionals are valid and certainly worthy of consideration, research has long supported the efficacy of combining medication with a variety of behavioral interventions in order to reduce or eliminate stereotyped self-injury in children with developmental disabilities.

Exercise

A review of interventions used to suppress the rate of stereotyped self-injury in children with autism spectrum disorder and mental retardation is not complete without reference to the use of physical exercise.[61] Exercise may act on dopamine receptors by increasing the dopamine metabolite norepinephrine, which, in turn, may serve to counterbalance the absence of dopamine and reduce the potential for supersensitivity, resulting in a decrease of stereotyped responding. However, rates of self-injury associated with exercise may be reduced simply because of extraneous factors, such as fatigue.

Need for Further Treatment Research

Controversy abounds for the small percentage of children with autism spectrum disorders and mental retardation whose stereotyped self-injury has been unresponsive to conventional treatment (behavior therapy, pharmacotherapy, or combinations of behavior therapy and pharmacotherapy), particularly when the self-injurious behavior has worsened to levels at which the child's life is at stake. Highly restrictive protective equipment is invariably applied in these cases, and in some instances, mechanical restraint is necessary to ensure the child's safety. These are safety management procedures, not treatment. It is unacceptable that nothing more can be done. Consequently, studies are needed that further explore and better delineate the causal mechanisms of intractable self-injury, especially when it is of the life-threatening variety, such as the forceful and repetitive striking of the knee to the face and head. Is there something different about these children in comparison with others within the same population of patients with developmental disabilities who also engage in stereotyped self-injury but respond well to treatment? Conducting large-scale, longitudinal research on intractable, life-threatening, stereotyped self-injury is difficult for a variety of reasons. First, autism spectrum disorders and mental retardation occur in low incidences. Second, stereotyped self-injury afflicts only a small percentage of the population of children with developmental disabilities. Finally, children with intractable, life-threatening forms of stereotyped self-injury are even rarer. A national, multicenter project is necessary to assemble an adequate sample size that will allow for the close and systematic examination of patient characteristics (e.g., genetics, neu-

ropsychological profiles), as well as the effects of various biological therapies designed to address the suspected dopaminergic, serotoninergic, and opioid peptide mechanisms involved in the onset and maintenance of the most severe forms of stereotyped self-injury. In this regard, a series of carefully conducted single-case studies that demonstrate improvement over a detailed baseline could provide instructive findings and pave the way for future larger multisite studies.

IMPULSIVE SELF-INJURY

Treatment of superficial impulsive self-injury, as it applies to adolescents with average or above-average intelligence, is confounded by the fact that the behavior is not considered a discrete disorder. Instead, it is viewed as a behavior that is characteristic of another disorder, principally borderline personality disorder and affective illness. There exist a number of theories regarding the origin of borderline personality disorder[10]; however, none are supported empirically. The symptoms of borderline personality disorder may include labile mood, irrational thoughts, erratic behavior, unstable interpersonal relations, and poor self-image. Most adolescents with borderline personality disorder cannot stand to be alone and constantly demand attention. They also are observed as chronically angry individuals who quickly become offended by the remarks or actions of others and can become depressed quite easily. Engaging in provocative social behavior, including suicidal threats and gestures; making unreasonable demands on friends and family members; and immature tantrum-like behavior are commonly exhibited traits.

Consequently, adolescents seeking treatment for impulsive self-injury are subjected to wide variety of therapies designed to treat the larger underlying personality and/or affective disorder. In this regard, cognitive behavior therapy and pharmacotherapy account for most of the treatment literature involving impulsive self-injury.[11]

Cognitive-Behavior Therapy

Cognitive-behavior therapy is a research-supported, short-term therapy that is systematic and instructive in nature. It is a deliberate therapy that is highly structured and very goal-oriented. Goals consist of meeting various objectives within therapy that, in turn, facilitates meeting objectives for successful daily living and, across time, results in the achievement of life goals. Penultimate success is defined by an increasing ability to engage daily in effective self-counseling.

Among the cognitive behavioral therapies, DBT has the most empirical support with regard to the treatment of borderline personality disorder.[11] DBT is described as a problem-solving approach to treatment in which contingency management strategies, exposure tactics, cognitive restructuring, and the development of social and life skills are used to effect behavior change. The core objective of DBT with regard to impulsive self-injury is to contract with the patient to recognize and accept the feelings and circumstances that are associated with the onset of the behavior and engage in a process of behavior change. A number of well-controlled studies have demonstrated marked decreases in the impulsive self-injury of adolescent girls, as well as young adult and older women with a diagnosis of borderline personality disorder. In one study,[62] 31 female patients with borderline personality disorder demonstrated significant improvement on 10 of 11 psychopathological variables, including self-injury, after 3 months of inpatient treatment with DBT. A remarkable finding was that 42% of the treatment group receiving DBT were judged clinically recovered on a general measure of psychopathology and no longer met diagnostic criteria for personality or affective disorder. In a similar randomized study,[63] 27 female patients with borderline personality disorder showed dramatic decreases to zero and near-zero rates of self-injury after 1 year of outpatient DBT treatment. An important additional finding associated with the use of DBT as a treatment for self-injury in adolescents with borderline personality disorder includes the high rate of retention of patients in treatment. In virtually all controlled studies employing DBT, researchers have commented on markedly decreased rates of attrition; most reported patient retention rates two to three times greater than those reported in other treatments. Some studies have reported dropout rates as small as 10%, a remarkable statistic because the patient population receiving DBT is well known, historically, for poor compliance with treatment protocols.

Despite the impressive achievements of DBT, the favorable clinical outcome associated with this approach to the treatment of impulsive self-injury has not been subjected to long-term follow-up evaluation. It is not known whether patients who received DBT and achieved zero or near-zero rates of self-injury upon conclusion of treatment were able to maintain these gains and continue to improve or whether they relapsed.

Pharmacotherapy

There is limited evidence to support the use of drug interventions in the management of impulsive self-injury in adolescents with comorbid personality or affective disorders.[11,12] Clinical studies typically consist of open-label medication trials and case reports. Low-dose neuroleptic drugs, such as haloperidol, have an extensive history of use in adolescents with a diagnosis of borderline personality disorder. Unfortunately, this history includes little treatment efficacy with regard to self-injury. The newer classes of medication, such as the SSRIs, appears to hold more promise and have proved useful in the treatment of the depressive symptoms and impulsivity that commonly accompany self-injury in adolescents with borderline personality disorder.

In this regard, a study[64] of 12 patients with active repetitive self-cutting were treated for 3 months with fluoxetine. Results of the study revealed that 10 of the 12 patients had stopped self-cutting by the end of the study and that the remaining 2 patients were self-cutting, on average, less than once a week. A similar result was forthcoming in a trial of sertraline in which, after 1 year of treatment, 9 of 11 patients were no longer actively engaged in self-injurious behavior.[65] Unfortunately, the high dosage requirements (fluoxetine, 60 to 80 mg/day; sertraline, 325 mg/day) have raised speculation over whether patients can tolerate the levels apparently necessary to achieve the desired results.

Naltrexone, an opiate antagonist, also has demonstrated some limited utility in the treatment of adolescents with borderline personality disorder and impulsive self-injury. Altered pain perception is prevalent in numerous psychiatric disorders, including borderline personality disorder. Several studies have included reports of patients with borderline personality disorder who claim to experience no pain when actively engaging in self-injury, which is suggestive of dysfunction of normal pain mechanisms.[66] Well-controlled experimental studies of such patients have confirmed their self-reports. Consequently, the use of naltrexone to antagonize the opioid peptide system has resulted in reports of increased pain perception and correspondent decreases in the magnitude of active self-injury. In this regard, a 3-week study of five female patients with borderline personality disorder and active self-injury demonstrated that all but one patient abandoned self-injury while being treated with naltrexone.[67] Patients in this study also reported significant decreases in self-injurious thoughts while receiving naltrexone. Similarly, of seven female patients with borderline personality disorder, six reported reversal of analgesia and ceased engaging in self-injury during treatment with naltrexone.[68] Interestingly, there are no published studies that address the popular notion that individuals with borderline personality disorder may engage in self-injury in order to gain access to the sensory consequence associated with the production of endogenous opiates, despite the vast number of self-reports indicating that among the potential consequences of their self-injury is a sense of relief and well-being.[10]

The use of atypical neuroleptic agents for the treatment of impulsive self-injury in borderline personality disorder was thought to hold promise equal to that of the SSRIs. However, the data in this regard are spotty, at best. There are a few scattered case reports and single subject studies that indicate the effectiveness of risperidone[69] and clozapine[70,71] in the remission of impulsive self-injury. The use of olanzapine, however, has not been reported as a useful treatment for impulsive self-injury associated with borderline personality disorder and appears to be far more useful in the treatment of impulsive aggressive behavior with this patient population.

Finally, it is important to note that there is no U.S. Food and Drug Administration–approved treatment for either impulsive self-injury or borderline personality disorder.[12] The consensus guidelines[72] for pharmacotherapy propose the use of SSRIs as the first line of line treatment. This recommendation is based on the well-documented connection of serotoninergic mechanisms to the regulation of both impulsivity and affect, two commonly associated features of self-injury in borderline personality disorder. Naltrexone is generally considered a second line of treatment. However, for patients with borderline personality disorder who report that they do not experience pain as a consequence of self-injury, a trial of naltrexone may be indicated. Atypical neuroleptic agents, such as risperidone and olanzapine, do not appear to have much utility in the treatment of impulsive self-injury. However, as noted earlier, case reports have indicated that a small percentage of selected individuals may respond quite favorably to risperidone or clozapine. The same is true for the use of the α_2 agonist clonidine: Several female patients with borderline personality disorder reported decreases in the subjective urge to engage in a self-injurious act.[73]

Future Directions of Research in Treatment

DBT for the treatment of adolescents with impulsive self-injury and borderline personality disorder has been available for nearly 15 years. It is a highly specialized and labor-intensive intervention that has produced a large number of successful outcomes. However, there are no long-term studies that demonstrate whether patients who respond favorably maintain their gains and continue to make progress across the lifespan. In addition, it is unknown whether the same population relapses and, if that is the case, what might be done to prevent it. Large-scale longitudinal research is clearly indicated. Similarly, successful outcomes related to the use of SSRIs and opiate antagonists lack adequate sample sizes, experimental control, and follow-up measures. Moreover, studies are needed to examine the utility of combining promising psychosocial treatments, such as DBT, with promising pharmacotherapies, such as SSRIs, as a means of exploring the potential for a synergistic outcome. Studies of combined use of DBT with naltrexone in cases in which altered pain perception is suspected also appear warranted.

PICA

Pica is a medical condition defined as the persistent ingestion of nonnutritive substances for at least 1 month without an accompanying aversion to food.[1] The condition is named for the magpie, one of numerous birds in the genus *Pica* that eats both food and nonfood items indiscriminately. Dirt, clay, pebbles, chalk, paper, string, wood, coffee grounds, cigarette butts, burnt matches, ashes, coal, coins, crayons, and plastic items (e.g., pen caps) are among the more common items ingested. However, ingesting sharp objects (such as nails, tacks, screws, nuts, bolts, glass, pins, and needles), potentially toxic substances (such as household cleaners, dishwashing fluid, laundry starch, medications (aspirin), house plants, and feces, and other poisonous substances such as gasoline, lead-based paint chips or plaster, and mercury) can lead to far more serious and potentially life-threatening consequences.[74-76]

Prevalence

The prevalence of pica is unknown, largely because it often goes unrecognized[20a] but also because of changing definitions and other methodological inconsistencies across studies of the disorder. However, some reviews[77] indicate that 10% to 32% of children aged 1 to 6 years exhibit this behavior. Many infants and toddlers routinely put nonfood substances in their mouths as a matter of exploration. Both intentional and accidental ingestions are common in this age group. These ingestions are not considered true pica. Typically, the early developmental habit of mouthing objects as an exploratory behavior does not persist beyond the age of 2 years. In children who engage in the behavior after age 2 years, there is a marked linear deceleration of the disorder across later childhood and adolescence; most individuals who remain afflicted have autism, mental retardation, or developmental disabilities. Children who continue to eat nonfood substances on a consistent basis after their second birthday should be evaluated for pica, as well as the presence of a developmental disability and a variety of medical conditions associated with the serious health risks that accompany chronic ingestion of nonfood substances.

Cause

The cause of pica is unknown. A number of theories have been proposed to account for the behavior, including hypotheses that promote cultural, ethnic, and familial origins, as well as nutritional issues and neuropsychiatric factors.

CULTURAL, ETHNIC, AND FAMILIAL THEORY

Ethnic and family customs, as well as folk traditions associated with a particular culture, are viewed as possibly playing a role in the development of pica in children. Geophagia, the eating of soil, particularly clay, is a well-known folk remedy thought to suppress morning sickness.[78] It is a reasonable assumption that families engaging in this activity may extend the practice to children and adolescents who complain similarly of abdominal pain, nausea, or diarrhea. The children, in turn, may learn to independently engage in the behavior whenever they feel ill; others may eat soils superstitiously with the hope of protecting themselves against sickness. The practice of pica also may have roots in religious ceremony and cult activities that center on magical beliefs.[79]

ORGANIC OR NUTRITIONAL THEORY

The possibility of iron deficiency anemia[80] and zinc deficiency[81] or substandard nutrition[82] that results in vitamin and/or mineral deficiency should be considered when a child with pica is evaluated. In this regard, it is hypothesized that children and adolescents with nutritional and/or mineral deficiencies experience cravings and engage in eating nonfood substances as a compensatory mechanism to eliminate the deficiency, as well as to satisfy the craving. The empirical data, however, are mixed; some studies suggest that the incidence of dietary and mineral deficiencies is not any greater in children and adolescents with the disorder than in children and adolescents who do not eat nonfood substances.[20a]

NEUROPSYCHIATRIC THEORY

Pica is overrepresented among children and adolescents with autism spectrum disorders, mental retardation, and developmental disabilities, including some children and adolescents with epilepsy.[20a] It is the most commonly observed eating disorder in these clinical populations. The incidence of pica in children and adolescents with developmental disabilities, comparable with the distribution of self-injurious behavior, is most frequently observed in those with severe and profound mental retardation. Like self-injurious behavior, pica in these populations is viewed as a subclass of stereotyped activity. Hypotheses identical to those proposed to explain stereotypic self-injury

are invoked to explain pica behavior. In this regard, children may learn to engage in pica because it provokes adult attention (positive reinforcement) or allows escape a nonpreferred activity (negative reinforcement). Pica also may be experienced as an activity that modulates arousal (homeostatic) or, in an uncomplicated manner, a sensory activity that the child experiences as stimulating or pleasant (e.g., lead paint chips are sweet and chewy; gasoline smells good). In addition, it may be viewed from a developmental perspective as a fixed circular reaction[22] or, more simply, reflective of something as straightforward as imitating the behavior of a family pet or a zoo or farm animal. Pica may also be explained by an organic hypothesis whereby the presence of a genetic disorder, such as Prader-Willi syndrome (a disorder characterized by hyperphagia), increases the risk of ingesting nonfood substances.[83] Finally, neurobiological theories[84] involving diminished dopaminergic neurotransmission, as well as elevated serotonin levels and the role of endogenous opiates, have been proposed to account for pica. Anxiety disorders, such as hysteria[20a] and obsessive-compulsive disorder,[85,86] as well as other forms of psychopathology, also have been hypothesized to explain pica from a psychological perspective.

Diagnosis and Assessment Issues

Toddlers who complain of abdominal pain and all children and adolescents with autism spectrum disorders and mental retardation, without exception, should be evaluated for the presence of pica. In addition, the developmental histories of these children should be carefully reviewed for any past evidence of the disorder. Although it is important to distinguish between stereotyped mouthing of objects by very young children who unwittingly or accidentally ingest them and genuine pica, it is more important to focus on the health risks, both immediate and long term, associated with the placing of nonfood substances in the mouth. The potential for parasitic infection with sequelae of myocarditis, encephalitis, hepatomegaly, and brain damage by intoxicants such as lead from paint and mercury from paper is of immediate concern, as are the life-threatening effects of frank poisons in petrochemical products and certain house plants, as well as obstruction from indigestible mass that may cause choking or perforate the stomach or intestine and result in peritonitis.

Except in circumstances involving children and adolescents with autism spectrum disorder and mental retardation, most cases of pica are easily diagnosed from self-report of the child or from interview with parents.[87] However, in some instances, child or parent reluctance to report the behavior makes diagnosis difficult. Children may not disclose pica for fear of being punished or, simply, because of embarrassment. Similarly, parents may contend that they are unaware of the behavior because they are embarrassed that their child eats dirt or feces or to safeguard cultural and familial secrets and to protect themselves against potential charges of child neglect.

The medical evaluation of a child or adolescent with real or suspected pica should begin with an interview with the patient, the patient's parent or parents, and (with parental permission) the patient's siblings. Brothers and sisters are an often overlooked source of information and may provide details regarding a sibling's habits that are otherwise unknown to a parent. A comprehensive physical examination should be performed, including laboratory studies to rule out dietary and/or mineral deficiency (complete blood cell count; iron, ferritin, and zinc measurements), as well as the presence of toxic substances such as lead and copper. Liver function tests, electrolyte measurements, and studies to rule out eosinophilia, as well as radiology and radiography studies for obstruction and parasites, should also be conducted, as indicated.

Treatment

The prevention of future occurrence is of the utmost importance when developing a treatment plan for a child or adolescent with pica. Parent and child education about the dangers associated with placing objects in the mouth is a crucial first step. This may be followed by instructions to parents for close supervision of the child and ways to ensure that the home environment is made as safe as possible. In the absence of effective prevention, there are many serious health risks associated with pica. Medical treatment is invariably required and often multimodal in nature. Treatment may include dietary supplements for mineral (iron or zinc) deficiencies, chelation therapy for children with clinical lead poisoning, therapy specific to the various sequelae of parasitic infection, and surgery to remove indigestible obstruction and repair dental injury. Psychological interventions also may be indicated, including learning-based behavior modification. In this regard, response blocking[88-90] is known to be effective. However, this procedure must be implemented with virtual perfection across an extended period if favorable results are to be gained and maintained. Children and adolescents with pica related to anxiety disorders, including obsessive-compulsive behavior, should be evaluated for possible treatment with SSRIs. Behavior modification procedures designed to positively reinforce the omission of placing nonfood substances in the mouth may be especially helpful in decreasing and eliminating the behavior in children and adolescents whose pica appears stereotypical or habitual in nature. In cases in which pica appears intractable, as may be the case in children and adolescents with a diagnosis of autism spectrum disorders and mental retardation, it may be necessary to increase the perceived magnitude of the reward associated with the absence of placing nonfood substances in the mouth by contrasting it against a mild punishment (such as loss of access to a preferred toy or removal from a preferred activity) when the behavior occurs. In cases in which pica has not responded favorably to either drug or behavioral treatments, a combination of approaches should be considered.

Future Directions of Research

Epidemiological research is crucial for a better understanding of pica. Studies are greatly needed in a variety of different areas, including establishing a true prevalence rate for the disorder and developing a risk profile of the children and adolescents most likely to be afflicted. The controversial nature of dietary or mineral deficiency in pica also needs to be established, specifically in terms of the role of iron and zinc. Treatment studies to examine the effectiveness of prevention protocols should be a primary concern. Anecdotal reports suggesting that stimulant drugs may decrease pica must be subjected to double-blind, placebo-controlled trials. Because of the obsessive quality typically associated with pica behavior, double-blind, placebo-controlled trials of SSRIs also are indicated. Studies such as these can eventually lead to the collaboration of pediatrics and child psychiatry on the development of a (greatly needed) best practice standard, for both medical evaluation and treatment of the child or adolescent with pica.

SUMMARY

Atypical behavior, in the form of self-injury and pica, are challenging forms of psychopathology in children and adolescents, in terms of both understanding the disorder and prescribing effective treatment. Although there are many theories as to why afflicted children and adolescents engage in self-mutilation and ingest nonfood substances, the truth remains a mystery. Despite a certain degree of homogeneity in terms of the diagnoses in the largest population of children and adolescents who are most likely to engage in these behaviors (i.e., developmental disabilities, borderline personality disorder), the children and adolescents themselves constitute a heterogeneous group. There is a great deal of variability between children within the diagnostic classification of pervasive developmental disorders, as well as across mental retardation subtypes and syndromes. The same may be said of adolescents with borderline personality disorder. It is highly unlikely that even children and adolescents sharing a identical diagnoses are engaging in the same type of self-injurious behavior or ingesting the same type of nonfood items or, if they are, that they are doing so for the same reason. Certainly, in some cases, the behavior in question is learned and can be treated with operant behavioral techniques. In cases in which the behavior appears impulsive with no apparent basis in learning, complex neurobiological hypotheses involving dopaminergic and serotoninergic mechanisms are offered as explanations. In still other cases, it may be learning in combination with a biological factor, such as neuropeptides, that is responsible for the origin and maintenance of the behavior.

Research on self-injury and pica has advanced greatly since the 1950s. Animal models and genetic studies have played a central role in facilitating an improved understanding of these behavioral phenomena. Self-injury and pica are no longer entirely incomprehensible. Unfortunately, much is still to be learned. No single treatment may be successful with either disorder. Moreover, it is likely that a panacea will never be identified. Children and adolescents engage in self-injury and pica for many different reasons. Consequently, each patient's case must be viewed without presumption of cause. The patient must be carefully assessed to determine which among many possible causal mechanisms, working alone or in concert with additional factors, are responsible for the resulting behavior. Finally, the clinician must make use of what is known about treating this class of behavior and develop an intervention that addresses proposed etiological mechanisms as comprehensively as possible. In this regard, combining learning-based approaches, such as behavior modification and DBT with pharmacotherapy, appears to be more efficacious than using one treatment independently of the other.

REFERENCES

1. American Psychiatric Association: Diagnostic and Statistical Manual of Mental Disorders, 4th ed. Washington, DC: American Psychiatric Association, 1994.
2. Schroeder SR, Oster-Granite ML, Thompson T: Self-Injurious Behavior. Washington, DC: American Psychological Association, 2002.
3. Linehan MM, Armstrong HE, Suarez A, et al: Cognitive behavioural treatment of chronically parasuicidal borderline patients. Arch Gen Psychiatry 48:1060-1064, 1991.
4. Hoch TA, Long KE, McPeak MM, et al: Self-injurious behavior in mental retardation. In Matson JL, Laud RB, Matson ML, eds: Behavior Modification for Persons with Developmental Disabilities, vol 1. New York: NADD Press, 2002, pp 190-218.
5. Matson JL, Bamburg JW, Mayville EA, et al: Psychotropic medications and developmental disabilities: A 10-year review. Res Dev Disabil 21:263-296, 2000.
6. King BH: Pharmacological treatment of mood disturbance, aggression, and self-injury in persons with pervasive developmental disorder. J Autism Dev Disabil 30:439-445, 2000.
7. Borrero JC, Vollmer TR, Wright CS, et al: Further evaluation of the role of protective equipment in the functional analysis of self-injury. J Appl Behav Anal 35:69-72, 2002.
8. Suyemoto KL: The functions of self-mutilation. Clin Psychol Rev 18:531-554, 1998.
9. Pattison EM, Kahan J: The deliberate self-harm syndrome. Am J Psychiatry 140:867-872, 1983.
10. Linehan MM: Cognitive Behavioral Treatment of Borderline Personality Disorder. New York: Guilford, 1993.
11. Paris J: Recent advances in the treatment of borderline personality disorder. Can J Psychiatry 50:435-441, 2005.
12. Smith BD: Self-mutilation and pharmacotherapy. Psychiatry (October):29-37, 2005.
13. Rojahn J, Esbensen AJ: Epidemiology of self-injurious behavior in mental retardation: A review. In Schroeder SR, Oster-Granite ML, Thompson T, eds: Self-Injurious Behavior Washington, DC: American Psychological Association, 2002, pp 41-77.
14. Favazza AR: The coming of age of self-mutilation. J Nerv Ment Dis 186:259-268, 1998.
15. Nock M, Prinstein M: A functional approach to the assessment of self-mutilative behavior. J Consult Clin Psychol 72:885-890, 2004.
16. Guertin T, Lloyd-Richardson E, Spirito A: Self-mutilative behavior in adolescents who attempt suicide by overdose. J Am Acad Child Adolesc Psychiatry 40:1062-1069, 2001.
17. Zlotnick C, Mattia JI, Zimmerman M: Clinical correlates of self-mutilation in a sample of general psychiatry patients. J Nerv Ment Dis 187:296-301, 1999.
18. Carr EG: The motivation of self-injurious behavior: A review of some hypotheses. Psychol Bull 84:800-816, 1977.
19. Winchel RM, Stanley M: Self-injurious behavior: A review of the behavior and biology of self-mutilation. Am J Psychiatry 148:306-317, 1991.
20. Favazza AR: Bodies under Siege: Self-Mutilation and Body Modification in Culture and Psychiatry, 2nd ed. Baltimore: Johns Hopkins University Press, 1996.
20a. Rose EA, Porcelli JH, Neale AV: Pica: Common, but commonly missed. J Am Board Fam Pract 13:356, 2000.
21. Sallustro F, Atwell CW: Body rocking, head banging, and head rolling in normal children. J Pediatr 93:704-708, 1978.

22. Piaget J: The Origins of Intelligence in Children. New York: International Universities Press, 1952.

23. Berkson G, Tupa M: Incidence of self-injurious behavior: Birth to 3 years. *In* Schroeder SR, Oster-Granite ML, Thompson T, eds: Self-Injurious Behavior. Washington, DC: American Psychological Association, 2002, pp 145-150.

24. Finncane B, Dirrigl KH, Simon EW: Characterization of self-injurious behaviour in children and adults with Smith-Magenis syndrome. Am J Ment Retard 106:52-58, 2001.

25. Hall S, Oliver C, Murphy G: Self-injurious behaviour in young children with Lesch-Nyhan syndrome. Dev Med Child Neurol 43:745-749, 2001.

26. Cassidy SB: Prader-Willi syndrome. Curr Prob Pediatr 14:1-55, 1984.

27. Berney TP, Ireland M, Burn J: Behavioral phenotype of Cornelia de Lange syndrome. Arch Dis Child 81:333-336, 1999.

28. Nomura Y, Segawa M: Characteristics of motor disturbances of the Rett's syndrome. Brain Dev 12:27-30, 1990.

29. Cohen DJ, Bruun RD, Leckman JF: Tourette's Syndrome and Tic Disorders: Clinical Understanding and Treatment. New York: Wiley, 1988.

30. Gedye A: Extreme self-injury attributed to frontal lobe seizures. Am J Ment Retard 94:20-26, 1989.

31. O'Reilly MF: Functional analysis of episodic self-injury correlated with recurrent otitis media. J Appl Behav Anal 30:165-167, 1997.

32. Kennedy CH, Thompson T: Health conditions contributing to problem behavior among people with mental retardation and developmental disabilities. *In* Weymeyer ML, Patton JR, eds: Mental Retardation in the 21st Century. Austin, TX: Pro-Ed, 2000, pp 211-231.

33. Taylor DV, Rush D, Hetrick WP, et al: Self-injurious behavior within the menstrual cycle of women with mental retardation. Am J Ment Retard 97:659-664, 1993.

34. Bohmer CMJ: Gastro-esophageal Reflux Disease in Intellectually Disabled Individuals. Amsterdam: VU University Press, 1996.

35. Symons FJ, Davis ML, Thompson T: Self-injurious behavior and sleep disturbance in developmental disabilities. Res Dev Disabil 21:115-123, 2000.

36. Turner CA, Lewis MH: Dopaminergic mechanisms in self-injurious behavior and related disorders. *In* Schroeder SR, Oster-Granite ML, Thompson T, eds: Self-Injurious Behavior. Washington, DC: American Psychological Association, 2002, pp 165-179.

37. Simeon B, Stanley B, Francis A, et al: Self-mutilation in personality disorders: Psychological and biological correlates. Am J Psychiatry 148:1665-1671, 1992.

38. Sandman CA, Touchette P: Opioids and the maintenance of self-injurious behavior. *In* Schroeder SR, Oster-Granite ML, Thompson T, eds: Self-Injurious Behavior. Washington, DC: American Psychological Association, 2002, pp 191-204.

39. Gunderson J: Borderline Personality Disorder. Washington, DC: American Psychiatric Press, 1984.

40. Rodham K, Hawton K, Evans E: Reason for deliberate self-harm: Comparison of self-poisoners and self-cutters in a community sample of adolescents. J Am Acad Child Adolesc Psychiatry 43:80-87, 2004.

41. Iwata BA, Dorsey MF, Slifer KJ, et al: Toward a functional assessment of self-injury. J Appl Behav Anal 27:197-209, 1992.

42. O'Neil R, Horner RH, Albin RW, et al: Functional Assessment and Program Development for Problem Behavior: A Practical Handbook, 2nd ed. Pacific Grove, CA: Brooks/Cole, 1999.

43. March RE, Horner RH: Feasibility and contributions of functional behavior assessment in schools. J Emotion Behav Disord 10:158-170, 2002.

44. Reed H, Thomas E, Sprague JR, et al: The Student Guided Functional Assessment Interview: An analysis of student and teacher agreement. J Behav Educ 7:33-49, 1997.

45. Matson JL, Vollmer TR: The Questions About Behavioral Function (QABF) User's Guide. Baton Rouge, LA: Scientific Publishers, 1995.

46. Durand VM, Crimmins DB: The Motivation Assessment Scale. Topeka, KS: Monaco and Associates, 1992.

47. Pyles DA, Riordan MM, Bailey JS: The stereotypy analysis: An instrument for examining environmental variables associated with differential rates of stereotypic behavior. Res Dev Disabil 18:11-38, 1997.

48. Groden G, Lantz S: The reliability of the Detailed Behavior Report (DBR) in documenting functional assessment observations. Behav Interv 16:15-25, 2001.

49. Nock M, Prinstein M: A functional approach to the assessment of self-mutilative behavior. J Consult Clin Psychol 72:885-890, 2004.

50. Gutierrez P, Osman A, Barrios F, et al: Developmental and initial validation of the Self-Harm Behavior Questionnaire. J Pers Assess 77:475-490, 2001.

51. Sansone R, Wiederman M, Sansone L: The Self-Harm Inventory (SHI): Development of a scale for identifying self-destructive behaviors and borderline personality disorder. J Clin Psychol 54:973-983, 1998.

52. Bongar B: Scale points for lethality assessment. *In* Bongar B, ed: The Suicidal Patient: Clinical and Legal Standards of Care. Washington, DC: American Psychological Association, 1991, pp 277-283.

53. Kahng S, Iwata BA, Lewin AB: Behavioral treatment of self-injury. Am J Ment Retard 107:212-221, 2002.

54. Reiss S, Aman MG: Psychotropic Medications and Developmental Disabilities: The International Consensus Handbook. Columbus, OH: Ohio State University Press, 1998.

55. Phelps L, Brown RT, Power TJ: Pediatric Psychopharmacology. Washington, DC: American Psychological Association, 2002.

56. Werry JS, Aman MG: Practitioner's Guide to Psychoactive Drugs for Children and Adolescents, 2nd ed. New York: Plenum Press, 1999.

57. Ricketts RW, Goza AB, Ellis CR, et al: Fluoxetine treatment of severe self-injury in adolescents and young

adults with mental retardation. J Am Acad Child Adolesc Psychiatry 32:865-869, 1993.

58. Barrett RP, Feinstein C, Hole W: Effects of naloxone and naltrexone on self-injury: A double blind, placebo-controlled analysis. Am J Ment Retard 93:644-651, 1989.

59. Aman MG, Singh NN, White AJ: Caregiver perceptions of psychotropic medication in residential facilities. Res Dev Disabil 8:449-465, 1987.

60. Singh NN, Watson JE, Winton ASW: Parents' acceptability ratings of alternative treatments for use with mentally retarded children. Behav Modif 1:17-26, 1987.

61. Baumeister AA, MacLean WE: Deceleration of SIB and stereotypic responding by exercise. Appl Res Ment Retard 5:385-394, 1984.

62. Bohus M, Haaf B, Simms T, et al: Effectiveness of inpatient dialectical behavioral therapy for borderline personality disorder: A controlled trial. Behav Res Ther 42:487-499, 2004.

63. Verheul R, Van Den Bosch LMC, Koeter MWJ, et al: Dialectical behaviour therapy for women with borderline personality disorder. Br J Psychiatry 182:135-140, 2003.

64. Markovitz PJ, Calabrese JR, Schulz SC, et al: Fluoxetine in the treatment of borderline and schizotypal personality disorders. Am J Psychiatry 148:1064-1067, 1991.

65. Zanarini MC: Update on pharmacotherapy of borderline personality disorder. Curr Psychiatry Rep 6:66-70, 2004.

66. Bohus M, Limberger M, Ebner U: Pain perception during self-reported distress and calmness in patients with borderline personality disorder and self-mutilating behavior. Psychiatry Res 95:251-260, 2000.

67. Sonne S, Rubey R, Brady K: Naltrexone treatment of self-injurious thoughts and behavior. J Nerv Ment Dis 184:192-194, 1996.

68. Roth AS, Ostroff RB, Hoffman RE: Naltrexone as a treatment for repetitive self-injurious behavior: An open label trial. J Clin Psychiatry 57:233-237, 1996.

69. Khouzam HR, Donnelly NJ: Remission of self-mutilation in a patient with borderline personality during risperidone therapy. J Nerv Ment Dis 185:348-349, 1997.

70. Chengappa KNR, Baker RW, Sirri C: The successful use of clozapine in ameliorating severe self-mutilation in a patient with borderline personality disorder. J Personal Disord 9:76-82, 1995.

71. Chengappa KNR, Ebeling T, Kang JS: Clozapine reduces severe self-mutilation and aggression in psychotic patients with borderline personality disorder. J Clin Psychiatry 60:477-484, 1999.

72. Soloff PH: Psychopharmacology of borderline personality disorder. Psychiatr Clin North Am 23:169-192, 2000.

73. Phillipsen A, Richter H, Schmal C: Clonidine in acute aversive inner tension and self-injurious behavior in female patients with borderline personality disorder. J Clin Psychiatry 65:1414-1419, 2004.

74. Keeling PJ, Ramsay J: Paper, pica and pseudoporphyria. Lancet 2:1095, 1987.

75. Olynyk F, Sharpe DH: Mercury poisoning in paper pica. N Engl J Med 306:1056-1057, 1982.

76. Needleman H, Schell A: The long term effects of exposure to low doses of lead in childhood: An 11-year follow up report. N Engl J Med 322:83-88, 1990.

77. Motta RW, Basile DM: Pica. *In* Phelps L, ed: Health Related Disorders in Children and Adolescents. Washington, DC: American Psychological Association, 1998, pp 524-527.

78. Dissanayake C: Of stones and health: Medical geology in Sri Lanka. Science 309:883-885, 2005.

79. Parry-Jones B, Parry-Jones WL: Pica: Symptom or eating disorder? An historical assessment. Br J Psychiatry 160:341-354, 1992.

80. Moore DF, Sears DA: Pica, iron deficiency, and the medical history. Am J Med 97:390-393, 1994.

81. Sayetta RB: Pica: An overview. Am Fam Physician 7:174-175, 1986.

82. Danford DE: Pica and nutrition. Annu Rev Nutr 2:303-322, 1982.

83. Dimitropoulis A, Blackford J, Walden T, et al: Compulsive behavior in Prader-Willi syndrome: Examining severity in early childhood. Res Dev Disabil 27:190-202, 2006.

84. Ellis CR, Schnoes CJ: Eating disorder: Pica. eMed J 2:1-8, 2001.

85. Luiselli J: Pica as an obsessive-compulsive disorder. J Behav Ther Exp Psychiatry 27:195-196, 1996.

86. Stein DJ, Bouwer C, van Heerden B: Pica and the obsessive-compulsive spectrum disorders. South Afr Med J 86:1586-1592, 1996.

87. Archer L, Rosenbaum P, Streiner D: The Children's Eating Behavior Inventory (CEBI): Reliability and validity results. J Pediatr Psychol 16:629-642, 1991.

88. McCord BE, Grosser JW, Iwata BA, et al: An analysis of response-blocking parameters in the prevention of pica. J Appl Behav Anal 38:391-394, 2005.

89. Rapp JT, Dozier CL, Carr JE: Functional assessment and treatment of pica: A single case experiment. Behav Interv 16:111-125, 2001.

90. Hagopian LP, Adelinis JD: Response blocking with and without redirection for the treatment of pica. J Appl Behav Anal 34:527-530, 2001.

Strategies to Enhance Developmental and Behavioral Services in Primary Care

MARTIN T. STEIN

The foundation of pediatric practice is child development. Knowledge and application of the principles of biological development and the interaction between biology and experience are concepts used by pediatricians each day in office and hospital practice. The momentum and focus of a comprehensive pediatric practice is captured in the term *biopsychosocial medicine,* in which biology, psychology, and social interactions mediate emerging developmental components of childhood, adolescence, and family life.[1]

Development, in the context of child and adolescent health, refers to the predictable emergence of specific milestones of growth. Pediatricians view these milestones from the perspective of predictable neuromaturational processes during fetal and postnatal brain growth. The interaction between genetic endowment and environmental experience mediates neuromaturation.[2]

Behavior refers to the way a person acts; it is conduct as experienced by others who interact with a person. Behavior is also influenced by neuromaturation in the brain during child and adolescent development, as well as by interpersonal experience with parents, other family members, peers, teachers and coaches. Behaviors are dependent on (1) temperament; (2) attainment of motor, language, social, and cognitive skills; and (3) the experience acquired from self-exploration and social interactions with others.

Development and behavior are shaped by transactions between genetic endowment and environmental influences. The interplay between the maturation of the developing brain and behavioral experiences is dynamic and present at each stage of child and adolescent development. The practice of biopsychosocial pediatrics during each well-child visit is ensured when the clinician's observations, questions, assessment, and management plan are based on a model that incorporates an understanding of neurological development and the spectrum of behavioral change.

The challenge for pediatricians is to adapt the principles of developmental and behavioral pediatrics to the practice of primary care. They strive to learn about the unique developmental pathway of each child and family, provide anticipatory guidance, and recognize early clues to developmental delays and behavioral problems. The conscientious practice of developmentally and behaviorally sophisticated primary care pediatrics supplies the fuel that sustains an intellectual interest in pediatric medicine.

Several innovative strategies to enhance the quality of developmental and behavioral practices have been described. The use of a group format for well-child care, collaborative care with a mental health professional or a child development specialist located in the office, and creating methods to encourage parents to model reading to young children are among a few of these new formats. Other innovations have involved new ways to screen for delays in development and behavior problems through more efficient and effective screening questionnaires, and the use of new information technologies. In this chapter, these strategies are explored and how they may enhance primary care practice is discussed.

WHY CHANGE AT THIS TIME?

More than half of the parents with children younger than 5 years old report that common developmental and behavioral topics were not discussed during well-child visits. Parents report that they would like more information and support about infant crying (23%), toilet training (41%), discipline (42%), sleep issues (30%), and ways to encourage a child to learn (54%).[3] Screening for developmental and behavioral conditions is highly variable, as reported by pediatricians. When asked about office screening practices in an American Academy of Pediatrics (AAP) Periodic Survey, 96% of pediatricians responded that they screen for these conditions, but only 71% reported using a structured clinical assessment, and only 23% reported using any standardized screening instrument.[4] Expanded screening that includes family issues is also variable. Ascertainment of parents' health by pediatricians is limited in areas of domestic violence, social support, depression, and alcohol or drug abuse.

Developmental and behavioral aspects of primary care practices have been affected by a change in the ecology of many office and clinic practices. For example, only 46% of parents reported that their child had seen the same pediatric clinician for well-child visits up to 3 years of age.[5] Continuity of care by one person, a fundamental principle of primary care, has been replaced by continuity within one clinic or office.[6] Many children do not even have the benefit of the number of well-child visits recommended by the AAP; nationally, only half of the well-child visits recommended by the AAP are completed in the first 2 years of life.[7]

At the same time, stress on families continues to grow. Poverty, lack of health insurance, unemployment, marital conflicts and divorce, community and family violence, and parental depression are among the many contemporary factors that potentially challenge a child's development. Many families are now without extended family supports. These social factors interact with biological vulnerabilities and may account for the growing number of children who display adverse effects in neurodevelopment and social interactions.

Two traditional roles of pediatric practice have been to focus on all aspects of growth and development and to provide scientifically sound primary prevention. The early assessment of maternal depression, school failure, substance abuse, and family violence is as important as an early diagnosis of short stature or the assurance of complete immunizations. This type of pediatric practice can be achieved by discovering effective methods to emphasize child development, behavior, and family functioning on an equal footing with biological aspects of pediatric care.

HISTORICAL PERSPECTIVE

Pediatrics has a long history of attention to preventive aspects of child health care. Nineteenth century pioneers of pediatrics in Europe and America focused on descriptions of childhood diseases, but they soon recognized the value and importance of prevention. Abraham Jacobi, one the founders of pediatrics as a specialty for children, devoted his work to the elimination of the deadly summer diarrhea epidemics in New York City by emphasizing prevention through

hygiene in the preparation of milk and other foods for young children.[8] At the opening of the 20th century, periodic and frequent weight determinations in infants and young children in public health clinics was a way to monitor children's general health and well-being. As a part of America's Progressive Movement from 1900 to 1920, the U.S. Children's Bureau proposed that monitoring the weight of young children should be the central activity for the National Year of the Child in 1918 in order to diagnose malnutrition.[9]

Nurses, social workers, and lay reformers planned and implemented these screening programs as a part of the child welfare movement in cities and small communities throughout the country. Eventually, physicians who cared for children adopted routine weight and height measurements in their offices and clinics as a part of overall supervision of a child's health. A major force that led to the establishment of the AAP in 1930 was a recognition that pediatric care would improve significantly when pediatricians adopted a prevention-oriented strategy and collaborated with the leaders of the child welfare movement. In 1933, the president of the AAP made the radical (for that time) proposition that pediatricians should begin to offer periodic health examinations. This may have marked the beginning of primary care pediatrics and standard well-child visits. In 1910, there were approximately 100 physicians who limited their practice to children. By 1930, there were several thousand; it is estimated that a third of their visits were for well-child care.[9] In 2000, the AAP had almost 60,000 members.

Developmental and behavioral health care for children in the context of pediatric practice was an outgrowth of these early events. Leaders in pediatrics wrote about the importance of attention to the social and psychological development of children during pediatric encounters. Significant contributions to the practice of well child care were made by many pioneers, including Anderson Aldrich, Edith Jackson, Morris Wessel, Milton Senn, Helen Goffman, and Benjamin Spock.[10] They increased the attention of pediatricians to motor, language, and social skill development of young children; the importance of assessing mother-child attachment and educational achievement; and the development of a therapeutic alliance in optimizing all aspects of pediatric care.

These historical trends are antecedents to the schedule of well-child visits used in contemporary pediatrics. The so-called periodicity schedule was established in the 1960s by a group of pediatricians working with the AAP. It was based on the best clinical judgment available at the time and guided by the immunization schedule. Since the 1950s, multiple additional topics for assessment and anticipatory guidance have been added to the initial template.[11] Unfortunately, developmental themes and psychosocial tasks among children and families that are unique to each age group have not led to specific recommendations and guidance about optimal structuring of well-child visits or to their increased frequency or duration.

WELL-CHILD VISITS: WHAT DO WE DO THAT IS EVIDENCE-BASED?

Medical care, including preventive medicine, strives for a foundation of evidence-based studies to support clinical practice. There are some areas of well-child care that are supported by strong evidence from randomized controlled studies. Examples of these practices include standard immunizations,[12] promoting good nutrition during infancy,[13] encouraging parents to put their infants to sleep on their backs,[14] and the judicious use of antibiotics for respiratory infections.[15]

Other components of well-child care practices that focus on the development and behavior of children have not been studied with large randomized trials. A careful review of published studies reveals support for some practices, suggestions for new directions, and opportunities for further research. Regalado and Halfon[16] reviewed published studies on evaluations of four areas of developmental and behavioral pediatric practice in children from birth to 3 years of age. These studies reflect the potential for current clinical practices. Regalado and Halfon's conclusions were the following:

1. Structured and systematic approaches to eliciting concerns of parents during well-child visits improve communication between parents and clinicians and are helpful in detecting developmental and behavioral problems.[17,17a]
2. Current developmental and behavioral screening in pediatric practice is not routinely performed, and as a result, children with mild and moderate conditions are not identified effectively during these years.
3. The use of a standardized questionnaire in conjunction with clinical observations and impressions is more effective in identifying psychosocial risk factors than simply clinical impressions alone. Parental risk factors such as depression, substance abuse, poor self-esteem, domestic violence, and abuse of a parent during childhood are all areas of relevance that can be identified with a questionnaire.
4. Only one study has supported the overall effectiveness of anticipatory guidance by showing that pediatricians may affect a child's development through

positive effects on the mother-child relationship.[17a] However, evidence does exist for the effectiveness of selected parts of the health supervision agenda:

A. Discussions or a videotape about infant social development during the postpartum period and during early well-child visits resulted in more favorable interactive behavior with infants, less reported maternal stress, and enhanced mother-infant interactions during feeding.
B. Parents report that a discussion of their infant's temperament during well-child visits is an effective method to inform them about approaches to child rearing.
C. Preventive counseling directed to parents of infants to inform them about caregiving practices that improve infant sleep habits has been demonstrated to be effective. Behavioral approaches include extinction (ignoring the child's crying for attention at bedtime), reinforcement, shaping (adjustments of the bedtime period), and cueing (institution of a bedtime routine).
D. Behavioral interventions and counseling that provide specific advice and strategies to parents to prevent and manage excessive crying have been demonstrated to be effective in comparison with empathic listening alone or no intervention.

Many components of well-child care need improvement in order to determine and maximize their effectiveness. Evidence-based studies of the effectiveness of pediatric well-child visits are insufficient with regard to the following:

- Promoting optimal nutrition after infancy: prevention of obesity and eating disorders.
- Safety issues: bicycle safety and helmets, accessible guns in homes, preventing burns and motor vehicle injuries.
- Substance abuse: education/prevention.
- Counseling parents about behavioral concerns: oppositional behaviors, feeding problems, bullying.
- Early detection and diagnosis of behavioral conditions: Autistic Spectrum Disorder, Attention-Deficit/Hyperactivity Disorder, Oppositional Defiant Disorder, Anxiety, Depression, Post-traumatic Stress Disorder, learning disabilities, and social dysfunction.

CLINICAL INTERVIEW AND THERAPEUTIC RELATIONSHIP

As in most areas of medical practice, clinicians rely on the medical interview to determine patients' (and parents') concerns. A detailed and focused medical history, including psychosocial and biological factors in an individual and family, suggests a diagnosis. The mutual trust that is the outcome of a therapeutic alliance between patient (parent and child) and clinician is the core of clinical practice.

In the early 1980s, a major shift occurred in the way pediatricians think about health care delivery. Before that time, models of care—especially primary care—were based largely on the relationship between a pediatrician and the parents and children in her or his practice. The pediatrician was given responsibility for all aspects of care: diagnostic, prescriptive, and preventive. The quality of the doctor-patient (and doctor-staff) relationship was the core ingredient of quality care.

After 1980, organized systems of health care delivery became prominent. Initially a public health concept, systems-based medicine attracted the leaders of clinical medicine: both inpatient and outpatient, both specialist and general care. Systems were created for screening for disease; monitoring chronic medical and psychological conditions; and maintaining efficiency, output, and patient satisfaction. Systems were also developed for guiding clinical practice patterns in developmental-behavioral pediatrics. This trend had a profound effect on the development of a multitude of time-saving techniques to increase the efficiency of well-child visits, including questionnaires (for parents, older children and adolescents, and teachers) to assess and monitor problems in child development and behavior.

Pediatricians in training have always been encouraged to develop interpersonal clinical skills that nurture the doctor-patient relationship. From that relationship, in the best of circumstances, a "therapeutic alliance" takes shape. Morris Green defined the therapeutic alliance as

> When pediatricians succeed in engaging parents and children as partners in health care. . . . The powerful therapeutic potential of the interactions of pediatricians with families is not always sufficiently realized. In order to achieve the most effective working relationship (i.e., therapeutic alliance) with parents, pediatricians must be responsive consistently to contributions of children and parents while being aware of their own resources and limitations.

—*Morris Green,[18] p 3*

Clinical strategies that enhance the therapeutic relationship include the following:

1. Communication of trust and respect; sensitive awareness of patients' needs, expectations, and concerns, as well as their resources and limitations.
2. Long-term comprehensive, personalized, family-centered care (see Chapter 8B).
3. Realistic recognition of limitations in self, patient, time, and environment.
4. Effectively planned use of time.
5. Respect for patients' agendas and solutions.

An effective therapeutic alliance is dependent on an informed communication process between child/parent and clinician/office staff that is developed over time. Clinicians should strive to be as careful with their use of words as in their prescription of medicine. When an office visit is viewed as an opportunity to teach parenting skills and convey knowledge that will promote health, the importance of both verbal and nonverbal components of communication is emphasized. *Nonverbal information* refers to observations about the style, timing, affect, and flow of information and even what is not said. The quality and tone of speech, facial expressions, posture, and body movements of parents and children often provide clues to critical aspects of a child's life and family. A few examples of nonverbal communication providing important clinical information follow:

- Entering the examination room, the pediatrician observes that the mother of a toddler appears sad and pale; eye contact with the pediatrician is minimal and difficult to encourage. The child plays in a corner of the room without mother-child interchange. *There is not enough information to suggest a diagnosis, but the initial impression is maternal depression. An empathic introductory comment, "You appear sad today" often opens a dialogue. If the mother does not respond, suggest, "Is there something you'd like to talk about—about your child or something in the family?"*

- A mother, father, and 5-year old come to the office for a 2-week well-child visit for the new addition to the family. Mother's facial appearance and minimal body movements suggest sleep deprivation. The father, in contrast, is ebullient about his new son. *The 5-year old draws a picture of his family that reveals these nonverbal communications* (Fig. 27-1).

- An 8-year-old girl sits in the chair biting her nails with slightly flexed truck and neck. She fidgets and responds to questions in short phrases. Inquiries about school and friends are followed by splotchy areas of erythema on her neck and face. *Nonverbal body language suggests an anxiety state and an opportunity to gently probe her concerns. If she remains silent, spending time with her parent alone while the child is asked to draw a picture of her family may be a good strategy to encourage communication.*

- A 4-year-old monitored since birth with a slow-to-warm-up temperament refuses to speak to the pediatrician. Her mother notes that she thinks his behavior is appropriate for a younger child; language acquisition continues to be delayed. A neuromaturational developmental screening test

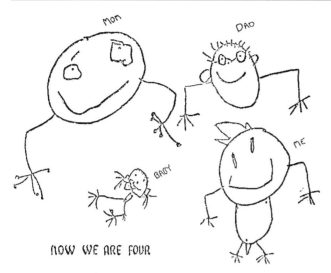

NOW WE ARE FOUR

FIGURE 27-1 Enhancing the communication process between pediatrician and parents during a well child visit (see text).

suggests global delay. *Mild or moderate cognitive delay may be missed when an attractive, nondysmorphic child with minimal social responsiveness is assumed to be shy and temperamentally slow to warm up.*

There are many opportunities to fine-tune a clinical interview with children and parents (Table 27-1). These methods have been studied and used by experienced clinicians who recognize the value of the clinical interview as a means of acquiring information and counseling children and families.[19] In addition, the physical proximity between the pediatrician, child, and family members may orchestrate the interview. Physical barriers to communication should be avoided (Table 27-2).

SCREENING FOR DEVELOPMENTAL AND BEHAVIORAL CONDITIONS WITH CHECKLISTS AND QUESTIONNAIRES

Developmental milestones (in the motor, language, and social domains according to the neuromaturational theory of child development) and behavior problems are assessed informally during a clinical interview and/or by use of an abbreviated checklist format. An individual clinician or practice group may develop these checklists by developing questions about selective developmental milestones and behaviors described in screening instruments. Monitoring development and behavior through a clinical interview or an informal checklist is dependent on the experience and skill of the clinician.

In contrast to informal screening, the advantage of a systematic screening questionnaire used in

TABLE 27-1 ■ **Fine-Tuning the Clinical Interview**

Open- and Closed-Ended Questions

Open-ended questions ("How is your baby doing?" or "What do you like about your baby?") encourage spontaneous, less structured responses than do closed-ended questions. They allow parents to express their concerns and an "explanatory model" of a problem or illness. Too many closed-ended questions, especially early in an interview, inhibit spontaneity and assessment of the parent's agenda for the visit.

Pauses and Silent Periods

Such periods provides time for a parent or child to collect thoughts and express feelings at moments when stressful or sad feelings emerge during an interview. They convey the message that the clinician cares enough to take the extra time.

Repetition of Important Phrases

Repeating or interpreting a statement made by the patient often encourages further clarification and exploration.

Active Listening

Most interviewing mistakes are caused by too much talking by the clinician. Active listening is the process of giving undivided attention to a patient's words and body language. The empathic clinician practices active listening through his or her facial expressions, posture, hand movements, and head nodding. It is a skill that can be learned.

Transference

On some occasions, a parent (or older child) may experience the pediatrician as someone who is symbolically and psychologically identified with another important person in his or her life. The symbolic attachment (to a mother, father, other relative, or person) is experienced by a parent or child at a time of deep emotional expression (joy, relief, anger, grief, or disappointment). Recognition of the transference process guides a clinician's insight and responses.

the course of a well-child visit is that predictable areas are assessed at each visit by asking a parent about specific neurodevelopmental achievements and behaviors. Many standardized questionnaires and observational tools have been developed for use in primary care pediatric practices[17a] (see Chapter 7B).

One innovation to incorporate developmental and behavioral issues into primary care is the Child Health and Development Interactive System (CHADIS). Parents complete questionnaires and computerized interviews online through an electronic decision support system, before a well-child care visit. The questionnaires are scored by the computer, which generates a list of prioritized parent concerns and scored questionnaires. These results provide evidence of behavioral and developmental concerns consistent with formats in the *Diagnostic and Statistical Manual of*

TABLE 27-2 ■ Positioning the Participants during a Pediatric Interview to Enhance Observations and Communications

The clinician and parent should be positioned at the same level to ensure eye contact and to prevent a subservient positioning effect. Both sit down or both stand up.

For a new patient or a new problem that requires an extensive history, sitting down with the parent and child may encourage greater information exchange, as well as allow the clinician to pay more attention to nonverbal cues.

For an established patient with an acute illness, the history may be taken while the parent and clinician are standing.

A young child who is ill may remain in the arms of the parent or with close physical contact.

The placement of chairs in an examination room and the proximity of clinician and patient influence the style and content of the interview.

A desk between a practitioner and the parent and child can be a barrier to optimal communication.

Picking up a chair and moving it closer to a parent may facilitate the exchange of information; the act itself may enhance a therapeutic relationship.

When interviewing a child or a teen, apply the same principles of spacing and eye contact.

A cautionary note on the use of the electronic medical record during an interview: Remember that you are interviewing the parent and child, not the computer screen. Frequently turn to the parent and child, make effective eye contact, and send a visual message that they are important. Or take notes and convert it to the electronic record later.

From Stein MT: Developmentally based office: Setting the stage for enhanced practice. *In* Dixon SD, Stein MT, eds: Encounters with Children: Pediatric Behavior and Development, 4th ed. Philadelphia: Elsevier, 2006, p 78.

Mental Disorders, 4th edition *(DSM-IV),*[19a] and the Diagnostic and Statistical Manual for Primary Care (DSM-PC): Child and Adolescent Version.[19b] The results are also linked to resources, including parent handouts, national level organizations, books, and videos, and local resources such as mental health clinicians, support groups, mentors, agencies, and activities.[20]

Screening questionnaires should be viewed as a supplemental aid to the clinical interview. When they are available before the interview, screening instruments may guide the clinician's area of inquiry, focus the visit on a particular topic that emerges from the questionnaire, or provide an opportunity for the parent or child to clarify a response on the questionnaire. They should not be used as a substitute for clinical observations, and interviewing must be tailored to the needs of each child and family. Patients and children need to "tell their own story"[21]—a process that is enhanced by the trust that develops through a therapeutic relationship based on sensitive interpersonal communication with children and parents (Table 27-3).

INNOVATIONS TO ENHANCE QUALITY AND BREADTH OF ATTENTION TO DEVELOPMENT AND BEHAVIOR IN OFFICE PRACTICE

In an effort to increase the efficient and effective delivery of developmentally sophisticated primary care, a number of innovative strategies have been considered and tried, with variable success.

Group Office Visits

The usual organization of medical practice is built on a model that attends to individual medical and psychological concerns. In an alternative model, the group process is used as a way to improve practice efficiency, get messages across to a larger number of patients, and encourage dialogue and support among patients with similar concerns or conditions.

PARENT GROUP DISCUSSIONS

Groups have been used to bring together individuals with similar problems. Parents of children with a chronic physical health condition, Down syndrome, attention-deficit/hyperactivity disorder, learning disabilities, mental retardation, cerebral palsy, and other conditions have been assembled for educational programs that enhance knowledge and skills in these specific areas. Parents who are negotiating similar life transitions (e.g., divorce, adoption, caring for aging parents) have also found group discussions helpful. These parent groups may be condition specific, especially those in specialty practices and children's hospitals, but more general groups have been successful in community practices. The clinician may be more or less directive in running these groups, taking the role of a teacher or a facilitator. As teacher, the leader of the group provides information that may be supplemented with written or audiovisual material. As facilitator, the leader encourages more dialogue among participants as a way to raise both individual and shared concerns and to provide an opportunity for parents to receive support and feedback from other parents who are (or who have children) in a similar circumstance.

In some primary care pediatric practices, the group discussion model has been adapted to address preventive topics. The focus can be on a developmental stage (e.g., in toddlers, school-aged children, adolescents), a particular topic (e.g., nutrition, tantrums and discipline, home safety, school underachievement, substance abuse), or a condition (e.g., asthma/allergies, recurrent ear infections, attention deficit/hyperactivity disorder, eating disorders, divorce). Some pediatricians have found the well-child visit before

TABLE 27-3 ■ Screening Checklists as Aids to Interview: Benefits and Risks
Selected screening checklists may supplement or focus the clinical interview. These tests, when administered before a child is seen, can trigger questions, raise issues, and prevent omissions in data collection. Most formal screening tests have been evaluated for validity, reliability, and predictive value. Be aware that a screening test is not diagnostic. Rather, it suggests a problem that must then be evaluated further through a comprehensive and focused interview by a primary care clinician. A referral for a developmental assessment or a mental health consultation may follow, depending on the clinician's interpretation of the screening test and clinical interview. Perrin and Stancin[17a] observed that "screening instruments are clinical tools that are useful to help identify and quantify parent's concerns and worrisome child behavior or feelings efficiently . . . as long as their limitations are recognized." Rating scales for behavioral conditions (e.g., depression) cannot take the place of a careful clinical interview. They are often helpful in the assessment of severity of symptoms and monitoring progress over time.
It is important to be informed about the advantages and limitations of these instruments. They provide a standardized database that serves to organize a health supervision visit. Screening tests prevent omissions that may occur during an interview alone. They provide potential educational value as a parent or older child answers questions that raise a concern that may not have been considered previously. They may help parents become better observers of their child's developmental changes and behaviors. Maintaining copies of the screening checklist in the medical record leads to quality assurance. A potential disadvantage of using a checklist alone is missing a parent's agenda for the visit by not permitting an individualized focus for the visit. A checklist without a therapeutic interview encourages an emphasis on content at the expense of process and a false sense of completeness.
When a screening test is used, it is the clinician's responsibility to interpret the results accurately and convey the information to the parents and/or child clearly. Screening for developmental and behavioral conditions should always be done with current knowledge about available referral sources in the community. Screening programs, whether for a biological, developmental, or behavioral condition, should be associated with a referral source for further evaluation and treatment when a positive test occurs. It is unethical to screen for a treatable condition without accurate interpretation, parent/child education, and an appropriate source for a more comprehensive assessment.[48]
Each opportunity to screen for developmental and behavioral problems is an interaction between the examiner and the child. The state, temperament, and availability of the child, as well as the training, ease, skill, and style of the examiner, influence it. The results of screening tests must always be interpreted with these factors in mind. They should never be a substitute for face-to-face clinical encounters in primary care practice.

Modified from Dixon SD, Stein MT: Encounters with Children: Pediatric Behavior and Development, 4th ed. Philadelphia: Elsevier, 2006, p 727.

kindergarten entry especially suitable for this format. Some practices are beginning to experiment with the notion of providing actual behavioral guidance to selected parents in groups.[21a]

GROUP WELL-CHILD CARE

An innovative use of the group process in pediatric practice has been the group well-child model.[22] In this model, children and their parents are seen for health supervision visits in the first few years of life, not individually but in small groups of parents and infants. Beginning usually with the first well-child visit after the child's birth, a group of infants and parents meet (usually 45 minutes) to discuss issues of general interest. The clinician is in the roles of both an educator and facilitator. Parent concerns guide the discussion. Because their children are of similar age, parents typically have similar concerns, and they learn from each other as well as from the clinician-facilitator. After the group discussion, each child is examined; the physical and developmental assessment can occur within the group or individually. Group well-child care was developed in an effort to find a method of delivering well-child care that includes more attention to development and behavior; is also cost effective, efficient, and satisfying to parents; and includes all the substantive content found in traditional individual care. It has the added advantage of creating a mutually

supportive group of parents who can share their parenting experiences while observing a range of developmental and behavioral characteristics.

Studies comparing group and traditional well-child care visits document several assets but also suggest limitations of the group process. A study of typically developing children in group well-child care found improved attendance at well-child visits, fewer calls between visits, more time for personal issues, and more open-ended questions.[23] In another study, more well-child care topics were discussed, including safety, nutrition, behavior, development, sleep, and parenting.[24] Parents' child care knowledge, social support, and maternal depressive symptoms were compared between groups and traditional models and found to be surprisingly similar.[25] Group well-child visits have been studied among high-risk families, for which higher no-show rates were found with group well-child care but no differences were seen in child development status, maternal-child interactions, home environment, provider time spent at visits, parental competence, social isolation, social support, and reports to child protective service.[26,27]

Teachable Moments

"Teachable moments" are opportunities for a clinician to comment about or demonstrate a response to a

TABLE 27-4 ■ Teachable Moments
Jake has been a healthy child before his health supervision visit at 18 months old. As you enter the examination room, you observe Jake playing on the floor with a plastic toy that has several movable parts. He appears engaged and intent on mastering the toy. You also notice that his fine motor skills are mature for his age when you observe Jake drawing. Jake appears not to notice you when you enter. Shortly after you begin to gather information from his mother, Jake's activity level and focus change dramatically. He starts hitting the toy, screams "bad . . . bad," and throws the toy into a wall. He starts to cry, resists his mother's attempt to hold him while she provides reassuring words, and hits her with his hand several times. His mother begins to cry and says, "He was such a good baby. In the last few months, he's a different child—selfish, angry, and always throwing a tantrum." You are faced with several options at this point:
1. Quickly perform a physical examination, check the growth chart, and order immunizations (and a blood lead and hematocrit if appropriate).
2. Talk to Jake's mother about tantrums and the need for discipline. Provide a handout on toddler development and discipline.
3. Attempt to engage Jake with words and a toy (i.e., sit down on the floor and play with the toy and say something like: "Gee, this is a great toy. I can make the door open so the boy can go inside."). Alternatively, address Jake and say, "It's real hard to come to the doctor!" or, "You are real upset at the doctor's office." Follow these words with silence and wait patiently for Jake's response.
The first option brings closure to the office visit but does not address Jake's behavior. The second option demonstrates recognition of a problem and expands the mother's knowledge about toddler behaviors and approaches to discipline. The third option illustrates immediate recognition of a "teachable moment." The pediatric clinician chooses to model an age-appropriate response to a tantrum through action and language. Engaging the child formulates the scene to the child's reality. The pediatrician's language is direct and brief; she tries to mirror the child's feelings with a few words and waits for a response. This technique, known as "active listening," encourages Jake's mother to learn that she can interact with her son at these difficult moments by feeding back to him the feelings he is experiencing. The clinician's modeling of the behavior can be followed by the information exchange illustrated in the second option.

From Stein MT: Developmentally based office: Setting the stage for enhanced practice. *In* Dixon SD, Stein MT, eds: Encounters with Children: Pediatric Behavior and Development, 4th ed. Philadelphia: Elsevier, 2005, p 80.

child's behavior or to communicate information during the physical, developmental, and behavioral examinations. They are *unplanned opportunities* to provide information, promote discussion, and support parents. Observation of a difficult temperament, a child's refusal to cooperate during a physical examination, and concern about maternal depression are examples of teachable moments. They occur frequently during both well-child and illness-related visits. In a busy practice, not every observed event that the clinician would like to comment on can be used as a teachable moment. Conscious vigilance for these opportunities and a commitment to responding to them several times each day enhance quality of care, satisfaction with the practice, and intellectual stimulation of the pediatrician (Table 27-4).

Teachable moments involve using experiences and questions that occur in the context of the visit to provide an opportunity for discussion, the exploration of parental feelings, modeling positive interactions, reframing negative parental attributions about their child, and providing specific information. A teachable moment capitalizes on the parent's immediate issues and concerns, when there is an increased desire to learn, rather than a preset list of anticipatory guidance issues, which may or may not coincide with parental priorities. Many teachable moments occur in response to a parent's questions but can also be found in the child's office behavior or in responses to written materials such as prompt sheets. Teachable moments provide a clinically effective and efficient

approach to anticipatory guidance so that parents can prevent problems.

—*Zuckerman et al,[28] p 822*

"Reach Out and Read"

This creative, office-based intervention was developed by a group of pediatricians to promote literacy, language skills, and a close parent-child attachment through reading to children at an early age. The rationale for the Reach Out and Read (ROR) program is that poor reading skill among many children in elementary school is associated with limited exposure to reading aloud during preschool years. A meta-analysis of 29 studies revealed a significant association between early reading aloud and later academic outcomes.[29]

The ROR program offers a developmentally appropriate book to a family at each well-child visit from 6 months to 5 years old. In some programs, a volunteer reads to children in the waiting room as a way to model reading aloud for parents. Clinicians are encouraged to demonstrate reading a book during an office visit. ROR has been used extensively in more than 2000 pediatric offices and clinics, especially (but not limited to) those serving underserved populations.

A number of studies have evaluated some form of the ROR program in pediatric settings; three of the studies are prospective controlled trials. Results of 12 studies support an association between ROR and increased reading aloud at home; four studies revealed that children in the program show increases in expressive and receptive language at 2 years of age in comparison with children in control groups.[30] In a large study including 730 parents who participated in ROR in 19 clinical sites in 10 states, and 917 parents from the same clinics who did not participate in the program, significant associations were found between exposure to ROR and reading aloud as a favorite parenting activity, reading aloud at bedtime, reading aloud 3 or more days per week, and ownership of 10 or more picture books.[31]

Co-location of Mental Health Clinicians

Effective professional relationships between pediatric clinicians and mental health professionals have been difficult to maintain because of very different training experiences, pacing, and different clinical languages. Traditional referrals to mental health clinicians have been successful only about half the time. Barriers such as stigma, financial constraints, and time limitations limit the effectiveness of the traditional referral procedure.

One solution that has been proposed to address this dilemma is to co-locate a mental health consultant in the pediatric office.[31a] A referral can be made more efficiently to "my colleague in the office" rather than to someone in another office building. Communication between the primary care clinician and the consultant, and common recordkeeping, are facilitated. For some families, the location of the mental health clinician in the pediatrician's office reduces the stigma associated with a mental health referral. Billing for mental health services may be done synchronously or independently, depending largely on the structure of health insurance plans in the community. In large staff-model health maintenance organizations and in some multispecialty community clinics, mental health services may be seamlessly included; however, the office of the mental health professional is still often physically distant from the primary care clinician, and some of the potential benefits of the collegial relationship are sacrificed.

Co-locating clinical care facilitates active communication through which referral history, psychopharmacological and psychotherapeutic treatments, and plans for follow-up are discussed in person. Joint care of some patients is facilitated: for example, when mental health professionals refer children to the pediatrician when they recognize the need for an updated or comprehensive medical assessment. The care of children with a chronic health or developmental condition is especially amenable to this form of teamwork.

Healthy Steps

An innovative form of co-locating care is the Healthy Steps model. The goal of this system of care is to increase a clinician's ability to address behavioral, emotional, and cognitive development in early childhood. To achieve this goal and create a strong bond between clinicians and parents, a specialist in child development—trained in pediatric nursing, early childhood education, or social work—is added to the practice staff to provide enhanced well-child care.[32] In this model, the child development specialist is an additional staff member whose role supplements those of the pediatrician and the office nurse. Her or his activities may include the following:

- Making home visits to the family, starting in the child's neonatal period.
- Focusing on promotion of children's development, including strategies to improve "the goodness of fit" between parent and child; paying closer attention to parental questions and concerns.
- Meeting with parents before, during, and after well-child visit to discuss behavioral and developmental concerns.
- Performing standardized developmental and behavioral screening tests.
- Providing written materials.
- Being accessible for questions and concerns through a child development telephone information line.
- Providing links to community resources.
- Initiating and managing parent groups to discuss common concerns.
- Coordinating early detection of substance abuse and domestic violence.

An evaluation of Healthy Steps included 5565 children and their parents at 15 sites.[28] Research demonstrated that parents in the program acquired more knowledge about child development and behavior and were better able to use community resources than control parents, who used traditional pediatric care. Families involved in the Healthy Steps program received significantly more preventive and developmental services than did families in the control group. They were *more likely* than nonparticipating families to

- Discuss with someone in the practice the importance to children of routines, discipline, language development, temperament, and sleeping patterns.
- Have greater adherence to visits, nutritional guidelines, developmental stimulation, and use of appropriate discipline techniques.
- Be highly satisfied with their care.
- Ensure that infants slept on their backs, to help reduce the risk of sudden infant death syndrome.
- Receive timely well-child visits and vaccinations.

■ Be more sensitive to their child's signals during play and more likely to match their interactions to their child's developmental level, interests, and capabilities.

The positive effects of the program were identified for all parents regardless of their income, parity, or maternal age. On the other hand, other measured outcomes showed no significant differences between the groups; these outcomes included initiation or duration of breastfeeding, child development knowledge, sense of competence, self-report of nurturing behavior and expectation of children, reports of children's language development at 2 years of age, and safety practices.[28]

Collaborative Office Rounds

Programs known as *collaborative office rounds* have been initiated in many communities to develop and support effective relationships between pediatricians and mental health professionals.[33] These group meetings consist of 8 to 12 pediatricians and one or two mental health clinicians who meet once or twice a month to discuss clinical cases that are challenging and engaging to the participants. Some of these groups also include a specific topic for discussion at some of the sessions. Supplementary readings, audio recording of office interviews with children and parents, invited experts from the community, and families invited to contribute to the discussion have been additional components. These ongoing group meetings have been evaluated and appear to provide

■ Enhanced understanding of psychosocial aspects of pediatrics.
■ Greater facility in dealing with developmental crises.
■ A more comprehensive approach to health supervision.
■ Fuller appreciation of psychosocial implications of chronic illness and disability.
■ Increased ability to advocate for families.
■ Expanded power to discriminate between transient disturbances and more serious psychiatric disorders.
■ More highly developed interviewing and counseling skills.
■ Heightened awareness of the scope of one's competency in the area of psychiatric disorders.
■ Increased effectiveness in making referrals to mental health colleagues.[34]

Building Consensus with Staff

A pediatric office or clinic is, in many ways, like a family. The individuals who work in a child health care setting bring a wide variety of personal, educa-

tional, and professional experiences to the work setting each day. Individually and collectively, they each affect quality of care. To achieve a developmental-behavioral focus in the office, it is crucial that the entire staff understand concepts of child development and behavioral interactions that are adaptive to pediatric practice.

In an office or clinic with more than one clinician, different opinions and perspectives on practice style and emphasis should be discussed. Formative pediatric training, prior practice experience, and temperament often shape a practice style. This is especially true in the area of development and behavior. Goals for developmental and behavioral monitoring should be outlined with enough specificity so that each clinician has a clear understanding of the group consensus. Each member of the staff should be given an opportunity to express her or his point of view and concerns. Research into alternative practice patterns and consultation with local experts should be encouraged. Pediatricians in some communities have found it valuable to meet periodically with colleagues from other offices to discuss practice patterns and strategies to improve care.

During meetings with the nurses and nonprofessional office staff and through selective printed material and videotapes, the clinic staff can receive education about major themes of development at each age group, developmental milestones, and common problems in development and behavior at specific ages. The goal of this educational process should be to empower the office staff to be sensitive "observers" of social interactions throughout the office visit and to prevent missed opportunities for important observations: when making an appointment by phone, at the time a parent and child check in with the office receptionist, when weighing and measuring a child, and when asking about a parent's concerns for the visit. These moments are opportunities to observe parent-child interactions in a context that may not be available to the pediatrician in the examination room. The office staff should be encouraged to communicate their observations to the child's clinician (Table 27-5). Periodic discussions during staff meetings with case examples from the office serve to reinforce the importance of staff observations.

COMMUNITY-BASED NEEDS ASSESSMENT

Pediatric practices might consider borrowing a public health method to assess the needs of a community with regard to behavioral and developmental concerns of parents who bring their children to the practice. Socioeconomic, educational, and ethnic differences create different concerns. Environmental

TABLE 27-5 ■ Notes from Medical Assistants Who Make an Important Observation while Preparing a Child or Youth for an Office Visit
2-Month-old's well-child visit: "Mom seems tired or depressed . . . few words and awkward when handling the baby."   5-Year-old's well-child visit: "I know this child . . . she is usually shy but cooperative. Today she resists weighing, blood pressure, and vision test. She won't talk to me."   12-year-old girl with a sore throat: "Very rude to her mom when checking in."

- Specialty medical consultations (e.g., neurology, genetics, audiology, speech therapy, occupational therapy, physical therapy, orthopedics).
- Psychological referrals (mental health professionals).
- Educational evaluation and services (school, community psychologists).
- Child care resources.
- Early intervention programs.
- Regional centers for children with neurodevelopmental disabilities.
- Families with children with chronic physical or developmental disabilities who agree to meet with other families to share their experiences.

To coordinate referrals in the community, it is useful to have one person in the office with the responsibility to assist parents with a community referral and to follow up to ensure that an appointment was made and kept. A coordinator can develop rapport with parents and act as an ombudsman to ensure that the care is received. The care coordinator can assist a parent with insurance eligibility, provide options for insurance coverage that may not be known to the parents, and act as a liaison between the referral source, parent, and pediatrician.

Some primary care practices have created a Parent Advisory Group made up of parents of children with a variety of chronic physical and developmental disabilities. The group provides ongoing suggestions about improvements in the care of children with chronic conditions. The parent group may also link with advocacy groups in the community bringing information and resources into the practice.[36a]

hazards, child care opportunities, and school curriculum and health services are among a few examples of community differences. An example of community-based needs assessment is evidenced in primary care family practice in Cuba, where a doctor and nurse are responsible for about 180 families surrounding the office neighborhood. An initial and ongoing assessment of health and psychosocial needs is the responsibility of the physician and nurse. Preventive programs and health education are formulated from the results of the assessments.[35]

A similar assessment of pediatric developmental and behavioral needs in the community would be a valuable exercise for a pediatric office staff member.

COORDINATION OF CARE AND LINKAGES WITH COMMUNITY RESOURCES

A primary care pediatric office should serve as the coordinator of care for the medical, educational, and psychosocial needs of children. These activities are a major component of the medical home (see Chapter 8B). An individual provider of care (or a single office) cannot fulfill all the needs of all children and families. Coordinated care with community resources is crucial for effective developmental and behavioral services for children and adolescents. Coordinated services for children with disabilities have been organized in some communities through a network whereby initial referrals and monitoring of referrals are organized by a central agency that works closely with each pediatric practice in the community to ensure access to appropriate services. An extensive outreach program links at-risk children and their families to programs and services.[36]

To achieve coordinated care for children with chronic physical and developmental conditions, pediatricians (and other office personnel) must be up to date on services available in a variety of areas, including the following:

FAMILY DRAWINGS: AN OPPORTUNITY FOR ENHANCED COMMUNICATION WITH PARENTS AND CHILDREN

Children naturally like to draw. The regular use of drawings can make a number of contributions to a child's visit to the pediatric office or clinic. The information obtainable from routinely asking a child to "draw a picture of your family" at all health supervision visits beginning at 4 or 5 years of age may be considerable. Drawing a picture may lessen the stress of a visit to the pediatric office; help the clinician assess fine motor and visual-perceptual abilities; and provide information about the child's sense of self, developmental status, family relationships, and adaptation to stress.[37]

Although a single figure in the drawing may be used as a screening test of visual-perceptual/fine motor maturation, there is often more to gain by using the family drawing as an opportunity to discuss issues about the child or family that do not surface during many pediatric office encounters. Asking a child to talk about the picture ("Tell me about the people you drew in your picture") or targeting a particular aspect of the drawing ("Where is your daddy . . . or your sister?") often provides an opportunity to engage a child or parent in a topic that may have been too difficult to talk about without the benefit of the drawing. At best, the dialogue generated by the drawing becomes a therapeutic discussion among the parents, child, and clinician. A sense of control and ownership in the visit to the pediatrician builds a foundation for involvement in and responsibility for health and health care. In addition, the drawings can also make parents aware of a stressful experience that has not been previously disclosed by the child. Sequential drawings should be part of the medical record to mark the child's development, to monitor both ordinary and extraordinary adaptive stress, and to serve as a developmental screen (Figs. 27-2 to 27-4).[38]

DEVELOPMENTAL AND BEHAVIORAL PEDIATRIC TRAINING FOR PEDIATRIC RESIDENTS

The specialty of developmental/behavioral pediatrics was supported by the recognition that pediatric training programs require a faculty member with knowledge, clinical skills and research programs in normal and abnormal development.[39] Teaching medical students, residents and practicing pediatricians remains a significant component of the specialty.

Primary care pediatrics is an office-based clinical practice. It follows that educational programs for primary care clinicians (including family physicians and pediatric nurse practitioners) are most effective when the curriculum is focused on outpatient pediatric practice. Residents in pediatrics and family medicine need information on normal development and behavior of children, adolescents, and families. In addition, they benefit from exposure to common developmental and behavioral conditions encountered in primary care practice. These functions are commonly provided for residents in the context of their continuity clinic and in developmental-behavioral pediatrics rotations.

Normal pathways of motor, social, language, and cognitive development are too often given short shrift in residency training programs. A list of developmental milestones often suffices. At least one textbook with a focus on resident education in normal development and behavior is available.[40] Reading, however,

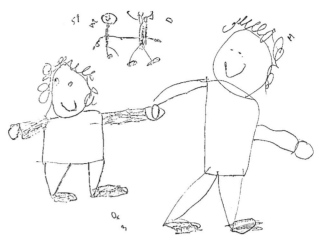

FIGURE 27-2 Drawing by a 5½-year-old girl of her family. The girl (depicted at upper left) drew a picture illustrating her close relationship with her father (typical parent choice for gender at this age) and her oversized 3-year-old sister holding the mother's hand. When the mother looked at the drawing at the end of the well-child care visit, she commented, "I forgot to ask you about the frequent arguing between my two daughters; they never seem to get along." The drawing was a prompt for the pediatrician to engage the mother in a brief discussion about sibling rivalry, place it in a developmental context, and suggest some reading material. A follow-up call was planned.

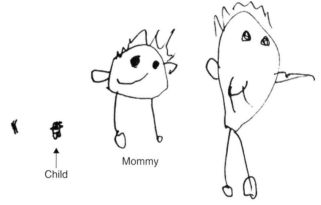

FIGURE 27-3 Drawing by a 6-year-old boy of his family. The boy was brought to the pediatrician because of a 3-month history of disruptive behavior in school and at home and refusal to participate in school activities. Three months ago, the parents separated after several years of marital disharmony. The child had not seen nor spoken to his father in 3 months. The mother was defiant in her refusal of the counseling recommended by the pediatrician. When she viewed her son's drawing (her son depicted as the second figure on the left), she cried for several minutes and then stated, "Now I understand what you mean. My son has no self-esteem when he draws himself so small—he's hardly recognizable." The mother immediately agreed to the counseling referral.

only begins the process of understanding developmental and behavioral differences among typically developing children. Supervised observations (in an office, child care center, school, or playground) are crucial for learning about children.

Pediatric residents and community-based pediatricians can be engaged in developmental theories as a method of discovering different perspectives on developing children, adolescents, and families and understanding unifying constructs of development adaptable to clinical practice. Theories of child development can assist pediatric clinicians in their understanding of variations in behavior and development from differ-

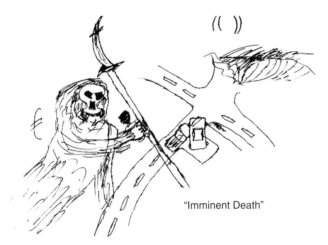

"Imminent Death"

FIGURE 27-4 A drawing by an 18-year-old boy. The adolescent was seen for a pre-college well visit. He was an excellent student with good social and athletic skills; the interim history and physical examination findings were normal. He had no specific concerns. At the end of the visit, the drawing he completed while waiting to be seen was reviewed. The drawing depicts his feelings about the recent death of his best friend as a result of an auto accident. This was the most significant recent event in this young man's life, an event that did not surface during the office visit. It encouraged the pediatrician to engage the patient in a discussion about loss and grief. Arrangements for a follow-up visit were made.

ent perspectives (see Fig. 27-5). Neuromaturational, cognitive, behavioral, psychoanalytic, and psychosocial theories each bring a unique language to the understanding of child development. The language in each theory can assist clinicians in helping parents gain insights into their children that may lead to alternative childrearing strategies.

Pediatric resident training should focus on common developmental and behavioral conditions seen in primary care practice and less common conditions that benefit from early recognition. In a resident curriculum that devotes extended time to rare neurological, genetic, and metabolic disorders, residents have limited opportunity to learn about more common conditions such as excessive crying in an infant, an evaluation of a child with language delay, oppositional behavior in a toddler, and the evaluation of a child with school underachievement. Attachment, parent-child interactional problems, and different family constellations are among the many topics that are useful to the next generation of pediatricians. Learning through clinical observations and incorporating standardized screening tests that lead to an early diagnosis of autistic spectrum disorder, learning disabilities, psychosocial risk factors, and other conditions should be a part of the curriculum.

Resident curricula in development and behavior vary among institutions and teachers, depending on resources and time. Some situations and tools available in most settings include the following:

1. Case-based learning.[41,42]
2. Videotapes of clinical problems.[43]

FIGURE 27-5 The progress of child development as described by several major theorists (John Bowlby, Margaret Mahler, D. W. Winnicott, Anna Freud, Erik Erikson, and Jean Piaget).

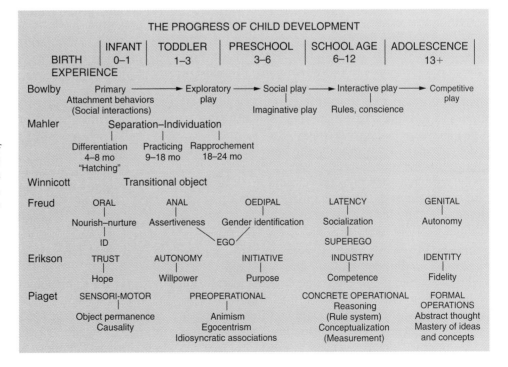

3. Developmental Behavioral Pediatrics Online, a Website with essential content for clinical practice: www.dbpeds.org.
4. Child care center observations.
5. School observations (typically developing children and those with learning and behavioral problems).
6. Observations in a primary care practice.
7. Observations in a developmental-behavioral pediatric specialty clinic.
8. Joint case conference with child psychiatry and/or psychology experts.

All students (including residents and pediatricians in practice) learn most effectively when they are challenged with new ideas. The innovations in office-based primary care discussed in this chapter offer opportunities for discussion, followed by active encouragement to adapt them in practice. Initiating a new program or method of practice in a continuity clinic is a good start. Examples of programs that residents can initiate to enhance their learning about children's development and behavior include developing a ROR program, initiating the use of a screening test not used previously in the practice, and visiting the classroom or preschool of a continuity clinic patient with a learning or behavioral problem.

RETHINKING WELL-CHILD CARE

The premise of the discussion in this chapter is the idea that incremental, focused innovations will enhance the quality of developmentally and behaviorally sophisticated pediatric care. Some of the suggestions (e.g., Healthy Steps) are costly and require structural change in the practice. Others (e.g., family drawings, screening procedures, and teachable moments) are inexpensive, may even save time, and may be added to existing practices with ease. Still others (e.g., group well-child care, parent groups, teen groups) do not add extra costs but do require a structural change in the office pattern of care. Of importance is that all are achievable and adaptable in a primary care pediatric setting.

Pediatricians are beginning the process of rethinking the format and content of well-child care, especially with regard to the prevention, identification, and treatment of developmental and behavioral conditions.[44] Many ideas are emerging. Some examples include the following:

1. Increased use of Internet technology to prepare parents and older children for well-child visits. These materials provide the developmental and behavioral content issues that may be discussed at an upcoming visit. Parents and children can select areas of concern and download the material to bring to the office visit.

2. Parent-child, age-specific guides to well-child visits, available from the AAP Bookstore and included in the *Guidelines for Health Supervision III* (American Academy of Pediatrics). These guides provide an opportunity to list concerns and review developmental, behavioral, and environmental issues.[45]

3. Selected topics to emphasize during several 1-week periods, which focus each well-child visit on that topic in the context of the child's age. Examples might include sleep patterns and disturbances; oppositional behavior in toddlers and preschool children; social development (including play, bullying, sports, and dating); educational competencies; tobacco, alcohol, and substance abuse; and television watching patterns in the family. Pediatricians (and the office staff) will be motivated to develop a level of expertise in an area that is discussed frequently in a short time frame.

4. A scheduled "shot clinic." As a way to permit more time for discussions and evaluations of developmental and behavioral problems during well-child visits, an immunization-only time period may be appropriate. The medical assistant or nurse may also perform growth measurements and ask whether there are any concerns, but the focus of the visit is on immunizations. This system may allow for *fewer and longer* well-child visits without additional expenditures.

5. Provision of developmental and behavioral surveillance at all office encounters, but selection of critical moments (especially in the first 3 years) to assess development and behavior in more detail through the use of a standardized screening test. An example of this idea has been proposed by the AAP with developmental and behavioral surveillance at all well-child and illness-related visits and the performance of a standardized screening test at the following ages:[46]
   A. Nine months: motor development and communication skills, including vision, hearing, eye contact, orienting to name, and pointing.
   B. Eighteen months: language and social development, including screening for autistic spectrum disorders.
   C. Thirty months: reassessment of language and cognitive development that is important in children with limited emerging language skills at 24 months (a recommendation for a 30-month well-child visit is currently under consideration by the AAP).

A logical extension of this model is the use of standardized screening at 5 years (school readiness), 7-8 years (problems associated with learning and social interactions), and 12 years (autonomy, peer relations, sexuality, academic achievement, substance abuse).

SUMMARY: ESSENTIAL COMPONENTS OF "THINKING DEVELOPMENTALLY" DURING PRIMARY CARE OFFICE PEDIATRIC ENCOUNTERS

Observing and Understanding the Parent-Child Relationship

Observing the quality of attachment between a child and parent in the first few years of life provides pediatricians with a valuable source of information. The enduring psychological connection between a child and parent (attachment) provides clues to subsequent social competence, self-reliance, school success, and emotional well-being. It begins with a pediatrician's observation of the quality with which parents read their baby's signals in early infancy. These observations of attachment inform anticipatory guidance during well-child visits.

"Biopsychosocial Pediatrics" Is a Useful Mantra

Pediatric medicine is practiced optimally with frequent considerations of biological, social, and psychological elements of care. Children with streptococcal tonsillitis, chronic recurrent asthma, attention-deficit/hyperactivity disorder, or anxiety all benefit from the biopsychosocial model of medical practice in that it links important aspects of a child's life with each other. Thinking biopsychosocially expands a clinician's care to include the whole patient and does not limit clinical thinking and patient interactions to an isolated disease process.[47]

Temperament

Temperament provides a language to describe a child's behavior and interactions with others. Consistent evaluations of temperament assist pediatricians when communicating with parents. They encourage reflections and guidance that is individualized and more accurate.

Brain Maturation and Plasticity

Advances in neuroscience provide pediatricians with objective evidence for a core principle of pediatric practice: that the social and psychological environment in which a child is raised has a significant effect on developmental achievements.

The structure of the human brain continues to change during childhood and adolescence through a process of synapse generation and pruning. Recogni-

tion that these changes are mediated by the quality of environmental experience has fueled pediatricians' goal to help families optimize the development of their children. Emotionally healthy conditions in the home, school, and neighborhood interact with genetic endowment to provide appropriate brain maturation and sustain adequate development.[2] Nature and nurture are always interacting as developmental and behavioral change occurs. The developmentally oriented pediatrician who is aware of this interaction usually conveys a more optimistic and realistic perspective at each clinical encounter.

Engaging Developmental Theory Wisely and Frequently

Theoretical ideas are the basis for medical practice whether they are derived quantitatively (e.g., biological experiments in a laboratory) or qualitatively (focused observations of children over time). Developmental theories provide a framework for understanding and interpreting psychological, social, neuromaturational, and cognitive development during childhood and adolescence. Theories provide clinically useful linkages between sequential stages in development and often guide clinicians' understanding of individual differences in behavior, learning, and social interactions. A conscious effort to correlate clinical observations in the office with a developmental theory has an added benefit: to enhance the intellectual stimulation of pediatricians who have the opportunity to witness the wide spectrum of normal and abnormal development.

REFERENCES

1. Engel GL: The need for a new medical model: A challenge for biomedicine. Science 196:129-136, 1977.
2. Shonkoff JP, Phillips DA, eds: From Neurons to Neighborhoods: the Science of Early Childhood Development Washington, DC: National Academies Press, 2000.
3. Young, KT, Davis, K, Schoen, C, Parker, S: Listening to parents: A national survey of parents with young children. Arch Pediatr Adolesc Med 152:255-262, 1998.
4. Sand N, Silverstein M, Glascoe FP et al: Pediatricians' reported practices regarding developmental screening: Do guidelines work? Pediatrics 116:174-179, 2005.
5. Inkelas M, Schuster MA, Olson LM, et al: Continuity of primary care clinician in early childhood. Pediatrics 113(6 Suppl):1917-1925, 2004.
6. Alpert JJ, Zuckerman PM, Zuckerman B: Mommy, who is my doctor? Pediatrics 113(6 Suppl):1985-1987, 2004.
7. Kogan MD, Schuster MA, Yu SM, et al: Routine assessment of family and community health risks: Parent views and what they receive. Pediatrics 113(6 Suppl):1934-1943, 2004.

8. Cone TE Jr: History of American Pediatrics. Boston, MA: Little, Brown, 1979.

9. Brosco JP: Weight charts and well-child care. Arch Pediatr Adolesc Med 155:1385-1389, 2001.

10. Baker JP, Pearson HA, eds: Dedicated to the Health of All Children. Elk Grove Village, IL: American Academy of Pediatrics, 2005.

11. American Academy of Pediatrics, Committee on Practice and Ambulatory Medicine: Recommendations for Preventive Pediatric Health Care. Elk Grove Village, IL: American Academy of Pediatrics, 2000.

12. Pickering LA, ed: Redbook, 27th ed. Elk Grove Village, IL: American Academy of Pediatrics, 2006.

13. Kleinman RE, ed: Pediatric Nutrition Handbook, 5th ed. Elk Grove Village, IL: American Academy of Pediatrics, 2004.

14. Task Force on Sudden Infant Death: The changing concept of sudden infant death. Pediatrics 116:1245-1255, 2005.

15. Siegel RM, Kiely M, Bien JP: Treatment of otitis media with observation and a safety-net antibiotic prescription. Pediatrics 112:527-531, 2003.

16. Regalado M, Halfon N: Primary care services promoting optimal child development from birth to age 3 years. Arch Pediatr Adolesc Med 155:1311-1322, 2001.

17. Glascoe FP: Collaborating with Parents: Using PEDS to Detect and Address Developmental and Behavioral Problems. Nashville, TN: Ellsworth VandeMeer Press, 1998.

17a. Perrin EC, Stancin T: A continuing dilemma: Whether and how to screen for concerns about children's behavior. Pediatr Rev 23:264-275, 2002.

18. American Academy of Pediatrics: Guidelines for Health Supervision III, 3rd ed. Elk Grove Village, IL: American Academy of Pediatrics, 2002, p 3.

19. Lipkin ML Jr, Putnam SM, Lazare A: The Medical Interview—Clinical Care, Education, and Research. New York: Springer-Verlag, 1995.

19a. American Psychiatric Association: Diagnostic and Statistical Manual of Mental Disorders, 4th ed–Primary Care Version. Washington, DC: American Psychiatric Press, 1995.

19b. American Academy of Pediatrics: The classification of child and adolescent Mental Diagnosis in Primary Care—Diagnostic and Statistical Manual for Primary Care (DSM-PC) Child and Adolescent Version. Elk Grove Villiage, IL: American Academy of Pediatrics, 1996.

20. Sturner R, Howard B: CHADIS. (Available at: www.childhealthcare.org; accessed 2/22/07.)

21. Cole R: The Call of Stories: Teaching and the Moral Imagination. Boston: Houghton Mifflin, 1990.

21a. Sheldrick R, McMenamy J, Kavanaugh K, Tannebring E, Perrin E: A Preventive Intervention for ADHD in Pediatric Settings [poster]. Pediatric Academic Societies, May 2005.

22. Stein M: The providing of well baby care within parent-infant groups. Clin Pediatr 16:825, 1977.

23. Osborn LM, Woolley FR: Use of groups in well child care. Pediatrics 67:701-706, 1981.

24. Dodds M, Nicholson L, Muse B, et al: Group health visits more effective than individual visits in delivering health care information. Pediatrics 9:668-670, 1993.

25. Rice RL, Miles CE, Slater CJ: An analysis of group versus individual health supervision visits. Am J Dis Child 146:488, 1992.

26. Taylor JA, Davis RL, Kemper KJ: A randomized controlled trial of group versus individual well child care for high-risk children: Maternal-child interaction and developmental outcomes. Pediatrics 99:e9, 1997.

27. Taylor JA, Kemper KJ: Group well-child care for high-risk families. Arch Pediatr Adolesc Med 152:579-584, 1998.

28. Zuckerman B, Parker S, Kaplan-Sanoff M: Healthy Steps: A case study of innovation in pediatric practice. Pediatrics 114:820-826, 2004.

29. Bus AG, van IJzendoorn M, Pelligrini A: Joint book reading makes for success in learning to read: A meta-analysis on intergenerational transmission of literacy. Rev Educ Res 65:1-21, 1995.

30. Needlman R, Silverman M: Pediatric interventions to support reading aloud: How good is the evidence? J Dev Behav Pediatr 25:352-363, 2004.

31. Needlman R, Toker KH, Dreyer BP, et al: Effectiveness of a primary care intervention to support reading aloud: A multi-center evaluation. Ambul Pediatr 5:209-215, 2005.

31a. Perrin EC: The promise of collaborative care. Dev Behav Pediatr 20:57-62, 1999.

32. Minkovitz CS, Hughart N, Strobino D, et al: A practice-based intervention to enhance quality of care in the first three years of life: Results from the Healthy Steps for Young Children Program. JAMA 290:3081-3091, 2003.

33. DeMaso DR, Knight JR: The Collaboration Essentials Office Rounds Case Manual. (Available at: http://collaborationEssentials.org/ce/using/index.html.)

34. Fishman ME, Kessel W, Heppel DE, et al: Collaborative office rounds: Continuing education in the psychosocial/developmental aspects of child health. Pediatrics 99:e5, 1997.

35. Swanson KA, Swanson JM, Gill AE, et al: Primary care in Cuba: A public health approach. Health Care Women Int 16:299-308, 1995.

36. Dworkin PH: Historical overview: From ChildServ to Help Me Grow. J Dev Behav Pediatr 27(1 Suppl):S5-S7, 2006 [discussion, J Dev Behav Pediatr 27(1 Suppl): S17-S21,S50-S52, 2006].

36a. Young M, McMenamy JM, Perrin EC: Parent advisory groups in pediatric practices: Parents' and professionals' perceptions. Arch Pediatr Adolesc Med 155:692-698, 2001.

37. Stein MT: The use of family drawings by children in pediatric practice. J Dev Behav Pediatr 18:334, 1997.

38. Welsh JB, Instone SL, Stein MT: Use of drawings by children at health encounters. In Dixon SD, Stein MT, eds: Encounters with Children: Pediatric Behavior and Development, 4th ed. Philadelphia: Elsevier, 2006, pp 98-121.

39. Haggerty RJ, Friedman SB: History of developmental-behavioral pediatrics. J Dev Behav Pediatr 24(Suppl): S1-S18.

40. Dixon SD, Stein MT: Encounters with Children: Pediatric Behavior and Development, 4th ed. Philadelphia: Elsevier, 2006.

41. Stein MT, ed: Challenging cases in developmental and behavioral pediatrics. J Dev Behav Pediatr Suppl 22: S1-S184, 2001. Suppl 25:1-111, 2004.

42. Pedicases: A series of primary care problems including development and behavior. (Available at: www.pedicases.org.)

43. Developmental and Behavioral Pediatrics: Training Modules on Clinical Issues in Primary Care [DVD]. New York: Commonwealth Fund, 2006. (Available at: http://www.cmwf.org/tools/tools_show.htm?doc_id=360961; accessed 2/22/07.)

44. Schor EL: Rethinking well-child care. Pediatrics 114:210-216, 2004.

45. American Academy of Pediatrics: Parent/child guides to pediatric visits. *In:* Guidelines for Health Supervision III. Elk Grove Village, IL: American Academy of Pediatrics, 2002, pp 247-256.

46. American Academy of Pediatrics: Identifying infants and young children with developmental disorders in the medical home: An algorithm for developmental surveillance and screening. Pediatrics 118:405-420, 2006.

47. Apley J, Ounsted C, eds: One Child. Philadelphia: JB Lippincott, 1982.

48. Perrin EC: Ethical questions about screening. Commentary. J Dev Behav Pediatr 19:350-352, 1998.

Ethical Issues in Developmental-Behavioral Pediatrics: A Historical Approach

JEFFREY P. BROSCO ■ PAUL STEVEN MILLER ■
KENNETH W. GOODMAN ■ SARAH R. FUCHS

Ethical issues in developmental-behavioral pediatrics (DBP) fall within the larger discipline of bioethics. Children with developmental or behavioral disorders may have unique needs or face end-of-life issues more frequently than do other children, but the fundamental approach to resolving ethical issues is and should be the same as for any other child. Philosophers have sought to ground clinical ethical decisions in theories of morality; in everyday practice, clinicians and families work together to determine the best interests of a particular child within the constraints of law and generally accepted social values. Consensus on ethical decisions has varied with time and place, as each community has struggled to define its core values in laws, words, and deeds. This is especially true with regard to ethical issues and persons with developmental disabilities, because the way clinicians understand and value the quality of life of people with disabilities has changed dramatically since the 1950s. The role of history is therefore critical in understanding ethical issues in DBP.

This chapter focuses on ethical issues of interest to DBP specialists. In accordance with the framework of this textbook, disorders of child development and behavior are viewed as on a continuum: On one end are children with classic neurodevelopmental disabilities such as mental retardation, hearing impairment, or cerebral palsy; on the other are children with disorders such as depression or attention-deficit/hyperactivity disorder (ADHD). In most affected children, of course, the disorders defy such simple categories and often occupy different points along that continuum. For example, a child with mental retardation may also have oppositional behavior. Another child with an apparent behavioral disorder may have subtle neurodevelopmental issues that influence his or her ability to cope with environmental demands. Because the special ethical issues of DBP tend to occur more commonly in children with developmental disabilities, many of the examples in this chapter focus on these children and their families.

The core task of this chapter on clinical bioethics is to attempt to define the areas of broad social consensus in North America. There are obviously many areas of controversy, but even with this objective, the range of choices is constrained by specific social and historical circumstances. Rather than attempt to cover all pertinent issues in brief sections in traditional textbook format, this chapter provides a framework for understanding clinical bioethics through four main sections: (1) an introduction to traditional bioethics; (2) a description of how the history of persons with developmental disabilities frames current issues, such as end-of-life decisions; (3) an overview of controversies in genetics and surgical cures of disability; and (4) some notes on how the DBP practitioner seeks to balance science, clinical practice, and advocacy, especially in the context of behavioral disorders.

OVERVIEW OF TRADITIONAL BIOETHICS

Professional Codes of Conduct

Guidelines for the professional behavior of medical practitioners have been promulgated for at least 4000 years, according to writings from ancient Egypt and Mesopotamia. The comparatively recent Oath attributed to Hippocrates (460-380 B.C.) is among the most famous, but other prominent medical writers such as Galen and Maimonides offered advice on privacy, duty to patients, and end-of-life issues.[1] Such guidelines express values common to medical practitioners, but they also serve to elevate the standing of medicine as a profession and not a mere vocation. For example, the American Medical Association was founded in 1847 in part to restrain unseemly competition among medical practitioners; that same year, the association's leadership disseminated a code of appropriate behavior for medical practitioners that included rules for referrals and fee splitting.[2]

Since the early 1980s, a surge of interest in professional behavior has led a number of organizations to develop codes of conduct for health care providers (Table 28-1). The European Federation of Internal Medicine, the American College of Physicians–American Society of Internal Medicine, and American Board of Internal Medicine, for example, collaborated to publish a physician charter outlining principles to which "all medical professionals can and should aspire."[3] As in similar documents since the 1950s, the physician charter focused on principles that many argue provide the foundation for medical practice: beneficence, autonomy, privacy, and social justice or equity. Rules of professional behavior described in these or similar principles are now being integrated more fully into the training and accreditation of physicians; examples include recommendations and requirements of the Accreditation Council for Graduate Medical Education, the Association of American Medical Colleges, and the National Board of Medical Examiners.[4]

The seemingly universal nature of ethical principles is underlined by their international scope. The Declaration of Geneva adopted in 1948 by the World Medical Association was an attempt to describe a world standard for medical professionals, and there is evidence that the professionals' beneficial influence extended beyond the physician-patient relationship to help shape humanistic and egalitarian features of the world's legal and political institutions.[5] Indeed, the United Nations General Conference began devising universal standards in the field of bioethics that extended far beyond professional conduct by physicians. The 2005 Universal Draft Declaration on Bioethics and Human Rights outlines the ethical practices expected of policymakers, health care providers, and professional groups (Table 28-2).[6]

TABLE 28-1 ■ Professionalism According to Medical Institutions[4]

Institution	Publication	Definition

ABIM, ACP-ASIM, EFIM	A Physician Charter (2002)[3]	Professionalism: a foundation of the social contract for medicine
		Principles: primacy of patient welfare, patient autonomy, social justice
		Commitments:
		    Professional competence
		    Scientific knowledge
		    Professional responsibilities
		    Managing conflicts of interest
		    Patient confidentiality
		    Honesty with patients
		    Improving quality of care
		    Improving access to care
		    Appropriate relationships
		    Just distributions of finite resources

General Medical Council	Good Medical Practice[54]	Make the care of your patient your first concern Treat every patient politely and considerately Respect patient's dignity and privacy Listen to patients and respect their views Give patients information in a way they can understand Respect the right of patients to be fully involved in decisions Keep your professional knowledge and skills up to date; recognize the limits of your competence Be honest and trustworthy Respect and protect confidential information Make sure that your personal beliefs do not prejudice your patients' care Act quickly to protect patients from risk (from unfit physicians) Avoid abusing your position as a physician Work with colleagues in the ways that best serve patients' interests
AAMC	Medical School Objectives (1999)[55]	Knowledgeable: scientific method, biomedicine Skillful: clinical skills, reasoning, condition managing, communication Altruistic: respect, compassion, ethical probity, honesty, avoidance of conflicts of interest Dutiful: population health, advocacy, and outreach to improve nonbiological determinants of health, prevention, information management, health systems management

AAMC, American Association of Medical Colleges; ABIM, American Board of Internal Medicine; ACP-ASIM, American College of Physicians–American Society of Internal Medicine; EFIM, European Federation of Internal Medicine.

TABLE 28-2 ■ Universal Draft Declaration on Bioethics and Human Rights[6,48]

Concept	Definition
Human dignity and human rights	Recognition that all persons have unconditional worth
Equality, equity and justice	Equality: equal treatment of individuals in a similar situation Equity: the use of discretion when examining special circumstances of particular cases; a correct mechanism to formal equality Justice: normative principle describing, how institutions, society, and other groups of people should act; implementing the balance between equality and equity
Benefit and harm	Any decision or practice shall seek to benefit the person concerned and to minimize the possible harm
Respect for cultural diversity and pluralism	Ethical standards must be interpreted and adapted to the manifold ways in which cultures of different social groups and societies find expression
Nondiscrimination and nonstigmatization	Nondiscrimination: prohibition of discrimination, which is treating a morally neutral and immutable characteristic as having a negative effect Nonstigmatization: elimination of stigma requires a longer process of social transformation in which ethics and ethics teaching can play a significant role
Autonomy and individual responsibility	Individuals cannot be instrumentalized and treated merely as a means to a scientific end; they should be granted the authority to make autonomous decisions in all aspects of their lives
Informed consent	A patient or potential research subject has to receive relevant, structured, and individually tailored information that makes it possible for him or her to make a decision whether or not to accept medical treatment, as well as to understand and cope with the diagnosis; also, special protection shall be given to persons who do not have the capacity to consent
Privacy and confidentiality	Privacy: guarantees a control over personal information Confidentiality: refers to the relationship between doctor and patient (or researcher and research subject); it provides that the shared information shall remain secret, confidential, and not disclosed to third person (unless strictly defined interest justifies disclosure under domestic law)
Solidarity and cooperation	Collective social protection and fair opportunity in access to health care worldwide, with special attention to vulnerable groups
Social responsibility	Takes into account the wider social dimension of the scientific process by specifying five elements of universal priority (access to quality health care, access to adequate nutrition and water, improvement of living conditions and the environment, elimination of marginalization and exclusions of persons on the basis of any ground, and reduction of poverty and illiteracy)
Sharing of benefits	Benefits from advances in biology, genetics, and medicine shall be made available to all
Responsibility for the biosphere	Recognizes that human beings are an integral part of the biosphere and have responsibilities toward other forms of life and future generations

Moral Theory

For centuries, many physicians have grounded ethical behavioral in their religious beliefs, whether invoking the gods of Hippocrates's Greece or the monotheism of today. Particularly in the United States, appeals to the Ten Commandments or especially the "golden rule"—"Do unto others as you would have them do unto you"—are especially common approaches to proscribing behavior. Other physicians and scholars have turned to secular theories of moral behavior. John Stuart Mill's and Jeremy Bentham's utilitarianism, commonly understood as the "greatest good for the greatest number," is one system that focuses on the consequences of given actions as the tool for making the best choice. Immanuel Kant held that moral behavior would follow from meeting the rational requirement to choose the course of action that a person would want everyone in a similar position to

follow, as if that person were setting the rules for behavior. In the 1970s, largely in response to reports of abuse of research subjects in the Tuskegee syphilis experiments, the U.S. federal government commissioned a group of scholars to provide a guide for the proper conduct of research, and the resulting Belmont Report focused on the principles of autonomy, beneficence, and justice. Further developed by Beauchamp and Childress, "principlism" has been widely applied to clinical ethics as well.[7]

Gert argued that these traditional systems of moral theory are generally not useful in resolving clinical and other ethics debates.[8] Each of these systems has noteworthy exceptions, and any system that sometimes produces the wrong answer cannot be relied upon to produce the right answer when faced with an ethical dilemma. Furthermore, Gert argued, moral theories that suggest that there is one right answer can actually impede resolution of ethical dilemmas by creating conflict among participants. Instead, according to Gert, most dilemmas can be resolved if there can be agreement on the facts, and in cases of true conflict on values, such as abortion, there can be more than one morally acceptable answer. He offered his own approach of moral rules and ideals and suggested that breaking the rules is appropriate when a person would be willing to describe publicly why he or she is breaking a rule and have it stand as policy. For example, breaking a promise of confidentiality is appropriate when a clinician learns that a patient plans to injure somebody.

Autonomy, Beneficence, and Justice

Despite the limits of principlism for resolving ethical dilemmas, it provides a useful framework for understanding clinical ethics.[9]

There are three basic elements to autonomy: agency (awareness of oneself, desires, and intentions), independence (absence of influences), and rationality (capacity for reflection on desires). Respect for a patient's autonomy is the fundamental principle underlying privacy, confidentiality, valid consent, and refusal of treatment. In the United States, the right to privacy was first recognized as protected by the Constitution in the 1965 U.S. Supreme Court ruling, *Griswold v. Connecticut,*[9a] a case involving use of contraception by married couples. In clinical practice, autonomy has come to mean that patients generally decide what medical care they receive, and their wish to refuse treatment should be respected if they are fully informed and appreciate the consequences of their refusal. Because of age and cognitive level, children are typically not deemed competent to make medical decisions. Parents or guardians are usually called upon to do what is in the best interests of the child. As children enter their teens, they begin to participate in health care decisions, especially when the issues involve pregnancy or treatment for sexually transmitted infections.

When the health care team believes that a family's wishes are not in the best interest of the child, they have an obligation to argue that a "reasonable person" would choose otherwise. When such conflicts cannot be resolved, even with help from social workers and pastoral care providers, the health care team can appeal to a state government to protect the interests of the child. The state typically intervenes on behalf of the child through the court system, for example, when parents refuse obviously lifesaving treatment on religious grounds. Most hospitals have bioethics committees that can help clarify ethical dilemmas and provide leadership in articulating a consensus on community values.

The twin principles of nonmaleficence and beneficence also focus on the individual patient's best interest. Nonmaleficence, the duty to do no harm to patients, is deeply rooted in the history of medicine. However, it is not enough to merely restrain from harmful acts; the physician must take active steps to contribute to the welfare of the patient. Deciding whether aggressive intervention at the end of life would produce more harm than benefit for a patient is a classic example of how the principle of beneficence may be applied. Constructing a risk : benefit ratio can operationalize the principle of beneficence: a favorable benefit : harm ratio is the prerequisite for any action to be ethically justified.

In attempting to follow the principles of autonomy and beneficence, the health care provider will confront inequities in the social and economic fabric of society. The philosopher John Rawls offered one way to describe such inequities: The "natural lottery" distributes properties through birth, and the "social lottery" distributes social assets through family property, social class, and education. The principle of justice holds that people do not deserve advantageous properties any more than they deserve disadvantageous properties.[7] In the United States, however, children living in poverty and those without health insurance are much more likely to experience poor heath than are those who are wealthier and those with health insurance. A just distribution of resources implies that all children, indeed all persons, should have equal access to medical treatment and adequate education, housing, and nutrition. Children with special health care needs are especially likely to suffer from inadequate access to beneficial medical care, and their families face substantial economic hardship.

Principlism, Historical Context, and the Role of the Bioethics Committee

Despite the popularity of principlism as a framework for clinical ethics, there is empirical evidence that education in such principles of ethics does not affect moral decision making as much as do culture, personal history, and social and institutional context.[10] Indeed, it is sometimes difficult in practice to balance all the principles equally and simultaneously, inasmuch as an emphasis on one principle often minimizes that on another. For example, in an effort to minimize harm to a patient with an aggressive medical intervention, the physician might indirectly diminish the patient's autonomy. Beneficence and autonomy often conflict with the principle of social justice, in the presence of finite resources in health care. An individual physician may advocate for a third liver transplantation for her patient, for example, but in the context of a long waiting list, social justice suggests that other patients should have an opportunity to benefit from that limited resource. Which principle takes precedence? Who is to decide which principle is most important in a given case?

The answers to these questions vary with time and place. Each society works out an approximate consensus for most ethical issues, and this consensus may shift over time. For example, during the 1950s in the United States, there was a general consensus that beneficence trumped autonomy: the physician knew best what to do at the end of life, and it was appropriate to withhold information from patients and families. Through the 1960s and 1970s, such "paternalism" came under attack as part of a larger movement questioning the beneficence of institutional authority, and today autonomy typically outweighs beneficence (see Chapter 8B).[11] This shift towards patient autonomy is embodied in the case of Nancy Cruzan* in 1990, when the U.S. Supreme Court recognized the right of competent persons to decline medical treatment even if it led to the person's death. Living wills and advanced directives now instruct the health care team to respect the wishes of the patient at the end of life.

One way of defining the social consensus on controversial ethical issues is through institutional bioethics committees. Since the 1970s, such committees have been increasingly active in the United States and elsewhere, in part to fulfill the requirement by the Joint Commission on Accreditation of Healthcare Organizations that hospitals have a mechanism for addressing ethical issues in patient care. One key role of an institutional bioethics committee is to define current standards of ethical practice: that is, to help the entire community understand what the social consensus is with regard to typical issues such as confidentiality and end-of-life decisions. The membership of a bioethics committee is therefore crucial for its success: Some members should be well trained in the philosophical principles of bioethics, some should be legal experts, some should have experience with pastoral care, some should have clinical experience with common ethical issues, and some, arguably, should have a personal experience of living with a disability.[12] Overall diversity of membership is crucial,

however, because the committee needs to be able to say that its deliberations reflect the broad consensus of a community. In this case, diversity refers to gender, age, disability, race/ethnicity, professional background, political viewpoints, and association with the hospital. The presence of at least one committee person with a developmental disability helps ensure that special issues related to persons with disabilities are appropriately considered. Table 28-3 describes the properties of an institutional ethics committee according to the United Nations Educational, Scientific, and Cultural Organization (UNESCO), the American Medical Association, and the American Academy of Pediatrics.

END-OF-LIFE DECISIONS AND THE HISTORY OF PERSONS WITH DEVELOPMENTAL DISABILITIES

End-of-life decisions constitute a critical area of bioethics and, for the purposes of this chapter, also provide a salient example of how the history of persons with developmental disabilities informs current ethical issues. Centuries of discrimination against persons with developmental disabilities, sterilization and euthanasia early in the 20th century, and the disability rights movement of the late 20th century are a few of the key points in this history. This brief historical overview is necessarily an oversimplification, and emerging evidence suggests that life for persons with disabilities before the modern period in particular was much more nuanced than previously acknowledged.[13] To understand how current ethical debates are informed by a popular understanding of history, however, this section focuses on major points in Western civilization that provide the context for ethical issues such as death and dying.

From Antiquity to the Enlightenment

Persons with disabilities have suffered from discrimination and abuse since antiquity, although such treatment was not universal. In ancient Greece and Rome, for example, most scholars attributed disabling condition to failure of parents to properly revere the gods. Hippocrates' hypothesis that epilepsy was a disturbance of the natural processes in the mind was a rare example of seeking material causes of disease. In their everyday lives, many persons with disabilities served as scapegoats for minor or major problems, and they typically pursued the only work available: as singers, dancers, musicians, jugglers, or clowns. Blind people were occasionally revered as poets and bards, but that was an exception to typical beliefs about the cognitive

---

*Nancy Cruzan nearly died in a car accident in 1983 but continued living in a persistent vegetative state. Her parents' request some years later that hydration and nutrition be withheld led the U.S. Supreme Court to rule that the due process clause of the U.S. Constitution allowed competent persons to refuse medical care. However, the Court also allowed states to determine what degree of evidence is necessary to determine a person's wishes, which led to nationwide interest in advanced directives. Cruzan died in 1990 when the state court ruled that there was sufficient evidence of her wishes to order the removal of her feeding tube.

TABLE 28-3 ■ Guidelines for Institutional Ethics Committees (IECs)

Organization	Publication	Definition

UNESCO	Universal Draft Declaration on Bioethics and Human Rights[6,46]	Necessity: independent, multidisciplinary, and pluralist ethics should be established, promoted, and supported at the appropriate level
		Functions:
		  Assess the relevant ethical, legal, scientific and social issues related to research projects involving human beings
		  Provide advice on ethical problems in clinical settings
		  Assess scientific and technological developments, formulate recommendations, and contribute to the preparation of guidelines
		  Foster debate, education, and public awareness of and engagement in bioethics

AMA	CEJA Report E-I-84: Guidelines for Ethics Committees in Health Care Institutions[47]	Size: consistent with the needs of the institution Function: to consider and assist in resolving complicated ethical problems involving patients and those responsible for their care within the health care institutions; the recommendations produced should be confined exclusively to ethical matters and should not violate applicable laws of jurisdiction Membership: the majority should consist of physicians, nurses, and health care providers. These members should be selected on the basis of perspective member's concern for the welfare of the sick, their interest in ethical matters, and their reputation in the community and among peers

AAP	Committee on Bioethics[48]	Recommendations for IECs:
		  Ethics consultations serve an advisory role only; all parties that disagree with committee's recommendation take full responsibility for their own actions
		  Membership should be diverse and reflect different perspectives within hospital and community; membership requires a commitment to acquire and maintain sufficient knowledge to address complex issues
		  Responsible for clinical ethics consultation, review of policies, and education of professional, administrative, and support staff
		  Policies and procedures should conform to ethical principles of fairness and confidentiality
		  IECs should establish continuing education and training programs to ensure that IEC members are qualified
		  Individual ethics committees should be dissolved or restructured to report to the larger IEC

AAP, American Academy of Pediatrics; AMA, American Medical Association; CEJA, (AMA) Council on Ethical and Judicial Affairs; UNESCO, United Nations Educational, Scientific, and Cultural Organization.

abilities of persons with disabilities. Deaf people, according to Aristotle, were incapable of learning. However, Aristotle also echoed Socrates in his admonition to "pity the weak," and thus the city of Athens provided some support to individuals with disabilities. In the warlike state of Sparta, in contrast, "deformed" and sickly infants were sometimes abandoned, because their continued existence threatened the strength of the state.

Christian religious authority and superstition reigned in the Middle Ages. Parents were still blamed for a child's disabilities, for example, but in the new religious context, explanations for disability were more likely to be found in the sins of the parents. St. Augustine, although generally progressive in his approach to persons with disabilities, also argued that disabilities represented proof of God's power over the natural world and that because the deaf could not hear the gospels, they were to be excluded from church activities. Other church officials sought to help people with mental illness by tying them up in the church in the belief that they could be improved by attending mass. In other parts of Europe, the teachings of Jesus set a new example of pity and sympathy toward the physically and mentally disabled. Some religious cloisters provided places of refuge, and persons with physical disabilities commonly traveled to pilgrimage sites such as Rome and Jerusalem in search of salvation.

During the Middle Ages, civil authority was deeply intertwined with the Christian religious hierarchy throughout Europe, which affected the civil rights of persons with disabilities. In early modern England, "poor laws" provided some material support to individuals unable to work because of a disability. In other places, however, the negative view of persons with disabilities meant that they were not allowed to inherit property; testify in court; or make a deed, contract, or will. Even worse, in 1484 Pope Innocent VIII proclaimed a war against witches, and during the next 300 years, there were more than 100,000 witch trials throughout Europe. People with disabilities were frequently accused of demonic possession, and tens of thousands were tortured, hanged, or burned at the stake.

Whereas Christian and lay authorities provided widely varying views on disability, Jewish teachers more consistently emphasized that all human life is to be considered a gift and that no form of life, even a disabled one, constitutes divine punishment. Thus, the principle of the sanctity of human life guided much of the treatment toward disabled children through Judaic history. For example, the revered 11th century Talmudic scholar Rashi wrote that no child should be abandoned to die but, rather, even children born with overwhelming abnormalities should be nursed by their mothers.

Similar to the teaching of prominent Jewish scholars, the Islamic tradition typically highlighted the sacredness of all human life.[9] Although the study of disability in the medieval Islamic world is only in its infancy, preliminary evidence suggests that Islamic society generally did not associate disabilities with moral or spiritual deficiencies.[14] However, the legal rights of persons considered to be incompetent were considerably curtailed, and they were typically entrusted to a legal guardian's care. Medical treatment for this population varied, including incantations, magic, exorcisms, and a physiological approach adopted from Galen: Like the famous physician, Islamic practitioners hoped to heal cognitive or physical disabilities by restoring the balance of humors.

From the Renaissance through the Enlightenment, religious authority was increasingly separated from civil authority, and governments slowly moved from monarchist to republican models with power invested in representative governments. Enlightenment philosophers argued for the rights of the individual, and through the 19th century, children in particular took on new cultural value as individuals, rather than mere small adults who were the property of their father. From Paris hospitals through German laboratories, the scientific model was applied to medicine, and the search for rational explanations to disease and medicine was reinvigorated.

Persons with disabilities benefited from these broader changes in society. Among richer families, for example, deaf first-born sons were taught to read and write in order to fulfill legal inheritance requirements. In Germany and France in particular, individuals with disabilities began to take part in community activities, and the discipline of physical therapy emerged to treat persons with physical disabilities. The most dramatic development was that

governments in Europe and the United States built large hospitals to treat mental retardation in the early 1800s. Founders of these institutions believed that special training programs and the appropriate environment could cure mental retardation. Optimism waned in the late 1800s, however, because discharges were rare and doctors began to recognize mental retardation as a chronic problem. Underfunded and overwhelmed, these institutions became custodial care centers, and reports of horrific conditions recurred throughout the 20th century.[15]

Twentieth Century and Eugenics

In 1915, H. F. Haiselden recommended not performing lifesaving surgery on a newborn boy because the procedure would not cure underlying physical and mental abnormalities. Baby Bollinger died 5 days after birth, with the parents' assent. This was probably a very common occurrence in the early 20th century, but in this case, Haiselden, the head of the German-American Hospital in Chicago, went public. He revealed that over the previous decade he had allowed many other infants to die because they were "defective." Haiselden even created a movie loosely based on the Bollinger baby case, the "Black Stork," in an effort to promote his beliefs. A substantial number of prominent Americans and established medical organizations, including the National Medico-Legal Society, endorsed Haiselden's position. Although some local officials criticized Haiselden's actions, no one concluded that a crime had been committed. Rather, it was determined that Dr. Haiselden was fully within his rights as a physician to refuse to perform an operation that his conscience would not sanction.

Pernick used this example to remind us that ethical issues regarding withholding of treatment from persons with disabilities are not the result of technological advances in the 20th century.[16] Decisions about what care to provide to persons with disabilities have a certain continuity throughout human history. Ancient Spartans believed that infants who survived exposure were fit to live; medieval Christians attempted religious cures of persons with mental retardation; early modern physicians hoped that by bleeding patients, they could restore humoral balance and thus health; Enlightenment scholars believed that properly constructed institutions could dispel mental afflictions. Although modern medicine may judge such practices as ineffective or barbaric, practitioners (and patients) understood them to be the standard of care, and hence decisions to apply or withhold them share common themes with such debates today.

As Pernick also pointed out, the specific historical context is critical for understanding how such ethical debates are resolved. Haiselden's actions took place at a time in American history, for example, when eugenics was an accepted social philosophy among many mainstream scholars, such as Judge Oliver Wendell Holmes, geneticist Charles Davenport, and other leaders across the political spectrum. By combining Darwin's theory of evolution with an emerging understanding of genetics, advocates of eugenics believed that they could eliminate pain from disease and inequity in U.S. society in a single generation. They understood human behavior in simple genetic terms: Characteristics such as intelligence, honesty, and sobriety were passed on according to mendelian genetics. The future therefore lay in encouraging "fit" couples to marry and discouraging others from parenthood. Mental retardation in particular was seen as an inherited condition that at best did not contribute to society and too often led to crime and general depravity. Advocates of eugenics believed that persons with mental retardation could not be trusted to refrain voluntarily from procreation; they persuaded many states to pass laws that led to the involuntary sterilization of adults with mental retardation. Upheld by the U.S. Supreme Court in their 1927 *Buck v. Bell*[16a] decision, such laws resulted in the sterilization of more than 60,000 individuals. In Nazi Germany, more than 200,000 individuals with disabilities were euthanized in that nation's atrocious effort to eliminate disability.

The Disability Rights Movement

The U.S. disability rights movement of the 1970s followed the model of similar struggles for civil rights by women in the 1970s and African-Americans in the 1960s and early 1970s. Disability rights leaders also owe much, however, to a long tradition of advocacy by relatively anonymous families, beginning in the early 1930s. Parents of children with mental retardation began to join together in local grassroots associations to challenge social prejudice and work collectively to improve the well-being of their children. By 1951 there were more than 125 such groups in the United States and Canada, loosely held together by the desire for peer support and the conviction that the public schools had a responsibility to aid children with disabilities. The National Association of Parents and Friends of Mentally Retarded Children was founded in 1950, with the common objective to further the movement for disability rights on the national level.

Despite the work of such advocacy groups, however, most disabled people remained hidden from public view, either in their homes or in institutions. Well into the 20th century, American society still treated its disabled population, especially those with mental disabilities, as a group that needed to be controlled by segregation, sterilization, and isolation. In the1950s more than 500,000 Americans were housed in overcrowded psychiatric hospitals with custodial care.[17] Mental retardation, like many chronic conditions, was associated with poverty, immorality, and racial or ethnic minority status.

The needs of persons with physical disabilities gained national attention with the return home of injured veterans after World Wars I and II and from impaired survivors of polio epidemics. War veterans and polio survivors did not fit simple stereotypes of disability, and their demands to be fully part of community activities challenged long-held attitudes toward persons with disabilities. Rehabilitation medicine grew as a medical discipline, and dramatic advances in assistive technological devices after World War II led to improved quality of life for persons with disabilities.

Public perception of developmental disabilities changed also because of the efforts of famous families who began to publicly discuss their experience of disability. Before the 1960s, most families hid any association with disability, and even today many people vaguely remember hearing about or visiting a family member who lived in an institution. President Franklin Roosevelt contracted polio long before he was president, for example, but in his years in office from 1932 until his death in 1945, not a single picture that revealed his disability was ever printed. An unspoken code of honor in the White House and among press photographers allowed the general public to believe that Roosevelt had fully recovered from polio. Roosevelt and his colleagues assumed that the American public could not accept a president with a disability.[18]

By the time that John F. Kennedy became president in 1960, the American people were ready to openly discuss disability. Largely through the urging of his sister Eunice, President Kennedy revealed that he had a sister Rose with mental retardation and argued that the nation had a responsibility to do more for persons with disabilities. Kennedy was following the example of other public figures such as author Pearl S. Buck* and entertainer Roy Rogers,† whose

---

*Buck is among the most famous and prolific writers in U.S. history; her work earned both Pulitzer and Nobel prizes for literature in the early 20th century. Buck's first daughter was born with phenylketonuria and developed profound mental retardation, and Buck wrote movingly and spoke publicly about her daughter at a time when shame was still common for parents.

†Rogers, the singing cowboy of movie and radio fame, was a childhood hero to many in the mid-20th century United States. His wife, actress Dale Evans, teamed up with him on popular entertainment shows to help explain the story of their daughter, Robin Elizabeth, who was born with Down syndrome.

personal stories helped many families overcome the shame commonly associated with mental retardation. As president, Kennedy had the ability to make an enormous difference. His expert President's Panel on Mental Retardation recommended investing in prevention, basic research, and training professionals to provide health and special education to persons with mental retardation and other developmental disabilities. Through legislation and federal directives, millions of federal dollars were allocated to support maternal and child health programs, train teachers and physicians, and investigate the causes of mental retardation (see Chapter 8A).[19] Today more than $40 billion per year in federal and state spending is devoted to education, health care, and other programs for persons with developmental disabilities. Nearly all large state institutions for persons with mental retardation/developmental disabilities have closed, and interdisciplinary outpatient care has been the recognized standard since the 1950s.

Despite such federal programs, however, most persons with developmental disabilities still faced many barriers to full participation in school, work, and community activities. In the 1970s, disability rights advocates used legislation, court rulings, and public acts of disobedience to claim full access to all aspects of American life. Ed Roberts* and Judy Heumann,[†] for example, each completed university degrees and joined the workforce despite prejudice and administrative roadblocks that prevented persons with disabilities from participating in public schools and the workplace. These two renowned leaders of the disability rights movement eventually held government posts designed to remove barriers to education and employment, thus helping to reform the very institutions that once tried to exclude them. Access to a "free appropriate public education" was ensured legally to all children with disabilities in 1975 when Congress passed Public Law 94-142 (Education of All Handicapped Children Act), now codified as the Individuals with Disabilities Education Act.[20]

More general access to public institutions was ensured in the aftermath of a critical incident in 1977,

when disability rights activists in nine cities staged demonstrations and occupied the offices of the federal Department of Health, Education, and Welfare. They also conducted a "sit-in" to force the President Carter's administration to enact Section 504 of the Rehabilitation Act of 1973, which made it illegal for any federal agency, public university, federal contractor, or any other federally funded institutions to discriminate on the basis of a disability. The demonstrations galvanized the disability community nationwide, particularly in San Francisco, where protests lasted for nearly a month. The legal protections of Section 504 were extended beyond federal institutions with the passing of Developmental Disabilities Act in 1990, and subsequent court decisions have affirmed that persons with disabilities must have the opportunity to participate fully in the community (Table 28-4).

The emergence of "disability culture" and acknowledgment of a disability history also suggest how persons with developmental disabilities have moved beyond previous notions of shame and pity. Within the diversity of physical and cognitive impairments that fit under the label "disability," there is a common experience of isolation, vulnerability, difference, and fear of discrimination or pity. With the disability rights movement came a willingness to challenge the status quo and build a unique collective identity that supports both the right to be different and the right to be included in all aspects of society. Disability culture is gaining increased acceptance in the academic world, in which disability studies scholars work to understand how myths, prejudice, and physical or cognitive limitations interact in American society. More broadly, disability culture implies that pity should be replaced with the understanding that doing something differently from the norm implies not necessarily an illness to be cured but simply a difference.

Disability culture has important implications for health care. Traditionally, disabled people were viewed by medical professionals through the prism of a "medical model of disability." Disabled people "suffered" from a reduced quality of life as a result of their impairments, which were medical problems that needed to be cured or obviated through medical interventions. The social model of disability challenges these assumptions by suggesting that there is nothing intrinsically "wrong" with a person with a disability. Rather, disability occurs as a natural part of life. The challenges and stigma confronting people with disabilities in society are the result of physical and social barriers and prejudices that exist in society. Thus, decisions about the medical treatment of people with disabilities should be grounded in an underlying assumption that a disabled life has inherent value and dignity and need not be unduly medicalized and

---

*Roberts was admitted to the University of California at Berkeley in 1962, despite administration concerns that his polio-related paralysis should disqualify him. Roberts became a leader in the disability rights movement and has been called the "father of independent living."

[†]After initially being discouraged from attending school because of her disability, Heumann became one of the key shaping forces of federal disability policy starting in the 1970s. By the end of the 20th century, she had become Assistant Secretary of Education; over the previous three decades, she had worked to develop the regulations (Section 504) and laws (Americans with Disabilities Education Act) that together help guarantee civil rights to persons with disabilities.

TABLE 28-4 ■ Key Disability Rights Laws in the United States in the Late 20th Century[49-51]

Law	Summary
The Rehabilitation Act of 1973 (Public Law 93-112)	Section 504 prohibits discrimination on the basis of disability in programs conducted by recipients of federal financial assistance and federal agencies This law has far-reaching effects on public education, providing special education programs, accessibility requirements for public buildings and transportation systems, and accessible information technology
Education for All Handicapped Children Act (Public Law 94-142), 1975	Guarantees that a "free appropriate education" is available to all children with disabilities while ensuring that their rights and their parent/guardians' rights are protected Federal funds are made available to assist state and local government efforts to provide these educational opportunities
Child Abuse Amendments of 1984 (Public Law 98-457)	Defines child abuse as the "withholding of medically indicated treatment" from children Under only three conditions is life-sustaining treatment recognized as optional: when a child is comatose, when treatment would merely prolong dying rather than correct the infant's life-threatening conditions, and when provision of such a treatment would be futile and inhumane
Developmental Disabilities and Bill of Rights Act Amendments of 1987	Provides finances to states in order to establish Developmental Disabilities Councils and to support the establishment and operation of state protection and advocacy systems Awards discretionary grants to support university-affiliated programs that provide training in the field of developmental disability Promotes projects aimed at increasing the independence, productivity, and community integration of person with developmental disabilities
Americans with Disabilities Act (ADA), 1990	Purpose: to provide a clear and comprehensive national mandate with enforceable standards for the elimination of discrimination against individuals with disabilities; this Act extends protections similar to those provided to individuals on the basis of civil rights, race, sex, national origin, and religion to individuals with disabilities Defines *disability* as a physical or mental impairment that substantially limits one or more life activities, a record of such impairment, or being regarded as having such an impairment "Guarantees equal opportunity for individuals with disabilities in employment, public accommodation, transportation, state and local government services, and telecommunications. The ADA is the most significant federal law ensuring the full civil rights of all individuals with disabilities" Mandates: Accessibility of local, state, and federal governments and programs Businesses with more than 15 employees make "reasonable accommodations" for disabled workers Private enterprises that provide public accommodations, such as restaurants and stores, make "reasonable modifications" to ensure access for disabled members of the public Establishment of telephone relay services for individuals who use telecommunications devices for deaf persons (TDDs) or similar devices
Developmental Disabilities Assistance and Bill of Rights Act of 1994	Defines *developmental disability* as a severe, chronic disability of an or older that individual 5 years of age 1. Is attributable to a mental or physical impairment or combination of mental and physical impairments 2. Is manifested before the person attains age 22 3. Is likely to continue indefinitely 4. Results in substantial functional limitations in three or more of the following areas of major life activity: (a) self-care, (b) receptive and expressive language, (c) learning, (d) mobility, (e) self-direction, (f) capacity for independent living, and (g) economic sufficiency 5. Reflects the individual's need for a combination and sequence of special, interdisciplinary, or generic services; supports; or other assistance that is of lifelong or extended duration and is individually planned and coordinated

cured. Just as most people of color living in a predominately white society do not yearn to be white, people with disabilities do not seek to be "cured" of their disability.[21]

Implications of the Disability Rights Movement for End-of-Life Decisions

In the early 1900s, the physician typically made nearly all end-of-life decisions. During the Bollinger case, for example, surveys demonstrated that only a minority of people favored allowing parents any say in the decision-making process. For most of the 20th century, the central role of the physician remained intact. As late as the 1970s, physicians routinely withheld necessary surgery from children with disabilities such as Down syndrome or spina bifida. At one prominent university's intensive care nursery in 1973, for example, 43 of the 299 consecutive deaths resulted from the health care team's decision to withhold treatment because of the infants' extremely poor prognosis for a "meaningful life."[22] As noted previously, able-bodied persons must be cautious when making judgments about quality of life for a person with a disability. Health care providers in particular prize superior cognitive ability and full control over all aspects of their lives, making it difficult for them to imagine the worth of a life with a cognitive or physical impairment.[23,24]

Through the 1970s and 1980s, physicians in the United States gradually moved away from taking primary responsibility for end-of-life decisions and began to involve patients and families. Autonomy in end-of-life decisions is now commonly granted to competent adults in North America, and most scholars of pediatric ethics believe that families should play a critical role in end-of-life decisions for children.[25] The American Academy of Pediatrics Committee on Bioethics, for example, endorsed "individualized decision making about life-sustaining medical treatment" and argued "these decisions should be jointly made by physicians and parents."[26] According to one formulation of the best-interest model of decision making, reasonable and informed people committed to the well-being of the child should consider the immediate and long-term interests of the child and then seek to maximize benefits and minimize burdens.[27]

Withholding medical treatment for infants younger than 1 year is more complicated because of the so-called Baby Doe regulations. In 1981 the parents of a newborn with Down syndrome and tracheoesophageal fistula refused to consent to a standard operation that would have enabled the child to take food and water by mouth. President Reagan, his Surgeon General C. Everett Koop, and other leaders of the right-to-life movement joined forces with disability rights leaders who feared that babies with disabilities were not getting appropriate treatment because of discrimination. The Child Abuse Amendments of 1984 defines one form of child abuse as the "withholding of medically indicated treatment" from children, and the statute recognizes only three conditions in which life-sustaining treatment is optional: when a baby is comatose, when treatment would merely prolong dying rather than correct the infant's life-threatening conditions, and when the provision of such a treatment would be futile and inhumane. Many neonatologists have interpreted these rules as forcing them to continue aggressive treatment of such newborns, although the American Academy of Pediatrics' guidelines suggest that the rules provide more discretion than is commonly assumed.[26] Although debate has persisted since the Baby Doe rules were effected, the general consensus among ethicists and state governments seems to be that all children, regardless of age, deserve the flexibility of individualized judgments through a best-interest model.[28]

As demonstrated by the case of Terri Schiavo,* however, there remains a strong current in American political and moral life that holds that life is worth preserving at all costs.[29] The dramatic showdown between the parents and spouse of Ms. Schiavo, a young woman in a permanent vegetative state, provoked responses from all levels of government and public life in the United States. Many medical ethicists viewed this case as reopening issues that seemed settled with the Cruzan case in 1990, and yet a variety of politicians, religious leaders, and disability rights advocates battled to preserve Ms. Schiavo's life despite testimony by expert witnesses and a multitude of court decisions. Those who believe that any life—even one of pain and suffering—is better than death typically reject withholding or withdrawing care at the end of life.

The history of persons with disabilities helps explain why many disability rights advocates are extremely cautious in debates about end-of-life decisions, including euthanasia and physician-assisted suicide. Even a charitable interpretation of disability history cannot ignore the forced sterilization of adults with mental retardation in the United States and the

---

*Schiavo suffered cardiopulmonary arrest in 1990 and eventually was determined to be in a persistent vegetative state. Her husband petitioned the Florida court system to remove her feeding tube in 1998, an action that was opposed by her parents. After more than a dozen court decisions supporting her husband's argument that Schiavo would not want to live in a persistent vegetative state, the tube was removed, and she died in March 2005. In the last 2 years of her life, President George W. Bush, the U.S. Congress, Florida Governor Jeb Bush, and the Florida state legislature attempted to prevent removal of the feeding tube.

euthanasia in Nazi Germany. Daily experience of discrimination adds to this understanding of disability history, and examples of more recent court decisions that undervalue a life with a disability are not hard to find.[30]

Although the older and more recent history of persons with disabilities provides reason for caution on end-of-life issues, a core principle of the disability rights movement—respect for self-determination—is that persons with disabilities should have the same rights as any able-bodied person to avoid pain and burdensome care. Scholars such as Beltran and Nelson[31] have argued that respect for persons with disabilities does not necessarily mean that life must be preserved at all costs. What it does suggest is that decisions should be based on the best interests of that particular individual, without preconceived notions about the quality of life with a disability. Thus, for example, if a child with Down syndrome has leukemia and has experienced relapse despite aggressive treatment, decisions about further intervention should be based on that particular child's quality of life, just as they would for any child with a similar prognosis. Similarly, medical interventions such as feeding tubes or antibiotics for pneumonia should be based on whether such interventions allow that child to continue participating in life activities that are meaningful to the particular family and child.

There are instances when a child's impairment may be a factor in deciding medical care. It could be argued that the outcome of heart transplantation or similar medical interventions rests in part on the ability of the person to follow complex medical regimens or at least understand the need for recurring painful procedures. Furthermore, there is some level of cognitive impairment so severe that most observers would agree that the child has virtually no purposeful interaction with the world and that recurring medical care leads to experiencing life as a series of painful procedures. In situations in which the presence of a disability is part of the decision to withhold medical care, institutional clinical ethics committees can support the family and the health care team by reviewing the case and offering the collective wisdom of an independent group. If the committee does not include at least one person with direct experience of disability, the members can consider bringing in a consultant for cases involving a child with developmental disabilities.

Reasonable people will always disagree on some end-of-life issues, but history teaches that there are some standards of care specific to time and place. In the early 1970s a physician may have may have recommended immediate institutionalization rather than trying to raise a child with Down syndrome at home, or a physician may have decided unilaterally to withhold surgical repair of duodenal atresia. Today, neither action is acceptable in the United States. Since the 1950s, patients and families have gained the right to participate in medical decisions, and the disability rights movement has taught physicians to value the life of every person, regardless of ability.

GENETICS, SURGICAL SHAPING, AND ASSUMPTIONS ABOUT DISABILITY

As medical science advances and is able to prevent or repair underlying impairments, there arise new ethical issues that are best understood in the context of the social model of disability. This section addresses two rapidly changing areas of medical care that affect particularly children with developmental disorders: genetics and surgery.

Surgical Shaping

Innovative surgical procedures hold promise to reduce impairment or at least the appearance of a disability. Although surgical repair of a cleft lip or cleft palate has long been well accepted, controversy surrounds procedures such as cochlear implants for profound hearing impairment, facial reconstruction for children with Down syndrome, and limb-lengthening for little people (defined as a person with a medical or genetic condition that usually results in an adult height of 4 feet 10 inches [147cm] or shorter). Cochlear implants are routinely performed in major medical centers, although some advocates of deaf culture continue to argue that such surgery is serving to eliminate a linguistic minority.[32] Surgery to repair a cleft lip is standard of care for functional and aesthetic reasons, but reconstructing the face of a child with Down syndrome is highly controversial because it suggests that there is something inherently wrong with having certain facial features. Limb-lengthening procedures are fraught with complications; most little people function well with assistive technology and environmental modifications.

There are obviously differences among these procedures. Limb-lengthening seems to have some functional significance, whereas facial surgery for children with Down syndrome seems purely cosmetic. There is evidence that some children with cochlear implants learn to hear and speak better than do hearing-impaired children who focus solely on sign language, although on average neither group of hearing-impaired children learn as well as their non–hearing-impaired peers. Cochlear implants also carry certain risks such as meningitis.[33] Despite these differences in functional significance, there is also a critical similarity among these sorts of procedures. They do not save or prolong life, and there is relatively little evidence that they improve function more than do less invasive approaches. Indeed, they are typically offered to parents with the goal of making the child appear less different, in hopes of reducing the societal stigma or environmental inconveniences associated with having a disability. Thus, a child is subjected to a surgical procedure in many cases simply because some adults are uncomfortable with the child's appearance. Such motivation conflicts with a basic tenet of the disability rights movement by suggesting that there is something inherently wrong with the disabled child that must be fixed.[34]

Because these procedures are elective and alter the natural identity of the child, traditional consent procedures may not be sufficient to protect the best interests of the child. As noted previously, parents have broad decision-making authority with regard to rearing children, including the obligation to look after their child's medical needs. Parents can give valid consent for their children to undergo a medical procedure if they have sufficient information, have the capacity to make decisions, and are free from coercion or undue influence. However, consent for surgical procedures too often focuses on parental understanding of the safety of the procedure itself, with less attention to alternatives and the long-term outcome for the child. For surgical "cures" of disability, it is crucial to examine these issues in the broadest possible context.

How should physicians counsel parents when presented with a surgical option to correct a physical anomaly that does not threaten the child's life or health? In general, acting in the best interests of a child means protecting the child's health and safety and creating an environment in which the child can achieve his or her full potential. For a child with a disability, is it best to leave the child alone and let him or her be potentially subjected to teasing, ridicule, and inconvenience because of the physical differences? Or is it better to allow surgery to normalize the difference and alter forever the body and thus the identity the child was born with, while potentially reducing the psychosocial trauma? The predicament is especially difficult because it is generally necessary to operate on children when they are young and their preferences are unknown.

The history of early surgery to augment gender assignment in children with ambiguous genitalia provides a cautionary example.[35,36] On the basis almost exclusively of the work of John Money, gender identity was thought to be malleable before age 2 years, and surgery was thus indicated to assign gender on the basis of appearance and chances for procreation. Since the 1980s, Money's thesis has been attacked—most famously, by the key patient who served to buttress his theory. Some evidence suggests that adults who were surgically assigned the "wrong" gender suffered because of the operation and subsequent treatment, and many have reportedly changed gender as adults. Furthermore, some authors have argued that minimal interventions in early childhood are most appropriate, especially as tolerance and understanding of intersex genitalia grows in the United States.

Even though societal norms about disability are changing, the birth of a child with a disability is often met by parents with alarm, confusion, disappointment, and anxiety. In general, parents make decisions in the best interest of a child, but able-bodied parents of a disabled child face an added challenge: They may not understand the disability and may not have any personal experience with other people who have the same condition. Such families often harbor fears, embrace myths, and accept stereotypes about their child with a disability. In this context, the idea of surgery to ameliorate the appearance of disability can be alluring. One way to help families understand their choices is link them to an affected adult (or disability rights advocate) who can provide an insider's view and help pierce the myths about disability. It may not be obvious how best to get input from the affected community, especially because affected persons have individual, varied opinions about their lives. One option is to consider parent support groups and adult advocacy associations, especially those devoted to specific disabling conditions. By employing a broader range of perspectives that includes the affected population, parents can better envision their child's best interests.

Genetic Information

New genetic techniques present many ethical issues in DBP. Perhaps the most obvious is that each year seems to bring new possibilities for prenatal diagnosis, giving parents an opportunity to exercise the option of terminating a pregnancy and preventing the birth of a child with a disability. Although a woman's right to an abortion has been protected by the 1973 Supreme Court ruling *Roe v. Wade*,[36a] there is widespread opposition to abortion in the United States. Reasonable people can disagree on whether prenatal testing and termination reduces human suffering or constitutes disrespect for life. Some people believe that a fetus is a human being entitled to the same protections as any other liveborn person, and because people in the United States have generally rejected arguments for active euthanasia in children with disabilities, it is wrong to terminate a pregnancy on the basis of prenatal diagnosis. Other people support U.S. laws and custom that define life as beginning approximately when a fetus is able to survive outside the womb; if a woman has the right to choose to carry a pregnancy to term, then certainly she and her family can decide whether to use prenatal testing to help ensure a healthy baby.

Philosopher Peter Singer and others have offered a third approach.[37] Singer argues that personhood does not begin until sometime in the first year of life, when a human being is capable of interacting purposefully with the environment and begins to recognize the self as an independent being. According to this definition of personhood, termination of pregnancy and active euthanasia in the neonatal period for a baby with profound disabilities may be morally appropriate actions. However, the current consensus in the United States is that brainstem activity is sufficient to define life: Babies with anencephaly and individuals in a persistent vegetative state—conditions in which brainstem function may be present—are considered live persons, and state laws for brain death require absence of brainstem function.

From a disability rights perspective, recommending the termination of a pregnancy on the basis of prenatal diagnosis of a disability suggests that a life with a disability is less valued and perpetuates eugenic myths about the perfectibility of humankind. Parents of a child with spina bifida, for example, may be offended during a subsequent pregnancy if they are offered termination of a fetus diagnosed with spina bifida. On the other hand, other approaches to preventing disability enjoy widespread support in the United States. Few argue that preventing neural tube disorders through preconception consumption of folic acid, for example, undermines persons already living with spina bifida. Other preconception and prenatal interventions such as rubella vaccination or medical treatment of human immunodeficiency virus infection similarly have become standard practice to prevent subsequent death or disability.

Universal neonatal screening programs to prevent the neurodevelopmental consequences of congenital hypothyroidism or phenylketonuria also have widespread support and have substantially reduced the prevalence of mental retardation.[38] As neonatal screening programs for genetic conditions expand, however, new ethical issues arise. Some authors have argued that the high number of false-positive results in universal screening programs constitutes unacceptable morbidity for affected families, whereas others are concerned that identifying conditions with no simple intervention is unfair. Genetic testing in general often reveals information not only about the patient, but about the patient's family and about future generations. As in genetic tests for specific individuals, universal neonatal screening often produces results that have implications for entire fami-

lies, many of whom may not have consented to revealing such information or wanting to know such information. Once predicative genetic information is known, it cannot be "un-known," and there is no simple way to offer extended family members individual testing without causing emotional discomfort or exposing the affected individual. This is a difficult situation particularly when the medical condition has no specific cure, and such issues are best considered *before* such diagnostic tests are offered. Currently in the United States, there is a consensus that universal neonatal screening should be restricted to conditions for which early interventions and treatments are available,[38a] though a strong argument can be made for newborn screening to understand the natural history of metabolic variants of rare conditions.[38b,38c] Furthermore, when a genetic diagnosis has implications for family members, physicians have some obligation to inform them of the possibility for testing and treatment.

Genetic information may also have implications outside of the strict health care context. For example, predictive genetic information can have negative implications in the areas of employment and insurance for patients and/or family members. Genetic discrimination can occur when either an employer or an insurance company uses an individual's predictive genetic information to refuse employment or insurance opportunities out of a fear that a genetic marker indicates a chance that the individual will become ill or disabled or will have a child with a disability.[39] Although many legal commentators agree that such treatment should be viewed as illegal discrimination, courts have not offered definitive rulings on the issue. This may also be interpreted as good news: in view of the technology that has been available at least since the 1990s, it is reassuring that there have been no major cases of genetic discrimination.

Research on genetic issues adds yet another level of complexity to all of these ethical issues. Informed consent is particularly difficult, and provisions for communicating with family members must be determined ahead of time. For example, at least one state has considered requiring consent from all family members when genetic research is undertaken. Furthermore, storing samples and maintaining privacy require careful consideration, and researchers need to determine what to do if new information that would affect former research subjects becomes available. Finally, researchers may confront social and political consequences of their research results. Identifying genetic predispositions for stigmatizing conditions, particularly in vulnerable populations, can harm an entire population. For example, the genetics of cognitive ability has been related to race or ethnicity in nefarious ways since the 19th century.[40]

SCIENCE, PRACTICE, AND ADVOCACY

In addition to classic developmental disabilities such as mental retardation, the developmental-behavioral practitioner is also responsible for a wide array of more common disorders such as ADHD and learning disabilities, as well as providing counsel on practices that promote normal development and appropriate behavior. Some ethical issues in this context arise because professionals providing mental health treatment are often subject to higher expectations in protecting confidentiality. Clinical responsibility for behavioral issues also leads to a variety of clinical, research, and advocacy issues related to society's high emotional stake in appropriate behavior. Last, the role of environmental conditions such as poverty and violence in child health suggests that DBP professionals have a critical role in advocating for broader social and political changes in their communities.

Privacy and Confidentiality

One essential component of being human is the ability to protect one's privacy. Although parents need to be deeply involved in the lives of their children, the need for privacy grows with age and independence through the school-age and teen years. One role of pediatric health providers is to help parents understand the developmental needs of growing children and adolescents. For medical professionals, there is the added responsibility first suggested by Hippocrates to protect the "sacred secrets" that patients reveal in the course of obtaining health care. Like all physicians, developmental-behavioral pediatricians must protect the confidentiality of patient and family information according to state and federal laws, such as the Health Insurance Portability and Accountability Act (HIPAA). As mental health professionals, however, developmental-behavioral providers may be held to a higher standard when and if they provide psychotherapy. HIPAA and most state laws include special protections for medical records of mental health therapists; for instance, only treatment summaries may be shared with insurers, families, and other members of the health care team.

More commonly, developmental-behavioral pediatricians face dilemmas in protecting the confidentiality of their adolescent patients.[41] In general, parents or guardians must consent to treatment for any person younger than 18 years, and such consent also brings the right to control medical information and make treatment decisions. Nearly every state provides exceptions for certain conditions regarding when adolescents can consent for care and thus control their own medical information. Such conditions typically include sexually transmitted infections, birth control,

pregnancy, and, in some states, substance abuse treatment. The public health rationale for such laws is that adolescents are more likely to seek appropriate care if they believe that medical professionals will protect their confidentiality; in most such case, the medical team cannot share information about these specific conditions with anyone, including parents, without the teenaged patient's consent. In practice, most adolescent patients are able to reveal such important diagnoses to their family with the practitioner's support, especially because medical bills may eventually reveal the nature of the diagnosis.

State law protects adolescents' confidentiality only for specific conditions, but it is typically in the best interest of the patient that he or she feels comfortable discussing any topic with the practitioner under the promise of confidentiality. Many parents recognize the value of their child's having access to accurate, professional medical advice and would agree to the practitioner's request to maintain confidentiality. Substance abuse is a particularly difficult issue, because the medical practitioner must balance preserving the adolescent's trust with the need to protect the adolescent's health by informing the parents of particularly dangerous behavior. Most practitioners will not respect the adolescent's request for confidentiality when suicide is a possibility, and most state laws either allow or compel the practitioner to break confidentiality when a patient reveals the intention to hurt another individual.

Developmental-behavioral practitioners are typically adept at handling complex family communication issues. However, in view of the legal and professional consequences of breaking confidentiality, it is crucial to understand state law and to work with legal and/or risk management professionals in difficult cases.

The Legitimacy of Behavioral and Learning Disorders

A distinction continues to be made between *developmental* disorders and *behavioral* disorders, despite ample evidence of their considerable overlap. After centuries of blaming parents for disabilities, nearly everyone today understands that Down syndrome and cerebral palsy are medical conditions caused by natural processes. Mental illness in the United States, on the other hand, continues to carry the stigma of personal responsibility; for example, depression is different from diabetes, or so it seems to many individuals, despite research establishing the biological basis of behavioral and learning disorders. The popular media both stimulate and reflect public opinion in articles that question the biological legitimacy of disorders such as ADHD or learning disabilities. Such opinions are fueled by relatively vague definitions and limited diagnostic techniques for many disorders, by the "hidden" quality of these disabilities in comparison with cerebral palsy or Down syndrome, and by the complex interplay between biomedical and psychosocial manifestations of these disorder.

There is public controversy over both the diagnosis and treatment of common developmental-behavioral disorders. Increases in the diagnosis and use of prescription medications for ADHD, for example, has led to concern that physicians are overmedicating children. Although there are certainly cases of inappropriate diagnosis and treatment, most evidence suggests that the rise in prescriptions in stimulant medications reflects improved diagnosis and access to care. Indeed, some children with ADHD do not receive proper medical care despite overwhelming evidence of the value of medication in treating the core symptoms of inattention, impulsivity, and hyperactivity (for more detail, see Chapter 16).[42] On the other hand, many children with behavioral disorders are being treated with four or five psychotropic medications; in view of the lack of data for such polypharmacy, the quality of care these children are receiving must be questioned.

Such unevenness in the diagnosis and treatment of developmental and behavioral disorders may reflect a critical national shortage in well-trained pediatric mental health professionals, particularly those who are bilingual and bicultural. According to the 1999 Report of the Surgeon General on Mental Health, 10% to 20% of children in the United States meet diagnostic criteria for a behavioral disorder, but fewer than one in every five of these children receive appropriate mental health treatment. On the other hand, access to services may partly account for the evidence that white boys attending private schools are particularly likely to receive a diagnosis of specific learning disabilities.[43] Families with resources to obtain proper evaluations are better able to aid their children in obtaining accommodations in school and on standardized tests.

Access to quality medical care in general remains a persistent and peculiar problem in the United States, where more than 16% of the gross national product is spent on health care and yet 46 million residents have no health insurance. Most other industrialized nations spend less than half per capita as the United States but manage to provide medical care to every resident. As many as 10 million children are not covered by health insurance in the United States, despite gains in the economy and expansions in state-funded health insurance programs since the 1990s. Such children are more likely to suffer from a variety of medical conditions than are their peers with adequate insurance, and mental health services are among the most difficult to secure. Even when children do have insurance, many parents lack access to health care and cannot provide an optimal home environment when they are struggling with chronic illness.

Partly because of poor access to care, children living in poverty are more likely to receive diagnoses of developmental and behavioral disorders. Poor child and family health are often compounded by inadequate nutrition, lead exposure, family violence, unstimulating environments, and low-quality child care and education settings. Discrimination on the basis of race, ethnicity, culture, and disability continue to disproportionately affect families struggling with poverty, and indeed such bias typically contributes to family circumstances in the first place.

Subtle and inadvertent discrimination may also play a role in the diagnostic labels applied to certain children. Because of the lack of biological markers for most developmental and behavioral disorders, clinical judgment may be subject to bias. For example, although the diagnosis of mental retardation includes the use of standardized testing instruments, it remains a clinical diagnosis,[44] and mental retardation is much more likely to be diagnosed in black boys than in children of other groups.[45,46] Although such diagnostic labels may lead to individualized educational services, such labels frequently lower expectations and contribute to poor achievement.[47]

More in general, there is considerable flexibility in the diagnosis of some developmental-behavioral disorders, and clinical decisions often have important implications because specific diagnoses led to access to educational and financial support. In some school districts in Florida, for example, a diagnosis of autistic disorder qualifies a student for services under the Individuals with Disabilities Education Act, whereas the diagnosis of Pervasive Developmental Disorder Not Otherwise Specified does not. Parents who recognize the value of a specific diagnosis may appropriately advocate for decisions that provide the most support for their child, and the developmental-behavioral practitioner must negotiate such diagnoses within the bounds of best practice.

Although diagnosis of developmental-behavioral disorders only occasionally requires negotiation with parents, treatment is often a matter of some contention. It is a relatively straightforward matter that the health care practitioner should refuse to prescribe medication when it is not indicated, even if the family or schoolteacher seems eager for the child to begin pharmacotherapy. The more difficult situation is that in which families oppose medication despite abundant evidence that the child would benefit from it. Physicians are obligated to report instances of medical neglect to state authorities, but whereas failure of a parent to give insulin for diabetes would prompt state intervention, it is unlikely that anyone would force a family to provide methylphenidate for ADHD. In the future, U.S. society may view behavioral disorders as sufficiently legitimate to require appropriate treatment in all cases; until then, the developmental-behavioral practitioner must educate the family and hope that patience and follow-up are sufficient.

Although some families refuse treatment with medications, many more seek complementary and alternative medical treatment. Parents are particularly eager for simple solutions to chronic conditions such as autism and cerebral palsy, and the desire for "natural" treatments appears strong for almost all behavioral and developmental disorders. For most alternative treatments, there is little evidence of safety or efficacy, and many are quite expensive. Complementary and alternative medicine is an area in which more evidence of benefits and adverse effects is needed, and some research is in progress (for more details, see Chapter 8E). Although the practitioner may be frustrated by family's attention to alternative treatments, it is important to remember that many improvements in diagnosis and treatment of developmental and behavioral disorders have resulted from families' advocating for their children and challenging the status quo. By keeping an open mind and working with families over time, the developmental-behavioral practitioner can help families conserve their resources and focus on treatments that are most likely to benefit their children.

Developmental-Behavioral Practitioner as Scientist and as Advocate

There can be little doubt that commitment to high-quality scientific research is one critical component to solving many of the dilemmas arising in the clinical practice of DBP. As the biological understanding of developmental and behavioral disorders grows, so should the legitimacy of diagnosis and treatment. Better diagnostic tools can reduce bias, and improved treatment can improve collaboration between parents and clinicians. Understanding specific causal mechanisms should lead to prevention and better treatment and can even help build a widespread consensus that every child and family deserves access to high-quality mental health treatment (for more detail, see Chapter 3). Even if not directly involved in research, practitioners can serve as an educator and ambassador: They are obligated to teach families and the public about scientific principles that guide their practice and to continue to better understand the causes and treatments of behavioral disorders.

Advances in science also lead to new ethical dilemmas, of course, as suggested by the possibilities of innovative genetic and surgical techniques. Furthermore, the advantages of new medical interventions tend to accrue to those who already enjoy the best health and most wealth, thus further exacerbating underlying inequities in U.S. society. This suggests a continuing role for the developmental-behavioral practitioner as an advocate for broader social change. For some practitioners, this may mean participating in local school and child care centers or providing community education opportunities. Others may engage the legislative process to improve access to health care, reduce economic inequity, or improve professional standards. Practitioners should at least be informed about critical child health issues and should recognize that advocacy can be learned just as can any other skill in medicine.[47a]

The roles of scientist and advocate can conflict in some cases. Developmental-behavioral practitioners are frequently called upon to provide objective opinions about social issues such as the effects of divorce, witnessing violence, corporal punishment, or being raised by same-sex parents on children. Such issues are highly emotional and are not easily subjected to prospective, double-blind, controlled trials. There is value in adhering to the limits of this profession in providing advice about topics, explaining the levels of confidence that practitioners can achieve in various study designs. On the individual level, it is critical to recognize how practitioners' life experiences and personal opinions can affect their advice to families, as well as their interpretation of scientific data. Furthermore, professional ethics call for placing the well-being of the patient before their own personal views about controversial topics. Despite holding strong opinions about abortion or homosexuality, for example, each developmental-behavioral practitioner is called upon to practice medicine in nonjudgmental ways that respect individual decisions.

This is not to suggest that practitioners are not also obligated at a policy level to work to build consensus on critical issues in DBP. For example, there is ample evidence that children who grow up in poverty experience profound developmental and behavioral consequences, and there seems to be broad social consensus that whatever the personal and social causes of family poverty, children should not suffer. Although much political and academic debate focuses on issues at the beginning and end of life, not nearly enough attention seems to flow to the children who grow up in poverty. For example, resources continue to be devoted to the criminal justice system, whereas prevention programs that support families, improve child care, and improve mental health are chronically underfunded. International comparisons are instructive: Most European nations, for example, have created public systems that provide high-quality medical care to all children and buffer the effects of poverty on most children. The increased burden of illness for children of low socioeconomic status and of ethnic or racial minorities is unacceptable, and it is only partly explained by decreased access to care. At the highest level of moral reasoning, the developmental-behavioral practitioner is an advocate not just for the child in the office but for the well-being of all children.

REFERENCES

1. Ad Hoc Committee on Medical Ethics: American College of Physicians Ethics Manual. Ann Intern Med 101:129-137, 263-274, 1984.

2. Starr P: The social transformation of American medicine: The rise of a sovereign profession and the making of a vast industry. New York: Basic Books, 1983.

3. American Board of Internal Medicine Foundation, American College of Physicians–American Society of Internal Medicine Foundation, European Federation of Internal Medicine: Medical professionalism in the new millennium: A physician charter. Ann Intern Med 136:243-246, 2002.

4. Inui TS: A Flag in the Wind: Educating for Professionalism in Medicine. Washington, DC: Association of American Medical Colleges, 2003.

5. Faunce TA: Will international human rights subsume medical ethics? Intersection in the UNESCO Universal Bioethics Declaration. J Med Ethics 31:173-178, 2005.

6. United Nations Educational, Scientific, and Cultural Organization (UNESCO): Universal Declaration on Bioethics and Human Rights. Paris: UNESCO, 2005. (Available at: *http://portal.unesco.org/shs/en/ev.php-URL_ID=1883&URL_DO=DO_TOPIC&URL_SECTION=201. html;* accessed 2/25/07.)

7. Beauchamp TL, Childress JF: Principles of Biomedical Ethics, 4th ed. New York: Oxford University Press, 1994.

8. Gert B: Morality: Its Nature and Justification, rev. ed. New York: Oxford University Press, 2005.

9. Post SG, ed: Encyclopedia of Bioethics, 3rd ed. New York: Macmillan, 2004.

9a. Griswold v. Connecticut, 381 U.S. 479, 1965.

10. Bardon A: Ethics education and value prioritization among members of U.S. Hospital Ethics Committees. Kennedy Inst Ethics J 14:395-406, 2004.

11. Siegler M: Searching for moral certainty in medicine: A proposal for a new model of the doctor-patient encounter. Bull N Y Acad Med 57:56-69, 1981.

12. American Society for Bioethics and Humanities: Core Competencies for Health Care Ethics Consultation. Glenview, IL: American Society for Bioethics and Humanities, 1998.

13. Walton O, Schalick I: History of disability: Medieval west. *In* Albrecht GL, Mitchell DT, Snyder SL, et al, eds: Encyclopedia of Disability, vol 5. London: Sage Publications, 2005.

14. Meri JW, ed: Medieval Islamic Civilization, An Encyclopedia, nos. 1 and 2. New York: Taylor & Francis, 2006.

15. James W, Trent J: Inventing the Feeble Mind: A History of Mental Retardation in the United States. Berkeley: University of California Press, 1994.

16. Pernick MS: The black stork: Eugenics and the death of "defective" babies in American medicine and motion pictures since 1915. New York: Oxford University Press, 1996.

16a. Buck v. Bell, 274 U.S. 200, 1927.

17. Braddock DL, Parish SL: An Institutional History of Disability. *In* Albrecht GL, Seelman KD, Bury M, eds: Handbook of Disability Studies. New York: Sage Publications, 2000, pp 11-68.

18. Fleischer D, Zames F: The disability rights movement: From charity to confrontation. Philadelphia: Temple University Press, 2001.

19. Shorter E: The Kennedy Family and the Story of Mental Retardation. Philadelphia: Temple University Press, 2000.

20. Shapiro JP: No pity: People with disabilities forging a new civil rights movement. New York: Times Books, 1994.

21. Liachowitz CH: Disability as a Social Construct: Legislative Roots. Philadelphia: University of Pennsylvania Press, 1988.

22. Robertson JA: Extreme prematurity and parental rights after Baby Doe. Hastings Center Rep 34(4):32-39, 2004.

23. Lee SK, Penner PL, Cox M: Comparison of the attitudes of health care professionals and parents toward active treatment of very low birth weight infants. Pediatrics 88:110-114, 1991.

24. Lee SK, Penner PL, Cox M: Impact of very low birth weight infants on the family and its relationship to parental attitudes. Pediatrics 88:105-109, 1991.

25. American Academy of Pediatrics Committee on Bioethics: Informed consent, parental permission, and assent in pediatric practice. Pediatrics 95:314-317, 1995.

26. American Academy of Pediatrics Committee on Bioethics: Ethics and the care of critically ill infants and children. Pediatrics 98:149-152, 1996.

27. Kopelman LM: Rejecting the Baby Doe rules and defending a "negative" analysis of the Best Interests Standard. J Med Philos 30:331-352, 2005.

28. Kopelman LM: Are the 21-year-old Baby Doe rules misunderstood or mistaken? Pediatrics 115:797-802, 2005.

29. Cerminara K, Goodman K: Key events in the case of Theresa Marie Schiavo. Miami: University of Miami Ethics Programs, Last updated 21-Aug-2006. (Available at: *http://www.miami.edu/ethics2/schiavo/timeline.htm;* accessed 2/25/07.)

30. Miller PS: The impact of assisted suicide on persons with disabilities—Is it a right without freedom? Issues Law Med 9:47-62, 1993.

31. Nelson LJ: Respect for the developmentally disabled and forgoing life-sustaining treatment. Ment Retard Dev Disabil Res Rev 9:3-9, 2003.

32. Balkany T, Hodges AV, Goodman K: Ethics of cochlear implantation in young children. Otolaryngol Head Neck Surg 121:673-675, 1999.

33. Reefhuis J, Honein MA, Whitney CG, et al: Risk of bacterial meningitis in children with cochlear implants. N Engl J Med 349:435-445, 2003.

34. Parens E, ed: Surgically Shaping Children: Technology, Ethics and the Pursuit of Normality. Baltimore: Johns Hopkins University Press, 2006.

35. Kipnis K, Diamond M: Pediatric ethics and the surgical assignment of sex. Clin Ethics 9:398-410, 1998.

36. Kuhnle U, Krahl W: The impact of culture on sex assignment and gender development in intersex patients. Perspect Biol Med 45:85-103, 2002.

36a. Roe v. Wade, 410 U.S. 113, 1973.

37. Singer P: Practical Ethics, 2nd ed. Cambridge, UK: Cambridge University Press, 1993.

38. Brosco JP, Mattingly M, Sanders LM: Impact of specific medical interventions on reducing the prevalence of mental retardation. Arch Pediatr Adolesc Med 160:302-309, 2006.

38a. Botkin JR, Clayton EW, Fost NC, Burke W, Murray TH, Baily MA, Wilfond B, Berg A, Ross LF: Newborn screening technology: proceed with caution. Pediatrics 117(5):1793-1799, 2006.

38b. Howell RR: We need expanded newborn screening. Pediatrics 117(5):1800-1805, 2006.

38c. Bailey DB, Jr., Skinner D, Warren SF: Newborn screening for developmental disabilities: reframing presumptive benefit. Am J Public Health 95(11):1889-1893, 2005.

39. Miller PS: Is There a pink slip in my genes? Genetic discrimination in the workplace. Health Care Law Policy 3:225-237, 2000.

40. Brosco JP: History and ethics in public health research. Prof Ethics 11(3):45-64, 2003.

41. Anderson SL, Schaechter J, Brosco JP: Adolescent patients and their confidentiality: Staying within legal bounds. Contemp Pediatr 22:54-64, 2005.

42. U.S. Department of Health and Human Services: Mental Health: A Report of the Surgeon General. Rockville, MD: National Institutes of Health, National Institute of Mental Health, Substance Abuse and Mental Health Services Administration, Center for Mental Health Services, 1999.

43. Weiss KR: New test-taking skill: Working the system. The Los Angeles Times, January 9, 2000, p A1.

44. American Association on Mental Retardation: Mental Retardation: Definition, Classification, and Systems of Supports, 10th ed. Washington, DC: American Association on Mental Retardation, 2002.

45. Yeargin-Allsopp M, Drews C, Decoufle P, et al: Mild mental retardation in black and white children in metropolitan Atlanta: A case-control study. Am J Public Health 85:324-328, 1995.

46. Naglieri JA, Rojahn JL Intellectual classification of black and white children in special education programs using the WISC-III and the Cognitive Assessment System. Am J Ment Retard 106:359-367, 2001.

47. Losen D, Orfield G, eds: Racial Inequity in Special Education. Boston: Harvard Education Publishing Group, 2002.

47a. Sanders LM, Robinson TN, Forster LQ, Plax K, Brosco JP, Brito A: Evidence-based community pediatrics: building a bridge from bedside to neighborhood. Pediatrics 115(4 Suppl):1142-1147, 2005.

48. UNESCO: Explanatory Memorandum on the Elaboration of the Preliminary Draft Declaration on Universal Norms of Bioethics. Paris: UNESCO, 2005.

49. American Medical Association: Guidelines for ethics committees in health care institutions. JAMA 253:2698-2699, 1985.

50. American Academy of Pediatrics Committee on Bioethics: Institutional ethics committees. Committee on Bioethics. Pediatrics 107:205-209, 2001.

51. National Dissemination Center for Children with Disabilities (NICHCY): The Education of Children and Youth with Special Needs: What Do the Laws Say? Washington, DC: NICHCY, October 1996.

52. U.S. Equal Employment Opportunity Commission: Americans with Disabilities Act: Questions and answers. Washington, DC: U.S. Department of Justice, Civil Rights Division, U.S. Equal Employment Opportunity Commission, 2002, pp 1-22.

53. Disability Programs and Resource Center: A Chronology of the Disability Rights Movement. San Francisco: San Francisco State University, 2006. (Available at: http://www.sfsu.edu/~hrdpu/chron.htm; accessed 2/22/07.)

54. General Medical Council. Good Medical Practice. London: General Medical Council; 1998. Booklet available at http://www. gmc-uk.org/guidance/good_medical_practice/GMC_GMP.pdf.

55. Anderson M, Cohen J, Hallock J, Kassebaum D, Turnbull J, Whitcomb M: Learning objectives for medical student education—guidelines for medical schools. Academic Medicine 74:13-18, 1999.

Appendix

CHAPTER 6

Diagnostic and Statistic Manual of Mental Disorders, 4th edition–Primary Care Version (DSM-PC) Coding Sheet

DSM PC			
CHILD MANIFESTATIONS			
	Variation	Problem	Disorder
Developmental Competency			
Cognitive Adaptive Skills/Mental Retardation	V65.49	V62.3	317 Mild Mental Retardation, 318.0 Moderate Mental Retardation, 318.1 Severe Mental Retardation, 318.2 Profound Mental Retardation, 319 Mental Retardation Severity Unspecified
Academic Skills	V65.49	V40.0	315.00 Reading Disorder, 315.1 Mathematics Disorder, 315.2 Disorder of Written Expression
Motor Development	V65.49	781.3	315.4 Developmental Coordination Disorder
Speech and Language	V65.49	V40.1	315.31 Expressive Language Disorder, 315.32 Mixed Receptive-Expressive Language Disorder, 307.9 Communication Disorder NOS, 307.0 Stuttering, 315.39 Phonological Disorder
Impulsive/Hyperactive or Inattentive Behaviors			
Hyperactive/Impulsive Behaviors	V65.49	V40.3	314.01 Predominantly Hyperactive-Impulsive Type, 314.01 Combined Type, 314.9 Attention-Deficit/Hyperactivity Disorder NOS
Inattentive Behaviors	V65.49	V40.3	314.00 Predominantly Inattentive Type, 314.01 Combined Type, 314.9 Attention-Deficit/Hyper-Activity Disorder NOS
Negative/Antisocial Behaviors			
Negative Emotional Behaviors	V65.49	V71.02	296.x Major Depressive Disorder, 300.4 Dysthymic Disorder, 309.0 Adjustment Disorder
Aggressive/Oppositional Behaviors	V65.49	V71.02	313.81 Oppositional Defiant Disorder, 312.81 Conduct Disorder Childhood Onset, 312.82 Conduct Disorder Adolescent Onset, 309.3 Adjustment Disorder With Disturbance of Conduct, 312.9 Disruptive Behavior Disorder NOS
Secretive Antisocial Behaviors	V65.49	V71.02	312.81 Conduct Disorder Childhood Onset, 312.82 Conduct Disorder Adolescent Onset, 309.3 Adjustment Disorder With Disturbance of conduct, 312.9 Disruptive Behavior Disorder NOS
Substance Use/Abuse			
Substance Use/Abuse	V65.49	V71.09	305.xx Substance Abuse Disorder, 303.xx Substance Dependence, 292.0 Substance Withdrawal

DSM PC—cont'd			
CHILD MANIFESTATIONS			
	Variation	**Problem**	**Disorder**
Emotions and Moods			
Anxious Symptoms	V65.49	V40.2	300.02 Generalized Anxiety Disorder, 300.23 Social Phobia, 300.29 Specific Phobia, 300.01 Panic Disorder, 309.21 Separation Anxiety Disorder, 308.3 Acute Stress Disorder
Sadness and Related Symptoms	V65.49	V40.3	296.2x, 296.3x Major Depressive Disorder, 300.4 Dysthymic Disorder, 309.0 Adjustment Disorder With Depressed Mood, 311 Depressive Disorder NOS, 296.0x Bipolar I Disorder, With Single Manic Episode, 296.89 Bipolar II Disorder, Recurrent Major Depressive Episodes With Hypomanic Episodes
Ritualistic, Obsessive, Compulsive Symptoms	V65.49	V40.3	300.3 Obsessive Compulsive Disorder, 300.00 Anxiety disorder NOS
Suicidal Thoughts or Behaviors	V65.49	V40.2	313.89 Suicide Ideation and Attempts
Somatic and Sleep Behaviors			
Pain/Somatic Complaints	V65.49	V40.3	300.82 Undifferentiated Somatoform Disorder, 307.80 Pain Disorder, 300.11 Conversion Disorder, 300.16 Factitious Disorder, 300.82 Somatofrom Disorder NOS, 300.19 Factitious Disorder NOS
Excessive Daytime Sleepiness	V65.49	V40.3	307.45 Circadian Rhythm Sleep Disorder-Delayed Sleep Phase Type, 307.44 Primary Hypersomnia, 347 Narcolepsy, 307.47 Dyssomnia NOS
Sleeplessness	V65.49	V40.3	307.42 Primary Insomnia, 307.47 Dyssomnia NOS, 307.45 Circadian Rhythm Sleep Disorder
Nocturnal Arousals	V65.49	V40.3	307.46 Sleep Terror Disorder, 307.46 Sleepwalking Disorder, 307.47 Parasomnia NOS
Feeding, Eating, Elimination Behaviors			
Soiling Problems	V65.49	V40.3	307.7 Encopresis Without Constipation and Overflow Incontinence, 787.6 Encopresis With Constipation and Overflow Incontinence
Day/Nighttime Wetting Problems	V65.49	V40.3	307.6 Enuresis
Purging/Binge Eating	V65.49	V69.1	307.51 Bulimia Nervosa, 307.50 Eating Disorder NOS
Dieting/Body Image Problems	V65.49	V69.1	307.1 Anorexia Nervosa, 307.5 Eating Disorder NOS
Irregular Feeding Behaviors	V65.49	V40.3	307.59 Feeding Disorder of Infancy or Early Childhood
Illness-Related Behaviors			
Psychological Factors Affecting Medical Condition	V65.49	V15.81	316 Psychological Factors Affecting Medical Condition
Sexual Behaviors			
Gender Identity Behaviors	V65.49	V40.3	302.6 Childhood Gender Identity Disorder, 302.85 Adolescent Gender Identity Disorder
Sexual Development Behaviors	V65.49	V40.3	302.9 Sexual Disorder NOS
Atypical Behaviors			
Repetitive Behavioral Patterns	V65.49	V40.3	307.3 Stereotypic Movement Disorder, 312.39 Trichotillomania, 307.21 Transient Tic Disorder, 307.22 Chronic Motor or Vocal Tic Disorder, 307.23 Tourette's Disease
Social Interaction Behaviors	V65.49	V40.3	299.00 Autistic Disorder/Pervasive Developmental Disorder, 299.80 Rett's Disorder/Asperger's Disorder/Pervasive Developmental Disorder NOS, 299.10 Childhood Disintegrative Disorder
Bizarre Behaviors			293.0 Delirium Due to a General Medical Concern
Overall Severity	**Mild**	**Moderate**	**Severe**

	CODES	PRESENT	PROBLEMATIC
Environmental Situations:			
Challenges to Primary Support Group	**V61.20**		
Challenges to Attachment Relationship	V61.20		
Death of a Parent/Other Family Member	V62.82		
Marital Discord	V61.1		
Divorce	V61.0		
Domestic Violence	V62.8		
Other Family Relationship Problems	V61.9		
Parent-Child Separation	V61.20		
Challenges in Caregiving	**V61.20**		
Foster Care/Adoption/Institutional Care	V61.29		
Substance Abusing Parents	V61.9		
Physical Absue	995.54		
Sexual Abuse	995.53		
Quality of Nurture Problem	V61.20		
Neglect	995.52		
Mental Disorder of Parent	V61.8		
Physical Illness of Parent	V61.4		
Physical Illness of Sibling	V61.4		
Mental or Behavioral Disorder of Sibling	V61.8		
Other Functional Change in Family	**V61.2**		
Addition of a Sibling	V61.8		
Change in Parental Caregiver	V61.0		
Community/Social Challenges	**V62.4**		
Acculturation	V62.4		
Social Discrimination and/or Family Isolation	V62.81		
Religious/Spiritual Problem	V62.89		
Educational Challenges	**V62.3**		
Illiteracy of Parent	V62.3		
Inadequate School Facilities	V62.3		
Discord With Peers/Teachers	V62.3		
Parent or Adolescent Occupational Challenges	**V61.20**		
Unemployment	V62.0		
Loss of Job	V62.0		
Adverse Effect of Work Environment	V62.1		
Housing Challenges	**V60.0**		
Homelessness	V60.0		
Inadequate Housing	V60.1		
Unsafe Neighborhood	V60.9		
Dislocation	V60.8		
Economic Challenges	**V60.2**		
Poverty	V60.2		
Inadequate Financial Status	V60.2		
Inadequate Access to Health and/or Mental Health Service	**V61.9**		
Legal System or Crime Problem	**V62.5**		
Health-Related Situations	**V61.4**		
Chronic Health Conditions	V61.49		
Acute Health Conditions	V61.49		
Other Environmental Situations	**V62.8**		
Natural Disaster	V62.8		
Witness of Violence	V62.8		

CHAPTER 8B

Desirable Characteristics of a Medical Home (52)

ACCESSIBLE

Care is provided in the child's or youth's community.

All insurance, including Medicaid, is accepted.

Changes in insurance are accommodated.

The practice is accessible by public transportation, where available.

Families or youth are able to speak directly to the physician when it is needed.

The practice is physically accessible and meets Americans with Disabilities Act (70) requirements.

FAMILY CENTERED

The medical home physician is known to the child or youth and family.

Mutual responsibility and trust exists between the patient and family and the medical home physician.

The family is recognized as the principal caregiver and center of strength and support for child.

Clear, unbiased, and complete information and options are shared on an ongoing basis with the family.

Families and youth are supported in playing a central role in care coordination.

Families, youth, and physicians share responsibility in decision making.

The family is recognized as the expert in their child's care, and youths are recognized as the experts in their own care.

CONTINUOUS

The same primary pediatric health care professionals are available to patients from infancy through adolescence and young adulthood.

Assistance with transitions, in the form of developmentally appropriate health assessments and counseling, is available to the child or youth and family.

The medical home physician participates to the fullest extent allowed in care and discharge planning when the child is hospitalized or care is provided at another facility or by another provider.

COMPREHENSIVE

Care is delivered or directed by a well-trained physician who is able to manage and facilitate essentially all aspects of care.

Ambulatory and inpatient care for ongoing and acute illnesses is ensured 24 hours a day, 7 days a week, 52 weeks a year.

TABLE A8-1 ■ Example Worksheet: Community Resources and Contacts for Referrals				
Center	Contact Person	Location/Address/Meetings	Phone/Fax	Email/Web Address
Family-to-Family Networking Resources				
Family Resource Centers				
1 e.g., Family Voices	National and state contacts available	2340 Alamo SE, Suite 102 Albuquerque, NM 87106	Phone: (888) 835-5669 Fax: (505) 872-4780	*www.familyvoices.org*
2				
3				
4				
Family Support Groups				
1 e.g., Down Syndrome Support Group of Anytown, Anystate	J. Smith	United Church of Christ North of Brown Rd. on Maple Ave. When: 3rd Tuesdays of month Time: 11:00 a.m–12 Noon	Phone: (405) 555-5555	
2				
3				
Parent-to-Parent Listserves				
1 Oklahoma Parent Network (OPN)				*http://www.okparentnetwork.org/*
2				

Preventive care is provided that includes immunizations; growth and development assessments; appropriate screenings; health care supervision; and patient and parent counseling about health, safety, nutrition, parenting, and psychosocial issues.

Preventive, primary, and tertiary care needs are addressed.

The physician advocates for the child, youth, and family in obtaining comprehensive care and shares responsibility for the care that is provided.

The child's or youth's and family's medical, educational, developmental, psychosocial, and other service needs are identified and addressed.

Information is made available about private insurance and public resources, including Supplemental Security Income, Medicaid, the State Children's Health Insurance Program, waivers, early intervention programs, and Title V State Programs for Children with Special Health Care Needs.

Extra time for an office visit is scheduled for children with special health care needs, when indicated.

COORDINATED

A plan of care is developed by the physician, child or youth, and family and is shared with other providers, agencies, and organizations involved with the care of the patient.

Care among multiple providers is coordinated through the medical home.

A central record or database containing all pertinent medical information, including hospitalizations and specialty care, is maintained at the practice.

TABLE A8-2 ■ Example Worksheet: Community Resources for Children with Developmental Delays					
	Center	Contact Person	Address/County	Phone/Fax	Email/Web Address
Early Intervention					
1	National Information Center for Children and Youth with Disabilities (NICHCY)			800-695-0285	*http://www.thearc.org/faqs/earlyintervention.doc*
2	In each state			Contact local school district	
3					
	Name or Group	Phone	Fax	Address	Information/Insurance Accepted, Other Information
Developmental and Behavioral or Neurodevelopmental Pediatricians					
1					
2					
Child Psychiatrists					
1					
2					
Child Psychologists					
1					
2					
Child Neurologists					
1					
2					
Pediatric Physiatrists					
1					
2					
PT/OT/ST/Audiology/Special Daycares/Schools/Other					
1					
2					

OT, occupational therapy; PT, physical therapy; ST, speech therapy.

Record#	Patient's Last Name	Patient's First Name	Referred to	Date Referred	Date Feedback Received	Feedback

TABLE A8-3 ■ Example Worksheet: Referral Tracking Sheet

The record is accessible, but confidentiality is preserved.

The medical home physician shares information among the child or youth, family, and consultant and provides specific reason for referral to appropriate pediatric medical subspecialists, surgical specialists, and mental health/developmental professionals.

Families are linked to family support groups, parent-to-parent groups, and other family resources.

When a child or youth is referred for a consultation or additional care, the medical home physician assists the child, youth, and family in communicating clinical issues.

The medical home physician evaluates and interprets the consultant's recommendations for the child or youth and family and, in consultation with them and subspecialists, implements recommendations that are indicated and appropriate.

The plan of care is coordinated with educational and other community organizations to ensure that special health needs of the individual child are addressed.

COMPASSIONATE

Concern for the well-being of the child or youth and family is expressed and demonstrated in verbal and nonverbal interactions.

Efforts are made to understand and empathize with the feelings and perspectives of the family, as well as the child or youth.

CULTURALLY EFFECTIVE

The child's or youth's and family's cultural background, including beliefs, rituals, and customs, are recognized, valued, respected, and incorporated into the care plan.

All efforts are made to ensure that the child or youth and family understand the results of the medical encounter and the care plan, including the provision of professional or paraprofessional translators or interpreters, as needed.

Written materials are provided in the family's primary language.

Helpful Web Sites from Supplement (71)

Institute for Family Centered Care

> http://www.familycenteredcare.org/
> The Institute for Family Centered Care is a national organization formed in 1992 through the col-

laboration of families and professionals. The Institute disseminates information to promote the practice of family-centered care through annual conferences, information publications, guidelines for hospitals, and consultations to individual health organizations.

National Center of Medical Home Initiatives for Children with Special Needs

> http://www.medicalhomeinfo.org
> The National Center of Medical Home Initiatives for Children with Special Needs provides support to physicians, families, and other medical and nonmedical providers who care for children with special health care needs so that they have access to a medical home.

The Medical Home Improvement Collaborative

> www.medicalhomeimprovement.org

Achieving and Measuring Success: A National Agenda for Children with Special Health Care Needs

> http://www.mchb.hrsa.gov/programs/specialneeds/measuresuccess.htm
> This includes the six critical indicators of progress.

President's New Freedom Initiative—Fulfilling America's Promise to Americans with Disabilities

> http://www.hhs.gov/newfreedom/

DisabilityInfo.gov

> http://www.disabilityinfo.gov/
> The comprehensive federal Web site of disability-related government resources.

The National Center on Financing for Children with Special Health Care Needs

> http://cshcnfinance.ichp.edu/

The Maternal and Child Health Policy Research Center

> http://www.mchpolicy.org

Family Voices

> http://www.familyvoices.org

National Center for Cultural Competence

> http://www.georgetown.edu/research/gucdc/nccc/

CHAPTER 10F

Information and Service Organizations for Patients with Hearing Impairment

Alexander Graham Bell Association for the Deaf and Hard of Hearing

> 3417 Volta Place NW
> Washington, DC 20007
> *www.agbell.org*

American Society for Deaf Children

> PO Box 3355
> Gettysburg, PA 17325
> *www.deafchildren.org*

American Speech-Language-Hearing Association

> 10801 Rockville Pike
> Rockville, MD 20852
> *www.asha.org*

Council for Exceptional Children

> 1920 Association Drive
> Reston, VA 22091
> *www.cec.sped.org*

Deafness Research Foundation

> 366 Madison Avenue
> New York, NY 10017
> *www.drf.org*

Laurent Clerc National Deaf Education Center

> Gallaudet University
> 800 Florida Avenue NE
> Washington, DC 20002
> *http://clerccenter.gallaudet.edu/*

National Association of the Deaf

> 814 Thayer Avenue
> Silver Spring, MD 20910
> *www.nad.org*

National Center for Hearing Assessment and Management

> Utah State University
> 2880 Old Main Hill
> Logan, UT 84322
> *www.infanthearing.org*

National Institute on Deafness and Other Communication Disorders

> 31 Center Drive, MSC 2320
> Bethesda, MD 20892-2320
> *www.nidcd.nih.gov*

National Technical Institute for the Deaf

> Rochester Institute of Technology
> Rochester, New York 14623
> *http://www.ntid.rit.edu/*

Resources and Publications for Parents and Other Caregivers of Visually Impaired Children

STUART TEPLIN

BROCHURES, ARTICLES, BOOKS, AND WEB SITES

Educational booklets and videos (in English and Spanish) from the Blind Children's Center (Los Angeles, CA; phone: 1-800-222-3566; Web site: *http://www.blindcntr.org/pubs.htm*):

- *Dancing Cheek to Cheek: Nurturing Beginning Social, Play, and Language Interactions* (available in English only).
- *Starting Points:* Intervention guidelines for helping young children with multiple disabilities including visual impairment. Good information for the classroom teacher of 3- to 8-year-olds with visual impairment (available in English only).
- *Fathers: A Common Ground:* Concerns and roles of fathers in early development of their children with visual impairments (available in English only).
- *First Steps: A Handbook for Teaching Young Children Who Are Visually Impaired:* Easy-to-understand handbook to assist professionals and parents working with children with visual impairment (available in English only).
- *Heart to Heart: Parents of Children Who Are Blind and Partially Sighted Discuss Their Feelings* (available in both English and Spanish)
- *Learning to Play: Common Concerns for the Visually Impaired Preschool Child:* Presents play activities for preschoolers with visual impairment (available in English only).
- *Let's Eat: Feeding a Child with a Visual Impairment:* Teaching competent feeding skills to children with visual impairment (a booklet and VHS video; available in either English or Spanish).
- *Move with Me: A Parent's Guide to Movement Development for Babies Who Are Visually Impaired* (booklet; available in English and Spanish).
- *Pediatric Visual Diagnosis Fact Sheets:* Addresses commonly encountered eye conditions, diagnostic tests, and materials (available in English only).
- Reaching, Crawling, Walking . . . *Let's Get Moving:* Orientation and mobility skills for preschool children (available in English only).
- *Selecting a Program: A Guide for Parents of Infants and Preschoolers with Visual Impairments:* Guide for parents in selecting the most appropriate program for their

infant or preschool who is visually impaired (available in English and Spanish)

- *Standing on My Own Two Feet:* Guide to designing and making simple, individualized mobility devices for preschool-age children who are visually impaired (available in English and Spanish).
- *Talk to Me* and *Talk to Me II:* Guide and sequel for facilitating language development for infants and preschool-age children who are visually impaired (available in English and Spanish).

Various resources, materials, and suggestions for advocacy from the American Foundation for the Blind (Louisville, KY; *www.afb.org*):

- Chen D, ed: Essential Elements in Early Intervention: Visual Impairment and Multiple Disabilities. Louisville, KY: AFB Press, 2000 ["comprehensive resource, provides range of information on effective, early intervention with young child who is blind/visually impaired and who has additional disabilities. Explanation of functional and clinical vision and hearing assessments, educational techniques, and suggestions for on working with families"].
- Corn AL, Huebner KM: Report to the Nation: National Agenda for Education of Children and Youth with Visual Impairments, Including Those with Multiple Disabilities. Louisville, KY: AFB Press, 1998 ["invaluable material and data for advocates working to improve educational services"].
- Dickerson ML: Small Victories: Conversations about Prematurity, Disability, Vision Loss, and Success. Louisville, KY: AFB Press, 2000 ["interviews with individuals who were born prematurely and with parents of children who were born prematurely who discuss the many issues they faced . . . contains a detailed resource guide"].
- Fazzi DL, Lampert JS, Pogrund RL: Early Focus: Working with Young Blind and Visually Impaired Children and Their Families. Louisville, KY: AFB Press, 1992 ["clear descriptions of early intervention techniques with blind and visually impaired children . . . stresses the benefits of family involvement and transdisciplinary teamwork"].
- Harrell L: Touch the Baby: Blind and Visually Impaired Children as Patients: Helping Them to Respond to Care. Louisville, KY: AFB Press, 1984 [useful pamphlet for health care providers].
- Holbrook C: Children with Visual Impairments—A Parent's Guide. Bethesda, MD: Woodbine House, 1996 [an excellent first book for parents and professionals previously unfamiliar with issues and stresses surrounding care of a young child with significant visual impairment].
- Sacks SZ, Wolffe K: Focused On: Social Skills for Teens and Young Adults with Visual Impairments. Louisville, KY: AFB Press, 2000.

OTHER USEFUL AGENCIES AND WEB SITES

National Association for Parents of Children with Visual Impairments (NAPVI): *http://www.spedex.com/NAPVI/*

National Federation for the Blind: *http://www.nfb.org/nfb/Default.asp*

National Library Services for Blind and Physically Handicapped: *http://www.loc.gov/nls/*

California Dept. of Education: *http://www.cde.ca.gov/spbranch/sed*

BOOKS AND WEB SITES REGARDING DEAF-BLIND CHILDREN

Miles B, Riggio M, eds: Remarkable Conversations—A Guide to Developing Meaningful Communication with Children and Young Adults Who Are Deafblind, Watertown MA: Perkins School for the Blind, 1999.

Welch TR: Hand in Hand. Louisville, KY: AFB Press, 1995 [20-volume self-study text that "explains how deaf-blind students learn (particularly with regard to) communication and mobility"]

DB-LINK (phone, voice: 800-438-9376; phone, TTY: 800-854-7013; Web site: *http://www.tr.wou.edu/dblink*) [national information clearinghouse on children who are deaf-blind, a federally funded information and referral service].

National Technical Assistance Consortium for Children and Young Adults Who Are Deaf-Blind (*http://www.tr.wou.edu/ntac/*)

CHAPTER 11

Listings for Organizations Discussed in Text

SANDRA A. PALOMO-GONZALEZ

Supports change over time. Community and private supports depend on dedicated parents and advocacy professionals, private foundation funding, and innovative networking. Public supports are dependent on federal laws, but these do not materialize into supports until state legislatures allocate funds to implement them. State budgets vary a great deal as a result of political climates. Thus, any index of supports available to families and individuals with mental retardation at the time this text is written may be nonexistent by the time it is published, distributed, and read.

Therefore, the authors, with the assistance of Dr. Sandie Palomo-Gonzalez, have agreed to update and keep current a document they have developed for national presentations titled "The Mental Retardation Toolkit." It includes other listings in addition to the ones included in this Appendix. It also provides useful forms, checklists, and parent handouts. This will be emailed to the reader, upon request. *(drchris@flash. net; william.walker@seattlechildrens.org)*

Note that the *Annual Resource Guide* of *Exceptional Parent* provides a much more extensive listing and is updated annually. Contact *www.eparent.com.*

American Association on Intellectual and Developmental Disabilities (AAIDD)

444 N. Capitol Street, NW
Suite 846
Washington, DC 20001-1512
Phone: 202-387-1968; toll-free phone: 800-424-3688
Web site: *www.aamr.org*
Formerly known as the American Association on Mental Retardation (AAMR), this organization conducts advocacy and sets policy regarding mental retardation.

The Arc of the United States

1010 Wayne Avenue
Suite 650
Silver Spring, MD 20910
Phone, voice: 301-565-3842
Fax: 301-565-5342
Email: *info@thearc.org*
Web site: *www.thearc.org/*
The Arc (formerly the Association for Retarded Citizens) promotes inclusion and conducts advocacy on behalf of persons with mental retardation.

The President's Committee for People with Intellectual Disabilities (PCPID)

The Aerospace Center
370 L'Enfant Promenade SW
Room 701
Washington, DC 20447
Email: *www.acf.hhs.gov/programs/pcpid/index.html*
The PCPID is a federal advisory committee that advises the President and Secretary of the Department of Health and Human Services with regard to mental retardation issues.

National Dissemination Center for Children with Disabilities (NICHCY)

PO Box 1492
Washington, DC 20013
Phone, voice/TTY: 202-884-8200, 800-695-0285
Email: *nichcy@aed.org*
Web site: *http://nichcy.org/*
This national clearinghouse specializes in disseminating information about disability and education issues for children birth to age 22 years.

National Organization for Rare Disorders (NORD)

55 Kenosia Avenue
PO Box 1968
Danbury, CT 06813-1968
Phone, voice: 203-744-0100; TDD: 203-797-9590
Toll-free voice mail only: 800-999-6673
Fax: 203-798-2291
Email: *orphan@rarediseases.org*
Web site: *www.rarediseases.org/*
NORD provides information and referral and offers a program that links individuals with the same or similar illnesses.

PACER Center

8161 Normandale Boulevard
Minneapolis, MN 55437-1044
Phone, voice: 952-838-9000; toll-free phone: 888-248-0222; TTY: 952-838-0190
Fax: 952-838-0199
Email: *alliance@taalliance.org*
Web site: *www.taalliance.org/*
This organization provides technical support for the development, coordination, and assistance of parent training and information.

National Down Syndrome Congress (NDSC): parents

1370 Center Drive
Suite 102
Atlanta, GA 30338
Phone: 770-604-9500; toll-free phone: 800-232-NDSC
Email: *info@ndsccenter.org*
Web site: *www.ndsccenter.org/*

National Organization on Fetal Alcohol Syndrome

900 17th Street, NW
Suite 910
Washington, DC 20006
Phone: 202-785-4585; toll-free phone: 800-66-NOFAS
Email: *info@nofas.org*
Web site: *www.nofas.org/*

National Fragile X Foundation (NFXF)

PO Box 190488
San Francisco, CA 94119
Phone: 925-938-9300; toll-free phone: 800-688-8765
Email: *NATLFX@FragileX.org*
Web site: *www.nfxf.org/*

Parent to Parent–USA (P2P-USA): parents

Web site: *www.p2pusa.org/*
P2P-USA is an alliance of statewide programs that matches trained, veteran parents of chil-

dren with disabilities with new ones for peer support.

Youth Leadership Forum for Children with Disabilities (YLF)

Office of Disability Employment Policy (ODEP)
1331 F. Street, NW
Washington, DC 2004
Phone: 202-693-7880
Fax: 202-693-7888
Email: *epstein.alicia@dol.gov*
Web site: *www.dol.gov/odep/*
YLF is a free 4-day career and leadership training program for junior and high school students with disabilities.

Best Buddies: peers

100 SE Second Street
Suite 2200
Miami, FL 33131
Toll-free phone: 800-89-BUDDY
Web site: *www.bestbuddies.org/*
Best Buddies is an international nonprofit committed to providing supportive employment opportunities and promoting friendships between persons with intellectual disabilities and their peers.

Sibling Support Project (SSP) of The Arc of the United States: siblings

6512 23rd Ave NW
#213
Seattle, WA 98117
Phone: 206-297-6368
Fax: 509-752-6789
Email: *donmeyer@siblingsupport.org*
Web site: *http://www.siblingsupport.org/*
Founded by Donald Meyer, the SSP is a national effort that provides support and information to siblings of persons with disabilities while helping caregivers understand the unique issues facing siblings.

ARCH National Respite Network and Resource Center

800 Eastowne Drive
Suite 105
Chapel Hill, NC 27514
Phone: 919-490-5577
Fax: 919-490-4905
Web site: *www.archrespite.org/*
ARCH helps families and professionals locate respite programs.

Partners for Youth with Disabilities (PYD) Access to Theatre

95 Berkeley Street
Suite 109
Boston, MA 02116
Phone: 617-556-4075; TTY: 617-314-2989
Email: *mgallagher@pyd.org*
Web site: *www.pyd.org/*
The Access to Theatre (ATT) program engages youth with and without disabilities from the Boston area, aged 13 to 24, to work collaboratively to create theatrical productions.

VSA Arts (formerly Very Special Arts)

1300 Connecticut Avenue
Suite 700
Washington, DC 20036
Toll-free phone: 800-933-8721
Fax: 202-737-0725
Email: *info@vsarts.org*
Web site: *www.vsarts.org/*
VSA Arts is an international nonprofit dedicated to ensuring that persons with disabilities have the opportunity to learn about, take part in, and enjoy the arts.

Special Needs Alliance (SNA): guardianship, special needs wills

Toll-free phone: 1-877-572-8472
Web site: *www.specialneedsalliance.com/*
SNA is a national network of lawyers specializing in disability and public benefits law. Families of children with disabilities can locate a SNA lawyer.

MassMutual SpecialCare[SM] Program: estate planning

1295 State Street
Springfield, MA 01111-0001
Toll-free phone: 800-272-2216
Web site: *www.massmutual.com/mmfg/prepare/ specialcare/index.html*

MetDESK: estate planning, life insurance

Phone: 877-MET-DESK (877-638-3375)
Web site: *www.metlife.com/desk*

Special Needs Advocate for Parents (SNAP)

11835 W. Olympic Boulevard
Suite 465
Los Angeles, CA 90045
Phone: 310-479-3755; toll-free phone: 888-310-9889
Email: *info@snapinfo.org*
Web site: *www.snapinfo.org/home.html*
This nonprofit organization provides parents with information, education, advocacy, networking, special needs wills, private medical insurance system.

CHAPTER 12

Resources: Advocacy, Legislation, Research, and Education

Council for Exceptional Children

Division of Learning Disabilities
1920 Association Drive
Reston, VA 22091
Phone: 703-620-3660
Web site: *www.cec.sped.org*
This organization deals with special education for exceptional children, including those with learning disabilities. It has a strong professional focus with regard to educational standards, professional roles, and professional development of different people who work with exceptional children.

International Dyslexia Association

8600 La Salle Road
Chester Building
Baltimore, MD 21286
Phone: 800-ABC-D123
Web site: *www.interdys.org*
This is the oldest learning disability organization, founded in memory of Dr. Samuel Orton. It provides information about legislation, advocacy, research, and education. It advocates on behalf of individuals with learning disabilities and covers learning disabilities in children and adolescents, as well as in adults in college and the workplace. It sponsors a large annual conference.

Learning Disabilities Association

4156 Library Road
Pittsburgh, PA 15234
Phone: 412-341-1515
Web site: *www.ldaamerica.org*
This nonprofit volunteer organization advocates for people with learning disabilities. It has more than 200 state and local affiliates, as well as international membership from 27 countries. It provides services, resources, and advocacy for children and adults with learning disabilities, for parents of individuals with learning disabilities, and for professionals who work with people with learning disabilities.

Learning Disabilities Association of Canada (national office)

250 City Centre Avenue
Suite 616
Ottawa, Ontario K1R 6K7

Canada
Phone: 613-238-5721
Web site: *www.ldac-taac.ca*
This organization provides contact information for provincial and regional chapters across the country with Web site information in English and French. The national office and provincial offices provide information on learning disabilities for parents, educators, and other professionals; resources; and information about legislation. Some chapters offer resources in terms of social skills groups and parent support groups and provide referral information.

National Center for Learning Disabilities

381 Park Avenue South
New York, NY 10016
Phone: 212-545-7510
Web site: *www.ncld.org*
This organization provides information, resources, and programs on learning disabilities as well as on early literacy. It provides advocacy tools for youth and adults with learning disabilities, as well as advocacy tools for parents, educators, and professionals. It provides updates on legislation affecting individuals with learning disabilities.

Research Works!

PAS 3269
200 University Avenue West
Waterloo, Ontario N2L 3G1
Canada
Phone: 519-888-4009
Web site: *www.research-works.ca*
A community-university research alliance designed to share and apply research knowledge in child literacy. The alliance provides systematic reviews of child literacy research in areas such as volunteer tutoring programs and literacy and autism.

Canadian Language and Literacy Research Network

c/o The University of Western Ontario
Elborn College
1201 Western Road
London, Ontario N6G 1H1
Canada
Phone: 519-661-4223
Web site: *www.cllrnet.ca*
This organization, a federal Network of Centres of Excellence, brings together leading scientists, clinicians, students and educators as well as public and private partners. The Network's mandate is to generate, integrate, and dissemi-

nate bias-free scientific research and knowledge that is focused on improving and sustaining children's language and literacy development in Canada. The Network is hosted by The University of Western Ontario.

Student Progress Monitoring

1000 Thomas Jefferson Street, NW
Washington, DC 20007
Phone: 866-770-6111
Web site: *www.studentprogress.org*
The National Center on Student Progress Monitoring is located at the American Institutes for Research, is funded by the Office of Special Education Programs, and works in conjunction with researchers from Vanderbilt University. Progress monitoring assesses student progress and evaluates the effectiveness of instruction. The Center provides technical assistance and dissemination of information pertinent to the implementation of scientifically based student progress monitoring practices across academic content areas from kindergarten and up.

What Works Clearinghouse
2277 Research Boulevard
MS 5M
Rockville, MD 20850
Phone: 866-992-9799
Web site: *www.whatworks.ed.gov*
This site was set up by the U.S. Department of Education's Institute of Education Services to provide educators, policymakers, researchers, and the public with a central source of scientific evidence of what works in education.

CHAPTER 16

Helpful Internet Resources for Attention-Deficit/Hyperactivity Disorder (ADHD)

Comprehensive Treatment for Attention Deficit Disorder, Inc.

http://ctadd.com/ctadd/aboutctadd.html

How to Establish a Daily Report Card

http://ctadd.com/ctadd/PDFs_CTADD/How_To_Establish_DRC.pdf

Parent and Teacher Behavior Rating Scales with Scoring Instructions

http://ctadd.com/ctadd/PDFs_CTADD/DBD.pdf
http://peds.mc.vanderbilt.edu/cdc/VTBES.html
http://peds.mc.vanderbilt.edu/cdc/ADTRS.htm

What Parents and Teachers Should Know About ADHD

http://ctadd.com/ctadd/PDFs_CTADD/What_Parents_Teachers.pdf

Children and Adults with Attention-Deficit/Hyperactivity Disorder

http://www.chadd.org/

Educational Materials List

http://www.mhmr.state.tx.us/centraloffice/medicaldirector/cmapadhded.html#self

ADHD Medication and You

http://www.mhmr.state.tx.us/centraloffice/medicaldirector/24a.pdf

Tips for Teachers: Medication and ADHD

http://www.mhmr.state.tx.us/centraloffice/medicaldirector/43a.pdf

Does My Child Have an Attention Disorder?

http://www.mhmr.state.tx.us/centraloffice/medicaldirector/11a.pdf

Teenagers and ADHD

http://www.mhmr.state.tx.us/centraloffice/medicaldirector/12a.pdf

ADHD Medications and Your Child How Do the Medications for ADHD Work?

http://www.mhmr.state.tx.us/centraloffice/medicaldirector/23a.pdf

Parenting the Child with ADHD

http://www.mhmr.state.tx.us/centraloffice/medicaldirector/61A.pdf

CHAPTER 18B

Publisher Information for Select Self-Report and for Parent and Teacher Rating Scales

Achenbach System of Empirically Based Assessment (ASEBA): *www.ASEBA.org*

- Teacher Report Form (TRF)
- Youth Self-Report (YSR)

Mind Garden: *www.mindgarden.com*

- Family Environment Scale (FES)

Multi-Health Systems, Inc.: *www.mhs.com*

- Multidimensional Anxiety Scale for Children (MASC)
- The Social Phobia and Anxiety Inventory for Children (SPAI-C)

National Center for Posttraumatic Stress Disorder (U.S. Dept of Veteran's Affairs): *www.ncptsd.va.gov/ncmain/index.jsp*

- Traumatic Events Screening Inventory for Children (TESI-C)

Pearson Assessments: *www.pearsonassessments.com*

- Behavior Assessment System for Children (BASC)

Psychological Assessment Resources (PAR) Inc.: *www.parinc.com*

- Child Behavior Checklist (CBCL)
- Conners' Parent and Teacher Rating Scales
- Revised Children's Manifest Anxiety Scale (RCMAS)
- State-Trait Anxiety Inventory for Children (STAI-C)

CHAPTER 19

Resources: Where to Go for Help

Al-Anon

Al-Anon Family Group Headquarters
1600 Corporate Landing Parkway
Virginia Beach, VA 23462
Phone: 888-425-2666; help line: 800-344-2666
Web site: *www.al-anon.alateen.org*
This organization supports spouses and other relatives and friends of alcoholic persons. Al-Anon Family Group Headquarters can assist in finding a local affiliate.

Alateen

Al-Anon Family Group Headquarters
1600 Corporate Landing Parkway
Virginia Beach, VA 23462
Phone: 888-425-2666; help line: 800-344-2666
Web site: *www.alanon.alateen.org*
Alateen is part of Al-Anon; it supports young people whose lives have been affected by the alcoholism of a family member or friend.

Alcoholics Anonymous (AA)

AA General Service Office
PO Box 459
Grand Central Station
New York, NY 10163
Phone: 212-870-3400

Web site: *www.alcoholics-anonymous.org*
This is the oldest of organizations designed to help alcoholic persons help themselves. The AA General Service Office can help locate a nearby affiliate.

The Center for Substance Abuse Prevention (CSAP)/ Substance Abuse and Mental Health Services Administration (SAMHSA)

One Choke Cherry Road
Rockwall II, 9th Floor
Rockville, MD 20857
Web site: *www.prevention.samhsa.gov*
These organizations provide national leadership in the federal effort to prevent alcohol, tobacco, and illicit drug problems.

Narcotics Anonymous

Narcotics Anonymous World Service Office
PO Box 9999
Van Nuys, CA 91409
Phone: 818-773-9999
Web site: *www.na.org*
This is an international, community-based association of recovering drug addicts.

National Association for Children of Alcoholics

11426 Rockville Pike
Suite 100
Rockville, MD 20852
Phone: 301-468-0985 or 888-554-COAS
Web site: *www.nacoa.org*
This is a membership organization and clearinghouse for information and support materials for children of alcoholics and for those in a position to assist them.

The National Student Assistance Association

4200 Wisconsin Avenue, NW
Suite 106-118
Washington, DC 20016
Phone: 800-257-6310
Web site: *www.nasap.org*
This organization represents interests of student assistance professionals across the United States.

National Clearinghouse for Alcohol and Drug Information

PO Box 2345
Rockville, MD 20852
Phone: 800-729-6686
Web sites: *www.health.org* (for youth: *www.health.org/kidsarea*)
This organization supplies relevant materials covering the gamut of alcohol- and drug-related issues.

National Council on Alcoholism and Drug Dependence

20 Exchange Place
Suite 2902
New York, NY 10005
Phone: 212-269-7797
Web site: *www.ncadd.org*

Through local affiliates, this organization provides information about treatment opportunities and, sometimes, counseling of alcoholics and their families.

National Institute on Alcohol Abuse and Alcoholism

5635 Fishers Lane
MSC 9304
Bethesda, MD 20892-9304
Phone: 301-443-3860
Web site: *www.niaaa.nih.gov*

This organization supports and conducts biomedical and behavioral research on the causes, consequences, treatment, and prevention of alcoholism and alcohol-related problems.

National Institute on Drug Abuse

Room 5213
6001 Executive Boulevard
Bethesda, MD 20892-9561
Phone: 301-443-1124
Web site: *www.nida.nih.gov*

This organization supports and conducts research and ensures the effective dissemination and use of the results of research to significantly improve drug abuse and addiction prevention, treatment, and policy.

Index

Note: Page numbers followed by the letter f refer to figures, those followed by the letter t refer to tables, and those followed by the letter b refer to boxed material.

A

Abdominal examination, metabolic disorders and, 340
Abdominal pain, recurrent, 712
  management of, 730
Abortion, ethical issues associated with, 917-918
Abstinence syndrome
  in heroin users, 674
  neonatal, opiate-induced, 690
Abuse. *See* Child maltreatment; *specific type of abuse.*
Academic achievement, eating disorders and obesity and, 786
Academic achievement tests, in assessment of behavior problems, 613t
Achenbach System of Empirically Based Assessment (ASEBA), 149, 159-160
Achievement tests, 155, 157
  academic, 613t
Acquired immunodeficiency syndrome (AIDS). *See also* Human immunodeficiency virus (HIV) infection.
  among gay youth, 850
Acupuncture, 270-271, 270t
  adverse effects of, 271
Acute alcohol overuse syndrome. *See also* Alcohol abuse (alcoholism).
  treatment of, 672
Acyl-carnitine profile, for metabolic disorders, 342-343
Adaptive behavior, limitations in, 406-407
Adaptive behavior scales, 151, 415
Adaptive domain, in Battelle Developmental Inventor-II, 151

Adaptive equipment, for cerebral palsy, 489
Adaptive skills, assessment of, in mental retardation, 413
Additive-free diet, 264t, 265
Adenotonsillectomy, for sleep-disordered breathing, 746
Adherence, medical. *See* Medical adherence.
Adolescence-limited delinquency, 31
Adolescent(s)
  academic achievement by, psychological adjustment and, 83-84
  compliance behavior by, 604
  conceptualization of illness by, 283
  decision making by, 294-295
  delayed sleep phase syndrome in, 749
  depression in, interpersonal therapy for, 243t, 244
  developmental changes in, framework for understanding, 35-36, 36f
  gay/lesbian identity in, development of, 842-847. *See also* Gay/lesbian *entries.*
  gender identity disorder in, treatment of, 835-836
  infections in, 352-357, 352t, 355t
  motor skills assessment in, 199
  normal sleep in, 744-745
  sexual behavior problems in, 814-815
    parent education and clinical management of, 816-817
  sexual development in, 808-809, 809t
  substance use/abuse by
    discussion of, 681-682
    identification of, 678-679
    screening for, 684, 684f

Adolescent(s)—cont'd
  with autistic spectrum disorders
    need of guardianship for, 558
    transition issues for, 551-552
  with mental retardation
    special health concerns in, 426-428
    supports for, 435-437
      development of plan in, 436-437, 436t
Adolescent Clinical Sexual Behavior Inventory (ACSBI), 815
Adolescent sexual offender, definition of, 806t
Adoption, by lesbian women, 857
Adrenal hyperplasia, congenital, gender role behavior and, 831
α-Adrenergic agonists
  for attention-deficit hyperactivity disorder, 229, 587t, 593
  for autistic spectrum disorders, 554-555, 554t
  for tone management, in cerebral palsy, 489, 489t
Adult care, transition of children with special needs to, 295-296
Adult Children of Alcoholics groups, attendance at, 684
Adult outcomes, of individuals with mental retardation, 437, 438t, 439f
Adult sexual behavior, definition of, 806t
Adult sexual offenders, vs. adolescent sexual behavior problems, 815
Advocacy, in developmental-behavioral pediatric research, 51